Textbook of
EMERGENCY AND TRAUMA CARE

Textbook of
EMERGENCY AND TRAUMA CARE

Editor-in-Chief

Devendra Richhariya
MBBS MD FICM
Senior Consultant
Department of Emergency and Trauma Care
Medanta—The Medicity
Gurugram, Haryana, India

Co-Editors

Saleh Fares
MD MPH FRCPC(EM) FAAEM FACEP
Consultant (Emergency Medicine)
EMS and Disaster Medicine
Deputy Commander
Zayed Military Hospital
Founder and Chairman
Trauma System Initiative
Emirate of Abu Dhabi
Founder and President
Emirates Society of Emergency Medicine
Abu Dhabi, UAE

Khusrav Bajan
MD EDIC
Consultant (Critical Care) and Head
Department of Emergency
PD Hinduja National Hospital and
Medical Research Center
Mumbai, Maharashtra, India

Sudhir S Pawaiya
MBBS Diploma in Emergency Medicine
Consultant
Department of Emergency and Trauma Care
Medanta—The Medicity
Gurugram, Haryana, India

Forewords

Naresh Trehan
Yatin Mehta
Ravi R Kasliwal

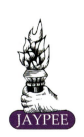

JAYPEE *The Health Sciences Publisher*
New Delhi | London | Panama

Jaypee Brothers Medical Publishers (P) Ltd.

Headquarters
Jaypee Brothers Medical Publishers (P) Ltd
4838/24, Ansari Road, Daryaganj
New Delhi 110 002, India
Phone: +91-11-43574357
Fax: +91-11-43574314
E-mail: jaypee@jaypeebrothers.com

Overseas Offices

J.P. Medical Ltd
83, Victoria Street, London
SW1H 0HW (UK)
Phone: +44 20 3170 8910
Fax: +44 (0)20 3008 6180
E-mail: info@jpmedpub.com

Jaypee-Highlights Medical Publishers Inc
City of Knowledge, Bld. 235, 2nd Floor, Clayton
Panama City, Panama
Phone: +1 507-301-0496
Fax: +1 507-301-0499
E-mail: cservice@jphmedical.com

Jaypee Brothers Medical Publishers (P) Ltd
17/1-B, Babar Road, Block-B, Shaymali
Mohammadpur, Dhaka-1207
Bangladesh
Mobile: +08801912003485
E-mail: jaypeedhaka@gmail.com

Jaypee Brothers Medical Publishers (P) Ltd
Bhotahity, Kathmandu
Nepal
Phone: +977-9741283608
E-mail: kathmandu@jaypeebrothers.com

Website: www.jaypeebrothers.com
Website: www.jaypeedigital.com

© 2018, Jaypee Brothers Medical Publishers

The views and opinions expressed in this book are solely those of the original contributor(s)/author(s) and do not necessarily represent those of editor(s) of the book.

All rights reserved. No part of this publication may be reproduced, stored or transmitted in any form or by any means, electronic, mechanical, photocopying, recording or otherwise, without the prior permission in writing of the publishers.

All brand names and product names used in this book are trade names, service marks, trademarks or registered trademarks of their respective owners. The publisher is not associated with any product or vendor mentioned in this book.

Medical knowledge and practice change constantly. This book is designed to provide accurate, authoritative information about the subject matter in question. However, readers are advised to check the most current information available on procedures included and check information from the manufacturer of each product to be administered, to verify the recommended dose, formula, method and duration of administration, adverse effects and contraindications. It is the responsibility of the practitioner to take all appropriate safety precautions. Neither the publisher nor the author(s)/editor(s) assume any liability for any injury and/or damage to persons or property arising from or related to use of material in this book.

This book is sold on the understanding that the publisher is not engaged in providing professional medical services. If such advice or services are required, the services of a competent medical professional should be sought.

Every effort has been made where necessary to contact holders of copyright to obtain permission to reproduce copyright material. If any have been inadvertently overlooked, the publisher will be pleased to make the necessary arrangements at the first opportunity. The **CD/DVD-ROM** (if any) provided in the sealed envelope with this book is complimentary and free of cost. **Not meant for sale**.

Inquiries for bulk sales may be solicited at: jaypee@jaypeebrothers.com

Textbook of Emergency and Trauma Care

First Edition: **2018**

ISBN: 978-93-5270-191-9

Printed at Sanat Printers

Dedicated to
My parents for providing me best education and values, they always inspire me.
My sisters Arti, Jyoti, and brother Rajendra for endless support and encouragement.
My wife Bhawna and daughter Avighna for unconditional love and affection.
All my friends of "the class 89", who continuously pampered me and supported me, when I need them most.

—**Devendra Richhariya**

Contributors

Abdul Muniem DM (Neurology)
Consultant
Medanta Institute of Neurosciences
Medanta—The Medicity
Gurugram, Haryana, India

Adarsh Kumar MBBS MD (Forensic Medicine)
Professor
Forensic Medicine and Toxicology
All India Institute of Medical Sciences
New Delhi, India

Aditi Gupta MBBS MD
Senior Resident
Pediatric Cardiology
Medanta—The Medicity
Gurugram, Haryana, India

Aditya Aggarwal MBBS MS MCh
DNB (Plastic Surgery) MNAMS
Director
Department of Plastic, Aesthetic and
Reconstructive Surgery
Medanta—The Medicity
Gurugram, Haryana, India

Ajeet Singh MD IDCCM EDICC
Senior Resident
Institute of Critical Care
Medanta—The Medicity
Gurugram, Haryana, India

Ali Zamir Khan MS FRCS (CTH) FRCS (Glasg)
Associate Director
Minimally Invasive and
Robotic Thoracic Surgery
Medanta—The Medicity
Gurugram, Haryana, India

Amit D Nabar MD DA FCPS
Consultant (Critical Care)
Head, Department of Accident and
Emergency Medicine
SL Raheja Hospital
Mumbai, Maharashtra, India

Anand Jaiswal MBBS MD
Director
Respiratory and Sleep Medicine
Medanta—The Medicity
Gurugram, Haryana, India

Anand Yadav MS
Fellow, Minimal Access Surgery (NBE)
Institute of Minimal Access
Metabolic and Bariatric Surgery
Sir Ganga Ram Hospital
New Delhi, India

Anil Bhan MBBS MS MCh
Vice Chairman
Cardiothoracic Surgery
Medanta Heart Institute
Medanta—The Medicity
Gurugram, Haryana, India

Anjan Shrestha MBBS MD
Consultant, Hemato-oncology and
Blood and Marrow Transplant
Rajiv Gandhi Cancer Institute and
Research Center
New Delhi, India

Archana Shrivastav MBBS MD
Associate Consultant Critical Care
PD Hinduja National Hospital and
Medical Research Center
Mumbai, Maharashtra, India

Arun Garg MD DM (Neurology)
Director
Medanta Institute of Neurosciences
Medanta—The Medicity
Gurugram, Haryana, India

Aseem K Tiwari MBBS MD (Pathology)
Associate Director
Transfusion Medicine
Medanta—The Medicity
Gurugram, Haryana, India

Ashish Kumar Prakash MBBS DNB (Resp Med) DTCO (European Diploma) FCCP (USA) FAPSR MNCCP
Associate Consultant
Respiratory Medicine
Medanta—The Medicity
Gurugram, Haryana, India

Ashish Nandwani DNB (Nephrology)
Consultant
Department of Nephrology
Medanta—The Medicity
Gurugram, Haryana, India

Ashok Mishra MBBS MD PhD FIAPSM
Professor
Department of Community Medicine
Gajra Raja Medical College
Gwalior, Madhya Pradesh, India

Ashok Kumar Puranik MBBS MS (Gen Surgery) Fellowship Trauma (Aust)
Trauma Surgeon and Surgical Intervention
All India Institute of Medical Sciences
Jodhpur, Rajasthan, India

Ashok Vaid MD DM
Chairman
Division of Medical
Oncology and Hematology
Medanta Cancer Institute
Medanta—The Medicity
Gurugram, Haryana, India

Atma Ram Bansal MD DM (Neurology)
Neurologist and Epileptologist
Senior Consultant
Medanta Institute of Neurosciences
Medanta—The Medicity
Gurugram, Haryana, India

Atul Bansal MRCEM FRCEM
Consultant Emergency Department
Frimley Health NHS Trust
Wexham Park Hospital
Slough SL2 4HL UK

Basar Cander MD
Professor
Department of Emergency Medicine
Okmeydani Training and
Research Hospital
Okmeydani, Istanbul, Turkey

Beena Bansal MD (Medicine) DM (Endo)
Associate Director
Endocrinology and Diabetes
Medanta—The Medicity
Gurugram, Haryana, India

Bhanu Prakash Zawar MBBS MD
Associate Consultant
Cardiac Anesthesia
Medanta—The Medicity
Gurugram, Haryana, India

Bhawna Sharma DNB (Respiratory Medicine)
Specialist Critical Care
Artemis Hospital
Gurugram, Haryana, India

Bornali Datta MBBS MD CSST (UK) MRCP
Associate Director
Respiratory Medicine
Medanta—The Medicity
Gurugram, Haryana, India

Brajesh Kumar Mishra MBBS MD (Med)
DNB (Cardio)
Fellowship in Cardiac
Electrophysiology and Intervention
Medanta Heart Institute
Medanta—The Medicity
Gurugram, Haryana, India

Chandrashekhar MBBS DA DNB
(Anesthesia) IDCCM
Consultant
Institute of Critical Care
Medanta—The Medicity
Gurugram, Haryana, India

Chitra Mehta DNB (Respiratory Medicine)
FNB (Critical Care Medicine)
Associate Director
Institute of Critical Care
Medanta—The Medicity
Gurugram, Haryana, India

Devendra Richhariya MBBS MD FICM
Senior Consultant
Department of Emergency and
Trauma Care
Medanta—The Medicity
Gurugram, Haryana, India

Devender Sharma MD PGDCR
Fellowship in Pain and
Palliative Medicine
Associate Consultant
Division of Medical
Oncology and Hematology
Medanta Cancer Institute
Medanta—The Medicity
Gurugram, Haryana, India

Dheeraj Kapoor DM (Endocrinology)
Senior Consultant Endocrinology
Artemis Hospitals
Gurugram, Haryana, India

Dhiren Gupta MD
Senior Consultant
Department of Pediatrics
Institute of Child Health
Sir Ganga Ram Hospital
New Delhi, India

Dinesh Arora DCP
Consultant
Transfusion Medicine
Endocrinology and Diabetes
Medanta—The Medicity
Gurugram, Haryana, India

Dinesh Bhurani DM (Clinical Hematology)
FRCPA
Director
Hemato-oncology and BMT
Rajiv Gandhi Cancer Institute and
Research Center
New Delhi, India

Dinesh Chandra MCh
Associate Consultant
Cardiothoracic Surgery
Medanta—The Medicity
Gurugram, Haryana, India

Ganesh Jevalikar MD DNB PDCC
Senior Consultant
Pediatric Endocrinologist
Medanta—The Medicity
Gurugram, Haryana, India

HR Tomar DM (Cardiology)
Principal and Consultant
Department of Cardiology
Medanta Heart Institute
Medanta—The Medicity
Gurugram, Haryana, India

Hashim Mozzam MBBS
Attending Consultant
Department of Emergency and
Trauma Care
Medanta—The Medicity
Gurugram, Haryana, India

Jamal Yusuf DM (Cardiology)
Professor
Department of Cardiology
Govind Ballabh Pant Institute of
Postgraduate Medical
Education and Research
New Delhi, India

JS Wasir MD (Medicine) DM (Endocrinology)
Consultant, Endocrinology and Diabetes
Medanta—The Medicity
Gurugram, Haryana, India

Jyoti Wadhwa MD DM (Medical Oncology)
Director
Division of Medical Oncology and
Hematology, Medanta Cancer Institute
Medanta—The Medicity
Gurugram, Haryana, India

Kalpesh Sanariya MD (Medicine) DNB
(Trainee)
Senior Resident
Medanta Institute of Neurosciences
Medanta—The Medicity
Gurugram, Haryana, India

Kartikeya Bhargava MD DNB (Cardiology)
FHRS FCSI
Associate Director—Cardiology (EPS)
Medanta Heart Institute
Medanta—The Medicity
Gurugram, Haryana, India

Keerti Khetan MS (Obs and Gyne)
Senior Consultant
Department of Obstetrics and Gynecology
BLK Superspecialty Hospital
New Delhi, India

Khusrav Bajan MD EDIC
Consultant (Critical Care) and
Head
Department of Emergency
PD Hinduja National Hospital and
Medical Research Center
Mumbai, Maharashtra, India

Kishalay Datta MD
Head
Department of Emergency
Max Super Speciality Hospital
New Delhi, India

Kulbir Ahlawat MD
Associate Director
Department of Radiology
Medanta—The Medicity
Gurugram, Haryana, India

Kushagra Mahansaria MD
Senior Resident
Medanta Heart Institute
Medanta—The Medicity
Gurugram, Haryana, India

Madhukar Shahi MBBS MD DM (Cardiology)
DNB (Cardiology)
Director, Interventional Cardiology
Medanta Heart Institute
Medanta—The Medicity
Gurugram, Haryana, India

Manish Vaish DNB (Neurosurgery)
International Fellow of American
Association of Neurological Surgeons
(IFAANS)
Associate Director
Department of Neurosurgery
Max Healthcare
New Delhi, India

Contributors

Manish Bansal MD (Medicine) (AIIMS) DNB (Cardiology) FACC FASE FISCU Fellowship in Cardiac Imaging (Australia)
Associate Director
Department of Cardiology
Medanta—The Medicity
Gurugram, Haryana, India

Manish Garg MBBS (Dip Anaesthesia)
Senior Anesthetist and Intensivist
North Delhi Nursing Home
New Delhi, India

Manish Jain MBBS MD (Internal Medicine) DM (Nephrology)
Senior Consultant
Department of Nephrology
Medanta—The Medicity
Gurugram, Haryana, India
Clinical Fellow, UBC, Vancouver, Canada

Mansi Kaushik MBBS PGDCC
Associate Consultant
Medanta Heart Institute
Medanta—The Medicity
Gurugram, Haryana, India

Manvendra Singh MCh
Consultant
Cardiac Thoracic Surgery
Medanta—The Medicity
Gurugram, Haryana, India

Mayank Jain MBBS MD
Attending Consultant
Medanta Heart Institute
Medanta—The Medicity
Gurugram, Haryana, India

Michael J Nolan MSc BSc (HONS) Dip IMC RCS Ed
Search and Rescue Flight Paramedic
UAE Air Force and
Air Defence/Abu Dhabi Aviation
Abu Dhabi, UAE

Mona Dhingra MBBS MD
Senior Registrar
Endocrinology
Artemis Hospitals
Gurugram, Haryana, India

Mrinal Sircar MBBS DTCD MD DNB EDIC EDRM
Director and Head
Pulmonology and Critical Care
Fortis Hospital
Noida, Uttar Pradesh, India

M Sai Surendar MD DEM FICM D (DIAB)
Head
Emergency Department
Chennai National Hospital
Chennai, Tamil Nadu, India

MS Kuchay MD (Medicine) DM (Endocrinology)
Associate Consultant
Endocrinology and Diabetes
Medanta—The Medicity
Gurugram, Haryana, India

Mukul Aggarwal MBBS MD
Consultant Hemato-oncology and
Blood and Bone Marrow Transplant
Rajiv Gandhi Cancer Institute and
Research Center
New Delhi, India

Mukund Khetan MS
Consultant
Institute of Minimal Access
Metabolic and Bariatric Surgery
Sir Ganga Ram Hospital
New Delhi, India

Munesh Tomar MD (Pediatrics) FNB (Ped Cardio)
Associate Director
Pediatric Cardiology and
Congenital Heart Disease
Medanta—The Medicity
Gurugram, Haryana, India

Nagendra Singh Chouhan DM (Cardiology)
Associate Director
Medanta Heart Institute
Medanta—The Medicity
Gurugram, Haryana, India

Narendra Agarwal MBBS MD
Consultant Hemato-oncology and
Blood and Bone Marrow Transplant
Rajiv Gandhi Cancer Institute and
Research Center
New Delhi, India

Narendra Nath Jena MBBS MD
Consultant and Head
Emergency Medicine
Meenakshi Mission Hospital
Madurai, Tamil Nadu, India

Naval Mendiratta MD (Fellowship in Rheumatology)
Associate Consultant
Department of Rheumatology
Medanta—The Medicity
Gurugram, Haryana, India

Neelam Sharma MD DM
Associate Director
Division of Medical Oncology and
Hematology
Medanta Cancer Institute
Medanta—The Medicity
Gurugram, Haryana, India

Neeraj Saraf DNB (Gastroenterology)
Fellowship in Advanced Clinical Hepatology
Director
Gastroenterology and Hepatology
Medanta—The Medicity
Gurugram, Haryana, India

Nishant Arora MD (Anesthesia) FIACTA
Specialist Cardiac Anesthesia
National Heart Center
Royal Hospital
Muscat, Oman

Nitin Sood MD DNB MRCP (UK) MRCPath FRC (Pathology) CCT (Hemato-oncology)
Associate Director
Division of Medical Oncology and
Hematology
Medanta Cancer Institute
Medanta—The Medicity
Gurugram, Haryana, India

Omar Ghazanfar MBBS EBBEM
Physician Emergency Medicine
Zayed Military Hospital
UAE

P Aggarwal MD Medicine
Fellow, Endocrinology and Diabetes
Medanta—The Medicity
Gurugram, Haryana, India

Pooja Kataria MBBS
Resident
Department of Emergency and
Trauma Care
Medanta—The Medicity
Gurugram, Haryana, India

Poulomi Chatterji MD DNB (Respiratory Medicine) FISDA NCCP
Associate Consultant
Department of Respiratory Medicine
Medanta—The Medicity
Gurugram, Haryana, India

Prabhat Maheshwari MD (Pediatrics)
Senior Consultant
Artemis Hospital
Gurugram, Haryana, India

Pratibha Dhiman DM (Clinical Hematology)
Consultant
Division of Medical
Oncology and Hematology
Medanta Cancer Institute
Medanta—The Medicity
Gurugram, Haryana, India

Prattay Guhasarkar DM
Fellow of Cardiology
Govind Ballabh Pant Institute of
Postgraduate Medical
Education and Research
New Delhi, India

Praveen Chandra DM (Cardiology)
Chairman
Intervention Cardiology
Medanta Heart Institute
Medanta—The Medicity
Gurugram, Haryana, India

Puneet Ahluwalia MCh
Attending Consultant
Urology, Robotics and Kidney Transplant
Medanta—The Medicity
Gurugram, Haryana, India

Rachit Saxena MBBS MS MCh (CTVS)
Consultant
Cardiothoracic Surgery
Medanta—The Medicity
Gurugram, Haryana, India

Rahul Mehrotra MBBS MD DNB (Cardiology)
Principal
Consultant and Head
Noninvasive Cardiology
Max Super Speciality Hospital
New Delhi, India

Rahul Rai MD DM
Transplant Hepatology
Medanta Institute of Digestive and
Hepatobiliary Sciences and Medanta
Institute of Liver Transplantation and
Regenerative Medicine
Medanta—The Medicity
Gurugram, Haryana, India

Rajani Yadav MBBS
Consultant Thyrocare Laboratory
Thyrocare Diagnostics
New Delhi, India

Rajeev Goyal MD (Medicine) DM (Neurology)
Fellow in Movement Disorders
Consultant
Medanta Institute of Neurosciences
Medanta—The Medicity
Gurugram, Haryana, India

Rajesh Chawla MD EDIC
Senior Consultant
Department of Respiratory and
Critical Care
Indraprashtha Apollo Hospital
New Delhi, India

Rajesh Puri MBBS MD DNB (Gastro) MNAMS
Director
Gastroenterologist and Hepatologist
Institute of Digestive and
Hepatobiliary Sciences
Medanta—The Medicity
Gurugram, Haryana, India

Rajiva Gupta MD DNB MRCP (UK) FACR (US)
FRCP (Glas) FRCP (Edn)
Director and Head
Rheumatology and Clinical Immunology
Medanta—The Medicity
Gurugram, Haryana, India

Rajiv Yadav MCh
Associate Director
Uro-oncology and Robotic Surgery
Medanta—The Medicity
Gurugram, Haryana, India

Rajneesh Kapoor MD DNB (Cardiology)
Senior Director
Interventional Cardiology
Medanta Heart Institute
Medanta—The Medicity
Gurugram, Haryana, India

Rakesh Khera MBBS MS (Surgery) MCh
(Urology) DNB (Urology)
Director
Urology, Robotics and Kidney Transplant
Medanta—The Medicity
Gurugram, Haryana, India

Rakesh K Khazanchi MBBS MS MCh
(Plastic Surgery)
Chairman
Department of Plastic Surgery
Medanta—The Medicity
Gurugram, Haryana, India

Ramanjit Singh MD
Visiting Consultant
Department of Dermatologist
Medanta—The Medicity
Gurugram, Haryana, India

Ram NG MBBS
Junior Consultant
BGS Global Hospitals
Bengaluru, Karnataka, India

Randhir Sud MD DM (Gastroenterology)
Chairman
Institute of Digestive and
Hepatobiliary Sciences
Medanta—The Medicity
Gurugram, Haryana, India

Rashmi Xavier MD
Associate Consultant
Medanta Heart Institute
Medanta—The Medicity
Gurugram, Haryana, India

Ratandeep Bose MBBS MS MCh
(Neurosurgery)
Associate Consultant
Medanta Institute of Neurosciences
Medanta—The Medicity
Gurugram, Haryana, India

Ravi C Dara MD (Transfusion Medicine)
Attending Consultant
Transfusion Medicine
Medanta—The Medicity
Gurugram, Haryana, India

Ravi R Kasliwal MD DM MNAMS FIMSA
Chairman
Clinical and Preventive Cardiology
Medanta Heart Institute
Medanta—The Medicity
Gurugram, Haryana, India

Rayaz Ahmed MD
Consultant
Hemato-oncology and
Bone Marrow Transplantation
Rajiv Gandhi Cancer Institute and
Research Center
New Delhi, India

Ritabh Kumar MBBS MS (Ortho)
Senior Consultant Orthopedics
Indian Spinal Injuries Center
New Delhi, India

Rohit Goyal MD
Attending Consultant
Medanta Heart Institute
Medanta—The Medicity
Gurugram, Haryana, India

Roop Sharma MD
Fellow in Pediatric Critical Care
Sir Ganga Ram Hospital
New Delhi, India

Ruchi Kapoor MD
Senior Consultant and
Chief of Lab Medicine
OncQuest Diagnostics
New Delhi, India

Sabhyata Gupta MD (Obs and Gyne)
Director and Head
Division of Gynecology
Gyne-Oncology and Robotic Surgery
Medanta—The Medicity
Gurugram, Haryana, India

Contributors **xi**

Safal DM
Assistant Professor
Department of Cardiology
Govind Ballabh Pant Institute of
Postgraduate Medical
Education and Research
New Delhi, India

Saibal Mukhopadhyay DM (Cardiology)
Professor
Department of Cardiology
Govind Ballabh Pant Institute of
Postgraduate Medical
Education and Research
New Delhi, India

Saleh Fares MD MPH FRCPC (EM) FACEP FAAEM
Consultant, Emergency Medicine
EMS and Disaster Medicine
Deputy Commander
Zayed Military Hospital
Founder and President
Emirates Society of Emergency Medicine
Abu Dhabi, UAE

Salil Jain MD DNB (Nephrology)
Additional Director
Nephrology and Kidney Transplant
Fortis Hospital
Gurugram, Haryana, India
Clinical Fellowship (Nephro)
Toronto, Canada

Sandeep Jain MS FNB (Trauma Care)
PGDMLS MEM
Senior Consultant and Head
Department of Emergency and Trauma
Max Super Speciality Hospital
New Delhi, India

Sangeeta Kaushik Sharma MS (Obs and Gyne) FCGP FIAMS
Senior Consultant Gynecologist
Director
Sharma Hospital
Bilaspur, Chattisgarh, India

Sanjiv Saigal MD DM MRCP
Director–Transplant Hepatology
Medanta Institute of Digestive and
Hepatobiliary Sciences and Medanta
Institute of Liver Transplantation and
Regenerative Medicine
Medanta—The Medicity
Gurugram, Haryana, India

Saurabh Mehra MBBS MD IDCC FNB EDIC
Associate Consultant
Pulmonology and Critical Care
Fortis Hospital
Noida, Uttar Pradesh, India

Shaiwal Khandelwal MS (Surgery) FIAGES FICS
Consultant
Minimally Invasive and
Robotic and Thoracic Surgery
Medanta—The Medicity
Gurugram, Haryana, India
Fellowship
Seoul National University
Seoul, South Korea

Sharad Manar MD (Physician)
Attending Consultant
Department of Emergency and
Trauma Care
Medanta—The Medicity
Gurugram, Haryana, India

Shashank Chauhan MBBS MEM
(Masters in EM)
Associate Consultant
Department of Emergency and
Trauma Care
Medanta—The Medicity
Gurugram, Haryana, India

Shradha Chaudhari MD (Obs and Gyne)
FCPS FICOG DGO
Consultant
Gyne-oncology and Robotic Surgery
Medanta—The Medicity
Gurugram, Haryana, India

Shruti Bajad MD
Attending Consultant
Department of Rheumatology
Medanta—The Medicity
Gurugram, Haryana, India

Sinoy Jose RN RM
Training Co-ordinator
Medanta—The Medicity
Gurugram, Haryana, India

Sonal Krishan MBBS MD (Radiology) FRCR
MSc (Radiology)
Consultant
Department of Radiology
Medanta—The Medicity
Gurugram, Haryana, India

Sonam Kaushika MBBS MEM
Attending Consultant
Department of Emergency and
Trauma Care
Medanta—The Medicity
Gurugram, Haryana, India

Sucheta Yadav MD DM (Nephrology)
Associate Consultant
Fortis Hospital
Gurugram, Haryana, India

Sudha Kansal MD IDCCM
Senior Consultant
Department of Respiratory and
Critical Care
Indraprastha Apollo Hospital
New Delhi, India

Sudhir BS MBBS (Dip Emergency Medicine)
Attending Consultant
Department of Emergency and
Trauma Care
Medanta—The Medicity
Gurugram, Haryana, India

Sudhir Dubey MCh
Director
Minimally Invasive Neurosurgery
Medanta Institute of Neurosciences
Medanta—The Medicity
Gurugram, Haryana, India

Sudhir S Pawaiya MBBS Diploma in
Emergency Medicine
Consultant
Department of Emergency and
Trauma Care
Medanta—The Medicity
Gurugram, Haryana, India

Sukhdeep Singh MBBS MS MCh
Consultant
Plastic, Aesthetic and
Reconstructive Surgery
Medanta—The Medicity
Gurugram, Haryana, India

Sunil Dubey MD (Physician) MBA MHA
Head
Air Ambulance Services
Pre-Hospital Care
Department of Emergency and
Trauma Care
Medanta—The Medicity
Gurugram, Haryana, India

Sunil Kumar Mishra MD DM
Associate Director
Endocrinology and Diabetes
Medanta—The Medicity
Gurugram, Haryana, India

Swarup S Padhi MBBS MD FNB
Senior Resident
Institute of Critical Care
Medanta—The Medicity
Gurugram, Haryana, India

Syed Ahmed Adil MD
Accident and Emergency
Consultant and Deputy Head
Department of Emergency
Dr Mehta's Multispecialty Hospital
Chennai, Tamil Nadu, India

Taif Nabi MD (Physician)
Clinical Associate
Emergency and Trauma Care
Medanta—The Medicity
Gurugram, Haryana, India

Tamorish Kole MBBS Fellowship in
Emergency Medicine
Chairman
Emergency and Trauma Care
VPS Rockland Hospital
New Delhi, India

Tarannum MD DNB
Senior Resident
Department of Endocrinology
Medanta—The Medicity
Gurugram, Haryana, India

Tariq Ali MBBS MD EDIC
Director
Institute of Critical Care
Medanta—The Medicity
Gurugram, Haryana, India

Tarun S FNB (Critical Care)
Consultant
Department of Respiratory and
Critical Care
Indraprashtha Apollo Hospital
New Delhi, India

TS Srinath Kumar MD
Head
Department of Emergency
Narayana Hrudayalaya
Bengaluru, Karnataka, India

Uday Aditya Gupta MBBS DTCD DNB
IDCCM FCCP(USA)
Associate Consultant
Max Super Speciality Hospital
Ghaziabad, Uttar Pradesh, India

Umang B Kothari MBBS MS
Senior Resident
Department of Plastic Surgery
Medanta—The Medicity
Gurugram, Haryana, India

Varun Mittal MBBS MS (Surgery)
MCh (Urology) DNB (Urology)
Consultant
Urology, Robotics and Kidney Transplant
Medanta—The Medicity
Gurugram, Haryana, India

Vikas Mudgal MD (Physician) PGDCC FNIC
Associate Consultant
Department of Cardiology
Medanta—The Medicity
Gurugram, Haryana, India

Vimalendu Brajesh MBBS MS MCh
Consultant
Plastic, Aesthetic and Reconstructive Surgery
Medanta—The Medicity
Gurugram, Haryana, India

Vinayak Agarwal MD DNB (Cardiology)
Associate Director
Noninvasive Cardiology
Medanta—The Medicity
Gurugram, Haryana, India

Vishal Saxena MD DNB (Nephrology)
Senior Consultant
Nephrology and Kidney Transplant
Fortis Hospital
Gurugram, Haryana, India

Vivekanshu Verma MBBS
Diploma in Forensic Medicine and Toxicology
Attending Consultant
Department of Emergency and Trauma Care
Medanta—The Medicity
Gurugram, Haryana, India

Vijay Kumar Chopra MD DM (Cardiology)
Director
Heart Failure Programme
Medanta Heart Institute
Medanta—The Medicity
Gurugram, Haryana, India

VV Pillay MD DCL
Chief
Poison Control Centre and
Clinical Forensic Unit
Professor and Head
Forensic Medicine Toxicology
Amrita Institute of Medical
Sciences and Research
Kochi, Kerala, India

Yatin Mehta MD MNAMS FRCA FAMS
FIACTA FICCM FTEE
Chairman
Medanta Institute of
Critical Care and Anesthesiology
Medanta—The Medicity
Gurugram, Haryana, India

Yeeshu Singh Sudan MD Fellow in
Pediatric Neurology
Associate Consultant
Pediatric Neurologist
Medanta Institute of Neurosciences
Medanta—The Medicity
Gurugram, Haryana, India

Foreword

As I write the foreword for the first edition for his book, I cannot help but reminisce Dr Devendra Richhariya's humble beginnings as a good emergency physician, managing emergencies efficiently, making practical protocols and updated guidelines for doctors and nurses in emergency department and beyond. I have been closely associated with emergency department since my days as a novice surgeon, than as a cardiothoracic surgeon, and now as a Chairman and Managing Director of Medanta—The Medicity.

Injury and illness are universal healthcare problems. All over the world, efforts are being made to curb the preventable diseases, which have devastating consequences for society, economy, and country. There has been gradual recognition worldwide that managing illnesses and injuries as disease processes managed by trained and qualified emergency physicians, and not just a nocturnal activity of young, novice untrained resident doctors in casualty improves outcome. India has been late in recognition of emergency medicine as a specialty, and trauma is becoming subspecialty of surgical sciences. The arrival of *Textbook of Emergency and Trauma Care* developed specifically for India is long overdue.

I have closely observed the struggle and stress of DNB and MD students in emergency, who during their graduation, find it difficult to read and learn from bulky textbooks of foreign authors, unrelated to Indian emergency scenarios, which is very nicely covered in the textbook. It describes the *know-how* of managing emergencies in prescriptive format, to facilitate the primary intention to be a *ready-reckoner*, and to empower the first responder with confidence and clarity. Therapeutic regimen and infusion protocols are deliberately kept simple for realistic application in rustic conditions. It is a multi-authored book, written by the experienced and expert authorities in the field, both at national and international levels. Their vision, thought process and knowledge get reflected in their writings. In addition, each one of them has added a flavor of their individual writing style, so reading through different chapters of the book is an interesting journey. It is a *must-read* textbook for every healthcare provider, making his/her entry in multispecialty hospital, before embarking his clinical activities. It can ease the problems of young ones, and keep the senior doctors abreast with current trends in emergency medical services. However, it is not a book to be read in one sitting. I advice them read slowly, assimilate, reflect, shape their day-to-day clinical practice, and provide feedback to the editor for the next edition. In case anyone wishes to delve deeply into any of the interest area, the list of authentic references provided at the end of each chapter will guide them. Dr Richhariya has used his academic and research experience to edit the detailed views of the authors, and presented a reliable emergency handy guide with a problem-solving approach.

Naresh Trehan
Diplomate
American Board of Cardiothoracic Surgery
Chairman
Medanta Heart Institute
Chairman and Managing Director
Medanta—The Medicity
Gurugram, Haryana, India

Foreword

Emergency medicine is a fast-growing specialty still in its infancy in India. Mushrooming of secondary and tertiary care hospitals in India particularly in the metropolitan cities, exponential increase in the number of highways, and high-end speeding cars with drunken drivers has led to sharp increase in admissions in emergency room (ER) or triage or/casualties of hospitals.

Existence of age-old systems or complete absence of standard operating procedures (SOPs) in these cases leads to confusion, chaos, and delay in life-saving procedures with huge escalation in morbidity, mortality, increased length of stay, cost, and subsequent medicolegal implications.

Poor prehospital transport and interventions lead to loss of precious initial golden hours in trauma, acute stroke, and myocardial infarction with catastrophic results.

Initial prehospital management which may be remote monitoring, thrombolytic or antiarrhythmics, advance cardiac life support (ACLS), and advanced trauma life support (ATLS) can save a lot of lives. India is just catching up with all these with national board starting DNB in Emergency Medicine and Society of Emergency Medicine in India already having Masters in Emergency Medicine (MEM), but these are just drops in ocean for the trained manpower requirement of ER. Also, these structured courses will lead to original Indian data and research done in India, so that clinical pathways for patients in ER can be designed specifically for Indian conditions rather than using extrapolated SOPs from the West.

Early goal-directed therapy for severe sepsis or septic shock was started in a study in ER of Detroit. So, initial ER care can lay the foundation for management strategies in the critical care.

In this context, the *Textbook of Emergency and Trauma Care* is a timely welcome addition to the current literature. It has 100 chapters with a large number of authors covering the whole spectrum of emergency medicine. I congratulate Dr Devendra Richhariya and the team of M/s Jaypee Brothers Medical Publishers (P) Ltd, New Delhi, India, for this commendable endeavor. This would be a valuable asset to any library of ER.

Yatin Mehta
MD MNAMS FRCA FAMS FIACTA FICCM FTEE
Chairman
Medanta Institute of Critical Care and Anesthesiology
Medanta—The Medicity
Gurugram, Haryana, India

Foreword

I, first congratulate Dr Devendra Richhariya, for an excellent book on emergency care. This is truly a *Textbook of Emergency and Trauma Care*. In this fast-moving world emergencies arise with alarming frequency—in the home, at the place of work and while travelling the busy highways not to mention natural disasters, calamities and accidents. To add to this burden of emergencies is the ever-increasing number of patients, who suffer from life style disease, and frequent the ERs with chest pain, strokes, uncontrolled hypertension to name a few.

In this background, the book is timely and much needed. With 100 chapters, it is also all encompassing and will be widely read and appreciated. In the plethora of books available in this field, it will stand out purely on the basis of the fact that its strength lies in that the authors are senior, savvy and seasoned professionals, who have spent hours working with their staff in the ER. Many of the authors are personally known to me, and I can say that they have impeccable credentials as authors and teachers. Hence, the strength of the book.

I have known Dr Devendra Richhariya from the past 8 years, and I can say that he is a sincere and dedicated individual, who cares for sick patients and above all as a team player.

Happy Reading!

Ravi R Kasliwal
MD DM MNAMS FIMSA
Chairman
Division of Clinical and Preventive Cardiology
Medanta—The Medicity
Gurugram, Haryana, India

Preface

"The life so short, the craft so long to learn" —*Hippocrates*

We have a passion for improving patient care. Our journey with *Textbook of Emergency and Trauma Care* began with superb mentors, who instilled in us a drive to become excellent clinicians and educators. We discovered imaging was a powerful tool to take the learner *to-the-bedside* and establish permanence, in a fashion unlike any other didactic technique.

Emergency care is defined by time, and the emergency department is the most diverse melting pot of acute conditions in the hospital. Diagnostic accuracy, prognostic prediction, and the treatment pathways rely heavily on typical clues.

We also strongly believe the emergency experience, while sometimes downplayed within the hectic and time-pressured environment of modern medicine, is critical to ideal education.

How do we identify the scope of practice, and knowledge that is today's specialty of emergency medicine? Is it through paper books, blogs, social networking, Google, journals, or clinical practice? While e-information is perfectly suited for multitasking, frequent-attention shifts of the emergency medicine environment may make it unsuitable at times. E-information provides information about snippets of care, but not about the comprehensive knowledge set that is our specialty. The practice of emergency medicine continues to evolve, bringing greater expectations of the physicians, who provide field care in interhospital shifting by ambulance and medical oversight.

There have been many milestones along the road of development of the specialty. The breadth of knowledge and skills required to serve as a competent emergency physician is unique and rapidly expanding. The advent of MD in Emergency Medicine, start of DNB-accreditation of emergency medicine programs, and the continuous broadening of the clinical practice of emergency medicine has made the formal study of the art and practice even more essential than ever before.

Emergency medicine has taken its place in the *House of Medicine*. Now, it is our duty to ensure we show our worth by never-ending commitment to improving patient care across the entire scope of our practice as emergency physicians. Now is the time of our "Renaissance" and it is our most sincere hope that this text serves you well on your journey, wherever the practice of emergency medicine may take you.

The audience for this text is all who provide emergency medical care including clinicians, educators, MD and DNB residents, nurses, prehospital caregivers, and medical students. Many have also found it extremely useful as a review for written pre-postgraduation examinations containing pictorial questions. Other healthcare workers, such as internists, family physicians, pediatricians, nurse practitioners, and physician assistants, will find this textbook a useful guide in identifying and treating many acute conditions, where clinical clues significantly guide, improve, and expedite diagnosis as well as treatment.

We thank many contributors and readers who have helped make this edition possible. We are especially grateful to three great educators who share our passion: Dr Naresh Trehan, Dr Yatin Mehta, and Dr Ravi R Kasliwal.

Devendra Richhariya
Saleh Fares
Khusrav Bajan
Sudhir S Pawaiya

Acknowledgments

We are grateful to Dr Naresh Trehan, Dr Yatin Mehta, and Dr Ravi R Kasliwal, for showing trust on us and giving us the opportunity to work in the state-of-the-art institution, *Medanta—The Medicity*, Gurugram, Haryana, India, and also for providing the best infrastructure and facilities in emergency department for the patients.

We are thankful to each and every member of the Medanta family.

Especially thankful to Dr Sudhir Singh Pawaiya and Dr Sunil Dubey for giving us encouragement and support over the period of more than a decade and the journey still continues. We would like to acknowledge all our seniors and emergency department colleagues for supporting us during the project.

We would like to sincerely thank all the authors for providing manuscripts in spite of their busy schedules.

Special thanks to publisher Shri Jitendar P Vij (Group Chairman), Mr Ankit Vij (Group President), Ms Chetna Malhotra Vohra (Associate Director–Content Strategy), Ms Heena Gogia (Development Editor), Mr Binay Kumar (Proofreader), Mr Chandra Dutt (Typesetter), Mr Ram Singh Pundhir (Graphic Designer), and all members of M/s Jaypee Brothers Medical Publishers (P) Ltd, New Delhi, India, for their invaluable contribution.

Contents

SECTION 1: ESSENTIALS FOR EMERGENCY PHYSICIAN

1. Essentials for Good Emergency Physician — 3
Devendra Richhariya, Vivekanshu Verma

Good Emergency Physician Must Demonstrate *3*

2. Emergency Design and Staffing — 6
Saleh Fares, Omar Ghazanfar

- Emergency Department Design *6* • Emergency Department Function *6*
- General Considerations for Designing an Emergency Department *6* • Patient Flow *7*
- Dedicated Areas within an Emergency Department *7* • New Concepts in Emergency Department Design *7* • Staffing Model *8* • Medical and Practitioner Staffing in Emergency Departments *8* • How to Staff an Emergency Department? *8*

3. Triaging — 10
Devendra Richhariya

- Emergency Department Triaging *10* • Requirements for Triaging *10*
- Triaging Process *11* • Early Warning Score in Triage *12* • Triage in Mass Casualty Incident *13*

4. Rapid Assessment and Treatment in Emergency — 17
Devendra Richhariya

- Benefits of Rapid Assessment *17* • Requirements for Rapid Assessment *17*
- Steps for Rapid Assessment and Treatment *17* • Components of Rapid Assessment and Treatment *18* • Clinical Quality Indicators for Rapid Assessment *19*
- Rapid Assessment, Early Interventions and Improving Outcome in Sepsis, Stroke and Trauma *19*

5. Point of Care Testing — 22
Shashank Chauhan, Rajani Yadav

- Point of Care Testing: Need of the Hour *22* • Challenges in Effective Implementation of Point of Care Testing *24*

6. Essentials of Medicolegal Case Writing — 25
Vivekanshu Verma, Devendra Richhariya

- Medicolegal Classification of Wounds *25* • Preparation of MLC Reports *27*
- Practical Tips for Medicolegal Case Writing *31*

7. Medicolegal Issues in Emergency — 35
Adarsh Kumar, Vivekanshu Verma

- Doctor: Working for the Law or Against the Law? *35* • What is Duty of Care Towards Patient? *37*
- What is Doctrine of *Res IPSA Loquitur*? *37* • Why Medical Services are included Under Consumer Protection Act, 1986? *39* • What Constitutes Medical Negligence? *41*

- What does not Constitute Medical Negligence? *41* • Mediclaims and Medicolegal Issues *43*
- Medicolegal Tips for Emergency by Dr RK Sharma *44* • Medicolegal Queries Answered by Dr MC Gupta *53*

8. Patient Safety and Quality in Emergency Department — 72
Devendra Richhariya, Sudhir S Pawaiya

- Triaging and Smooth Flow of Emergency Department *72* • Good Quality Trained Emergency Team *72*
- Timely Support by Specialties *74* • Important Diagnostics Areas Near Emergency Department *74*
- Observation Areas *74* • Medications and Sedation Safety *75*

9. Standards of Care during Air Transfer — 78
Saleh Fares, Michael J Nolan

- Pathophysiology *79* • Standards of Care *80* • Special Considerations *81* • Recent Advances *82*

10. Standards of Care during Road Transfer — 83
Sunil Dubey, Sudhir S Pawaiya, Vivekanshu Verma

- Standard ABCDE Approach *83* • What you Need to Know before You Go!! *85*
- Factors Associated with Fewer Adverse Events during Ambulance Transfer *85*
- Advantages of 'Specialized Teams' for Transportation *85* • Recommendations for the Transfer of Critically Ill Patients *85* • Clinical Handover Process for Ambulance Transfer *85*
- National Standard for Ambulances in India *86* • Medicolegal Issues in Ambulance Transfer *86*

SECTION 2: RESUSCITATION AND CRITICAL CARE IN EMERGENCY

11. Management of Cardiac Arrest in Adults — 91
Uday Aditya Gupta, Sinoy Jose

- Pathophysiology *91* • Chain of Survival *91*

12. Airway Management — 99
Amit D Nabar

- Applied Anatomy *99* • Causes of Airway Obstruction in Emergency Department *100*
- Objective Signs of Airway Obstruction *100* • Clinical Assessment of the Airway *101*
- Preparation *101* • Management *102*

13. Management of Critically Ill Patient in Emergency — 110
Chandrashekhar, Swarup S Padhi, Ajeet Singh, Tariq Ali, Yatin Mehta

- Body Fluid Compartments *110* • Principles of Fluid Therapy in Critically Ill *110*
- Vasoactive Agents *113* • Assessment *115*

14. Overview of Shock — 117
Khusrav Bajan, Archana Shrivastav

- What is Shock? *117* • Etiopathophysiology of Shock *117* • Clinical Presentation *118*
- Management of Shock *118*

15. Sepsis and Septic Shock — 122
Chandrashekhar, Swarup S Padhi, Ajeet Singh, Tariq Ali, Yatin Mehta

- Clinical Criteria for Sepsis *122* • Tool for Screening Out Sepsis *124* • Management of Septic Shock and Sepsis Protocols *125* • Fluid Therapy of Sepsis: Use of Vasopressors, Inotropes and Corticosteroids *129* • Supportive Therapy *130*

16. Noninvasive Ventilation — 135
Kishalay Datta

- Noninvasive Positive-Pressure Ventilation *135* • How does NIPPV Work? *136*
- What Type of Ventilators can be used for NIPPV? *137* • What Modes of Ventilator can be used for Noninvasive Ventilation? *137* • How to Set the Ventilator for NIPPV? *137*
- Selection Criteria for NIPPV *137* • Contraindications for NIPPV *137*
- How to Initiate NIPPV in Patients? *137* • Monitoring of Patients on NIPPV *138*
- Predictors of Success of NIPPV *138* • Weaning *138* • Complications of NIPPV *138*

17. Mechanical Ventilation — 142
Mrinal Sircar, Saurabh Mehra

- Physiology of Breathing *142* • Mechanical Determinants of Patient-Ventilator Interactions *143*
- Indications of Mechanical Ventilation *143* • Types of Mechanical Ventilation *144*
- Modes of Ventilation *144* • Initiation of Ventilation *147* • Ventilation in Special Conditions *148*
- What to do after Initiating Ventilation? *150* • Transporting Intubated Patients *150*
- Complications and Side Effects of Intubation and Ventilation *150*

18. Use of Blood and Blood Products in Emergency — 153
Aseem K Tiwari, Ravi C Dara, Dinesh Arora

- Responsibility of Emergency and Blood Bank Team *153* • Transfusion Approach in Emergency and Massive Transfusion Protocol *154* • Role of Specific Blood Components *155*

19. Arterial Blood Gas Analysis — 158
Sudha Kansal, Rajesh Chawla, Tarun S

- Indications *158* • Absolute Contraindications *158* • Definitions of Acid–base Disorders *158*
- Nomenclature *159* • pH and Partial Pressure of Carbon Dioxide Relationship in Respiratory Disorders *159*
- Equations for Analysis of Acid–base Disorders—Compensations *159* • Anion Gap Concept *160*
- Interpretation of Arterial Blood Gas *160* • Seven Steps of Analysis of Arterial Blood Gas *160*
- Strong Ion Difference versus Traditional Approach *162*

20. Oxygen Therapy — 164
Poulomi Chatterji, Bhawna Sharma

- Indications *164* • Types of Hypoxia *164* • Oxygen Devices *164* • Long-term Oxygen Therapy *169* • Hyperbaric Oxygen Therapy *169* • Which Oxygen Delivery System to Use? *169* • Goals of Oxygen Therapy *169* • Monitoring *169*
- Oxygen Toxicity *169*

21. Acute Pain Management in Emergency Department — 172
Sonam Kaushika, Devendra Richhariya, Manish Garg

- Pain Categories *172* • Mechanism Involved in Nociceptive Pain *172* • Assessment of Pain in Emergency Department *173* • Indications of Urgent Pain Management in Medical Emergencies *173* • Potential Causes for Pain Control Failure *174* • Treatment of Pain in Emergency Department *174*

SECTION 3: CARDIAC EMERGENCIES

22. Chest Pain — 183
Rohit Goel, Rashmi Xavier, Nagendra Singh Chouhan, Praveen Chandra

- Causes of Chest Pain *183* • Evaluation *185* • Diagnostic Approach *188*
- Evaluation of Chest Pain of Cardiac Origin *188* • Evaluation of Chest Pain of Various Causes *188*

23. Palpitations 193
Shashank Chauhan, Ram NG, HR Tomar
- Etiology *193*
- Differential Diagnosis of Palpitations *193*
- Managing Palpitations *194*
- Management Pearls *195*

24. Syncope 196
Brajesh Kumar Mishra
- Epidemiology *196*
- Pathophysiology or Mechanism *196*
- Classification *196*
- Management *198*
- Investigation *199*
- Treatment *201*
- Future Perspective and Advancement *203*

25. Acute Coronary Syndrome: Risk Stratification 205
Mayank Jain, Rajneesh Kapoor
- Risk Stratification after ST-elevation Myocardial Infarction *205*
- Risk Stratification of Unstable Angina and Non-ST-segment Elevation Myocardial Infarction *207*

26. Cardiogenic Shock 216
Devendra Richhariya, Vikas Mudgal, Madhukar Shahi
- Definition *216*
- Etiology *216*
- Pathophysiology *217*
- Diagnosis *218*
- Management *219*
- Intensive Care Unit Support *220*
- Special Situation *223*

27. Heart Failure 226
Vijay Kumar Chopra
- Initial Clinical Assessment *226*
- Specific Agents used during Hospitalization *228*
- Escalating Support *230*

28. Bradyarrhythmias 233
Jamal Yusuf, Safal, Saibal Mukhopadhyay
- Etiology *233*
- Symptoms *233*
- Classification *233*
- Management *236*

29. Tachyarrhythmia 238
Jamal Yusuf, Prattay Guhasarkar, Saibal Mukhopadhyay
- Electrocardiographic Features *238*
- Supraventricular Tachycardias *239*
- Ventricular Tachycardias *240*

30. Temporary Pacing 244
Kartikeya Bhargava
- Types of Temporary Pacing *244*
- Indications of Temporary Pacing *245*
- Temporary Pacing Procedure *245*
- Complications of Temporary Pacing *246*
- Post-Procedure Care *247*

31. Hypertensive Emergency 248
Ravi R Kasliwal, Kushagra Mahansaria
- Classification *248*
- Epidemiology *249*
- Pathogenesis *249*
- Clinical Presentation *249*
- Assessment *249*
- Initial Therapeutic Approach *250*
- Pharmacological Therapy for Hypertensive Crisis *250*

32. Aortic Dissection 256
Rachit Saxena, Manvendra Singh, Dinesh Chandra, Anil Bhan

- Definition *256* • Classification *256* • Pathophysiology *257* • Clinical Implications *257*
- Clinical Features *258* • Symptoms *259* • Clinical Signs *259* • Investigations *260*
- Diagnostic Strategy *262* • Aims of Treatment *263* • Exceptions *263*
- Management of Type A Aortic Dissection *263* • Management of Type B Aortic Dissection *263*

33. Care of Patient on Anticoagulation 266
Vinayak Agarwal, Devendra Richhariya

- Types of Anticoagulants *266* • Advantages *266* • Disadvantages *266* • Medicines that Increase the Risk of Bleeding in Patients on Oral Anticoagulants *267* • Heparin and Low Molecular Weight Heparin *267* • Monitoring Anticoagulation Therapy: Target INR *267*
- Blood Tests used in Emergency Department to Monitor Anticoagulants *267*
- Management of Over Anticoagulation *267* • Education to Patient about Anticoagulation *267*

34. Cardiac Biomarkers 269
Rahul Mehrotra

- The Ideal Cardiac Biomarker *269* • Acute Coronary Syndrome *270* • Deep Vein Thrombosis and Pulmonary Embolism *270* • Cardiac Biomarkers in Heart Failure *271*
- Multimarker Strategy *271* • Summary and Future Perspective *271*

35. Electrocardiogram Interpretation in Emergency 273
Kartikeya Bhargava

- Cardiac Arrhythmias *273* • ST-Segment Deviation *277* • T Wave Changes *278*
- QRS Morphology, Amplitude and Duration and Axis Patterns *279*
- Miscellaneous Electrocardiogram Findings in Emergency *280*

36. Role of Echocardiography in Emergency Room 281
Mansi Kaushik, Manish Bansal, Ravi R Kasliwal

- Patients Presenting with Acute Chest Pain *281* • Dyspnea/Shortness of Breath *285*
- Hypotension and Hemodynamic Instability *287* • Echocardiography in Stroke Patients *289*
- Syncope *290* • Fever of Unknown Origin *291*

37. Coronary Computed Tomography in Emergency 294
Kulbir Ahlawat, Devendra Richhariya

- Indications of Coronary Computed Tomography Angiography (CT Angiography of Heart) *294*
- Contraindications for Coronary CT in the ED *295* • Preparation for Coronary CT *295*
- Interpretation and Reporting of Coronary CT *296* • Factors Affecting the Quality of Coronary CT Images *297* • Advantages of Coronary CT in Emergency Department *297*
- "Triple Rule Out" Protocol *297*

38. Precardiac Surgery Evaluation 299
Bhanu Prakash Zawar, Yatin Mehta

- Physical Examination *299* • Investigations *300*
- Risk Assessment and Stratification *300*

39. Postcardiac Surgical Emergencies — 301
Nishant Arora, Yatin Mehta

- Postcardiac Surgical Emergencies *301* • Immediate Postoperative Complications *301*
- Early Postoperative Complications *304*

SECTION 4: RESPIRATORY EMERGENCIES

40. Hemoptysis — 315
Poulomi Chatterji, Bhawna Sharma

- Massive Hemoptysis *315* • Pulmonary Circulation *316* • Evaluation *316*
- Risk Factors *316* • Family History *316* • Physical Examination *316* • Investigations *316*
- Initial Resuscitation *317* • Localization of Site *318* • Topical Bronchoscopic Therapy *318*
- Medical Treatment *319* • Bronchial Artery Embolization *319* • Surgery *319* • Clinical Pearls *320*

41. Acute Respiratory Failure — 322
Chitra Mehta, Yatin Mehta

- Definition *322* • Epidemiology *322* • Classification *322* • Pathophysiology *323*
- Clinical Presentation *324* • Diagnostic Approach *324* • Management *325*

42. Acute Exacerbation of Asthma and Chronic Obstructive Pulmonary Disease — 328
Ashish Kumar Prakash, Bornali Datta, Anand Jaiswal

- Bronchial Asthma *328* • Chronic Obstructive Pulmonary Disease *328*
- Acute Exacerbation of COPD and Acute Asthma in Emergency *329*

43. Pneumonia — 336
Ashish Kumar Prakash, Bornali Datta, Anand Jaiswal

- Pneumonia in Emergency *336* • Clinical Evaluation *336* • Diagnostic Approach *337*
- Treatment of Pneumonia *337* • Initial Empiric Antimicrobial Therapy for Cap *338*

44. Pneumothorax and Insertion of Chest Tube — 340
Shaiwal Khandelwal, Ali Zamir Khan

- Classification and Etiology *340* • Pathophysiology *340* • Clinical Features *340*
- Imaging Modalities *341* • Treatment of Pneumothorax *341* • Chest Drain Insertion *342*

45. Pulmonary Embolism — 345
Saleh Fares, Omar Ghazanfar

- Pathophysiology of Pulmonary Embolism *345* • Clinical Signs and Symptoms *345*
- Scoring Systems for Risk Stratifying Pulmonary Embolisms *347*

SECTION 5: NEUROLOGICAL EMERGENCIES

46. Vertigo — 353
Kalpesh Sanariya, Abdul Muniem

Approach to the Patient with Acute Vertigo *354*

47. Acute Headache — 360
Devendra Richhariya, Rajeev Goyal

- Objectives for Emergency Physician in Acute Headache Patients *360* • Primary Headache *360*
- Secondary Headache *362* • Approach to Acute Headache in Emergency Department *362*
- Alarming Signs and Symptoms in Acute Headache *363* • Neuroimaging in Acute Headache *363*
- Laboratory Investigations *363* • Disposition *363*

48. Acute Confusional State — 364
Devendra Richhariya, Rajeev Goyal

- Risk Factors for Acute Confusional State/Delirium *364* • Etiology of Acute Confusional State/Delirium *365* • Life-threatening Causes of Acute Confusional State/Delirium *365*
- Clinical Presentation of Acute Confusional State/Delirium in Emergency Department *365*
- Pathophysiology: Acute Confusional State/Delirium *365* • Differential Diagnosis *365*
- Workup for Acute Confusional State/Delirium in Emergency Department *365*
- Acute Confusional State/Delirium Assessment Tools *367* • Management of Agitation in Emergency Department *367* • Effects of Acute Confusional State/Delirium *369*

49. Acute Stroke — 370
Arun Garg, Devendra Richhariya

- Risk Factors *370* • Ischemic Stroke *370* • Presentation of Acute Stroke in Emergency Department *371* • Types of Stroke Syndromes and their Symptoms *372*
- Approach to Stroke Patient in Emergency Department *372* • Transient Ischemic Attack *374*
- Radiological Investigations in Acute Stroke *375* • Treatment of Acute Stroke in Emergency Department *376* • Concept of Thrombolysis *377* • Types of Hemorrhagic Stroke *380*
- Cryptogenic Stroke *383*

50. Status Epilepticus and Refractory Status Epilepticus — 386
Atma Ram Bansal, Yeeshu Singh Sudan

- Definition of Status Epilepticus *386* • Diagnosis of Status Epilepticus *386*
- Management of Status Epilepticus *387* • How to do Electroencephalogram Monitoring in a Patient with Status Epilepticus? *388* • Reasons for Failure of Treatment in Status Epilepticus *389* • Clinical Tips in Managing Status Epilepticus *389*

SECTION 6: GASTROINTESTINAL EMERGENCIES

51. Gastrointestinal Bleed in Emergency — 393
Neeraj Saraf

- Approach to the Patient *393* • Diagnostic Testing *395* • Upper Gastrointestinal Bleed *395*
- Lower Gastrointestinal Bleed *395*

52. Hepatic Encephalopathy — 399
Rahul Rai, Sanjiv Saigal

- Pathophysiology *399* • Clinical Presentation *400* • Diagnosis *400* • Management *401*
- Treatment *401* • Intensive Care Management *401* • Management of Precipitating Factors *402*
- Reduction of the Nitrogenous Load from the Gut *402* • Modulation of Fecal Flora *402*
- Long-term Management of Hepatic Encephalopathy *402* • Liver Transplantation *402*

53. Acute Pancreatitis — 404
Rajesh Puri, Randhir Sud

- Etiology, Pathophysiology, and Definition *404* • Clinical Presentation *405*
- Risk Factors to Consider *405* • Assessing Severity of Acute Pancreatitis *405*
- Management of Acute Pancreatitis *407*

54. Acute Appendicitis — 410
Mukund Khetan, Anand Yadav

- Anatomy *410* • Etiology and Pathophysiology *411* • Presentation *412*
- Diagnosis *412* • Special Considerations *413* • Differential Diagnosis *414*
- Treatment *415* • Postoperative Care *415* • Special Considerations during Appendectomy *415*
- Recent Advances *416*

55. Perforation Peritonitis — 419
Sharad Manar, Hashim Mozzam, Sudhir BS

- Classifications *419* • Stages of Perforation Peritonitis *419* • Clinical Manifestation of Perforation Peritonitis *420* • Physical Examination *420* • Investigation and Radiological Imaging in Patient with Perforation Peritonitis *420* • Differential Diagnosis *420* • Treatment *420*

56. Intestinal Obstruction — 423
Ashok Kumar Puranik, Devendra Richhariya

- Definition *423* • Classification *423* • Pathophysiology *424* • Investigations *425*
- Treatment of Acute Intestinal Obstruction *427*

SECTION 7: RENAL AND GENITOURINARY EMERGENCIES

57. Electrolyte Imbalance — 431
Vishal Saxena

- Hyponatremia *431* • Hypernatremia *432* • Hyperkalemia *432* • Hypokalemia *433*
- Hypercalcemia *434* • Hypocalcemia *434* • Hypophosphatemia *438* • Hyperphosphatemia *438*

58. Acute Kidney Injury in Sepsis — 441
Manish Jain, Ashish Nandwani

- Sepsis *441* • Incidence *441* • Risk Factors *441* • Pathophysiology *442*
- Diagnostic Markers *442* • Treatment *442*

59. Emergencies in Renal Failure and Dialysis Patients — 445
Salil Jain, Sucheta Yadav

- No Known Renal Dysfunction in Past *445* • Chronic Kidney Disease/On Hemo/Peritoneal Dialysis *450* • Renal Allograft Recipients *451*

60. Urinary Tract Infections — 452
Ashish Nandwani, Manish Jain

- Incidence and Epidemiology *452* • Classification and Definitions of Urinary Tract Infections *452*
- Pathogenesis *453* • Microbiology *453* • Host Factors Predisposing for Urinary Tract Infection *453*
- Clinical Manifestations of Urinary Tract Infection *453* • Management of Urinary Tract Infections *454*

Contents xxxi

61. Hematuria 456
Puneet Ahluwalia, Varun Mittal, Rajiv Yadav

- Definition of Hematuria *456*   • Confirmation of Hematuria *456*   • History and Initial Evaluation *457*
- Some Clues *458*   • Stepwise Approach for Evaluation *458*   • Role of Cystoscopy *459*
- Follow-up after Initial Negative Evaluation *459*

62. Acute Urinary Retention 463
Rakesh Khera, Varun Mittal, Puneet Ahluwalia

- Epidemiology *463*   • Etiopathogenesis *463*   • Clinical Presentation *466*   • Evaluation *466*
- Initial Management of Acute Urinary Retention *467*   • Label Acute or Acute on Chronic Retention *467*
- What to do Next? *467*

SECTION 8: ENDOCRINAL EMERGENCIES

63. Hypoglycemia 473
JS Wasir, MS Kuchay, P Aggarwal

- Pathophysiology *473*   • Clinical Presentation *475*   • Management *475*   • Treatment in Emergency Settings *476*   • Preventing Future Hypoglycemia *477*

64. Diabetic Ketoacidosis in Adults 478
Beena Bansal, Tarannum

- Epidemiology *478*   • Precipitating Factors *478*   • Pathogenesis *479*
- Clinical Presentation *479*   • Treatment *481*   • Complications *482*

65. Thyroid Emergencies 483
Dheeraj Kapoor, Ruchi Kapoor, Mona Dhingra

- Thyroid Storm *483*   • Hypothyroid Coma (Myxedema Coma) *486*   • Hashimoto's Encephalopathy *488*

66. Acute Adrenal Crisis 490
Devendra Richhariya, Sunil Kumar Mishra

- Basic Anatomy and Physiology of Adrenal Gland *490*   • Factors Contributing to Shock in Acute Adrenal Crisis *491*   • Diagnosis *492*   • Treatment *493*   • Differential Diagnosis *493*

SECTION 9: OBSTETRICS AND GYNECOLOGY

67. Vaginal Bleeding 497
Sabhyata Gupta, Shradha Chaudhari

- Initial Assessment *497*   • Initial Assessment *498*   • Blood Investigations *499*
- Imaging Studies *499*   • Treatment *499*   • Therapeutic Measures *500*
- Treatment of Bleeding Per Vaginum in Hemodynamically Stable Patients *501*

68. Ectopic Pregnancy 502
Sabhyata Gupta

- Etiology and Risk Factors *502*   • Signs and Symptoms of Ectopic Pregnancy *503*
- Differential Diagnosis of Ectopic Pregnancy *503*   • Diagnosis of Ectopic Pregnancy *503*

- Management of Ectopic Pregnancy *503* • Surgical Management for Ectopic Pregnancy *503*
- Medical Management for Ectopic Pregnancy *504* • Ovarian Pregnancy *505*
- Cervical Pregnancy *506* • Interstitial Pregnancy *506*

69. Emergency Delivery — 508
Sangeeta Kaushik Sharma, Keerti Khetan

- Prehospital Care *508* • Emergency Department Care *508* • Medicolegal Issues in Emergency Obstetric Care *517*

SECTION 10: PEDIATRIC EMERGENCIES

70. Fever in Children — 521
Dhiren Gupta, Roop Sharma

- The Age Groups *521* • Presentation *522* • Physical Examination *522* • Management *523*
- Treatment of Fever *524*

71. Vomiting, Diarrhea and Dehydration in Children — 526
Prabhat Maheshwari, Devendra Richhariya

- Common Causes of Vomiting *526* • Diarrhea *526* • Management of Diarrhea and Dehydration *528*
- Persistent Diarrhea *529*

72. Febrile Seizure and Status Epilepticus in Children — 531
Yeeshu Singh Sudan, Devendra Richhariya

- Classification *531* • Febrile Seizure *532* • Status Epilepticus *532*
- Localization Features and Common Causes of Seizures *534* • Antiepileptic Drugs *534*

73. Central Nervous System Infections in Children — 536
Yeeshu Singh Sudan

- Clinical History, Approach, and Initial Management in Emergency *536*
- Acute Bacterial Meningitis *536* • Subacute Meningitis *537* • Chronic Meningitis *537*
- Adjunctive Corticosteroid Therapy *538* • Repeat Cerebrospinal Fluid Analysis *538*
- Differential Diagnosis *540* • Recommended Diagnostic Studies for Viral Meningitis *540*
- Recommendations for Initial Empiric Therapy of Meningitis in the Neonate *540*

74. Diabetes Management in Children — 541
Ganesh Jevalikar

- Diagnosis and Classification *541* • Management of Type 1 Diabetes *542*
- Management of Type 2 Diabetes *548*

75. Pediatric Cardiac Emergencies: Evaluation and Management — 552
Aditi Gupta, Munesh Tomar

- Cardiac Diseases Presenting as Emergency *552* • Neonatal Cardiac Emergencies: an Overview *552*
- Pediatric Cardiac Emergencies *557* • Commonly used Drugs in Cardiac Emergencies *562*

SECTION 11: DERMATOLOGICAL EMERGENCIES

76. Dermatologic Emergencies — 567
Ramanjit Singh, Devendra Richhariya

- Acute Skin Failure *567* • Stevens-Johnson Syndrome and Toxic Epidermal Necrolysis *568*
- Pyoderma Gangrenosum *569* • Staphylococcal Scalded Skin Syndrome *570*
- Necrotizing Fasciitis *570* • Urticaria (Hives), Angioedema, and Anaphylaxis *570*
- Pemphigus Vulgaris *570* • Vasculitis *571* • Lepra Reaction *571*

SECTION 12: RHEUMATOLOGICAL EMERGENCIES

77. Rheumatological Emergencies — 575
Shruti Bajad, Naval Mendiratta, Rajiva Gupta

- Pathogenesis *575* • When to Suspect? *575* • How to Evaluate and Manage? *576*
- Treatment Guidelines *577*

SECTION 13: HEMATOLOGIC AND ONCOLOGICAL EMERGENCIES

78. Evaluation and Management of Oncological Emergencies — 581
Devender Sharma, Pratibha Dhiman, Nintin Sood, Neelam Sharma, Jyoti Wadhwa, Ashok Vaid

- Superior Vena Cava Syndrome *581* • Spinal Cord Compression *582* • Hyperviscosity Syndrome *583*
- Cardiac Tamponade *583* • Malignant Pleural Effusion *584* • Brain Metastasis *584*
- Tumor Lysis Syndrome *584* • Hypercalcemia of Malignancy *584* • SIADH *585*

79. Care of Patients with Hematological Malignancies and Bone Marrow Transplantation — 587
Mukul Aggarwal, Anjan Shrestha, Narendra Agrawal, Rayaz Ahmed, Dinesh Bhurani

- Neutropenic Care *587* • Tumor Lysis Syndrome and Dyselectrolytemia *588* • Leukostasis *588*
- Bleeding (Thrombocytopenic and Coagulopathy) *589* • Cord Compression *590* • Graft Versus Host Disease *590* • Graft Failure and Relapse *590*

SECTION 14: TRAUMA

80. Basics of Trauma System — 595
Sandeep Jain

- Definition *595* • System *595* • Mechanism of Injury *596* • Trauma Scoring System *599*

81. Code Trauma — 601
M Sai Surendar

- Statistics *601* • What is Golden Hour? *601* • Code Trauma *602*
- Advantages of Code Trauma *604* • Goals to Keep in Mind in Code Trauma *604*

82. Trauma: Initial Assessment and Management 605
Khusrav Bajan, Archana Shrivastav

- Trauma Mortality: A Trimodal Distribution *605* • Systematic Approach for Management of Trauma Patient *606*

83. Facial Trauma 612
Syed Ahmed Adil

- Approach and Management *612* • Investigation *619*

84. Head Trauma 622
Devendra Richhariya, Manish Vaish

- Epidemiology *622* • Pathophysiology of Traumatic Brain Injury *622* • Modes of Trauma and Pattern of Brain Injuries *623* • Head Trauma According to Severity *623* • Resuscitation and Management of Head Trauma in Emergency Department *624* • Guidelines for Management of Head Injuries *626*

85. Spinal Trauma 629
Sudhir Dubey, Ratandeep Bose, Devendra Richhariya

- Modes of Spinal Injuries *629* • Various Syndromes in Spinal Cord Injury *629*
- Types of Fractures *630* • Prehospital Care and Spine Immobilization *632*
- Management in Emergency Department *634* • Treatment *635*

86. Thoracic Trauma 637
Shaiwal Khandelwal, Ali Zamir Khan

- Chest X-ray *637* • Computerized Tomography Scan *637* • Focused Assessment with Sonography for Trauma *638* • Angiography *638* • Chest Wall Injuries *638*
- Lung Injuries *639* • Cardiac Injuries *640* • Esophageal Injuries *641*
- Diaphragmatic Injuries *641* • Pneumothorax *642* • Hemothorax *642*
- Emergency Department Thoracotomy *643*

87. Abdominal Trauma 646
Ashok Kumar Puranik, Devendra Richhariya

- Penetrating Abdominal Trauma *646* • Blunt Abdominal Trauma *648* • Management of Abdominal Trauma *653* • Laparoscopy in Penetrating and Blunt Abdominal Traumas *653*

88. Extremity Trauma and Management of Fractures in Emergency 656
Ritabh Kumar

Fracture Care *656*

89. Emergency Wound Management and Closure 670
Aditya Aggarwal, Vimalendu Brajesh, Sukhdeep Singh, Umang B Kothari, Rakesh K Khazanchi

- What is a Wound? *670* • Initial Assessment of the Patient *671* • Investigations *672*
- Pain Relief *672* • Wound Management Plan *673* • Specific Wound Sites *674*
- Bites *681* • Wound Care *684* • Summary Wound Triage *689*

90. Radiology in Emergency and Trauma — 692
Sonal Krishan

- Abdominal Emergencies *692* • Ultrasound and Plain Abdominal Radiographs *694*
- Chest and Cardiovascular Emergencies *697* • Neurologic and Spinal Emergencies *698*
- Abnormal Vaginal Bleeding *698* • Multidetector Computed Tomography in a Polytrauma Patient *699*
- Plain Radiography in Common Fractures: Must for Every Trauma Physician *700*

91. Disaster and Mass Casualty Management in Emergency — 704
Devendra Richhariya, TS Srinath Kumar, Tamorish Kole

- Definitions *704* • Examples of Disasters *704* • Classification of Disasters *704*
- Terminology Related to Disaster *704* • Factors Contributing to Disaster *705*
- Disaster Management Cycle *706* • Disaster Management *706* • Incident Command System *707*
- Mass Casualty *709* • Emergency Department Preparedness for Chemical and Radiological Disaster *710*

SECTION 15: TOXICOLOGY

92. Assessment and Management of Poisoning — 717
VV Pillay

- Diagnostic Considerations *717* • General Management of Poisoning *720* • Stabilization *721*
- Evaluation *727* • Decontamination *734* • Elimination *740* • Alkaline Diuresis *740*
- Extracorporeal Techniques *741* • Antidote Administration *746* • Nursing and Psychiatric Care *748*
- Special Precautions in Poisoned Pregnant Patient *750* • Glasgow Coma Scale *752*

93. Organophosphate and Carbamate Insecticides Poisoning — 753
VV Pillay

- Pesticides *753* • Classification *753* • Organophosphorus Insecticide Poisoning *753*
- Carbamates *765*

94. Aluminum Phosphide Poisoning — 771
Vivekanshu Verma, Devendra Richhariya

- Peculiar Features *771* • Mechanism *772* • Clinical Features *772* • Diagnosis *772*
- Laboratory Investigations in Aluminum Phosphide Poisoning *774* • Management *774*
- Intra-aortic Balloon Pump in Aluminum Phosphide Poisoning *775*

SECTION 16: ENVIRONMENTAL EMERGENCIES

95. Management of Animal Bite Cases — 779
Ashok Mishra

- Current Scenario *779* • Pathophysiology of the Condition *780* • Clinical Presentation *781*
- Rabies in Dogs *783* • Management of a Case of Human Rabies (Hydrophobia) *783*
- Control of Rabies *785*

96. Snake Bite — 788
Narendra Nath Jena, Devendra Richhariya

- Facts about Snake Bite *788* • Identification of Venomous and Nonvenomous Snake *788*
- Classification of Venomous Snake *788* • Components of Snake Venom *788*

- Clinical Features of Snake Bite *790* • Management of Snake Bite *790* • Specific Treatment *791*
- Recent Advances in Snake Bite Management *792*

97. Heat Stroke 793
Sharad Manar, Taif Nabi, Pooja Kataria

- Classical Heat Stroke *793* • Exertional Heat Stroke *793* • Risk Factors for Heat Stroke *793*
- Pathophysiology *793* • Laboratory Findings *794* • Complications *794* • Treatment *794*
- Heat Exhaustion *795* • Prognosis *795* • Prevention *795*

98. Drowning 797
Vivekanshu Verma, Atul Bansal, Devendra Richhariya

- Stages in Drowning *798* • Symptoms in Drowning *798* • Complications of Drowning *798*
- Management of Drowning *798* • Prevention of Drowning *799*

99. Emergency Management of Burns 801
*Aditya Aggarwal, Vimalendu Brajesh, Sukhdeep Singh,
Umang B Kothari, Rakesh K Khazanchi*

- Classification *801* • Assessment and Management *802*
- Criteria for Referral to a Specialized Burn Center *809*

100. Electrical Injuries 811
Basar Cander

- Pathophysiology of the Condition or Description *811* • Clinical Presentation *812*
- Management *813*

Index *817*

SECTION 1

Essentials for Emergency Physician

- **Essentials for Good Emergency Physician**
  Devendra Richhariya, Vivekanshu Verma

- **Emergency Design and Staffing**
  Saleh Fares, Omar Ghazanfar

- **Triaging**
  Devendra Richhariya

- **Rapid Assessment and Treatment in Emergency**
  Devendra Richhariya

- **Point of Care Testing**
  Shashank Chauhan, Rajani Yadav

- **Essentials of Medicolegal Case Writing**
  Vivekanshu Verma, Devendra Richhariya

- **Medicolegal Issues in Emergency**
  Adarsh Kumar, Vivekanshu Verma

- **Patient Safety and Quality in Emergency Department**
  Devendra Richhariya, Sudhir Singh Pawaiya

- **Standards of Care during Air Transfer**
  Saleh Fares, Michael J Nolan

- **Standards of Care during Road Transfer**
  Sunil Dubey, Sudhir Singh Pawaiya, Vivekanshu Verma

CHAPTER 1

Essentials for Good Emergency Physician

Devendra Richhariya, Vivekanshu Verma

INTRODUCTION

Emergency medicine is a relatively new academic field in India. As the medical field is an ever growing field, and emergency medicine is rapidly progressing, a good emergency physician is a need of Indian health care. A dedicated emergency medicine faculty will be the key factor in developing emergency care workforce.

Emergency is a situation or condition of any life-threatening consequences requiring immediate intervention. It is unreasonable to expect that every patient in emergency department is diagnosed in one day, even specialty departments take days for final diagnosis.

Good emergency faculty should be expert in resuscitation and able to treat each and every disease of almost every specialty.

GOOD EMERGENCY PHYSICIAN MUST DEMONSTRATE

- Ability to triage the patient appropriately
- Ability to obtain an adequate history related to specific complaints and focus physical examination to decide whether the patient is stable or unstable
- Ability to provide adequate care for both emergent and non-emergent conditions
- Sound knowledge to treat emergency aspects of medical and surgical problems, and its application within the golden hour
- Knowledge of advanced cardiac life support (ACLS), advanced trauma life support (ATLS), pediatric advanced life support (PALS) and neonatal advanced life support (NALS)
- Ability to implement appropriate investigation and therapeutic plan
- Ability to write appropriate discharge summary
- Ability to interpret various laboratory results and diagnostic test and able to perform lifesaving procedures like endotracheal intubations promptly
- Ability to perform various procedures, like lumbar puncture, bone marrow aspiration/biopsy, liver/nerve/muscle/skin/kidney/pleural biopsy, fine needle aspiration cytology of palpable lumps, pleural/pericardial/abdominal/joint fluid aspiration
- Appropriate knowledge of biochemical, clinical, epidemiological of disease
- Familiar with the fundamentals of clinical research and recent development
- Ability to apply fundamentals of evidence-based medicine
- Ability to explain the cost of various test and treatment to the patient and having sound knowledge of principles of cost benefit analysis
- Ability to serve as an advocate for the patient in view of complex health care system
- Ability to use published studies and information technologies to improve patient's care
- Ability to demonstrate good time management and able to attend several patients at a time
- Ability to demonstrate good knowledge to handle mass casualty and must participate in mass casualty disaster drill
- Ability to understand the value of good documentation
- Ability to file cases properly and documents should be correct, clear, comprehensive and in chronological order
- Document should be relevant and legible. All important positive and negative findings in complicated cases with reasons for procedure and surgery failure, and follow-up advices given to patient should be noted with date and time.
- Weak record means weak defense, no record means no defense

- Before discharging the patient, ask two questions to yourself, "why the patient come to emergency and have I made the patient feel better?" and be ready with their answers
- Ability to understand responsibility towards community
- Always carry a stethoscope, symbol of a doctor and a healer
- Respect patient privacy
- Sensitivity and responsiveness to patient culture, age, gender and disabilities
- Commitment to sound ethical principles regarding the patient care
- Respect for dignity and colleagues as persons
- Ability to train the juniors and assist them in training
- Ability to be up-to-date with the recent advances in the field of emergency
- Ability to show humanity which is necessary to develop good doctor–patient relationship **(Fig. 1)**
- Effective interpersonal and communication skills with patients and their families, other physicians and healthcare providers **(Fig. 2)**
- Ability to show professionalism **(Fig. 3)**

Being an emergency doctor is not easy because of:
- Too much work
- Too much hassle
- Too much paperwork
- Irritated patient
- Too much competition.

So emergency physician must be **(Fig. 4)**:
- Calm
- Logical
- Approachable
- Imaginative
- Passionate
- Knowledgeable
- Role model
- Enthusiastic leader
- Reliable mentor
- Efficient
- Learner flexible
- Facilitator.

Things that require zero talent in emergency department:
- Being on time
- Work ethics
- Effort
- Body language
- Energy
- Attitude
- Passion
- Being coachable

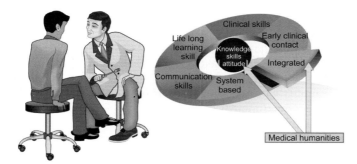

Fig. 1 Skills to develop good doctor–patient relationship

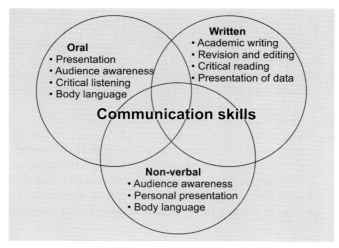

Fig. 2 Ways to develop communication skills

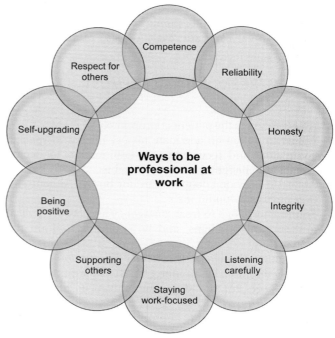

Fig. 3 Ten ways to be professional at work

Good emergency physician should be creative by adopting these ways:
- Carry a notebook everywhere
- Make notes
- Be open
- Know your roots
- Surround yourself with creative people
- Get feedback
- Collaborate
- Do not give up
- Practice
- Follow rules of disciplines
- Keep your workplace clean
- Get lots of rest
- Listen to music.

CONCLUSION

"Do Not Neglect" "Protect"

> *"There are three factors in the practice of medicine: the disease, the patient, and the physician. The physician is the Servant of Science, and the patient must do what he can to fight the disease with the assistance of the physician."*
> —Hippocrates, The Epidemics, Book I

BIBLIOGRAPHY

1. Good Medical Practice 2013, GMC, 2013 http://www.gmc-uk.org/guidance/good_medical_practice.asp.
2. Managing shift work: Health and Safety guidance, Health and Safety Executive, HSG256 2006, http://www.hse.gov.uk/pubns/books/hsg256.htm.
3. Promoting Mental Health Wellbeing at Work—NICE Public Health Guideline 29, NICE, November 2009 http://www.nice.org.uk/nicemedia/live/12331/45893/45893.pdf.
4. Strategies for coping with stress in emergency medicine: Early education is vital. Schmitz et al. J Emerg Trauma Shock. 2012;5(1):64-9 http://www.ncbi.nlm.nih.gov/pmc/articles/PMC3299157/.
5. Workplace-Wellness-Sep10.pdf Physician burnout, Burger E. Annals of Emergency Medicine Volume 61,No 3: March 2013 http://www.annemergmed.com/article/S0196-0644%2813%2900002-4/abstract.

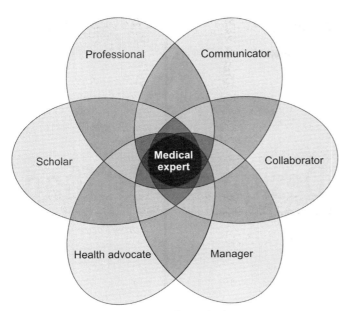

Fig. 4 Qualities of a medical expert

Box 1 Do's and don'ts for emergency physician

Doctor should avoid	Doctor should
• Advertising • Agents for procuring patients • Assisting unqualified • Association with patient • Association with drug manufacturing firm • Adultery arising out of professional relationships • Addiction • Alcohol consumption on duty	• Attend and give first aid in all types of medical emergencies • Attend court on being summoned in MLC • Authorities of state should be informed in epidemic, fatal communicable disease

- Doing extra
- Being prepared.

Box 1 is showcasing do's and don'ts for emergency physician as per Indian code of medical ethics by Medical Council of India (MCI)—Mnemonic of All As.

CHAPTER 2

Emergency Design and Staffing

Saleh Fares, Omar Ghazanfar

EMERGENCY DEPARTMENT DESIGN

INTRODUCTION

The emergency department (ED) plays a central role in providing vital access to acute healthcare to the public. An ED is also an important gateway to many inpatient and outpatient services offered by the hospital. In addition, a major proportion of acute admissions to inpatient beds are via ED.

The major characteristics which make the ED unique include the following points:
- Emerging and novel models of ED care and design
- Varying levels and types of staffing models
- Undifferentiated case mix including critical and life-threatening illnesses, major trauma, dependent on the hospital status and a wide spectrum of age groups from pediatrics to geriatrics
- The presence of patients, carers and relatives with varying levels of anxiety
- High patient turnover
- Variable admission and discharge pathways
- Medical services provided by largely specialist emergency physicians, supported by junior doctors and allied nursing and other health professionals.

EMERGENCY DEPARTMENT FUNCTION

The primary function of the ED is to receive, resuscitate and provide acute healthcare to patients. It should also be equipped to handle disasters and mass causalties.

Varied patient population requiring varying medical inputs include the following, but the list is not exhaustive:
- Major trauma
- Geriatrics
- Pediatrics
- Mental health disorders
- Patients with abuse (any age group)
- Custodial patients
- Patients with infectious diseases
- Mass causalties (to include chemical, biological and radiological contaminants).

GENERAL CONSIDERATIONS FOR DESIGNING AN EMERGENCY DEPARTMENT

There are a number of factors which must be considered when structuring an ED. This will include both, staff requirements and patient needs, and demographics.

The needs of these varying patient groups can be addressed through, for example, suitably placed furniture and art, adequate access to information and communications technology, and appropriately designed rooms and equipment that are suitable for use by particular patient populations.

While the needs of patients, carers and relatives are highly important, it is also necessary that a healthy working environment for staff is facilitated by the design of the ED. These needs can be catered to through the use of well-placed staff bases, staff rooms large enough to accommodate the maximum number of possible users, and ensuring that staff facilities are located separately from clinical areas, in order to promote effective breaks from patient care.

Designing of an efficient ED should look at certain elements which will aim to make the department efficient, reliable and cost effective.

The design needs to be practical and reflect the needs of the professionals who run the department and treat patients with varied needs and requirements.

The structure and design should reflect the spatial relationships between staff and patients, and improve the flow and continuity of care from the front door of the hospital to admission or discharge of patients. It should be kept in mind that the ED functioning is very fluid with ebb and flow of patients changing during the 24 hours or a 7-day week, and flexibility is needed to enable reallocation of treatment spaces as required.

The ED should aim to create a healthy environment through proper application of occupational health standards to ensure a safe working environment. The well-being of patients and staff should be an important consideration through proper and safe use of design and space.[1-3]

PATIENT FLOW

The ED has a wide case mix and varying volume of patients presenting with varies pathologies at different part of the day and week. Many different models have been used successfully, internationally, taking into account both staff and patients to aid the flow of care through the emergency service. No single system works for all hospitals as this is largely dependent on patient needs and adequate and safe staffing.

Some of the concepts of patient care that affect flow within the ED include the following:
- Medical-led triage with senior nursing staff
  - Triage done by senior nurse to make definitive investigations and decision-making on the patient's arrival to the ED.
- Traditional models of care which filtered patient on the basis of their primary complaint. This was a medical-surgical model which still exists in some healthcare systems
- Rapid Assessment Team (RAT) for critically ill patients
  - Senior doctor
  - Nursing staff
  - Administrative staff
  - Phlebotomist
  - Scribe

This team may either be mobile within the department or be stationed in specific assessment areas and can be mobilized as per needs and requirements.[3-5]

DEDICATED AREAS WITHIN AN EMERGENCY DEPARTMENT

As part of the structural design of an ED a variety of considerations need to be taken into account. These include dedicated clinical areas for ED staff, access to the main hospital, multidisciplinary team areas, staff facilities, and areas for special and specific clinical requirements. These are summarized in **Table 1**.

Patient and staff experience is essential in designing and developing an ED and various factors need to be taken into account to facilitate this. These are summarized in **Table 2**.

Table 1 The dedicated areas within an emergency department

Hospital access areas	Clinical areas
Proximity to main entrance	Entrance, waiting room and reception area
Streamlined access to investigative areas	Triage
Close or cohabited areas for other acute services	Resuscitation area
Helipad	Mental health assessment area
Angiography	Clinical consultation area to include fast-track, subacute minors or ambulatory care
HDU/CCU/ICU	Acute treatment area
Operating theater	Investigative areas: Z-Ray, short stay, investigation room, etc.
Clear route to wards	
Outpatient access	
Communication hub	
Areas for disaster management	
Multidisciplinary team areas	**Special areas**
Equipment storage	Eye/ENT/Gyne/Plaster rooms
Refreshment areas	Storage areas
Physio- and OT-assessment area	Disposal room
	Medication room
	Office space
	Staff room
Staff and amenities areas	Ambulance offloading area
	Decontamination area
	Ambulatory or urgent care
Administrative areas	
Storage	
Drug preparation room	
Sluice and dirty utility	
Patient amenities	
Toilets	
Teaching and research areas	

Abbreviations: CCU, coronary care unit; ENT, ear, nose and throat; HDU, high dependency unit; ICU, intensive care unit; OT, operation theater.

NEW CONCEPTS IN EMERGENCY DEPARTMENT DESIGN

The Breathing Emergency Department

Studies conducted to determine the benchmark size for an ED patient unit indicate that smaller EDs with fewer visits function more efficiently and have higher patient satisfaction rates than larger EDs. These studies suggest that the

Table 2 Factors to consider in the design to improve staff and patients experience in the emergency department (ED)

Staff experience	Patient experience
• Comfortable seating areas at staff bases and bedside • Easy and ready access to equipment • Efficient workflow design with good access to all work space areas • Design which limits overcrowding • Confidential discussion rooms • Air quality with ventilation control • Good staff rest facilities with appropriate amenities and storage facilities • Overnight facilities for staff	• Clear signs for pathways and facilities • Information about ED process to include triage and/or waiting times • Multilingual signs • Public health educations leaflets • Friendly staff • Security personnel • Clean and well presented • Information desks • Appropriate waiting areas ideally with color coding • Availability of refreshments

functional ED patient unit should be 13 beds to enable better management of patients and tasks.[6-9] However, as patient visits increase, the majority of EDs increase their footprint and number of beds, decreasing efficiency. There are a few models designed to divide the department into smaller, more manageable units, including the Fast-Track approach (focused on lower acuity flow, discussed later). This design divides an ED into two separate departments based on patient acuity. Another option to help reduce unit size is the breathing emergency department, which subdivides the department into smaller units and opens and closes them based on the cyclical cycle of peak patient visit times.[6]

STAFFING MODEL

MEDICAL AND PRACTITIONER STAFFING IN EMERGENCY DEPARTMENTS

Correct staffing is the key to delivering timely and high-quality care in the ED. There is no one-size-fits-all staffing model for EDs. Intelligent staffing models will also allow for rota patterns that are realistic and sustainable and will involve the use of clinicians from a range of professional backgrounds. A tiered approach to staffing is therefore necessary, with consideration of sustainability for each tier.

Correct staffing in EDs results in safer care with improved quality, better performance, increased efficiency, and happy and resilient workforce.

HOW TO STAFF AN EMERGENCY DEPARTMENT?

Staffing an emergency department is a complex and demanding job and requires input from a variety of different internal and external factors. In essence, staffing is a function of the following:
- Capacity
- Capability
- Sustainable working
- Resilience

Capacity

Required capacity can be calculated on the basis of predicted demand. Demand needs to be considered in terms of volume, case mix and segregated work streams. Capacity calculations need to be considered. EDs should be staffed to meet variation in demand, aiming to cope with normal demand variation.

Capability

A capable system does what it is supposed to do. This essentially means that the right number of clinicians with the appropriate skill mix is needed at the right time.

There is a natural desire to specify the productivity of different groups of clinicians. The best estimate of local productivity is local data **(Table 3)**.

Tier 1 clinicians (interns) or clinicians with enhanced supervision requirements, e.g. doctors in difficulty, may have minimal or even negative productivity due to the senior input required on cases they see. Tier 2 doctors (junior residents or rotating doctors) are generally thought to see about one patient per hour, perhaps slightly more on minors although this depends on the case mix seen. A consultant (tier 5) supervising a department may see no new patients, in order to maximize their efficacy in the command and control role, and to avoid potentially disadvantaging patients, they do see through interruptions and multitasking. The productivity of the remaining groups (senior residents and other senior

Table 3 The different tiers working in an emergency department

Tier	Classification
Tier 1	Require complete supervision. All patients must be signed off before admission or discharge, e.g. interns or junior residents
Tier 2	Require access to advice or direct supervision, or practice independently but with limited scope, e.g. doctors, some primary care clinicians, junior residents
Tier 3	More senior or experienced clinicians, requiring less direct supervision. Generally, fewer limitations in scope of practice, e.g. senior residents, experienced practitioners
Tier 4	Senior clinicians able to supervise a department alone with remote support, possess some extended skills. Full scope of practice
Tier 5	Senior clinicians with accredited advanced qualifications in EM; or full set of extended skills, e.g. consultants in EM

Abbreviation: EM, emergency medicine.

ED physicians) will vary between about 0.5 patients per hour and 3 patients per hour, depending on such variables as experience, professional development, case mix, the effectiveness of efforts to maximize workforce efficiency, the requirement to move between physical areas, procedures undertaken and supervisory demands.

- All EDs require a senior doctor, immediately available, at all times
- Larger departments will require several senior doctors on duty to manage the supervisory workload, to see the sickest and most complex patients and to undertake dedicated tasks such as rapid assessment
- Larger departments may be able to develop specific areas led predominantly by tier 2 or tier 3 clinicians.

Sustainable Working and Sustainable Staffing

There are significant concerns around attrition rate in emergency departments. Sustainable working requires attention to specific details taking into account work-life balance due to the antisocial nature of shift work. These include the following:

- Workload and work intensity, when on duty
- A balanced mix of clinical, nonclinical and academic activity, particularly for senior clinicians
- Professional development
- Physiological and physical limitations of staff (e.g. age, chronic illness or disability)
- Compensation for late night or overnight working.

Rota's for individual tiers can be combined provided attention is paid to skill-mix. Sustainable working leads to more effective working. Tired or burned-out staffs are less safe, less efficient and less effective. Sustainable working is also the key to building an emergency medicine workforce for the future.

Furthermore, many emergency physicians are concerned about how they will work in an ED as they get older, and in particular how they will cope with intense, late and overnight working. Constructing sustainable working for an aging workforce, while ensuring development within the consultant role into the third and fourth decades of consultant life, are key considerations for workforce planning.

Alongside sustainable working, consider sustainable staffing. This means paying attention to recruitment and retention.

Retention is the first part of recruitment. Permanent workforces are safer and more efficient than using locums or relying on staff to internally cover gaps and vacancies.

Consider how to keep your staff happy and fulfilled. This is partly about how you set up the work force in general:

- Enough staff of the right skill mix, doing work they enjoy
- Develop a culture that genuinely values staff (rather then paying lip service to the concept)
- Provide a reasonable and healthy working environment
- Offer terms and conditions that recognize the intensity and demands of ED shift work
- Invest in professional development.

Resilience

This contributes towards sustainable working recommendations for action and research from others.

Further research is needed into the following:
- Staffing models for EDs of different sizes
- The relationship between appropriate staffing and patient safety
- Decision-making density and interruptions within EDs
- The combined effects of age, time of day and shift patterns on safe decision-making in clinicians
- Recruitment and retention in acute specialties.

Action is needed to build an emergency medicine workforce fit to meet the demands of the future. This includes attracting people into emergency medicine, and then retaining them. This comes down to providing professionally satisfying workplaces, sustainable working patterns, attractive terms and conditions, and professional development.

CONCLUSION

Emergency department design and structure works hand in conjunction with the staffing structure to provide a safe, productive, efficient and reliable service to provide ultimate and immediate care to the unscheduled and undifferentiated patient population which presents to the emergency healthcare services.

REFERENCES

1. The Royal College of Emergency Medicine. Safe Staffing. Available from *http://www.rcem.ac.uk/Shop-Floor/Safer Care/Safety in your ED/Safe staffing* [Accessed November, 2016].
2. Collins M. 2009. Staffing an ED appropriately and efficiently. [online] Available from *http://www.acep.org/Clinical-Practice-Management/Staffing-an-ED-Appropriately-and-Efficiently/* [Accessed November, 2016].
3. Gilinson D. Emergency physicians monthly. Building a smarter staffing model. Available from *http://epmonthly.com/article/building-a-smarter-staffing-model/*[Accessed November, 2016].
4. Wang X. Emergency department staffing: A separated continuous linear programming approach. Mathematical Problems Eng. 2013;doi:10.1155/2013/680152.
5. HSK. 2012. Data Driven EDs. [online] Available from *http://www.hksinc.com/insight/data-driven-eds/* [Accessed November, 2012].
6. The Royal College of Emergency Medicine. Medical and Practitioner Workforce Guidance. [online] Available from *http://www.rcem.ac.uk/Shop-Floor/Service Design & Delivery/The Emergency Medicine Workforce/Medical and Practitioner Workforce Guidance* [Accessed November 2016].
7. Hoot NR, Aronsky D. Systematic review of emergency department crowding: causes, effects, and solutions. Ann Emerg Med. 2008;52(2):126-36.
8. Flanagan T, Haas AJ. Planning a new emergency department: from design to occupancy. J Ambul Care Manage. 2005;28(2): 177-81.
9. Broderick KB, Ranney ML, Vaca FE, et al. Study designs and evaluation models for emergency department public health research. Acad Emerg Med. 2009;16(11):1124-31.

CHAPTER 3

Triaging

Devendra Richhariya

INTRODUCTION

Triage is derived from French word "trier" which means to sort out or to pick. This process was used in 18th century Napoleonic wars where injured are removed rapidly from battlefield to safe places for care. This process become more refined and used in established healthcare setting and in modern medicine this system is known as triaging system. Nowadays triaging area and triage process is important function in modern emergency department. Emergency department is a place where many patients may present simultaneously and available resources become inadequate to provide quality care. Thus, it is both clinically and ethically important to identify those patients who need most urgent emergency care. Mass casualty incident triaging also evolving to achieve maximum good for maximum number of the patients.

EMERGENCY DEPARTMENT TRIAGING

With increasing awareness among public about emergency care, number of patients visiting the emergency department are increasing day-by-day. Various triaging strategies are used in emergency department for clinical service development, patient safety, and clinical risk management. The purpose of triage system is to deliver quality health services across the population rather than administrative or organizational compulsion.

REQUIREMENTS FOR TRIAGING

- Triaging area must be easily approachable, well illuminated and clearly sign posted.
- All patient should enter through single entry point so that they all go through similar process
- Special area for examination of patient and privacy should be maintained
- Appropriate communication system between entrance and triage area
- Emergency lifesaving equipment
- Universal protective facilities, e.g. hand washing and gloves
- Strategies to protect staff
- Trauma victim should be prioritize in specific area
- Document for recording the triage information
- Level of urgency must be noted at the entry point of emergency department
- Triaging should be based on clinical condition only, should not be influenced by any other factors
- Primary triaging task consists of chief complaints and assessment of urgency
- Secondary triaging task is consists of diagnostic investigations, emergency care, and disposition.
- There should be well-organized processing system from triage point to disposition.

Triaging Scales

Various triaging scales **(Table 1)** are being used internationally. These include five-tier, four-tier, and three tier scales. Valid and reliable scale should have following characteristics.
- Easy to understand and simple to apply by emergency nurses and doctors
- It should measure clinical urgency
- Triage scale must be sensitive enough to register clinical urgency with accuracy.

Five-tier triage **(Table 2)** scales are more reliable, valid, and internationally accepted.

Table 1 Various triage scales

Five-tier triage scales	Four-tier triage scales	Three-tier triage scales
• Australasian triage scale • Manchester triage scale • Canadian triage scale • Emergency severity index • Cape triage score	Hong Kong four level field triage system	Simple triaging and rapid treatment (START) Field triaging, mass causality triaging

Table 2 Five-tier triage scales

Triage scale	Level	Time to attend by physician	Color coding
Australasian triage scale	1. Resuscitation 2. Emergency 3. Urgent 4. Semiurgent 5. Nonurgent	1. 0 min 2. 10 min 3. 30 min 4. 60 min 5. 120 min	none
Manchester triage scale	1. Immediate 2. Very urgent 3. Urgent 4. Standard 5. Nonurgent	1. 0 min 2. 10 min 3. 60 min 4. 120 min 5. 240 min	1. Red 2. Orange 3. Yellow 4. Green 5. Blue
Canadian triage scale	1. Resuscitation 2. Emergent 3. Urgent 4. Less urgent 5. Nonurgent	1. 0 min 2. 15 min 3. 30 min 4. 60 min 5. 120 min	None

TRIAGING PROCESS

Assessment of patient: All patients coming to emergency department should be triaged on arrival by trained nurse or physician. Diagnosis making should not be the priority. Vitals measurement should be done to estimate the urgency. Other parameters should be noted for estimation of urgency are general appearance, chief complaints, and physiological observation. Standing order should be followed by treatment nurse and immediate care need should be fulfilled. As per hospital protocol initiate appropriate investigations and treatment.

Triage assessment should be completed within 3–5 minutes.

Documentation details in the patient assessment notes:
- Patient name, age, and sex
- Date and time of assessment, name of triage nurse and doctor
- Chief complaints
- Relevant history
- Relevant assessment findings (appearance of patient, airway breathing circulation disability)
- Vitals signs and random blood sugar
- Initial triage category
- Assessment of alertness [Glasgow Coma Scale/Alert Verbal Painful Unresponsiveness (GCS/APVU scale)]
- Assessment of pain (various pain scale implementation)
- Initiation of any treatment measures
- Care plan and discharge plan if patient is discharged from emergency
- Retriaging if any parameter changes
- Trauma record should be used in trauma patient
- Other consideration like pediatric age group, elderly group, and high-risk features (comorbidities, poisoning, severe pain, rashes), and history of violence medicolegal cases.

Triaging in Pediatric Age Group

Children are usually uncooperative during examination and gives poor history; so, it is very important to recognize markers of serious illness.

Useful signs are drowsiness, hypotonic, respiratory grunt, wheeze, crepitation, stridor, tachypnea, pallor, fever, signs of dehydration, abnormal posture, cold periphery, vomit or less urination, and convulsion tender abdomen.

Assessment of Pain in Triage

Pain is one of the most common symptoms for which people visit to emergency and pain influences the triage category. Pain description and pain assessment should be included in triage assessment as physiological and behavioral indicator.

Description about factors influencing the pain, various pain assessment scales and pain management strategies should be included in triage document.

Pain assessment should include:
- Location, intensity, time of onset, duration of pain, and aggravating and relieving factors
- Heart rate, respiratory rate, and blood pressure
- Facial expression and body language
- Various pain scales are used in triage setting:
  - Verbal pain score
  - Visual analogue scale
  - Numerical rating scale
  - Wong-baker FACES rating scale
  - Abbey pain scale.

Triaging and Medicolegal Issues

Following documentation is required:
- Patient name, age, sex, and address
- Name of accompanying person
- Date, time, and place of event
- Name of examining physician
- Documentation of injuries
- Management details
- Legal responsibility to report to relevant authorities and jurisdiction
- Preservation of forensic evidence (in case of poisoning assault rape).

Triage and Pregnancy

Pregnant women are at increased risk of various conditions and may present with variety of serious situation **(Table 3)**. Triage nurse and physician should aware of normal physiological and adaptive changes during pregnancy. Pregnant women may present with any disease in emergency department. Cerebral hemorrhage, cerebral thrombosis, severe pneumonia, venous thrombosis, and embolus pyelonephritis are more common in pregnant women than nonpregnant women of child bearing age. Triaging should focus on wellbeing of mother and fetus.

Benefits of Triage

Life threatening, limb threatening, and time critical emergencies (like stroke and myocardial infarction) are treated on priority basis.
- Triaging improves the patient flow
- Triaging improves the patient satisfaction
- Triaging decrease the overall length of hospital stay.

EARLY WARNING SCORE IN TRIAGE

In many triage system various warning scales are used to identify the patients who are at risk of clinical deterioration and who need hospitalization, so these warning scales are beneficial for quality improvement. Early warning score is based on vital sings: respiratory rate, heart rate, blood pressure, temperature, oxygen saturation, and level of consciousness (AVPU).

Various warning score are developed according to the need:
- Modified early warning score (MEWS)
- Triage early warning score (TEWS)
- Modified pediatric early warning score (MPEWS)
- Modified early obstetrics warning score (MEOWS).

Modified Early Warning Score

Modified early warning score is based on blood pressure, heart rate, respiration oxygen saturation, and alertness. In some triage scale urine output and pain score is also taken into consideration. Patient's clinical deterioration can be anticipated by this score and requirement of hospitalization can also be assessed. MEWS score uses basic equipment and simple parameter so it is easy to use by junior most staff also. MEWS useful for triaging of medical emergencies but not for trauma patient triaging. MEWS score more than 5 considered as risk of clinical deterioration and need of hospitalization **(Table 4)**.

Triage Early Warning Score

Triage early warning score is described in **Tables 5 and 6**.

Table 3 Problems occurring during gestational age		
Less than 20 weeks	More than 20 weeks	Postnatal problems
• Vaginal bleeding (common cause in miscarriage) • Abdominal pain (ruptured ectopic pregnancy, torsion or ruptured cysts) • Domestic violence common in pregnancy	• Antepartum hemorrhage • Pre-eclampsia • Preterm rupture of membranes and labor	• Postpartum hemorrhage • Puerperal sepsis • Wound infection • Mastitis • Eclampsia • Postpartum cardiomyopathy • Postpartum psychosis

Table 4 Modified early warning score

Vital signs	3	2	1	0	1	2	3
Systolic BP	<70	71–80	81–100			>200	
Heart rate		<40	41–50	51–100	101–110	111–129	>130
Respiratory rate		<9		9–14	15–20	21–29	>30
Temperature		<35		35–38.4		>38.5	
AVPU				Alert	React to voice	React to pain	No response

In some triaging system urine output and pain sore is also added in early warning score.
Abbreviations: BP, blood pressure; AVPU; alert, response to voice, response to pain, unconscious.

Table 5 Triage early warning score

Parameters	3	2	1	0	1	2	3
Mobility				Walking	With help	Immobile	
Respiratory rate		<9		9–14	15–20	21–29	>29
Heart rate		<40	41–50	51–100	101–110	111–129	>129
Systolic BP	<70	71–80	81–100	101–199		>199	
Temperature		<35		35–38.4		>38.5	
AVPU				Alert	React to voice	React to pain	No response
Trauma				No	Yes		

Abbreviations: BP, blood pressure; AVPU; alert, response to voice, response to pain, unconscious.

Table 6 Correlating the triage early warning score (TEWS) with color code triaging

Color	Red	Orange	Yellow	Green	Blue
TEWS score	7 or more	5–6	3–4	0–2	

Early warning scores are the important tool for appropriate risk management, and also helpful in improving the safety and quality of patient in emergency department. Measurement of physiologic parameter and early recognition of warning signs and timely action would add value to patient care in emergency department and can lead to improved quality of care and decreased morbidity and mortality.

TRIAGE IN MASS CASUALTY INCIDENT

In mass casualty situation number of patients and their severity are much more than the existing capability for management. Triage is most important part of any disaster response. The main objective of mass casualty or disaster triage is to do the maximum help to maximum number of people. Following are the incidents which cause the mass casualty:
- Road traffic accident
- Building collapse
- Earthquake
- Flood
- Major fire
- Train derailment
- Explosion
- Air crash
- Terrorist attack
- Hazardous material release.

Main objectives of triaging in disaster and mass casualty are:
- To decompress the disaster area
- Most critical casualty should get best care
- Special care for burn and crush injuries.

Triaging Scales for Mass Casualty Incident

Triaging scales for mass casualty incident are:
- START (simple triaging and rapid treatment)
- SALT triaging.

Components of START Triaging (Respiration, Perfusion, Mental Status)

Components of START triaging have been described in **Flow charts 1 and 2**.

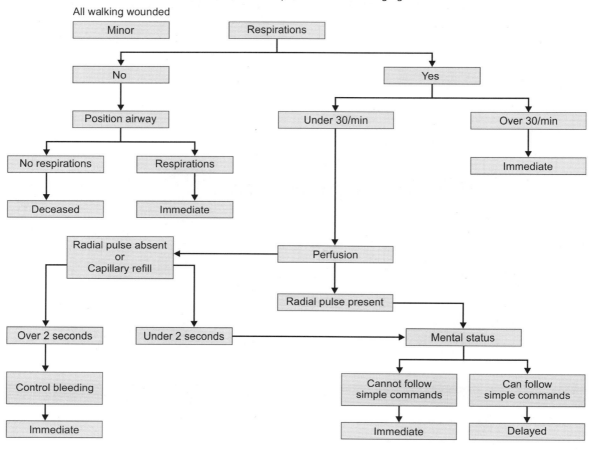

Flow chart 1 Components of START triaging

Components of SALT Triaging

Components of SALT triaging have been described in **Flow chart 3**.

CONCLUSION

Triage is an essential first step in efficient and effective emergency department. A use of comprehensive triage tool will help to save lives and reduce the mortality.

BIBLIOGRAPHY

1. Australasian College for Emergency Medicine. A National Triage Scale for Australian Emergency Departments (position paper). 1993b.
2. Australasian College for Emergency Medicine. Guidelines for implementation of the Australasian Triage Scale in Emergency Departments.
3. Australasian College for Emergency Medicine. Policy Document—The Australasian Triage Scale.
4. Australasian College for Emergency Medicine. Triage (policy document). 1993a.
5. Brillman JC, Doezema D, Tandberg D, et al. Triage: limitations in predicting need for emergent care and hospital admission. Ann Emerg Med. 1996;27(4):493-500.
6. Buist MD, Jarmolowski E, Burton PR, et al. Recognising clinical instability in hospital patients before cardiac arrest or unplanned admission to intensive care. A pilot study in a tertiary-care hospital. Med J Australia. 1999;171(1):22-5.
7. Cioffi J. Triage decision making: educational strategies. Accid Emerg Nurs. 1999;7:106-11.
8. Commonwealth Department of Health and Family Services and the Australasian College for Emergency Medicine. The Australian National Triage Scale: a user manual 1997.
9. Considine J, Ung L, Thomas S. Clinical Decisions using the National Triage Scale: how important is postgraduate education? Accid Emerg Nurs. 2001;9(2):101-8.
10. Considine J, Ung L, Thomas S. Triage nurses' decisions using the National Triage Scale for Australian emergency departments. Accid Emerg Nurs. 2000;8(4):201-9.
11. Deane SA, Gaudry PL, Woods P, et al. The management of injuries—a review of deaths in hospital. Aust N Z J Surg. 1988;58(6):463-9.
12. Dubois RW, Brook RH. Preventable deaths: who, how often, and why? Ann Intern Med. 1988;109(7):582-9.

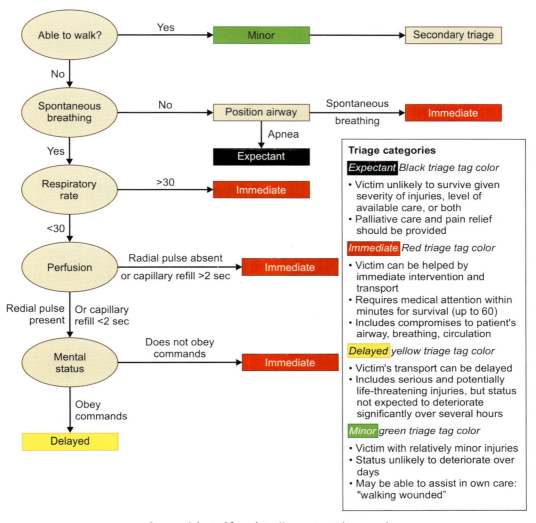

Flow chart 2 START triage algorithm for adult patient

Source: Adapted from *http://www.start-triage.com/*

13. Edwards B. Telephone triage: how experienced nurses reach decisions. J Adv Nurs. 1994;19(4):717-24.
14. Emergency Nurses' Association of Victoria (Inc). Position Statement: Educational preparation of triage nurses. 2000b.
15. Emergency Nurses' Association of Victoria (Inc). Position Statement: Triage. 2000a.
16. Ferraris VA, Propp ME. Outcome in critical care patients: a multivariate study. Crit Care Med. 1992;20(7):967-76.
17. Franklin C, Mamdani B, Burke G. Prediction of hospital arrests: toward a preventative strategy. Clin Res. 1986;34:954A.
18. Franklin C, Matthew J. Developing strategies to prevent in hospital cardiac arrest: analyzing responses of physicians and nurses in the hours before the event. Crit Care Med. 1994;22(2):244-7.
19. George S, Read S, Westlake L, et al. Nurse triage in theory and in practice. Arch Emerg Med. 1993;10(3):220-8.
20. Geraci EB, Geraci TA. An observational study of the emergency triage nursing role in a managed care facility. J Emerg Nurs. 1994;20(3):189-94.
21. Gerdtz M, Bucknall T. Australian triage nurses' decision making and scope of practice. Aust J Adv Nurs. 2000;18(1):24-33.
22. Gerdtz MF, Bucknall TK. Why we do the things we do: Applying clinical decision making frameworks to practice. Accid Emerg Nurs. 1999;7(1):50-7.
23. Hollis G, Sprivulis P. Reliability of the National Triage Scale with changes in emergency department activity level. Emerg Med. 1996;8:231-4.
24. Hourihan F, Bishop G, Hillman K, et al. The Medical Emergency Team: a new strategy to identify and intervene in high risk patients. Clin Intensive Care. 1995;6:269-272.

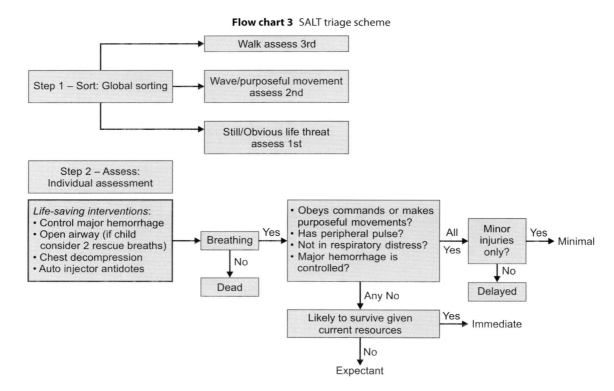

Flow chart 3 SALT triage scheme

25. Knaus W, Draper E, Wagner D, et al. APACHE II: a severity of disease classification system. Crit Care Med. 1985;13(10):818-22.
26. Mallett J, Woolwich C. Triage in accident and emergency departments. J Adv Nurs. 1990;15(12):1443-51.
27. McQuillan P, Pilkington S, Allan A, et al. Confidential inquiry into quality of care before admission to intensive care. Brit Med J. 1998;316(7148):1853-8.
28. Monitor L. Triage dilemma and decisions: A tool for continuing education. J Emerg Nurs. 1985;11(1):40-2.
29. Purnell LDT. A survey of emergency department triage in 185 hospitals: physical facilities, fast-track systems, patient classification, waiting times, and qualification, training, and skills of triage personnel. J Emerg Nurs. 1991;17(6):402-7.
30. Rowe JA. Triage assessment tool. J Emerg Nurs. 1992;18(6):540-4.
31. Sax FL, Charlson ME. Medical patients at high risk for catastrophic deterioration. Crit Care Med. 1987;15(5):510-5.
32. Whitby S, Ieraci S, Johnson D, et al. Analysis of the process of triage: the use and outcome of the National Triage Scale. Liverpool: Liverpool Health Service; 1997.
33. Williams G. Sorting out triage. Nursing Times. 1992;88(30):34-6.
34. Wuerz R, Fernandes C, Alarcon J. Inconsistency of emergency department triage. Ann Emerg Med. 1998;32(4):431-5.
35. Zwicke DL, Bobzien WF, Wagner EH. Triage nurse decisions: a prospective study. J Emerg Nurs. 1982;8:132-8.

CHAPTER 4

Rapid Assessment and Treatment in Emergency

Devendra Richhariya

INTRODUCTION

Emergency department has challenging working environment; most of the patients present with acute illness, severe pain and in great discomfort, and often these patients do not get appropriate privacy and empathy what they deserve. Emergency department system is not uniform across the country so that different triaging scales are used by various emergency departments for assessing the severity of illness. Patients admitted to emergency with wide variety of complaints like simple fever pain to severe sepsis shock, polytrauma, stroke, exacerbation of asthma, and chronic obstructive lung disease and also as mass casualties. Various assessment tools like ABCDE (airway, breathing, circulation, disability, exposure) approach, START (simple triaging and rapid treatment for disaster) and various *triage* methods are based on time, make the patient to wait according to categories, makes delay in treatment and increase in errors and cost of unnecessary tests. Since different disease presentations in emergency has different requirements so that superior method should be applied in which care plan (including investigation; treatment chart, admission requirement and referral) is initiated only by experienced qualified emergency team then instruction should be followed by rest of the team. Rapid assessment and treatment of patient by *experienced and qualified team* in emergency increases the patient safety and satisfaction as well as improves patient flow and also solve the problem of emergency department overcrowding.

BENEFITS OF RAPID ASSESSMENT

- Team lead by senior doctor attend the patient
- Appropriate investigation of blood, electrocardiogram (ECG), X-rays, computed tomography (CT), urinalysis (unnecessary investigations can be avoided) and early treatment plan like analgesia, antibiotics, and intravenous infusion can be decided in early stage. Investigations and treatment are initiated in early stage in time bound emergencies like stroke and myocardial infarction
- Early identification of patients for admission, prompt bed requests and for discharge after treatment
- Risk stratification can be done to identify patients for resuscitation or for transfer to high dependency unit or ward thus clinical risks are minimized
- Improves patient safety, quality and outcome
- Reduces the overcrowding, and provide learning experience for junior doctors.

REQUIREMENTS FOR RAPID ASSESSMENT

- Dedicated team consists of senior doctor consultant, attending consultant, qualified nurse, social worker, general duty attendant
- Manager to arrange bed and manage patient flow
- Point-of-care testing devices like arterial blood gas (ABG), glucometer and card test.

STEPS FOR RAPID ASSESSMENT AND TREATMENT

- All patients are changed into gowns on arrival and given identification bands
- A brief history (allergy history), examination, and documentation of management plan
- Assessment and resuscitation of patient as soon as they arrive in emergency by senior doctor and nurse
- On the basis of presenting complaints, investigations are decided
- Point-of-care testing like blood sugar, ABG, card test, D dimer is used
- Medications are prescribed and delivered as per guidance
- Necessary referral should be taken from the specialty if required

- Nonmedical need should be assessed by social worker.
- Patient should be admitted or discharged on the basis of comprehensive assessment.

COMPONENTS OF RAPID ASSESSMENT AND TREATMENT (FLOW CHART 1)

Resuscitation and Assessment

Resuscitation should be started within minutes of arrival of the patient. Assessment starts with shaking hands with the patient as it provide many clinical informations like level of consciousness, airway patency and peripheral perfusion of the patient, along with this it also provide confidence to patient and attendant. Focused history, examination and investigation history from the patient and attendant should be obtained.

Assessment of Airway

Complete airway obstruction leads to death within minutes but partial airway obstruction is quite common and can be recognized by noisy breathing such as snoring or gurgling which causes reduced level of consciousness (due to reduced airway muscular tone, loss of protective airway reflexes, principally the gag and cough reflexes, retention of oropharyngeal secretions and tongue malposition). Level of consciousness can be rapidly assessed using the AVPU method (alert, responds to voice, responds to pain, unresponsive). If the patient can talk, then this usually implies that the airway is safe. Simple maneuver such as jaw thrust or a chin lift can relieve the partially obstructed airway. Airway adjuncts such as oropharyngeal or nasopharyngeal devices can also be useful.

Assessment of Breathing

Increased respiratory work commonly associated with severity of illness as a result of an increased metabolic rate and oxygen consumption. This may lead to respiratory distress, signs of which include inability to complete sentences, high respiratory rate, diaphoresis, accessory muscle use and cyanosis. Focused clinical examination including tracheal palpation, percussion and auscultation may pinpoint the diagnosis (tracheal deviation and hyperresonance chest indicate tension pneumothorax, dull percussion note indicate pleural effusion or empyema, wheeze/silent chest indicate acute severe asthma, bronchial breath sound indicates pneumonia). High flow oxygen should be administered to all acutely ill patients; the effects of therapy should be assessed using pulse oximetry, and the target oxygen saturations should be 94–98%. The appropriate oxygen delivery device to use is a mask with a reservoir bag. It is vital that the reservoir is kept inflated at all times; this is usually achieved by setting the flow rate of oxygen to 15 L/min. This mask will usually deliver an inspired oxygen concentration (FiO_2) of 60–85%.

Assessment of Circulation

Assess the radial pulse, rate, rhythm and character. Attach cardiac monitor, note the blood pressure. Clinical signs that are common to hypovolemic, obstructive and cardiogenic shock include confusion or agitation, cold extremities, reduced capillary refill, tachycardia, absent or small volume peripheral pulses, hypotension and oliguria. The jugular venous pulse assessment is useful in distinguishing between hypovolemic states (low) and cardiogenic or obstructive shock (elevated). Circulatory features of septic shock include warm peripheries (vasodilatation) and a bounding pulse. Peripheral cannula can usually be inserted into antecubital fossa or external jugular veins and central lines can be inserted into internal jugular, subclavian and femoral veins. Sizes of peripheral cannula are determined by gauge (16 largest, to 26 smallest). Two 16-gauge lines are recommended for resuscitation.

Assessment of Disability

Assessment of neurological status, relevant clinical examination would include level of consciousness (LOC), focal and localizing neurological signs, pupillary reflexes and signs of meningism. Rapid assessment of neurosurgical status can be done by using AVPU scale.

Pain Management and Patient Needs Assessment

Pain management is an important aspect in the emergency department and described in another chapter while assessment of nonmedical need of the patient is equally important and involvement of social worker is helpful.

Investigations and Intervention

Important relevant investigations are carried out once the assessment part is over, e.g. blood tests, X-ray, ultrasound, CT scan, while point of care testing is helpful in rapid assessment of critically ill patient. Other interventions like specialty reference should be taken on the basis of investigations result for definitive care.

Diagnosis, Definitive Treatment and Disposition

Once a diagnosis is certain or the causes understood, definitive treatment can be started. This may require transfer

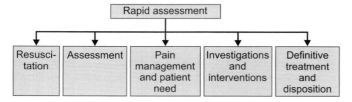

Flow chart 1 Components of rapid assessment

of the patient to the operating theater, interventional cardiology, laboratory, endoscopy suite, intensive care unit (ICU) or high dependency unit. Proposed management should be carefully communicated to the patient and close relatives of the patient. If patient is discharged to home, medication prescription, indicating diagnosis, follow-up test, and consultation should be clearly mentioned on the discharge summary.

CLINICAL QUALITY INDICATORS FOR RAPID ASSESSMENT

- Time to analgesia
- Time to delivering urgent medication, including antibiotics and bronchodilators
- Time to starting intravenous fluids
- Time to blood tests
- Time to imaging
- Time to specialty referral and assessment.

RAPID ASSESSMENT, EARLY INTERVENTIONS AND IMPROVING OUTCOME IN SEPSIS, STROKE AND TRAUMA

Timely recognition and intervention are important in reducing the morbidity and mortality due to sepsis and shock. Clinical suspicion, thorough physical examination, and laboratory screening using base deficit or lactate can improve outcome **(Tables 1 and 2)**.

Sepsis: Improving Outcome through Early Recognition

Improving outcome has been described in **Table 1**.

Stroke: Improving Outcome through Early Recognition

Improving outcome has been described in **Flow chart 2**. **Table 3** shows neurology assessment in stroke patient (stroke syndrome).

Trauma: Improving Outcome through Early Recognition

Blunt injury: Nonpenetrating but including crush laceration amputation

Penetrating: Bullet knife or spike

Long bone injury: Fracture or dislocation of femur, tibia, humerus, ulna, radius, and fibula

Polytrauma or multiple trauma: Injury to one body cavity (head, thorax, and abdomen) + two long bone or pelvic fracture or injury of two body cavities.

Trauma Team

Trauma team includes:
- Emergency team
- Neurosurgery
- Orthopedics
- Surgery/gastrointestinal (GI) surgery
- Critical care
- Thoracic surgery, vascular surgery.

Criteria for Trauma Team Activation

Criteria include:
- Blunt trauma, penetrating injury, gunshot wounds, stab wounds with systolic blood pressure (SBP) less than 90 mm Hg, require endotracheal intubation
- Mechanically unstable pelvic injury (open or obvious by physical examination)
- Respiratory compromise, obstruction, or intubation with presumed thoracic, abdominal, or pelvic injury
- Glasgow coma scale or score (GCS) less than 8 with presumed thoracic, abdominal, or pelvic injury, amputation proximal to the ankle or wrist
- Transfer patients from other facilities receiving blood to maintain vital signs or suspicion that patient likely will require urgent operative intervention.

Primary Survey (ABCDE)

It includes:
- Check patency of airway and clear secretion
- Oropharyngeal airway
- High concentration oxygen
- Intubation and initial normal-ventilation of trauma patient
- Cervical spine stabilization (c-spine collar)
- Two large bore cannula simultaneously obtain blood for analysis; complete blood count (CBC), blood grouping and typing
- Initial fluid therapy normal saline (NS) or Ringer's lactate (RL), control bleeding
- GCS score, pupil size, assess spinal injury
- Prevention of hypothermia
- *Adjuncts*: ABG, cardiac monitoring and insertion of urinary and gastric catheters
- Consider need for chest X-ray, pelvic X-ray and focused assessment with sonography for trauma (FAST).

Secondary Survey

This survey includes:
- Detail history and examination
- Obtain history of injury producing event and mechanism of injury

SECTION 1 Essentials for Emergency Physician

Table 1 Sepsis: Improving outcome through early recognition

Sepsis cascade			
SIRS (systemic inflammatory response syndrome)	Sepsis (SIRS + infection)	Severe sepsis (sepsis with organ dysfunction)	Shock (severe sepsis and shock)
• Temperature >100.4 and <96.8°F • Heart rate >90 beats/min • Respiratory rate >20 • WBC >12,000 or <4,000	• Fever • Cough • Dysuria • Documented positive culture for blood, urine, and sputum	• Fluid-responsive hypotension • Hypoxia • Low urine output • Rise in creatinine • Lactate liver enzyme • Low platelet • Altered sensorium	• Not responding to fluid (30 mL/kg)

Table 2 Early recognition of sepsis and shock improve outcome

Early recognition of sepsis	Early recognition of shock	Priorities in severe sepsis
• White blood cells (WBC) high/low • Temperature high/low • High heart rate • High respiratory rate • Infection	• Tachypnea • Tachycardia • Weak or bounding peripheral pulses • Delayed capillary refill (>2 seconds) • Pale or cool skin • Narrowed pulse pressure • Oliguria • Lactic acidosis • Elevated base deficit	• Oxygenation and airway management • Fluid resuscitation • Hemodynamic stability • Blood culture • Lactate levels • Antibiotics • Intensive care admission when lactate >2

Table 3 Clinical features of stroke

Focus neurology assessment in stroke patient (stroke syndrome)	
Carotid	• Aphasia (dominant hemisphere) or neglect (nondominant hemisphere) • Contralateral homonymous hemianopsia • Contralateral motor/sensory loss of face, arm, and leg • Conjugate ipsilateral eye deviation
MCA	• Aphasia (dominant hemisphere) or neglect (nondominant hemisphere) • Contralateral homonymous hemianopsia • Contralateral motor/sensory loss face/arm > leg
ACA	• Apathy, abulia, disinhibition • Conjugate eye deviation • Contralateral motor/sensory loss leg > arm
PICA	• Ipsilateral palatal weakness, Horner's syndrome • Wallenberg syndrome • Ipsilateral limb ataxia • Decreased pain/temperature contralateral body
AICA	• Ipsilateral deafness • Ipsilateral facial motor/sensory loss • Ipsilateral limb ataxia • Decreased pain/temperature contralateral body
Basilar	• Altered consciousness • Oculomotor difficulties, facial nerve paresis • Ataxia, quadriparesis

Abbreviations: MCA, middle cerebral artery; ACA, anterior cerebral artery; PICA, posterior inferior cerebellar artery; AICA, anterior inferior cerebellar artery.

Flow chart 2 Stroke: Improving outcome through early recognition

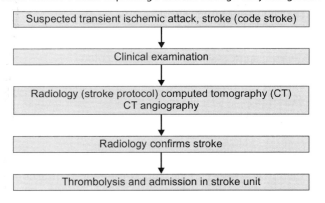

- Re-evaluation and detail examination of head, face, cervical, spine, chest, abdomen, perineum, rectum, vagina, and musculoskeletal **(Table 4)**
- Re-evaluation of neurological status and GCS score.

Management of Shock in Trauma

Shock can be managed by:
- Fluid therapy initiation in hypotensive trauma patient
- Recommendation crystalloid
- *Rapid responder* require only crystalloid fluid
- *Transient responder* may need addition of colloids and blood
- Target systolic blood pressure (BP) 80–90 mm Hg and urinary output 0.5 mL/kg/h in adult and 1.0 mL/kg/h in children
- Addition of vasopressors and inotropic agents, if not responding to fluid therapy, norepinephrine is often used.

Blood and Blood Products and Control of Bleeding

- Target hemoglobin is 7–9 g/dL
- Use of blood and blood products
- Type specific blood is preferred, but type O negative blood indicated in massive hemorrhage (which is available within 10 min in most of the blood banks)

Table 4 Assessment, findings and investigations of system

Assessment of system	Findings	Investigations to confirm
Consciousness, pupil, head, cervical spine tenderness	GCS, <8 mass effect, scalp laceration, skull fracture	CT head and cervical spine
Maxillofacial area	Facial fracture and soft tissue injury	CT scan of facial bone
Neck and thorax	s/c emphysema, tenderness, hematoma, muffled breath sound and heart sounds	CECT thorax, angiography, bronchoscopy, tube thoracostomy
Abdomen and flank pelvis	Bruising, deformity, visceral injury, pelvic fracture, hematuria, perineal injuries	Ultrasound, CECT abdomen, angiography, laparotomy, pelvic X-ray urethrogram cystogra, IVP
Vertebral column and spinal cord	Quadriplegia, paraplegia nerve root injury, fracture dislocation	Plain spine X-ray CT/MRI
Extremities	Swelling bruising pain tenderness absent/ diminished pulse tense muscular compartment neurological deficit	Specific X-ray Doppler examination angiography
Polytrauma (mandatory investigations)	Injury to one body cavity (head, thorax, abdomen) + two long bone or pelvic fracture OR injury of two body cavities	CT head and cervical spine, screening of whole spine CECT chest and abdomen CT pelvis

Abbreviations: GCS, Glasgow coma scale; s/c, subcutaneous; CT, computed tomography; CECT, contrast-enhanced computed tomography; IVP, intravenous pyelogram; MRI, magnetic resonance imaging

- Early use of red blood cells (RBCs) and fresh frozen plasma (FFP) improves the outcome (initial recommendations 10–15 mL/kg, additional dose depends on coagulation parameters PT or APTT 1.5 times the normal values)
- *Platelets* transfusion is recommended when platelets counts are <50,000
- *Tranexamic acid* 1 g over 10 minutes then 1 g over 8 hour
- *Rapid control of bleeding*—by local hemostatic procedures, packaging, direct surgical bleeding control, and angiographic embolization.

Disaster: Rapid Assessment

Mass casualty incident: An incident whenever the number of victims is greater than resource capability to provide usual standards of care. Situations when standard triage methods may be inadequate:
- Treat as many as possible who have a chance of survival
- Focus on easily treated conditions
- Perform rapid act accurate assessment
- Reassess and re-triage.

START (Simple Triage and Rapid Treatment)

Only two treatments are allowed:
1. Open and clear airway
2. Control of major external hemorrhage:
   - *Respiration*: Airway breathing
   - *Pulse*: Circulation
   - *Mental status*: Disability

All patients are reassessed at treatment areas.
- Actions which save lives (early)
  - ABC
  - Control of hemorrhage
  - Chest decompression
- Actions which save lives (delayed)
  - Intravenous (IV) antibiotics
  - Dressings and splints

CONCLUSION

Rapid assessment and formulation of care of plan by senior doctor ensure the patient's safety. Any important emergency or time critical interventions are instituted (blood tests/X-rays/ultrasounds/CT, etc.). Initial clinical assessment and plan clearly documented and communicated with nursing staff. This system improves the outcome of many critical illnesses like sepsis, trauma and stroke.

BIBLIOGRAPHY

1. Frost PJ, Wise MP. Early management of acutely ill ward patients. BMJ. 2012;24;345:e5677.
2. Frost PJ, Wise MP. Recognition and early management of the critically ill ward patient. Br J Hosp Med (Lond). 2007;68(10):M180-3.
3. Frost PJ, Wise MP. Recognition and management of the patient with shock. Acute Med. 2006;5(2):43-47.
4. Hostutler JJ, Taft SH, Snyder C. Patient needs in the emergency department: nurses' and patients' perceptions. J Nurs Adm. 1999;29(1):43-50.
5. Muntlin A, Gunningberg L, Carlsson M. Patients' perceptions of quality of care at an emergency department and identification of areas for quality improvement. J Clin Nurs. 2006;15(8):1045-56.
6. NICE. (2013). Intravenous fluid therapy in adults in hospital. Clinical guideline 174. [online] NICE website. Available from https://www.nice.org.uk/guidance/cg174?unlid=724084. [Accessed January 2017].
7. NICE Short Clinical Guidelines Technical Team. (2006). Acutely ill patients in hospital: recognising and responding to deterioration. Clinical guideline [CG50]. [online] NICE website. Available from https://www.nice.org.uk/guidance/cg50. [Accessed January 2017].
8. O'Driscoll BR, Howard LS, Davison AG, et al. BTS guideline for emergency oxygen use in adult patients. Thorax. 2008;63:vi1-68.
9. Wilson JE, Pendleton JM. Oligoanalgesia in the emergency department. Am J Emerg Med. 1989;7(6):620-3.

CHAPTER 5

Point of Care Testing

Shashank Chauhan, Rajani Yadav

INTRODUCTION

Emergency departments (EDs) around the world frequently experience prolonged waiting times and extended periods of overcrowding. Minimizing the delay between the onset of symptoms and the initiation of treatment is both, critical and lifesaving in dealing with the life-threatening conditions as well as in improving the outcomes for critically ill patients.

Point of care testing (POCT) refers to any diagnostic test administered at or near the site where the patient is located, that do not require permanent dedicated space, and that are performed outside the physical facilities of the clinical laboratories. With advances in technology, it has become increasingly possible to perform common clinical investigations outside the laboratory at the point of care with a dependable level of accuracy. The main advantages of POCT devices are increased level of portability, thus making it possible to perform vital POCT at remote locations with accuracy and the significantly decreased turnaround times (TAT), which are of utmost importance in dealing with the life-threatening conditions. Using POCT, healthcare professionals can perform, analyze, obtain and act on test results at the patient's bedside in a matter of minutes. Thus, judicious use of POCT has the potential to decrease the delays for diagnosing a clinical condition and treatment initiation, increase the efficiency of ED working, enhance the quality care to the patients and alleviate the negative effects of ED overcrowding, thus imposing a positive outcome in patient care and job satisfaction of healthcare professionals.

POINT OF CARE TESTING: NEED OF THE HOUR

The question arises, why POCT is becoming the gold standard of care in EDs around the world? Answer to this lies in meeting the growing need of better healthcare, by rapidly diagnosing and treating the real emergent conditions, to tackling the overcrowded EDs by enhancing the patient turnover due to decreased TAT of the investigations. When used in appropriate scenarios, POCT is an effective tool to minimize the time to diagnose and treatment initiation, thus improving the patient outcome.

Available literature shows that the real-life impact of POCT in the ED can vary greatly and often serves a lifesaving tool in conditions in which:
Delays in the treatment of at least 1 hour can have significant effects on outcomes
- Delays in test results are the primary determining factor holding up patient management decisions and there appropriate dispositions
- Remote areas of healthcare operations without a dedicated centralized laboratory imposing a challenge in patient management.

Common instances in which evidence supports the use of POCT in EDs can be summarized as:

Acute Coronary Syndrome

Chest pain grabs a major chunk of presentations to the ED at any given point of time. As per the statistics, around 35% of patients presenting to the ED with complains of chest pain turn out to be acute coronary syndrome (ACS), conversely a large number of patients of ACS were mistakenly discharged home from the ED, leading to increased mortality rate. Thus, a means of rapidly assessing a patient with chest pain with an increased sensitivity would increase the efficiency of ED along with the quality care management of patients, as the patient benefits the most from early and aggressive treatment.

Biochemical evaluation of ACS with cardiac biomarkers, specifically cardiac troponins has become the base of ACS management in EDs around the world in last few years. It would not be an exaggeration to label these biomarkers as being abused by the ED personnel's in almost all patients coming with the chest pain, the high level of sensitivity and specificity of these biomarkers makes them the initial investigation of choice to rule in or out the ACS in a rapid and accurate manner. Since troponins are the markers of myocardial necrosis, current guidelines recommends that the initial titre of troponin-I should be made available to the physicians within the first 30 minutes of sample collection, as delay increases the probability of adverse outcomes. Several POCT technologies exist for cardiac troponin-I testing with TATs of not more than 20 minutes. A rapid rule-out protocol using a combination of high-sensitivity (hs) troponin-I, risk score and electrocardiogram was recently shown to be safe and effective in identifying low-risk patients. The new hs troponin-T (hs-TnT) assay is a modification of the fourth generation cTnT, which has a high analytical performance as compared to the conventional cTnT. The diagnostic accuracy for acute myocardial infarction (AMI), as quantified by the area under the receiver-operating characteristic curve was significantly higher with the hs-cTnT assay than the standard assay. The superiority of hs-cTnT assay in diagnosing myocardial infarction within the first 3 hours of onset of symptoms is now making it the investigation of choice for diagnosing ACS in leading EDs worldwide. Thus, hs-cTnT as a POCT is now gaining popularity in early diagnosis of AMIs, providing an opportunity in extending early treatment options, as more rapid diagnosis of AMI may reduce complications by facilitating earlier revascularization, earlier transfer to the coronary care units, and earlier initiation of evidence-based treatment for AMIs.

Venous Thromboembolic Disease

Venous thromboembolic disease, including pulmonary embolism and deep venous thrombosis (DVT), is a life-threatening condition accounting to high mortality rates. Sometimes, the subtle symptoms of pulmonary embolism makes it liable to be missed in the initial patient assessment, therefore the availability of a sensitive method for a reliable identification of patients with suspected venous thromboembolic disease is critically important. D-dimer is used widely as a diagnostic aid in low- and moderate-risk patients with suspected venous thromboembolism. Many EDs use D-dimer as a POCT to facilitate patient management with an increased pace. A multicentric study in the USA showed shorter TATs of D-dimer than the central lab. A negative D-dimer result can be used to safely rule out DVT, thus eliminating the need to waste time and resources on further investigations. Therefore, using POCT in the evaluation of suspected thromboembolic disease can rule in or out the life-threatening pulmonary embolism with a fast and accurate method, thus improving the patient prognosis, decreasing the waiting time in the ED and judicious use of the ED resources for the better caring of the needful.

Severe Sepsis

Probable or documented presence of infection together with systemic manifestations is defined as sepsis.

In 1904, Sir William Osler was quoted as saying that, "except on few occasions, the patient appears to die from the body's response to infection rather than from it".

Sepsis, after ACS remains the leading cause of death in critically ill patients around the world. The high variability and nonspecific nature of signs and symptoms of sepsis, makes it very difficult to identify patients with sepsis for timely intervention. "Time is money" in the management of sepsis, and has a very important role in patient prognostication. As per the "Surviving Sepsis" study done by the European Intensive Care Society, every hour of delayed diagnosis of sepsis decreases the survival rate by 7.6%.

Keeping in view the profound effect of delayed diagnosis and treatment of sepsis, the Society of Critical Care Medicine, the European Intensive Care Society and the International Sepsis Forum launched the "Surviving Sepsis Campaign" with a founding statement that became known as the "Barcelona Declaration". Hemodynamic resuscitation to normal physiological parameters has been trialed as early goal-directed therapy (EGDT) in sepsis, published in 2001 and formed the backbone of Surviving Sepsis Campaign. Though a latest study called as Australasian Resuscitation in sepsis evaluation (ARISE) trials had contradicted the benefit outcomes of EGDT in sepsis, but it is still being practiced in various emergency and critical care departments worldwide. The grassroot level of successful treatment of sepsis remains the timely intervention. Therefore, an accurate and immediate means of identifying patients with severe sepsis is critically important for minimizing delays to resuscitation. These days the use of serum biomarkers as a point of care in diagnosing, risk stratifying and monitoring response to therapy in patients of sepsis is being widely used in EDs and ICUs equipped with cutting-edge technology. The timely assessment of these biomarkers, as a POCT may improve diagnosis and therapeutic decision-making, thus impacting patient's prognostication. Presently, more than 170 biomarkers have been assessed for sepsis prognosis and diagnosis, of which the ones used widely are as follows:
- Serum lactate
- Serum procalcitonin
- Serum C-reactive protein
- Interleukins (IL-6).

Elevated serum lactate levels have been shown to be a sensitive marker of global tissue hypoxia in patients with suspected sepsis. Lactate levels are particularly useful when measured serially, to guide response to resuscitation and fluid therapy. Lactate clearance in the first 6 hours of initiation of treatment has been shown to be a better prognostic factor than a single lactate determination. Serum lactate must be available with rapid TAT (within minutes) to effectively treat severely septic patients. An arterial blood gas analyzer located in the EDs usually accomplishes this. These days many EDs are utilizing valid POCT technologies for measuring whole blood and fingertip lactate levels, providing almost immediate feedback of the sick patients. Therefore, while dealing with a septic patient, utilizing serum lactate levels as a POCT in EDs aids in rationalizing the treatment protocol and have a positive effect on risk stratification and prognostication of the patient. Hospitals should invest in point of care devices to meet the present standards of care for septic patients.

Likewise lactates, serum procalcitonin induction is very rapid in sepsis. Initially the level increases within 2–6 hours, reaching plateau after 6–12 hours. The concentration remains high for up to 48 hours after contacting infection, which returns to baseline within the following 2–3 days. This characteristic rise and fall pattern of procalcitonin (PCT) has been used for the early detection of sepsis. Evolving technology has devised many POCT for PCT, utilizing it as an early marker of sepsis. There are various cut-offs for PCT titers in POCT. It can also be a guide for antibiotic regimen and can be a prognostic indicator for morbidity and mortality.

Stroke

During recent years, thrombolysis by intravenous tissue plasminogen activator (rtPA) has revolutionized the treatment of ischemic stroke, increasing long-term survival and reducing mortality. The clinical benefit in acute ischemic stroke is time-dependent. The statement "Time is Neuron", in the management of acute ischemic stroke is not an exaggeration. Reducing the door to needle time in acute ischemic stroke has been shown to have positive outcomes in terms of the degree of disability or the residual deficits, thus reducing the morbidity and mortality of the patient.

As per the international guidelines practiced for stroke thrombolysis, the "Window Period" of 4.5 hours is taken as an appropriate for thrombolyzing a proven stroke. With such a narrow range of time for diagnosing and thrombolyzing a stroke, it becomes utmost important to have a POCT at hand before even shifting a patient for neuroimaging. This cannot be achieved by running a sample for standard analytic techniques, which are time-consuming. It will kill the precious time of salvaging the brain parenchyma, thus deteriorating the prognosis of the patient. This can only be done with the POCT for the coagulation status international normalized ratio (INR) and serum creatinine value of the patient. Various studies say that the POCT of the INR are sufficiently precise for emergency management of thrombolysis in acute stroke. Moreover, it substantially reduces the time interval until INR values are available and therefore may hasten initiation of thrombolysis, positively impacting the patient care.

CHALLENGES IN EFFECTIVE IMPLEMENTATION OF POINT OF CARE TESTING

Clinical pathways and ED logistics may need substantial modification to maximize the clinical and economic benefits of rapid TATs provided by the POCT since the average cost per POCT is more than the conventional testing. But, the monetary burden is to be weighed against the clinical benefit outcomes both in and out of hospital. Secondly, a rapid turnover of noncritical patients will help to reduce the overcrowding, and more time at hand, of the care givers for the high-risk patients in the EDs.

As the technology advances further, development of new and novel POCT tools for infectious diseases and cancer screening are in the pipeline, which would change the way emergency medicine is practiced.

CONCLUSION

Points of care testing are the tests done outside the lab, but within the health care setup. Test are performed near the patient's location where the patient are being treated. POCT results makes positive changes in the management strategies. POCT results are used to make decision and take appropriate action which will lead to improved health care outcome.

BIBLIOGRAPHY

1. Australian General Practice POCT Study. (2012). Policies, procedures and guidelines for point-of-care testing. [online] Available from *www.health.gov.au/internet/main/publishing.nsf*. [Accessed November, 2016].
2. Boran G, Collier J, Hurley T, et al. Guidelines for Safe and Effective Management and Use of Point of Care Testing. Ireland: Academy of Medical Laboratory Science, Association of Clinical Biochemists in Ireland, Irish Medicines Board and RCPI Faculty of Pathology; 2007.
3. World Health Organization. (2011). Guidelines for point of care testing. [online] WHO website. Available from *http://whqlibdoc.who.int/php*. [Accessed November, 2016].

CHAPTER 6

Essentials of Medicolegal Case Writing

Vivekanshu Verma, Devendra Richhariya

INTRODUCTION

Medicolegal case (MLC) can be expressed as any case of injury, disease or infirmity, or death in which law enforcing agencies have to enquire into the matter and fix the responsibility of a person or a group of persons responsible for causing the said injury, disease or infirmity, or death and penalize as per the existing law of land **(Box 1)**.[1]

Medicolegal reports (MLRs) are documents prepared by a government or private doctor, pertaining to injury, sexual offence, poisoning or unexplained death. It contains all the facts, observed by the doctor and his opinion drawn therefrom. His opinion must be based upon the observations made by him and not on hearsay evidence.[2]

Medicolegal case writing comprises of 3 parts, namely:[3]
1. *Preamble*: It includes the date, time and place of examination, name of the patient, his residential address, occupation; name of the person or police official accompanying, daily diary register or first information report number, informed consent of the person being examined, two marks of identification, thumb impression, etc. wherever applicable.
2. *Findings or observations*: It includes a complete description of the injuries or any other findings present; any investigations or referrals, etc. asked for.
3. *Opinion*: It includes the following:
   - *Nature of the injury*: Whether simple or grievous
   - *Weapon or force used*: Whether blunt or sharp or firearms or burns, etc.
   - *Duration of the injuries*: Based on the characteristics of the external injuries.[3]

In the casualty, while attending to an emergency, the doctor should understand that his first priority is to save the life of the patient. He should do everything possible to resuscitate the patient and ensure that he is out of danger. All legal formalities stand suspended till this is achieved.

Box 1 Cases that are to be treated as medicolegal

- All cases of injuries and burns the circumstances of which suggest commission of an offence by somebody (irrespective of suspicion of foul play)
- All vehicular, factory or other unnatural accident cases specially when there is a likelihood of patient's death or grievous hurt
- Cases of suspected or evident sexual assault
- Cases of suspected or evident criminal abortion
- Cases of unconsciousness where its cause is not natural or not clear
- All cases of suspected or evident poisoning or intoxication
- Cases brought dead with improper history creating suspicion of an offence
- Cases of suspected self-infliction of injuries or attempted suicide
- Any other case not falling under the above categories but has legal implications

This has been clearly exemplified by the Honorable Supreme Court of India in Parmanand Katara versus Union of India.[4]

MEDICOLEGAL CLASSIFICATION OF WOUNDS[5]

The wounds or injuries may be classified as follows:

Mechanical injuries
- Those caused by hard blunt weapons, fall or friction with rough surface, etc.:
  - Abrasion
  - Bruise or contusion
  - Laceration
- Those caused by sharp-cutting and/or sharp edge of sharp-cutting pointed weapons: Incised wound.
- Those caused by pointed tip of sharp cutting or blunt weapon:
  - *Stab wound*: It may again be subclassified as follows:
    - Punctured
    - Penetrating
    - Perforating

- Those caused by firearms (**Box 2**), e.g.
  - Shotguns
  - Rifled gunshot weapons
  - Improvised country made weapons

Thermal injuries
- *Dry heat*: Burns
- *Moist heat*: Scalds and blisters

Chemical injuries: These are caused by corrosive acids or alkalis.

Legally on the Basis of Gravity of Injury

- Simple hurt
- Grievous hurt
- Dangerous to life

Section 319 and 320 of the Indian Penal Code (IPC) define hurt and grievous hurt, respectively:

Section 319 Indian Penal Code

Hurt: Whoever causes bodily pain, disease or infirmity to any person is said to cause hurt.

Section 320 Indian Penal Code

Grievous Hurt[6]

First: Emasculation (penis or testis amputated or erectile dysfunction after spine injury).[6]

Second: Permanent privation of the sight of either eye (corneal opacity by injury/optic nerve damage/retinal detachment).[6]

Third: Permanent privation of the hearing of either ear (tympanic membrane rupture or auditory nerve damage). Audiometry is needed to prove the loss.

Fourth: Privation of any member or joint (limb amputation or kidney rupture).

Fifth: Destruction or permanent impairing of the powers of any member or joint (muscle and tendon cut or post-traumatic contractures in limb muscles).

Sixth: Permanent disfiguration of the head or face (acid vitriolage/cutting nose/permanent scar on face).

Seventh: Fracture or dislocation of a bone or tooth. X-ray of dislocation and repeat X-rays after reduction of dislocated joint are necessary, as it is unique reversible grievous hurt, which cannot be proved in court without X-ray of patient.

Eighth:
- Any hurt which endangers life (dangerous to life).
- Any hurt which causes the suffered to be during the space of 20 days in severe bodily pain or unable to follow his ordinary pursuits.
- Any hurt which sufferer unable to follow his ordinary pursuits.

Dangerous to life injuries are those which may be fatal, if no surgical aid is available. For example, tension pneumothorax, cardiac tamponade, liver and splenic laceration, deep incised wound in slit throat, stab wound in chest and abdomen, traumatic extradural hematoma, and acute subdural hematoma with midline shift.

Time Since Injury

Time since wounded
- *Time since abrasion* (**Table 1**):
- *Time since bruise* (**Table 2**):
- *Time since burn injury* (**Table 3**):

Table 1	Time since abrasion
Abrasion of fresh duration	Abrasion is red with evidence of oozing of serum and a little blood. There is no scab
12–24 hours	The exudation dries up and reddish soft scab formation
By 2nd/3rd day	The scab is brownish
By 4th–5th day	The scab is dark brown and hard
By 6th–7th day	The scab blackish, dries up, shrinks and starts falling off from the margin which is completed within next 7 days

Box 2 Dangerous weapons or means

Dangerous weapon is defined under section 324 and 326 of Indian Penal Code (IPC), as any instrument, used for shooting, stabbing or cutting, or any instrument which, when used as weapon of offence, is likely to cause death, or by means of fire or any heated substance, or by means of any poison or any corrosive substance, or by means of any explosive substance, or by means of any substance which it is deleterious to human body to inhale, to swallow or to receive into the blood, or by means of any animal.

Table 2	Time since bruise
Fresh bruise	Skin is intact and reddish in color
Next 3 days	Within a few hours it becomes bluish and remains bluish for about up to three days
By 4th day	It becomes brownish/bluish black—hemosiderin
By 5th/6th day	It changes to greenish discoloration—hematoidin
By 7th/8th day	It becomes yellowish-bilirubin and gradually fades away

Table 3 Time since burn injury

Fresh burn	Erythematic and formation of blister
2nd day	Erythematic around a blister or deep injury passes off
3rd day	Pus formation
4th to 6th day	Slough formation which is shed off by the end of the first week

PREPARATION OF MLC REPORTS

Medicolegal cases (MLC) are like any other injured patients and doctor duty is to treat as well as document the details of injuries and communicating to investigation officer of law enforcing agencies under section 39 of CrPC and failure to do so will attract legal penalty and liable to be prosecuted under Section 201 of IPC.

Any doctor who possess permanent registration with medical council and who has first contact with patient should prepare an ML case report and in rape victims the examination and preparation of MLC is done by female doctors.

Emergency Department is the area where majority of ML reports are prepared, but sometimes may be in wards after detection of new findings. Initiation of MLC is required in following cases.

Consent for medicolegal examination to be taken in written in all cases except in cases brought by police being arrested on charge of committing an offence and person below 12 years/unsound mind- consent of guardian is to be taken.

The institution of proper treatment to the patient and life saving is the prime responsibility of doctor and the hospital in accident or medicolegal cases (MLC). No delay for providing first aid. Doctor to complete the injury sheet, which is a part of the assessment of the patient.

Situations when a Doctor Prepare a Medicolegal Report

- Brought by the police for examination and reporting.
- Already registered MLC referred from other health care system for expert management/advice
- After history taking and thorough examination, if the doctor suspects that the circumstances/ findings of the case are such that registration of the case as an MLC is warranted RTA's, Rail accidents, factory accidents or any other unnatural mishap
- Suspected or evident homicides or suicides
- Suspected or evident poisoning
- Burn injuries due to any cause
- Injury cases where foul play is suspected
- Injury cases where there is likelihood of death in near future
- Sexual assault cases
- Suspected or evident criminal abortions
- Unconscious cases where cause of it is not clear
- Brought in dead cases where suspicion of foul play
- As per directive of court.

Completion of Medicolegal Record

- Documentation is done in duplicate/triplicate in a set performa as per hospital policy
- Separate performas may be available for medical examination, examination of drunkenness, etc.
- All columns are filled up carefully and by the same doctor who had examined the patient
- Each MLC is given a fresh MLC number sequentially or parallel series as per hospital policy
- The details are completed then and there only, leaving no provisions as to be completed later on.
- After completion doctors sign and mention his/her name in full below it with designation
- Police constable on duty informed in each case
- After registration of a case as MLC, thereafter all documents and requisition forms bear the same MLC number including the discharge slip.
- The details are completed then and there only, leaving no provisions as to be completed later on
- After completion doctors sign and mention his/her name in full below it with designation
- Police constable on duty informed in each case
- After registration of a case as MLC, thereafter all documents and requisition forms bear the same MLC number including the discharge slip.

Components of Medicolegal Record (Format for Medicolegal Report)

General Details

- Registration number
- MLC no.
- Name and S/D/W of
- Age sex religion
- Occupation
- Residential address
- Details of person who brought the victim
- Mark of identification are noted and documented
- Date and time of examination
- Name of police station informed

Examination Details

- Alleged history to be precise and to the point, legible and clearly written
- Description of injuries like minor injuries and multiple injuries in poly trauma
- Specialist consultation obtained

- Abbreviation should be avoided
- As a part of documentation of MLC report or whenever the investigative officer requests the doctor for certifying fitness of the patient to make a statement the examining doctor will certify the same on the original MLC sheet. He/she will mention date and time clearly with signature, name in full with designation below the certification.
- Opinion regarding injuries whether simple, under observation and reference for specialist opinion, grievous (after all findings/investigation/X-ray), caused by sharp or blunt objects
- A doctor cannot refuse to examine medicolegal case on the basis of being a private practitioner or citing a jurisdiction problem.
- Patient can be discharged after initial treatment or admitted in hospital, referred to other hospital after providing first aid/stabilization for expert management after completion of all necessary documentation.

Time Limit for Registering a Medicolegal Case

- There is no time limit for preparing an MLR or registering a case as MLC
- A case which otherwise qualifies to be an MLC was not registered earlier is to be registered as MLC by the concerned doctor
- A case due to unraveling of new findings—history/clinical examination, etc. later on qualifies to be an MLC to be registered by the concerned doctor
- A medicolegal case is registered as soon as a doctor suspects foul play or feels it necessary to inform the police, at any time after admission
- A case is registered as an MLC even if it is brought several days after the incident
- If the case brought is a referred case and is already registered as medicolegal case fresh report is not required.
- A case that is admitted and on treatment, later on found out be MLC, is made MLC by the concerned doctor
- If death is inevitable, arrangement to take the dying declaration is made
- All the materials such as vomit, gastric lavage sample, blood urine, etc. in poisoning cases, vaginal swab and pubic hair in sexual offences, foreign bodies found in the wounds, etc. are collected.
- Samples are properly preserved, packed and sealed then handed over to the police.

Admission and Discharge of MLC

- Whenever a medicolegal case is admitted the same is documented in admission papers and hospital records
- When discharged, the same should be intimated to the police authorities of the hospital
- Police is informed if a MLC is taking discharge against medical advice
- At the time of discharge, detailed instructions to the patient regarding treatment, follow-up general care, diet, exercise, etc. are given in writing.

Death of a Person Admitted as a Medicolegal Case

The following are the do's and don'ts in case a person admitted as a medicolegal case expires.
- Police informed immediately.
- Body sent to the hospital mortuary for preservation, till the legal formalities are completed and the police releases the body to the lawful heirs.
- Death certificate not issued—even if the patient was admitted.
- Dead body never released to the relatives directly.

Brought in Dead Patient

- Police to be informed
- Number of injuries noted in MLC record
- Article in possession to be documented and handed over to police/relatives
- Dead body to be sent to hospital mortuary and handed over to police.

Medical Examination of Victims of Sexual Assaults (Section 164A of CrPC)

- Examination only by female registered medical practitioner
- Without delay
- Consent—documented
- Note down particulars
- Complete history
- Examination—Genital examination and injuries:
- Standard protocols and guidelines
- Preserve samples—DNA profiling
- Emergency contraception if required
- Treatment/prophylaxis as required
- Opinion

How does the Law Protect the Victim in Medicolegal Cases?

The law states that concerns like legal formalities, monetary considerations or even the infrastructural restraints of the institution should not prohibit the institution or hospital from providing basic and emergency medical treatment. Here are a few things everyone should know:
- A hospital cannot deny emergency medical care to an accident victim under Article 21.
- It cannot deny treatment on the alleged reason of lack of facilities. The hospital has to provide emergency care and then transfer the patient safely in their ambulance to

CHAPTER 6 Essentials of Medicolegal Case Writing

Medicolegal Report (Form-II)

Serial. No.....................

MEDICOLEGAL REPORT NUMBER... DATED ....
Consent for medicolegal examination (in case of accused, consent is not required u/s 53CrPC)

I, Dr.. Designation...
PHC/CHC/Hospital/Deptt...
examined Sh/ Smt/Miss (First name).................................... (Last Name)...
s/o,d/o,w/o.. Age..................... Sex............................ Occupation........................
Address... PS.. Distt..............................
as per particulars given below:
(A) Date and time of arrival:..
(B) Date and time of examination:..
(C) Place of examination: Casualty/Ward/OPD/Deptt:...
(D) Police request Number and Date (if brought by police):..
     Police informed (if coming direct) vide No:.. Date.................... Time...........................
(E) Brought by Police Official... No...
     PS..Distt..
(F) Accompanied by: Name... Relation......................................
     Address.. PS........................
     District..
(G) Name and Address of the Female Attendant (in case of Female Patient).....................................
(H) Identification marks of the patient   (1)
                                            (2)
(I) OPD No.. Referred to...
    If admitted: (i) C.R.No........................... Date................................. Ward...
               (ii) Date of Discharge...
              (iii) Where Dying Declaration is necessary, indicate steps taken:
    (a) Whether the Magistrate was informed for recording Dying Declaration............................
    (b) Name and Address of the Magistrate..
         ....
    (c) Time at which the Magistrate arrived on the spot..
    (d) If Magistrate not available, details of witnesses in whose presence the Dying declaration was recorded:
        1. ....
        2. ....
    (e) Dying declaration handed over to Police official: Name...
        No......... PS.. District..
(J) Material collected, preserved and handed over to police for chemical analysis, etc. (write complete detail)

Amount of fee paid (if any) Rs.................to......................................vide No................................

SECTION 1 Essentials for Emergency Physician

I. Gist of incident as stated by the injured/accompanying person.
II. General condition of the person, clothing, etc.
III. Particulars of injuries, viz. type, dimension, shape, location, nature, duration, etc. and kind of weapon used:

1. Nature of injuries _____
   (Simple, Grievous, Dangerous or pending for observation)
2. Probable duration of injuries_____
3. Kind of weapon used (Sharp, Blunt, Firearm, Fire, Position, etc.) _____

Signature of the Examining Medical Officer
Name (In capital letters).…..........................……....
Designation…...…...

CHAPTER 6 Essentials of Medicolegal Case Writing 31

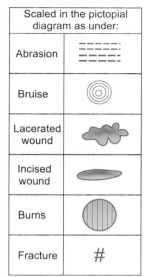

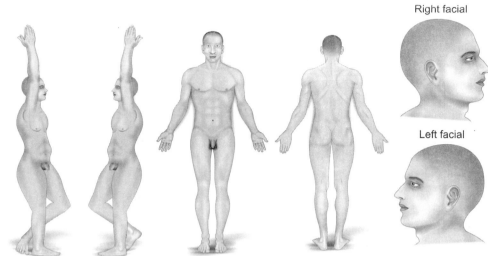

Right facial

Left facial

Guidelines

As per Section 320 IPC, any injury falling under following clauses is grievous:
1. Emasculation.
2. Permanent privation of the sight of either eye.
3. Permanent privation of the hearing of either ear.
4. Privation of any member or joint.
5. Destruction or permanent impairing of the powers of any member or joint.
6. Permanent disfiguration of the head or face.
7. Fracture of dislocation of a bone or tooth.
8. Any hurt (i) which endangers life or (ii) which causes the suffer to be during the space of 20 days.
   a. In serve bodily pain, or
   b. Unable to follow his ordinary pursuits.

At the end in column No.7 opine whether multiple injuries, individually simple, are collectively dangerous to life.

- the nearest facility. This includes government and private hospitals. It also includes private clinics and nursing homes
- The hospital cannot deny a patient emergent treatment on the basis that he/she is unable to pay the required fees or that there is no close relative to sign for consent (Consent is overridden in an emergency)
- In the case of a rape or criminal abortion the lady cannot be examined by a doctor without written consent from the victim
- In both cases—rape and criminal abortion the doctor is bound by law to keep the patients information including her name confidential
- In cases where a woman is being examined another woman must be present during the examination. In the case of males, a male has to be present at all times
- In the case of suicide causing death, the doctor is obligated to report the matter to the police for further investigation
- If the patient is alive and suicide is suspected the doctor is not obligated to report the matter to the police
- Please remember, on visiting a hospital for a medicolegal case, after the patient has received treatment, the doctor or hospital must inform the police about the case, it's advised to take an acknowledgment of receipt for future reference. If the intimation is given orally or via the phone, a docket number is provided which can be used as proof of intimation and is documented in the patient's records.
- Once the patient is stabilized and fit to give statement to police the patient required to authenticate the information that has been provided and the victim/patient will be visited by the police. They will take down the statement of the victim, and confirm if a case needs to be filed or not. The doctor is responsible to give accurate information to the police which will assist them in their investigation. After the case is filed the victim will get a receipt stating the file number and case number. If required the victim can employ a lawyer to take the case forward.

PRACTICAL TIPS FOR MEDICOLEGAL CASE WRITING

Ques. *How to describe gunshot and shotgun wound in an MLC report?*

Ans. Gunshot is single bullet injury by rifled firearm; Shotgun is multiple pellets injury by *desi katta* or improvised revolver.

Indian law enquires in firearm wound description—number of wounds and type of firearm projectile (bullet or multiple pellets), nature of injury (simple or grievous), killing range of firearm by blackening and tattooing; length × breadth × depth, location and direction (circular or oval) of entry wound (inverted margins, blackening, tattooing, abrasion collar) or exit wound (everted), fresh duration or not.

For example, one gunshot in back, described as follows:
Single gunshot entry wound 1 cm in diameter, circular in shape, deep on the right side back of the chest, 16 cm below the tip of acromion process and 8 cm lateral to the midline with fresh bleeding blood oozing out of wound with inverted margins.

Blackening and tattooing present around the wound in an area of 8 cm in diameter.

Opinion reserved: *Surgeon's opinion for depth and grievousness. Near shot range of firearm.*[7]

Ques. *How to describe a shotgun wound on right lower limb in an MLC report?*
Ans. Multiple punctured lacerated wounds of varying size 0.2 cm × 0.2 cm × muscle deep present in a diameter of 10 cm on the back of right thigh 7 cm above the knee, circular in shape, with blackening and tattooing around the wounds, margins are inverted with active bleeding present.

Opinion reserved: X-ray and surgeon's operative notes for depth and grievousness.

Opinion is reserved, as not all firearm wounds on limbs are dangerous to life. In distant range of firearm, it is just a laceration, if no fracture or vascular/nerve injury caused.[6]

Ques. *How to describe 90% burn caused by kerosene?*
Ans. Indian law enquires in burn severity: Type of burn (dry heat/scald), depth of burn, nature of injury (simple/grievous/dangerous to life), location and percentage of burn and its duration.

It should be described—superficial to deep burns with blackening and peeling of skin with singeing of hair with red line of demarcation over the following parts of the body. Head as whole with singeing of scalp hair, face as a whole with singeing of eyebrows and eyelashes, neck and chest as a whole, abdomen in its whole circumference and genitalia in patches and both buttocks in patches with singeing of pubic hair, both upper limbs and both lower limbs at places, sparing the soles. Total burnt surface area is about 90%.

Opinion of injury: Dry heat flame burn of fresh duration and dangerous to life.[8]

Ques. *How to describe chopped wound upper limb by wooden axe in an MLC report?*
Ans. Indian law enquires in wound description: Type of wound to know the weapon (sharp or blunt and heavy or light), nature of injury (simple or grievous) length × breadth × depth, location, margins of wound, fresh duration or not.

So we can write—Chop wound 5 cm × 4 cm × through and through deep, with clean cut regular margins, and fresh blood oozing out, present over left forearm mid part with missing of distal part of left of upper limb.

Opinion: Grievous, advice X-ray for record or sharp heavy weapon.

Ques. *How to write MLC findings of acute poisoning case by suspected celphos pesticide* (**Box 3**)?
Ans. Patient is conscious, oriented restless, vomiting of greyish color, intense thirst, burning epigastric pain and dizziness with alleged history of pesticide poisoning. Celphos, amounting three tablets, ingested 1 hour ago at his home, as told by the conscious patient himself.
On examination: Glasgow coma scale = 15/15, moving all four limbs. Pupils are bilaterally equal in size and reactive to light. Blood pressure is 90 mm Hg systolic. Pulse rate is 160 beats/min on cardiac monitor, and carotids feeble on palpation. Respiration rate is 40 breaths/min. Chest—bilateral air entry present. Temperature is 97°F. Face is greyish blue (cyanosed). Tongue is dry. Garlicky odor of breath. Abdomen—soft, tenderness in epigastrium.

Gastric aspiration samples and clothes of patient sent for Forensic Science Laboratory analysis.

Ques. *How to write injuries in MLC report of sexual assault or rape?*
Ans. Patient is conscious, oriented with complaints of severe pain in genitals and bleeding per vagina with alleged history of sexual assault 1 hour ago at her home, as told by conscious patient herself.

Injuries on the body (examined in presence of female staff): Stains over external genitalia, matted pubic hair, vagina bruised in the posterior wall, labia majora and minora both are contused, edematous and inflamed, hymen torn at 6 o'clock position with fresh bleeding present.

Written consent of patient for examination of genitalia is mandatory in sexual assault cases, take consent of parents in minors (less than 18 years). Note marks of identification on victim's face: Black mole, or any permanent tattoo mark on limbs or old scar mark for future identification in court evidence.

Box 3 Ten Ks mnemonic for medicolegal case writing in poisoning

- K – Kaun hai victim (Name, age, gender, address)
- K – Konsa occupation (High risk in housewife/spy/banker/policeman/Journalist/politician/witness of heinous crime)
- K – Kya khaya (than call poison center to know antidote)
- K – Kitna khaya (fatal dose)
- K – Kab khaya (fatal period)
- K – Kese khaya (ingestion/inhalation/injection - S/c, I/M, I/V)
- K – Kahan khaya (place of crime)
- K – Kitne patients (mass poisoning)
- K – Kisne diya (suicidal/attempt to murder)
- K – Kyun khaya (Intention-accidental/homicidal/suicidal)

Vaginal swabs of patient, preserved, sealed and labeled as follows:
- One glass slide (sealed in envelope) smeared with first swab from vagina
- One swab from cervix
- One swab from posterior fornix
- One sealed glass vial containing vaginal swab in normal saline
- One sealed test tube containing air dried vaginal swab
- One sealed test tube containing air dried swab of blood for blood grouping and DNA matching
- One sealed test tube containing air dried swab of saliva for blood grouping and DNA matching.[9]

Ques. *How to send samples to police forensic laboratory for chemical analysis?*

Ans. Samples are preserved in sterile transparent container, sealed and labeled about details of patient and handover to police with forwarding letter enlisting samples and patient's details.

Samples include clothes and gastric aspiration samples in suspected poisoning, impregnated bullets, pellets, knife removed from wound of patient, clothes and vaginal swabs from sexually assaulted victim.[9]

Ques. *During court evidence, most common question of defense lawyer to a doctor (who made MLC) in injury case: Can this injury be caused by falling of victim by self, on hard and blunt surface?*

Ans: *First case*: Nitish Katara case—homicidal physical assault by blunt weapon, comminuted depressed skull fracture of frontal bone by hammer.[10]

Defense lawyer proposed that it was a case of high speed road traffic accident (RTA) as victim was found by police in the bushes near roadside.

Now defense lawyer asked first question: Can skull fracture be caused by falling on hard and blunt surface?

Doctor replied: No. Wound of this nature could be caused only when a moving person hits a stationary hard surface, results in *contrecoup injury* and will result in a lesion in an area opposite to the point of impact. But no contercoup lesions found in Nitish Katara's head. Lawyer lost the case.[10]

Second case: Road traffic accident of a 30-years-old pedestrian, crossing road and hit by vehicle on right lower limb of victim, sustaining primary impact injury—right lower limb deformity with fracture of femur, tibia and fibula.

Now, when the defence lawyer asked first question: Can this injury be caused by falling on hard and blunt surface?

Doctor replied: No. If the victim would have fallen from height, than his both lower limbs would have got injured, there's not even an abrasion on left side.

Lawyer asked: If victim fell on his right side laterally?

Doctor replied: Then he would have got injury over right side upper limbs or trunk too, along with lower limb.

Lawyer lost the case.

Third case: Road traffic accident of a car driving 25-year-old male, taking a turn over a crossing, hit by another car coming in high speed, sustaining whiplash injury of cervical spine, leading to paraplegia of both lower limbs.

Now the defense lawyer asked: Can this injury be caused by falling on hard and blunt surface?

Doctor replied: No. Victim had no abrasions or bruises, on any part of body. If he would have fallen, than these injuries would be sustained along with, for getting deep injury over neck. Lawyer lost the argument again.

So, I will request doctors to go through all the medical documents of the victim, before facing a defense lawyer; whose goal is to prove that accused has not directly injured the victim, the victim fell by self—so no proven crime and no financial claim for compensation to be paid by accused **(Box 4)**.

By using common sense during court proceedings, genuine victim gets justice and compensation demanded.

Always refer to your medical records when preparing the report.

Doctors often perform a detailed physical examination, but make the mistake of not thoroughly documenting the examination. The old medical maxim, "If it is not documented, it was not done," should be remembered.

Remember that you may be cross-examined on your report; only write what you would be prepared to say under oath in court.

Medicolegal case reports should be prepared in duplicate preferably with ball pen.

Do not alter your report at the request of your patient or a third party- if you receive additional information, or you have made a mistake, provide a supplementary report.

Do not record the patient's history of events as "fact", e.g. "When asked what happened, Mr A said he was hit by a

---

Box 4 Do's and don'ts in medicolegal case (MLC) writing to avoid legal punishment

- No overwriting in MLC, if any word corrected, it should be initialed by signature of doctor
- MLC reports are confidential legal document, any tempering or alteration in entries, antedate entries—fabricating false evidence of crime–S.191 IPC– punishable–7 years
- Issuing or signing false injury certificate–S.197 IPC–3 years Jail
- Don't miss the court date on summons—arrest warrant will be issued—Contempt of court–S.228 IPC–Punished for 6 months
- Don't state false findings—giving false evidence under oath –S.199 IPC–punishable–3 years
- Always intimate the Police about MLC promptly—Not informing police–to screen o'fender–S.201 IPC–punishable–3 years
- MLC report should be kept in safe custody—if lost/stolen-destruction of evidence–S.204 IPC punishable–3 years
- Don't rely on memory either in writing MLC reports or in giving court evidence-always review and reply

car" not "Mr A was hit by a car"; and "In my opinion, Ms B's depression has been caused by the reported behavior of her husband" not "the behavior of Ms B's violent and aggressive husband has caused her depression".[11]

Common mistakes in MLC writing is wrong side of body mentioned: Left limb fracture, noted as right side, relying on memory–creating confusion and ground for discrediting MLC reports by courts, disciplinary action, suspension from job and Medical Council of India (MCI) notice for doctor's negligence. This can be prevented by properly proofreading their reports. Doctor should take all the steps necessary to catch and correct all the following: Misspelled words, transcription errors, and grammatical mistakes.

When writing your MLC report it is important to remember that how you say it is just as important as what you are saying.

- Doctors, often inadvertently, use hedge words such as "it seems", "I think", "I believe", "it appears", "it could", "apparently", etc. in their MLC reports. These hedge words lessen the impact of their findings and conclusions.
- "Complete", "thorough", "meticulous", "exhaustive" and other such words to describe the examiner's chart review, research, or examination: These self-serving words will hold the doctor and his MLC report to an extremely high standard.
- "Appears", "presumably", "supposedly", "is said", and "evidently": These terms imply uncertainty.
- "Obviously" and "clearly": These terms can be used to make the doctor appear patronizing or presumptuous.
- "Malingering": Sometimes police asks for opinion on "generalized body ache to victim patient of assault". In the majority of cases, it is usually better for the doctor to merely document exaggerated pain behaviors, inconsistencies, nonorganic findings and lack of objective findings rather than making a diagnosis of malingering.
- "Alleged", "credible", and other words that directly or indirectly opine on the credibility of the doctor. The doctor is a medical expert, not a credibility expert.
- "Dictated but not read" and "electronic signature": These practices make the examiner appear to be more interested in cranking out reports and collecting fees than in precision and accuracy.
- Using incorrect, imprecise, or confounding language in a report will raise red flags and result in uncomfortable and unnecessary cross-examination by lawyer.[12]

SUMMARY

Writing a medicolegal report is important legal responsibility for doctors in prescribed cases which is helpful for investigating authority. In medicolegal report relevant details noted legibly and confidentially without abbreviation. Giving Life saving treatment is priority in any medicolegal case. Remain nonjudgemental about any case, doctor duty is to examine the patient and document the injuries and findings and management. The onus of fixing responsibility of guilt is for investigating authorities and court.

REFERENCES

1. Kochar SR. Practical Book on MLC writing, 1st edition; 2010.
2. Pillay VV. Textbook of Forensic Medicine and Toxicology, 17th edition. India: Paras Publishers; 2016.
3. Harish D, Chavali KH. The Medico-legal case—Should we be afraid of it? Anil Aggrawal's Internet Journal of Forensic Medicine and Toxicology. [online]. Available from: *http://www.anilaggrawal.com/ij/vol_008_no_001/others/pg/pg001.html* [Accessed November, 2016].
4. Pt. Parmananda Katara vs Union of India and Ors on 28 August, 1989. 1989 AIR 2039, 1989 SCR (3) 997.
5. Karmakar RN. Procedures For MLC Report writing, 1st edition. Kolkata: Academic Publishers; 2009.
6. Saraswat PK. Manual of MLC practice, 1st edition. New Delhi: Unique Books; 1996.
7. Reddy KSN, Murty OP. Reddy's Forensic Medicine and Toxicology, 33rd edition. New Delhi: Jaypee Brothers Medical Publisher's; 2014.
8. High Court of Delhi. Court Rules. (2010). Medico-legal Work. [online] Available from *http://delhihighcourt.nic.in/CourtRules.asp?currentPage=5* [Accessed November, 2016].
9. Mathiharan K, Patnaik AK. Modi's Medical Jurisprudence and Toxicology, 23rd edition. India: Lexis Nexis; 2012.
10. Infamous Nitish Katara case: Delhi High court judgment in Vishal Yadav vs State of UP on 2 April, 2014.
11. Bird S. How to write a medico-legal report. Australian Family Physician. 2014;45(11):773-852.
12. Babitsky S. (2012). The 10 Biggest Mistakes Physicians Make in Writing Their Medical Reports.

CHAPTER 7

Medicolegal Issues in Emergency

Adarsh Kumar, Vivekanshu Verma

DOCTOR: WORKING FOR THE LAW OR AGAINST THE LAW?

If a doctor works for the law by reporting a crime, the doctor can safeguard his career and his reputation during false allegations. If the doctor works against the law by not reporting crime, by doing illegal abortions, or by doing illegal transplantation, the doctor can be arrested and punished.

Whenever a patient is injured with suspicion of intention of foul play it becomes a medicolegal case (MLC). When a patient is injured outside the hospital and is brought for treatment, then the doctor has to inform the police and prepare MLC **(Fig. 1)**.

And when a patient is injured inside the hospital either due to slipping on wet floor in the bathroom or due to lack of proper medical care, then it becomes a medicolegal issue for medical negligence. This adverse event should be reported to the legal department by the treating doctor so that proper documentation is implemented for future court litigation **(Figs 2 and 3; Flow chart 1; Boxes 1 and 2)**.

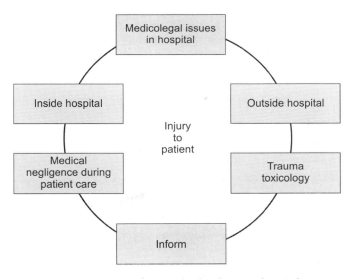

Fig. 2 Procedure for a medicolegal issue in hospital

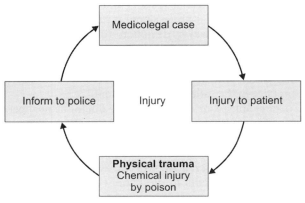

Fig. 1 Procedure of a medicolegal case

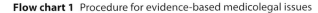

Flow chart 1 Procedure for evidence-based medicolegal issues

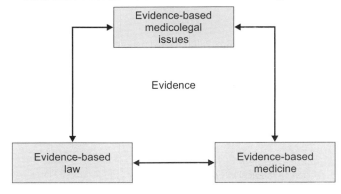

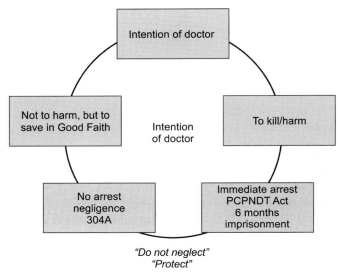

Fig. 3 Intention of a doctor
Abbreviations: JCI, Joint Commission International; PCPNDT, Pre Conception, Pre Natal Diagnostic Technique
Do not neglect patient's rights and protect patient's safety (JCI guidelines for International Patient Safety Goals).

Box 1 Goals of JCI and NABH for patient safety

Providing patient safety protects doctors from malpractice suits
Goals of JCI and NABH for patient safety
6 goals of IPSG
IPSG. 1 Identify patients correctly
IPSG. 2 Improve effective communication
IPSG. 3 Improve the safety of high-alert medication
IPSG. 4 Ensure correct-site, correct-procedure, correct-patient surgery
IPSG. 5 Reduce the risk of health care-associated infections
IPSG. 6 Reduce the risk of patient harm resulting from falls

Abbreviations: JCI, Joint Commission International; NABH, National Accreditation Board for Hospitals and Healthcare Providers; IPSG, International Patient Safety Goals

Box 2 Rights of a patient

Following are the rights of a patient:
- Right to medical care
- Information on identity of the staff taking care of them
- A second opinion
- Dignity
- Confidentiality
- Privacy
- Informed consent
- Access to medical information

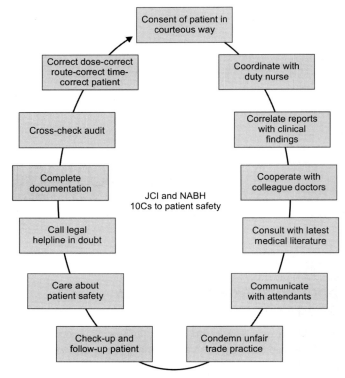

Fig. 4 Ten Cs to patient's safety

The issue of medical negligence is one of the most distressing medicolegal topics for the medical practitioners. To face the problem head on, it is extremely important to thoroughly understand the concept. Medical negligence may be defined as an "act of omission which a reasonably competent medical practitioner, guided by such medical knowledge and practice as is commonly known at the time and at the place where he practices and further guided by such other considerations which ordinarily regulate the conduct of a reasonably competent medical practitioner, would do, or doing something which a reasonably competent medical practitioners would not do". It is the failure on the part of a doctor to exercise his skill and diligence, which are required of a medical professional resulting in harm to the patient **(Fig. 4)**. However, deviation from common practice is not necessarily an evidence of negligence. Similarly, a mere accident or error of judgment is also not evidence of negligence. Medical negligence is termed as medical malpractice in the American legal system.

To label any act or omission by the doctor as negligence, all the essential ingredients of medical negligence must be presented **(Fig. 5)**. The essential constituents of negligence include: (1) duty of care towards patient (doctor-patient relationship), (2) dereliction or breach in duty of care, (3) damage that results to the patient must be reasonably foreseeable, and (4) direct causation (direct relation between the breach in duty of care and the damage) **(Table 1)**.

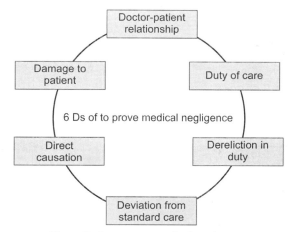

Fig. 5 Six Ds to prove medical negligence

Table 1	Laws providing legal protection to doctors
88–93	IPC – Legal protection to doctor
88	Act not intended to cause death, done by consent in good faith for peron's benefit
89	Guardian consent taken for surgery of child/insane
90	Consent to surgery is not valid, if it given under fear/unsoundness of mind/intoxication/misconception
92	Emergency surgery without consent
93	Privileged communication

Abbreviation: IPC, Indian Penal Code

WHAT IS DUTY OF CARE TOWARDS PATIENT?

In order to charge a medical practitioner with negligence, the complainant must prove that the practitioner owed a duty of care to the person complaining of negligence. When a patient enters the clinic or hospital and the doctor starts examining the patient, the duty begins. Even in charitable hospitals where no money is charged, a doctor can be charged of medical negligence. Not charging a professional fee does not protect the doctor from criminal negligence. Where no duty of care existed towards the person complaining of negligence, there would be no liability on the part of the medical practitioner, even where his action or conduct has caused damage to the complainant.

In *Laxman Balkrishna Joshi versus Trimbak Bapu Godbole and Another*, the Apex Court has held that a person who holds himself out ready to give medical advice and treatment impliedly undertakes that he is possessed of skill and knowledge for the purpose. Such a person when consulted by a patient owes him certain duties, viz. (1) duty of care in deciding whether to undertake the case, (2) duty of care in deciding what treatment to give, (3) duty of care in the administration of that treatment. A breach of any of these duties gives a right of action for negligence to the patient.

The practitioner must bring to task a reasonable degree of skill and knowledge and must exercise a reasonable degree of care. Neither the very highest degree nor a very low degree of care and competence judged in the light of the particular circumstances of each case is what the law requires.

Doctor-patient relationship is absent with doctors in radiology, pathology, microbiology, and biochemistry. Because these doctors do not consult or examine patients, they just report the investigations. But in recent times, in intervention radiologic procedures like ultrasound-guided stenting, radiologists examine and interact with patients, and do procedures, so a doctor-patient relationship exists.

Doctor-patient relationship is not formed when the doctor sees the acutely ill patient for the first time in emergency room. So, doctors giving lifesaving drugs in an emergency are protected by law from allegations of using dangerous drugs without discussing with patient (**Fig. 6**).

What is Breach in Duty of Care?

It is expected of the doctor that once he has obtained requisite qualification, he will acquire skill to treat the patient and exercise good care. It is assumed that he will exercise reasonable degree of skill and care. He may not be the best in the community of doctors, but it is assumed that he is average and his expertise should be at least average in his peer group. It is also understood that a doctor may not always know the latest in his field, but it is expected that he is aware of new techniques that are coming to his specialty.

Whenever a patient gets injured during patient care either by wrong drug, wrong route, wrong site, wrong time, or wrong dose; it leads to medical negligence (**Fig. 7**). When a surgeon operates at wrong site, by wrong procedure, on wrong patient, at wrong time, or in wrong surroundings; it leads to surgical negligence.

In *Dr Ganesh Prasad and Another versus Lal Janamajay Nath Shahdeo*, National Commission held that, "where proper treatment is given, death occurring due to process of disease and its complication, it cannot be held that doctors and hospital are negligent. Though death of the child is unfortunate, it cannot be said that there was negligence on the part of doctor".

WHAT IS DOCTRINE OF *RES IPSA LOQUITUR*?

Under certain exceptional circumstances where the doctrine of *res ipsa loquitur* applies, the patient is freed from responsibility of providing the evidence to prove negligence by the defendant. The burden of proof shifts from the complainant to the medical practitioner who has to prove that damage did not occur from his conduct of negligence. The maxim *res ipsa loquitur* is derived from Latin which literally means "the thing speaks for itself". In context to medical negligence, this maxim applies where it is improbable that the damage complained of could have happened without the wrong of the medical practitioner.

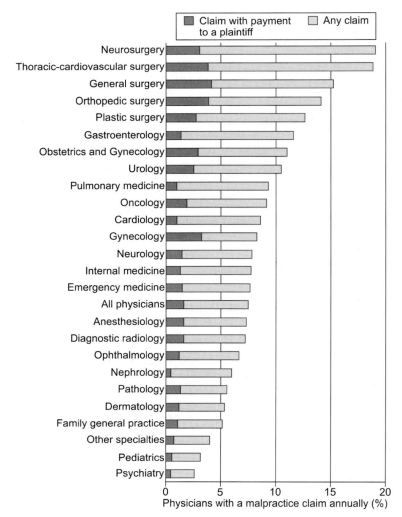

Fig. 6 Malpractice claims in multidisciplinary hospital in 2013 in United States of America
Source: www.kevinmd.com/blog/2013/08/medical-malpractice-claims-drag-long.html

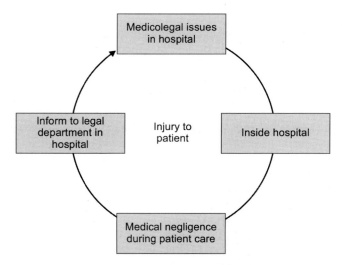

Fig. 7 Procedure of medical negligence during patient care in hospital

In *Dr G Vivekananda Verma versus Chinta Bharamaramba and Others*, National Commission held that, "the petitioner Surgeon gave anesthesia himself and has not shown how "anoxic encephalopathy" occurred and whether immediate action was taken to avoid the complication and whether timely treatment was imparted to the patient to avoid anoxic encephalopathy. From the records of the Swatantra Hospital and National Institute of Medical Statistics (NIMS) it is seen that the patient died due to anoxic encephalopathy suffered during tonsillectomy. We agree with the findings of the state commission that there is deficiency in service and negligence by the petitioner. It is clear that the doctrine of *res ipsa loquitur* applies in the present case".

In *baby Geeta and Others versus Cosmopolitan Hospitals (P) Ltd. and Others*, facts of the case are that, a post-term baby was delivered after administering "Pitocin" to induce labor. The delivered child suffered high fever, convulsions and breathing difficulties, and within 16 hours of discharge, tests revealed birth asphyxia resulting in lifelong mental retardation, epilepsy and physical disability of the child. National Commission observed that proper antenatal monitoring was not done by the respondent hospital and the doctors. Admittedly, special care was required but the case was treated as a normal delivery. No appropriate care was taken despite the request of the mother that the baby was suffering from tremors at times during the night and was not drinking milk actively. From the facts and the medical literature produced, the National Commission held that failure to take into account all warning signals and take immediate steps to prevent birth asphyxia, indicates a clear case of deficiency in service and medical negligence. There is enough evidence to show case of *res ipsa loquitur*.

If it can be proved that the damage suffered by the patient was the possible consequence and is consistent with due care provided by the medical practitioner, then maxim of *res ipsa loquitur* can de refuted. Medical practitioner has to prove that due care was shown towards the patient. In that case, the court will infer that the damage suffered by the patient was the result of misadventure or error of judgment and not due to negligence.

In *Jaswinder Singh versus Santokh Nursing Home and Others* (2012) 12 SCC 550, a case where two mops or gauges were left in the abdominal cavity and the patient died due to septicemia. *Gossypiboma* (retained foreign object) is the technical term for a surgical complication resulting from foreign materials, such as a surgical sponge, accidentally left inside a patient's body.

WHY MEDICAL SERVICES ARE INCLUDED UNDER CONSUMER PROTECTION ACT, 1986?

In a landmark case of *Indian Medical Association versus VP Shanta and Others*, the Honorable Supreme Court (SC) laid to rest the controversy whether the services rendered by the doctors or hospitals are covered under the Consumer Protection Act (CPA) or not. The Apex Court held that the services rendered by the doctors or hospitals are covered by the CPA unless such services are rendered by them entirely free of charge or to all the patients.

To clarify the concept and coverage of such services under CPA the Apex Court has clarified the definition of "service" under Section 2 (1)(o) into three parts, namely:
1. *Main part which says*: Service means service of any description
2. *Inclusionary part which includes*: The provision of facilities in connection with banking, finance, house construction and entertainment
3. *Exclusionary part which does not include*: rendering of any service free of charge or under contract of personal service.

Supreme Court further observed that, "Contract for personal service implies a contract whereby one party undertakes to render services (professional or technical) to or for another in the performance of which he is not subject to detailed direction and control but exercises professional or technical skill and uses his own knowledge and discretion". Control of personal service implies a relation of master and servant, and there is an obligation to obey the orders in the work to be performed as to the manner in which the work is to be performed. Services rendered by the doctors cannot be termed as personal service.

A personal service necessarily implies that service is not only provided at the behest of the master but also that service is provided as per the direction of the master; whereas in case of professional service, a professional such as a doctor advises his patient on the nature of disease and the treatment required to be obtained. A professional may not necessarily follow the advice of his client while performing his functions **(Fig. 8)**.

What Kind of Medicolegal Issues are Faced in Dealing with International Patients?

Presently, India is seeing a boom in the medical tourism industry and gets patients from various countries who seek better medical facilities here. When a hospital deals with an international patient, it must ensure that detailed records are kept including reason for admission, transfer, and plan of care, if required. Insurance companies have experts in their panel to cross verify the line of treatment, and hence it is a good practice to have a team of specialists attending a patient instead of looking at him individually. When any international patient is injured inside Indian territory, then intimation to local police and MLC report is done, as we do for all injured patients.

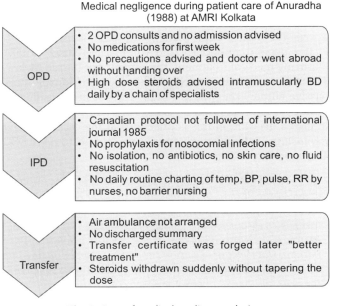

Fig. 8 Case of medical negligence during patient care of Anuradha in 1988

When an injured patient is having injury out of India (e.g. Gunshot in spine with paraplegia, refer for surgical removal), then doctor needs to inform legal department of the hospital, who will coordinate with the concerned embassy for the collection of material, evidence of bullet, etc. to be sent back in chain of custody.

When any person is injured or poisoned onboard an international flight, then medicolegal formalities need to be done according to the jurisdiction, as mentioned in contract of flight carrying the person.

What are the Medicolegal Guidelines for Managing Terminally Ill-patient in Emergency Room?

Regulation 6.7 of the Indian Medical Council Regulations (Professional Conduct, Etiquette, and Ethics), 2002 provides:

> "Practicing Euthanasia shall constitute unethical conduct. However, on specific occasion, the question of withdrawing supporting devices to sustained cardiopulmonary function even after brain death shall be decided only by a team of doctors, and not merely by the treating physician alone. A team of doctors shall declare withdrawal of support system. Such team shall consist of the doctor in charge of the patient, Chief Medical Officer or Medical Officer in charge of the hospital, and a doctor nominated by the incharge of the hospital from the hospital staff or in accordance with the provisions of the Transplantation of Human Organ Act, 1994."

In India, active euthanasia and assisted death continue to be illegal. Active euthanasia entails the use of lethal substances or forces which would cause the death of a person, e.g. a lethal injection given to a person with terminal cancer who is in terrible agony. Active euthanasia is a crime all over the world except where permitted by legislation.

If a person consciously and voluntarily refuses to take lifesaving medical treatment, the same is not barred by law. The SC has laid down guidelines with respect to nonvoluntary passive euthanasia (where a person is not in a position to decide for himself, e.g. if he is in coma, and is incompetent to take a decision in this connection) in the case of *Aruna Ramachandra Shanbaug versus Union of India*, (2011) 4 SCC 454, which are as follows:

> "A decision has to be taken to discontinue life-support either by the parents or by the spouse or other close relatives and in the absence of any of them, such a decision can be taken even by a person or a body of persons acting as a next friend. It can also be taken by the doctors attending the patient. However, the decision should be taken bona fide in the best interests of the patient. Even if a decision is taken by the near relatives or doctors or next friend, to withdraw life-support, such a decision requires approval from the High Court concerned".

What are Medicolegal Issues of Patients who are Below Poverty line and how to Manage Patients with weak Financial Background in a Private Hospital?

The Honorable SC in the landmark judgment of *Parmanand Katara versus Union of India*, 1989 (4) SCC 286, has held that every doctor whether in a government hospital or private hospital is under a professional obligation to provide immediate medical aid to an injured person to save human life. However, the treatment should be supplemented by the same process of reporting to the authorities, as undertaken vis-à-vis any other patient of the hospital. Cost of treatment is covered under corporate social responsibility (CSR).

How to Face a Medicolegal Complaint?

Medicolegal complaints are to be dealt with due caution and care. Facing a medicolegal complaint is something that needs preparation prior to visit of the patient to the doctor, wherein, however small might be a doctor's setup, there has to be a provision in the system of the clinic or the hospital for appropriately facing the MLC/s that might come up in the future. The key to fearlessly facing the cases is proper documentation.

The legal counsel (in-house or external) should be immediately informed and provided copies of the relevant complaint/notice/summon/warrant. In a multidisciplinary hospital, it is necessary that there is a coordination between the various departments and when a case arises, they should not get into a blame-game.

How to Prevent Medical Negligence?

At the time of the admission of a patient, it must be ensured that all forms are properly filled and signed by the patient or by a first-degree relative. Uniform fact sheets and consent forms must be used by all the departments in a multidisciplinary hospital. Also, history of the patients should be accurately recorded. Proper and accurate records are a must in preventing the chances of medical negligence. A doctor, from the treating team, must explain the risks and benefits of any surgical procedure or treatment that a patient has to undergo in that hospital. Doctor-patient or attendant communication must take place between a doctor from the treating team and the family and should be recorded by the nurses. Patient's family education is also crucial.

What are the Common Causes of Medical Negligence?

It is important to understand the difference between medical negligence and medical malpractice as the two terms are at times used interchangeably. Medical negligence is an inadvertent medical misconduct which may occur due to technical insufficiency of the practitioner or due to lack of complete knowledge of a particular case or out of plain ignorance, whereas medical malpractice is a misconduct done on purpose and generally involves unethical behavior on the part of medical practitioner. In the hospital and the likes of its setups, delayed medical attention, overdose, wrong medication, wrong surgical interventions, etc. lead to medical negligence. However, in medical streams of other than allopathic system of medicine where patients turn to more as a last option rather than system of choice, which is of course a changing trend nowadays, medical negligence has a higher chance of occurrence. Existence of multidisciplinary treatment options has increased the risk to which any person might be exposed to. Failure on the part of the doctors to inform or interact with or procure informed consent from, the patients or attendants is the most common cause of claims of medical negligence. Discrepancy in the documentation, for instance, billing documents, discharge summary, doctor's notes, nurse's chart, etc. also result in claims for medical negligence. One of the common complaints in MLCs is that the patient or his/her family was not explained of the risks involved prior to the procedure being undertaken.

WHAT CONSTITUTES MEDICAL NEGLIGENCE?

In *Poonam Verma versus Ashwin Patel*, while deliberating on the absence of basic qualification of homeopathic doctor to practice allopathic system of medicine, SC held that a person who does not have knowledge of a particular system of medicine but practices in that system is a quack. That person is guilty of negligence per se, and no further proof is needed.

In *Nihal Kaur versus Director, PGIMER*, a patient died the next day after surgery and the relatives found scissors while collecting last remains. A compensation of Rs 1.20 lakhs was awarded by state commission Chandigarh on the ground that negligence was proved in handling the case.

WHAT DOES NOT CONSTITUTE MEDICAL NEGLIGENCE?

In *Mrs Shantaben Muljibhai Patel and Others versus Breach Candy Hospital and Research Centre and Others*, National Commission dismissed the complaint filed by wife and two sons of the deceased Mr MM Patel who died in Breach Candy Hospital alleging negligence by staff and treatment administered by surgeon and anesthetist. Deceased had undergone bypass surgery in 1988, mitral valve replaced. Deterioration of 15% ejection fraction (pumping efficiency) found in 1996. Operation was performed successfully. While undertaking postoperative treatment there was extubation. As per medical literature such chances of extubation are between 8.5% and 13%. Extubation was swift and sudden and immediately noticed by a nurse. Expert doctor was called but intubation was found difficult and patient died due to cardiac arrest. Hospital was equipped with necessary equipment and doctors performed their duties to the best of ability with due care and caution. Deceased was a high-risk case and such accidental eventualities cannot be controlled. Every surgical operation is attended by risk. If something goes wrong, conclusion of deficiency in service cannot be drawn. Reasonable care was exercised by nursing staff. No negligence or deficiency in service proved. While delivering its judgment, the National Commission approvingly referred to the observations of *Lord Denning in Roe and Woolley versus the Ministry of Health and an Anesthetist 75*, which stated, "Every surgical operation is attended by risks. We cannot take the benefits without taking the risks. Every advance in technique is also attended by risks. Doctors like the rest of us, have to learn by experience; and experience often teaches in a hard way".

Query: *What is Bolam's Test and why emergency doctors should know about it* **(Fig. 9)**?

Answer: *Bolam's Test defines medical negligence*: A reference made to observations of justice McNair in *Bolam versus Friern Hospital Management Committee* wherein a patient suffering from mental illness was advised to undergo electroconvulsive therapy, though the therapy has risk of fracture, "In the case of a medical man, negligence means failure to act in accordance with the standards of reasonably competent medical men at the time. This is a perfectly accurate statement, as long as it is remembered that there may be one or more perfectly proper standards; and if a medical man confirms to one of those proper standards then he is not negligent. Patient's lawyer was right in saying that mere personal belief that a particular technique is best is no defense, unless that belief is based on reasonable grounds. That again is unexceptionable". A doctor is not guilty of negligence if he has acted in accordance with a practice accepted as proper by a reasonable body of medical men skilled in that particular art.

Query: *How to prevent medical negligence during patient care in emergency?*

Answer: When a doctor consults a patient and admits him under his care, then the doctor should take informed valid consent from the patient and advice investigations and medications which are to be administered by the duty nurse.

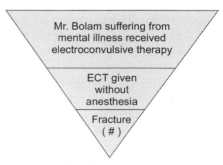

Fig. 9 Bolam's test

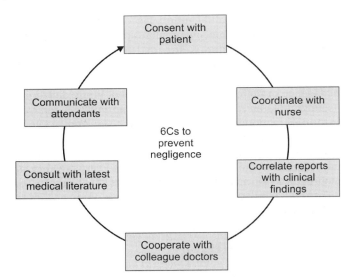

Fig. 10 Simplified strategies to prevent medical negligence during patient care

Flow chart 2 Steps for illness and injury insurance

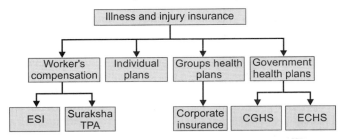

Negligence starts when the doctor carelessly prescribes management verbally without written orders, nurses forget in-between the chaos of multiple emergency patients and the individual patient does not get the appropriate treatment **(Fig. 10)**. Timely and correct documentation of advice by doctor is the key to correct treatment.

Query: What is medical malpractice stress syndrome?
Answer: If a doctor is sued for negligence is dismissed from a private hospital as it brings bad name in media. Doctor loses job and is harassed financially; he/she loses precious time in attending courts on dates of hearing and loses time in waiting for his/her turn that could be used in making progress in medicine. Doctor is stressed socially and psychologically. So, prevention of negligence is better than facing the allegations in court.

Query: What is medical indemnity insurance?
Answer: Medical indemnity insurance is provided by insurance companies to doctors, nursing homes, or hospitals to pay compensation to patients claiming for medical negligence and malpractice **(Flow chart 2)**.

Query: Do cashless mediclaims and accidental claims cover the expenses of patients in MLCs?
Answer: Mediclaim is a health insurance product with legal contract between patient and insurance company. Mediclaim insurance is a cover which takes care of the hospitalization expenses subject to maximum sum insured of the insured person in respect of the following situations:
- In case of a sudden illness
- In case of an accident
- In case of any urgent surgery which is required in respect of any disease that was not pre-existing and has arisen during the policy period.

Insurance cover for "Risk" to Health: Insurance covers the involuntary risks but does not cover voluntary risks.
- *Risky activities:* Entertainment acrobatics in circus, TV shows
- *Risky games:* Adventure sports, racing, jumping, ice skating, boxing, wrestling, cricket, football, tennis, parachuting, flying, professional sports, etc.
- *Risky jobs:* Military, security and police service, noise-induced hearing loss, gas-welding vision loss, coal dust-induced lung disease, construction, etc.
- *Risky physical behavior:* Promiscuous behavior leading to- human immunodeficiency virus (HIV) or sexually transmitted disease (STD)
- *Risky mental behavior:* Suicidal, schizophrenia
- *Risky lifestyle:* Smoking, drinking alcohol, drugs abuser, etc.

Exclusion list: Voluntary acts of injury not covered in mediclaim are as follows:
- Intentional criminal act of violence
- Intentional self-injury or suicide attempt
- Influence of intoxicating drugs or alcohol
- Substance abuse and addiction
- War, invasion and war-like operation
- Injury by nuclear weapons or material
- Speed contest, racing and adventure sports.

So assault is a voluntary act of violence—so not covered in mediclaim.

And to rule out assault and alcohol abuse, mediclaims rely on medicolegal injury report and opinion of treating doctor and the police, before paying for mediclaim to the insured.

All roadside accidents are covered in mediclaim bought as accidental claim cover by the patient, unless the patient was not intoxicated during the accident and did not attempt suicide or suffered assault. An accident is a sudden, unforeseen, and involuntary event caused by external and visible means.

Following is the exclusion list of therapies not covered under mediclaim:
- Diseases not life-threatening
- Cosmetic surgeries, liposuction, bariatric surgery, circumcision, sex change surgery, and dental surgeries are generally not covered.

- *Therapies not lifesaving*: Tonics, cosmetic, ayurvedic, massage, and acupuncture
- *Not a disease*: Natural physiology, pregnancy, and abortion
- Vaccination or inoculation except postbite.

MEDICLAIMS AND MEDICOLEGAL ISSUES

Mediclaim Issues

Mediclaim covers **(Flow chart 3)** for unexpected critical illnesses (predecided diseases) like the following:
- Cancer of specified severity
- *Cardiac illness*: Angioplasty, coronary artery bypass grafting (CABG), and valve repair
- Cerebral and cerebellar stroke
- Critical sickness requiring intensive care unit (ICU) care
- Critical polytrauma requiring ICU care
- Critical burn requiring ICU care
- Coma of specified severity
- Chronic kidney disease (CKD) requiring regular dialysis
- Critically vital organ or bone marrow transplant.

Court Evidence of Doctors in MLCs

Query: *What is the first question asked to a doctor by a lawyer in MLC evidence?*
Can this injury be caused by falling?
Answer:
- *First case*: Nitish Katara case—homicidal physical assault by blunt weapon—comminuted depressed skull fracture of frontal bone by hammer—postmortem burned by accused to destroy identity of victim.

Defense lawyer proposed that it was a case of high-speed road traffic accident (RTA) followed by petrol tank burn as victim was found by police in the bushes near roadside.

The defense lawyer asked first question to the doctor, "Can skull fracture be caused by falling on hard and blunt surface?"

Doctor replied "No. Wound of this nature could be caused only when a moving person hits a stationary hard surface—results in "contrecoup injury" and will result in a lesion in an area opposite to the point of impact".

But no contrecoup lesions were found in Nitish Katara's head.

Lawyer lost the case.

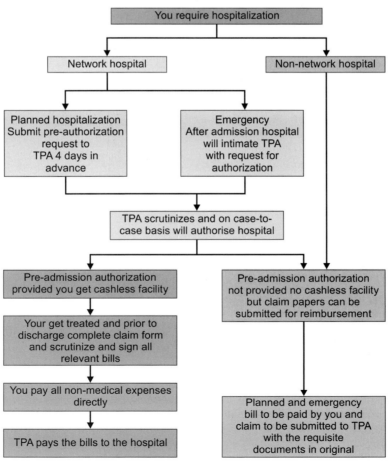

Flow chart 3 Steps for mediclaim

- *Second case*: RTA of a 30-year-old pedestrian, crossing road and hit by a vehicle on right lower limb, sustaining primary impact injury—right lower limb deformity with fracture of femur, tibia, and fibula.

  When the defense lawyer asked the first question, "Can this injury be caused by falling on hard and blunt surface?" The doctor replied, "No. If the victim would have fallen from a height, then both his lower limbs would have gotten injured, there is not even an abrasion on the left side".

  Lawyer asked, "If the victim fell on his right side laterally?" Doctor replied, "Then he would have gotten injury over right side upper limbs or trunk too, along with lower limb." Lawyer lost the case.

- *Third case*: RTA of a car driven by a 25-year-old male, taking a turn over a crossing, hit by another car coming in high speed, driver sustained whiplash injury of cervical spine, leading to paraplegia of both lower limbs.

  The defense lawyer asked, "Can this injury be caused by falling on hard and blunt surface?"

  Doctor replied, "No. Victim had no abrasions or bruises, on any part of body. If he would have fallen, than these injuries would be sustained along with, deep injury over neck".

  Lawyer lost the argument again.

  So, I will request doctors to go through all the medical documents of the victim, before facing a defense lawyer, whose goal is to prove that accused has not directly injured the victim, the victim fell by himself, so no crime is proven and no financial claim for compensation is to be paid by accused.

Query: *How to interpret summon of witness?*
- I happened to observe that mostly odd numbers of last digit, with regard to Indian Penal Code (IPC) sections are safer in law and bailable than even numbers, which are nonbailable.
- It is helpful in interpreting summon of witness or warrant received by doctors, to appear after making medicolegal report (MLR).
- In even number IPCs in summon **(Box 3)**, doctors need to be ready to answer in court to defense lawyer and judge, whether the injuries were dangerous to life or not?

MEDICOLEGAL TIPS FOR EMERGENCY BY DR RK SHARMA

Query: *How an emergency doctor can give information to police regarding MLCs?*

Answered by Dr RK Sharma: Following are the ways you can choose what is best for you:
- You can call number 100 and give information, note down in your register the day and the exact time of information.
- You can call local police station and inform.
- Ask for daily diary number.

Box 3 Even numbers Indian Penal Code (IPC) and nonbailable offences in Indian Law

124-A IPC – Sedition	354 – Outrage modesty of woman
148 IPC – Riot by dangerous weapon	354B – Intent to disrobe woman
232 IPC – (adulteration of drugs)	364 – Kidnapping for murder/ransom
302 IPC – (Murder)	370 – Human trafficking
304 IPC – Culpable homicide	372 – Selling/hiring minor for prostitution
304A – Death due to negligence	376 – Punishment of sexual assault
304B – Dowry death	384 – Extortion
306 IPC – Abetment of suicide	386 – Extortion by threat of death/grievous hurt
308 IPC – Attempt to commit culpable homicide	392 – Robbery
314 – Causing Death by Act with Intent of Miscarriage	406 – Criminal breach of trust
316 – Causing Death of a Quick Unborn Child	420 – Cheating
324 – Dangerous weapon causing hurt	436 – Mischief by fire/explosive
326 – Dangerous weapon/means causing grievous hurt	466 – Forgery of a record of—court/Birth and Death register/kept by public servant
326A – Grievous hurt by use of acid	498A – Cruelty to married woman
326B – Voluntarily throwing acid or attempting to throw	
328 – Criminal poisoning	
332 – Voluntarily causing hurt to deter public servant from duty	

- Note down this in your register.
- You should maintain a register of information to the police.
- Note all details of patient, time, and day of information to the police.
- Remember after this you have done your legal duty, so there is no need to worry any further. It is the job of the police to investigate, not yours.

Query: *I understand that there is confusion between MLC and the police information. All our examinations are valid as an MLC. Only question is having proper record. It is not necessary to have MLC record on figured medicolegal register or it can be our plain paper with stamp and signatures. The basic issue is whether to inform police or not.*

Answered by Dr RK Sharma: You are right. Nursing homes and hospitals have MLC register but general practitioners do not have it. An MLC can also be made on prescription. Police information is must. The police can be informed either on dialing 100 or by contacting a local police station. Always ask for daily diary number of your information. Maintain a register which you can show later on that you have informed the police on the particular day, time, and with daily diary number.

Query: *If following an RTA, a patient has sustained a fracture but the patient and his/her relatives are not interested in informing the police and are ready to give it in written, then, is it still mandatory for the doctor to inform the police? Is that written statement by the patient party valid in the court if patient goes on to file a case against the third party after few days?*

Answered by Dr RK Sharma: If the patient is conscious and does not want an MLC in an RTA case, then you can treat it as a non-MLC, but get his statement recorded in your records to avoid future litigations. If patient in unconscious, even if relatives ask you to treat the case as a non-MLC, do not listen to them and make the case as an MLC. Ask relatives to contact the police, who may drop proceedings, if facts of the case warrant so. Medical officer has no choice but to make it a MLC.

Written statement that he does not want a MLC is valid in law only when he says so in the court of law. Patient may deny it later also. But, doctor is safe if it is signed by the patient himself.

Query: *I worked as a junior resident in a government hospital and made an MLC on behalf of the Chief Medical Officer (CMO), now a summons has been issued to me regarding that MLC. Currently, I am not working in that hospital and resigned a long time ago. So, I want to ask:*
- *Whether I should accept that summons or not?*
- *How can I escape going to court for that MLC?*
- *In hospitals of Delhi, CMO forces junior residents to make MLCs, is it legal or not?*

Answered by Dr RK Sharma: Please understand that making an MLC is as important as giving treatment. In hospitals, most of the time, making an MLC is entrusted to the most junior doctor. It has to be done as it is part of training.

If you have made an MLC, then a summons from court will also come. Attending court is a statutory duty besides being our professional duty. If you refuse a summons continuously, warrant can be issued by court to arrest you and produce you before the court. Even if you have left that hospital, where you made the MLC, you will have to attend court on summons. You can apply for duty leave to attend court which cannot be refused by any organization. If any organization refuses, attend the court and bring it to knowledge of court which will take action against such organization.

Query: *I want to ask you that I used to work at a tertiary care hospital, I used to receive summon from different nearby districts and attend them regularly. Previously, court used to give me diet money and travelling allowance, which they have stopped. Now, they tell us to collect it from the hospital. The hospital says you are not working with us why should we pay you diet money and travelling allowance?*

Answer: Your problem is genuine and it has no solution. In fact, many doctors are suffering from it. Once you leave a hospital and join another one, the previous hospital refuse to pay. Even if court pays, it will only give you bus fare. I, myself, have suffered from this problem many times after I took retirement from All India Institute of Medical Science (AIIMS). Imagine the plight of witnesses who repeatedly have to come to court and nobody pays them. They even lose wages for the day. None of the witnesses want to come to court only because of this harassment. It will not improve till we change our law system.

Query: *I treated one patient with injury in a finger after assault. MLC was made. It was just a hairline fracture at the base of proximal phalanx. Radiologist reported it as normal. But in my opinion it was a hairline fracture, moreover, there was one dot of radio-opaque artifact. Now the investigating police officer is asking for a final opinion. What opinion should I give; simple based on the radiologist's report or grievous? Should I also ask for the treatment papers from the patient?*

Answered by Dr RK Sharma: Please note that you can always review a case if you have any doubts regarding a fracture. Call the patient again after 2 weeks and get an X-ray done again. Please note that hairline fracture is a grievous injury. If still in doubt, get an magnetic resonance imaging (MRI) done.

Query: *A female patient was brought to our hospital on 14th April 2015 after sustaining scalp injury, pain, and swelling on the left shoulder following an RTA. She was crossing the road and was hit by a biker. The biker brought the patient in the emergency room of our hospital. X-ray of her left shoulder showed fracture of clavicle and 2nd, 3rd, 4th, 5th ribs and of the scapula. Computed tomography (CT) scan of the head was normal. Patient left the hospital after initial management in stable condition. All the expenses for X-ray and management were paid by the biker and no MLC was registered in the hospital nor was the police informed, because attendants of the patient and biker agreed for the same by mutual consent. The left shoulder X-ray (referred above) was not reported by the radiologist and the X-ray was issued to the attendants of the patient without report. The biker later refused to pay expenses for subsequent follow-up treatment. Patient's attendants then lodged an FIR (First Information Report) with the police and filed the case in court. After filing the FIR, the attendants of the patient approached the hospital with the said radiograph of her left shoulder and were asking for its report. Can this X-ray be reported by the present radiologist and if so, what procedure is to be followed?*

No thumb impression was taken nor was any mark of identification noted on the radiograph on X-ray register of radiology department on 14 April 2015. Please advise if it is important to put these on the X-ray film following the examination in cases of all types of injuries, particularly the road accidents where no MLC is recorded nor the police FIR is lodged?

Answered by Dr RK Sharma: Please note, it is quite common that initially patients do not want MLC and give it in writing, but later change their mind and report it. Be wiser in such cases, documentation should be proper with due signatures and declaration that "I do not want an MLC". In your case, X-ray should be reported and report given preferably by radiologist who was present at that time. If he is not there, another radiologist can give opinion, and reason of absence of first radiologist should be documented like he has left, moved somewhere, etc. If patient has consented for non-MLC, formalities like taking his/her thumb impression and marks of identification need not be done on the X-ray requisition form.

Query: *I have received a summon as expert witness for a patient I attended 4 year back in emergency, details I do not remember due to frequent posting to new places. I do not have any details or any paper for that patient. In that case, what should I answer in court? Please guide me what I should do?*

Answered by Dr RK Sharma: No need to worry, you should go to the court and ask for seeing the record on which you are summoned. Original record would be there in the court in case file. Review your hospital records in that case file and answer logically.

Query: *As we know that hospitals do not handover all original documents to patients at the time of discharge, but patients' attendants are asking for them, saying "when we are paying money to the hospital, we have right to get all original documents for our further reference and any other medical reimbursement. But hospital is not giving original documents and giving Xerox copies. Please advise us which is the correct way?*

Answered by Dr RK Sharma: Please note, a patient does not have any rights over original documents of the hospital. You can give duly certified photo copies. In case of investigation, patient is entitled to have copy of CD or imaging films. Custody of original documents belongs to the hospital and they have to produce them when ordered by court or police. Court has power to retain original documents and the police have power to seize original documents, if required by law.

Query: *Is there any law against patient and patient's attendants who abuse the hospital staff and damage the hospital property, if so please send me the details, and can it be pasted in the hospital surroundings?*

Answer by Dr RK Sharma: Yes, there is a law against patient and patient's attendants who abuse hospital staff and damage the hospital property. Now almost all states in India have their own law. I am giving you here a link of the Delhi law which you can read yourself.

The Delhi Medicare Service Personnel and Medicare Service Institutions (Prevention of Violence and Damage to Property) Act, 2008

"Medicare service personnel" shall include,
- Registered medical practitioners
- Registered nurses, nursing aids, midwives
- Paramedics
- Ambulance service providers.

"Violence" means activities of causing any harm or injury or endangering life, or intimidation, obstruction or hindrance to any medicare service personnel in discharge of duty in hospital or damage to property in such institution.

Penalty: Any offender, who commits any act in contravention of Section 3, shall be punished with imprisonment for a term which may extend to 3 years, or with fine which may extend to Rs. 1,000, or with both.

It is advisable that **Figure 11** should be pasted in hospital premises to deter violence.

Query: *Can we allow relatives of an unconscious patient admitted in hospital to take thumbs impression of the patient for encashing the patient's fixed deposits?*

Answered by Dr RK Sharma: Please remember, a patient who is admitted in a hospital is in lawful custody of the hospital. If patient is unconscious, responsibility is even more. You should never allow relatives to take thumb impression of unconscious patients for any purpose as it amounts to fraud. Doctor may later be sued in court by legal heir for assisting and conniving in crime which is punishable by jail sentence.

Can Doctor Dispense Medicine in Emergency?
Query: *I am a practicing pediatrician for more than 30 years. Rules are being revised and people are more inquisitive, so I want to know the law of dispensing medicines or vaccines. This*

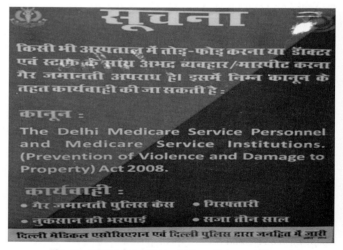

Fig. 11 Notice for damage to hospital property and violence against hospital staff

will help all doctors, especially, in rural areas where they have to or are dispensing practice. What about giving medicines in emergency at night when no nearby chemists are open. Please elaborate and oblige.
Answered by Dr RK Sharma: Please note, license is not required for a doctor who is dispensing medicines for his own patients. But, there are a number of instances where drug inspectors have harassed doctor. Please adhere to the following instructions to keep out of harassment:
- Doctor should not run an open shop
- Preferably no board should be there of pharmacy
- Stocks of medicines should not be more than 1 month old
- No separate bills of medicines should be given.
- Medicines kept should be related to the specialty practiced
- In emergency, you can give medicines at maximum retail price (MRP), if it is not available.

But please do not issue separate bill for drugs. It may be billed in consultancy charges.

Who is qualified to thrombolysis the acute thrombus in ischemic stroke in emergency?
Query: *Thrombolytic therapy is an established form of treatment for acute ischemic stroke; in emergency, when a patient arrives in hospital duty doctors, who are MD (medicine) or pursuing DNB (Diplomate of National Board) in cardiology assess the patient and invite the neurologist after CT scan. Sometimes neurologists are not available physically. Medico-legally, is it safe and justified for them to thrombolyze a stroke patient without the physical presence of a neurologist?*
Answered by Dr RK Sharma: It is always assumed that a full-time neurologist (being super specialist) would not be available in emergency 24 hours but should be on-call. Till he comes and reviews the treatment, emergency room team is fully authorized to give standard and established form of treatment to save the life of patient.

In the above mentioned case, thrombolytic treatment is a standard and established treatment for acute ischemic shock and resident who is already a medical specialist and doing major in cardiology is quite competent to administer it.

Query: *I am a practicing gynecologist at Nasik, and my hospital is on the road with heavy traffic. One evening, a lady was brought to my hospital, who was injured due to a dash given by an unknown vehicle. We immediately gave first aid, and sent her to another accident hospital before the relatives arrived, to save the time. The patient had filed a complaint against her husband, saying that the accident was carried out by him, as there is dispute going on between them. Now, the police is asking us, why we had not informed them and why an MLC was not done?*

As the patient had acute pain in the right hypochondriac region with severe breathlessness and ours being maternity hospital, we referred her to a critical care hospital for further care. Please guide us. What answer we should give them in reply?

Answered by Dr RK Sharma: It is a common mistake committed by nursing homes and small hospital that they do not make MLCs and do not inform the police. Even if you have no time for making MLC, you should note down all the particulars of patient and enter them into a medicolegal register and later inform the police in writing; it is legally required.

Please note that due to the presence of a large number of closed-circuit television (CCTV) cameras present in the vicinity, it can be easily proved that patient was brought to the hospital. In this particular case, you can tell the police that due to emergency condition of the patient, you simply could not take details as the patient needed transfer immediately and regret the mistake.

Query: *What is the order of priority in legal guardians for giving consent in cases of minor or incompetent patients?*
Answered by Dr RK Sharma: Legal guardian is father, then mother, then other relatives, then friends and even accompanying person(s), especially, in case of unconscious or emergency patient or patient under influence of alcohol or drugs.

Query: *What is the legal status of "Do-not-resuscitate policy" in India?*
Answered by Dr RK Sharma: "Do-not-resuscitate (DNR) policy" has no legal status in India; till a person is conscious, he/she has command over his/her body, but the moment the person becomes unconscious, next of kin is empowered to make any decision. Even consent given during lifetime for organ donation can be over-turned by next of kin. After death, a dead body becomes property of the next of kin and he is the absolute owner.

Query: *Is a doctor legally safe if he/she does not resuscitate a patient just because relatives have given DNR consent?*
Answer: The "DNR policy" has no legal status in India, relatives cannot give consent for not to resuscitate his patient. Doctor has to provide basic life-support to patient by providing cardiopulmonary resuscitation (CPR). Doctor can be held negligent, if he fails to provide CPR. After CPR, if the patient is not revived, doctor did his job in trying best to save patient's life, so he is legally safe.

Query: *I would like to ask, does a doctor have the right to refuse to treat a patient and when?*
Answered by Dr RK Sharma: Yes, doctors too have the right to refuse treatment to any patient they do not want to treat, provided
- The patient must not be in need of emergency treatment
- The refusal cannot be done in case you are duty bound to see patient just like in government hospital
- Refusal should not be done on the basis of caste, religion, gender, or community
- Refusal should be documented with reason, if patient is admitted.

Query: *Suppose a patient of any age is hospitalized in emergency, on life-support measures or not and not brain dead but incompetent to give valid consent due to age or illness and probably will not survive without hospital support. Can his/her guardians ask for the patient to be discharged in such a condition?*

Answered by Dr RK Sharma: Yes, next of kin or guardian has full legal rights to get any patient who is incompetent to give consent due to any reason discharged at any stage of treatment knowing fully that he/she might not survive, if discharged. In all such cases, the discharge must be made on request with full declaration from next of kin or guardian in following language "I am withdrawing my patient who is related to me from hospital against medical advice. I will not hold hospital or doctors responsible for any untoward incident happening to my patient after discharge. Doctors have explained me all consequences." Get this declaration in local language and get it witnessed by two more relatives of the patient.

Query: *I am a senior physician in a private hospital, many a times a situation arises when a patient is terminally ill and relatives ask you to withdraw the blood pressure support inotropes and intra-aortic balloon pump (IABP) machines or sometimes even they refuse for continuation of ventilator support for their patient, especially when the patient is elderly and in terminal illness where they know that there is no use for continue life-support. How should we make ourselves clear and immune to such situation; I know there is no provision in Indian law where a doctor is authorized to pull out life-support of a patient even if his/her dear ones push him to do so. What should we do if they take him leave against medical advice (LAMA); how to transport such case out of hospital if they take LAMA and we know the patient will die on removing inotropes and ventilator?*

Answer: It is a very tricky problem but keeps on occurring. My advice is as follows:
- Remember very well that relatives have right to take away patient any time
- Get a request in writing from next of kin that he/she wants to take away the patient LAMA even knowing well that it may cause death of patient
- Get it witnessed by two more relatives
- Discharge patient LAMA and make LAMA discharge summary showing vital parameters that patient is alive on ventilator and inotropic support.
- Shift the patient to ambulance with bag-mask or Bain's Breathing Circuit or Versamed (portable ventilator).
- Let the ambulance go with a doctor to their home and then remove it.
- This will take care of all legalities.

Query: *What is the legal position in India with force feeding a patient, who is on hunger strike? Many times people on hunger strike are brought by the police for first aid and treatment, or sometimes ambulance with doctor is called from nearby hospital, on the site of people sitting on hunger strike for first aid. He/she is effectively refusing treatment.*

Answered by Dr RK Sharma: As per human rights, nobody can be force fed if on hunger strike till he/she is conscious. But sometimes, in cases where hunger strike is for political motives, government has intervened and force fed the person.
- Irom Sharmila from Manipur was force fed for 16 years as her hunger strike was for repeal of Armed Forces Special Power Act
- Many leaders in India sat on hunger strike but not force fed
- Irish prisoners did hunger strike for political reasons and many died while on hunger strike but not force fed.
- It is government's prerogative to act.

Query: *I would like to ask that if any general practitioner (GP) asks any emergency consultant any opinion on phone or on WhatsApp by sending document, then can the opinion be given online. And, if yes, is it valid medicolegally.*

For example, if a case of accelerated hypertension comes to a GP and he/she send an ECG, vital parameters and history to me. Can I advise him/her the drugs and can he/she prescribe the drugs by writing on paper with due online discussion?

Answered by Dr RK Sharma: Please note that any conversation on SMS and WhatsApp is encrypted and can be produced in court of law as evidence. It is perfect and medicolegally correct if you give advice on WhatsApp and SMS. Please add the following at the end to protect you from future litigation.
- The information provided is provisional in nature as it is based on limited information given to me.
- It is better if I can see patient at the earliest.
- The information is confidential in nature and for the recipient use only.

Query: *In emergency conditions, can we collect blood and crossmatch and test by rapid methods? Can hospital purchase blood illegally in private healthcare set-ups? In blood banks in view of HIV, they have stopped doing rapid method sampling doing only ELISA for HIV, Hepatitis C, and HBs Ag—they are doing TriDot only. In towns, getting blood products (platelets) become difficult during dengue season in emergency conditions. Is there any provision or if recipient gives consent for rapid method for tests in lifesaving conditions?*

Answered by Dr RK Sharma: In emergency, any step to save life of a person is justified and person doing it is protected in good faith. But, it has been seen quite often in small places that procedures are routinely flouted in the name of emergency. Emergency is only on paper. If there is a dispute, doctor would be held responsible for fraud too.

Query: *If a patient is under treatment of a doctor, can doctor charge money for issuing certificate for medical bed-rest and* thereafter certificate of fitness for resuming duties on job by patient after recovery?

Answered by Dr RK Sharma: Yes, you can charge for a medical certificate, fitness certificate, or any certificate issued on request. But you should not charge for death certificate. Premier institute like AIIMS charges for medical certificate and fitness certificate.

Query: *My question is that one patient came to a hospital as a case of RTA. MLC was made and the patient required multiple surgeries, the patient was in critical condition when brought to the hospital, but because of doctor's work, the patient responded well and revived, and was discharged after 10 days in stable condition. The patient was again admitted after the 10th day because he needed debridement of wounds done and next day the patient was again discharged; after 3 days the patient was again brought in with septicemia to the hospital. This time the patient died after 6 days. In this case, postmortem is to be done or not since last two admissions were non-MLC?*

Answered by Dr RK Sharma: Always remember the golden rule, "if MLC has been made in a case and patient dies due to injuries even after a longtime, postmortem must be conducted." It has been seen that after death, patient's relatives files for compensation in courts and postmortem report is required in such cases.

Query: *A child was admitted in a hospital with diarrhea and dehydration, which turned out to be full-blown septic shock after 2 days. The child was intubated and referred to another hospital with an accompanying doctor without intimation and status of bed and at arrival the child was in shock and sick. I assessed the child in ambulance and advised admission; on explaining the parents about the cost and treatment, the parents said that they cannot afford the treatment at the corporate hospital and decided to take the child to another hospital. Is it right to send a patient without making any documentation which in corporate would be no less than Rs. 500 for emergency visit and more over take essential minutes from the child's treatment adding nothing, meanwhile the accompanying doctor would drop the patient and wash his hand off him/her. Also, if sent from outside without documentation and the accompanying doctor leaves the child halfway to other hospital, who gets the onus?*

Answered by Dr RK Sharma: This is a routine problem. Once the patient is referred to another hospital, Medical Superintendent of that hospital should talk to Medical Superintendent of the other hospital about bed position. This is in reference to following guidelines issued by SC. Accompanying doctor cannot leave unless patient is transferred to other hospital. All cases coming to emergency services should be registered and stabilized before retransfer to other hospital. As per Clinical Establishment Act (CEA), emergency treatment is free and cannot be charged; CEA has been notified in many states.

The Honorable SC in their judgment dated 06-05-1996 in SLP (C) No.796/92 – *Paschim Banga Khet Mazdoor Samity and Others versus State of West Bengal,* suggested remedial measures to ensure immediate medical attention and treatment to persons in real need.

The following guidelines may be kept in view while dealing with emergency cases in addition to the existing guidelines:

- In the hospital, the Medical Officer in the emergency or casualty services should admit a patient whose condition is morbid or serious in consultation with the specialist concerned on duty in the emergency department.
- In case the vacant beds are not available in the concerned department to accommodate such patient, the patient has to be given all necessary attention.
- Subsequently, the Medical Officer will make necessary arrangement to get the patient transferred to another hospital in the ambulance. The position as to whether there is vacant bed in the concerned department has to be ascertained before transferring the patient. The patient will be accompanied by the resident medical officer in the ambulance.
- In no case the patient will be left unattended for want of vacant beds in the emergency or casualty department.
- The services of Centralized Ambulance Trauma Services (CATS) should be utilized to the extent possible in Delhi.
- The efforts may be made to monitor the functioning of the emergency department periodically by the Heads of the institution.
- The medical record of patient attending the emergency services should be preserved in the medical record department.
- The medical superintendents may coordinate with each other for providing better emergency services.

Query: *I would like to know your opinion about the right practice if a patient got discharged at request or against medical advice.*
1. *Do we need to give discharge summary or a simple reference letter will suffice?*
2. *If we give discharge summary, do we need to give prescription for discharge medications?*

Answered by Dr RK Sharma: Your liabilities are different in each case and are summarized as follows:

- Patient absconding (patient went away without informing): Just note down in case file that patient has absconded and inform the police in writing.
- Patient want discharge against medical advice (LAMA): Patient has the right to take discharge summary. Record in case sheet that patient or relatives want discharge against medical advice and take their signature.
- Discharge on request (DOR) as they want to take patient to another hospital: Give discharge summary, arrange for ambulance and doctor, if patient is critically ill. Record in case sheet that patient or relatives want discharge and take their signature.
- Discharge on request when patient gets relief from pain, but doctor wants the patient to stay for definitive care: Give

discharge summary and discharge medication. Record in case sheet that patient or relatives want discharge and take their signature.

Query: *If a patient wants to leave the hospital against medical advice (LAMA), can he insist for discharge and treatment summary or clinical or operative notes? I have noticed, majority of times, this is not done specially in government setups and small nursing homes.*

Answered by Dr RK Sharma: I have seen that doctors become uncomfortable when a patient decides to use his fundamental right, right to choose doctor, whether to accept treatment, or not, from a particular doctor or hospital. It is labeled as LAMA. Patient is denied treatment papers and discharge slip. It is wrong. You can record it in case sheet that risk and prognosis of delaying treatment has been explained to the patient in his own language and the patient has gone on his/her own and that you have taken signature of the patient on LAMA intimation form. Hospital should provide discharge summary along with copy of all investigation reports, and keep the health records for future reference. As per SC guidelines, a patient has the fundamental right to get a copy of his treatment records, and hospital has to provide it within 72 hours.

Query: *Sometimes when relatives of a child patient want to take the child against medical advice, whose signature is required on documents for going LAMA? If father is not available in that case, please advise.*

Answered by Dr RK Sharma: Please understand that a father is the first legal guardian, then a mother. If the father is not there, get signatures of the mother, positively. If the mother is also not there, then grandfather or grandmother, brother or sister (must be major) and then other relatives like uncles and aunts. Please take copy of ID proof of relative, in doubt.

Query: *A patient needs to be admitted for giving intravenous (IV) medication like IV antibiotics or antifungal, in which no oral alternative is available. But after 1st dose, the patient wants DOR and requested for IV medication from home. Is it medicolegally correct to discharge and advice IV medication at home or not?*

Answered by Dr RK Sharma: Patient has a right to seek DOR, when he/she is clinically stable with normal range of vital parameters. In the case mentioned, since patient requires IV medication, doctors have to mention special precautions while making discharge summary. Mention in discharge summary that patient has been advised to take IV medicines under supervision of doctor. Mention specifically that patient has been discharged on request and has been advised how to take IV medicines under supervision, and to report to nearby hospital in emergency, if any adverse reaction happens during drug administration.

Query: *I am working in a public sector undertaking (PSU) hospital in a semi-rural location. The project is close to a big city and patients are frequently taking treatment for various ailments from the private practitioners. Very frequently they turn up at our hospital demanding administration of injectable medicines as advised by their treating doctors. Many times we may not agree to the medication being administered and being a PSU/government hospital, it leads to confrontations. My query is, "Do we have to prescribe the injection again on our prescription slip for it to be given?" It has already been prescribed by a qualified doctor elsewhere. Can the injection be administered with request and undertaking of the patient as "I XYZ, hereby give my request and consent towards administration of the injection to me/my patient as advised and prescribed by Dr ABC. I have been explained the side effects and adverse effects of the injection to be administered by my treating and prescribing doctor. The entire responsibility towards the administration of the injection including adverse effects shall lie on me. This hospital, its doctors, and staff shall not be responsible of any adverse reaction or event that may occur subsequent to administration of such an injection".*

Do such consents carry any validity in case of any adverse reactions? Can the injection be simply given with this consent and original prescription of private practitioner? In case of any adverse reaction, who would be responsible? In certain cases we may agree to the injectable to be administered. Is there a boundation on a doctor to prescribe that medicine? The patient has already bypassed our hospital and available specialist services citing various reasons and has merely come back for essentially nursing services.

Answered by Dr RK Sharma: Every medical practitioner is independent to follow his own treatment policy. You may or may not agree with your colleague or another qualified doctor. In your case, if you think, injection is required in this case; you can endorse it on your own letter head so that it can be given by a nurse. If you think, it is not required, just refuse it. If any reaction or negligence occurs, you would be held liable, if injection has been prescribed by you.

Please remember that your hospital is a PSU which is manned by qualified doctors and patients have no right to treat it as injection facility center where they can get any injection at will.

Your hospital is well within rights to refuse injections not prescribed by doctors of your hospital. The consent from patients, which you mentioned, has no legal value.

Query: *I am an emergency physician at a government hospital in Delhi. Recently, the state government has issued a diktat to all government hospitals to not prescribe or advise any medicine for the patient which is not available in the hospital. In other words, patients "cannot" be asked to buy any medicine from outside, "under any circumstances". My query is what to do in cases where medicine is necessary and irreplaceable for treatment of patient and is unavailable in the hospital pharmacy. Please consider that many drugs or instruments are lifesaving and essential for patient treatment, yet they are unavailable in hospital pharmacy or wards.*

In such circumstances, how to balance patient concerns and our own legitimate concerns about victimization at the

hands of the administration, if these diktats are not followed?
Answered by Dr RK Sharma: This is most unfortunate as government direction is illogical. Surprisingly, none of the top doctors like Directorate General of Health Services (DGHS), Medical Superintendent of hospitals must have not objected to it. All doctors who are in administration seats fear politicians and do not raise a voice even on wrong advisories by government as they fear victimization.

The best way is to deal with it through association. Please ask your doctors association to take up this matter directly with Chief Minister and issue press statements. Please keep the Indian Medical Association (IMA) in loop too, if needed, a writ petition in court may be filled in the Delhi High Court. If you go through association, individual victimization would not be there.

Query: *I am a working orthopedic surgeon in a corporate hospital. We get frequent orthopedic emergencies like acute dislocation, compound fracture, and vascular injuries. These are orthopedic emergencies as per my knowledge. But, we cannot deliver treatment due to financial clearance from hospital. In case of any delay in delivering the treatment who will be responsible—me, hospital, or patient himself? And how should I protect myself legally? Kindly advice.*
Answered by Dr RK Sharma: Please bring it to the knowledge of hospital authorities, like Medical Superintendent or Medical Director, immediately for issues of financial clearance in acute surgical emergencies. It is difficult to say who will be responsible in case of negligence and delay in treatment—either hospital or doctor or both, as it will depend on circumstances. If hospital authorities do not respond and correct the system, change the hospital.

Query: *Is it medicolegally mandatory for an emergency physician to call on an obstetrician and pediatrician to attend all child deliveries.*
Answered by Dr RK Sharma: It all depends on what level of care you are providing:
- If you are posted in a village primary health center, facility of an obstetrician and pediatrician may not be there.
- If you are working in a district hospital where an obstetrician and pediatrician are posted, you should call.
- If you are working in private nursing home or corporate hospital, where facility of an obstetrician and pediatrician is always there, you must call.
- If any problem occurs during childbirth like birth asphyxia, emergency physician may be held responsible if he or she has not called an obstetrician and pediatrician.

Query: *I am a government doctor, if any patient comes to my home for any emergency, what to do since I do not have any emergency kit at home? If I write any prescription to him, will it be taken as breach of contract with employer and can it be used against me as a proof of private practice?*
Answered by Dr RK Sharma: Since you are not doing open practice, you are not covered by CEA, so there is no reason that you are under any obligation to provide emergency care and stabilize the patient as per provisions of CEA. Try to help him as much as you can either by assistance in calling ambulance or correct referral.

You are legally right in giving prescription also, but since you are in government service, you cannot charge.

All government doctors are free to write prescription and help in emergency situation which is brought before them at home or on road. No action can be taken if you have not charged the patient. If you desire, you can inform your employer in writing about any case seen in emergency although it is not legally binding.

Query: *Casualty medical officer working in government hospital had referred an RTA case to an orthopedician of the same hospital for opinion. Final wound certificate was given by the CMO. Now the case has come to the court but the X-ray is missing (the constable of the concerned police station took it without permission). Sir, since the judge is insisting to produce X-ray, what can be done (case is 5 years old and X-ray is not traceable as it was not digital X-ray).*
Answered by Dr RK Sharma: It is quite deplorable to know that the X-ray has been taken away by constable without permission. You can bring it to the knowledge of senior police officers to take action against him. You can request the court to order re-X-ray of the patient to verify that fracture sustained by patient and request the court to take old report cognizance in view of findings of re-X-ray. Extend apology for lapse. Record keeper or medical record section incharge is fully responsible for it. Ask medical superintendent to take administrative action against the record keeper.

Query: *We are working in a corporate hospital situated in a remote and tribal area of India. Sometimes, we come across some so called high social status patients who are from larger cities of India and consider this area and its people to be backward. Whenever we suggest certain treatment or investigations they want us to seek approval from their doctor relative or friends. Although we do not mind discussing their health problem with their doctor relative or friend, but when the issue of seeking approval for initiating treatment or investigation comes we feel offended.*

What we should do in such cases when the patient's condition is an emergency and is life-threatening? In routine cases, can we politely refuse consultation and advise them to go elsewhere.
Answered by Dr RK Sharma: The problem referred by you is very common in all hospitals. Whenever any procedure is planned, patient may ask doctor to speak with family physician or doctor friend. You should politely refuse all such requests. You should know that there is a clinical discretion where one doctor may follow one school of treatment while the other may follow another and both are right as per standard medical practice. Difference of opinion in treatment is quite common. One may recommend surgery and another may not.

In life-threatening situations, refuse with firmness and explain urgency. If patient insists and refuses treatment, discharge the patient with proper procedure to declare him LAMA. Do not go overboard to please him. It may prove costly at any day.

Query: *What is the legal policy for "Brought Dead" patient? Should an MLC be lodged? Is MCD registration of death a liability of hospital? Can hospital charge towards services provided?*
Answered by Dr RK Sharma: As a rule, all patients brought to hospital as dead on arrival should be made medicolegal and death certificate should not be issued. But in following cases, where the patient is your old patient or getting treatment from some other hospital, you may adhere to following guidelines and issue death certificate at your own risk.
- Just check carefully all treatment papers and be convinced that they are genuine.
- See whether illness was severe enough to cause death.
- Check whether person is quite old to die naturally.
- Examine the body in detail for injury, ligature marks, anything strange to point toward unnatural death. If you are convinced and do not suspect foul play then you can issue death certificate at your own risk.

Please be careful, in the following conditions of brought dead, under no circumstances death certificate should be issued.
- Death of young woman.
- Child of any age.

There is no harm making a case as MLC. The police have power to waive off postmortem. In Delhi, this power rests with the Assistant Commissioner of Police (ACP).

Yes, information to MCD is hospital liability in all cases of death occurring or announced in hospital. Ideally, hospital should not charge for such services from patient.

Query: *Is online video consultation legal in India where in you give your opinion online through a video consultation and can advise the patient to come to your clinic, if necessary. What is the legal status and liability?*
Answered by Dr RK Sharma: Online video consultation is legal and is now becoming routine. It is a good medium where consultation can be taken at a distance. Liability is same as you are seeing a patient at your own clinic.

Query: *I am a senior specialist, working in community health center. I was on leave and out of station for 4 days. On 2nd day of my leave there was an assault case. In spite of leave, my district in-charge doctor has given me a memo stating that I am irresponsible and have not done my duty and proved to be negligent. I do not know where I have gone wrong.*
Answered by Dr RK Sharma: Let me tell you the legal position in your case. Please know that leave is not a matter of right as per Central Civil Services (CCS) rules. Any leave (even casual) can be refused. Leaves are granted by employer at discretion.

In your case, issue of memo was unjustified as you have already applied for leave as per procedure and was sanctioned. Memo should be issued to a doctor who fails to attend call when he agreed to do so.

Please form an association of doctors and then represent to concerned authorities for improving leave sanctioning procedure. You can threat of strike from association level. Individual efforts are not successful and sometimes harassment is done by sanctioning authority.

Query: *Who can waive off postmortem in MLCs like RTA, poisoning, etc.? Today there was a case of death allegedly due to snake bite poisoning. He was a 15-year-old boy. The police papers were ready and postmortem was about to start. But relatives forwarded a request to hand over the body without postmortem examination. But doctor on postmortem duty and Investigating Officer (IO) showed their inability. Both said that this power of waiving of postmortem lies with the sub-divisional magistrate (SDM) only. Then the relatives went to SDM and got the permission and body was handed over to relatives without postmortem.*

Second case was of a young male and the police had requested an MRI scan, CT scan, bone scan, chemical test, and pathological test of the body to ascertain the cause of death. The MRI and CT facility are not there at most of the civil hospital setup. MRI facility is even not there at some of the Government Medical colleges and bone scan in my view is not possible on dead body. Can the CT and MRI facility of a private diagnostic center be used? And if yes, whole body scan would have to be done? And who will pay for all this (relatives)?
Answered by Dr RK Sharma: Please remember that the police also have the power to waive off any postmortem. Doctor conducts postmortem only on request of the police or magistrate. Doctor cannot do postmortem on his/her own. Even for pathological autopsy, he needs consent from relatives of deceased.

The police rarely use its power to waive off postmortem, normally they approach SDM or Deputy Commissioner of Police (DCP) to exercise magisterial powers vested in them. I have seen many cases in my professional life where the police has withdrawn request for postmortem at last minute and handed over dead body to relatives without postmortem.

Nowadays, postmortems are waived off in mass tragedy like railway accidents, airline crashes (except crew) by the police on orders of government.

It is government purview to decide whether postmortem is needed or not, doctor has no role except giving advice which is not binding on state.

Query: *There is news that a renowned pulmonologist has been arrested by the police in Kolkata based on the complaint lodged by a lady at local police station in a charge of molestation during medical examination of the lady herself. Can a doctor be arrested by a mere complain of alleged molestation? What Indian law says, as there was a Honorable SC judgment, a* *doctor cannot be arrested unless a medical board is set into confirm the incident?*

Answered by Dr RK Sharma: Yes, the doctor can be arrested on a mere complain of alleged molestation as according to new Rape Law, even touching of private parts constitutes rape. The SC in case *State versus Jacob Mathew* has ordered that doctor may not be arrested, in case of medical negligence till a board of doctors or medical council gives a verdict of negligence. But, it does not give doctor immunity in other cases like molestation, murder, or other serious offences.

Query: *Further to your advice, what do you say if a male examines a female breast even though a nurse is present, the patient can say that no female was present. We do not take videos of the examination. Similarly, a male cannot do a vaginal examination. What law is this? Please clarify.*

Answered by Dr RK Sharma: Please remember that false allegations are possible in every case as examination done may be thought as unnecessary and demeaning. We can take only precautions and take everything as way of life. We should contest these cases and put a defamation suit after winning court battle. There is no law that a male cannot do vaginal examination. West Bengal has highest number of male gynecologists and they are quite successful.

Query: *I am not clear about what you say regarding death on operation table. I was under the impression that death on table (irrespective of having explained beforehand to the relatives) should be informed to the police and body sent to the government (civil) hospital for postmortem. Please clarify.*

Answered by Dr RK Sharma: Please remember that we are doing a lot of surgeries nowadays, where risk of death is higher as people are living in their 80s and 90s where even natural death is possible during operation. So, all deaths in operation theater need not be labeled as MLC and forwarded for postmortem. It would appear as an insult to human body and inconvenience to relatives. Make only those deaths MLC where relative put a label of medical negligence.

Answered by Dr Lalit Kapoor: Any death on operation theater table comes under the category of "unnatural" death. Ideally one cannot give a death certificate in any such death and cause of death has to be established by postmortem. Relatives are always reluctant to have postmortem. Also, postmortem has its own implications for the concerned doctors and hospital. At the same time one should not avoid MLC just because relatives are not alleging negligence. After funeral they show their true colors.

In Mumbai, we take the middle path. Earlier, in times of coroner he had power to waive postmortem. Now same power is vested in ACP of the area. It is safe to give death certificate with no objection certificate (NOC) from the police which they give after taking statements from relatives. We have done this many times and it has worked well. But operation theater death should always be informed to the police.

MEDICOLEGAL QUERIES ANSWERED BY DR MC GUPTA

Query: In every road traffic accident, MLC to be made compulsory, if attendant of patient denies for making MLC, and is quarreling for making MLC. What should be done?

Answered by Dr MC Gupta:
- Whether or not to make an MLC is the sole prerogative and discretion of the medical officer concerned.
- Doctor should, when in doubt, opt for the MLC.
- Making an MLC means informing the police about the incident, inviting the police to come and take necessary steps, such as registering a complaint or FIR, etc., recording statements of the concerned individuals and collecting necessary samples, etc.
- The medical officer does not need the attendants' permission to inform the police or make an MLC.
- If the medical officer wants to make an MLC but does not do so because of any other factors or ground, situation, he should keep safely detailed records of the incident, history, and examination, etc., almost as if in a regular MLC, so that such records should be made available later to the police or court, as necessary.

Query:
1. If a resident doctor treats a patient in the emergency before the patient has been admitted under any department and something goes wrong, then who is responsible—the consultant of the emergency or the concerned resident doctor?
2. Another scenario is that if in a case while treating a patient in the emergency we give a call to the concerned department and by the time the concerned team arrives, the patient expires. Then who is responsible?

In both these scenarios does the responsibility lie with the resident emergency doctor or the consultant responsible for the emergency?

Answered by Dr MC Gupta:
1. This is a theoretical or imaginary question. Theoretical or imaginary questions often do not merit a detailed legal answer. It is not a must that somebody must be held responsible if something goes wrong. Proper answers can be given only when complete details of the case are given. Primarily, the hospital would be responsible. It does not appear that the consultant would be held responsible. The responsibility, if any, of the resident would depend upon the facts of the case.

Query: *Can a Medical Superintendent appear in court on behalf of the hospital doctors? What to do if his expenses are not paid for such appearance?*

Question: An RTA case was admitted in a private hospital. He had intestinal perforation. The following specialists had examined or treated the patient—surgeon, orthosurgeon, anesthesiologist, Medical Superintendent, and physician.

Finally, the wound certificate was written by medical transcriptionist and issued by the Medical Superintendent under his signature. My questions are as follows:
a. Whether the Medical Superintendent is competent to attend the court as an expert witness?
b. If there is question related to the fracture or perforation by the advocate, is it necessary to call all the doctors to give answer when superintendent is able to give a reasonable reply?
c. Is it necessary that the wound certificate should be written by the same doctor who is attending the court?
d. To whom one should complain about not getting the compensation (Travelling allowance-Dearness Allowance), etc. as per rules on the ground that no funds were available (the Medical Superintendent travelled in his own car at a distance of 50 km)?

Answered by Dr MC Gupta:
a. Yes, the Medical Superintendent is competent.
b. If the Medical Superintendent is able to give reasonable replies to the questions asked, it is not necessary to call all the doctors. But, with the permission of the court, there is nothing to prevent the other doctors from being called. Likewise, with the permission of the court, there is nothing to prevent the other doctors from being presented as witnesses by the defendant hospital.
c. It is natural that a person can testify only that document which he has written or signed himself.
d. It appears that it was a police case and the information about nonavailability of funds was given informally by the court staff. The complaint should be made to the court itself.

Answered by Dr Narayan Reddy:
1. In this case the Medical Superintendent signed the wound certificate.
2. As a result the court summoned the Medical Superintendent.
3. The Medical Superintendent is under legal duty to attend the court.
4. The Medical Superintendent has to take prior permission of the court to depute some other doctor to attend the court on his behalf.
5. The summons is neither a requisition nor an invitation. It is an order to be obeyed. Without reasonable cause, if a witness does not attend the court, the court is at liberty to punish the witness under Section 350 of the *Code of Criminal Procedure* (CrPC), 1973: Summary procedure for punishment for nonattendance by a witness.
6. In majority of the criminal cases the prosecutor is the government of that state, and for prosecution witnesses, the concerned State Government adopts its own mode of payment of travelling allowance and dearness allowance.

Query: *How to proceed with medical negligence in treatment of a snake bite patient? What action can be taken to improve the following situation?*

"On 4th October 2011, patient, 53 years, Male of Haldia, an industrial town, was bitten by a viper snake. He was taken to the Haldia State General Hospital. No treatment was given there and he was referred to the Tamluk district hospital about 60 km away. There he was given only 5 vials of anti-viper serum (AVS) and was transferred to the NRS Medical College Hospital at Kolkata, where, on 5th October (Nabami of Durgapuja), he was admitted in the Male Medical Ward and had to purchase 10 vials of AVS from outside."

Answered by Dr MC Gupta: This is a disappointing and unacceptable situation that should not be quietly and silently accepted without protest if any change has to be brought about. I suggest the following:
- Write letters to the three hospitals concerned under the Right to Information (RTI) Act to get relevant information.
- At the same time, without waiting for RTI replies, send a proper (legally drafted) complaint to the state health authorities under the West Bengal Clinical Establishments Act, 1950.
- Send a complaint to the West Bengal Medical Council against doctors of the Haldia State General Hospital who sent away a viper snake bite patient without proper treatment. Even if the hospital did not have the medicine, the hospital should have procured the same urgently and administered it to the patient without loss of time.
- Most likely, the Haldia State General Hospital and the NRS Hospital would be covered under the CPA, 1986. A consumer complaint seeking compensation can be filed there.
- Later, at an appropriate stage, a writ petition or public interest litigation (PIL) may be filed in Calcutta High Court.
- All the above should be done with legal guidance.

Query: *Is there some difference in the nature of claims made in case of death or injury incurred because of vehicle accident or because of medical treatment?*

Answered by Dr MC Gupta: Yes. There are many differences. A claim arising out of medical treatment compensates the claimant for medical negligence that caused the death or injury. A claim arising out of a vehicle accident compensates the claimant for the loss due to the death or injury.
- A claim of medical negligence concerns professional negligence which is of such a character that cannot be decided by a nonprofessional person and for determination and punishment of which statutory professional councils in the nature of medical councils have been established whose opinion (or opinion of other professional experts) is almost a must in medical negligence cases except when the nature of negligence is such that it is palpably visible even to a layman.
- A claim in vehicular accident cases is decided by laymen because it is not a matter of professional negligence. Driving is not a profession and there is no professional Driving Council like the Dental, Medical, Nursing, or Bar Councils.

- Payment in a medical negligence case is made only if medical negligence is established. Payment in a motor vehicle accident case is made if injury is established, irrespective of the fact whether there was negligence on the part of the driver or not. Even if there is no negligence whatsoever, payment is made from the Solatium Fund established under the Motor Vehicles Act, 1988.
- Payment in a motor accident case is made by the insurance company concerned, it being illegal to ply a vehicle which is not insured. Payment in a medical negligence case is primarily payable by the medical person concerned except when a part or whole is payable by an insurance company from which the doctor might have optionally bought insurance.

Query: *Can a Department of Ayurveda, Yoga and Naturopathy, Unani, Siddha and Homoeopathy (AYUSH) doctor prepare an MLC report or perform an autopsy?*
Answered by Dr MC Gupta: No. This can be done only by an MBBS doctor.

This is supported by the following legal provisions:
- Indian Medical Council Act, 1956–Clauses (c) and (d) of Section of 15(2) of the Indian Medical Council Act, 1956, read as follows:

  "No person other than a medical practitioner enrolled on a State Medical Register:

  (c) Shall be entitled to sign or authenticate a medical or fitness certificate or any other certificate required by any law to be signed or authenticated by a duly qualified medical practitioner.

  (d) Shall be entitled to give evidence at any inquest or in any court of law as an expert under Section 45 of the Indian Evidence Act, 1872 on any matter relating to medicine.
  Note:
- Section 45 of the Indian Evidence Act, 1872 reads, "When the Court has to form an opinion upon a point of foreign law, or of science, or art, or as to identity of hand writing or finger-impressions, the opinions upon that point of persons specially skilled in such foreign law, science or art, or in questions as to identity of handwriting[1] or finger impressions, are relevant facts. Such persons are called experts".
- Section 53 of the *CrP, 1973* reads, "Examination of accused by medical practitioner at the request of police officer.
  1. When a person is arrested on a charge of committing an offence of such a nature and alleged to have been committed under such circumstances that there are reasonable grounds for believing that an examination of his person will afford evidence as to the commission of an offence, it shall be lawful for a registered medical practitioner, acting at the request of a police officer not below the rank of sub-inspector, and for any person acting in good faith in his aid and under his direction, to make such all examination of the person arrested as is reasonably necessary in order to ascertain the facts which may afford such evidence, and to use such force as is reasonably necessary for that purpose.
  2. Whenever the person of a female is to be examined under this section, the examination shall be made only by, or under the supervision of a female registered medical practitioner.
  Explanation: In this Section and in Sections 53A and 54,
  (a) "Examination" shall include the examination of blood, blood stains, semen, swabs in case of sexual offences, sputum and sweat, hair samples, and finger nail clippings by the use of modern and scientific techniques including DNA profiling and such other tests which the registered medical practitioner thinks necessary in a particular case;
  (b) "Registered medical practitioner" means a medical practitioner who possess any medical qualification as defined in clause (h) of section 2 of the Indian Medical Council Act, 1956 and whose name has been entered in a State Medical Register."

Query: *A nursing home employs homeopaths as registered medical officers (RMOs). Can it be held liable in law?*
Question: A nursing home, claiming to provide allopathic services, employs RMOs who are homeopaths. When questioned, the nursing home argues, "We are not committing any irregularity. The RMOs never claim to be MBBS. They do not prescribe any medicines. They only observe the patients and relay their observations to the consultant in modern medicine who alone is responsible for all clinical decisions". Will such argument succeed in a court of law in view of the *Thakur versus Han Charitable Trust judgment*?
Answered by Dr MC Gupta:
1. The National Consumer Commission observed as follows in *Prof PN Thakur versus Hans Charitable Hospital*, NC, 16 August 2007 *http://ncdrc.nic.in/op21497.html*, "We feel, it is high time that hospital authorities realize that the practice of employing nonmedical practitioners such as doctors specialized in Unani system and who do not possess the required skill and competence to give allopathic treatment and to let an emergency patient be treated in their hands is a gross negligence."
2. The word treatment means as follows:
   - "Treatment" means the provision of specific physical, mental, social interventions, and therapies which halt, control or reverse processes that cause, aggravate or complicate malfunctions or dysfunctions.
   - "Treatment includes not only medical treatment in the sense that the patient or subject is looked after and attended to by a doctor, but also nursing in the sense that the subject or patient is looked after and attended to by persons professionally trained to look after and attend to the sick".

Minister of Health versus Royal Midland Counties Home for Incurables, etc. (1954) 1 All ER 1013, 1017.

- In terms of the *Coal Mine Health and Safety Regulation 2006, made under the Australian Coal Mine Health and Safety Act 2002*, "Medical treatment means the carrying out, by or under the supervision of a registered medical practitioner, of an operation, the administration of a drug or other like substance, or any other medical procedure (not including diagnostic tests or advice that do not lead to treatment)."

3. Whether an argument succeeds in a court depends upon many factors, such as:
   - The nature and level of court
   - The nature and level of the advocate
   - The nature and facts and circumstances of the case.
4. I think I will succeed if I argue as follows:
   - The word "treatment" in the quote from the Thakur judgment has to be interpreted as per the definitions given above. This means that "Medical treatment means the carrying out, by or under the supervision of a registered medical practitioner". Carrying out some function under the supervision of a registered medical practitioner does not mean to independently observe the patients and relay their observations to the consultant in modern medicine.
   - That nowhere in the hospital is it displayed that the RMOs are homeopathy graduates.
   - That the name plates of the RMOs working in the hospital only read as "Dr ABC" and not as "Dr ABC, BHMS".
   - That in view of the above, there is no information to the patients that in its real meaning of the term "treatment", they are being treated by non-MBBS persons.
   - "That patients come to the hospital because the nursing home claims to offer and the patients want treatment by practitioners of modern medicine and, in the circumstances, the practice of employing non-MBBS practitioners such as doctors specialized in homeopathic system who do not possess the required skill and competence to give allopathic treatment amounts to gross negligence" in terms of the judgment in *Prof PN Thakur versus Hans Charitable Hospital*.

Query: *Is the hospital management liable to pay compensation when the negligence in surgery or treatment is, in fact, committed by a consultant?*

Question: I am Director (Medical Services) in a 350 bed hospital. I read an article in The Times of India last year which stated that the hospital management does not have any responsibility if treating consultant is negligent. Is this correct?

Answered by Dr MC Gupta:
1. No. This is not correct.
2. The reasons why it is not correct are as follows:
   - There is no contract between the patient and the consultant. The contract is between the patient and the hospital. Fees are paid to the hospital. The ward where the patient is admitted is owned by the hospital. The operation theater where he is operated is owned by the hospital. The owner of a vehicle pays the damages, not the driver.
   - Let us look at it more analytically. There are three essential ingredients of a contract: (1) offer; (2) acceptance; and (3) consideration. In the present case:
     – Offer to treat is made by the hospital by way of advertisements, etc. and not by the consultant physician (as a matter of fact, it is against the Code of Ethics Regulations, 2002, for a physician to advertise himself).
     – The patient accepts an offer made by the hospital. He does not accept any offer made by the consultant whom he even does not know.
     – Consideration by way of advance deposit and payment of bill, prepared by the hospital, is made to the hospital and not the physician.

   Hence, there is no way that there can be a legal contract between the physician and the patient.
   - The consultant has no independent entity. He works as a part or agent of the hospital. The principal is responsible for the acts of the agent. This is as per the principle of vicarious liability according to which, when negligence is committed by an employee such as a resident or a nurse or a ward assistant, the responsibility lies upon the hospital which is the principal under whom they work.
   - If negligence occurs and the court awards compensation, the patient or complainant has a right to recover it. He cannot exercise his right if the consultant is dead, untraceable or a pauper. The complainant cannot be left uncompensated. That is why a hospital has to be made liable. A hospital cannot be dead, untraceable or pauper. Even if the hospital ceases to exist or becomes insolvent, its assets can be attached for payment of compensation.
3. The above statements are supported by the decision in *Shri Naresh Mehra versus Dr AP Choudhary*, decided by The Delhi State Consumer Commission on 31 October 2008, as follows:

"We have taken a view that whenever any patient lands in any hospital or nursing home, medical center, his direct relationship of consumer for hiring or availing the medical services is with the said hospital or nursing home or medical center and not with the treating doctors and other personnel; secondly, the entire consideration in the form of expenses including the component of charges or fees of the operating doctor and other junior doctors and staff engaged in pre- or postoperative care or any other kind of care are paid to the Nursing Home or Hospital or Medical Center directly; and thirdly, there is totality or compendium of various services including medical and those of para staff and other conveniences and the privity of contract is not with the operating or treating or attending doctors, nurses, and other staff.

Thus, if a patient suffers due to the medical negligence or carelessness of doctors and staff of the hospital or nursing home or medical Center whose services he avails against consideration, said hospital or nursing home or medical center alone is liable to compensate the patient as to loss or injury suffered by him, and nursing home or hospital or medical center has independent remedy to take any kind of action against such doctors or staff but no doctor or staff has a joint or several liability qua the patient.

Similarly nursing homes or medical centers or hospitals alone are liable for the acts of omission or commission or medical negligence of visiting or consulting doctors as the patient has no direct contract with such doctors and services of such doctors are availed by the hospital or nursing home or medical center and not the patient.

Query: *I am an orthopedician. I want to get training in musculoskeletal ultrasonography and use the ultrasound machine in my clinic? Will I face some legal problem?*
Answered by Dr MC Gupta: As a first step, you will have to get registered under the Pre-Conception and Pre-Natal Diagnostic Techniques (PCPNDT) Act, 1994, by submitting a proper application along with a non-refundable application fee of Rs 25,000/-
- Then you will have to buy the machine
- Then you will have to maintain records in a strict manner and will have to send a monthly report to the authorities as per the given proforma
- Also, you will have to be prepared for surprise inspections of your clinic by the authorities.
- If you are comfortable with the above, you may go ahead.
- Two of my doctor clients have surrendered their PCPNDT registration because they did not find the restrictions worth it.

Query: *Patients asking for doctor's mobile number for emergency, should we give it or not?*
Answered by Dr MC Gupta: It has become the norm for patients to ask for the doctor's mobile phone number. Doctors accede to the request because they do want patients to be able to contact them in case of an emergency. Unfortunately in India emergency services are not accessible to many patients easily, even in cities; thus it does become difficult for patients at times. However, most patients have a family physician or general practitioner who is accessible to them in their area, so ideally he should be the one attending to a real or perceived emergency. Or, if the emergency seems to be of a serious nature, one just has to rush to the nearest hospital.

Unfortunately, however, the vast majority of phone calls we receive are not emergencies. They are usually for trivial reasons (forgot the timing of the medicine; does it matter if I use a different brand; I am with the chemist and want to clarify something; should I give the blood sample in a fasting state; my TSH report is XYZ; I saw you today but forgot to tell you that I have occasional knee pain; suddenly my sugar level is 180 today!; can I have carrots? I could not sleep last night, etc.) Others are more complicated, such as reading out the laboratory results, several pages long, complex numbers or descriptions, and expecting you to prescribe on phone or detailed clinical description of problems, again expecting telephonic prescriptions. If you tell them that you do not actually remember the details of their case they either get offended or start explaining their problem in even more detail. All this might be happening when you are actually in the middle of an actual physical consultation with a patient, in a seminar or meeting or having dinner or trying to sleep or with your family or out for dinner, etc. Quite often, the patient may not have seen you for years, but will start a conversation as if he or she saw you yesterday.

The problem is you cannot decide whether a call is for an actual emergency or not till you have answered it and the moment you do that, the damage is done. What remains unclear to me is the following:
- Are doctors supposed to answer calls round the clock from their patients, or is it ok to give the assistant's number for routine queries, and the hospital number for emergencies?
- Are doctors supposed to give out our mobile numbers or do we have a choice in the matter?
- What is the value of telephonic advice from a legal point of view? Can we get caught on the wrong side of the law for advice given over the phone that leads to a complication?
- Can doctors refuse to talk to a patient?

I know the answers seem very simple, it is a matter of personal choice for the doctor, you may or may not give your number; may choose not to take phone calls; advice given over the phone has no legal validity; doctors have a right to refuse.

Query: *What all legal formalities are required or adhered to when we get any "Brought Dead Patient". Should we issue Death Certificate if cause of death is not known to the hospital?*
Answered by Dr MC Gupta: The standard guidelines by DGHS are that when a patient is brought dead, police should be informed and postmortem should be done. Your job is to inform the police. If the police decide to waive the postmortem, it is OK and it is not your headache. If you do not inform the police, there may be complications later. Death certificate can be issued if you have informed the police.

Query: *What can we write for cause of death in death certificate in brought dead patient?*
Answered by Dr MC Gupta: Cause of death: Not known.

Query: *If patient is not signing the discharge against Medical Advice consent in DAMA cases, what document are to be completed by the hospital for legal compliance and safety against future litigation of malpractice.*

Answered by Dr MC Gupta: A note should be made in the case sheet that the patient LAMA and refused to sign the papers. This note should be countersigned by two more witnesses or doctors or staff members.

Proper discharge slip should be given to even LAMA patients. If the relatives receive the discharge summary but do not sign acceptance or acknowledgment, a note as above should be made on the office copy.

Query: *Can you suggest me if MLC is required in all these cases:*
- *A relative falling in patient unit in hospital following seizure*
- *Child coming with injury in hand while playing in school*
- *Fall at home as claimed*
- *Fall from height.*

Answered by Dr MC Gupta:
- Making an MLC means informing the police. The discretion lies with the medical officer. If there is a possibility of foul play, MLC must be made.
- Even if there is minimal or low possibility of foul play, MLC may not be made but full and proper details, almost on the lines required in an MLC, must be recorded and preserved so that they may be made available to the police or court if such a demand is made at a later stage.

Query: *A patient refusing medically necessary cesarean in obstructed labor. A competent 30-year-old patient who is 38 weeks pregnant refuses to have a cesarean delivery despite the fact that without the surgery the fetus will probably die. Both her surgeon and psychiatrist have failed to convince her to have the surgery. What would be the most appropriate action for the surgeon to take at this time?*

Answered by Dr Pratibha Kane: A pregnant woman who is competent can refuse surgery even if it means injury to the fetus. The fetus is viable so fetal rights will get violated. There must be documentation of all the explanation, given to the patient by the surgeon and psychiatrist. Refusal for surgery must be clearly documented, witnessed by husband and any close relative. As the surgeon is not bound to treat this patient he/she must ask the patient to seek treatment with some other doctor. In case there is fetal distress, one can take the plea of an emergency life-saving procedure and continue with the cesarean.

Answered by Dr MC Gupta: If the patient does not follow the treatment advised and does not go back home or to another hospital and insists on staying in the hospital with the sure consequence of death of the child and fatal or nonfatal adverse consequences in the mother (with likely legal complications or violence afterwards), it would be best to inform the police. All this must be properly documented.

Query: *I am doing Doctorate in Medicine (DM). I feel sad that doctors in India face so many problems. I am planning to do Bachelor of Laws (LLB) after my DM. What are your suggestions?*

Answered by Dr MC Gupta:
- I am very glad that you have a perceptive, logical and realistic mind. What you wrote is correct. Main causes of the problems enumerated by you are as follows:
  - Very low health budget.
  - Promotion of quackery by the government by allowing AYUSH to practice allopathy.
- The above problems can be fought by two means:
  1. Through law
  2. Through mobilizing mass opinion, channeled through IMA, that forces the government to change or enforce laws and to increase health budget.
- I have no hope regarding the second. The first is workable through genuine persons like you who take to law to improve national health care.
- Doing LLB is not difficult. But you must hurry up because the Bar Council of India wants to close evening law colleges. You should enroll for an evening law course even while doing DM or as soon as possible after that.
- Possible ways how LLB can be useful to you:
  - You can join the bar and practice as an advocate
  - You can go on to do LLM and PhD in law and become a Professor of law
  - You may one day become a member of a consumer forum or commission, almost like a judge. Minimum age is 50 years. LLB is not a requirement but will make you all the more eligible. Appointment is for 5 years, renewable.
  - If you are in service (especially with administrative responsibilities), a law degree always helps.
  - If you become an advocate, you have to give up medical practice. If you want to continue medical practice, you may get registered as an accredited agent with a Consumer Commission. This will entitle you to argue cases in consumer courts (LLB is not a requirement for this).
- What matters is commitment. You already have high IQ, knowledge, analytical skills, and capacity to do hard work, as also a good knowledge of english. All these will be helpful in the legal career. There are increasing numbers of MLCs in courts nowadays. You will never lack work.
- *Summary*: Go ahead. Do LLB. All the best. You will never regret following my advice. That is a personal guarantee.

Query: *What are the laws against quackery?*

Answered by Dr MC Gupta: There is no specific antiquackery law in India at present. However, quackery is illegal in view of the following legislations or judgments:
- Section 15(2)(b) read with section 15(3) of the Indian Medical Council Act, 1956, whereby imprisonment up to 1 year or fine up to Rs 1,000 or both are provided for quacks.
- Section 23 of the Punjab Medical Registration Act, 1916, as amended in 2010, whereby a quack can "be liable to be punished on conviction by a magistrate of the first class

with a sentence of imprisonment for a term, not exceeding three years and with fine, not exceeding ten thousand rupees".
- Section 27 of the Delhi Medical Council Act, 1997. However, this section is so badly drafted that it seems to be meaningless.
- *Indian Penal Code*: The words quack and quackery do not find a place in the IPC. Thus, there is no crime like quackery as per the IPC. The only way to book a quack under IPC is under sections like:
  – IPC 419 Attempt of cheating
  – IPC 420 Cheating
  – IPC 338 Inject drugs causing damage to the body
  – IPC 471 Keeping fake documents.

The IMA has demanded that quacks must be booked under IPC 307 (Attempt to murder).
- *Poonam Verma versus Ashwin Patel and Others*, decided by the SC on 10th May 1996, reported as 4 SCC 332.
- *Dr Mukhtiar Chand and Others versus State of Punjab and Others*, decided by the SC on 8th August 1998, reported as AIR 1999, SC 468 [1998 (7) SCC 579].

Query: *Is it unethical to complain to the medical council against doctors supporting illegal pathology laboratories?*

I think that in order to curb the menace of illegal pathology laboratories, complaints should be lodged with the medical council against doctors supporting such laboratories. Other members of the local IMA action committee oppose this, saying that it is unethical to complain against our colleagues. What are your comments?

Answered by Dr MC Gupta: My comment is that you are right and the views of the IMA action committee are wrong.
- The IMA action committee is expected to be aware of Regulation 1.7 of the Indian Medical Council (Professional conduct, Etiquette, and Ethics) Regulations, 2002, which reads as follows:
  "1.7 Exposure of Unethical Conduct: A physician should expose, without fear or favor, incompetent or corrupt, dishonest or unethical conduct on the part of members of the profession".
- The incompetent or corrupt, dishonest or unethical conduct can be alleged on the following grounds:
  – Associating with quacks by referring cases to them and by relying on reports given by them (those who practice pathology without having a medical qualification are quacks).
  – Mechanical signing of illegal pathology laboratory reports by pathologists.
  – Running a pathology laboratory without having a qualification in pathology.
- If the action committee is afraid to take action, it has no right to call itself an action committee.
- As a matter of fact, nothing prevents the medical council from taking action against quacks on its own, without any complaint, but inaction is the name of the game played by all.
- My suggestion is that you should go ahead filing such complaint on your own.

Query: *Is it required to take specific informed consent for blood transfusion? Will this not be covered by the doctrine of implied consent?*

Answered by Dr MC Gupta: The short answer to this question is that there must be a written informed consent from the patient before blood transfusion is given. However, if more than 1 unit of blood is to be given, there need not be detailed informed consent each time and the former proper informed consent would suffice. There is nothing like implied consent in the context of blood transfusion.

The question of consent is very often ignored by doctors. It is necessary for them to understand the legal principles behind informed consent. These principles have been explained in detail in paras 16–26 of the order dated 29 March 2016 passed by the National Consumer Commission in *Sulochana Lad versus Dr Mohan Gerra and Another* (Appeal No. 138 of 2008), reproduced below.

Para 16: The doctrine of consent, stems from the notion that every adult human body, with a sound mind, has a right of self-determination and personal autonomy to decide what shall be done with his own body, a fundamental aspect of the right to health, the basic principle, which permeates through all cases. As we shall notice hereafter, Consent is not mere acceptance of a medical intervention, but a voluntary informed decision by the patient, whether or not to opt for a particular medical procedure. It may be conceded that while consent by the patient for simple procedures may sometimes be implied but it needs little emphasis that invasive treatments do require explicit consent. Therefore, in so far as the first limb of the question, viz. whether blood transfusion is an invasive procedure, is concerned, internationally blood transfusion is considered as a medical invasive procedure, performed on a live body. That being so, undoubtedly the doctor is bound to disclose to the patient the associated benefits, risks and alternatives to blood transfusion, and it is now an accepted medical norm to obtain informed consent of the patient before its transfusion, albeit in a legally recognized emergency on the facts of each case, an aspect, which shall be dealt with in the later part of this order. Nevertheless, depending on the medical procedure, the consent can be either combined with consent for other procedures or on its own. In fact, the National AIDS Control Organization, under the Ministry of Health and Family Welfare, while prescribing the Standards for Blood Banks and Blood Transfusion Services, specifically states, "Informed Consent: The patient should be informed about his/her need for blood, alternatives available, as well as risks involved in transfusion and non-transfusion. His/her written consent should be taken in the language he/she understands best only after providing information. For minors and unconscious patients the next of kin should sign the informed consent." Similarly, the DGHS, Ministry of Health and Family Welfare, Government of India, in its Transfusion Medicine Technical Manual, requires that "Informed consent for transfusion of blood and its products should be taken. The physician should explain the risks and alternatives of transfusion to the recipient or responsible family." With respect to multiple transfusions, it states "One-time consent for repeated transfusions will suffice".

Para 17: In the United Kingdom, consent for transfusion is considered a best medical practice, though it is subject to debate as to whether it is a legal requirement. As a result of an extensive consultative process, an Advisory Committee on the Safety of Blood, Tissues and Organs (SaBTO) has made its recommendations, inter-alia, recommending the need for informed consent in the case of blood transfusions. Various bodies of medical professionals have issued guidelines to its members. One such organization is the Royal College of Surgeons which issued an advisory in September 2010 stating, "The College recognizes that patients should be fully informed of the likelihood of blood (and blood product) transfusion as well as the reasons, benefits, risks and alternatives, before they consent to their operation. The consent process is fundamentally one of patient education and understanding, which should begin in the outpatient department and continue right through the pre-operative discussion…" The National Health Services in the UK website also provides some guidance, wherein it states on its webpage titled "Preparing for a blood transfusion", "If you are going to receive a blood transfusion as part of a planned course of treatment, the doctor, nurse, or midwife planning your transfusion will usually obtain your informed consent for the procedure. In obtaining consent, they should: explain why a blood transfusion is required and if there are any alternatives, explain potential risks or complications associated with the transfusion. There may be circumstances when it is not possible to obtain consent before a transfusion – for example, if someone is unconscious after a major accident".

Para 18: In the US, for all planned transfusions informed consent is required. An article from the American Journal of Clinical Pathology, titled "Informed Consent for Blood Transfusion: What do medicine residents tell?" What do patients understand? Sets forth the standards of informed consent from the American Association of Blood Banks, as "(1) a description of the risks, benefits, and treatment alternatives (including non-treatment), (2) the opportunity to ask questions, and (3) the right to accept or refuse transfusion".

Para 19: In the light of overwhelming literature on the point, our answer to the first limb of the question, formulated above, is that before blood transfusion, Consent of the patient is required to be taken.

Para 20: Now time to advert to the pivotal question, viz. the basic doctrine of informed consent, as understood in the legal parlance, to be borne in mind while deciding whether in a given case a legally valid consent of the patient had been taken or not?

Para 21: Fundamentally, the law requires the disclosure to the patient, information relating to the diagnosis of the disease; nature of the proposed treatment; potential risks of the treatment and the consequences of the patient refusing the suggested line of treatment. Disclosure of such information is the basic attribute of an informed consent and is considered mandatory in every field of medicine or surgical procedure. The only exception to the general rule is the emergency medical circumstances, where either the patient is not in a medical condition or mental stage to take a conscious decision in this regard. In India, the standard of disclosure of information to the patient regarding ailment and recommended treatment, with attendant risks of treatment, necessary to secure his informed consent, as enunciated in Bolam versus Friern Hospital Management Committee— (1957) 2 All ER 118, commonly referred to as the Bolam test, is being applied. The standards laid down in Bolam, were: (i) when a doctor dealing with a sick man strongly believed that the only hope of cure was submission to a particular therapy, he could not be criticized if, believing the danger involved in the treatment to be minimal, did not stress them to the patient. In other words, what degree of disclosure of risks, is best calculated to assist a particular patient to make a rational choice as to whether or not to undergo a particular treatment must primarily be left to clinical judgment of the doctor; and (ii) in order to recover damages for failure to give warning about the danger, the complainant must show not only that the failure was negligent but also that if he had been warned, he would not have consented to the treatment.

Para 22: In *Malay Kumar Ganguly versus Dr Sukumar Mukherjee and Others* – (2009) 9 SCC 221 dealing with the question of right of the patient to be informed about the recommended treatment for the ailment he is suffering from and the risks involved in the treatment, while observing that the only reasonable guarantee of a patient's right of bodily integrity and self-determination is for the courts to apply a stringent standard of disclosure in conjunction with a presumption of proximate cause, at the same time, a reasonable measure of autonomy for the doctor is also pertinent to be safeguarded from unnecessary interference, the Honourable Supreme Court said as follow:

> "142. Patients by and large are ignorant about the disease or side or adverse effect of a medicine. Ordinarily the patients are to be informed about the admitted risk, if any. If some medicine has some adverse effect or some reaction is anticipated, he should be informed thereabout. It was not done in the instant case. In *Sidaway versus Board of Governors of Bethlem Royal Hospital the House of Lords*, inter alia held as under: (WLR pp. 504 H-505 C)
> The decision what degree of disclosure of risks is best calculated to assist a particular patient to make a rational

choice as to whether or not to undergo a particular treatment must primarily be a matter of clinical judgment. An issue whether non-disclosure of a particular risk or cluster of risks in a particular case should be condemned as a breach of the doctor's duty of care is an issue to be decided primarily on the basis of expert medical evidence. In the event of a conflict of evidence the judge will have to decide whether a responsible body of medical opinion would have approved of nondisclosure in the case before him.

A judge might in certain circumstances come to the conclusion that disclosure of a particular risk was so obviously necessary to an informed choice on the part of the patient that no reasonably prudent medical man would fail to make it, even in a case where no expert witness in the relevant medical field condemned the nondisclosure as being in conflict with accepted and responsible medical practice.

143. The law on medical negligence also has to keep up with the advances in the medical science as to treatment as also diagnostics. Doctors increasingly must engage with patients during treatments especially when the line of treatment is a contested one and hazards are involved. *Standard of care in such cases will involve the duty to disclose to patients about the risks of serious side effects or about alternative treatments. In the times to come, litigation may be based on the theory of lack of informed consent.*

144. A significant number of jurisdictions, however, determine the existence and scope of the doctor's duty to inform based on the information a reasonable patient would find material in deciding whether or not to undergo the proposed therapy". (Emphasis supplied)

Para 23: At this juncture, it would be apposite to briefly refer to the subsequent developments on the point, after Bolam. In *Sidaway versus Board of Governors of Bethlem Royal Hospital* – (1985) 1 All ER 643 (HL), per majority, the House of Lords preferred Bolam test as a measure of doctor's duty to disclose information about potential consequences and risks of proposed medical treatment. The stringent standards regarding disclosure laid down in *Canterbury versus Spence* - 150 US App. DC 263 (1972) were not accepted. In Canterbury (Supra), the US Court of Appeal had observed that it is normally impossible to obtain Consent worthy of the name unless the physician first elucidates the options and the perils for patient's edification. Thus, the physician has long borne a duty, on pain of liability for unauthorized treatment, to make adequate disclosure to the patient. However, after the majority opinion in Sidaway (Supra), rendered in the year 1985, much water has flowed down the River Thames. Very recently in *Montgomery versus Lanarkshire Health Board, Scotland*—(2015) UK SC 11, the question of a doctor's duty to advise a patient of risks involved in treatment came up for consideration before the United Kingdom Supreme Court.

Making a significant departure from the majority opinion of the House of Lords in Sidaway (Supra), by a unanimous opinion, the Court has now approved the following minority opinion of Lord Scarman in Sidaway, which was earlier rejected:

"To the extent that I have indicated I think that English Law must recognize a duty of the doctor to warn his patient of risk inherent in the treatment which he is proposing: and especially so, if the treatment be surgery. The critical limitation is that the duty is confined to material risk. The test of materiality is whether in the circumstances of the particular case the court is satisfied that a reasonable person in the patient's position would be likely to attach significance to the risk. Even if the risk be material, the doctor will not be liable if upon a reasonable assessment of his patient's condition he takes the view that a warning would be detrimental to his patient's health".

Para 24: Inter-alia, observing that the paradigm of the doctor-patient relationship, implicit in the speeches in Sidaway has ceased to reflect the reality and complexity of the way in which, healthcare services are now provided, or the way in which, the providers and recipients of such services view their relationship, as also a wider range of healthcare professionals now provide treatment and advice of one kind or another, it has been opined as under:

"86. It follows that the *analysis of the law by the majority in Sidaway is unsatisfactory, in so far as it treated the doctor's duty to advise her patient of the risks of proposed treatment as falling within the scope of the Bolam test, subject to two qualifications of that general principle, neither of which is fundamentally consistent with that test*. It is unsurprising that courts have found difficulty in the subsequent application of Sidaway, and that the courts in England and Wales have in reality departed from it; a position which was effectively endorsed, particularly by Lord Steyn, in Chester versus Afshar. *There is no reason to perpetuate the application of the Bolam test in this context any longer.*

87. The correct position, in relation to the risks of injury involved in treatment, can now be seen to be substantially that adopted in Sidaway by Lord Scarman An adult person of sound mind is entitled to decide which, if any, of the available forms of treatment to undergo, and her consent must be obtained before treatment interfering with her bodily integrity is undertaken. *The doctor is therefore under a duty to take reasonable care to ensure that the patient is aware of any material risks involved in any recommended treatment, and of any reasonable alternative or variant treatments.* The test of materiality is whether, in the circumstances of the particular case, a reasonable person in the patient's position would be likely to attach significance to the risk, or the doctor is or should reasonably be aware that the particular patient would be likely to attach significance to it.

88. The doctor is however entitled to withhold from the patient information as to a risk if he reasonably considers that its disclosure would be seriously detrimental to the patient's health. *The doctor is also excused from conferring with the patient in circumstances of necessity, as for example where the patient requires treatment urgently but is unconscious or otherwise unable to make a decision."* (Emphasis supplied by us)

Para 25: In view of the aforenoted significant development on the issue of informed consent in the country of origin of Bolam, as also adherence to Montgomery (Supra) approach by the Apex Courts in other Countries, including the SC of Canada and High Court of Australia, which seem to have also moved closer to Canterbury (supra) principle, perhaps, it is high time when the Honorable SC of India may have to take a relook at the concept or principle of "consent", "informed consent", or "real consent", whatever expression one may like to use. However, till the occasion arises, we shall examine the present case on the touchstone of the principles lucidly enunciated by a three-judge Bench of the Honorable SC in *Samira Kohli versus Dr Prabha Manchanda and Another* – (2008) 2 SCC 1, presently in vogue and has been applied subsequently by yet another three-judge Bench of the SC in *Nizam's Institute of Medical Sciences versus Prasanth S Dhananka and Others* – (2009) 6 SCC 1. On a bare reading of Samira Kohli (supra), we feel that it already has the flavor of Montgomery (Supra). Significantly, while rendering the decision in Samira Kohli (Supra) in the year 2008, the Honorable Bench had envisioned that in due course of time, Lord Scarman's minority view in Sidaway (Supra) would ultimately become the law in England and a beginning in that direction had already been made in *Bolitho versus City and Hackney Health Authority* – (1997) 4 All ER 771 (HL) and *Pearce versus United Bristol Healthcare NHS Trust* – (1999) ECC 167, which has now come true in Montgomery (Supra).

Para 26: In Samira Kohli (Supra), the principles, relating to consent, have been summarized as follows:
i. A doctor has to seek and secure the consent of the patient before commencing a 'treatment' (the term "treatment" includes surgery also). The consent so obtained should be real and valid, which means that: the patient should have the capacity and competence to consent; his consent should be voluntary; and his consent should be on the basis of adequate information concerning the nature of the treatment procedure, so that he knows what he is consenting to.
ii. The "adequate information" to be furnished by the doctor (or a member of his team) who treats the patient, should enable the patient to make a balanced judgment as to whether he should submit himself to the particular treatment or not. This means that the doctor should disclose (a) nature and procedure of the treatment and its purpose, benefits and effect; (b) alternatives if any available; (c) an outline of the substantial risks; and (d) adverse consequences of refusing treatment. But, there is no need to explain remote or theoretical risks involved, which may frighten or confuse a patient and result in refusal of consent for the necessary treatment. Similarly, there is no need to explain the remote or theoretical risks of refusal to take treatment which may persuade a patient to undergo a fanciful or unnecessary treatment. A balance should be achieved between the need for disclosing necessary and adequate information and at the same time avoid the possibility of the patient being deterred from agreeing to a necessary treatment or offering to undergo an unnecessary treatment.
iii. Consent given only for a diagnostic procedure, cannot be considered as consent for therapeutic treatment. Consent given for a specific treatment procedure will not be valid for conducting some other treatment procedure. The fact that the unauthorized additional surgery is beneficial to the patient, or that it would save considerable time and expense to the patient, or would relieve the patient from pain and suffering in future, are not grounds of defense in an action in tort for negligence or assault and battery. The only exception to this rule is where the additional procedure though unauthorized, is necessary in order to save the life or preserve the health of the patient and it would be unreasonable to delay such unauthorized procedure until patient regains consciousness and takes a decision.
iv. There can be a common consent for diagnostic and operative procedures where they are contemplated. There can also be a common consent for a particular surgical procedure and an additional or further procedure that may become necessary during the course of surgery.
v. The nature and extent of information to be furnished by the doctor to the patient to secure the consent need not be of the stringent and high degree mentioned in Canterbury but should be of the extent which is accepted as normal and proper by a body of medical men skilled and experienced in the particular field. It will depend upon the physical and mental condition of the patient, the nature of treatment, and the risk and consequences attached to the treatment".

Query: *An X-ray in an MLC has been reported 5 months after head injury as "of poor, un-reportable quality". Should I recall the patient for a fresh X-ray?*

Question: I was asked to report on the X-ray skull of an MLC. I am not a radiologist. I sent the X-rays to a radiologist in March. The radiologist received and reported the same in June. I received the report in August. The report said that the quality of the X-rays was too poor to be worth reporting.

CHAPTER 7 Medicolegal Issues in Emergency

My questions are:
- Have I acted in a proper manner?
- Should I recall the patient and get him re-X-rayed? Please note that 5 months have passed and any fracture, if present, would have fused by now.

Answered by Dr MC Gupta: It is not clear why the X-rays sent by you in March should have reached the radiologist in June. I assume that you sent the X-rays through the police and the delay was on the part of the police. I also assume that the police collected the X-ray report from the radiologist in June and brought it to you in August.
- It is possible that a radiologist would be able to find evidence of a fracture that has healed.
- What you should do is to send the final report to the police saying that the X-rays are of poor quality and cannot be reported upon. No further action lies on your part. If you wish, you may add, if so advise in writing by the radiologist, that a fresh X-ray can be performed and reported if the police gets a fresh X-ray done (it is not your responsibility to locate the patient and get an X-ray done and reported by the radiologist).
- You seem to be assuming the role of the investigating agency by offering to recall the patient for a fresh X-ray. You are assuming that you have such a right. You do not have such a right. As a doctor, your right and duty is to treat a patient when he presents for treatment. You have no right to ask a patient to make himself/herself available at your bidding for an X-ray. He is not your patient.
- If the above assumptions are correct, you have acted properly so far. You should not act proactively now by recalling the patient on your own.

Query: *I have been called by the court for an MLC with which I was not involved. The summons should have gone to another doctor. What should I do?*

Question: I was summoned to appear in the Magistrate's court for appearing as a witness in an MLC because I had allegedly reported an X-ray. The fact is that I was never involved in this case and I was summoned mistakenly. It seems that I share my first name (though not the surname) with the doctor who was actually involved in this case. When I went as summoned, the magistrate did not appear in the court that day. The public prosecutor told me that he would apprise the magistrate that I had attended the court and that he would apprise him of the concerned facts. I was summoned again, and I refused to accept the summons. My questions are:
- Did I do something illegal? If so, what are the implications?
- What is the way out?

Answered by Dr MC Gupta:
- Summon are issued by the court under court seal and are court's orders. The courts are very sensitive towards their power and respect. You did the right thing by appearing the first time. Verbal statements and assurances do not have any value in legal situations. You should have submitted to the court a written application, addressed to the court for being discharge as a witness in the case in view of the factual situation. You could have given the application, under acknowledgement, both to the court reader and the public prosecutor.
- As regards the second summons, it would have been better to accept it and do as told above. In the alternative, you could have written at the back of the summons as follows: "Not accepted because nobody by the name (say) Dr Arvind Kalra lives here. My name is Dr Arvind Sharma and I was never concerned with this case. It may be sent to the person concerned at his proper address".
- Now that you have refused to accept the summons, you need not fret about it. Nothing great will happen. It is possible you may be called by the court again. If you are so called, do as above.
- If you are in service, it is best to keep your boss in the picture and ask for his instructions.

Query: *Does free treatment in terms of the recent SC judgment include free treatment and medicines, etc.?*

Question: Please tell me what the implications of the recent SC judgment regarding free treatment of poor persons as regards the following are:
- Is it applicable all over India?
- Besides free indoor stay, does it also imply free investigations, medicines, implants, disposables, and diet?

Answered by Dr MC Gupta: I have not seen the full judgment. I believe the following is the correct response to your question:
- The judgment arose out of appeal by about 10 hospitals against the Delhi High Court order that hospitals which have been established with government subsidy like concessional land allotment should provide free treatment to poor patients subject to a limit of 10% for indoor and 25% for outdoor patients. Thus, it appears that the judgment is only in respect of the concerned hospital. However, the principles of the judgment may be relied upon by other States and High Courts.
- The judgment makes it clear that free means free in all respects. I am not sure whether the judgment specifically says anything about diet. As per legal principles and common sense, diet of a diseased person needs medical supervision and is part of treatment and hence should be free like the rest of the treatment.

Query: *When can a copy of the MLC report be issued to the accused?*

Please answer the following question. I have asked three different legal experts and they have given three different answers:

An *accused* wants an attested copy of MLR from the doctor. The doctor will issue the report:
A. On court order only
B. On order of the hospital higher authority only (Medical Superintendent/Head of Department)
C. Under the RTI Act
D. Can issue the report directly on application and deposit of fee
E. Any of the above
F. Any other procedure under law.

- **Answered by Dr MC Gupta:** As per rules, the MLR is prepared by the doctor for the police at the specific or deemed request of the police. To quote Modi, "MLRs are the documents prepared by medical officers in obedience to a demand by an authorized police officer or a magistrate". The original is to be given to the police and the copy is to be retained by the hospital. It is clear that the transaction is between the police and the hospital or doctor. All other parties are strangers to this transaction. The MLC report is an important document for investigation of crime and cannot be revealed to others without the permission of the authorities concerned, which are the state or the police and the court.
- As a matter of fact, if the applicant accused wants a copy of the MLC, it stands to common sense that the copy should be made from the original and not from a copy of the original. It is again logical that that the holder of the original should provide the copy. The practice of the hospital telling the accused to bring an NOC from the police before issuing a copy to the applicant is questionable. Since the original is supposed to be in the possession of the police, the police themselves should give a copy of the original to the applicant.
- None of the responses A to E is really correct. The logically correct answer is that "If an accused wants attested copy of the MLR, he should apply for such a copy to the holder of the original. The original is supposed to be with the police. However, if the original is with the hospital or doctor, a copy can be supplied as per court orders or on production of a No Objection Certificate from the police".

Refer: *The Public Information Officer (PIO) has to cite the Section under which an information is exempted under RTI. He is not supposed to verify the identity of the applicant (cannot ask whether the applicant is an accused or victim or else). I do not find any merit in the argument "It is again logical that the holder of the original should provide the copy and that the copy should be made from the original and not from a copy of the original"*

- I did not make any reference to the RTI in what I wrote. It is natural that all provisions or rules under the Act need to be followed.
- It is a matter of common sense and general legal principles, practice and conventions that a certified copy means a copy of the original and not a copy of another copy.

Query: *What are your comments about the Delhi Government's recent so called "Antiquackery advertisement"?*
The Directorate of Health services, Delhi Government, has recently published an advertisement titled "neem hakimon se saavadhaan". What are your comments about it?
Answered by Dr MC Gupta: My comments are as follows:
- This advertisement says the following two things:
  1. The public should get treatment for their diseases from qualified practitioners of allopathy, homeopathy, Ayurveda, Unani, or Dentistry.
  2. The list of such practitioners can be had from the Registrars of the respective Councils.
- I wonder what purpose this advertisement can serve in view of the following:
  - Even a moron knows that if he is feeling sick and is paying from his own pocket, he should get treatment from a qualified doctor if he can afford the same (if he cannot afford to pay, he will do one of the two things: (1) Firstly, he may go to a government facility where no quacks are employed, hence this advertisement does not help him. (2) Secondly, if the government services are not affordable, accessible, available, or satisfactory, he may have no option but to go to a quack who might provide cheaper services. In this case also this advertisement does not help him).
  - It is supposed to be an advertisement against quackery. It makes no mention and gives no caution regarding the biggest quackery prevalent in Delhi today—the practice of allopathy or modern medicine by Ayush practitioners.
  - A simple device to help people locate a qualified doctor in their area would be to refer them to a website where such information may be available, rather than the telephone numbers of departmental officials.
  - The simplest thing for the government would be to ensure that every practitioner displays clearly the following on his letterhead, etc. and in his clinic: "His authorized qualification; registration number; name of the registering council; specialty practiced (allopathy, homeopathy, Ayurveda, or Unani)". This can be enforced as per existing law. Is the IMA prepared to demand this from the government and to take necessary legal action regarding the same? The answer, apparently, is an obvious – No.

Query: *The CMO has the habit of "inspecting" all the case sheets written by other doctors. Is it legal?*
Question: The CMO of a private hospital has this habit of "inspecting" all the case sheets (OPD and IPD) of all other physicians claiming that she has ultimate authority to do so. Is it legal?
Answered by Dr MC Gupta: There is no illegality here. It is the right as well as duty of the CMO to ensure that all medical records are kept as per proper standards. Those doctors who do not keep proper records can thus be appropriately

advised or disciplined, if needed. After all, it is the CMO or hospital which will have to face the music when a case is filed in the court by a patient.

Query: *Digital signature in pathology report is valid or not? Many laboratory issues report on digital signature. Is it valid?*
Answered by Dr MC Gupta: I think it is valid as per IT Act, 2000.

I think people get confused in between digital signature and electronic signature. Normally, pathology laboratory reports have electronic signature only which is nothing but copy paste of a picture of the signature. Copy paste signature means nothing. It has no legal validity.

Technically the legal signature is a digital signature as per IT Act 2000, which is different. Digital signatures are of three types: Type 1, 2, and 3. It has a dongle and validity which needs to be renewed after that period. It can be issued by only two to three companies authorized by the government like TCS, etc. It is required by IT department to file returns online and also required in online trademark registration applications. This real digital signature is seldom used by pathology laboratories. I am yet to see any pathology report "digitally signed". These we can see normally in insurance policies, etc.

Query: *Is a postmortem necessary in proving death due to alleged medical negligence?*

Due to recent awareness in media about possible alleged medical negligence in many cases almost on a day-to-day basis from various corners in India, I would like to know what protocol is to be followed when a doctor handles any routine death which may later be claimed to be due to negligence.

What if patient party claims negligence say 1 month after cremation of body, without doing a postmortem? Can an FIR be filed without postmortem?

Is it the duty of treating doctor to counsel (and record in case paper) the patient party regarding need for postmortem in cases where the doctor feels or has high suspicion of possible claims for medical negligence by the party at a later date? What if party refuses to allow postmortem but still claims later of negligence? Is it not a win-win situation for patient party in cases of alleged medical negligence?

The name and fame of doctor is already at stake and lost, whereas the party has nothing to lose. Can there be a defamation case or something of that sort against the patient party?

Will courts decide on the number of patients lost by the doctor or percentage of practice lost by the doctor (due to alleged negligence) on a yearly basis, apart from tremendous mental agony or stress, till the number of years of practice available with the doctor in giving compensation to the doctor?

Has any doctor won a defamation suit in such cases and what is the amount?

In which situations do the patient's kins, the police, and treating doctors have the right to deny postmortem examination?

What are the conditions in which postmortem is mandatory and none of the above can deny it?

If patient's relatives or the police refuse postmortem examination, what losses patient party and treating doctor suffer or what benefits do they get in subsequent trial?
Answered by Dr MC Gupta:
- A dead body is nobody's property. This is a principle of law.
- There is no question of anybody having a right to refuse permission to the police to do a postmortem. If the police want to get postmortem done, relatives, etc. cannot object. The police are competent to get the postmortem without such objection.
- Whether a postmortem is needed or not will be decided by the police, not by others.
- The question of the police refusing to do a postmortem does not arise. They are not there to follow the wishes of a relative who wants the police to get postmortem done. It is the police who decide about the need or otherwise for the postmortem.

Query: *When postmortem should be avoided?*
Answered by Dr MC Gupta: When the cause of death has been given by the attending or treating medical practitioner in the Government Format of Medical Certification of Cause of Death (MCCD Form 4/4A). This will happen only when the police, *panch*, as well as relatives have no doubt in the cause of death given by the treating doctor.

Query: *When is a postmortem mandatory?*
Answered by Dr MC Gupta: When there is a doubt about the cause of death. All unnatural or suspicious deaths of a female who has died within 7 years of marriage (even though the treating doctor has given the cause of death in Form 4/4A).
- As per provisions under the Maharashtra Medical Civil Code and Hospital Manual, in any death reported within 24 hours of admission, it is mandatory to do a postmortem. This is a foolproof method that is in practice since 1870 and the proposal mooted has lot of gray areas, which cannot be accepted in totality. Also medical negligence cases will go unchallenged, without an autopsy.
- Medical board needs to be constituted to examine possible negligence in the case. The medical board will be constituted by the District Medical Officer (DMO), based on the request of the investigation officer. After checking evidence, the medical board will file a report stating whether the death occurred due to negligence on the part of the hospital authorities, doctors or medical staff, and then the police will register a case under Section-304 A of the IPC.

Query: *"What is the position in different states as with regards to section 10(1) (iii) of the Registration of Births and Deaths Act, 1969"?*

As per Section 10(1) of the Registration of Births and Deaths Act, 1969, "10(1). It shall be the duty of:

- The midwife or any other medical or health attendant at a birth or death,
- The keeper or the owner of a place set apart for the disposal of dead bodies or any person required by a local authority to be present at such place, or
- Any other person whom the State Government may specify in this behalf by his designation, to notify every birth or death or both at which he or she attended or was present, or which occurred in such areas as may be prescribed, to the Registrar within such time and in such manner as may be prescribed".

The above means that the hospital is not empowered to issue a death certificate to a person brought dead to the hospital unless any person in the hospital has been specified in this behalf by his designation in accordance with clause (iii) above.

The position as to whether any person in the hospital has been specified in this behalf by his designation in accordance with clause (iii) above the hospital can vary from state-to-state because "*Vital statistics including registration of births and deaths*" is, by virtue of entry 30, a subject included in list III (Concurrent list) of Schedule 7 of the Constitution.

Answered by Dr SK Roy Chaudhary: Attendant at a birth or death, law is same in every state for registration of birth and death. In a case where a person is brought dead to the hospital, there is no attendant of death and hence no reporting of death by the hospital. It will be done by the autopsy surgeon.

Query: *Is it the duty of the hospital authorities to issue a death certificate and send the death information to the Birth and Death Registrar when a patient is brought dead?*

A patient was brought to a private hospital. The hospital recorded the case as "Brought dead." No police information, MLC, or autopsy were done and the body was handed over to the relatives. The relatives demand that the hospital should issue a death certificate for their legal requirements pertaining to bank accounts and other money matters. My question is, "Is it the duty of the hospital in this case to issue a death certificate and to send the information about death to the Registrar of Births and Deaths?"

Answered by Dr MC Gupta : It was wrong on the part of the hospital not to inform the police and, having informed the police, not to register it as an MLC.

- Even otherwise, if a patient is brought dead to the hospital and the police is not informed and an MLC is not prepared for whatsoever reason, the hospital should maintain proper record of the case almost on the same lines as an MLC so that if at some time in future legal issues crop up and the hospital gets a notice in this regard, it should be able to give a proper and satisfactory reply.

- The hospital is not legally competent to issue a death certificate unless it is so authorized in terms of section 10(1) (iii) of the Registration of Births and Deaths Act, 1969. Section 10(1) is reproduced below:

  "10. (1) It shall be the duty of:
  i. The midwife or any other medical or health attendant at a birth or death,
  ii. The keeper or the owner of a place set apart for the disposal of dead bodies or any person required by a local authority to be present at such place, or
  iii. Any other person whom the State Government may specify in this behalf by his designation, to notify every birth or death or both at which he or she attended or was present, or which occurred in such areas as may be prescribed, to the Registrar within such time and in such manner as may be prescribed."

- Whether the hospital is thus empowered or not should be known to the hospital. If the hospital is not sure about this position, it should make necessary inquiry from the state health directorate to get a realistic official answer. The position can vary from state to state because "Vital statistics including registration of births and deaths" is, by virtue of entry 30, a subject included in list III (Concurrent list) of Schedule 7 of the Constitution.

The relatives' demand is without basis. They are trying to avoid their legal duty cast upon them in terms of section 8(1)(a) of the Registration of Births and Deaths Act, 1969. Section 8(1)(a) is reproduced below:

"8(1) It shall be the duty of the persons specified below to give or cause to be given, either orally or in writing, according to the best of their knowledge and belief, within such time as may be prescribed, information to the Registrar of the several particulars required to be entered in the forms prescribed by the State Government under sub-section (1) of section 16:

(a) in respect of births and deaths in a house, whether residential or non-residential, not being any place referred to in clauses (b) to (e), the head of the house or, in case more than one household live in the house, the head of the house-hold, the head being the person, who is so recognized by the house or the house-hold, and if he is not present in the house at any time during the period within which the birth or death has to be reported, the nearest relative of the head present in the house, and in the absence of any such person, the oldest adult male person present therein during the said period."

Query: *What is meant by a death certificate?*
Answered by Dr MC Gupta: The Registration of Births and Deaths Act, 1969, do not have the words "Death certificate".
- The above Act talks of two things:
  1. Notification of death
  2. Certificate as to the cause of death.

- The provisions of the Act concerning these two terms are reproduced below:

"10(1) It shall be the duty of:
(i) The midwife or any other medical or health attendant at a birth or death,
(ii) The keeper or the owner of a place set apart for the disposal of dead bodies or any person required by a local authority to be present at such place, or
(iii) Any other person whom the State Government may specify in this behalf by his designation, to notify every birth or death or both at which he or she attended or was present, or which occurred in such areas as may be prescribed, to the Registrar within such time and in such manner as may be prescribed".

10(2) In any area, the State Government, having regard to the facilities available therein in this behalf, may require that a certificate as to the cause of death shall be obtained by the Registrar from such person and in such form as may be prescribed.

10(3) Where the State Government has required under sub-section (2) that a certificate as to the cause of death shall be obtained, in the event of the death of any person who, during the last illness, was attended by a medical practitioner, the medical practitioner shall, after the death of that person, forthwith, issue without charging any fee, to the person required under this Act to give information concerning the death, a certificate in the prescribed form stating to the best of his knowledge and belief the cause of death; and the certificate shall be received and delivered by such person to the Registrar at the time of giving information concerning the death as required by this Act".

- The above means that in areas covered by section 10(2), the so called death certificate actually means, in terms of the Act, "Notification of death and certificate as to the cause of death". In other areas, what is required is merely a notification or information of death.

Query: *What is the definition of a consultant and the criteria for appointment and responsibilities in respect of a unit head?* Please answer the following queries:
a. Is there any legal definition of a consultant?
b. Is there any rule as to who can be appointed as the head of a ward or clinical unit in a hospital?
c. Under whose name a patient is supposed to be admitted?
d. Is it permissible to appoint as head of a clinical toxicology unit a person having the qualification of MBBS and the experience of heading an ICU unit for 12 years (please note that there is no Medical Council of India (MCI) recognized MD degree in Toxicology)?
e. What would be the legal liability of such person?

Answered by Dr MC Gupta : Legally speaking, as per http://definitions.uslegal.com/c/consultants/
1. "A consultant is someone who gives expert or professional advice".
2. "A consultant is an individual who possesses special knowledge or skills and provides that expertise to a client for a fee".
   a. Whom the employer can appoint as the head of a unit would be defined in the recruitment rules or eligibility criteria developed by the employing institution itself as per relevant norms and guidelines which can vary from place to place.
   b. As per the MCI guidelines, a patient is supposed to be admitted in the name of and under the unit incharge.
   c. The answer, read with (b) above, would be in the affirmative.
   d. The legal responsibility of any head of a unit in a hospital would include the fact that he/she would be answerable whenever an allegation of negligence in treatment is made in respect of a patient admitted in his unit.

Even an MBBS doctor is also entitled to call himself a "Physician" as per MCI definition.

Query: *What is the legal status of a foreign surgeon who comes for camps and conferences and does surgery there? What will be their responsibility regarding complications or misconduct? Should they take prior permission from MCI or local authority?*

Answered by Dr MC Gupta: Nobody can treat a patient in India unless he is registered with the medical council here. The foreign surgeons need to take a special short time or temporary registration with the MCI. Operating without such permission would be illegal.

- Foreigners should not venture illegally in their own interest. If they operate and a police complaint or FIR is registered against them for criminal negligence, they may have problem leaving the country and may even be arrested.
- Hospitals sponsoring such surgery will be fully liable in law for compensation and also for criminal negligence for allowing an unlicensed person to operate and causing harm.
- It is also possible, depending upon legal provisions, that a complaint alleging negligence may be made or referred to the foreign medical council where the surgeon is registered and the council may decide upon the complaint and take action against him.
- If a hospital thinks that getting a patient operated by the foreign surgeon but not showing his name as the person conducting the surgery in the medical records will save the hospital or the surgeon from the requirements or consequences mentioned above, this is a fallacy. It would be deemed as fraudulent on the part of the hospital.

Query: *What is the legal responsibility of an ambulance driver, especially when doing the following:*
- Doing rash driving and violating speed limits or crossing red lights, etc.
- Hitting any vehicle and no casualty happened

- Hitting any vehicle and injury to a man or death of a person.

What are the privileges to him/her?

Query: *Are there any special requirements for ambulance driver license or some extra qualification needed?*
Can he use mobile while driving?
Answered by Dr MC Gupta: Ambulance driver is licensed to drive heavy motor vehicles; he should be trained in basic life-support.
If he jumps red light and injures someone, than he is liable to pay the compensation as per Motor Vehicles Act. Mobile can be used in speaker mode on screen stand in car screen, for getting directions to reach the patient.

Query: *Is consent of the patient or relatives required for labeling the case as MLC?*
Answered by Dr MC Gupta: Consent of the patient or relatives is not required for labeling the case as MLC. In fact, even if the patient is stressing that he does not want an MLC, it should still be made.

For example, consider a case of suicidal poisoning. Suicide is an offence u/s 309 IPC. Patient insists that he/she does not want an MLC. If the doctor agrees to the patient's request, it is like agreeing to a criminal requesting him not to give evidence regarding his crime to the police. Doctor's MLC with relevant history from the patient is a piece of evidence that a crime u/s 309 IPC has been committed. If the doctor does not inform the police, and does not hand over the MLC to the police, he may be sued u/s 201 IPC (causing disappearance of evidence of an offence). However, consent for examination would still be required because the patient is not arrested at that point in time.

Thus a possibility exists, when a person reports to a doctor after, say, failing in an attempt to commit suicide → insists that he does not want an MLC → the doctor, however, proceeds to inform the police → Patient begins to leave → Doctor cannot legally stop him → Since in this situation, the doctor has not treated him, nor has he collected any evidence from his person, he is now a member of general public and must act in accordance with Section 39(1) in (CrPC), and may not inform the police. If, however, the patient stays on and the doctor collects evidence from his person (gastric lavage, etc.), it becomes his duty to pass on this evidence to the police (s201 IPC).

Query: *Can private practitioners (PPs) make an MLC?*
Answered by Dr MC Gupta: Private practitioners can make an MLC. The practice by PPs of sending patients to government hospitals for getting registered as MLCs is wrong. If the patient is serious, and dies on the way to government hospital, the PPs can be sued u/s 304A IPC. Treatment in serious cases must take precedence over completion of the injury report. Injury report can be completed after patient has stabilized **(Table 2)**.

Table 2 Distinction in the process of medicolegal case (MLC) and nonmedicolegal case (non-MLC)

MLC	Non-MLC
Information to police must be sent	No such information to police
Report must be made in duplicate, one copy of which is handed over to the police, and his signatures taken on doctor's copy. The other copy is retained with the doctor, which he may have to produce before the court. This copy is retained in a register called a "Medicolegal Register." This register is a confidential record, and should be in the safe custody of the doctor only	Report made as a single copy only
Both copies of the report must be marked "medicolegal case" in bold. In X-ray requisition slips and other lab report slips, similar markings should be made	No such mark made
Report, X-rays, etc., not to be handed over to the patient. They are handed over to the police	Report, X-rays etc., handed over to the patient
Detailed personal entries must be made. Please see below under the column "Entries to be made in an injury report"	Not required
Example: Stab wounds, lacerated wounds, fractures, bruises, abrasions, etc.	Example: Asthmatic attack, myocardial infarction (MI), status epilepticus, etc.

Referral to a second hospital: If a case has been labeled as MLC, and has been referred to another hospital, it is in second doctor's interest to make a fresh MLC (second MLC), so as to record meticulously his own findings. It is because when he is summoned in the court, he has to go by his own findings.

Dead on arrival ("brought dead" cases): All cases which are pronounced dead on arrival at hospital must be labeled as MLC and the police should be informed.

Query: *I am an anesthetist. A stillbirth occurred. An FIR has been filed against me and the gynecologist alleging that cesarean should have been done. Should I apply for an anticipatory bail?*
On 18 August 2011, a nonrailway woman was admitted, without permission, under the gynecologist at Railway Divisional Hospital where I am working as an anesthetist. On 19th August, an ultrasound revealed mild fetal ascites. On 20th morning, the treating gynecologist was out of station on leave and I was away on official training at Railway HQ. Another gynecologist examined the patient and could not find fetal heart sound (FHS) and referred the patient to an outside or nonrailway hospital where stillbirth took place on 20th night. An allegation of negligence was made because

cesarean section delivery was not done, though it should have been done and the baby could have been saved. An FIR was registered against the gynecologist who was on leave and against me.

What are the legal aspects? Should I Seek an anticipatory bail?

Answered by Dr MC Gupta: The first legal aspect is that of an anticipatory bail.

1. The SC held as follows in the Jacob Mathew case [*Jacob Mathew versus State of Punjab and Another, SC, decided on 05/08/2005 (by CJI RC Lahoti, GP Mathur and PK Balasubramanyan, reported as 2005), 6 SCC 1*, 2005 SCCL. COM 456]

   In view of the principles laid down hereinabove and the preceding discussion, we agree with the principles of law laid down in Dr Suresh Gupta's case (2004) 6 SCC 422 and reaffirm the same. Ex-abundanti cautela, we clarify that what we are affirming are the legal principles laid down and the law as stated in Dr Suresh Gupta's case. We may not be understood as having expressed any opinion on the question whether on the facts of that case the accused could or could not have been held guilty of criminal negligence as that question is not before us. We also approve of the passage from Errors, Medicine and the Law by Alan Merry and Alexander McCall Smith which has been cited with approval in Dr Suresh Gupta's case (noted vide para 27 of the report).

   As we have noticed hereinabove that the cases of doctors (surgeons and physicians) being subjected to criminal prosecution are on an increase. Sometimes such prosecutions are filed by private complainants and sometimes by the police on an FIR being lodged and cognizance taken. The investigating officer and the private complainant cannot always be supposed to have knowledge of medical science so as to determine whether the act of the accused medical professional amounts to rash or negligent act within the domain of criminal law under Section 304-A of IPC. The criminal process once initiated subjects the medical professional to serious embarrassment and sometimes harassment. He has to seek bail to escape arrest, which may or may not be granted to him. At the end, he may be exonerated by acquittal or discharge but the loss which he has suffered in his reputation cannot be compensated by any standards. We may not be understood as holding that doctors can never be prosecuted for an offence of which rashness or negligence is an essential ingredient. All that we are doing is to emphasize the need for care and caution in the interest of society; for, the service which the medical profession renders to human beings is probably the noblest of all, and hence there is a need for protecting doctors from frivolous or unjust prosecutions. Many a complainant prefers recourse to criminal process as a tool for pressurizing the medical professional for extracting uncalled for or unjust compensation. Such malicious proceedings have to be guarded against.

   Statutory Rules or Executive Instructions incorporating certain guidelines need to be framed and issued by the Government of India and/or the State Governments in consultation with the MCI. So long as it is not done, we propose to lay down certain guidelines for the future which should govern the prosecution of doctors for offences of which criminal rashness or criminal negligence is an ingredient. A private complaint may not be entertained unless the complainant has produced prima facie evidence before the court in the form of a credible opinion given by another competent doctor to support the charge of rashness or negligence on the part of the accused doctor. The investigating officer should, before proceeding against the doctor accused of rash or negligent act or omission, obtain an independent and competent medical opinion preferably from a doctor in government service qualified in that branch of medical practice who can normally be expected to give an impartial and unbiased opinion applying Bolam's test to the facts collected in the investigation. A doctor accused of rashness or negligence, may not be arrested in a routine manner (simply because a charge has been leveled against him). Unless his arrest is necessary for furthering the investigation or for collecting evidence or unless the investigation officer feels satisfied that the doctor proceeded against would not make himself available to face the prosecution unless arrested, the arrest may be withheld.

2. Please note specifically the following in the above quotation, "The investigating officer should, before proceeding against the doctor accused of rash or negligent act or omission, obtain an independent and competent medical opinion preferably from a doctor in government service qualified in that branch of medical practice who can normally be expected to give an impartial and unbiased opinion applying Bolam's test to the facts collected in the investigation. A doctor accused of rashness or negligence, may not be arrested in a routine manner (simply because a charge has been leveled against him). Unless his arrest is necessary for furthering the investigation or for collecting evidence or unless the investigation officer feels satisfied that the doctor proceeded against would not make himself available to face the prosecution unless arrested, the arrest may be withheld".

3. In view of the above, if the FIR has been registered by the police without getting expert opinion, it is in violation of the law as laid down by the SC and this should be an adequate ground to get the FIR quashed.

4. Anticipatory bail is meant for arrest by the police to be prevented even before court orders it. In view of the above judgment, you should not be arrested, and hence

the question of applying for anticipatory bail should not arise. You do not need to apply for anticipatory bail. You will simply be wasting your money and making the lawyer richer.
5. If the FIR does not get quashed, the case will come up for hearing in the court. When the case comes for hearing in the court, you should tell the court as follows:
"I have been wrongly implicated in this case. I am an anesthetist. My job is to give anesthesia when a surgeon operates upon a patient. No surgery was done in this case and therefore I had no role and I was never called to give anesthesia. The question of my negligence does not arise. The FIR has been wrongly filed against me. In the circumstances of the case that I had no role in the treatment of this patient, it is requested that I may be given exemption from personal appearance in this case".

The second legal aspect is that of medical negligence.
1. It will depend upon what expert report is available to the police. The usual practice is that the police may seek opinion from a government hospital or the medical council. It is possible that adverse opinion may be given by the experts because:
   a. No action was taken by the hospital even though ultrasound was abnormal.
   b. When no FHSs were heard, it was an emergency. The other gynecologist should have taken necessary measures. If she was not sure or confident, and the patient needed to be sent to some other hospital, she should have arranged emergency treatment at the other hospital and the railway hospital should have made arrangements for emergency transfer to the other hospital.
2. It appears that the hospital or doctors were not serious about performing their duties because of the reasons that she was a nonrailway patient and had been admitted without necessary formalities. These reasons are not valid in law and the court is likely to hold the hospital or its doctors guilty.

Query: *What are the legal aspects of a robotic surgery done upon a patient in India by a foreign surgeon sitting abroad in his chamber?*

Answered by Dr MC Gupta: Since the patient is admitted in India in a hospital under the care of a surgeon who is present in the operation theater to carry out: preoperative management; intraoperative management including necessary surgery and coordination and assistance in collaboration with the foreign expert; and, postoperative management, the patient will be entitled to sue the hospital and the surgeon in India for compensation, etc.

- The consent should be obtained after giving necessary information to the patient about the name of the foreign surgeon and the nature of the surgery.
- Necessary permission from the MCI should be taken because this would involve surgery in India by a doctor not registered with the MCI.
- The hospital and the surgeon should be adequately covered by professional indemnity insurance.

CONCLUSION

There is no doubt that advances in medicine have improved the quality of healthcare being provided to the patients. However, there has also been rise in unrealistic expectations from the physicians. Many times patients are not willing to accept anything less than complete recovery. The allegation of medical negligence is a stressful event for every physician, and even if the physician is not found guilty of medical negligence, a lot of suffering has already occurred. It is extremely important for physicians to understand the meaning, scope and legal interpretation of the term "medical negligence" so as to face the problem head on.

BIBLIOGRAPHY

1. Aggrawal A. Salient features regarding medicolegal certificate. MAMC J Med Sci [serial online]. 2015;1:45-51.
2. Baby Geetha and Ors. vs Cosmopolitan Hospitals (P) Ltd. III CPJ 89 (NC). 2006.
3. Bernard Knight. Knight's Forensic Pathology, 4th edition. New Delhi: Jaypee Brothers Medical Publishers (P) Ltd; 2016.
4. G Vivekananda Varma vs Chinta Bharamaramba and Ors. III CPJ 104 (NC). 2006.
5. Ganesh Prasad and Anr. vs Lal Janamajay Nath Shahdeo. I CPJ 117 (NC). 2006.
6. Indian Medical Association vs V.P. Shantha and Ors. 1996 AIR 550, 1996 AIR 550, 1995 SCC (6) 651. 1996.
7. Joint Commission International (JCI). International Patient Safety Goals. [online] Available from *http://www.jointcommissioninternational.org/improve/international-patient-safety-goals/* [Accessed January, 2017].
8. Laws of India. (2008). Delhi Medicare Service Personnel and Medicare Service Institutions (Prevention of Violence and Damage to Property) Act, 2008. [online] Available from http://www.lawsofindia.org/statelaw/2819/The Delhi Medicare Service Personnel and Medicare Service Institutions Prevention of Violence and Damageto Property Act 2008.html [Accessed January, 2017].
9. Laxman Balkrishna Joshi versus Trimbak Bapu Godbole and Anr. 1969 SCR (1) 206.
10. Medicolegal Queries answered by Dr MC Gupta. (2011). [online] Available from *https://in.groups.yahoo.com/neo/groups/medico-legal-queries* [Accessed January, 2017].

11. Mrs. Shantaben Muljibhai Patel and others vs Breach Candy Hospital & Research. 4 SCC 332. 1996.
12. Nihal Kaur vs Director, PGIMER. 1996 (3) CPJ 112. 1996.
13. Peter Ubel. (2013). Malpractice claims in multidisciplinary hospital in 2013 in USA. [online] Available from *www.kevinmd.com/blog/2013/08/medical-malpractice-claims-drag-long.html* [Accessed January, 2017].
14. Poonam Verma vs Ashwin Patel & Ors. 1996 SCC (4) 332. 1996
15. Satish Tiwari. Medicolegal Issues Related to Various Medical Specialties. New Delhi: Jaypee Brothers Medical Publishers (P) Ltd; 2012.
16. Sharma RK. Medicolegal Tips of Day [online]. Available from *www.smlps.in* [Accessed February 2017].
17. Sharma RK. Textbook of Medicolegal Aspects of Patient Care. New Delhi: PeePee Publishers; 2008.
18. Singh VP, Vivekanshu. Legal issues in Medical Practice: Medicolegal Guidelines for Safe Practice, 1st edition. New Delhi: Jaypee Brothers Medical Publishers (P) Ltd; 2016.

Disclaimer: Although every effort is made to give correct knowledge but legality of every answer cannot be guaranteed, all answers are based on our professional knowledge. It is brought to notice that since health is on concurrent list and both central government and state government can legislate on it, there are many variations in different states on health policy.

CHAPTER 8

Patient Safety and Quality in Emergency Department

Devendra Richhariya, Sudhir S Pawaiya

INTRODUCTION

Patient safety means safety within the entire healthcare system or in other words "the prevention of errors and adverse effects to patients associated with health care". Patient safety is a serious topic for all healthcare system around the globe. In any healthcare system, patient safety is the fundamental of good patient care. Health care can harm as well as heal so that patient safety is the key of healthcare quality system. Patient safety and good quality are interrelated.

Awareness about patient safety is the basic of all patient care. This is much more important for emergency department (ED) because of high numbers of different categories of patients, staff and various dramatic situations.

Emergency department provides, 24 hours a day, timely care to seriously ill or injured patient. The main aim is to provide safe care to patients and maintain efficient patient flow. Poor patient flow can compromise patient safety.

Working in ED is unique experience because of several diagnostic and therapeutic challenges. Most patients come to an ED having symptoms with complex diagnosis and need immediate lifesaving intervention. So, it is very necessary that professionals working in ED should be highly qualified and well trained so that high-quality safe care can be delivered. The high number of patient's inflow increases the probability of poor treatment and long waiting periods, compromise patient safety and reduces patient satisfaction. Crowding makes the working environment poor and is related to high staff mobility and turnover rate; both adversely affect patient safety and quality.

TRIAGING AND SMOOTH FLOW OF EMERGENCY DEPARTMENT

Aim is to prioritize the medical or surgical condition of the patient according to severity and to provide appropriate lifesaving care **(Flow chart 1 and Fig. 1)**.

Objectives are:
- To triage all incoming patients
- To have patients assessed by qualified individuals
- To diagnose, treat, admit and provide appropriate referral and follow-up
- To ensure critically ill patients receive the top priority care as determined by triage guidelines
- To initiate lifesaving treatment
- To provide end of life care
- To identify the common errors in emergency department described in **Table 1**.

GOOD QUALITY TRAINED EMERGENCY TEAM

Implementing the skilled triage team with a specialist emergency physician in the front line provides the best quality and safety to patients. Role of the emergency physician is to rule out serious or life-threatening cause and consequences of patient presentation not to arrive at the definitive diagnosis **(Fig. 2)**. Emergency team should have sound knowledge and skills of emergency aspect of medical and surgical specialties and their application within golden hour, competent in life saving emergency interventions and appropriate use of various diagnostic tests and interpret their results intelligently and promptly. Implementation of clear and short decision pathways improves the understanding between physicians and other team members lead to increased patient safety. Relieve the physical, physiological and psychological pain before discharge. Discharge summary should have specific follow-up instruction.

Teamwork

Improvement in efficiency and quality measures can be seen when the staff works in team. Teamwork has positive effects on the work environment by reducing stress. Improvement in safety and quality when staff members know their roles

CHAPTER 8 Patient Safety and Quality in Emergency Department

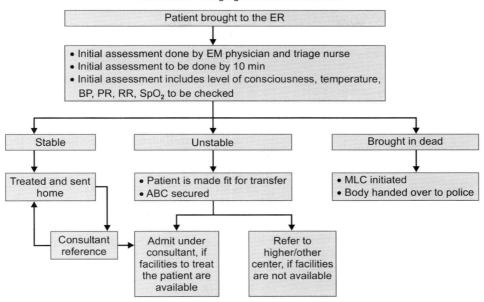

Flow chart 1 Triaging and smooth flow of ED

Abbreviations: ED, emergency department; ER, emergency room; BP, blood pressure; PR, pulse rate; RR, respiratory rate; SpO$_2$, peripheral capillary oxygen saturation; ABC, airway, breathing, circulation; MLC, medicolegal cases; EM physician, emergency physician.

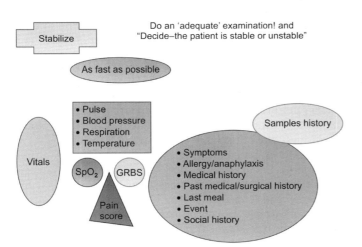

Fig. 1 Flow of care in emergency department

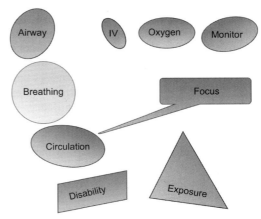

Fig. 2 Identification of life-threatening signs

and team communicate in a proper way. Team training is needed to develop efficient and effective teams.

Role of a Team Leader

- The team leader gives a message, order, or assignment to a team member.
- By receiving clear response and eye contact, the team leader confirms that the team member heard and understood the message.
- The team leader listens for confirmation of task performance from the team before assigning another task.
- The team leader organizes the group and monitors individual performance of team members.
- He should back up members of his team, models excellent team behavior and should train and give coaching to his team members.
- He should facilitates understanding and focuses on comprehensive patient care.

Table 1 Common errors and their conditions in emergency department (ED)

Common errors in ED	Conditions in which high possibilities of errors
• Delay in diagnosis • Failure to diagnose • Misdiagnosis • Failure to monitor patients • Discharging patient who need emergency care • Prescribing wrong medicine or treatment • Misinterpretation of the laboratory reports and medical records	• Heart attack • Aneurysm • Aortic dissection • Pulmonary embolism • Stroke • Appendicitis • Pancreatitis • Ectopic pregnancy • Missed injuries in polytrauma

- He must be clear about role assignment and always be prepared to fulfill their role responsibilities.
- He should be well practiced in resuscitation skills and must be knowledgeable about algorithms.
- He should be committed to success.

TIMELY SUPPORT BY SPECIALTIES

Timely clinical opinion by specialist to patient ensure a high-quality and safe ED. Prolong waiting time in the ED (on hospital trolleys) due to delay in laboratory report or radiology investigations or waiting for specialist opinion or lack of inpatient beds can increase morbidity and mortality. Emergency physician must ensure timely appropriate referral to senior clinical decision makers, to improve the flow of the ED. Good relationship with supporting specialties is the key for ED.

Ten most important supporting specialties for ED are critical care team, chest pain unit, stroke team, trauma team, pediatrics, orthopedics, general surgery, radiology, laboratory services and blood bank. Ideally these specialties should be on speed dial for quick communication. There should be clear policies and procedures to ensure rapid access to senior clinical decision maker of that particular speciality and after assessment transfer to inpatient bed as soon as possible.

IMPORTANT DIAGNOSTICS AREAS NEAR EMERGENCY DEPARTMENT

To provide better quality and better outcomes in ED to patients, it is important that the key diagnostic area, like laboratory, blood bank, and radiology area are situated near the ED.

The quality of ED depends on timely access to diagnostics and investigations which are essential for clinical diagnosis. Early access to appropriate imaging [computed tomography (CT), ultrasound and plain radiography] allows immediate investigation of potentially life-threatening conditions and timely intervention if needed. Immediate reporting by radiologist and laboratory is a key in decision making.

OBSERVATION AREAS

Observation areas in ED improve patient care and nowadays these facilities are an integral part of emergency medicine. Observation unit allows time to investigate the patient in a better way. Observation unit is used as an alternative to inpatient admission for a period of 4–12 hours so that patients with shorter expected recovery time can be investigated and treated. These units also allow time to investigate and to safely rule out serious diagnoses preventing both unsafe discharges and inpatient admissions. Overall, observation areas can provide patients with cost-effective shorter lengths of stay. These areas are most effective when they are exclusively managed by emergency medicine doctors and nurses with clear protocols.

Reception, Administration and Information Technology Support

Reception and administrative support should be available all the time in EDs as these require rapid registration and timely recording of information and electronic access to previous records to ensure high-quality service. EDs should have the latest and adequate information technology (IT) systems to support this. It is essential that every patient who attends an ED should have an electronic patient attendance and discharge summary.

Transfer Policy

Clear referral and transfer policy for patients improve quality of ED and provide safety to the patient. Extra care should be given to the critically ill patient while transferring to CT, magnetic resonance imaging (MRI) or intensive care unit. Adverse events like dislodgement of endotracheal tube can occur. Ambulance transfer of patient is also integral but challenging part for the ED. Ambulance handover delay can cause an adverse impact on patient's experience and may increase the risk to patient safety **(Flow chart 2)**.

Communication

Communication failure is the common risk for patient safety, especially during change in shift duties, handover and transfer of patient to ward, ICU or operation theater, and shift change is a critical moment. Good communication steps are listening, explaining, asking, recommending and negotiating. Implementing the various checklist and handover document reduces the communication-failure risk. Effective communication is fundamental for good quality health care. Positive exchange of information and feelings develops good

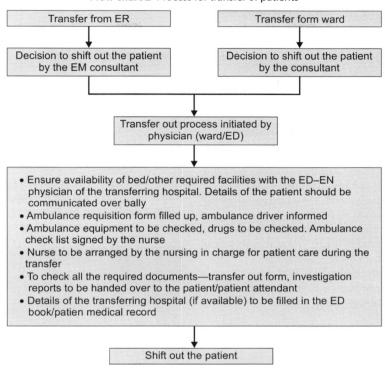

Flow chart 2 Process for transfer of patients

Abbreviations: ED, emergency department; ER, emergency room; EM physician, emergency physician.

relationship between the patient and ED staff. Patient-centered approach and proper dissemination of specific information about ED services are good communication strategies. Regular training session for emergency staff should be conducted about active listening, understanding, nonverbal and verbal messages, and building *trusting relationships and open communication* with patients. Training sessions for improving verbal communication (spoken word, spoken language) and nonverbal communications (voice quality like manner of speaking and loudness, and gesture like body language and posture) are helpful in improving patient satisfaction rate in ED.

Overcrowding

Overcrowding is the most common leading problem and patient safety risk at the ED. When an extreme number of persons or patients are present in treatment areas beyond the capacity and demand for emergency service exceeds the existing capabilities within reasonable amount of time. Crowding increases the workload and limits the ability to monitor the patients and compromise patient safety. There should be adequate space for all members of the ED team and patients; to protect, confidentiality, privacy and dignity. There should be separate areas within the ED for children, both for waiting and treatment. Poor patient flow associated with a lack of support from inpatient specialties. Overcrowding has a significant impact on critically ill patients. Crowding can result in a dysfunctional ED and is associated with longer waiting time, increased delays in admission and transmission of infectious diseases.

Confidentiality and Privacy

> *"What I may see or hear in the course of treatment or even outside of treatment in regard to the life of men, I will keep to myself."*
> —**Hippocrates**

MEDICATIONS AND SEDATION SAFETY

- High-risk medication should be kept under double lock
- Preparation and administration of drug only after verification by another nurse or doctor
- Verbal order for administration of drugs to be followed only in code blue or life-threatening situation. Follow "read back" procedure in verbal orders.

Monitoring of patient during and post-sedation:
- Patient should be on continuous vitals monitoring device during sedation
- Vitals to be documented during sedation
- Post-sedation vitals to be monitored till patient meets discharge criteria and is discharged
- To be discharged after sedation only if discharge criteria met.

Infection Control in Emergency Department

- All emergency physician and nursing staff should undergo training and follow infection control procedures laid down by the infection control department
- Since ED is one of the high-risk area, standard precautions should be taken by the staff at all times
- Equipment cleaning and sterilization should be supervised. Swabs should be taken from the different areas and screened for nosocomial pathogens
- Follow hand-wash procedure regularly (**Fig. 3**).

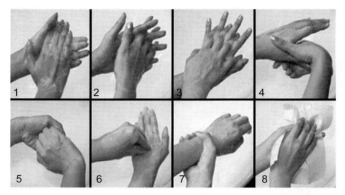

Fig. 3 Procedure of hand wash. 1. Palm to palm; 2. Between fingers; 3. Back of hands; 4. Base of thumbs; 5. Back of fingers; 6. Fingernails; 7. Wrists; 8. Rinse and wipe dry

Others Steps to Improve Safety in ED

- *Correct identification of patient*: Use two identifiers but should not include room number or bed number; use white band with specific information (**Fig. 4**)
- Consent with patient for every new procedure, treatment, intervention and surgery
- *Comprehensive prescription*: Avoid writing short terms in prescription
- Coordinate with duty nurse for administration of written orders
- Correct dose, correct route, correct time, correct patient
- Carefully correlate laboratory and radiology reports with clinical findings
- Cooperate with colleagues by proper handover of patient's condition during duty change
- Consult with latest medical literature
- Communicate with patient's attendants about line of treatment
- Complimenting the patient's efforts in following doctor's advice honestly
- Counseling patient and their attendants while breaking bad news
- Confidentiality about discussing patient's personal details in public place
- Condemn unfair trade practice
- Checkup and follow-up patient regularly
- Call patients to emergency, if laboratory or radiological findings are critical in outpatient department check-up
- Care and concern about patient safety, privacy and security
- Call legal helpline—police in doubt of suspected medico-legal case
- Complete documentation of medical records timely

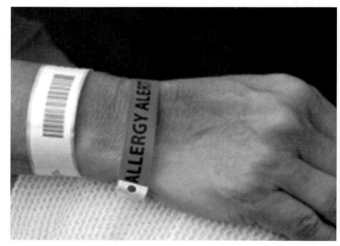

Fig. 4 Identification band for patients
Courtesy: To Patients and attendants, while meeting first time.

- Cross check audit daily to prevent missing out illnesses and injuries
- Conflict resolution with agitated patients by negotiation
- Continue medical training regularly to promote use safe techniques (workshops)
- *Correct disposal of waste*: Using colored biomedical waste disposal bags (**Fig. 5**).

Safety and Quality in ED and Medicolegal Aspect

Over the years, there are lots of changes in the medical practice in the ED; these changes are due to various reasons like consumerization of patient, commercialization of medical education, corporatization of hospitals, commodification of healthcare. All these changes lead to malpractice allegations. Providing safety and quality care to patients protect doctors from malpractice suits.

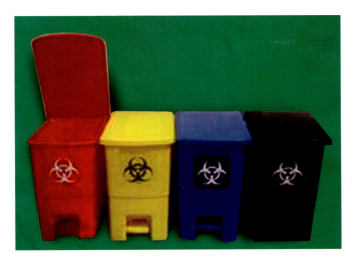

Fig. 5 Implementation of various color codes for waste disposal

Box 1 List of Indian laws

Promote ethical practice	Regulate unethical practice
• Epidemic Diseases Act, 1897 • Mental Health Act, 1987 • CEA 2010 • Medical Council Act, 1956 • Nursing Council Act, 1946 • Pharmacy Act, 1948 • Drug and Cosmetic Act, 1940 • Infant Milk Substitutes, 1992 • Biomedical Waste Management 1998 • Environment Protection Act, 1986 • Registration of Birth and Death Act 1969	• Medical Termination of Pregnancy Act, 1971 • Pre-conception and Pre-natal Diagnostic Techniques Act, 1994 • Human Organs Transplantation Act, 1994 • Narcotic Drugs and Psychotropic Substance, 1985 • Drugs and Magical Remedies Act, 1954 • Consumer Protection Act, 1986 • Indian Medical Council Regulation, 2002

Indian Medical Acts and Patient's Safety

- Drugs and Cosmetics Act, 1940: Quality of drugs, stents
- Drugs and Magic Remedies Act, 1954 (Objectionable Advertisements)
- Medicinal and Toilet Preparations Act, 1955
- Indian Medical Council Act, 1956—Quackery
- Consumer Protection Act, 1986 (COPRA)—Negligence
- Narcotic Drugs and Psychotropic Substances Act, 1985 (Narcotics)
- Transplantation of Human Organs Act, 1994
- Persons with Disabilities Act, 1995
- Clinical Establishments Act, 2010.

Indian Laws for Patient's Safety

Indian laws have been listed in **Box 1**.

CONCLUSION

The ED is the first impression of a hospital for patients and their relatives, in view of high-risk specialty implementing the various measures that ensures the patient safety in ED.

BIBLIOGRAPHY

1. Berwick DM. Continuous improvement as an ideal in health care. N Engl J Med. 1989;320:53-6.
2. Brook RH. Quality—can we measure it? N Engl J Med. 1977;296:170-2.
3. Chassin MR, Galvin RW. The urgent need to improve health care quality. Institute of Medicine National Roundtable on Health Care Quality. JAMA. 1998;280: 1000-5.
4. Donabedian A. Evaluating the quality of medical care. Milbank Q. 1966;44(3, suppl):166-206.
5. Eddy DM. Clinical decision making: from theory to practice. Guidelines for policy statements: the explicit approach. JAMA. 1990;263:2239-40, 2243.
6. James BC. Improving quality can reduce costs. Qual Assur Rev. 1989;1(1):4.
7. Millenson ML. Demanding Medical Excellence. Chicago: University of Chicago Press, 1997. p. 142.
8. Milstein A, Galvin RS, Delbanco SF, Salber P, Buck CR Jr. Improving the safety of health care: the Leapfrog Initiative. Eff Clin Pract. 2000;3(6):313-6.
9. ORYX requirements simplified. Jt Comm Perspect. 1999; 19(3):4.
10. Schneider EC, Riehl V, Courte-Wienecke S, Eddy DM, Sennett C. Enhancing performance measurement: NCQA's road map for a health information framework. National Committee for Quality Assurance. JAMA. 1999; 282:1184-90.

CHAPTER 9

Standards of Care during Air Transfer

Saleh Fares, Michael J Nolan

INTRODUCTION

The use of rotary wing and fixed wing aircraft in the transfer of patients has increased in popularity in recent years. The utilization of helicopters as air ambulances is beneficial due to the speed of transfer of a specialist medical team to the scene of the patient and subsequent transport to specialist hospital. This is especially important in urban areas where traffic congestion may hamper necessary resources **(Fig. 1)**. The use of fixed wing aircraft to transfer patients is required where the distance is greater and is advantageous due to the ability of longer distance and speed, however disadvantages include secondary transfers from airport and landing strip to hospital.

The air transfer of patients can generally be described into three phases (Martin, 2003):

1. *Primary transfer*: An air ambulance is used to transport a medical team to the scene of an accident or location of a patient. The patient is then transferred to an appropriate facility dependent on specific patient requirement and local specialist centers. This air transfer is usually undertaken by helicopter and flight times are usually short.
2. *Secondary transfer*: Fixed wing or rotary wing aircraft are used to transfer patients who require an advanced level of care. This transfer is usually from a clinic or hospital where medical treatment has been started but the patient requires treatment or intervention at a specialist facility. Fixed wing or rotary wing aircraft can undertake this.
3. *Tertiary transfer*: A patient is transferred by air from one facility to another usually for definitive care. This includes international transfer of patients who require repatriation to their home country after illness or injury. This is usually undertaken on fixed wing aircraft including commercial jets.

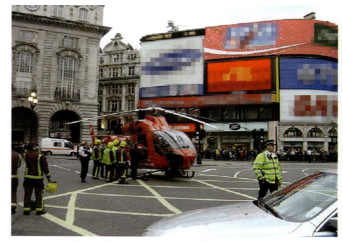

Fig. 1 Rotary wing air transfer in urban area
Source: London's air ambulance.

The decision to transfer a patient by air has several factors, including the current pathophysiology of the patient/intervention requirements, the training and expertise of the medical transport team, location of the aircraft and distance to the patient and hospitals or facilities. Patients who have time-critical injury or illness and require life-saving interventions can benefit most from air transfer. These include conditions such as polytrauma, myocardial infarction, severe burns, surgery, premature neonates, intra-aortic balloon pump, extracorporeal membrane oxygenation and many more.

Many important equipment are required for transfer of the critically ill patients, and these equipment ensure safe transfer of the patient. **Boxes 1 and 2** show various important equipment.

Box 1 Supplementary equipment for use during transport

Airway
- Guedel airways (assorted sizes)
- Laryngeal masks (assorted sizes)
- Tracheal tubes (assorted sizes)
- Laryngoscopes (spare bulbs and battery)
- Intubating stylet
- Lubricating gel
- Magill's forceps
- Tape for securing tracheal tube
- Sterile scissors
- Stethoscope

Ventilation
- Self-inflating bag and mask with oxygen reservoir and tubing
- High flow breathing circuit
- Spare valves for portable ventilator
- Chest drains (assorted sizes)
- Heimlich flutter valves

Suction
- Yankauer sucker
- Suction catheters (assorted sizes)
- Nasogastric tubes (assorted sizes) and drainage bag

Circulation
- Syringes (assorted sizes)
- Needles (assorted sizes)
- Alcohol wipes
- IV cannulae (assorted sizes)
- Arterial cannulae (assorted sizes)
- Central venous cannulae
- Intravenous fluids
- Infusion sets/extensions
- 3 way taps
- Dressings
- Tape
- Minor instrument/cut down set

Box 2 Important emergency medical equipment available in the air ambulance

- Stretcher
- Mattress
- Sheets, pillows, and towels
- Earplugs for patient
- Electrocardiographic equipment
- Blood-pressure monitors, including electronic monitor with liquid crystal display (LCD) screen
- Capnograph
- Pulse oximeter
- Thermometers
- Defibrillator with pads
- External cardiac pacing device
- Cervical spine collars
- Fracture immobilizers (not air splints)
- Portable oxygen with regulator
- Backup oxygen tanks
- Airframe-compatible ventilator
- Suction device with catheters and drainage-collection units
- Tubing with connections
- Bag-valve-mask systems
- Nasal cannulae
- Continuous positive airway pressure systems
- Intubation equipment
- Endotracheal tubes
- Oropharyngeal airway
- Tracheotomy kit
- Nebulizer
- Nasogastric tubes
- Jaw wire cutter
- Intravenous needles and tubing
- Intravenous fluids in bags (not glass)
- Infusion device (not dependent on gravity)
- Intraosseous needles
- Point-of-care laboratory kits
- Fetal Doppler monitor
- Delivery kit
- Neonatal resuscitation kit
- Battery packs with spares
- Power inverter for use of aircraft power source
- Satellite telephone
- Nutrition and hydration supplies for patient and crew
- Survival gear
- Reference materials
- Medication kit with drugs for resuscitations, anxiety, airsickness, and condition-specific uses
- Bandages and dressings
- Wound-treatment kit
- Gloves
- Small surgical kit
- Cleaning and disinfection material
- Bedpan, urinal, and emesis basin
- Sharps disposal system
- Waste containers

advanced medical team to the patient, where treatment/intervention can be initiated at the scene and en route to a specialist facility. Area C shows the distance that rotary wing aircraft will time beneficial over other forms of transport. Area D is the distance where fixed wing transfer would be the most beneficial regardless of necessary secondary transfers.

PATHOPHYSIOLOGY

The air transfer of patients creates many considerations for the medical team including the effects of altitude on the physiology of the patient. Any medical crew involved in air transfer should have advanced knowledge of flight physiology in order to be aware and subsequently deal with any situations that may arise due to the stressors of flight. This is especially pertinent when transferring critically ill patients who may already be at the upper end of their physiological reserve as physiological deterioration may occur more rapidly from the stresses of flight. These stressors would mainly be associated

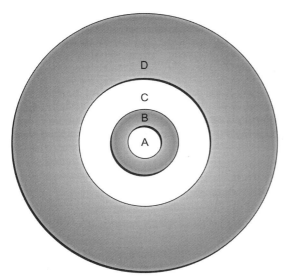

Fig. 2 Donut model of air transfer distances

A "donut model" (**Fig. 2**) has been created to display the benefits of using different modes of transport for air transfer over variant distances (Munford, 1996). The area marked *A* will provide minimal assistance using air transfer (ground transfer is quicker), whereas area *B*, is superior when using rotary wing air transfer to transport an

with fixed wing transfer due to the higher altitude however; patients transferred in helicopters may also suffer from the stresses of flight. It is important to note that these stressors are not limited to the patient but may also affect the medical crew. Some air transfer physiological considerations include:

- From sea level to 5,000 ft represents significant change in barometric pressure and temperature for a patient
- Trapped air will increase 20% in size
- Temperature will decrease by approximately 10°C
- Ambient oxygen pressure will decrease by almost 17%
- Arterial oxygen pressure will decrease by 23%
- Alveolar oxygen pressure will decrease by 21%
- Alveolar CO_2 pressure will decrease by 6.5%.

This will have a direct impact on air transfer patient care, and thus the medical crew must preempt these physiological changes that may occur and be prepared to treat accordingly (Blumen, 2006).

- *Effects of hypothermia*:
  - Increase in oxygen demand and consumption
- *Effects of hypoxic hypoxia*:
  - Good oxygen saturation and arterial blood gas (ABG) preflight may change at altitude
- *Effects of noise*:
  - Patient may become panicked/distressed/combative
  - Monitoring audible alarms may not be heard
  - Communication with awake patient may be difficult
- *Effects of vibration*:
  - Increase in pain at fracture sites
  - May exacerbate nausea and vomiting
  - Higher amounts of analgesia and sedation is required
  - Inaccurate electrical artifacts on monitoring machines.

STANDARDS OF CARE

The standards of care of the medical team will differ vastly across the globe. The medical team performing air transfer of patients should be highly qualified and competent within their respective field. A mix of medical teams exists, but is usually made up of doctors, paramedics, nurses and respiratory therapists. There is no ideal medical team, but should ideally be made up of clinical specialists who have undergone extra training in the air transfer of patients including postgraduate study. It may prove beneficial to have some heterogeneity within the medical team by mixing doctor/nurse or doctor/paramedic teams where each team member can bring their own specialist skills to the transfer and work together to provide optimal patient care. The skillset of the medical team should always match the potential needs of the patient. Air transfer of patients can be high risk for errors to occur, such as airway problems, detached intravenous lines, equipment failure, etc. so the medical team should be competent in skills/treatment for problems, which may arise during transfer.

Irrespective of the type of transfer, e.g. primary, tertiary or type of aircraft used, the medical approach to the patient should be similar. Standard operating procedures are an excellent tool in the transfer of patients by air as it gives an objective guide and provides "checklists" (**Boxes 3 and 4**) to ensure essential tasks have been completed. This mitigates potential problems that may occur during flight where these tasks are difficult and sometimes impossible to carry out in a moving and sometimes cramped aircraft (**Fig. 3**). An example of this would be a patient who has suffered burns including facial/airway burns. During assessment, it may be obvious the patient has facial/airway burns but not displaying any symptoms of airway swelling or obstruction. However, problems arise during air transfer where the patient becomes distressed with respiratory difficulty and impeding airway obstruction ensues due to swelling of the airway. It would prove beneficial to ensure that this potential complication is treated on the ground by identifying possible issues in flight and securing the airway beforehand with anesthesia and mechanical ventilation. This ensures a more comfortable environment to carry out this procedure and not in the back of an aircraft where conditions and space are limited.

The air transfer of patients is often most beneficial for critical care patients requiring specialist treatment/intervention. While it is necessary to stabilize certain types of patients, it may also be required to expedite patient transfer

Box 3 Checklist for transfer of a patient through air ambulance

Patient
- Stable on transport trolley
- Appropriately monitored
- All infusions running and lines adequately secured
- Adequately sedated and paralysed
- Adequately secured to trolley
- Adequately wrapped to prevent heat loss

Staff
- Adequately trained and experienced
- Received appropriate handover
- Adequately clothed and insured

Equipment
- Appropriately equipped ambulance
- Appropriate equipment and drugs
- Batteries checked (spare batteries available)
- Sufficient oxygen supplies
- Portable phone charged and available
- Money/credit cards for emergencies

Organization
- Case notes, X-rays, results, blood collected
- Transfer documentation prepared
- Location of bed and receiving doctor known
- Receiving unit advised of departure time and estimated time of arrival
- Telephone numbers of referring and receiving units available
- Relatives informed
- Return travel arrangements in place
- Ambulance crew briefed
- Police escort arranged, if appropriate

Departure
- Patient trolley secured
- Electrical equipment plugged into ambulance power supply where available
- Ventilator transferred to ambulance oxygen supply
- All equipment safely mounted or stowed
- Staff seated and wearing seat belts

Box 4 Checklist for transfer of a patient through air ambulance before departure

Is the patient stable for transport?

Airway
- Airway safe or secured by intubation
- Tracheal tube position confirmed on chest X-ray

Ventilation
- Paralyzed, sedated and ventilated
- Ventilation established on transport ventilator
- Adequate gas exchange confirmed by arterial blood gas

Circulation
- Heart rate, BP stable
- Tissue and organ perfusion adequate
- Any obvious blood loss controlled
- Circulating blood volume restored
- Hemoglobin adequate
- Minimum of two routes of venous access
- Arterial line and central venous access, if appropriate

Neurology
- Seizures controlled, metabolic causes excluded
- Raised intracranial pressure appropriately managed

Trauma
- Cervical spine protected
- Pneumothoraces drained
- Intra-thoracic and intra-abdominal bleeding controlled
- Intra-abdominal injuries adequately investigated and appropriately managed
- Long bone/pelvic fractures stabilized

Metabolic
- Blood glucose >4 mmol/L
- Potassium <6 mmol/L
- Ionized calcium >1 mmol/L
- Acid-base balance acceptable
- Temperature maintained

Monitoring
- ECG
- Blood pressure
- Oxygen saturation
- End-tidal carbon dioxide
- Temperature

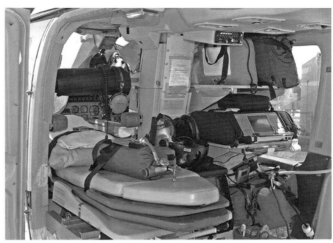

Fig. 4 Rotary wing air transfer—limited space and access to patient

to definitive intervention. This is the case in patients with noncompressible hemorrhage where the definitive treatment is surgery (penetrating/blunt injury). Minimal delay on scene should be advocated and solutions for any issues that arise en route to definitive care should be instigated.

The air transfer of patients in cardiac arrest should not be advocated due to several potential issues. The ability to perform cardiopulmonary resuscitation in the back of an aircraft is impractical due to limited space, crew restraint in the aircraft and safety issues **(Fig. 4)**. Advanced life support treatment should be instigated according to standard operating procedures at the scene of the patient where space and resources may not be limited.

SPECIAL CONSIDERATIONS

During the air transfer of patients, there are some special considerations that clinicians must be aware of to mitigate problems due to altitude. Any patient that may have trapped air in pathological airspaces can have possible catastrophic reaction to altitude. The conservative management of any condition with trapped air such as pneumothorax, intraocular air and pneumocephalus must be handled with extreme caution. The insertion of a chest drain in the restricted space of an aircraft if a patient deteriorates is impractical due to patient accessibility and limited space/resources. During the air transfer of psychiatric patients, special considerations are mandatory before placing the patient in the aircraft. The preferential use of ground transport is always advocated but certain instances may arise where air transfer is the only option. Patients experiencing psychiatric illness may appear docile on the ground, but become agitated due to the stressors of flight and the claustrophobic environment. This can have potential to jeopardize the safety of the crew and the flight.

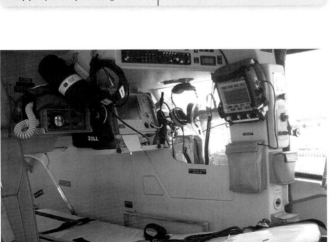

Fig. 3 Fixed wing air transfer—limited space and access to patient

Box 5 Advantages and disadvantages of road and air ambulance

Road ambulance	Air ambulance
Advantages	*Advantages*
• Door-to-door transfer, rapid mobilization time • No landing zone required • Few weather restrictions • Mostly affordable-low overall cost • Less potential for physiological disturbance • Staff are more familiar with the environment	• Rapid transfer • Long distance where road access is difficult • May carry more medical personnel
Disadvantages	*Disadvantages*
• Motion sickness • Traffic delays • Restricted to 150–200 km only	• Physiologic effect of high altitude, if not pressurized • Require assistance to load patient into aircraft • Require runway of certain length • Cost is substantially higher

All efforts must be made to carefully plan and adhere to local standard operating procedures while maintaining legal and ethical consideration in respect of pharmacological sedation of psychiatric patients.

Individual attention should be given to each and every conditions before air transfer of the patient as few advantages and disadvantages are associated with air transfer **(Box 5)**.

RECENT ADVANCES

The most recent advance in the air transfer of patients is the increasing number of rotary wing air ambulances. In the UK, there are approximately 20 civilian air ambulances providing life-saving care to the public. Most of these air ambulances are funded by charity and rely on public donations. With the introduction of major trauma centers, injured patients may have to travel further to access this specialist facility. Air ambulance helicopters are the fastest way to deliver patients to life-saving specialist intervention and play a key part in the 20% increase in patient survival since the introduction of major trauma centers in the UK *(http://www.associationofairambulances.co.uk/news/15/)*.

A recent advance in the USA enforced federal rules to air ambulance operators specifically rotary wing after several fatal crashes. These rules aim to increase the safety of air ambulance missions by implementing the latest technology and flight data monitoring systems to assist flying in challenging weather, at night and in remote locations *(https://www.faa.gov/news/press_releases/news_story.cfm?newsId=15795)*.

CONCLUSION

The air transfer of patients poses risks for the patient, medical and flight crew due to several reasons including altitude, environment and severity of patient's condition. Most situations that arise can be mitigated by careful planning and utilizing standard operating procedures, which ensure medical crews develop motor programs so that working in changing environment can be completed safely and successfully. Below are some helpful rules for the air transfer of patients:

- Most complications that occur were not anticipated by the air medical crew. Large problems are usually small ones that were not planned for
- The ability to competently deal with any situation that arises is mandatory. No one can run for help while in the sky!
- Make sure to spend extra time securing all tubes and infusion lines. These extra few minutes will payoff, as loading/unloading patients can be haphazard for accidental removal
- Treat the patient as well as the monitor. The environment of air transfer can be noisy and distracting. Ensure good clinical observation.

BIBLIOGRAPHY

1. Association of Air Ambulances. (2013). Air ambulances key part of 20% increase in patient survival rates. [online] Available from *http://www.associationofairambulances.co.uk/news/15/* [Accessed November, 2016].
2. Blumen IJ, Lemkin DL. Principles and Direction of Air Medical Transport: Previously the Air Medical Physician Handbook. Salt Lake City: Air Medical Physician Association; 2006.
3. Cong ML, Ramin G. (2014). Preperation of the critical patient for aeromedical transport. [online] Available from *http://prehospitalmed.com/2014/06/17/preparation-of-the-critical-patient-for-aeromedical-transport/* [Accessed November, 2016].
4. Federal Aviation Administration. (2014). FAA Issues Final Rule to Improve Helicopter Safety. [online] Available from *https://www.faa.gov/news/press_releases/news_story.cfm?newsId=15795* [Accessed November, 2016].
5. Martin TE. Practical aspects of aeromedical transport. Curr Anaesth Crit Care. 2003;14(3):141-8.
6. Milligan JE, Jones CN, Helm DR, et al. The principles of aeromedical retrieval of the critically ill. Trends Anaesth Crit Care. 2011;1(1):22-6.

CHAPTER 10

Standards of Care during Road Transfer

Sunil Dubey, Sudhir S Pawaiya, Vivekanshu Verma

INTRODUCTION

The standards of care of the medical team should be universal across the globe. The medical team performing road transfer of patients should be highly qualified and competent within their respective field. A mixture of medical teams exists, but is usually made up of doctors, paramedics, nurses, and driver. There is no ideal medical team but should ideally be made up of clinical specialists who have undergone extra training in the transfer of patients including postgraduate study. It may prove beneficial to have some heterogeneity within the medical team by mixing doctor/nurse or doctor/paramedic teams where each team member can bring their own specialist skills to the transfer and work together to provide optimal patient care. The skillset of the medical team should always match the potential needs of the patient. Road transfer of patients can be high-risk for errors to occur such as airway problems, detached intravenous (IV) lines, equipment failure, etc., so the medical team should be competent in skills or treatment for problems, which may arise during transfer.

Irrespective of the type of transfer, e.g. primary, tertiary, or type of vehicle used, the medical approach to the patient should be similar. Standard operating procedures are an excellent tool in the transfer of patients by road as it gives an objective guide and provides "checklists" to ensure essential tasks have been completed.

STANDARD ABCDE APPROACH

Use the Standard ABCDE Approach for Adequate Preparation for Transport of Critically-ill and Injured Patient

A-Airway (with cervical spine protection)
- A patent airway is the key goal.
- Use an oropharyngeal or nasopharyngeal airway, or consider intubation.
- If intubated, secure the endotracheal tube (ETT) and note and document its position. Use air in the cuff not fluid. This is a change from traditional practice based on research that air-filled cuffs are safer as the pressure can be measured with a manometer. Ensure that tube is well-secured. Pediatric patients can extubate from simple neck extension or neck flexion. Very difficult airways may require consideration of strong sedation with paralysis to ensure that the patient does not rouse and self-extubate as monitoring in the transport environment is challenging and unpredictable stimuli may occur.
- If unable to achieve tracheal intubation, a laryngeal mask airway is acceptable.
- Consider possible spine and/or significant head injury and apply a cervical or towel tolls, more comfortable to either side of the head.

B-Breathing
- Maintain adequate oxygenation—all patients requiring oxygen on the ground will require more oxygen at higher altitude. Anticipate what oxygen supply will be required for the transport and ensure there is enough for reserve. Conserve portable oxygen supplies whenever possible by using wall oxygen of sending facilities until ready to move. Conserve batteries of ventilators whenever possible
- Manual ventilation can be given and an Air Viva bag should be accessible
- Ideally, insert an intercostal catheter for all proven hemopneumothoraces. Attach either a Heimlich valve (a flutter one-way valve to prevent air travelling back along a chest tube) or emergency chest drainage bag, e.g. Portex.

C-Circulation
- Control any hemorrhage
- Ensure IV access with a minimum of two cannulas (Large bore IV trauma or hemorrhage present)
- An intraosseous needle is acceptable as reliable access

- Make sure all lines and tubes are well-secured, with an accessible injection port and a needle-free system (if available).

D-Disability and disturbed behavior
- Note that an adequate trial of preflight sedation is vital and best conducted at the remote hospital facility. Acute sedation during flight is risky (in terms of oversedation or failed sedation) with little margin for error. Disturbed patients can put the safety of staff, patient, and aircraft at risk. Identifying and managing this issue prior to departure is essential. An uncooperative or combative patient is a contraindication to transport and must be adequately managed prior to transport. If patient cooperation cannot be achieved through negotiation and communication there must be consideration of the need for transport balanced with the interventions that might be required to make a safe transport, including physical and chemical restraints as well as adequate numbers of team members.
- Police escort may be necessary and local involuntary mental health certification may be required.
- Document the level of consciousness using the Glasgow Coma Score (GCS).
- Report evidence of dementia, delirium, or confusion to the transporting team.
- Warning the retrieval team in advance of any anxiety or aggression is paramount. A clinical pearl here is to consider acute nicotine withdrawal that may reveal itself during an air evacuation flight of significant duration (>1 hour). Early institution of nicotine replacement therapy may markedly reduce the need for sedation during retrieval. Fear of travelling should be addressed with reassurance, explanation, and education about the medical retrieval process. Steps to mitigate stressors include use of antiemetics, safety restraints, etc. Oral sedation (e.g. diazepam) is acceptable (see below).

E-Extended care considerations: consider the need for other care specific to your patient's illness
- Adequate analgesia and/or sedation.
- Use of antiemetics (e.g. prochlorperazine, ondansetron, metoclopramide).
- Spinal immobilization, e.g. vacuum mattress.
- Immobilization of fractures (e.g. splinting with a backslab or traction splints).
- Tetanus prophylaxis or antibiotics or wound dressings.
- IV infusions refilled for journey (no burettes).
- Rationalize therapies and minimize number of infusions.
- Consider thermal control—space blankets, limit exposure.
- Secure all tubing and empty all drainage bags before flight.
- Minimize contamination—removes wet or soiled clothes.
- Complete documentation or transport notes.

Principles of Safe Transfer
- Experienced staff
- Appropriate equipment and vehicle
- Full assessment
- Extensive monitoring
- Careful stabilization of patient
- Reassessment
- Continuing care (**Fig. 1**).

Safety during Transport
- Patient should be wrapped in blanket and adequately strapped to trolleys
- All equipment should be securely wall mounted
- Staff should remain seated all the time and wear seatbelts
- Interventions should not be attempted in moving ambulances
- Vehicles should be stopped in safe place and high visibility clothing must be worn by staff, if they move out of ambulance.

Training of Ambulance Team
- "Team members should be chosen for both their medical skills and their ability to behave responsibly when interacting with personnel at him referring and receiving hospital, patient or family and one another."
- Advanced cardiac life support (ACLS) and Advanced trauma life support (ATLS) trained
- Team members should be trained and competent in resuscitation, critical care procedures and transport medicine, recognizing limitation of and managing supplies or equipment, and physiologic effect of transport on the patient.

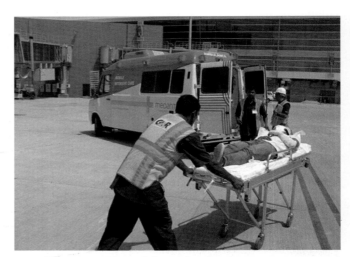

Fig. 1 Safe transfer of patient

WHAT YOU NEED TO KNOW BEFORE YOU GO!!

"ACCEPT" APPROACH
A: Assessment
C: Control
C: Communication
E: Evaluation
P: Preparation
T: Transportation

Rights of Safe Transport

The 6Rs of safe transport are:
1. The right patient
2. At the right time
3. By the right people
4. To the right place
5. By the right transport
6. With right care throughout (**Fig. 2**).

FACTORS ASSOCIATED WITH FEWER ADVERSE EVENTS DURING AMBULANCE TRANSFER

Factors associated are:
- Good crew skills or teamwork,
- Daily morning checking of equipment by checklist,
- Checking the patient's status from treating doctor before mobilizing ambulance,
- Regular checking of patient monitors
- Good interpersonal communication in ambulance team members—doctors, nurses, paramedic, and driver.

ADVANTAGES OF 'SPECIALIZED TEAMS' FOR TRANSPORTATION

Ambulance transport team is incomplete without a transport physician, just as an intensive care unit (ICU) would be incomplete without an intensivist. The advantage of a specialized transfer team is that it is more familiar with transport-specific procedures and equipment. Establishment of a specialized transfer team associated with a decline adverse events. "Specialized teams" are better able to stabilize the patient prior to the transfer. A specialized teams better deal with logistic problems.

RECOMMENDATIONS FOR THE TRANSFER OF CRITICALLY ILL PATIENTS

Recommendations and opinions include:
- Critically ill patients should be transferred by a specialized retrieval team
- Intensive care should not be interrupted by transportation of the patient
- Specialized retrieval teams should receive transfer training
- Specific training programs should be developed
- Specialized retrieval teams should be staffed by a physician, preferably an intensivist and an ICU nurse
- The accompanying physician makes the final decision whether the patient is transferrable and which treatment is given during the transport
- Experience and training are more important than speed
- Transfer organizations should have a quality management system
- Incident reporting should be standardized and mandatory
- Equipment used should conform with transfer standards
- Adults can learn from children (in the organization of transport).

CLINICAL HANDOVER PROCESS FOR AMBULANCE TRANSFER

A number of steps can be undertaken to ensure an effective clinical handover processes and limit variability of practice.
- Establishing and maintaining structured and documented processes for clinical handover, including policy, procedures and protocols, and tools and guides for localized use
- Regular monitoring and evaluation of clinical handover processes, tools, and guides
- Establishing a supportive culture which values clinical handover
- Provision of training to all relevant staff in clinician handover processes.

Clinical handover should be more complete and concise, utilize effective communication, in order to provide high quality patient care and reduce adverse events (**Box 1**). A standard clinical handover process improves patient safety (**Box 2**). The clinician receiving handover should be clearly identifiable and prepared to receive the handover uninterrupted. This is particularly important in the case of

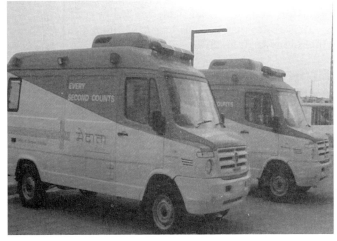

Fig. 2 Ambulance for safe transport

Box 1 Handover principles

- Appropriate environment
- Staff availability
- Agreement
- Concise
- Consistent structure and content

Box 2 Effect of standard handover process on patient clinical outcome

Standardized clinical handover of ambulance patients arriving in the ED impacts positively on:
- Patients outcomes and safety
- Timely and high quality care
- Paramedic and ED staff collaboration
- Paramedic availability to meet community needs

Box 3 Components used by nursing staff and doctors for ambulance patient handover

Ambulance Handover Mnemonic (IMIST_AMBO)	
I	– Identification (e.g. patient's name, age, sex)
M	– Mechanism of injury or medical complaint (e.g. presenting) problem, how it happened
I	– Injuries or information related to the complaint (e.g. symptoms and/or injuries)
S	– Signs (e.g. vital signs, such as HR, RR, BP, Temp, BGL, GCS, etc.)
T	– Treatment and trends (e.g. treatment administered and patient's response to treatment, trends in vital signs)
A	– Allergies
M	– Medications (e.g. patient's regular medications)
B	– Background history (e.g. patient's medical history)
O	– Other information (e.g. social, scene, relatives present, EAR result)

Abbreviations: HR, heart rate; RR, respiratory rate; BP, blood pressure; Temp, temperature; BGL, blood glucose level; GCS, Glasgow Coma Scale; EAR, enquiry about result.

trauma or time criticality when multiple clinicians may be in the receiving area. Clinical ambulance handover **(Box 3)** information should be timely, accurate, and completed only once and use an easily understood language with minimal accepted abbreviations.

NATIONAL STANDARD FOR AMBULANCES IN INDIA

National Ambulance Code (Automotive Industry Standard No. 125-Part 1) finally notified by Government of India. A journey which we began in 2012 has finally culminated into a National Standard for Ambulances which shall become mandatory w.e.f. 1st April 2018. National Standard for Ambulances, notified by Government of India in Gazette dated 8th September 2016.

"Road Ambulance" means a specially equipped and ergonomically designed vehicle for transportation and/or emergent treatment of sick or injured people and capable of providing out-of-hospital medical care during transit or when stationary commensurate with its designated level of care when appropriately staffed.

"Special Purpose Vehicle (SPV)" means a vehicle of category L [only in case of Road Ambulance complying with Automotive Industry Standard (AIS)-125 (Part l)-2014], M N, or T having specific technical features in order to perform a function which requires special arrangements and/or equipment.

Blinker type of red light with purple glass fitted to an ambulance van used for carrying patients or the warning lamps fitted on Road Ambulance in accordance with annexure-1 of AIS-125 (Part-1)-2014.

On and after the 1st April, 2018, the top lights (warning lamps) fitted on Road Ambulances, shall be in accordance with AIS-125 (Part 1)-2014, as amended from time to time, for all types of ambulances specified therein, till the corresponding Bureau of Indian Standards (BIS) specifications are notified under the Bureau of Indian Standards Act, 1986 (63 of 1986).

"Provided that requirements for sirens of Road Ambulances shall be in accordance with AIS-125 (Part 1)-2014, as amended from time to time, till the corresponding BIS specifications are notified under the Bureau of Indian Standards Act, 1986 (63 of 1986)".

Road Ambulances of categories L and M manufactured on and after the 1st April, 2018, shall be in accordance with AIS-125 (Part 1)-2014 as amended from time to time, for all types of ambulances specified therein. Till the corresponding BIS specifications are notified under the Bureau of Indian Standards Act, 1986 (63 of 1986).

These rules may be called *Central Motor Vehicles* (Ninth Amendment,) Rules 2016.

MEDICOLEGAL ISSUES IN AMBULANCE TRANSFER

Supreme Court of India Ruling

On being approached by the patient, if a medical profession person feels that standard of care that he could give is not really sufficient to save the life of the person, and some better assistance is necessary, it is the duty of the doctor to render all help that he can and also see that the person reaches the proper expert as early as possible.

The majority of doctors are worried when transferring accident or serious patients, for fear of the legal process.

However, in the strict sense, the law requires that the victim be transferred even by nonmedical persons. The transfer will be better if accomplished with medicos or even with paramedical staff. If a doctor is present during transportation it will be legally tenable to certify the death, in case it occurs during the transfer. Even if a patient dies during the transfer, the law just requires that the matter be informed to the police, whether the death occurred under suspicious circumstances or if it was Medical Law Case (MLC).

Many times, Ambulance is called by the police or attendants of the injured patients at scene of crime to shift a medicolegal case in ambulance to nearby hospital. Sometimes, we receive a vague urgent phone call in midnight for ambulance by nearby resident neighbors of victim, that a sick dying patient needs to be shifted urgent medical attention, and when we reach to pick up patient, we come to know that it is a gunshot, strangulation, or rape. We cannot just leave a rape victim and run away, as its offence in recent Anti-rape Laws of India [376 Indian Penal Code (IPC) Criminal Law (Amendment) Act, 2013], and we cannot refuse medical treatment to sexual assault victim, acid attack victim [326A IPC Criminal Law (Amendment) Act, 2013]. Then it becomes legal duty of every medical personnel to report medicolegal case and preserve the evidence of crime, otherwise he can be punished for not reporting crime and not giving first aid medical treatment, since we are on record by phone calls and closed-circuit television (CCTV) camera installed in most of residential buildings.

Later we are summoned to court for medical evidence, in which we become the first independent witness of scene of crime. Save our self as doctors by proving accused's crime by meticulous medical documentation in MLC and urgent ambulance transfer to higher center for "saving innocent lives of victims from knives of autopsy" to establish accused's crime.

In current scenario of medicolegal litigation against doctors for extortion of money, as courts are giving hefty amounts in crores in medical negligence but give meager amounts in thousands to victims of crime as per IPC, e.g. a victim of acid burn will get fixed amount for covering treatment expenses as per 326A IPC of grievous hurt, but if acid attack victim patient files negligence suit against doctor, who has treated his best facility, but scar will remain on face, and consumer court will find fault in medical documentation of consent or records and award hefty amounts to be paid by doctor to victim.

Many times, during investigation, it was found that the sexual assault and trauma victims go for out-of-court settlement with accused by taking money and then file medical negligence case against doctor to claim compensation for alleged negligence in reporting crime, or for permanent damages due to injury.

CONCLUSION

If an ambulance doctor works for the law by reporting crime, he/she can safeguard his career and his reputation during false allegations. If the doctor works against the law, by not reporting crime, by doing illegal abortions, by doing illegal transplantation, doctor can be arrested and punished.

BIBLIOGRAPHY

1. Barry PW, Ralston C. Adverse events occurring during interhospital transfer of the critically ill. Arch Dis Child. 1994;71:8-11.
2. Droogh JM, Smit M, Absalom AR, et al. Transferring the critically ill patient: are we there yet? Crit Care. 2015;19(1):62.
3. Golestanian E, Scruggs JE, Gangnon RE, et al. Effect of interhospital transfer on resource utilization and outcomes at a tertiary care referral center. Crit Care Med. 2007;35:1470-6.
4. Govt. of India in Gazette, National Standard for Ambulances, 2016.
5. Govt. of India. IPC Criminal Law (Amendment) Act, 2013. Section 376 & 326A 2013.
6. Haji-Michael P. Critical care transfers-a danger foreseen is half avoided. Crit Care. 2005;9:343-4.
7. Indian gazette notification (2015). Ministry of Road Transport and Highways (MoRTH) notified the "Good Samaritan" guidelines [Online]. Available from *www.egazette.nic.in/WriteReadData/2015/164095.pdf* [Accessed February 2017].
8. Kanter RK, Tompkins JM. Adverse events during interhospital transport: physiologic deterioration associated with pretransport severity of illness. Pediatrics. 1989;84:43-8.
9. Kumbar, SK. Legal binding of transportation of the patient to anaesthesiologist. Ind J Anaes. 2010;54(4):367-8.
10. Singh J. Medical negligence and compensation. Jaipur: Bharat Law Pub. 2015
11. The Department of Health, Victoria (2015). Ambulance handover, VEMD manual (2014-15) [Online] Available from *www.health.vic.gov.au/hdss/vemd/index.htm* [Accessed February 2017].
12. Waddell G, Scott PD, Lees NW, et al. Effects of ambulance transport in critically ill patients. BMJ. 1975;1:386-9.
13. Whiteley S, Macartney I, Mark J, et al. Guidelines for the transport of the critically ill adult. 2011.

SECTION 2

Resuscitation and Critical Care in Emergency

- **Management of Cardiac Arrest in Adults**
  Uday Aditya Gupta, Sinoy Jose

- **Airway Management**
  Amit D Nabar

- **Management of Critically Ill Patient in Emergency**
  *Chandrashekhar, Swarup S Padhi,
  Ajeet Singh, Tariq Ali, Yatin Mehta*

- **Overview of Shock**
  Khusrav Bajan, Archana Shrivastav

- **Sepsis and Septic Shock**
  *Chandrashekhar, Swarup S Padhi, Ajeet Singh,
  Tariq Ali, Yatin Mehta*

- **Noninvasive Ventilation**
  Kishalay Datta

- **Mechanical Ventilation**
  Mrinal Sircar, Saurabh Mehra

- **Use of Blood and Blood Products in Emergency**
  Aseem K Tiwari, Ravi C Dara, Dinesh Arora

- **Arterial Blood Gas Analysis**
  Sudha Kansal, Rajesh Chawla, Tarun S

- **Oxygen Therapy**
  Poulomi Chatterji, Bhawna Sharma

- **Acute Pain Management in Emergency Department**
  Sonam Kaushika, Devendra Richhariya, Manish Garg

CHAPTER 11

Management of Cardiac Arrest in Adults

Uday Aditya Gupta, Sinoy Jose

INTRODUCTION

In the United States of America, in the 2013, American Heart Association (AHA) statistical update,[1] there were 359,400 out-of-hospital cardiac arrests (OHCA) and 209,000 in-hospital cardiac arrests (IHCA) reported. In OHCA bystanders gave cardiopulmonary resuscitation (CPR) in about 40% of patients and survival to hospital discharge was 9.5%.[1] In IHCA, overall survival was about 21%.[2] In India, the data is extremely limited.[3-5] We found that in India, in indexed literature, the total number of CPR resuscitations reported is less than 800. OHCA has been included by two studies only and a total of less than 100 OHCA have been mentioned.[3,4] Further, in different subgroups, up to 60% of data of arrests has been rejected as mentioned in these studies.[3-5] In India, the overall survival to hospital discharge in predominantly IHCA patients is 7–14%.[3-5] The bystander CPR rate in India is dismal and is reported as rare in one study.[3]

PATHOPHYSIOLOGY

Cardiac arrest can be due to various causes. A popular acronym to remember common causes is "5H 5T". A healthcare worker (HCW) should identify these in an arrest scenario as soon as possible but without compromising on CPR quality.[6]

- 5Hs
  - Hypothermia
  - Hypovolemia
  - Hypoxia
  - *Hydrogen ion*: Acidosis or alkalosis
  - Hypo- or hyperkalemia
- 5Ts
  - Tamponade cardiac
  - Tamponade lung or tension pneumothorax
  - Thrombosis cardiac
  - Thrombosis pulmonary
  - *Toxins*: Drugs or poisoning

CHAIN OF SURVIVAL

Health administrators can designate resources for cardiac arrest management with *Chain of Survival* as a policy framework **(Fig. 1)**. Broadly, there are two settings for cardiac arrest management: (1) in hospital, and (2) out of hospital. For OHCA, emergency medical systems of community are needed and for IHCA rapid response team or code team is needed.[2,7]

First Response[8,9]

When responders arrive on scene, the first response is as follows:

- Verify scene safety. Save yourself first
- If victim is unconscious, use basic life support (BLS) survey
- If victim is conscious, or you are part of emergency medical system (EMS) and BLS is ongoing, use advanced cardiac life support (ACLS) survey.

Basic Life Support Survey (1-2-3-4)

1. Assess responsiveness
2. Activate EMS and send someone to get automated external defibrillator (AED)
3. Check breathing and pulse simultaneously, if pulse is not definitely felt in less than 10 seconds, start CPR immediately
4. *Defibrillate*: Use AED when available.

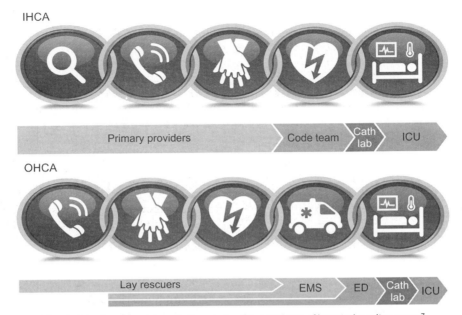

Fig. 1 American Heart Association chain of survival out of hospital cardiac arrest[7]
Note: Chain of Survival: The "Chain of Survival" is a metaphor which is used to summarize timely, coordinated and necessary actions in a cardiac arrest scenario[7]
Abbreviations: IHCA, in-hospital cardiac arrest; OHCH, out-of-hospital cardiac arrest; ICU, intensive care unit; EMS, emergency medical system; ED, external defibrillator.

Advanced Cardiac Life Support Survey (A-B-C-D)

A. *Airway*: Look for patency of airway, use airway adjuncts: oropharyngeal airway or nasopharyngeal airway. Is an advanced airway needed? Has placement of advanced airway been confirmed and it is secured in place?
B. *Breathing*: Is ventilation and oxygenation adequate? Look for chest rise or cyanosis. If feasible, see end-tidal continuous waveform capnography or pulse-oximetry.
C. *Circulation*: Attach ECG monitor. Identify basic pattern of ECG and check pulse, based on these two criteria use the ACLS algorithm as appropriate.
D. *Differential diagnosis*: Why did the victim suffer this arrest? Remember the "5Hs and 5Ts". See pathophysiology vide supra.

Out-of-Hospital Arrest[10-12]

In an OHCA scenario, CPR may be started by a lay rescuer or an EMS responder. AHA recommends that lay rescuers should identify unresponsiveness and lack of breathing but should not check for pulse. Identification of pulse by rescuers is not reliable. After identifying nonresponsiveness, immediate activation of EMS should be done and chest compressions started. One may use a mobile device and leave it on speaker mode so that if feasible, the EMS call center personnel can guide the lay rescuer to carry out CPR. AHA recommends at the minimum lay rescuers should provide chest compressions, if unable or unwilling to provide ventilations.[10] An HCW should check for responsiveness, activate EMS and check for abnormal or absent breathing and pulse simultaneously. HCW should provide ventilations and compressions or if infeasible, provide compressions only CPR at least.[10]

American Heart Association—Basic Life Support Algorithm for Healthcare Worker[10]

For adults follow adult BLS algorithm[10] **(Flow chart 1)**. For children and infants, follow children and infant BLS algorithm[11] **(Flow chart 2)**. Maintain five points of high-quality chest compressions **(Box 1)**.

Identify Unresponsiveness

- Adult or child
  - Tap on shoulder and shout "are you OK"
  - *Lack of breathing*: See by observing for chest rise from sides. Agonal breaths are insufficient breaths or impending cessation of breathing, hence are deemed as no breathing.
- Infant
  - Tap or slap on sole of foot and shout "baby, baby"

Check for Breathing and Pulse Simultaneously

Check for breathing and pulse simultaneously. Take less than 10 seconds. If pulse definitely not felt in less than 10 seconds, then start CPR immediately.

Flow chart 1 American Heart Association (AHA) adult basic life support (BLS) algorithm for healthcare worker (HCW): 2015 update[10]

```
                          Verify scene safety
                                  │
                                  ▼
                    • Victim is unresponsive
                    • Shout for nearby help
                    • Activate emergency
                      response system via mobile        ┌─────────────────────────┐
                      device (if appropriate)           │ Provide rescue breathing:│
                      Get AED and emergency             │ 1 breath every 5–6 seconds,│
                      equipment                         │ or about 10–12 breaths/min.│
                      (or send someone to do so)        │ • Activate emergency     │
                                  │                     │   response system (if not│
                                  ▼                     │   already done) after    │
              Normal        Look for no breathing  No normal 2 minutes.           │
              breathing,    or only gasping and    breathing, • Continue rescue   │
              has pulse     check pulse            has pulse   breathing:         │
           ┌──────────────  (simultaneously).  ──────────▶│   check pulse about   │
           │                Is pulse definitely           │   every 2 minutes. If │
           ▼                felt within 10 seconds?       │   no pulse, begin CPR │
   Monitor until                    │                     │   (go to "CPR" box).  │
   emergency                        │                     │ • If possible opioid  │
   responders                       │                     │   overdose administer │
   arrive                           │                     │   naloxone if available│
                                    │                     │   per protocol        │
                           No breathing                   └─────────────────────────┘
                           or only gasping,
                           no pulse
                                    │          ┌──────────────────────────────┐
                                    │          │ By this time in all scenarios,│
                                    │          │ emergency response system or  │
                                    │          │ backup is activated, and AED  │
                                    ▼          │ and emergency equipment are   │
                               CPR             │ retrieved or someone is       │
                       Begin cycles of 30      │ retrieving them.              │
                       compressions and        └──────────────────────────────┘
                       2 breaths. Use AED
                       as soon as it is available
                                    │
                                    ▼
                             AED arrives
                                    │
                                    ▼
                       Check rhythm shockable
                ┌────────▶     rhythm?     ◀────────┐
                │              │        │           │
           Yes, shockable      │        │     No, nonshockable
                │              │        │           │
                ▼                                    ▼
    • Give 1 shock. Resume CPR            • Resume CPR immediately for
      immediately for about 2 minutes       about 2 minutes (until prompted
      (until prompted by AED to allow       by AED to allow rhythm check)
      rhythm check)                       • Continue until ALS providers take
    • Continue until ALS providers take     over or victim starts to move
      over or victim starts to move
```

Abbreviations: AED, automated external defibrillator; ALS, advanced life support; CPR, cardiopulmonary resuscitation.
Note: Remember to maintain five points of high-quality chest compressions (Box 1).

- Breathing
  - *Adult or child or infant*: Observe for chest rise from sides. Agonal breaths are insufficient breaths or impending cessation of breathing, hence are deemed as no breathing
  - *Pulse check*: Look for carotid pulse.
- Pulse check
  - *Adult or child*: Look for carotid pulse
  - *Infant*: Look for brachial or femoral pulse.

Cycles of Cardiopulmonary Resuscitation

If pulse is definitely not felt, then start CPR within 10 seconds. Cycles of CPR include three skills:
1. Chest compression. Ensure high-quality chest compressions all the time **(Box 1)**. This is essential.
2. Ventilation **(Box 2)**.
3. Automated external defibrillator (*see* **Box 3**).

After every five CPR cycles or about 2 minutes or when AED prompts *analyzing rhythm*:
- Change rescuer doing chest compressions
- Check for rhythm with AED or check for pulse for return of spontaneous circulation (ROSC).
  Continue CPR till EMS arrives or victim starts to move.

In-hospital Arrest[13,14]

First responders will usually be the nurses. Verify scene safety and use BLS or ACLS survey as needed (vide supra). Continue CPR as needed till code team arrives.

SECTION 2 Resuscitation and Critical Care in Emergency

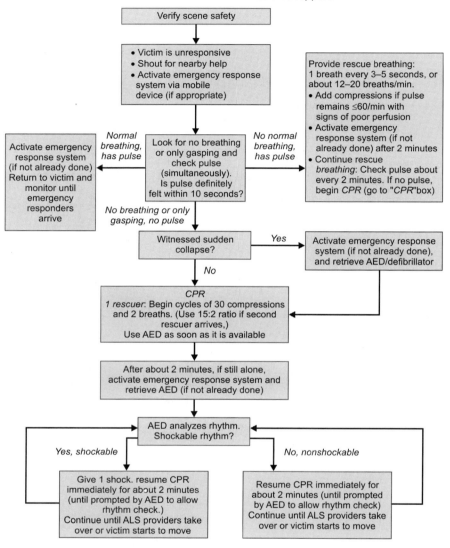

Flow chart 2 Use of AED in basic life support

Box 1 The five points of high-quality chest compressions[12]

Maintain these five points at all times when chest compressions are going on. Interruptions for anything, e.g. IV line, endotracheal intubation should be <10 seconds. If advanced airway is in place, continue chest compressions continuously for about 2 minutes till reassessment of patient by AED or HCW is done. The five points of high-quality chest compressions are as follows:
1. *Push hard, push fast*:
   - *Push hard*:
     – *Adults*: Push to depth of at least 2 inch or 5 cm. Without special devices, it may not be possible to limit chest compression depth to 2.4 inch or 6 cm deep, hence aim for at least 2 inch or 5 cm deep
     – *Children*: At least one-third anteroposterior diameter of chest or about 2 inch or 5 cm deep
     – *Infants*: At least one-third anteroposterior diameter of chest or about 1.5 inch or 4 cm deep
   - *Push fast*:
     – About 100–120 compressions per minute
2. Allow complete chest recoil after compression
3. Change chest compressor every 2 minutes
4. Minimum interruptions in chest compressions <10 seconds
5. Avoid excessive ventilations **(Box 2)**

Contd...

Contd...

Hand position for chest compression (Figs 2A to C).
- *Adult or child*: Place heel of one hand on lower half of sternum, just below the line joining two nipples, place other hand on top of the first, you may interlock fingers, bend from wrist to avoid rib fracture.
- *Infant*:
  - *Single rescuer*: Compress with index and middle finger on lower half of sternum, just below line joining two nipples.
  - *Two rescuers*: Encircle infant's chest with hands, compress sternum with thumbs at lower half of sternum, just below line joining two nipples.

Abbreviations: AED, automated external defibrillator; HCW, healthcare worker; IV, intravenous.

Box 2 Ventilation[9,12]

- In BLS or if advanced airway is not in place:
  - *Compression*: Ventilation ratio. Adult victim, single or >1 rescuers 30:2; child victim, single or >1 rescuers 30:2, infant victim, single rescuer 30:2; infant victim, >1 rescuers 15:2.
  - At all times interruptions in chest compressions <10 seconds.
  - Use mouth-to-mouth or mouth to mask or bag mask whatever is available.
  - Give inspiration over 1 second, not faster.
  - It is reasonable that HCW provide both compression and ventilations.
  - Lay rescuers may continue with chest compression only if they are unable or unwilling to provide ventilation.[8]
- In ACLS or if advanced airway is in place:
  - Give one breath every 6 seconds.
  - Give inspiration over 1 second not faster.
  - You may count out loud, "one one thousand, two one thousand, three one thousand, four one thousand, five one thousand, breath" to estimate 6 seconds interval.

Abbreviations: ACLS, advanced cardiac life support; BLS, basic life support; HCW, healthcare worker.

Box 3 Automated external defibrillator[12]

The steps of AED operation are in the following order:
1. Open lid
2. Switch on AED. Some AEDs will switch on automatically when lid is opened
3. Attach pads **(Fig. 3)**
4. Plug in connectors or wires.

Position of pads **(Fig. 3)**
- *Preferred for ease of access*: Upper right of bare chest, to the right of sternum, directly below clavicle and left of left nipple with top margin of pad few centimeters below armpit.
- *Other acceptable positions are*:
  - Anterior-left infrascapular
  - Anterior-right infrascapular

Precautions
- Shout out loud and visibly verify, no one is touching the patient when shock is delivered. You may say "All clear, shocking on 3, 1...2...3...shocking...shock delivered"
- Do not use AED inside water. Remove victim from water. If water over chest, wipe with cloth if available.
- If victim is in snow or puddle, use AED anyway.
- If victim has hairy chest, and AED shows pads not connected, jerk pads off the chest, few hairs will be plucked off with pads, and put pads again. If available, use razor to shave off hairs at areas of pads.
- Avoid oxygen flowing directly over AED pads.

Abbreviation: AED, automated external defibrillator.

American Heart Association—Advanced Cardiac Life Support Cardiac Arrest Algorithm [13]

If victim has no definite palpable pulse, then follow cardiac arrest algorithm[13] **(Flow chart 3)**.

Measures of CPR quality:
- *If available*: Markers of poor quality CPR
  - *Quantitative waveform capnography*: Partial pressure of end-tidal carbon dioxide ($PETCO_2$) less than 10 mm Hg
  - *Intra-arterial pressure*: Diastolic pressure less than 20 mm Hg.
- If not available, then ensure
  - *Compressions*: Five points of high-quality chest compressions
  - *Ventilations*: Chest rise.

Energy for shock:
- Biphasic
  - See manufacturer recommendation, if recommendation unknown, use maximum strength available
  - First dose, e.g. 120–200 J
  - Second and subsequent doses
    - Equivalent, and higher doses may be considered. Usually 200 J for first and subsequent doses
- *Monophasic*: 360 J

Drug Doses

After any drug, flush intravenous or intraosseous (IV/IO) with 20 mL fluid bolus and raise arm above body for 10–20 seconds.

Epinephrine:
- *Dose*: 1 mg IV or IO push.
- *Precautions or use*: Use every 3–5 minutes. In pulseless electrical activity or asystole, use as soon as available.

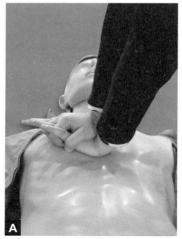
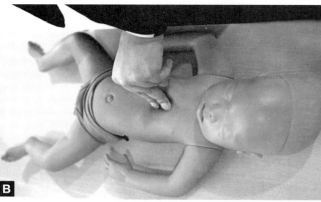
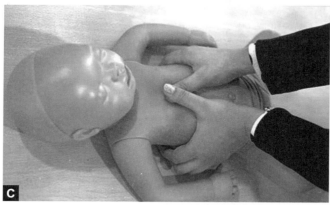

Figs 2A to C Position of hands for chest compression. (A) Adult victim; (B) Infant victim, one rescuer; (C) Infant victim, two rescuers

Amiodarone:
- *Dose*: First dose 300 mg, second or subsequent dose 150–300 mg.
- *Precautions or use*: In cardiac arrest scenario, given by IV or IO push.

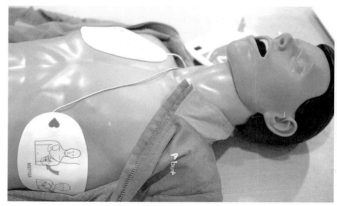

Fig. 3 Position of pads for automated external defibrillator (AED) or defibrillator
Note: One pad below right clavicle, its center is in midclavicular line. Second pad below and side of nipple, below armpit, its center is in midaxillary line.

Postcardiac Arrest Care[15-17]

If during CPR, at the end of any 2 minute cycle, there is any organized rhythm, and the pulse is definitely palpable, this is ROSC. Follow the ROSC algorithm **(Flow chart 4)**.[10,11]

Oxygenation and Ventilation

- Maintain airway, use advanced airway like endotracheal tube or others as feasible.
- Target SpO_2 greater than 94%; target PET CO_2 35–40 mm Hg.

Circulation

- Target systolic blood pressure greater than 90 mm Hg; use as available.
  - IV or IO bolus of 1–2 L normal saline or Ringer's lactate
  - *Epinephrine*: 0.1–0.5 µg/kg/min
  - *Dopamine*: 5–10 µg/kg/min
  - *Norepinephrine*: 0.1–0.5 µg/kg/min.

Advanced Critical Care

- Shift to advanced critical care as soon as possible
- Treat for possible causes (*see* pathophysiology 5Hs and 5Ts)
- Target temperature for targeted temperature management is 32°C–36°C for at least 24 hours. Use core temperature monitoring. Induce target temperature in 4 hours after arrest
- Use ice packs in groin and axillae with wet sheet over bare body and fan. Better still, use skin cooling pads with electronic temperature control if available

CHAPTER 11 Management of Cardiac Arrest in Adults **97**

Flow chart 3 American Heart Association (AHA) advanced cardiac life support (ACLS) cardiac arrest algorithm: 2015 update[13]

① Start CPR
- Give oxygen
- Attach monitor/defibrillator

Rhythm shockable?
- Yes → ② VF/pVT
- No → ⑨ Asystole/PEA

② VF/pVT
③ Shock
④ CPR 2 min
- IV/IO access

Rhythm shockable?
- No → (to ⑩ path)
- Yes → ⑤ Shock

⑥ CPR 2 min
- Epinephrine every 3–5 min
- Consider advanced airway, capnography

Rhythm shockable?
- No → (to ⑫)
- Yes → ⑦ Shock

⑧ CPR 2 min
- Amiodarone
- Treat reversible causes

⑨ Asystole/PEA
⑩ CPR 2 min
- IV/IO access
- Epinephrine every 3–5 min
- Consider advanced airway, capnography

Rhythm shockable?
- Yes → (Go to 5 or 7)
- No → ⑪ CPR 2 min, Treat reversible causes

Rhythm shockable?
- No → ⑫
- Yes → Go to 5 or 7

⑫
- If no signs of return of spontaneous circulation (ROSC), go to *10* or *11*
- If ROSC, go to post-cardiac arrest care

Abbreviations: CPR, cardiopulmonary resuscitation; IV, intravenous; IO, intraosseous; PEA, pulseless electrical activity; ROSC, return of spontaneous circulation; VF/Pvt, ventricular fibrillation/pulseless ventricular tachycardia

- Rewarming is passive, simply stop hypothermic interventions. Prognosticate about neurological recovery no sooner than 72 hours postarrest.

CONCLUSION

Chest compression and early defibrillation is the two most important aspect of basic as well as advanced life support during cardiac arrest. Good quality CPR improves the survival, minimum or no interruption of chest compression is required to improves the survival in cardiac arrest patient.

FURTHER READING/VIEWING

1. American Heart Association. (2015). AHA guidelines: Web based AHA guidelines for CPR ECC. [online] Guidelines for

Flow chart 4 American Heart Association (AHA) return of spontaneous circulation: 2015 update[10,11]

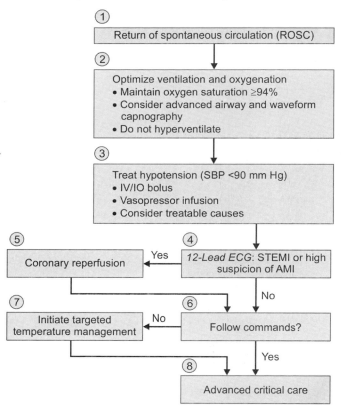

Abbreviations: AMI, acute myocardial infarction; ROSC, return of spontaneous circulation; SBP, systolic blood pressure; STEMI, ST-segment elevation myocardial infarction.

CPR and ECC website. Available from *https://eccguidelines.heart.org/index.php/circulation/cpr-ecc-guidelines-2*. [Accessed November, 2016].
2. American Stroke Association. (2015). CoSTR: The International Consensus on CPR and ECC Science with Treatment Recommendations. [online]. American Stroke Association website Available from *http://circ.ahajournals.org/content/132/16_suppl_1.toc*. [Accessed November, 2016].
3. European Resuscitation Council. (2015): Guidelines and science behind the ERC guidelines for CPR and ECC. Largely similar to AHA guidelines for CPR and AHA. [online]. ERC website. Available from *http://www.cprguidelines.eu/*. [Accessed November, 2016].
4. International Liaison Committee on Resuscitation. (2015). A group of 7 international professional bodies, publishes cardiopulmonary resuscitation (CPR) and emergency cardiovascular care (ECC) guidelines. [online] ILCOR website. Available from *www.ilcor.org*. [Accessed November, 2016].
5. YouTube. (2016). This website is an aggregator of private video clips. Useful academic videos are also found here. Discretion is warranted. [online] YouTube website. Available from *https://www.youtube.com/*. [Accessed November, 2016].

REFERENCES

1. American Heart Association. (2013). Statistical Update-Heart disease and stroke. AHA. [online] AHA website. Available from *http://cpr.heart.org/AHAECC/CPRAndECC/General/UCM_477263_Cardiac-Arrest-Statistics.jsp*. [Accessed November, 2016].
2. American Heart Association (AHA). Systems of Care. In: Advanced Cardiovascular Life Support Provider Manual. Texas: AHA; 2011.
3. Rajaram R, Rajagopalan RE, Pai M, et al. Survival after cardiopulmonary resuscitation in an urban Indian hospital. Natl Med J India. 1999;12(2):51-5.
4. Joshi M. A prospective study to determine the circumstances, incidence and outcome of cardiopulmonary resuscitation in a referral hospital in India, in relation to various factors. Indian J Anaesth. 2015;59(1):31-6.
5. Singh S, Namrata, Grewal A, et al. Evaluation of Cardiopulmonary Resuscitation (CPR) for Patient Outcomes and their Predictors. J Clin Diagn Res. 2016;10(1):UC01-4.
6. American Heart Association (AHA). Pulseless electrical activity. In: Advanced Cardiovascular Life Support Provider Manual. Texas.
7. International Liaison Committee on Resuscitation (ILCOR). (2015). Systems of care and continuous quality improvement. [online] ILCOR website. Available from *www.ilcor.org*. [Accessed November, 2016].
8. American Heart Association (AHA). The expanded systematic approach. In: ACLS for experienced providers: Manual and resource text. Texas: AHA; 2013.
9. American Heart Association (AHA). Respiratory Arrest. In: Advanced Cardiovascular Life Support: Provider Manual. Texas: AHA; 2016.
10. Kleinman ME, Brennan EE, Goldberger ZD, et al. Adult BLS & CPR quality. AHA 2015 CPR ECC guidelines. Circulation. 2015;132:S414-S435.
11. Pediatric Basic Life Support and Cardiopulmonary Resuscitation Quality. (2015). 2015 CPR ECC guidelines. Available from *www.ilcor.org*. [Accessed November, 2016].
12. American Heart Association (AHA). BLS for healthcare providers student manual. Texas: AHA;2016.
13. Advanced Cardiac Life Support. AHA 2015 CPR ECC guidelines. Circulation. 2015;132(suppl 2):S444-64.
14. American Heart Association (AHA). VF/pulseless VT. In: ACLS provider manual. Texas: AHA;2016.
15. International Liaison Committee on Resuscitation. (2015). Post Cardiac Arrest Care CPR ECC guidelines. [online] ILCOR website.Available from *www.ilcor.org* [Accessed November, 2016].
16. Callaway CW, Donnino MW, Fink EL, et al. Part 8: Post–Cardiac Arrest Care. 2015 American Heart Association Guidelines Update for Cardiopulmonary Resuscitation and Emergency Cardiovascular Care. Circulation. 2015;132:S465-S482.
17. Nolan JP, Morley PT, Vanden TL, et al. Therapeutic hypothermia after cardiac arrest. Circulation. 2003;108:118-121.

CHAPTER 12

Airway Management

Amit D Nabar

INTRODUCTION

Airway management is an essential skill and is fundamental to the practice of emergency medicine.

Hypoxia and airway compromise contribute significantly to prehospital deaths. Hypoxemia prevention needs an unobstructed and protected airway with adequate ventilation that takes precedence over management of all other clinical conditions.

The challenges facing an emergency physician are augmented in acute settings, and respiratory management demands higher level of competency and composure.

There has been a significant progress in effective airway management in emergencies and a lot of efforts are going into training and auditing these core skills.

APPLIED ANATOMY

The emergency physicians should possess a good knowledge of airway anatomy enabling them to build a mental image of the airway structure through which they pass.

A clear three-dimensional image of the upper airway is the cornerstone for a successful airway management.

This knowledge of airway helps in the following:
- Fast and focused assessment of the patient's airway and planning airway management
- Appropriate performance of airway opening skills
- For optimal laryngoscopy and intubation
- Assisting in planning for blind intubation and surgical airway.

Nasal Cavity

Presence of deviation of the nasal septum and hypertrophy of the turbinate's can lead to obstruction in the flow of the air as well as it can lead to difficulty in inserting a nasal airway or removal of a foreign body.

Oropharynx and Nasopharynx

These are the most common sites of narrowing and complete airway obstruction.

The three places where obstruction may be commonly encountered include:
1. The point where the soft palate meets the posterior pharyngeal wall in the nasopharynx.
2. In the oropharynx where the posterior movement of the tongue brings it near the soft palate and the posterior pharyngeal wall.
3. Point where the epiglottis moves posteriorly towards the posterior pharyngeal wall in the laryngopharynx.

Mandible

Mandible has an important role in opening of the airway.

Anterior translocation of the jaw elevates the tongue from the posterior pharyngeal wall, helping to clear the airway in obtunded patient or obese patients with history of obstructive sleep apnea.

Receding mandible can present difficulty in laryngoscopy.

Laryngopharynx

Cricoid Cartilage

It is the narrowest point of the airway in pediatric group of patients and is the site for performance of "BURP" maneuver (B: Backwards, U: Upwards, R: Rightwards and P: Posteriorly). Along with thyroid cartilage, it helps in locating the cricothyroid membrane for performing emergency surgical airway.

Laryngeal Inlet

In cases of difficult airways, the interarytenoids notch may be the only landmark to identify the glottic opening **(Fig. 1)**.

- *Valleculae*: It is the site where tip of laryngoscope is advanced into until it engages the underlying hypoepiglottic ligaments.
- *Epiglottis*: It is an important landmark during laryngoscopy and in assessment of the airway helping in predicting the difficulty in securing the airway.
- *Trachea*: The depth of the trachea from the skin tends to increase as it tends to descend downwards.

It comprises of cartilaginous rings that can be felt when advancing the bougie.

Right main bronchus is wider, shorter and more vertical than the left bronchus and can result in inadvertent endobronchial intubation to the right in emergencies.

Axis

An alignment of the pharyngeal and tracheal axis can be made by the flexion of the lower cervical spine. Similarly, the oral axis can be aligned to the pharyngeal or tracheal axis by extension at the atlanto-occipital joint (sniffing position) **(Fig. 2)**.

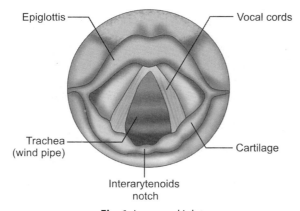

Fig. 1 Laryngeal inlet

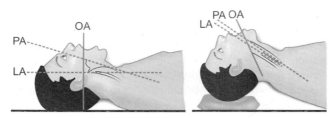

Fig. 2 Sniffing position

CAUSES OF AIRWAY OBSTRUCTION IN EMERGENCY DEPARTMENT

The most common causes of airway obstruction in patients presenting to the emergency department include infections of the oral cavity, trauma, burns and pregnancy.

A list of other causes is as follows:
- Congenital
    - Obstruction above the larynx
        - Choanal atresia
        - Skeletal malformations, e.g. micrognathia, Treacher Collins syndrome.
    - Obstruction in the larynx
        - Atresia
        - Webs
    - Tracheal obstruction
        - Web
        - Tracheomalacia
- Infections
    - Nose
        - Septal abscess
        - Rhinosporidiosis
    - Oral cavity
        - Peritonsillar abscess
        - Infection of floor of mouth
    - Pharynx
        - Adenoids
        - Retropharyngeal abscess
    - Larynx
        - Epiglottis
        - Laryngotracheobronchitis
        - Diphtheria
    - Neck
    - Ludwig angina
- *Tumor and benign masses*: The following conditions may lead to internal and external narrowing of the airway
    - Papilloma
    - Cyst
    - Hygroma
- Burns
    - Scarring
- Trauma
    - Maxillofacial trauma
    - Neck trauma
    - Laryngeal trauma
- Radiation
    - Edema of surrounding tissue
- Others
    - Pregnancy
    - Obtunded patient
    - Obese individuals.

OBJECTIVE SIGNS OF AIRWAY OBSTRUCTION

Recognition of an *obstructed airway* is the first step towards successful airway management.

The presentation may be as follows:
- Sudden in onset with complete obstruction
- Gradual onset with partial obstruction
- Progressive and recurrent
- Unobstructed respiration is always *quiet*, it is never silent or noisy
- Total respiratory obstruction may usually have a *silent* (due to absence of breath sounds and movement of air) presentation
- Partial respiratory obstruction is noisy
- Snoring which may be due to tongue fall
- Gurgling sounds due to collection of fluids or secretions in the pharynx
- Stridor due to glottic or supraglottic obstruction
- Tachypnea may be an early sign of airways and ventilatory compromise. Severely compromised airways may lead to the use of accessory muscles of respiration, sternal retraction, cyanosis, anxiety, sweating, tachycardia, etc.

CLINICAL ASSESSMENT OF THE AIRWAY

Emergent situations demand a fast and focused airway evaluation for patients requiring airway management.

Talking to patient is an important early measure in assessment of the airway for obstruction.

An affirmative and proper verbal response suggests an unobstructed airway with intact ventilation and an adequate brain perfusion in the patient.

A difficult airway cannot be essentially predicted always.

Mnemonic: LEMON highlights patient who may have difficulty in intubation.

L: Look externally (Inspect the patient for—foreign body, facial trauma, dental issues, anatomical variation, etc.)

E: Evaluate 3-3-2 **(Figs 3A to C)**
- 3-finger breadths between incisors
- 3 fingers from the tip of the chin to the neck
- 2 fingers from the chin or neck junction to the thyroid cartilage.

M: Mallampati classification **(Fig. 4)**

SUFA is a mnemonic for the same
- Class 1: The soft palate, uvula, fauces and anterior pillar can be seen completely
- Class 2: The soft palate, uvula and fauces can be seen completely
- Class 3: The soft palate and base of the uvula can be seen
- Class 4: Only the hard palate can be seen.

O: Obesity or obstruction, e.g. epiglottis, trauma, etc.

N: Neck mobility.
- None of the predictors are particularly sensitive
- The airway has to be evaluated prior to every intervention to predict the likelihood of difficulty in management.

PREPARATION

Emergency department is a time critical environment and preplanning for airway management is essential.

A checklist can aid in preparation and maintenance of airway assist devices **(Figs 5A to C)**.

Equipment for Airway Management

- Oxygen source
- Nasal prongs
- Clear face mask of various sizes
- Ambu bag
- Bag value mask
- *Laryngoscope*: Handle and blades
- Endotracheal tubes
- *Oropharyngeal airways*: Small, medium, large
- *Nasopharyngeal airways*: Small, medium, large
- Suction apparatus with suction catheter
- Magills forceps
- Stylets
- Bougie
- Anesthetic or lubricating gel
- *Rescue devices*: Laryngeal mask airway (LMA), combitube, laryngeal tube airway, etc.

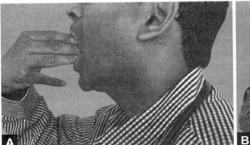 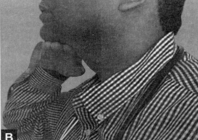 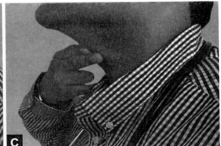

Figs 3A to C Airway assessment

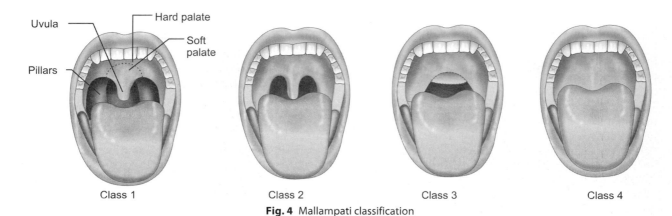

Fig. 4 Mallampati classification

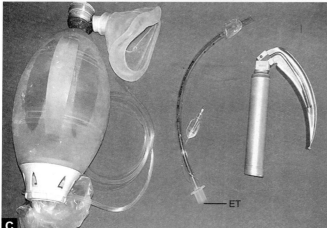

Figs 5A to C Equipment for airway management. (A) Laryngeal mask airway, oropharyngeal airway, nasopharyngeal airway; (B) Suction apparatus with suction catheter, magills forceps, stylets, anesthetic or lubricating gel; (C) Ambu bag, laryngoscope and endotracheal tubes
Abbreviation: ET, endotracheal tubes; LMA, laryngeal mask airway; OPA, oropharyngeal airway; NPA, nasopharyngeal airway.

- *Surgical airway*: Cricothyroidotomy kit
- Medications for rapid sequence intubation and topical airway anesthesia.

Monitors: A multipara monitor is ideal for the emergency department. It should comprise of the following variables:
- Pulse oximetery
- Noninvasive blood pressure monitoring
- Electrocardiogram
- End-tidal CO_2 or continuous wave capnography

A *portable* ventilator having invasive as well as noninvasive modes is preferred for the emergency department.

Difficult Airway Trolley

A difficult airway trolley may comprise of the following (Fig. 6):
- *Oropharyngeal airways of all sizes*: 1, 2, 3 and 4
- *Nasopharyngeal airway of sizes*: 5, 6, 7, 8 and 9
- Laryngoscope with a straight blade
- Macintosh blade with FlexiTip
- Short handle, slim handle laryngoscope, pediatric handle laryngoscope, magills forceps medium and large
- *Stylet*: Small, medium and large
- *Laryngeal mask airway*: Size 2, 3, 4 and patented versions of LMA are also available. For example, supreme and ProSeal. A type of LMA also exists which is known as an intubating LMA (LMA Fastrach) which serves as a conduit for intubation.
  - Light Wand
- *Endotracheal tube introducer*: Frova intubating introducer
- Bougie
- Video laryngoscope
- Fiberoptic bronchoscope
  - Cricothyroidotomy kit
- Surgical cricothyroidotomy set
- Jet ventilator.

The detailed description of all the above instruments are outside the scope of discussion in this chapter.

MANAGEMENT

The priority in patients with obstructed airway is to relieve the obstruction, if any, ensure adequate oxygenation or ventilation and protect the airway. Appropriate airway evaluation, clinical judgment, experience and preparation are the final determinant for the appropriate route of airway management.

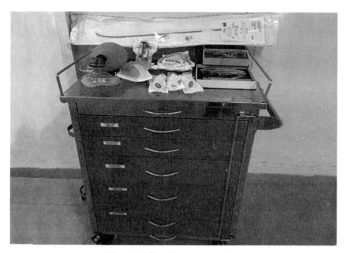

Fig. 6 Difficult airway trolley

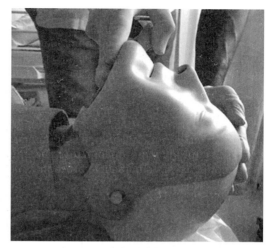

Fig. 7 Head tilt-chin lift maneuver

- Nonsurgical
  - Bag mask ventilation (BMV)
  - Rapid sequence intubation
  - Extraglottic and supraglottic devices
- Surgical airway
  - Needle cricothyroidotomy
  - Surgical cricothyroidotomy
  - Percutaneous cricothyroidotomy
- Newer techniques
  - Video laryngoscope
  - Fiberoptic intubation
  - Ultrasound.

Opening the Airway

- *Head tilt-chin lift maneuver*: Finger placed behind the mandible displace it upwards so as to bring the chin anterior (**Fig. 7**).
- *Jaw thrust*: It is accomplished by grasping the angle of jaw and lifting it with both hands, one on each side, moving the jaw forward. The patient's lips are opened by lowering the lip with the thumb.
  Care must be taken to avoid neck extension (**Figs 8A and B**).

Bag-mask Ventilation

It is an essential emergency skill that is mandatory to every member of the emergency team.

Following are the predictors of difficult bag mask ventilation:
- Higher body mass index or weight
- Older age
- Limited mandibular protrusion
- Decreased thyromental distance
- Mallampati score of three or four
- Beard
- Edentulous patient
- History of radiation to neck
- History of snoring or sleep apnea
- Facial trauma.

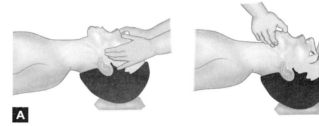

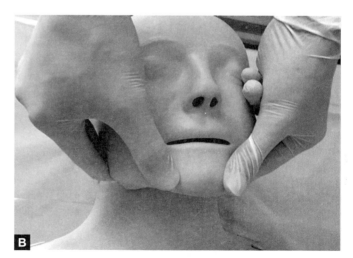

Figs 8A and B Jaw thrust

Techniques

- *One-hand Technique*: E-C technique **(Fig. 9)**
  - Place mask on the face with the narrow portion at the bridge of the nose
  - Make a complete seal by using the index finger and thumb of one hand on the side of the mask
  - Pull the face into the mask
  - Angle of jaw is lifted using the remaining fingers, opening the airway and pressing the face against the mask
  - The Ambu bag is squeezed gently to ensure adequate chest rise.
- *Two-hand Technique* **(Fig. 10)**
  - Two opposing semi circles are created with the thumb and index finger of each hand to form a ring around the mask connector and to hold the mask on the patients face
  - The mandible is lifted with the remaining digits
  - Choosing appropriate size of mask as it helps to create a good seal and provides effective ventilation.

Airway Adjuncts

Oropharyngeal Airway

- Used in unresponsive patients with absent gag reflex
- It helps to relieve obstruction caused by tongue fall by lifting the tongue from the back of hypopharynx
- *Optimum size*: Distance between angle of mouth and angle of jaw.

Nasopharyngeal Airway

- Inserted via the nose and can be used in both conscious and unconscious patients
- Does not stimulate gag reflex
- It helps to relieve obstruction caused by tongue fall
- *Size*: Distance between ala of the nose to the tragus.
  Contraindication:
  - Patients on anticoagulants
  - Fracture base of skull
  - Nasal deformity
  - Nasal infection
  - Pediatric patients.

Endotracheal Intubation

Rapid sequence intubation is the preferred mode of intubation in emergency department.

It is a process in which potent sedatives and rapidly acting neuromuscular blocking agents are administered simultaneously to induce unconsciousness and motor paralysis for tracheal intubation.

Seven P's of "Rapid sequence intubation":
1. *Prepare*: Organize and prepare the airway management plan with backup.
2. *Preoxygenation*: 100% oxygen is used along with non-rebreathing mask. This also helps in denitrogenation.
3. *Pretreatment*: With appropriate drugs
   - Lignocaine
   - Opiates
   - Anticholinergic agents
4. *Putting to sleep*:
   - The administration of induction and paralytic agent in rapid succession to induce sleep in the patient
   - Apply cricoid pressure until airway is protected with endotracheal tube
   - Inducing agents are as follows—
     - Etomidate
     - Ketamine

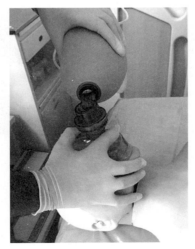

Fig. 9 One-hand technique

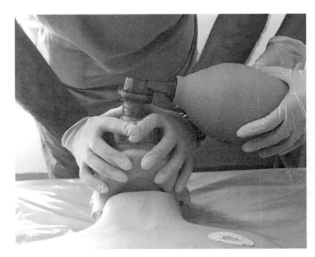

Fig. 10 Two-hand technique

- Midazolam
- Fentanyl
- Paralytic agents are as follows:
  - Succinylcholine
  - Rocuronium.
5. *Place the tube*:
   - Endotracheal tube is placed under vision.
   - Cricoid pressure is applied—BURP (B-backwards, u-upwards, r-rightwards and p-posteriorly) maneuver that minimizes the risk of aspiration.
   - The endotracheal tube cuff has to be inflated and placement of tube confirmed before releasing the cricoid pressure.
6. *Prove placement*: Placement of the tube can be confirmed by the following:
   - Auscultation
   - Capnography
   - Esophageal detectors
   - X-ray chest
   - Ultrasound
7. *Post-intubation management*:
   - Patient is sedated with appropriate drugs and placed on mechanical ventilation.
   - In event of an inability to secure the airway or intubate after administration of a sedative and neuromuscular blocking agent, the patient should be ventilated with bag mask and the *failed intubation protocol* in accordance with the available resources and expertise should be followed.

Failed Intubation Drill

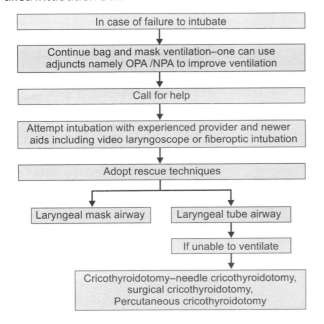

Extraglottic and Supraglottic Devices

Features

These devices are placed inside the oropharyngeal and esophageal area but outside the glottis, i.e. they do not pass through the vocal cords.
- Anatomical and technical factors have a lesser influence on their placement.
- They can be used for both ventilation and as intubation assist device.
- Ideal for short-term assistance until definitive airway is secured.

Laryngeal Mask Airway

- These devices are relatively easier to insert.
- Laryngeal mask airway can be used as a conduit for intubation especially in cases of failed or difficult intubations.
- It is designed like an endotracheal tube with a large elliptical mark on the distal end which is placed over the hypopharynx and covers the supraglottic structures, thereby allowing relative isolation of the trachea.
- However, aspiration prevention is not guaranteed by LMA **(Fig. 11)**.

Laryngeal Tube Airway

- These are double-balloon airway devices
- The provider can blindly insert the device and confirm placement by auscultation
- Used as a resuscitation rescue device
- It needs minimum manipulation of head and neck for its placement **(Fig. 12)**.

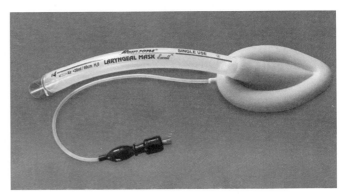

Fig. 11 Laryngeal mask airway

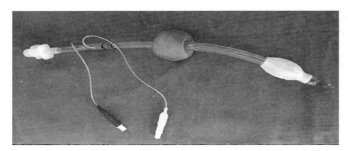

Fig. 12 Laryngeal tube airway

Surgical Airway

A surgical airway can be established in an emergent situation by the following:
- Needle cricothyroidotomy
- Surgical cricothyroidotomy
- Percutaneous cricothyroidotomy, using Seldinger technique.

Cricothyroidotomy

Cricothyroidotomy is an emergency procedure whereby a tube is placed through the cricothyroid membrane to establish a patent airway for oxygenation and ventilation.

This technique is adopted when there is failure to secure the airway using nonsurgical techniques or when other rescue devices have failed.

Needle cricothyroidotomy: It is the least of the invasive emergency airway surgical procedure that can be performed within a short time in event of an emergency. It needs minimal manipulation of the cervical spine.

A needle is inserted through the cricothyroid membrane in order to provide oxygenation until a definitive airway can be established.

It is then connected to an oxygen source with a flow rate of 15 L/min using a "Y" connector and 1 second on and 4 seconds off technique.

Patients with normal pulmonary functions can be ventilated for about 30–45 minutes with this technique.

Surgical cricothyroidotomy: The landmarks, namely the thyroid and cricoid cartilage as well as the cricothyroid membrane are palpated.

A vertical incision is made through the skin and further dissection is carried vertically until the cricothyroid membrane is identified.

A horizontal incision is made through the cricothyroid membrane and then widened with a hemostat or an artery forceps.

A small endotracheal tube or tracheostomy tube is then placed through the opening.

Percutaneous cricothyroidotomy: This is performed by using *cricothyroidotomy kit* available commercially and by using a Seldinger technique **(Figs 13A and B)**.

No significant difference has been demonstrated in outcomes or complications by use of any of the above techniques.

Cricothyroidotomy should not be performed in children less than 12 years of age, as the cricothyroid membrane is quite narrow resulting in an increased risk of permanent laryngeal injury. Other contraindications included are as follows:
- Obstruction distal to cricoid membrane.
    - Infection or lesion at site of incision
    - Lack of expertise

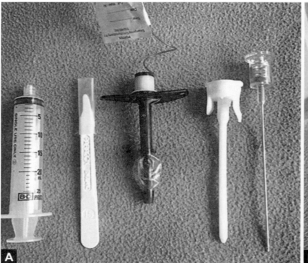
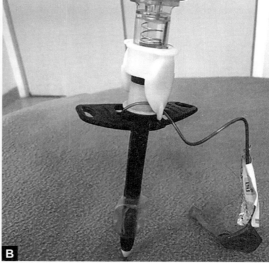

Figs 13A and B Percutaneous cricothyroidotomy

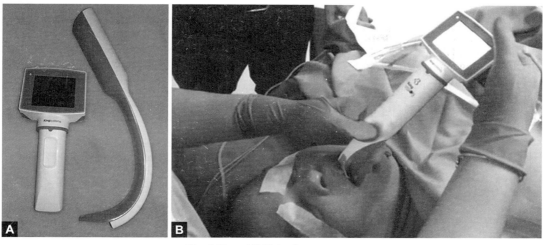

Figs 14A and B Video laryngoscope

- History of neck surgery
- Hematoma
- Obesity which may make localization of landmark difficult
- Trauma or burns.

Newer Techniques

Video Laryngoscope

- It works like a traditional laryngoscope with an angulated blade. The video images are captured and projected back on the monitor screen.
- It improves visualization of the larynx and reduces the time to tracheal intubation (**Figs 14A and B**).

Indications:
- Morbid obesity
- Trauma or anatomical limitation
- Restricted mouth opening
- Limited neck extension
- Suspected cervical spine injury.

Fiberoptic Intubation

- It is used in an emergency situation with a difficult airway to facilitate tracheal intubation in an awake patient, via the oral or nasal route.
- It is a technique that can be adopted in cases of anticipated difficult airways.
- This is a technique which requires arrangement of the instruments and apparatus so it is a time consuming process (**Fig. 15**).

Ultrasound

Bedside ultrasound is showing a promise in emergent airway management.

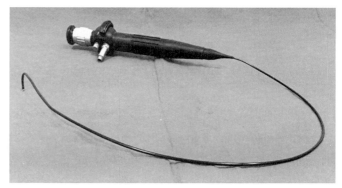

Fig. 15 Fiberoptic intubation

It may help in the following:
- Identify key landmarks and help in confirmation of tube placement
- Localization of trachea and tracheal ring interspaces for tracheostomy and percutaneous dilatational tracheostomy.

Ultrasound is useful for prediction of difficult airway and diagnosing pathology that can affect airway management. It helps to measure gastric content prior to airway management and for confirmation of gastric tube placement.
- For airway related nerve blocks.
- It is used for identification of the appropriate diameter of endotracheal, endobronchial or tracheostomy tubes.
- Ultrasound differentiates between tracheal versus esophageal intubation or tracheal versus endobronchial intubation.
- Ultrasound is helpful in bed diagnosing of pneumothorax.

CONCLUSION

Airway management in emergency department is a challenging procedure. Every emergency physician should be competent to perform it. Airway management is vital procedure and this is not a "one size fit to all" procedure. Emergency physician should be trained and expertise in managing the difficult airway. Patient with respiratory distress often need airway management. Systematic approach is needed for airway management.

BIBLIOGRAPHY

1. Abdelmalak B, Makary L, Hoban J, et al. Dexmedetomidine as sole sedative for awake intubation in management of the critical airway. J Clin Anesth. 2007;19(5):370-3.
2. Adnet F, Baillard C, Borron SW, et al. Randomized study comparing the "sniffing position" with simple head extension for laryngoscopic view in elective surgery patients. Anesthesiology. 2001;95(4):836-41.
3. Adnet F, Minadeo JP, Finot MA, et al. A survey of sedation protocols used for emergency endotracheal intubation in poisoned patients in the French prehospital medical system. Eur J Emerg Med. 1998;5(4):415-9.
4. Albanese J, Arnaud S, Rey M, et al. Ketamine decreases intracranial pressure and electroencephalographic activity in traumatic brain injury patients during propofol sedation. Anesthesiology. 1997;87(6):1328-34.
5. Altermatt FR, Munoz HR, Delfino AE, et al. Pre-oxygenation in the obese patient: effects of position on tolerance to apnoea. Br J Anaesth. 2005;95(5):706-9.
6. Aroni F, Iacovidou N, Dontas I, et al. Pharmacological aspects and potential new clinical applications of ketamine: reevaluation of an old drug. J Clin Pharmacol. 2009;49(8):957-64.
7. Baraka A, Salem MR, Joseph NJ. Critical hemoglobin desaturation can be delayed by apneic diffusion oxygenation. Anesthesiology. 1999;90(1):332-3.
8. Benumof J. Airway management: principles and practice. St Louis (MO): Mosby; 1996.
9. Burkle CM, Walsh MT, Harrison BA, et al. Airway management after failure to intubate by direct laryngoscopy: outcomes in a large teaching hospital. Can J Anaesth. 2005;52(6):634-40.
10. Carollo DS, Nossaman BD, Ramadhyani U. Dexmedetomidine: a review of clinical applications. Curr Opin Anaesthesiol. 2008;21(4):457-61.
11. Christian S, Manji M. Indications for endotracheal intubation and ventilation. Trauma. 2004;6(4):249-54.
12. Cook TM, Woodall N, Frerk C. 4th National Audit Project of The Royal College of Anaesthetists and the Difficult Airway Society. London: The Royal College of Anaesthetists; 2011. ISBN 978-1-900936-03-3.
13. de Boer HD, Driessen JJ, Marcus MA, et al. Reversal of rocuronium-induced (1.2 mg/kg) profound neuromuscular block by sugammadex: a multicenter, dose finding and safety study. Anesthesiology. 2007;107(2):239-44.
14. Dronen SC, Merigian KS, Hedges JR, et al. A comparison of blind nasotracheal and succinylcholine-assisted intubation in the poisoned patient. Ann Emerg Med. 1987;16(6):650-2.
15. El-Khatib MF, Kanazi G, Baraka AS. Noninvasive bilevel positive airway pressure for preoxygenation of the critically ill morbidly obese patient. Can J Anaesth. 2007;54(9):744-7.
16. El-Orbany M, Connolly LA. Rapid sequence induction and intubation: current controversy. Anesth Analg. 2010;110(5):1318-25.
17. Gudzenko V, Bittner EA, Schmidt UH. Emergency airway management. Respir Care. 2010;55(8):1026-35.
18. Hohl CM, Kelly-Smith CH, Yeung TC, et al. The effect of a bolus dose of etomidate on cortisol levels, mortality, and health services utilization: a systematic review. Ann Emerg Med. 2010;56(2):105-13.e105.
19. Janssens M, Hartstein G. Management of difficult intubation. Eur J Anaesthesiol. 2001;18(1):3-12.
20. Kulstad EB, Kalimullah EA, Tekwani KL, et al. Etomidate as an induction agent in septic patients: red flags or false alarms? West J Emerg Med. 2010;11(2):161-72.
21. Mallon WK, Keim SM, Shoenberger JM, et al. Rocuronium vs. succinylcholine in the emergency department: a critical appraisal. J Emerg Med. 2009;37(2):183-8.
22. McCafferty MH, Polk HC Jr. Patient safety and quality in surgery. Surg Clin North Am. 2007;87(4):867-81, vii.
23. McIndewar IC, Marshall RJ. Interactions between the neuromuscular blocking drug Org NC 45 and some anaesthetic, analgesic and antimicrobial agents. Br J Anaesth. 1981;53(8):785-92.
24. Minton MD, Grosslight K, Stirt JA, et al. Increases in intracranial pressure from succinylcholine: prevention by prior nondepolarizing blockade. Anesthesiology. 1986;65(2):165-9.
25. Morris C, Perris A, Klein J, et al. Anaesthesia in haemodynamically compromised emergency patients: does ketamine represent the best choice of induction agent? Anaesthesia. 2009;64(5):532-9.
26. Mort TC, Waberski BH, Clive J. Extending the preoxygenation period from 4 to 8 mins in critically ill patients undergoing emergency intubation. Crit Care Med. 2009;37(1):68-71.
27. Mort TC. Preoxygenation in critically ill patients requiring emergency tracheal intubation. Crit Care Med. 2005;33(11):2672-5.
28. Ong JR, Chong FC, Chen CC, et al. Comparing the performance of traditional direct laryngoscope with three indirect laryngoscopes: a prospective manikin study in normal and difficult airway scenarios. Emerg Med Australas. 2011;23(5):606-14.
29. Pagel PS, Kampine JP, Schmeling WT, et al. Ketamine depresses myocardial contractility as evaluated by the preload recruitable stroke work relationship in chronically instrumented dogs with autonomic nervous system blockade. Anesthesiology. 1992;76(4):564-72.
30. Ramachandran SK, Cosnowski A, Shanks A, et al. Apneic oxygenation during prolonged laryngoscopy in obese patients: a randomized, controlled trial of nasal oxygen administration. J Clin Anesth. 2010;22(3):164-8.
31. Reber A, Engberg G, Wegenius G, et al. Lung aeration. The effect of preoxygenation and hyperoxygenation during total intravenous anaesthesia. Anaesthesia. 1996;51(8):733-7.
32. Reynolds SF, Heffner J. Airway management of the critically ill patient: rapid sequence intubation. Chest. 2005;127(4):1397-412.
33. Riker RR, Shehabi Y, Bokesch PM, et al. Dexmedetomidine vs midazolam for sedation of critically ill patients: a randomized trial. JAMA. 2009;301(5):489-99.
34. Robinson N, Clancy M. In patients with head injury undergoing rapid sequence intubation, does pretreatment with intravenous lignocaine/lidocaine lead to an improved neurological outcome? A review of the literature. Emerg Med J 2001;18(6):453-7.

35. Sagarin MJ, Barton ED, Chng YM, et al. Airway management by US and Canadian emergency medicine residents: a multicenter analysis of more than 6,000 endotracheal intubation attempts. Ann Emerg Med. 2005;46(4):328-36.
36. Sagarin MJ, Barton ED, Sakles JC, et al. Underdosing of midazolam in emergency endotracheal intubation. Acad Emerg Med. 2003;10(4):329-38.
37. Salhi B, Stettner E. In defense of the use of lidocaine in rapid sequence intubation. Ann Emerg Med. 2007;49(1):84-6.
38. Santoni BG, Hindman BJ, Puttlitz CM, et al. Manual in-line stabilization increases pressures applied by the laryngoscope blade during direct laryngoscopy and orotracheal intubation. Anesthesiology. 2009;110(1):24-31.
39. Schofer JM. Premedication during rapid sequence intubation: a necessity or waste of valuable time? Cal J Emerg Med. 2006;7(4):75-9.
40. Sivilotti ML, Filbin MR, Murray HE, et al. Does the sedative agent facilitate emergency rapid sequence intubation? Acad Emerg Med. 2003;10(6):612-20.
41. Sparr HJ, Leo C, Ladner E, et al. Influence of anaesthesia and muscle relaxation on intubating conditions and sympathoadrenal response to tracheal intubation. Acta Anaesthesiol Scand. 1997;41(10):1300-7.
42. Stirt JA, Grosslight KR, Bedford RF, et al. "Defasciculation" with metocurine prevents succinylcholine-induced increases in intracranial pressure. Anesthesiology. 1987;67(1):50-3.
43. Thiboutot F, Nicole PC, Trepanier CA, et al. Effect of manual in-line stabilization of the cervical spine in adults on the rate of difficult orotracheal intubation by direct laryngoscopy: a randomized controlled trial. Can J Anaesth. 2009;56(6):412-8.
44. Turner CR, Block J, Shanks A, et al. Motion of a cadaver model of cervical injury during endotracheal intubation with a Bullard laryngoscope or a Macintosh blade with and without in-line stabilization. J Trauma. 2009;67(1):61-6.
45. Vaillancourt C, Kapur AK. Opposition to the use of lidocaine in rapid sequence intubation. Ann Emerg Med. 2007;49(1):86-7.
46. Walls RM, Brown CA 3rd, Bair AE, et al. Emergency airway management: a multicenter report of 8937 emergency department intubations. J Emerg Med. 2011;41(4):347-54.
47. Weingart SD. Preoxygenation, reoxygenation, and delayed sequence intubation in the emergency department. J Emerg Med. 2011;40(6):661-7.
48. Wilbur K, Zed PJ. Is propofol an optimal agent for procedural sedation and rapid sequence intubation in the emergency department? CJEM. 2001;3(4):302-10.
49. Wong E, Ng YY. The difficult airway in the emergency department. Int J Emerg Med. 2008;1(2):107-11.
50. Zvara DA, Calicott RW, Whelan DM. Positioning for intubation in morbidly obese patients. Anesth Analg. 2006;102(5):1592. The Difficult Airway 417

CHAPTER 13

Management of Critically Ill Patient in Emergency

Chandrashekhar, Swarup S Padhi, Ajeet Singh, Tariq Ali, Yatin Mehta

INTRODUCTION

With all its complexities, the human body runs incessantly with heart as the engine, blood as the fuel and traversing the entire body, the blood vessels acting like pipelines that distribute the fuel to all the organs. But due to illnesses, one or all of these mechanisms gets altered and becomes unsteady, resulting in slowing down of the body as a whole in its functioning.

BODY FLUID COMPARTMENTS

The body fluid is divided into extracellular and intracellular compartments. The extracellular compartment is further divided into plasma and interstitial fluid. If we consider a 70 kg healthy individual, the total body water (TBW) comprises of 60% of body weight or almost 42L **(Flow chart 1)**.

PRINCIPLES OF FLUID THERAPY IN CRITICALLY ILL

There arises times, when the body requires fluid from outside, as in various conditions viz., vomiting, diarrhea, blood loss, sepsis, shock, diabetic ketoacidosis, sweating, ascites, gastrointestinal fistula (GIF), fever, ascites, etc. To know which fluid is appropriate for a given clinical condition is imperative. So for the right therapy, it is necessary to know the reason behind the fluid deficit and the concurrent illnesses like renal condition, diabetes or any liver affection. This is necessary, as the clinician has to decide which fluid is to be infused in a specific condition and which fluid to avoid, how much fluid to give and at what rate the correction should go on and whether there is associated electrolyte imbalances that may necessitate a particular fluid therapy at a particular rate.

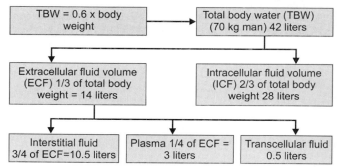

Flow chart 1 Distribution of fluid volume in a 70 kg man

Type	Total	ICF	ECF	Interstitial	Plasma
% of body weight	60%	40%	20%	15%	5%
Volume	42L	28L	14L	10.5L	3.5L

Extracellular fluid deficit indicates loss from the interstitial and intravascular compartments. The loss can be either equiproportion of solutes and water or water in excess of solutes leading to terminologies like iso-osmolar deficit and hyperosmolar deficit, respectively.

Table 1 is showcasing components of physical examination of septic shock and hypovolemic shock.

Hypovolemia has been classified in many ways. It can be classified clinically as mild, moderate and severe depending on the amount lost from the body. Fatal dehydration which is 20–30% of body weight leads to anuria and coma leading to death **(Table 2)**.

Indications of Fluids

- Severe vomiting and diarrhea
- Dehydration and shock

Table 1 Differentiation between septic shock and hypovolemic shock based on the components of traditional physical examination

Septic shock	Hypovolemic shock
Vasodilatation and a high-cardiac output state	Reduced cardiac output
• Warm extremities • Bounding pulse • Low diastolic blood pressure • Wide pulse pressure	• Cold extremities • Thready pulse • Narrow pulse pressure
Patients typically manifest early with mental status changes, tachypnea fever, and a toxic appearance	Mental status changes and a toxic appearance do not typically develop until the patient is severly shocked

Table 2 Clinical evaluation of fluid deficit and its signs and symptoms

Severity	Fluid deficit	Signs and symptoms
Mild	<2 L	Thirst, concentrated urine
Moderate	2–3 L	Weakness, oliguria, postural hypotension, low jugular venous pressure (JVP)
Severe	>3 L	Confusion, hypotension, tachycardia, cold extremities, reduced skin turgor

Table 3 Clinical usage and examples of intravenous fluids

Fluids	Examples	Clinical usage
Replacement fluid	Isotonic saline, Ringer's lactate (RL), dextrose normal saline (DNS), Isolyte-G (Iso-G)	Vomiting, diarrhea, infections, trauma, burns
Maintenance fluid	5% dextrose, dextrose with half normal saline	Fluids lost normally in urine, sweat, feces and via lungs
Special fluids	25% dextrose, 3% saline	Hypoglycemia, hyponatremia

- During surgery
- Hypoglycemia
- As a carrier for various drugs and as infusions like using antibiotics and vasopressors
- Total parenteral nutrition.

Fluids should be cautiously used in congestive conditions and in volume overload situations.

Therapy can be given both orally and intravenously but intravenous route is preferred for critically ill patients as it has various advantages over the oral route like prompt correction of fluids and electrolytes with immediate response to administration of fluids.

Out of all the fluids available with the clinician, Ringer's lactate (RL) happens to be the most physiological fluid as its components are similar to the extracellular fluid.

Classification of Intravenous Fluids (Table 3)

- Replacement fluids
- Maintenance fluids
- Special fluids

Replacement Fluids

- Isotonic saline, RL, dextrose normal saline (DNS)
- They are most commonly used and their usage is for correction of conditions like vomiting, diarrhea, infections, trauma, and burns.

Maintenance Fluids

- 5% dextrose, dextrose with half normal saline
- They are used to replenish the fluids that are lost normally in urine, sweat and feces.

Special Fluids

- 25% dextrose, 3% saline
- Used in conditions like hypoglycemia, hyponatremia, etc.

Fluids can also be classified into crystalloids and colloids. Commonly used crystalloids are RL, normal Saline and DNS whereas colloids are albumin, hetastarch, gelatin and dextran. **Table 4** indicates the fluids their composition, indications and contraindications.

Monitoring Fluid Therapy

How much fluid exactly a critically ill patient needs is difficult to define on clinical grounds alone. There are various modalities to assess the severity and need of fluid infusion in these patients.

Clinically regaining skin turgor, improvement in sensorium, moist tongue, capillary refill, increase in urine output, improvement in blood pressure, settling of tachycardia, improvement in acidosis suggest that fluid

Table 4 Composition, indications and contraindications of intravenous fluids

Fluids	Composition	Indications	Contraindications
5% dextrose	1L contains 50g glucose	Prevention and treatment of dehydration, to provide calories, IV administration of various drugs, correction of hypernatremia, pre- and postoperative fluid replacement	Cerebral edema, ischemic stroke, neurosurgeries, hyponatremia, diabetes
Normal saline	1L contains 154 mEq of Na and Cl each	Water and salt depletion, alkalosis with dehydration, diarrhea, vomiting, sweating, hyponatremia, initial therapy in diabetic ketoacidosis, ARF, vehicle for drugs, hypercalcemia	Hypertensive patients, hypernatremia, congestive heart failure, dehydration with severe hypokalemia
Dextrose normal saline (DNS)	1L contains 50g glucose, 154 mEq of Na and Cl each	Salt depletion and hypovolemia, vomiting along with supply of calories	Generalized edema as in liver and kidney disease, hypovolemic shock
Ringer's lactate	1L contains Na: 130 mEq, Cl: 109 mEq, K:4 mEq, Ca: 3 mEq, HCO_3: 28 mEq	Severe hypovolemia, postoperative patients, burns, diabetic ketoacidosis, diarrhea induced hypovolemia	Liver disease, and in shock patients, congestive heart failure, severe metabolic acidosis, along with blood transfusion
25% dextrose	1L contains 250g glucose	Rapid correction of hypoglycemia, treatment of hyperkalemia along with insulin	Dehydration and anuric patients, diabetes
Albumin	5% (50 g/L), 25% (250 g/L)	Plasma volume expansion, in plasmapheresis as an exchange fluid, correction of hypoproteinemia	Rapid infusion can cause pulmonary edema, caution in low cardiac reserve, severe anemia, cardiac failure
Dextran	Dextran 70 and dextran 40	Hypovolemia, as in burns, trauma and surgery, prophylaxis in DVT and to improve blood flow and microcirculation	Renal failure, hypersensitivity to dextran, severe dehydration, bleeding disorders
Gelatin (Haemaccel)	1L contains gelatin: 35 g, Na: 145 mEq, Cl: 145 mEq, Ca: 12.5 mEq, K: 5.1 mEq	Rapid expansion of intravascular volume as in shock, trauma, burns and blood loss	Hypersensitivity, bronchospasm
Hetastarch (HES)	6% solution in normal saline	Plasma expansion for hypovolemia	Bleeding disorders, congestive heart failure and renal failure

Abbreviations: Na, sodium; Cl, chlorine; K, potassium; Ca, calcium; HCO_3, bicarbonate anion; DVT, deep vein thrombosis; ARF, acute renal failure; IV, intravenous.

replenishment is adequate and hypovolemia is getting corrected.

The concept of preload, afterload and contractility is essential as they determine the cardiac output. Preload is defined as the load imposed on resting muscle that stretches the muscle to a new length. Contractility is defined as the velocity of muscle contraction when the muscle load is fixed. The total load that must be moved by a muscle when it contracts is the afterload.

But hemodynamic instability is very common in patients who are critically ill and might look normal deceptively, based on these parameters alone. This may result in false impression of a critically ill patient being stable. Thus there is a need for accurate hemodynamic monitoring surfaced resulting in interventions like central venous pressure (CVP) monitoring, pulmonary capillary wedge pressure (PCWP) monitoring for hemodynamic stability. But again pulmonary artery catheter fell into disrepute due to lack of much benefit with this intervention. CVP and PCWP were found to be a static marker of volume responsiveness. So newer modes or dynamic modes of volume responsiveness were included. These assessment methods are possible bedside.

Dynamic Markers of Volume Responsiveness

The principle of these markers is to induce a change in preload and see the response by monitoring changes in stroke volume and cardiac output (**Flow chart 2**).

Change in preload can be accomplished by either infusing a fluid bolus or passive leg raise that will autotransfuse around 200–300 mL of blood from lower limbs to the central circulation.

- *Monitoring of cardiac output or stroke volume with transesophageal Doppler*: If cardiac output or stroke volume increases by more than 15% with the above mentioned maneuver then the patient is fluid responsive

and if it is less than 10% then the patient would not benefit from fluid therapy.
- Changes in descending aortic blood flow velocity with similar cut-offs.
- Pulse pressure variation or stroke volume variation using arterial pulse tracing. More than 12% indicates fluid responsiveness.

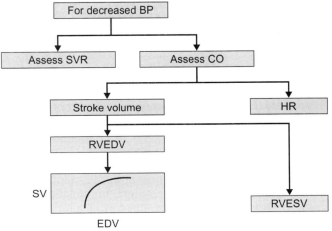

Flow chart 2 Overview of management of shock

Abbreviations: BP, blood pressure; SVR, systemic vascular resistance; CO, cardiac output; HR, heart rate; RVEDV, right ventricular end-diastolic volume; RVESV, right ventricular end-systolic volume; SV, stroke volume; EDV, end-diastolic volume.

These parameters are to be used when the patient is hemodynamically unstable as indicated by mean arterial pressure (MAP) of less than 65 mm Hg or when there is evidence of tissue hypoperfusion like decrease in urine output, confusion, tachycardia, and increase in lactate concentration.

If the blood pressure or cardiac output does not improve with fluid therapy then some form of inotropic support or vasopressors are required to augment them.

VASOACTIVE AGENTS

Vasopressors

These are drugs that cause the constriction of blood vessels, i.e. vasoconstriction resulting in increase in blood pressure, systemic and pulmonary vascular resistance, e.g. norepinephrine, epinephrine, vasopressin, dopamine, phenylephrine and dobutamine.

Inotropes

Inotropes are drugs or agents that increase myocardial contractility. These increase cardiac output, chronotropy and decrease afterload, e.g. epinephrine, dobutamine, isoprenaline and ephedrine.

Flow chart 3 is show casing vasopressor titration algorithm for septic shock.

The drugs mentioned in **Tables 5 and 6** affect various receptors in the body to show their effects.

Flow chart 3 Vasopressor titration algorithm for septic shock

Abbreviation: BP, blood pressure.

Epinephrine

- Naturally occurring, circulating catecholamine which is synthesized from the adrenal medulla
- *Uses*: During hemodynamic instability where it increases myocardial contractility and vascular resistance, during life-threatening anaphylaxis, asthma, during cardiopulmonary resuscitation, and as an additive to local anesthesia to prolong the action
- *Cardiovascular system*: Stimulates both alpha- and beta-receptors
- *Metabolic*: Beta-1 stimulation causes glycogenolysis and lipolysis, alpha-1 stimulation inhibits release of insulin resulting in hyperglycemia
- *Airway smooth muscles*: It is a bronchodilator by acting on the beta-2 receptors in the airways.

Norepinephrine

- Naturally occurring, synthesized in postganglionic sympathetic nerve endings
- *Uses*: Stimulates alpha receptors and produces a dose dependent increase in the systemic vascular resistance (SVR) and MAP. It is a very potent vasoconstrictor. It is the preferred agent for hypotension in sepsis when it is not adequately corrected by volume resuscitation. Its potent vasoconstriction causes decrease in blood flow to kidneys but this effect is not seen during sepsis where it increases the blood pressure without compromising on the renal function.

Dopamine

- It is an endogenous catecholamine that acts as a neurotransmitter and also regulates cardiac and vascular effects. It has dose-dependent effects. The effect cannot be predicted only on dose and needs to be titrated to desired effect.
- *Cardiovascular system*: It increases cardiac output in patients with decreased contractility and low blood pressure, i.e. it is used in conditions where both cardiac contractility and peripheral vasoconstriction is required. It also has a shorter half-life like epinephrine and norepinephrine demanding its use as a continuous infusion. Its dosing is based on ideal body weight.
- Renal dose of dopamine is now obsolete. At lower doses it acts on the dopamine receptors, intermediate doses (5–10 μg/kg/min) causes stimulation of beta receptors resulting in increase in myocardial contractility and at higher doses (>10 μg/kg/min) stimulates alpha receptors causing an increase in pulmonary and systemic vasoconstriction.
- *Caution*: Not to be used with any alkaline solutions as the drug gets inactivated in alkaline preparations. Tachyarrhythmias are common.

Dobutamine

- It is a synthetic catecholamine derived from isoprenaline. It is used an inotrope to increase cardiac output in decompensated heart failure. Dobutamine has potent beta-1 effects and weak beta-2 activity. Its effect on

Table 5 Receptors stimulated by vasoactive drugs

Drugs	Alpha	Beta-1	Beta-2	Dopamine receptors
Epinephrine	+	+++	++	
Norepinephrine	+++	++	0	
Phenylephrine	+++	0	0	
Ephedrine	++	+	+	
Dopamine	++	++	+	++
Dobutamine	0	+++	+	
Isoprenaline	0	+++	+++	

Abbreviations: +, minimal increase; ++, moderate increase; +++, marked increase; 0, no change.

Table 6 Pharmacology of vasoactive drugs

Drugs	Cardiac output	Heart rate	Dysrhythmias	Mean arterial pressure	Renal blood flow	Peripheral vascular resistance	Infusion dose
Epinephrine	++	++	+++	+	--	+-	1–20 μg/min
Norepinephrine	-	-	+	+++	---	+++	4–16 μg/min
Phenylephrine	-	-	NC	+++	---	+++	20–50 μg/min
Ephedrine	++	++	++	++	--	+	Not used
Dopamine	+++	+	+-	+	+++	+	2–20 μg/kg/min
Dobutamine	+++	+	+-	+	++	NC	2–20 μg/kg/min
Isoprenaline	+++	+++	+++	+-	-	---	1–5 μg/min

Abbreviations: NC, no change; +, minimal increase; ++, moderate increase; +++, marked increase; -, minimal decrease, --, moderate decrease; ---, marked decrease.

receptors increases at higher doses. Dobutamine does not produce vasoconstriction, so it is not effective in patients who require increased SVR to increase systemic blood pressure. Dobutamine affects heart rate through its action on beta-1 receptors. Rapid metabolism (half-life of 2 minutes) necessitates its usage as a continuous infusion.

- *Uses*: It produces potent beta agonistic effects at doses less than 5 µg/kg/min increasing myocardial contractility (beta-1 and alpha-1 receptors) and causing a modest degree of peripheral vasodilation (beta-2 receptors). Dobutamine is used to improve cardiac output in patients with congestive heart failure.
- *Side effects*: Tachyarrhythmias occur more frequently at higher dosages or in patients with underlying arrhythmias or heart failure. Ventricular ectopic is common. It is contraindicated in hypertrophic cardiomyopathy.

Phenylephrine

- It acts similar to norepinephrine but is long-lasting and less potent. It acts directly on alpha-1 receptors and it stimulates it at low doses as compared to its action on alpha-2 receptors. It primarily causes venoconstriction.
- *Uses*: It is primarily used to increase systemic blood pressure which has been decreased by sympathetic nervous system blockade. It is especially beneficial in patients with coronary artery disease and those with aortic stenosis as it increases coronary perfusion pressure without the chronotropic action. It reflexly causes decrease in heart rate.

Ephedrine

It acts both directly (by stimulating alpha and beta receptors) and indirectly (by releasing norepinephrine). Similar to phenylephrine, it is used to increase systemic blood pressure in the presence of sympathetic nervous system blockade. The action lasts longer although the increase in blood pressure is modest.

Isoprenaline

- It has action only on beta receptors. It is two to three times more potent than epinephrine and almost 100 times more potent than norepinephrine in terms of its action as a sympathomimetic.
- *Cardiovascular system*: It activates beta-1 receptors in the heart and beta-2 receptors in the skeletal muscle. Cardiac output increases, thereby increasing systolic blood pressure but the MAP may decrease due to decrease in SVR and diastolic blood pressure. Baroreceptor-mediated reflex slowing of the heart rate does not occur during infusion of isoproterenol because MAP is not increased.
- It increases the heart rate in presence of heart block, so it is used as a bridge in these patients till temporary or permanent pacemaker is not there in place.
- *Side effects*: The combination of decreased diastolic blood pressure, increased heart rate and arrhythmias may lead to myocardial ischemia.

ASSESSMENT

Question 1: For emergency department (ED) patients in shock, what are the side effects of vasopressors and inotropes?
- Dopamine increases the risk of tachyarrhythmia compared to norepinephrine
- Dopamine use in septic shock increases mortality compared to norepinephrine
- Vasopressin as a first line vasopressor may be associated with cellular ischemia and skin necrosis, particularly when combined with sustained moderate to high-dose infusions of norepinephrine
- Epinephrine increases metabolic abnormalities compared to norepinephrine
- Epinephrine increases metabolic abnormalities compared to norepinephrine–dobutamine in cardiogenic shock without acute cardiac ischemia.

Question 2: Which vasopressors and inotropes should be used in the treatment of ED patients with cardiogenic shock?
- *Recommendation*: Cardiogenic shock patients in the ED should receive norepinephrine as the first-line vasopressor. (Strong)
- *Recommendation*: Cardiogenic shock patients in the ED should receive dobutamine if an isotope is deemed necessary. (Conditional)

Question 3: Which vasopressors and inotropes should be used in the treatment of ED patients with hypovolemic shock?
- *Recommendation*: Routine vasopressor use in hypovolemic shock is not recommended. (Conditional)
- *Recommendation*: Vasopressin may be indicated in hemorrhagic or hypovolemic shock if a vasopressor is deemed necessary. (Conditional)

Question 4: Which vasopressors and inotropes should be used in ED patients with obstructive shock?
- *Recommendation*: If obstructive shock is not responding to indicated treatment, a systemically active vasopressor should be instituted. (Conditional)
- *Recommendation*: For patients with known or suspected hypertrophic obstructive cardiomyopathy (HOCM) or dynamic outflow obstruction, inotropic agents should be avoided. Judicious use of vasoconstrictive agents can be considered. (Conditional)

Question 5: Which vasopressors and inotropes should be used in ED patients with distributive shock?

- *Recommendation*: Norepinephrine is the first line vasopressor for use in septic shock. (Strong)
- *Recommendation*: Vasopressin should be considered in catecholamine refractory septic shock. (Conditional)
- *Recommendation*: Dobutamine should be used for septic shock with low cardiac output despite adequate volume resuscitation. (Strong)

Question 6: Which vasopressors and inotropes should be used in ED patients with undifferentiated shock?

- *Recommendation*: In undifferentiated shock, a second vasopressor should be added if a goal MAP >70 mm Hg is not being achieved. (Conditional)

Question 7: How should vasopressors and inotropes be administered to ED patients?

- *Recommendation*: Short-term vasopressor infusions (<1–2 hours) or boluses via properly positioned and functioning peripheral intravenous catheters are unlikely to cause local complications. (Conditional)
- *Recommendation*: Vasopressor infusions for prolonged periods (>2–6 hours) should preferentially be administered via central venous catheters. (Conditional)
- *Recommendation*: Inotropes can be given via peripheral catheters (short-term) or central venous catheters (prolonged period) with a similarly low incidence of local complications. (Conditional)
- *Recommendation*: The administration of vasopressors via intraosseous lines is safe in adults. (Conditional)
- *Recommendation*: Vasopressor choice in distributive shock secondary to adrenal insufficiency not responding to steroid replacement is not clear. Patient response to chosen agents should guide therapy. (Conditional)
- *Recommendation*: Epinephrine infusion is the preferred agent for anaphylactic shock that does not respond to intramuscular or intravenous bolus epinephrine. (Strong)
- *Recommendation*: Vasopressor choice in neurogenic shock is not clear. The agent should be determined by patient characteristics and response to treatment. (Conditional)
- *Recommendation*: Epinephrine infusion is the preferred agent for anaphylactic shock that does not respond to intramuscular or intravenous bolus epinephrine. (Strong)
- *Recommendation*: If undifferentiated shock is not responding to fluid resuscitation, norepinephrine should be the first-line vasopressor. (strong)

BIBLIOGRAPHY

1. Clark K, Normile LB. Patient flow in the emergency department: is timeliness to events. Nelson M, Waldrop RD, Jones J, Randall Z (Eds): Critical care provided in an urban emergency department. Am J Emerg Med. 1998;16(1):56-9.
2. Fromm RE, Gibbs LR, McCallum WG, Niziol C, Babcock JC, Gueler AC. Critical care in the emergency department: a time-based study. Crit Care Med. 1993;21(7):970-6.
3. Lambe S, Washington DL, Fink A, Herbst K, Liu H, Fosse JS. Trends in the use and capacity of California's emergency departments, 1990-1999. Ann Emerg Med. 2002;39(4):389-96.
4. McCaig LF, Nawar EW. National Hospital Ambulatory Medical Care Survey: 2004 emergency department summary. Adv Data. 2006;1-29:372.
5. Meggs WJ, Czaplijski T, Benson N. Trends in emergency department utilization, 1988-1997. Acad Emerg Med. 1999;6(10):1030-5.
6. Nelson M, Waldrop RD, Jones J, Randall Z. Critical care provided in an urban emergency department. Am J Emerg Med. 1998;16(1):56-9.
7. Rady MY, Rivers EP, Nowak RM. Resuscitation of the critically ill in the ED: responses of blood pressure, heart rate, shock index, central venous oxygen saturation, and lactate. Am J Emerg Med. 1996;14(2):218-25. 10.1016/S0735-6757(96)90136-9.
8. Rivers E, Nguyen B, Havstad S, Ressler J, Muzzin A, Knoblich B. Early Goal-Directed Therapy in the Treatment of Severe Sepsis and Septic Shock. N Engl J Med. 2001;345(19):1368-77.
9. Saukkonen KA, Varpula M, Rasanen P, Roine RP, Voipio-Pulkki LM, Pettila V. The effect of emergency department delay on outcome in critically ill medical patients: evaluation using hospital mortality and quality of life at 6 months. J Intern Med. 2006;260(6):586-91.
10. Trzeciak S, Dellinger RP, Abate NL, Cowan RM, Stauss M, Kilgannon JH. Translating research to clinical practice: a 1-year experience with implementing early goal-directed therapy for septic shock in the emergency department. Chest. 2006;129(2):225-32.

CHAPTER 14

Overview of Shock

Khusrav Bajan, Archana Shrivastav

WHAT IS SHOCK?

The word *shock* is derived from a French word *choc* coined by French surgeon Henri LeDran. In 1827, an English surgeon, George Guthrie, first used the word *shock* in association with a physiological response to injury.

Shock is best defined as a physiological state of circulatory failure, resulting in insufficient tissue perfusion and oxygenation.

The diagnosis of shock is based on *hemodynamic parameters, clinical findings and abnormal laboratory values*. Typically, hemodynamic parameters include systolic blood pressure greater than 90 mm Hg, mean blood pressure greater than 60 mm Hg; clinical findings include altered mentation, decreased urine output, etc. and abnormal laboratory values include elevated serum lactate and metabolic acidosis. *The skin, the kidneys and the brain* provide us with three types of *windows* through which we can visualize the effects of impaired tissue perfusion **(Fig. 1)**.

ETIOPATHOPHYSIOLOGY OF SHOCK

Shock state can result from four potential pathophysiological mechanisms:
1. *Hypovolemia*: Due to internal or external body fluid losses.
2. *Cardiogenic factors*: Myocardial infarction, myocarditis, etc.
3. *Obstruction*: Pulmonary embolism, cardiac tamponade and tension pneumothorax.
4. *Distributive*: Septic shock, anaphylactic shock.

Skin	Kidneys	Brain
Cold and clammy skin	Decreased urine output <0.5 mL/kg/hr	Altered mental status, obtundation, disorientation and confusion

Fig. 1 The skin, the kidneys and the brain provide us with three types of windows

To understand these mechanisms, we need to revise basic physiological equation of cardiac output (CO). The blood pressure (BP) is a product of cardiac output and systemic vascular resistance and CO is product of stroke volume and heart rate, thus:

$$BP = CO \times SVR$$
$$BP = (SV \times HR) \times SVR.$$

In this equation, BP represents contractility, SV represents preload and SVR represents afterload. Hence, the forces which determine CO are preload, contractility and afterload, and pathophysiological mechanisms of shock affect one of these factors. For example, in hypovolemic shock, there is reduced preload; in cardiogenic shock there is decrease in cardiac contractility; in obstructive shock there is increase in afterload and in distributive shock, there is decrease in SVR and CO is high, although CO may be low due to myocardial depression **(Flow chart 1)**.

We need to discuss the concept of oxygen delivery to tissues to better understand the concept of shock. Oxygen delivery to the tissues depends on CO, hemoglobin concentration of blood and the saturation of hemoglobin with oxygen,

$$DO_2 = CO \times CaO_2 = CO \times (1.34 \times Hb \times SaO_2) \times 10$$
$$VO_2 = CO \times 13.4 \times Hb \times (SaO_2 - SvO_2)$$

Flow chart 1 Basic pathophysiological mechanisms

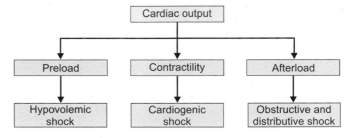

Where, DO_2 is oxygen delivery, CO is cardiac output, CaO_2 is oxygen content of blood, VO_2 is oxygen consumption, Hb is hemoglobin concentration, SaO_2 is % saturation of hemoglobin and SvO_2 is % saturation of mixed venous blood.

Oxygen delivery to tissues is reduced in hypovolemic, obstructive and cardiogenic shock, as a result of anemia, hypoxemia and low CO. In hypovolemic shock, reduction in CO is due to decrease in preload. In obstructive shock, venous return to left ventricle is reduced, while in cardiogenic shock, impaired contractility predominates. In septic shock, there is profound inflammatory response, which leads to vasodilation, increased CO despite impaired myocardial contractility and relative hypovolemia. There are abnormalities in perfusion at microcirculatory level resulting in locally reduced DO_2 despite global supranormal values. In addition, sepsis-induced myocardial dysfunction prevents oxygen utilization at cellular level **(Table 1)**.

CLINICAL PRESENTATION

Early signs include orthostatic hypotension, mild tachycardia, diaphoresis and late signs are hypotension, significant tachycardia, tachypnea and altered mental status. There may be signs of vasoconstriction (narrow pulse pressure and cool extremities) or vasodilation (wide pulse pressure and warm extremities) depending on the type of shock. The following table **(Table 2)** will offer an easy approach to determine the cause of shock **(Flow chart 2 and Fig. 2)**.

Other significant systemic manifestations are altered mentation, decreased urine output (<0.5 mL/kg/hr).

If Swan–Ganz catheter placement is used, then type of shock can be identified as given in **Table 3**.

MANAGEMENT OF SHOCK

Management of shock may be considered in terms of general measures that are applicable to all shock patients and specific measures as per the type of shock.

General Measures

Airway, breathing, circulation and O_2, (Intravenous) IV, monitor are two simple basic rules.

Airway or Breathing

Every shock patient should be given supplemental oxygen through face mask with the aim of improving arterial oxygen saturation and oxygen delivery to tissues. In cases of major hemodynamic instability, intubation and mechanical ventilation should be considered so as to reduce oxygen consumption by respiratory muscles and reduce work of breathing. Intubation at an early stage also facilitates insertion of invasive lines for hemodynamic monitoring and vasoactive drug administration, which is otherwise difficult and may be risky in confused and agitated patient.

Circulation

The primary aim is restoration of adequate tissue perfusion and IV fluid administration is the initial treatment in all types of shock and if fluid therapy is not sufficient then vasopressors and inotropes need to be added.

The initial fluid resuscitation is done through two large bore (16G or 18G) IV cannulae. If needed, then insertion of

Table 1 The four pathophysiological types of shock and their causes

Pathophysiological type	Causes
Hypovolemic	Hemorrhagic, trauma, dehydration
Cardiogenic	Myocardial infarction, cardiomyopathy, valvular disease, arrhythmias
Obstructive	Pulmonary embolism, tamponade, tension pneumothorax
Distributive	Sepsis, anaphylaxis

Table 2 Approach to determine causes of shock

Signs	Cardiogenic	Hypovolemic	Distributive
Pulse pressure	↓	↓	↑
Diastolic pressure	↓	↓	↓↓↓
Extremities	Cool	Cool	Warm
Nail bed blood return	Slow	Slow	Rapid
Jugular venous pressure (JVP)	Raised	Low	Low
Respiratory crepts	+++	–	–
S3, S4 gallop	+++	–	–
Chest X-ray	Cardiomegaly, pulmonary edema	Diminished cardiac size	Normal or with pneumonia
Site of infection	–	–	+++

Flow chart 2 Algorithm for initial assessment of shock

```
Cold,        Tachypnea    Tachycardia,    Decreased    Altered
clammy                    hypotension     urine        mentation,
skin                                      output       obtundation
```

↓
Elevated serum lactate
↓
Shock
↓
Estimate CO or SvO₂
├── N or high → CVP → Low → Distributive shock
│   → (via High path)
└── Low → CVP → Low → Hypovolemic shock
              → High → Cardiogenic shock
              → High → Obstructive shock

Abbreviations: CO, cardiac output; CVP, central venous pressure; SvO$_2$, oxygen saturation.

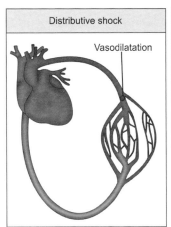
Distributive shock — Vasodilatation

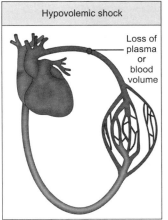
Hypovolemic shock — Loss of plasma or blood volume

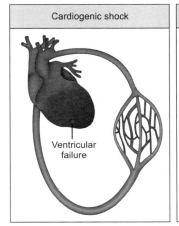
Cardiogenic shock — Ventricular failure

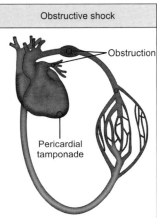
Obstructive shock — Obstruction; Pericardial tamponade

Fig. 2 Schematic representation of types of shock

Table 3 Types of shock					
Type of shock	*Cardiac index*	*SVR*	*PVR*	*SvO$_2$*	*Wedge pressure*
Cardiogenic	↓	↑	N	↓	↑
Hypovolemic	↓	↑	N	↓	↓
Distributive	N-↑	↓	N	N-↑	N-↓
Obstructive	↑	N-↑	↑	N-↓	N-↓

Abbreviations: SVR, systemic vascular resistance; SvO$_2$, oxygen saturation; PVR, pulmonary vascular resistance.

invasive lines should be considered for better hemodynamic monitoring and vasoactive drug administration.

Fluid therapy: Optimizing cardiac preload and restoring circulating volume are the basic aspects of correcting tissue hypoxia, increasing cardiac output and re-establishing perfusion in shock patients. Even patients with cardiogenic shock may benefit from initial fluid resuscitation, since acute edema may result in decrease in effective intravascular volume.

The replacement fluid should be chosen so as to replace the type of fluid lost, for example in hemorrhagic shock, patient clearly requires blood. Crystalloids, colloids and blood are the usual replacement fluids.

The fluid resuscitation should be optimized as per the hemodynamics, urine output and ongoing losses.

Vasoactive drugs: Vasopressors are indicated in cases of persistent hypotension despite fluid resuscitation. It is reasonable to use vasopressor temporarily, while fluid resuscitation is ongoing in cases of major hemodynamic instability.

Noradrenaline is the first choice; it has predominantly α-adrenergic properties and its modest β-adrenergic effects help in maintaining CO. Other vasopressors are adrenaline and dopamine. In randomized controlled trials, dopamine had no advantage over noradrenaline as first-line vasopressor and was found to be more arrhythmogenic. Adrenaline has predominantly β-adrenergic action at low doses, with α-adrenergic effects becoming more prominent in high doses. It is also more arrhythmogenic, decreases splanchnic circulation and increases lactate levels. Trials have not shown beneficial effects of adrenaline over nor adrenaline. Vasopressin deficiency can develop in patients with hyperkinetic forms of distributive shock and administration of low-dose vasopressin can lead to substantial increase in BP.

Amongst inotropes, dobutamine is the agent of choice, it has predominantly β actions. Other agents are phosphodiesterase III inhibitors, such as milrinone and newer agent like levosimendan, which acts primarily by binding to cardiac troponin C and increasing the calcium sensitivity of cardiac myocytes.

Specific Measures (Flow chart 3)

Hypovolemic Shock

Fluid administration is the first intervention, but in some trauma patients, it can be delayed until bleeding is controlled. Hemorrhagic shock warrants to identify the source of bleeding and appropriate control by surgical, radiological or endoscopic intervention. Hypovolemic shock due to intra-abdominal pathologies such as perforation and obstruction also needs surgery.

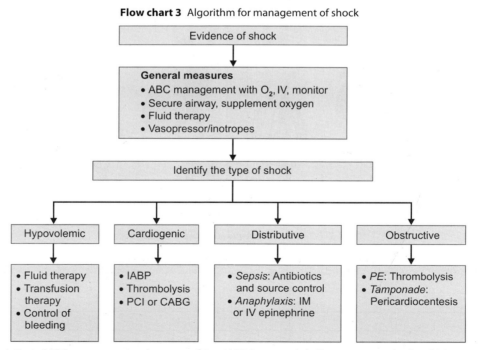

Flow chart 3 Algorithm for management of shock

Abbreviations: CABG, coronary artery bypass grafting; IABP, intra-aortic balloon counterpulsation; IV, intravenous; IM, intramuscular; PCI, percutaneous coronary intervention; PE, pulmonary embolus.

Cardiogenic Shock

If evidence of acute myocardial infarction with cardiogenic shock, then along with ventilator and inotropic support, intra-aortic balloon counterpulsation (IABP) is of great help. With IABP support, immediate reperfusion therapy in the form of either thrombolysis (if catheter laboratory is not available) or immediate cardiac catheterization followed by percutaneous coronary intervention or emergency coronary artery bypass surgery should be done.

Distributive Shock

The management of septic shock consists of early goal-directed therapy and administration of antibiotics within 1 hour after sending cultures. Source of sepsis should be sought for with appropriate source control.

Obstructive Shock

The main causes are pulmonary embolism and cardiac tamponade. In case of pulmonary embolism, thrombolysis or embolectomy are the options, while in cardiac tamponade, urgent pericardiocentesis will lead to relief of symptoms.

CONCLUSION

Shock is a medical emergency and resuscitation should begin immediately with simultaneous investigations to achieve good outcome. Correction of tissue hypoxia and restoration of adequate perfusion are of prime importance. It is very necessary to determine the type of shock to implement specific measures and correct the cause. The patient should be optimized with prompt resuscitation in emergency room to achieve reasonable hemodynamic stability before shifting to operation room, radiology or intensive care unit.

BIBLIOGRAPHY

1. Caterino JM, Kahan S. In a Page Emergency Medicine. Oxford: Blackwell; 2003.
2. Kelley DM. Hypovolemic shock: an overview, critical care nursing. Crit Care Nurs Q. 2005;28(1):2-19.
3. Nunez TC, Cotton BA. Transfusion therapy in hemorrhagic shock. Curr Opin Crit Care. 2009;15(6):536-41.
4. Vincent JL, De Backer D. Circulatory shock, review article, critical care medicine. N Engl J Med. 2013;369(18):1726-34.
5. Vincent JL, Ince C, Bakker J. Clinical review: Circulatory shock – an update: A tribute to Professor Max Harry Weil. Crit Care. 2012;16(6):239.
6. Worthley L. Shock: a review of pathophysiology and management. Part I. Crit Care Resusc. 2000;2(1):55-65.

CHAPTER 15

Sepsis and Septic Shock

Chandrashekhar, Swarup S Padhi, Ajeet Singh, Tariq Ali, Yatin Mehta

INTRODUCTION

The branch of critical care medicine has always eluded a satisfactory clinical definition of sepsis. Sepsis definition should be able to achieve two very important goals. One is to provide a rapid screening test and the other is to give a definitive diagnosis.

The original definitions of sepsis, systemic inflammatory response syndrome (SIRS), severe sepsis, and septic shock are now obsolete as SIRS as a criteria was far too sensitive to be followed in patients in the intensive care set up.

The earlier definition had reigned for almost two and a half decade. Severe sepsis ceased to be a concept and only concepts which exist are "sepsis" and "septic shock".

Sepsis is a life-threatening organ dysfunction due to a dysregulated host response to infection **(Flow chart 1 and Figs 1 to 3)**.

CLINICAL CRITERIA FOR SEPSIS

Organ dysfunction is defined as an increase of two points or more in the sequential organ failure assessment (SOFA) score, for patients with infections, an increase of two SOFA points gives an overall mortality rate of 10% **(Fig. 4)**.

The q-SOFA score (also known as quick-SOFA) is a bedside score that could identify patients with suspected infection who are thought to have a greater risk for a poor outcome outside the intensive care unit (ICU).

Patients with suspected infection whose ICU stay is likely to be prolonged or those who might succumb to their illness in the hospital can be identified at the bedside with the help of q-SOFA score.

q-SOFA score includes these three:
1. Hypotension which is defined as systolic blood pressure (SBP) less than or equal to 100 mm Hg
2. Altered mental status: Glasgow Coma Scale less than 15
3. Tachypnea defined as respiratory rate greater than or equal to 22.

If two or more of this score is positive, it suggests patient's outcome is poor **(Figs 5 and 6)**.

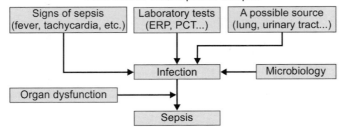

Flow chart 1 Development of sepsis

Abbreviations: CRP, C-reactive protein; PCT, procalcitonin.

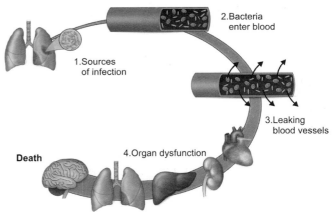

Fig. 1 Severe sepsis

CHAPTER 15 Sepsis and Septic Shock

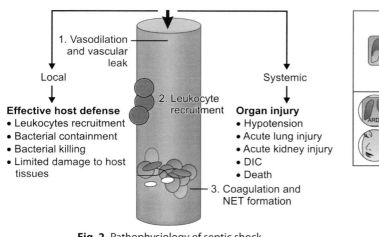

Fig. 2 Pathophysiology of septic shock
Abbreviations: DIC, disseminated intravascular coagulation; NET, neutrophil extracellular trap.

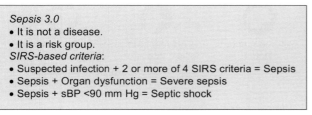

Sepsis 3.0
- It is not a disease.
- It is a risk group.

SIRS-based criteria:
- Suspected infection + 2 or more of 4 SIRS criteria = Sepsis
- Sepsis + Organ dysfunction = Severe sepsis
- Sepsis + sBP <90 mm Hg = Septic shock

Fig. 3 Sepsis definitions

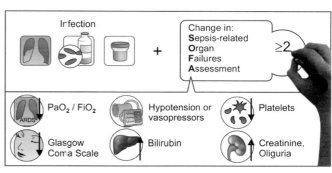

Fig. 4 Sepsis clinical criteria
Abbreviations: PaO$_2$, partial pressure of arterial oxygen; FiO$_2$, fraction of inspired oxygen.

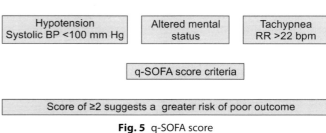

Fig. 5 q-SOFA score
Abbreviations: BP, blood pressure; RR, respiratory rate.
q-SOFA, quick, sepsis-related organ failure assessment

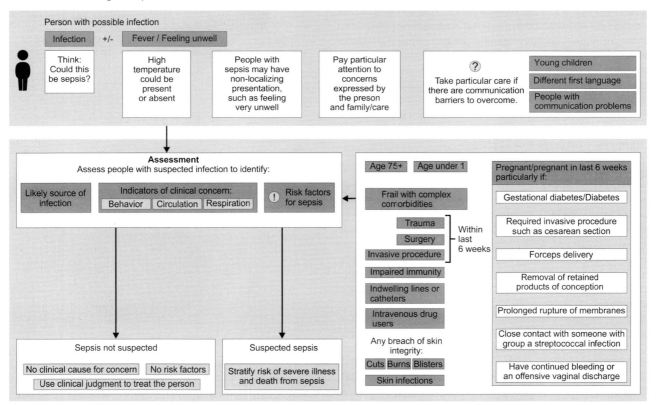

Fig. 6 Approach to assessment of sepsis

Where did q-SOFA come from?

More than 800,000 electronic health record encounters at 177 hospitals worldwide including community and academic, rural, suburban, urban public and private, and federal hospitals **(Fig. 7)**.

Septic shock is a subset of sepsis in which underlying circulatory and cellular or metabolic abnormalities are profound enough to substantially increase mortality. The difference between septic shock and sepsis is that the complications are more severe and the risk of patient death is greater in patients who are in septic shock **(Fig. 8; Flow chart 2)**.

Septic Shock Clinical Criteria

Sepsis despite adequate volume resuscitation with persistent hypotension requiring vasopressors to maintain mean arterial pressure (MAP) greater than or equal to 65 mm Hg, and lactate greater than or equal to 2 mmol/L.

With these criteria, mortality exceeds to more than 40%. Sepsis as an entity is a dynamic condition with clinical and laboratory manifestations that can vary over time. It is not necessary that all criteria be present at a single time.

To predict the mortality of any critically ill patient SOFA score can be used **(Table 1)**. qSOFA (quick-SOFA) was designed to predict mortality. Thus, q-SOFA and SOFA are not tests of sepsis but are predictors of mortality **(Algorithm 2)**. q-SOFA should not be thought to be a "sepsis screen" as anyone with positive q-SOFA should not be treated directly for sepsis, as they actually might require a careful investigation for other illnesses like cardiogenic shock or pulmonary embolism. Same mistake can also happen when lactate is interpreted.

Every emergency department (ED) should have a screening tool to evaluate sepsis and septic shock and to treat these patients before shifting them to a definitive place like the intensive care **(Figs 9 to 11)**.

TOOL FOR SCREENING OUT SEPSIS

This is a simplified tool that can be used to screen patients for sepsis in the ED or in the critical care.
1. *Obtain proper history for any potential source of infection*: Lung infections, kidney infections like urinary tract infection, infection lingering in the abdomen, meningitis and endocarditis, skin and soft tissue infection, wound infection, catheter-related infections, blood stream infections. ___ Yes ___No
2. *Search for signs and symptoms that would indicate*: Fever greater than 38.3°C or temperature less than 36° C, altered mental status with a Glasgow Coma Scale (GCS) less than 15, heart rate greater than 90 bpm (tachycardia), respiratory rate greater than 20 bpm (tachypnea), leukocytosis or leukopenia [white blood cell (WBC) count >12,000 μL or <4000 μL, respectively]. ___ Yes ___No

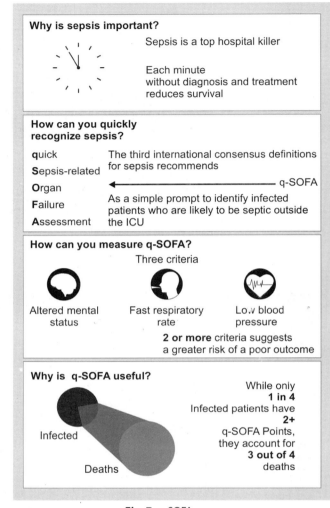

Fig. 7 q-SOFA score

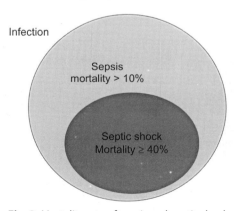

Fig. 8 Mortality rate of sepsis and septic shock

If both the above are *yes*, suspicion of infection is present. Laboratory investigations that should be ordered are complete blood count with differential, blood lactate and cultures, and basic metabolic panel.

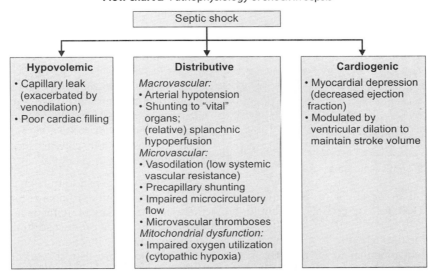

Flow chart 2 Pathophysiology of shock in sepsis

Table 1 Sequential organ failure assessment score					
	Score				
System	0	1	2	3	4
Respiration					
PaO_2/FiO_2, mm Hg (kPa)	≥400 (53.3)	<400 (53.3)	<300 (40)	<200 (26.7) with respiratory support	<100 (13.3) with respiratory support
Coagulation					
Platelets × $10^3/\mu L$	≥150	<150	<100	<50	<20
Liver					
Bilirubin, mg/dL (mmol/L)	<1.2 (20)	1.2–1.9 (20–32)	2.0–5.9 (33–101)	6.0–11.9 (102–204)	>12.0 (204)
Cardiovascular	MAP ≥70 mm Hg	MAP <70 mm Hg	Dopamine <5 or dobutamine (any dose)	Dopamine 5.1–15 or epinephrine ≤0.1 or norepinephrine ≤0.1	Dopamine >15 or epinephrine >0.1 or norepinephrine >0.1
Central nervous system					
Glasgow Coma Scale score	15	13–14	10–12	6–9	<6
Renal					
Creatinine, mg/dL (µmol/L)	<1.2 (110)	1.2–1.9 (110–170)	2.0–3.4 (171–299)	3.5–4.9 (300–440)	>5.0 (440)
Urine output, mL/d				<500	<200

Abbreviations: FiO_2, fraction of inspired oxygen; PaO_2, partial pressure of arterial oxygen; MAP, mean arterial pressure.

Ultrasound abdomen, CT scan, chest X-ray, amylase, lipase, arterial blood gas (ABG), procalcitonin should be obtained according to the signs and symptoms and according to physician discretion.

3. Whether organ dysfunction criteria present? ___ Yes ___ No. If suspicion of infection and organ dysfunction are present, the patient's condition is labeled as *septic shock* and should be entered into the protocol **(Flow charts 3 and 4)**.

MANAGEMENT OF SEPTIC SHOCK AND SEPSIS PROTOCOLS

- To be completed within first 3 hours:
  - Obtain serum lactate level
  - Obtain blood cultures prior to administration of broad-spectrum antibiotics
  - Administer broad-spectrum antibiotics to cover likely pathogens

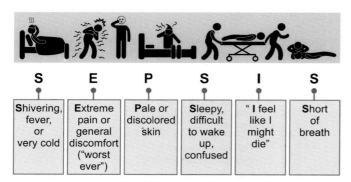

Fig. 9 Sepsis symptoms

- If lactate greater than or equal to 4 mmol/L and hypotension then 30 mL/kg crystalloid should be administered.
- To be completed within next 6 hours:
  - If MAP greater than or equal to 65 mm Hg is not maintained despite volume resuscitation, vasopressors should be administered to maintain the mentioned MAP
  - If hypotension (MAP <65 mm Hg) persists despite volume resuscitation and lactate continues to remain high, i.e. greater than or equal to 4 mmol/L, then volumes status and tissue perfusion should be reassessed.
  - Lactate to be measured again if initial lactate were elevated.

How to reassess volume status and tissue perfusion?

Vital signs, cardiopulmonary status, capillary refill time, pulse in terms of rate, rhythm and character, and skin findings should be meticulously examined after initial fluid resuscitation.

Or

Two of the following: CVP (central venous pressure), $ScvO_2$ (central venous oxygen saturation), cardiovascular ultrasound at the bedside, dynamic parameters of fluid responsiveness with passive leg raise or fluid challenge be used to reassess the volume status and tissue perfusion **(Flow chart 5)**.

The Surviving Sepsis Campaign Guidelines apart from the 3 hours and 6 hours protocol recommend these additional therapies for the care of septic patients with septic shock.
- Blood and blood product administration
- Lung protective mechanical ventilation of sepsis-induced acute respiratory distress syndrome (ARDS)
- Sedation, analgesia, and neuromuscular blockade in sepsis
- Glycemic control
- Renal replacement therapy
- Prophylaxis for deep vein thrombosis
- Prophylaxis for stress ulcer
- Nutrition.

Also note that the following modalities as therapy are now obsolete—intravenous immunoglobulin, selenium, and bicarbonate therapy.

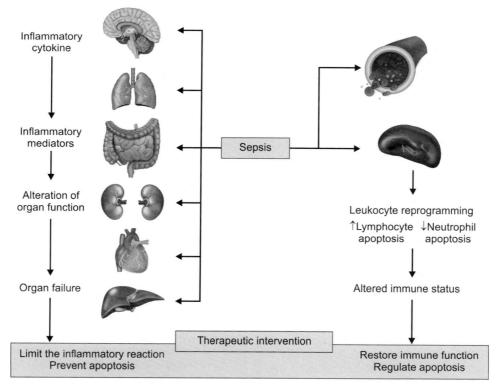

Fig. 10 Therapeutic intervention in sepsis

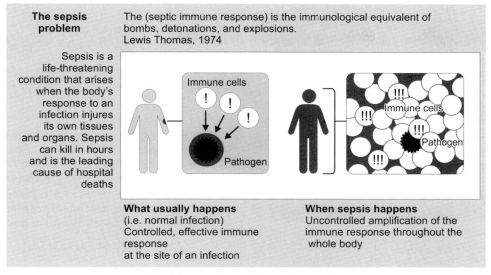

Fig. 11 Screening tool to evaluate sepsis

Flow chart 3 Operationalization of clinical criteria identifying patients with sepsis and septic shock

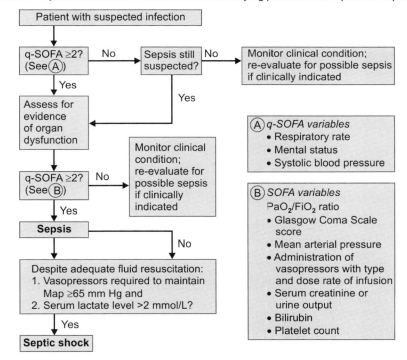

Abbreviations: FiO_2, fraction of inspired oxygen; PaO_2, partial pressure of arterial oxygen.

Stepwise Approach for Management of Sepsis

Stepwise approach for management of sepsis is given in **Box 1**.

Initial Resuscitation

- Sepsis causes hypotension that leads to hypoperfusion of tissues. To manage hypotension fluids especially

Flow chart 4 Approach to treatment of septic shock

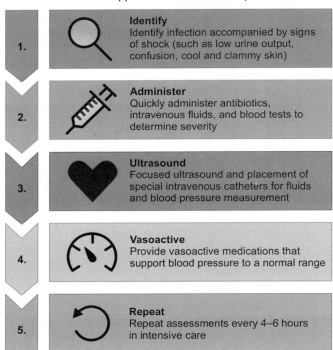

Box 1 Stepwise approach for management of sepsis

- Initially resuscitate the patient
- Screen for sepsis and performance improvement
- Diagnosis
- Broad-spectrum antimicrobial therapy
- Control the source of infection
- Infection prevention

crystalloids are infused at the rate of 30 mL/kg. Goals of resuscitation are to maintain a MAP of around 65 mm Hg, urine output of at least 0.5 mL/kg/hr, CVP of 8–12 mm Hg, SvO_2 and $ScvO_2$ of 65% or 70%, respectively.
- Patients who on admission are found to have elevated lactate levels (more than equal to 4 mmol/L) resuscitation should be done at the earliest to normalize it.

SEPSIS KILLS
TIME IS LIFE
Recognize Resuscitate Refer

Screening for Sepsis and Performance Improvement

- Routine screening for potentially infected seriously ill patients is of utmost importance for sepsis so that early therapy can be started to prevent worsening of the condition

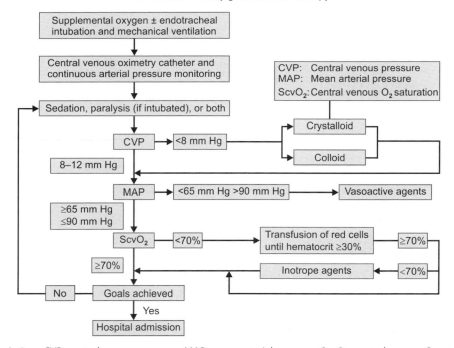

Flow chart 5 Early goal-directed therapy

Abbreviations: CVP, central venous pressure; MAP, mean arterial pressure; $ScvO_2$, central venous O_2 saturation

- Hospital-based performance improvement efforts in sepsis.

Diagnosis

Diagnosis can be made by culture and imaging studies. Before administering antibiotics at least two sets of blood cultures for aerobic and anaerobic bottle should be drawn out of which one should be a peripheral sample and one sample through each vascular access device. If the vascular access was recently (<48 hrs) inserted then sample might not be taken from the site. Fungal infections can be potential source of sepsis which in majority goes unrecognized. So, if the suspicion of fungal infection is there, 1,3 beta-D-glucan assay, and anti-mannan antibody assays be performed so that antifungal therapy can be started.

Antimicrobial Therapy

As soon as a diagnosis or assumption of sepsis or septic shock is made intravenous broad-spectrum antibiotics should be initiated within the first hour. Initial empiric anti-infective therapy should always include a broad-spectrum antibiotic that has the ability to cover the common organisms that play a role in sepsis. De-escalation is very important when broad-spectrum antimicrobials were started initially and the antibiotics should be reassessed on a daily basis. Procalcitonin levels, if low can be used to stop empirical antibiotics in patients who were assessed to be septic, but have no subsequent evidence of infection. Combination empirical therapy is used nowadays for patients who are neutropenic with severe sepsis and for those patients who are infected with multidrug-resistant pathogens. If risk factors for health care associated infections are present and suspicion of *Pseudomonas aeruginosa*, Acinetobacter or methicillin-resistant *Staphylococcus aureus* (MRSA) is high then a combination therapy is preferred—broad-spectrum cephalosporins like cefepime or carbapenems or BL-BLI (β-lactam-β-lactamase inhibitor) combination with an aminoglycoside or fluoroquinolone with an MRSA directed agent like vancomycin, tigecycline or linezolid be used. If community-acquired infection is thought to be the source of sepsis like *Streptococcus pneumoniae*, single agent is preferred like ceftriaxone or macrolide or fluoroquinolone or ertapenem be used as therapy.

Empiric combination therapy at best should be continued for 3–5 days. We usually administer drugs for 7–10 days and longer courses are reserved for patients who did not show adequate response from the initial therapy or were slow to respond, infection focus that could not be drained, neutropenic patients, patients with immune deficient condition, infection with *S. aureus*, fungal and viral infections. Antiviral therapy should be added to the regimen as early as possible, if virus is thought to be the offending pathogen.

Source Control

After identifying the potential source that had led to the infection, attempts to control it should be undertaken within 12 hours if feasible. The modality with least invasiveness should be undertaken like rather than a surgical drainage, a percutaneous approach should be done if an abscess is found. Intravascular devices are potential sources of infection and attempt to remove it should be done at the earliest after securing another access.

Infection Prevention

Apart from simple handwashing that prevents infection, selective oral decontamination with the use of chlorhexidine should be used to decrease the incidence of ventilator-associated pneumonia.

FLUID THERAPY OF SEPSIS: USE OF VASOPRESSORS, INOTROPES AND CORTICOSTEROIDS

Crystalloids: It is given at a dose of 30 mL/kg preferably should be used as the initial fluid of choice in the resuscitation. Avoid colloids like starches for fluid resuscitation. Albumin can be used as an alternative when amount of crystalloids for resuscitation is thought to be substantial.

Vasopressors: Vasopressors are almost required when the patient does not respond with initial fluid replacement when a diagnosis of septic shock is made. MAP of 65 mm Hg is targeted with noradrenaline as the first choice among the vasopressor. Adrenaline can be used when blood pressure is not adequately maintained with noradrenaline. If the requirement of noradrenaline is high or the need to raise the MAP rises then vasopressin at a dose of 0.03 units/min can be added. Dopamine is to be used in highly selected patients as they are arrhythmogenic. So, patients who are not prone to arrhythmias can be offered dopamine. Phenylephrine is used where noradrenaline would cause serious arrhythmias or when cardiac output is high and blood pressure is low or as a salvage therapy where everything else has failed to raise the blood pressure. Low-dose dopamine is now obsolete. Arterial cannula should be placed when the need of vasopressor is there.

If intravascular volume is maintained with fluids and target MAP is achieved but signs of inadequate perfusion and myocardial depression with low cardiac output with high filling pressures are found then dobutamine infusion can be tried up to a dose of 20 μg/kg/min.

Corticosteroids: Intravenous hydrocortisone as a therapy in a dose of 200 mg/day in divided doses or as an infusion has a role in septic shock when despite adequate fluid replenishment and vasopressor use blood pressure is not

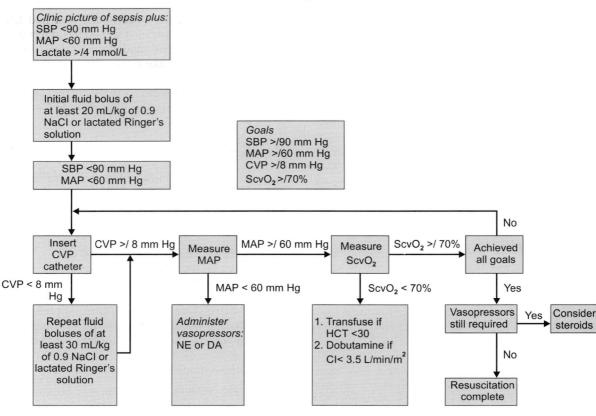

Flow chart 6 Fluid management of septic shock

Abbreviations: SBP, systolic blood pressure; MAP, mean arterial blood pressure; NaCl, sodium chloride; CVP, central venous pressure; NE, norepinephrine; DA, dopamine; ScvO$_2$, oxygen saturation of central venous pressure; CI, cardiac index; HCT, hematocrit

maintained or hemodynamic stability is not achieved. It has no role otherwise in sepsis and septic shock **(Flow chart 6)**.

SUPPORTIVE THERAPY

Blood and Blood Product Administration

This modality is used if hemoglobin is less than 7 g/dL and should be targeted to 7–9 g/dL, or platelet count of less than 10,000/mm^3 even in the absence of bleeding or as a prophylaxis when platelet count is less than 20,000 with risk of bleeding. In selected conditions a higher target of hemoglobin is targeted like myocardial ischemia, severe hypoxemia, and acute hemorrhage. Platelet counts greater than or equal to 50,000/mm^3 are targeted when there is active bleeding or a surgery or any invasive procedure where bleeding is anticipated.

Lung Protective Mechanical Ventilation of Acute Respiratory Distress Syndrome in Sepsis

Low-tidal-volume ventilation using 6 L/min tidal volume should be used for these subgroup of patients and methods to decrease aspiration like head end of bed elevation should be used. Noninvasive ventilation can be used in selected patients in mild ARDS.

Sedation in Sepsis

Paralyzing agents should be avoided if possible in the septic patient without ARDS as they might be at high-risk of myopathy and neuropathy. Paralytic agents are not contraindications and can be used but care to be taken that it should not be continued for more than 48 hours in sepsis-induced ARDS.

Glycemic Control

Glucose control also holds importance when managing sepsis and septic shock. Insulin should be administered and in most cases as an infusion when two consecutive blood glucose levels are greater than 180 mg/dL. Blood glucose values should be monitored every 1–2 hours until glucose values and insulin infusion rates are stable and then every 4 hours.

Renal Replacement Therapy

To manage the fluid balance continuous renal replacement therapies are recommended in patients who are hemodynamically unstable as they cause less fluctuation in hemodynamic parameters.

Prophylaxis for Deep Vein Thrombosis

Low-molecular weight heparin (LMWH) subcutaneously is used for prophylaxis against venous thromboembolism (VTE). If renal parameters are grossly deranged, dalteparin or unfractionated heparin (UFH) should be used. Intermittent pneumatic compression devices can also be used along with the earlier mentioned therapies whenever possible.

Patients who have a contraindication for heparin use like low platelet counts or coagulopathies and intracerebral bleed graduated compression stockings should be used.

Proton pump inhibitor should be started for patients who are at a high-risk for bleeding.

Total Parenteral Nutrition

Oral or enteral feedings should be initiated if patient can tolerate them. Total parenteral nutrition alone should not be started if possible and use along with intravenous glucose and enteral nutrition is beneficial in these patients. Parenteral nutrition in conjunction with enteral feeding in the first 7 days after a diagnosis of sepsis or septic shock can also be initiated.

CONCLUSION

Initial management of patients with septic shock appears to be critical in determining outcome. The key principle being "time is life" and practicing to recognize, resuscitate, refer (to critical care specialist). Institution of standardized, protocolized approach appears to consistently improve delivery of recommended therapies and, as a result may improve patient outcome. A protocolized, multidisciplinary approach and an evidence based practice should become standard of care for management of septic shock.

To summarize, the initial management of septic shock is very crucial and successful implementation of therapy as mentioned will help to improve the outcome in patients with sepsis and septic shock **(Fig. 12)**.

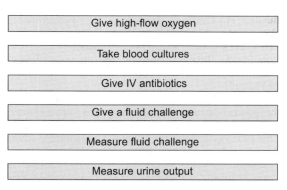

Fig. 12 Six simple things for sepsis patients

BIBLIOGRAPHY

1. Ali MZ, Goetz MB. A meta-analysis of the relative efficacy and toxicity of single daily dosing versus multiple daily dosing of aminoglycosides. Clin Infect Dis. 1997;24:796-809.
2. Allolio B, Dorr H, Stuttmann R, et al. Effect of a single bolus of etomidate upon eight major corticosteroid hormone and plasma ACTH. Clin Endocrinol (Oxf). 1985;22:281-6.
3. Amsden GW, Ballow CH, Bertino JS. Pharmacokinetics and pharmacodynamics of anti-infective agents. In: Mandell GL, Bennett JE, Dolin R (Eds). Principles and Practice of Infectious Diseases. Fifth edition. Philadelphia, Churchill Livingstone. 2000. pp. 253-61.
4. Angus DC, Linde-Zwirble WT, Lidicker J, et al. Epidemiology of severe sepsis in the United States: Analysis of incidence, outcome, and associated costs of care. Crit Care Med. 2001; 29:1303-10.
5. Annane D, Sebille V, Charpentier C, et al. Effect of treatment with low doses of hydrocortisone and fludrocortisone on mortality in patients with septic shock. JAMA. 2002;288:862-71.
6. Bellomo R, Chapman M, Finfer S, et al. Low-dose dopamine in patients with early renal dysfunction: A placebo-controlled randomised trial. Australian and New Zealand Intensive Care Society (ANZICS) Clinical Trials Group. Lancet. 2000;356: 2139-43.
7. Bendjelid K, Romand JA. Fluid responsiveness in mechanically ventilated patients: A review of indices used in intensive care. Intensive Care Med. 2003;29:352-60.
8. Bendjelid K. Right arterial pressure: Determinant or result of change in venous return? Chest. 2005;128:3639-40.
9. Blot F, Schmidt E, Nitenberg G, et al. Earlier positivity of central venous versus peripheral blood cultures is highly predictive of catheter-related sepsis. J Clin Microbiol. 1998;36:105-9.
10. Boldt J. Clinical review: Hemodynamic monitoring in the intensive care unit. Crit Care Med. 2002;6:52-9.
11. Bollaert PE, Bauer P, Audibert G, et al. Effects of epinephrine on hemodynamics and oxygen metabolism in dopamineresistant septic shock. Chest. 1990;98:949-53.
12. Bollaert PE, Charpentier C, Levy B, et al. Reversal of late septic shock with supraphysiologic doses of hydrocortisone. Crit Care Med. 1998;26:645-50.
13. Bone RC, Balk RA, Cerra FB, et al, and members of the ACCP/SCCM Consensus Conference: Definitions for sepsis and organ failure and guidelines for the use of innovative therapies in sepsis. Chest. 1992;101:1644-55 and Crit Care Med. 1992;20:864-74.
14. Briegel J, Forst H, Haller M, et al. Stress doses of hydrocortisone reverse hyperdynamic septic shock: A prospective, randomized, double-blind, single-center study. Crit Care Med. 1999;27:723-32.
15. Briegel J, Vogeser M, Annane D, et al. Measurement of cortisol in septic shock: Interlaboratory harmonization. Am Rev Respir Crit Care Med. 2007;175:A436.

16. Bufalari A, Giustozzi G, Moggi L. Postoperative intra-abdominal abscesses: Percutaneous versus surgical treatment. Acta Chir Belg. 1996;96:197-200.
17. Buwalda M, Ince C. Opening the microcirculation: Can vasodilators be useful in sepsis? Intensive Care Med. 2002;28:1208-17.
18. Centers for Disease Control and Prevention: Guidelines for the prevention of intravascular catheter-related infections. Morbid Mortal Wkly Rep. 2002;51(RR-10):1-29.
19. Choi PTL, Yip G, Quinonez LG, et al. Crystalloids vs. colloids in fluid resuscitation: A systematic review. Crit Care Med. 1999;27:200-10.
20. Cook D, Guyatt G. Colloid use for fluid resuscitation: Evidence and spin. Ann Intern Med. 2001;135:205-8.
21. Day NP, Phu NH, Bethell DP, et al. The effects of dopamine and adrenaline infusions on acid-base balance and systemic haemodynamics in severe infection. Lancet. 1996;348:219-23.
22. De Backer D, Creteur J, Dubois MJ, et al. The effects of dobutamine on microcirculatory alternations in patients with septic shock are independent of its systemic effects. Crit Care Med. 2006;34:403-8.
23. De Backer D, Creteur J, Silva E, et al. Effects of dopamine, norepinephrine, and epinephrine on the splanchnic circulation in septic shock: Which is best? Crit Care Med. 2003;31:1659-67.
24. Dellinger RP, Carlet JM, Masur H, et al. Surviving Sepsis Campaign guidelines for management of severe sepsis and septic shock. Crit Care Med. 2004;32:858-73.
25. Dellinger RP, Carlet JM, Masur H, et al. Surviving Sepsis Campaign guidelines for management of severe sepsis and septic shock. Intensive Care Med. 2004;30:536-55.
26. Dellinger RP. Cardiovascular management of septic shock. Crit Care Med. 2003;31:946-55.
27. Djillali A, Vigno P, Renault A, et al. The CATS STUDY Group: Norepinephrine plus dobutamine versus epinephrine alone for management of septic shock: A randomized trial. Lancet. 2007;370:676-84.
28. Dombrovskiy VY, Martin AA, Sunderram J, et al. Rapid increase in hospitalization and mortality rates for severe sepsis in the United States: A trend analysis from 1993 to 2003. Crit Care Med. 2007;35:1414-15.
29. Dünser MW, Mayr AJ, Tura A, et al. Ischemic skin lesions as a complication of continuous vasopressin infusion in catecholamine- resistant vasodilatory shock: Incidence and risk factors. Crit Care Med. 2003;31:1394-98.
30. Dünser MW, Mayr AJ, Ulmer H, et al. Arginine vasopressin in advanced vasodilatory shock: A prospective, randomized, controlled study. Circulation. 2003;107:2313-9.
31. Evans A, Winslow BH. Oxygen saturation and hemodynamic response in critically ill mechanically ventilated adults during intra-hospital transport. Am J Crit Care. 1995;4:106-11.
32. Finfer S, Bellomo R, Boyce N, et al. A comparison of albumin and saline for fluid resuscitation in the intensive care unit. N Engl J Med. 2004;350:2247-56.
33. Garnacho-Montero J, Sa-Borges M, Sole-Violan J, et al. Optimal management therapy for *Pseudomonas aeruginosa* ventilator associated pneumonia: An observational, multicenter study comparing monotherapy with combination antibiotic therapy. Crit Care Med. 2007;25:1888-95.
34. Gattinoni L, Brazzi L, Pelosi P, et al. A trial of goal-oriented hemodynamic therapy in critically ill patients. N Engl J Med. 1995;333:1025-32.
35. Giamarellos-Bourboulis EJ, Giannopoulou P, Grecka P, et al. Should procalcitonin be introduced in the diagnostic criteria for the systemic inflammatory response syndrome and sepsis? J Crit Care. 2004;19:152-7.
36. GRADE working group: Grading quality of evidence and strength of recommendations. BMJ. 2004;328:1490-8.
37. Gregory JS, Bonfiglio MF, Dasta JF, et al. Experience with phenylephrine as a component of the pharmacologic support of septic shock. Crit Care Med. 1991;19:1395-400.
38. Guidelines for the management of adults with hospital-acquired, ventilator-associated, and healthcare-associated pneumonia. Am J Respir Crit Care Med. 2005;171:388-416.
39. Guyatt G, Gutterman D, Baumann MH, et al: Grading strength of recommendations and quality of evidence in clinical guidelines: Report from an American College of Chest Physicians task force. Chest. 2006;129:174-81.
40. Guyatt G, Schünemann H, Cook D, et al. Applying the grades of recommendations for antithrombotic and thrombolytic therapy: The seventh ACCP conference of antithrombotic and thrombolytic therapy. Chest. 2004;126:179S-87S.
41. Hatala R, Dinh T, Cook DJ. Once-daily aminoglycoside dosing in immunocompetent adults: A meta-analysis. Ann Intern Med. 1996;124:717-25.
42. Hayes MA, Timmins AC, Yau EHS, et al. Elevation of systemic oxygen delivery in the treatment of critically ill patients. N Engl J Med. 1994;330:1717-22.
43. Hollenberg SM, Ahrens TS, Annane D, et al. Practice parameters for hemodynamic support of sepsis in adult patients: 2004 update. Crit Care Med. 2004;32:1928-48.
44. Holmes CL, Patel BM, Russell JA, et al. Physiology of vasopressin relevant to management of septic shock. Chest. 2001;120:989-1002.
45. Holmes CL, Walley KR, Chittock DR, et al. The effects of vasopressin on hemodynamics and renal function in severe septic shock: A case series. Intensive Care Med. 2001;27:1416-21.
46. Hughes WT, Armstrong D, Bodey GP, et al. 2002 Guidelines for the use of antimicrobial agents in neutropenic patients with cancer. http://www.idsociety.org. Accessed July 10, 2007.
47. Hyatt JM, McKinnon PS, Zimmer GS, et al. The importance of pharmacokinetic/pharmacodynamic surrogate markers to outcomes: Focus on antibacterial agents. Clin Pharmacokinet. 1995;28:143-60.
48. Ibrahim EH, Sherman G, Ward S, et al. The influence of inadequate antimicrobial treatment of bloodstream infections on patient outcomes in the ICU setting. Chest. 2000;118:146-55.
49. Jimenez MF, Marshall JC. Source control in the management of sepsis. Intensive Care Med. 2001;27:S49-S62.
50. Keh D, Boehnke T, Weber-Carstens S, et al. Immunologic and hemodynamic effects of "low-dose" hydrocortisone in septic shock: A double-blind, randomized, placebocontrolled, crossover study. Am J Respir Crit Care Med. 2003;167:512-20.
51. Kellum J, Decker J. Use of dopamine in acute renal failure: A meta-analysis. Crit Care Med. 2001;29:1526-31.

52. Klastersky J. Management of fever in neutropenic patients with different risks of complications. Clin Infect Dis. 2004;39 (Suppl 1):S32-S37.
53. Kortgen A, Niederprum P, Bauer M. Implementation of an evidence-based "standard operating procedure" and outcome in septic shock. Crit Care Med. 2006;34:943-9.
54. Kreger BE, Craven DE, McCabe WR. Gram negative bacteremia: IV. Re-evaluation of clinical features and treatment in 612 patients. Am J Med. 1980;68:344-55.
55. Kumar A, Roberts D, Wood KE, et al. Duration of hypotension prior to initiation of effective antimicrobial therapy is the critical determinant of survival in human septic shock. Crit Care Med. 2006;34:1589-96.
56. Landry DW, Levin HR, Gallant EM, et al. Vasopressin deficiency contributes to the vasodilation of septic shock. Circulation. 1997;95:1122-5.
57. Lauzier F, Levy B, Lamarre P, et al. Vasopressin or norepinephrine in early hyperdynamic septic shock: A randomized clinical trial. Intensive Care Med. 2006;32:1782-9.
58. Le Tulzo Y, Seguin P, Gacouin A, et al. Effects of epinephrine on right ventricular function in patients with severe septic shock and right ventricular failure: A preliminary descriptive study. Intensive Care Med. 1997;23:664-70.
59. LeDoux D, Astiz ME, Carpati CM, et al. Effects of perfusion pressure on tissue perfusion in septic shock. Crit Care Med. 2000;28:2729-32.
60. Leibovici L, Shraga I, Drucker M, et al. The benefit of appropriate empirical antibiotic treatment in patients with bloodstream infection. J Intern Med. 1998;244:379-86.
61. Levy B, Bollaert PE, Charpentier C, et al. Comparison of norepinephrine and dobutamine to epinephrine for hemodynamics, lactate metabolism, and gastric tonometric variables in septic shock: A prospective, randomized study. Intensive Care Med. 1997;23:282-7.
62. Levy MM, Fink MP, Marshall JC, et al. 2001 SCCM/ESICM/ACCP/ATS/SIS International Sepsis Definitions Conference. Crit Care Med. 2003;31:1250-6.
63. Linde-Zwirble WT, Angus DC. Severe sepsis epidemiology: Sampling, selection, and society. Crit Care. 2004;8:222-6.
64. Mackenzie SJ, Kapadia F, Nimmo GR, et al. Adrenaline in treatment of septic shock: Effects on haemodynamics and oxygen transport. Intensive Care Med. 1991;17:36-9.
65. Magder S. Central venous pressure: A useful but not so simple measurement. Crit Care Med. 2006;34:2224-7.
66. Malay MB, Ashton RC, Landry DW, et al. Low-dose vasopressin in the treatment of vasodilatory septic shock. J Trauma. 1999; 47:699-705.
67. Malbrain ML, Deeren D, De Potter TJ. Intraabdominal hypertension in the critically ill: It is time to pay attention. Curr Opin Crit Care. 2005;11:156-71.
68. Martin C, Papazian L, Perrin G, et al. Norepinephrine or dopamine for the treatment of hyperdynamic septic shock? Chest. 1993;103:1826-31.
69. Martin C, Viviand X, Leone M, et al. Effect of norepinephrine on the outcome of septic shock. Crit Care Med. 2000;28:2758-65.
70. Martin GS, Mannino DM, Eaton S, et al. The epidemiology of sepsis in the United States from 1979 through 2000. N Engl J Med. 2003;348:1546-54.
71. McCabe WR, Jackson GG. Gram negative bacteremia. Arch Intern Med. 1962;110:92-100.
72. Mermel LA, Maki DG. Detection of bacteremia in adults: Consequences of culturing an inadequate volume of blood. Ann Intern Med. 1993;119:270-2.
73. Micek SST, Roubinian N, Heuring T, et al. Before-after study of a standardized hospital order set for the management of septic shock. Crit Care Med. 2006;34:2707-13.
74. Mier J, Leon EL, Castillo A, et al. Early versus late necrosectomy in severe necrotizing pancreatitis. Am J Surg. 1997;173:71-5.
75. Moran JL, O'Fathartaigh MS, Peisach AR, et al. Epinephrine as an inotropic agent in septic shock: A dose-profile analysis. Crit Care Med. 1993;21:70-7.
76. Morrell M, Fraser VJ, Kollef MH. Delaying the empiric treatment of candida bloodstream infection until positive blood culture results are obtained: A potential risk factor for hospital mortality. Antimicrob Agents Chemother. 2005; 49:3640-5.
77. Moss RL, Musemeche CA, Kosloske AM. Necrotizing fasciitis in children: Prompt recognition and aggressive therapy improve survival. J Pediatr Surg. 1996;31:1142-6.
78. Nguyen HB, Corbett SW, Steele R, et al. Implementation of a bundle of quality indicators for the early management of severe sepsis and septic shock is associated with decreased mortality. Crit Care Med. 2007;35:1105-12.
79. O'Brien A, Calpp L, Singer M. Terlipressin for norepinephrine-resistant septic shock. Lancet. 2002;359:1209-10.
80. O'Grady NP, Alexander M, Dellinger EP, et al. Guidelines for the prevention of intravascular catheter-related infections. Clin Infect Dis. 2002;35:1281-307.
81. Oppert M, Schindler R, Husung C, et al. Low dose hydrocortisone improves shock reversal and reduces cytokine levels in early hyperdynamic septic shock. Crit Care Med. 2005;33:2457-64.
82. Pappas PG, Rex JH, Sobel JD, et al. Guidelines for treatment of candidiasis. Clin Infect Dis. 2004;38:161-89.
83. Patel BM, Chittock DR, Russell JA, et al. Beneficial effects of short-term vasopressin infusion during severe septic shock. Anesthesiology. 2002;96:576-82.
84. Paul M, Silbiger I, Grozinsky S, et al. Beta lactam antibiotic monotherapy versus beta lactam-aminoglycoside antibiotic combination therapy for sepsis. Cochrane Database Syst Rev. 2006;(1):CD003344.
85. Pinsky MR, Payen D. Functional hemodynamic monitoring. Crit Care. 2005;9:566-72.
86. Regnier B, Rapin M, Gory G, et al. Haemodynamic effects of dopamine in septic shock. Intensive Care Med. 1977;3:47-53.
87. Reincke M, Allolio B, Würth G, et al. The hypothalamic-pituitary-adrenal axis in critical illness: Response to dexamethasone and corticotropin-releasing hormone. J Clin Endocrinol Metab. 1993;77:151-6.
88. Reinhart K, Kuhn HJ, Hartog C, et al. Continuous central venous and pulmonary artery oxygen saturation monitoring in the critically ill. Intensive Care Med. 2004;30:1572-8.
89. Rivers E, Nguyen B, Havstad S, et al. Early goal-directed therapy in the treatment of severe sepsis and septic shock. N Engl J Med. 2001;345:1368-77.
90. Sackett DL. Rules of evidence and clinical recommendations on the use of antithrombotic agents. Chest. 1989;95:2S-4S.

91. Safdar N, Handelsman J, Maki DG. Does combination antimicrobial therapy reduce mortality in Gram-negative bacteraemia? A meta-analysis. Lancet Infect Dis. 2004;4:519-27.
92. Sakr Y, Payen D, Reinhart K, et al. Effects of hydroxyethyl starch administration on renal function in critically ill patients. Br J Anaesth. 2007;98:216-24.
93. Schierhout G, Roberts I. Fluid resuscitation with colloid or crystalloid solutions in critically ill patients: A systematic review of randomized trials. BMJ. 1998;316:961-4.
94. Schortgen F, Lacherade JC, Bruneel F, et al. Effects of hydroxyethyl starch and gelatin on renal function in severe sepsis: A multicentre randomised study. Lancet. 2001;357:911-6.
95. Schünemann HJ, Jaeschke R, Cook DJ, et al, on behalf of the ATS Documents Development and Implementation Committee: An official ATS statement: Grading the quality of evidence and strength of recommendations in ATS guidelines and recommendations. Am J Respir Crit Care Med. 2006;174:605-14.
96. Sebat F, Johnson D, Musthafa AA, et al. A multidisciplinary community hospital program for early and rapid resuscitation of shock in nontrauma patients. Chest. 2005;127:1729-43.
97. Shapiro NI, Howell MD, Talmor D, et al. Implementation and outcomes of the Multiple Urgent Sepsis Therapies (MUST) protocol. Crit Care Med. 2006;34:1025-32.
98. Sharshar T, Blanchard A, Paillard M, et al. Circulating vasopressin levels in septic shock. Crit Care Med. 2003; 31:1752-8.
99. Shorr AF, Micek ST, Jackson WL Jr, et al. Economic implications of an evidence-based sepsis protocol: Can we improve outcomes and lower costs? Crit Care Med. 2007;35:1257-62.
100. Sprung CL, Annane D, Briegel J, et al. Corticosteroid therapy of septic shock (CORTICUS). Abstr. Am Rev Respir Crit Care Med. 2007;175:A507.
101. Sprung CL, Bernard GR, Dellinger RP (Eds). Guidelines for the management of severe sepsis and septic shock. Intensive Care Med. 2001;27(Suppl 1):S1-S134.
102. Tenover FC. Rapid detection and identification of bacterial pathogens using novel molecular technologies: Infection control and beyond. Clin Infect Dis. 2007;44:418-23.
103. Trzeciak S, Dellinger RP, Abate N, et al. Translating research to clinical practice: A 1-year experience with implementing early goal-directed therapy for septic shock in the emergency department. Chest. 2006;129:225-32.
104. Trzeciak S, Dellinger RP, Parrillo JE, et al. Early microcirculatory perfusion derangements in patients with severe sepsis and septic shock: Relationship to hemodynamics, oxygen transport, and survival. Ann Emerg Med. 2007;49:88-98.
105. Varpula M, Tallgren M, Saukkonen K, et al. Hemodynamic variables related to outcome in septic shock. Intensive Care Med. 2005;31:1066-71.
106. Vincent JL, Weil MH. Fluid challenge revisited. Crit Care Med. 2006;34:1333-7.
107. Weinstein MP, Reller LP, Murphy JR, et al. The clinical significance of positive blood cultures: A comprehensive analysis of 500 episodes of bacteremia and fungemia in adults. I. Laboratory and epidemiologic observations. Rev Infect Dis. 1983;5:35-53.
108. Yamazaki T, Shimada Y, Taenaka N, et al. Circulatory responses to afterloading with phenylephrine in hyperdynamic sepsis. Crit Care Med. 1982;10:432-5.
109. Yildiz O, Doganay M, Aygen B, et al. Physiologic-dose steroid therapy in sepsis. Crit Care. 2002;6:251-9.
110. Zhou SX, Qiu HB, Huang YZ, et al. Effects of norepinephrine, epinephrine, and norepinephrine-dobutamine on systemic and gastric mucosal oxygenation in septic shock. Acta Pharm Sin. 2002;23:654-8.

CHAPTER 16

Noninvasive Ventilation

Kishalay Datta

NONINVASIVE POSITIVE-PRESSURE VENTILATION

In early 90s, increasing experience with positive-pressure ventilation led to development of a ventilatory strategy, where ventilation could be delivered through a well-fitted mask in patients of obstructive sleep apnea (OSA). Increasing success of noninvasive ventilation (NIV) in cases of OSA led to its adoption in ventilatory management of patients with chronic obstructive pulmonary disease (COPD). Finally, in the next ensuing 20 years, noninvasive positive-pressure ventilation (NIPPV) delivered via a mask widely became adopted as the first-line ventilatory management in many medical centers over the whole world.

Noninvasive ventilation (NIV/NIPPV) refers to the administration of ventilatory support through the patients upper airways using an oronasal or nasal or similar masks without using an invasive artificial airway (endotracheal or tracheostomy tube). Noninvasive ventilation has now become an integral tool in the management of both acute and chronic respiratory failure, in both hospital and home settings. Noninvasive ventilation is being used as a replacement for invasive ventilation in many cases due to its advantages and flexibility.

The basic concept of NIPPV is the application of positive pressure during the respiratory cycle (inspiration and expiration). The simplest application of that is a continuous positive pressure throughout the respiratory cycle, which is named continuous positive airway pressure (CPAP*). The next application is administration of two different levels of pressure, one for inspiratory phase and another for the expiratory phase, otherwise known as bilevel positive airway pressure (BiPAP†).

Continuous Positive Airway Pressure (CPAP)
This mode can be used in patients, who are breathing spontaneously (a must). At end expiration, pressure in airways equals to pressure at mouth and both equates with normal atmospheric pressure. Surfactant prevents collapse of the alveoli which would have otherwise collapsed at this low end-expiratory pressure.

In diseased state, the alveoli collapse at low end-expiratory pressures due to lack of surfactant. So, hypoxia occurs as a result of ventilation/perfusion (V/Q) mismatch and shunting.

Large number of alveoli collapses during disease process in lungs leading to decreased lung compliance. Once lung compliance decreases, more energy is needed to inflate the alveoli. So, higher inflation pressures are needed to open the diseased alveoli. Thus "WOB" (work of breathing) increases.

Such high pressures needed to open diseased alveoli may also result in alveolar rupture leading to barotrauma.

Continuous positive airway pressure and positive end-expiratory pressure (PEEP) both thus act as "internal splints" for unstable alveolar units. CPAP also elevates end-expiratory pressure above atmospheric pressure thus keeping unstable alveolar units from collapsing and then finally "recruiting" them for useful ventilation. CPAP also helps in the recruitment of collapsed alveoli thereby increasing functional residual capacity of lung.

Continuous positive airway pressure thus decreases "work of breathing". CPAP can reverse hypoxia by restoration of ventilation to perfused areas (recruitment) thereby improving lung compliance. Stabilization of upper airways is also a purpose of this mode.

†*Bilevel Positive Airway Pressure (BiPAP)*
Continuous positive airway pressure does not provide support during inspiration as it only maintains positive pressure in airways. So, pressure support ventilation (PSV) was added to provide pressure support during inspiration in patients with poor respiratory effort. This resulted in creation of a new mode called BiPAP.

So, BiPAP has two components providing pressures at two levels, i.e. inspiratory and expiratory level.
1. PSV—which provides inspiratory pressure.
2. PEEP—which provides expiratory pressure.

BiPAP and CPAP both have disadvantage of propensity toward hyperinflation of lung.

Noninvasive positive-pressure ventilation operates with application of positive pressure to upper airway (via masks) either by using a conventional ventilator or specialized equipment like BiPAP/CPAP machines. NIPPV can also be given by volume cycled or pressure cycled ventilators. CPAP/BiPAP/pressure support ventilation (PSV)/other modes can all be used in NIV, as per ventilatory needs of the patient.

HOW DOES NIPPV WORK?

Noninvasive positive-pressure ventilation (NIPPV) works by
- Decreasing inspiratory work of breathing (WOB)
- Decreasing inspiratory muscles work
- Decreasing "pressure time product" (PTP) of inspiratory muscle—an index for muscle O_2 consumption. (PTP of diaphragm is reduced by 25% with PSV alone, while with PSV + positive end-expiratory pressure (PEEP), it goes down to 40%).

Interface

Interface or masks are devices, which connect ventilator tubings to facial region of the patient, during NIV. Patient-ventilator interfaces available for NIPPV include a full face mask/oronasal mask/nasal mask/nasal prongs/helmets. The full face mask includes the eyes, nose, and mouth, while the oronasal mask includes the nose and mouth, but not the eyes. A simple nasal mask is also available.

Straps hold the interface in place and should be adjusted to avoid excess pressure on the nose or the face. The straps should be loose enough to allow one or two fingers to pass between the face and the strap. When a nasal mask is used, a chin strap is usually necessary to maintain closure of the mouth.

The efficacy of the various interfaces has been debated over years. The face mask confers physiologic improvement, but the nasal mask is better tolerated. Whichever mask is selected, it is helpful to keep the following points in mind **(Fig. 1)**:
- Most patients with acute respiratory failure are mouth breathers; therefore, NIPPV delivered by a nasal mask may result in a larger air leak through the mouth thus leading to a bad outcome.
- The nasal air passages offer significant resistance to airflow, which can reduce the beneficial effects of NIPPV, if low positive pressure is used.
- The monitoring for aspiration in NIPPV patients is often difficult.
- Humidification of the inspired air is difficult through any form of masks.

The helmet interface has been used to improve patient tolerance in many cases. Moreover, the helmet interface allows patients to talk, read, and drink through a straw, while minimizing complications, such as skin necrosis, gastric distension and eye irritation. But, this interface may cause accumulation of CO_2 within the helmet, may produce noise

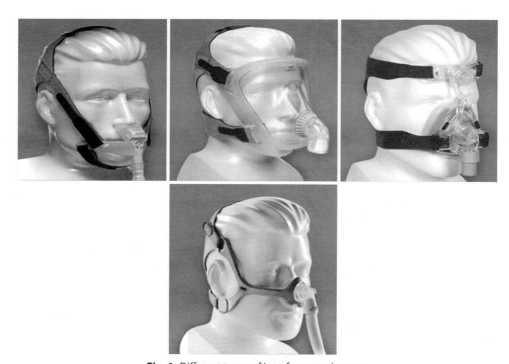

Fig. 1 Different types of interface attachments

sufficiently high enough to cause hearing damage, and may also to lead to more patient-ventilator asynchrony and less relief of inspiratory effort of the patient.

WHAT TYPE OF VENTILATORS CAN BE USED FOR NIPPV?

Noninvasive ventilation can be delivered via all standard type of ventilators found in most intensive care units of hospitals or by a portable ventilator. Nowadays "hybrid ventilators" offering both forms (invasive and noninvasive) of ventilatory support are also available. However, the standard invasive intensive care unit (ICU) ventilator has numerous advantages over the BiPAP/CPAP machines. The advantages are:
- A precise concentration of oxygen can be delivered, i.e. FiO_2 can be set.
- Separate inspiratory and expiratory tubing minimizes the rebreathing of carbon dioxide.
- Large mask leaks or patient's disconnection can be readily detected.
- Better monitoring and alarm features are present in standard ventilators.
- Higher inspiratory pressures (>20 cm H_2O) can be given if need arises.
- Backup ventilation is present when needed.

In addition, certain modes can only be delivered by a standard ICU ventilator (e.g. volume-controlled, pressure-controlled, and time-limited PSV, etc.).

WHAT MODES OF VENTILATOR CAN BE USED FOR NONINVASIVE VENTILATION?

Noninvasive positive-pressure ventilation can be delivered using the same modes that are used for invasive mechanical ventilation, although certain modes may be used more frequently:
- Assist control mode is the most common mode chosen by doctors who want a guaranteed minute ventilation.
- Pressure support ventilation is the most common mode chosen by doctors who focuses on patient's comfort and synchrony.
- Continuous positive airway pressure/BiPAP is used for patients with acute respiratory failure.
- Proportional assist ventilation delivers an inspiratory pressure that is proportional to patient effort. This allows better patient-ventilator synchrony.

HOW TO SET THE VENTILATOR FOR NIPPV?

The selected mode determines which parameters need to be set during the initiation of NIV, e.g. assist control mode requires a tidal volume, respiratory rate, inspiratory flow rate, PEEP, and (FiO_2) to be set.

Bilevel positive airway pressure mode delivers both inspiratory positive airway pressure (IPAP) and expiratory positive airway pressure (EPAP) like invasive ventilation.

SELECTION CRITERIA FOR NIPPV

First and foremost criteria is patient should be *conscious and spontaneously breathing*.

Patient should have the ability to protect airway himself, be cooperative and also should be hemodynamically stable. Care should be taken that there are no excessive respiratory secretions present in such patients undergoing a trial of NIPPV.

Selecting patients for NIPPV requires careful consideration of its indications and contraindications. A trial of NIPPV is worthwhile in most patients who do not require emergent intubation and have a disease known to respond to NIPPV, assuming that they lack contraindications.

Conditions known to respond to NIPPV are as follows:
- Exacerbations of COPD, where arterial carbon dioxide tension ($PaCO_2$) greater than 45 mm Hg or pH less than 7.30.
- Cardiogenic pulmonary edema.
- Acute hypoxemic respiratory failure.
- Obstructive sleep apnea-hypopnea syndrome.
- Congestive heart failure.
- Obesity hypoventilation syndrome.
- Acute exacerbations of COPD.
- Immunocompromised host with acute respiratory failure.
- Postextubation and respiratory failure after extubation.
- Facilitate weaning.
- Asthma and status asthmaticus.

CONTRAINDICATIONS FOR NIPPV

The need for emergent intubation is an absolute contraindication to NIPPV.

Noninvasive positive-pressure ventilation is also contraindicated in following conditions:
- Patients having no spontaneous breathing
- Unconscious patient
- Severe hemodynamic instability of the patient
- Upper airway obstruction
- Facial trauma in a patient
- Pneumothorax
- Inability to cooperate, protect the airway, or clear secretions
- High aspiration risk
- Prolonged duration of mechanical ventilation anticipated
- Recent esophageal anastomosis.

HOW TO INITIATE NIPPV IN PATIENTS?

1. It should be done through graded steps which are as follows: selection of proper interface is foremost followed by acclimatization of the patient with the interface.
2. Start with low pressure/volume in spontaneous mode.
3. O_2 supplementation should be continued at the rate of 3–5 L/min and adjusted as per pressure changes.
4. Initial IPAP should be started at 8–10 cm H_2O while EPAP at 3–4 cm H_2O.

5. An IPAP: EPAP ratio should be kept constant at 2.5:1.
6. Gradual increase of both pressures at 1–3 cm H_2O increments can be done.
7. Care should be taken that pressure should not exceed more than 20 cm H_2O.

MONITORING OF PATIENTS ON NIPPV

After NIPPV is initiated, the patient should be observed closely for the first 4–6 hours to troubleshoot, provide reassurance, and look for deterioration of clinical condition of the patient. Improvement of the pH and $PaCO_2$ within one and a half to 2 hours predicts success. In contrast, conditions like worsening encephalopathy or agitation, inability to clear secretions, inability to tolerate any of the interfaces, hemodynamic instability or decreased oxygenation may indicate towards failure.

The use of sedatives and analgesics is sometimes employed by clinicians to increase tolerance and comfort of NIPPV as well as to treat comorbid anxiety or pain.

PREDICTORS OF SUCCESS OF NIPPV

One of the most consistent signs of favorable response to NIPPV is drop in respiratory rate within 1st to 2nd hour of starting of NIPPV.

The following parameters should be considered for successful NIPPV trial:
- $PaCO_2$ greater than 45 and less than 90 mm Hg at initiation of NIPPV
- pH greater than 7.1 at initiation of NIPPV
- Less air-leakage via interface during NIPPV
- Ability of the patient to coordinate breathing with the ventilator
- Lower severity of illness (APACHE scores) and young age of the patient.

WEANING

Weaning from NIPPV may be accomplished by progressively decreasing the amount of positive airway pressure, permitting the patient to be disconnected from the NIPPV for progressively longer durations, or a combination of both.

COMPLICATIONS OF NIPPV

These are common complications:
- Leakage via mask leading to multiple adjustments
- Intolerance of positive pressure by patient
- Gastric distention due to positive pressure
- Aspiration (rare)
- Facial skin breakdown (long-term use)
- Increased gastric pressure may lead to abdominal compartment syndrome
- Hypotension
- Barotrauma.

BIBLIOGRAPHY

1. Ahmed A, Fenwick L, Angus RM, et al. Nasal ventilation vs doxapram in the treatment of type II respiratory failure complicating chronic airflow obstruction. Thorax. 1992;1:858.
2. Amato MB, Barbas CS, Medeiros DM, et al. Effect of a protective-ventilation strategy on mortality in acute respiratory distress syndrome. N Engl J Med. 1998;338(6):347-54.
3. Ambrosino N, Foglio K, Rubini F, et al. Non-invasive mechanical ventilation in acute respiratory failure due to chronic obstructive airways disease: correlates for success. Thorax. 1995;50(7):755-7.
4. Angus RM, Ahmed AA, Fenwick LJ, et al. Comparison of the acute effects on gas exchange of nasal ventilation and doxapram in exacerbations of chronic obstructive pulmonary disease. Thorax. 1996;51(10):1048-50.
5. Antonelli M, Conti G, Bufi M, et al. Noninvasive ventilation for treatment of acute respiratory failure in patients undergoing solid organ transplantation: a randomized trial. JAMA. 2000;283(2):235-41.
6. Antonelli M, Conti G, Rocco M, et al. A comparison of noninvasive positive-pressure ventilation and conventional mechanical ventilation in patients with acute respiratory failure. N Engl J Med. 1998;339(7):429-35.
7. Appendini L, Patessio A, Zanaboni S, et al. Physiologic effects of positive end-expiratory pressure and mask pressure support during exacerbations of chronic obstructive pulmonary disease. Am J Respir Crit Care Med. 1994;149(5):1069-76.
8. Barbe F, Togores B, Rubi M, et al. Noninvasive ventilatory support does not facilitate recovery from acute respiratory failure in chronic obstructive pulmonary disease. Eur Respir J. 1996;9(6):1240-5.
9. Benhamou D, Girault C, Faure C, et al. Nasal mask ventilation in acute respiratory failure. Experience in elderly patients. Chest. 1992;102(3):912-7.
10. Bersten AD, Holt AW, Vedig AE, et al. Treatment of severe cardiogenic pulmonary edema with continuous positive airway pressure delivered by face mask. N Engl J Med. 1991;325(26):1825-30.
11. Bolliger CT, Van Eeden SF. Treatment of multiple rib fractures. Randomized controlled trial comparing ventilatory with nonventilatory management. Chest. 1990;97(4):943-8.
12. Bott J, Baudouin SV, Moxham J. Nasal intermittent positive pressure ventilation in the treatment of respiratory failure in obstructive sleep apnoea. Thorax. 1991;46(6):457-8.
13. Bott J, Carroll MP, Conway JH, et al. Randomised controlled trial of nasal ventilation in acute ventilatory failure due to chronic obstructive airways disease. Lancet. 1993;341(8860):1555-7.
14. Brett A, Sinclair DG. Use of continuous positive airway pressure in the management of community acquired pneumonia. Thorax. 1993;48(12):1280-1.
15. Brochard L, Isabey D, Piquet J, et al. Reversal of acute exacerbations of chronic obstructive lung disease by inspiratory assistance with a face mask. N Engl J Med. 1990;323(22):1523-30.
16. Brochard L, Mancebo J, Wysocki M, et al. Noninvasive ventilation for acute exacerbations of chronic obstructive pulmonary disease. N Engl J Med. 1995;333(13):817-22.
17. Brown JS, Meecham Jones DJ, Mikelsons C, et al. Using nasal intermittent positive pressure ventilation on a general respiratory ward. JR Coll Physicians Lond. 1998;32(3):219-24.

18. Bunburaphong T, Imanaka H, Nishimura M, et al. Performance characteristics of bilevel pressure ventilators: a lung model study. Chest. 1997;111(4):1050-60.
19. Celikel T, Sungur M, Ceyhan B, et al. Comparison of noninvasive positive pressure ventilation with standard medical therapy in hypercapnic acute respiratory failure. Chest. 1998;114(6):1636-42.
20. Chevrolet JC, Jolliet P, Abajo B, et al. Nasal positive pressure ventilation in patients with acute respiratory failure. Difficult and time-consuming procedure for nurses. Chest. 1991;100(3):775-82.
21. Clinical indications for noninvasive positive pressure ventilation in chronic respiratory failure due to restrictive lung disease, COPD, and nocturnal hypoventilation—a consensus conference report. Chest. 1999;116(2):521-34.
22. Confalonieri M, Parigi P, Scartabellati A, et al. Noninvasive mechanical ventilation improves the immediate and long-term outcome of COPD patients with acute respiratory failure. Eur Respir J. 1996;9(3):422-30.
23. Confalonieri M, Potena A, Carbone G, et al. Acute respiratory failure in patients with severe community-acquired pneumonia. A prospective randomized evaluation of noninvasive ventilation. Am J Respir Crit Care Med. 1999;160(5 Pt 1):1585-91.
24. Conway JH, Hitchcock RA, Godfrey RC, et al. Nasal intermittent positive pressure ventilation in acute exacerbations of chronic obstructive pulmonary disease—a preliminary study. Respir Med. 1993;87(5):387-94.
25. Cowan MJ, Shelhamer JH, Levine SJ. Acute respiratory failure in the HIV-seropositive patient. Crit Care Clin. 1997;13(3):523-52.
26. de Lucas P, Tarancon C, Puente L, et al. Nasal continuous positive airway pressure in patients with COPD in acute respiratory failure. A study of the immediate effects. Chest. 1993;104(6):1694-7.
27. Delclaux C, L'Her E, Alberti C, et al. Treatment of acute hypoxemic nonhypercapnic respiratory insufficiency with continuous positive airway pressure delivered by a face mask: A randomized controlled trial. JAMA. 2000;284(18):2352-60.
28. Department of Health. Comprehensive critical care: a review of adult critical care services. London: Department of Health, 2000.
29. Doherty MJ, Greenstone MA. Survey of non-invasive ventilation (NIPPV) in patients with acute exacerbation of chronic obstructive pulmonary disease (COPD) in the UK. Thorax. 1998;53(10):863-6.
30. Edenborough F, Wildman M, Morgan D. Management of respiratory failure with ventilation via intranasal stents in cystic fibrosis. Thorax. 2000;55(5):434-6.
31. Elliott MW, Simonds AK. Nocturnal assisted ventilation using bilevel airway pressure: the effect of expiratory airway pressure. Eur Respir J. 1995;8(3):436-40.
32. Elliott MW, Steven MH, Phillips GD, et al. Non-invasive mechanical ventilation for acute respiratory failure. BMJ. 1990;300:358-60.
33. Ellis ER, Bye PT, Bruderer JW, et al. Treatment of respiratory failure during sleep in patients with neuromuscular disease. Positive-pressure ventilation through a nose mask. Am Rev Respir Dis. 1987;135(1):148-52.
34. Ferguson GT, Gilmartin M. CO_2 rebreathing during BiPAP ventilatory assistance. Am J Crit Care Med. 1995;151(40:1126-35.
35. Gachot B, Clair B, Wolff M, et al. Continuous positive airway pressure by face mask or mechanical ventilation in patients with human immunodeficiency virus infection and severe *Pneumocystis carinii pneumonia*. Intensive Care Med. 1992;18(3):155-9.
36. Girault C, Daudenthun I, Chevron V, et al. Noninvasive ventilation as a systematic extubation and weaning technique in acute-on-chronic respiratory failure. Am J Respir Crit Care Med. 1999;160(1):86-92.
37. Girault C, Richard JC, Chevron V, et al. Comparative physiologic effects of noninvasive assist-control and pressure support ventilation in acute hypercapnic respiratory failure. Chest. 1997;111(6):1639-48.
38. Goldberg P, Reissmann H, Maltais F, et al. Efficacy of noninvasive CPAP in COPD with acute respiratory failure. Eur Respir J. 1995;8(11):1894-900.
39. Gregg RW, Friedman BC, Williams JF, et al. Continuous positive airway pressure by face mask in *Pneumocystis carinii* pneumonia. Crit Care Med. 1990;18(1):21-4.
40. Haworth CS, Dodd ME, Atkins M, et al. Pneumothorax in adults with cystic fibrosis dependent on nasal intermittent positive pressure ventilation (NIPPV): a management dilemma. Thorax. 2000;55(7):620-2.
41. Hilbert G, Gruson D, Vargas F, et al. Noninvasive ventilation in immunosuppressed patients with pulmonary infiltrates, fever, and acute respiratory failure. N Engl J Med. 2001;344(7):481-7.
42. Hilbert G, Gruson D, Vargas F, et al. Noninvasive ventilation for acute respiratory failure. Quite low time consumption for nurses. Eur Respir J. 2000;16(4):710-6.
43. Hodson ME, Madden BP, Steven MH, et al. Non-invasive mechanical ventilation for cystic fibrosis patients—a potential bridge to transplantation. Eur Respir J. 1991;4(5):524-7.
44. Hoffmann B, Welte T. The use of noninvasive pressure support ventilation for severe respiratory insufficiency due to pulmonary oedema. Intensive Care Med. 1999;25(1):15-20.
45. Hurst JM, DeHaven CB, Branson RD. Use of CPAP mask as the sole mode of ventilatory support in trauma patients with mild to moderate respiratory insufficiency. J Trauma. 1985;25(11):1065-8.
46. Kerby GR, Mayer LS, Pingleton SK. Nocturnal positive pressure ventilation via nasal mask. Am Rev Respir Dis. 1987;135(3):738-40.
47. Kesten S, Rebuck AS. Nasal continuous positive airway pressure in *Pneumocystis carinii* pneumonia. Lancet. 1988;332(8625):1414-5.
48. Kramer N, Meyer TJ, Meharg J, et al. Randomized, prospective trial of noninvasive positive pressure ventilation in acute respiratory failure. Am J Respir Crit Care Med. 1995;151(6):1799-806.
49. Lapinsky SE, Mount DB, Mackey D, et al. Management of acute respiratory failure due to pulmonary edema with nasal positive pressure support. Chest. 1994;105(1):229-31.
50. Leung P, Jubran A, Tobin MJ. Comparison of assisted ventilator modes on triggering, patient effort, and dyspnea. Am J Respir Crit Care Med. 1997;155(6):1940-8.
51. Lim TK. Treatment of severe exacerbation of chronic obstructive pulmonary disease with mask-applied continuous positive airway pressure. Respirology. 1996;1(3):189-93.
52. Lin M, Yang YF, Chiang HT, et al. Reappraisal of continuous positive airway pressure therapy in acute cardiogenic pulmonary edema. Short-term results and long-term follow-up. Chest. 1995;107(5):1379-86.

53. Linton DM, Potgieter PD. Conservative management of blunt chest trauma. S Afr Med J. 1982;61(24):917-9.
54. Lofaso F, Brochard L, Hang T, et al. Home versus intensive care pressure support devices. Experimental and clinical comparison. Am J Respir Crit Care Med. 1996;153(5):1591-9.
55. Martin TJ, Hovis JD, Costantino JP, et al. A randomized, prospective evaluation of noninvasive ventilation for acute respiratory failure. Am J Respir Crit Care Med. 2000;161(3 Pt 1):807-13.
56. Masip J, Betbesé AJ, Páez J, et al. Non-invasive pressure support ventilation versus conventional oxygen therapy in acute cardiogenic pulmonary oedema: a randomized trial. Lancet. 2000;356(9248):2126-32.
57. Medical Devices Agency. Medical device and equipment management for hospitals and community-based organizations (MDA DB9801). London: Medical Devices Agency, 1999.
58. Meduri GU, Abou-Shala N, Fox RC, et al. Noninvasive face mask mechanical ventilation in patients with acute hypercapnic respiratory failure. Chest. 1991;100(2):445-54.
59. Meduri GU, Conoscenti CC, Menashe P, et al. Noninvasive face mask ventilation in patients with acute respiratory failure. Chest. 1989;95(4):865-70.
60. Meduri GU, Cook TR, Turner RE, et al. Noninvasive positive pressure ventilation in status asthmaticus. Chest. 1996;110(3):767-74.
61. Meduri GU, Fox RC, Abou-Shala N, et al. Noninvasive mechanical ventilation via face mask in patients with acute respiratory failure who refused endotracheal intubation. Crit Care Med. 1994;22(10):1584-90.
62. Meduri GU, Turner RE, Abou-Shala N, et al. Noninvasive positive pressure ventilation via face mask. First-line intervention in patients with acute hypercapnic and hypoxemic respiratory failure. Chest. 1996;109(1):179-93.
63. Meecham Jones DJ, Paul EA, Grahame-Clarke C, et al. Nasal ventilation in acute exacerbations of chronic obstructive pulmonary disease: effect of ventilator mode on arterial blood gas tensions. Thorax. 1994;49(12):1222-4.
64. Mehta S, Jay GD, Woolard RH, et al. Randomized, prospective trial of bilevel versus continuous positive airway pressure in acute pulmonary edema. Crit Care Med. 1997;25(4):620-8.
65. Meyer T, Hill N. Noninvasive positive pressure ventilation to treat respiratory failure. Ann Intern Med. 1994;120:760-70.
66. Miller RF, Semple SJ. Continuous positive airway pressure ventilation for respiratory failure associated with Pneumocystis carinii pneumonia. Respir Med. 1991;85(2):133-8.
67. Miro AM, Shivaram U, Hertig I. Continuous positive airway pressure in COPD patients in acute hypercapnic respiratory failure. Chest. 1993;103(1):266-8.
68. Nava S, Ambrosino N, Bruschi C, et al. Physiological effects of flow and pressure triggering during non-invasive mechanical ventilation in patients with chronic obstructive pulmonary disease. Thorax. 1997;52(3):249-54.
69. Nava S, Ambrosino N, Clini E, et al. Noninvasive mechanical ventilation in the weaning of patients with respiratory failure due to chronic obstructive pulmonary disease. A randomized, controlled trial. Ann Intern Med. 1998;128(9):721-8.
70. Nava S, Evangelisti I, Rampulla C, et al. Human and financial costs of noninvasive mechanical ventilation in patients affected by COPD and acute respiratory failure. Chest. 1997;111(6):1631-8.
71. Newberry DL 3rd, Noblett KE, Kolhouse L. Noninvasive bilevel positive pressure ventilation in severe acute pulmonary edema. Am J Emerg Med. 1995;13(4):479-82.
72. Pang D, Keenan SP, Cook DJ, et al. The effect of positive pressure airway support on mortality and the need for intubation in cardiogenic pulmonary edema: a systematic review. Chest. 1998;114(4):1185-92.
73. Patrick W, Webster K, Ludwig L, et al. Noninvasive positive-pressure ventilation in acute respiratory distress without prior chronic respiratory failure. Am J Respir Crit Care Med. 1996;153(3):1005-11.
74. Plant PK, Owen JL, Elliott MW. Early use of non-invasive ventilation for acute exacerbations of chronic obstructive pulmonary disease on general respiratory wards: a multicentre randomised controlled trial. Lancet. 2000;355(9219):1931-5.
75. Plant PK, Owen JL, Elliott MW. One year period prevalence study of respiratory acidosis in acute exacerbations of COPD: implications for the provision of non-invasive ventilation and oxygen administration. Thorax. 2000;55(7):550-4.
76. Prevedoros HP, Lee RP, Marriot D. CPAP, effective respiratory support in patients with AIDS-related *Pneumocystis carinii* pneumonia. Anaesth Intensive Care. 1991;19(4):561-6.
77. Räsänen J, Heikkilä J, Downs J, et al. Continuous positive airway pressure by face mask in acute cardiogenic pulmonary edema. Am J Cardiol. 1985;55(4):296-300.
78. Rennotte MT, Baele P, Aubert G, et al. Nasal continuous positive airway pressure in the perioperative management of patients with obstructive sleep apnea submitted to surgery. Chest. 1995;107(2):367-74.
79. Rocker GM, Mackenzie MG, Williams B, et al. Noninvasive positive pressure ventilation: successful outcome in patients with acute lung injury/ARDS. Chest. 1999;115(1):173-7.
80. Royal College of Physicians. Oxygen therapy services guidelines. London: Royal College of Physicians, 2000.
81. Rusterholtz T, Kempf J, Berton C, et al. Noninvasive pressure support ventilation (NIPSV) with face mask in patients with acute cardiogenic pulmonary edema (ACPE). Intensive Care Med. 1999;25(1):21-8.
82. Schönhofer B, Sonneborn M, Haidl P, et al. Comparison of two different modes of noninvasive mechanical ventilation in chronic respiratory failure: volume versus pressure controlled devices. Eur Respir J. 1997;10(1):184-91.
83. Sharon A, Shpirer I, Kaluski E, et al. High-dose intravenous isosorbide-dinitrate is safer and better than Bi-PAP ventilation combined with conventional treatment for severe pulmonary edema. J Am Coll Cardiol. 2000;36(3):832-7.
84. Shivaram U, Cash ME, Beal A. Nasal continuous positive airway pressure in decompensated hypercapnic respiratory failure as a complication of sleep apnea. Chest. 1993;104(3):770-4.
85. Simonds AK, Elliott MW. Outcome of domiciliary nasal intermittent positive pressure ventilation in restrictive and obstructive disorders. Thorax. 1995;50(6):604-9.
86. Simonds AK. Equipment. In: Simonds AK (Ed). Non-invasive Respiratory Support. London: Chapman and Hall; 1996. pp. 16-37.
87. Smith IE, Shneerson JM. A laboratory comparison of four positive pressure ventilators used in the home. Eur Respir J. 1996;9(11):2410-5.
88. Soo Hoo GW, Santiago S, Williams AJ. Nasal mechanical ventilation for hypercapnic respiratory failure in chronic

89. Teschler H, Stampa J, Ragette R, et al. Effect of mouth leak on effectiveness of nasal bilevel ventilatory assistance and sleep architecture. Eur Respir J. 1999;14(6):1251-7.
90. Vitacca M, Clini E, Rubini F, et al. Non-invasive mechanical ventilation in severe chronic obstructive lung disease and acute respiratory failure: short- and long-term prognosis. Intensive Care Med. 1996;22(2):94-100.
91. Vitacca M, Rubini F, Foglio K, et al. Non-invasive modalities of positive pressure ventilation improve the outcome of acute exacerbations in COLD patients. Intensive Care Med. 1993;19(8):450-5.
92. Wood KA, Lewis L, Von Harz B, et al. The use of noninvasive positive pressure ventilation in the emergency department. Chest. 1998;113(5):1339-46.
93. Wysocki M, Tric L, Wolff MA, et al. Noninvasive pressure support ventilation in patients with acute respiratory failure. A randomized comparison with conventional therapy. Chest. 1995;107(3):761-8.
94. Younes M. Proportional assist ventilation, a new approach to ventilatory support. Theory. Am Rev Respir Dis. 1992;145(1):114-20.

CHAPTER 17

Mechanical Ventilation

Mrinal Sircar, Saurabh Mehra

INTRODUCTION

Mechanical ventilation and intubation are an indispensable part of emergency room (ER) management. The indication for mechanical ventilation is either to provide assistance in breathing and/or airway protection. This applies to diverse conditions including trauma, sepsis, exacerbations of asthma and chronic obstructive pulmonary disease (COPD), severe pneumonia, congestive cardiac failure and neurological disorders associated with low Glasgow Coma Scale (GCS) or loss of protective airway reflexes, etc. All those working in ER need to be well versed in providing mechanical ventilation in ER as also during transport to intensive care unit (ICU), operating theaters or for imaging or while transporting patients by ambulance.

PHYSIOLOGY OF BREATHING

Spontaneous breathing involves contraction of diaphragm and intercostal muscles to cause expansion of thorax and movement of air into lungs. Physiologically, development of a pressure gradient (ΔP) between the alveoli and the atmosphere causes air movement into lungs. Since this involves generation of a negative pressure, spontaneous ventilation is negative pressure ventilation. The expiration is a passive phenomenon, however; in diseased states, it may require active contraction of accessory muscles.

The ventilation involves a number of pressures and ΔPs **(Fig. 1)**, which must be understood to know the physiology of breathing. Four different pressures are:

1. *Airway opening pressure (P_{awo}) or airway pressure or mouth pressure*: It is zero or atmospheric pressure unless a positive pressure is applied.
2. *Pressure at body surface (P_{bs})*: It is zero or atmospheric pressure.

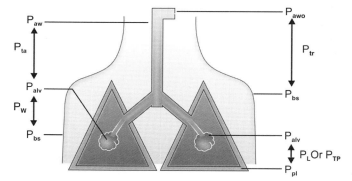

Fig. 1 Various pressures and pressure gradients of the respiratory system
Abbreviations: P_{aw}, airway pressure; P_{awo}, airway opening pressure; P_{ta}, transairway pressure; P_{tr}, transrespiratory pressure; P_{alv}, alveolar pressure; P_{bs}, body surface pressure; P_w, transthoracic pressure; P_{pl}, pleural pressure; P_{TP}, transpulmonary pressure.

3. *Intrapleural pressure (P_{pl})*: It is the pressure in the pleural space, i.e. space between the parietal and visceral pleurae. It is negative as there is no air in the pleural space. At the end of expiration in a spontaneously breathing person, it is about -5 cm H_2O. However, in an upright lung, it varies depending upon where it is measured. P_{pl} increases by 0.3 cm H_2O/cm vertical distance of lung. The cause of this vertical gradient is the weight of the lung itself. So, it is around -3 cm H_2O at the lung base and -7 cm H_2O at the lung apex.
4. *Alveolar pressure (P_A or P_{alv}) or intrapulmonary pressure or lung pressure*: It also varies with the phase of ventilation. P_A is -1 cm H_2O during spontaneous inspiration and becomes positive during expiration ($+1$ cm H_2O).

Four gradients are derived from these four pressures **(Table 1)**.

Table 1 Pressure gradients during spontaneous breathing	
Transairway pressure (P_{ta})	Airway pressure – alveolar pressure ($P_{aw} - P_{alv}$)
Transpulmonary pressure (P_{TP} or P_L) or transalveolar pressure	Alveolar pressure – pleural pressure ($P_{alv} - P_{pl}$)
Transthoracic pressure (P_w)	Alveolar pressure – body surface pressure ($P_{alv} - P_{bs}$)
Transrespiratory pressure (P_{tr})	Airway opening pressure – body surface pressure ($P_{awo} - P_{bs}$)

MECHANICAL DETERMINANTS OF PATIENT-VENTILATOR INTERACTIONS

To understand the interaction between a ventilator and a patient, we assume that lung may be represented as a simplified linear model with a tube (T) and a balloon or hollow sphere (S).[1,2] The sphere is inflated by applying a pressure (Pi) near the tube inlet **(Figs 2A and B)**.

The pressure applied to the tube inlet Pi is equal to the sum of two pressures, (1) an elastic pressure of the sphere (P_{el}) and (2) a resistive pressure of the tube (P_{res}).

$$Pi = P_{el} + P_{res} \text{ (Equation 1)}$$

P_{el} reflects the elastic properties of lungs and chest wall, whereas P_{res} reflects the resistive properties of endotracheal tube and airways.

We know from principles of physics that

Elastic recoil pressure (P_{el}) = Elastance × Volume = E × V

and

Flow resistance pressure (P_{res}) = Resistance × Flow = R × V̇ (Ohm's law)

So, equation 1 can be stated as:

$$Pi = EV + RV̇ \text{ (Equation 2)}$$

For a patient on ventilator, Pi has two components, i.e. P_{mus} (pressure generated by the respiratory muscles) and P_{vent} (pressure delivered by the ventilator)

So, equation 2 can be written as:

$$P_{mus} + P_{vent} = EV + RV̇ \text{ (Equation 3)}$$

Compliance (C) of the respiratory system is determined by measuring the change of volume (ΔV) that occurs when ΔP is applied to the system:

$$C = ΔV/ΔP$$

It is inversely proportional to elastance.

Resistance of respiratory system includes resistance to the flow of gases in airways [airway resistance (R_{aw})] or resistance offered by the lung tissue and the chest wall (tissue resistance) **(Table 2)**.

$$R_{aw} = \text{Transairway pressure/flow}$$

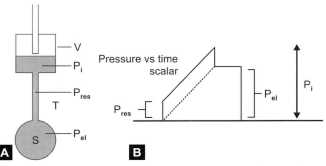

Figs 2A and B (A) It shows a simple linear system with a ventilator (V) applying a pressure (P_i) to the inlet of tube (T) leading to inflation of hollow sphere (S); (B) It shows the resulting pressure versus time waveform
Abbreviations: P_{res}, flow resistance pressure; P_{el}, elastic recoil pressure.

Table 2 Normal values of compliance and resistance		
Parameters	Compliance (mL/cm H_2O)	Resistance (cm H_2O/L/s)
Spontaneously breathing	100 (range 50–170)	0.6–2.4 (at 0.5 L/s flow)
Intubated and mechanically ventilated	40–50 (males) 35–45 (females) Can vary up to 100 in either gender	5–7 Can be higher depending on patients clinical condition or circuit determinants

Time constant: It tells us the time lung units or the acini take to fill and empty. It is the product of the C and resistance.

One time constant = 0.1 L/cm H_2O (C) × 1 cm H_2O/L/s (R)

Normally, one time constant is 0.1 second. One time constant means the time to exhale 63% of volume, similarly two, three, four and five time constants are the time to exhale 86, 95, 98 and 100% volume.[3,4]

Because lung is a heterogeneous structure, time constants can vary in different regions of lungs. This is exacerbated in diseased states such acute severe asthma or acute respiratory distress syndrome (ARDS).

The clinical importance of time constant lies in the fact that inspiratory time less than three time constants will lead to incomplete delivery of tidal volume (V_T). Similarly, if the expiratory time is less than three time constants, it will lead to incomplete exhalation.[3]

INDICATIONS OF MECHANICAL VENTILATION

Tracheal intubation with cuffed endotracheal/tracheostomy tubes protects from aspiration and ventilation supports the

Box 1 Common indications of mechanical ventilation

Cardiopulmonary arrest:
- Neurological problems (stroke, myasthenia gravis, meningitis, encephalitis, tumors, high intracranial pressure, drug overdoses causing unconsciousness, etc.)
- Pulmonary problems—asthma, COPD, ARDS and pneumonia

Trauma
- Congestive cardiac failure
- *Shock*: Septic shock, cardiogenic shock, hemorrhagic shock, etc.

Abbreviations: ARDS, acute respiratory distress syndrome; COPD, chronic obstructive pulmonary disease.

breathing. Patients, who have diminished airway reflexes or have respiratory insufficiency as evident by hypoxemia, hypercarbia or severe respiratory distress are the likely candidates to receive mechanical ventilation. Common indications are given in **Box 1**.

TYPES OF MECHANICAL VENTILATION

Mechanical ventilation can be categorized as following:
- Invasive or noninvasive
- Positive pressure or negative pressure
- Pressure control (PC) or volume control (VC) or dual mode.

Positive pressure ventilators are the ones used in clinical practice. A positive (higher than the atmospheric) pressure is applied to the patient's airway, which creates a flow of gases into the lungs. Such a pressure can be applied to endotracheal tube, tracheostomy tube or noninvasively to the face of the patient. However, in this chapter we will limit our discussion to the invasive mechanical ventilation only.

Volume control ventilation is the one in which volume is set and pressure is the independent variable, while in PC ventilation, pressure is set and volume is an independent variable.

Before moving on we will discuss about the "variables" in the ventilation.

Control Variables

Control variables are the main variables the ventilator adjusts to produce inspiration.[5] They include pressure, volume, flow and time.

Phase Variables

Phase variables control the four phases of a breath (i.e. beginning of inspiration, inspiration, end inspiration). Types of phase variables include:
- *Trigger variable*: It is a preset variable, which decides the beginning of inspiration. It can be pressure (pressure triggering), flow (flow triggering), volume (volume triggering) or time (time triggering). Traditionally pressure has been used, but modern ventilators have flow triggering, which is now considered better for patients.[6] Patients who have a spontaneous effort should generate the set amount of pressure or flow or volume that can be sensed by ventilator as a patient effort and then it can be supported by a positive pressure breath. When the ventilator starts inspiration according to the set rate and the duration of inspiration to the duration of expiration (I:E) ratio, it is called time triggering
- *Target variable (limit variable)*: A target variable is one that can reach and maintain a preset level before inspiration ends. It can be flow, volume or pressure. Achieving the target of limit does not mean end of inspiration. Some use the term limit variable; however, limit is a term which is generally used in reference to alarm settings.
- *Cycle variable*: It decides the cycling (termination of the inspiration and beginning of the expiration). It can be time, flow, pressure or volume cycled, e.g. decrease in flow to a particular proportion of the peak flow will cause the ventilator to cycle to expiration.
- *Baseline variable*: It is the parameter controlled during exhalation. The pressure level from which a ventilator breath begins is called the baseline pressure. Baseline pressure can be zero (atmospheric), which is also called zero end-expiratory pressure, or it can be positive if the baseline pressure is above zero [positive end-expiratory pressure (PEEP)].

Types of Breaths during Mechanical Ventilation

- *Mandatory breaths*: They are time triggered, volume or pressure limited and time cycled
- *Assisted breaths*: They are patient triggered, limited by the ventilator (volume or pressure limiting) and cycled by ventilator (time cycling)
- *Spontaneous breaths*: They are triggered limited and cycled by the patient. The variables, however, can be pressure, flow or volume.

MODES OF VENTILATION

The relationship between various possible types of breath and the inspiratory phase variables is called a mode of ventilation. Mode can be volume targeted, pressure targeted or combined.

Volume-targeted Mode

In this mode, the machine delivers a volume set on the control panel by the physician irrespective of the pressure generated within the system. There are several inspiratory flow profiles, e.g. square wave, sine wave, ascending ramp and descending ramp (decelerating) patterns **(Fig. 3)**. Descending ramp pattern is associated with lower peak airway pressure and higher mean airway pressure.[7]

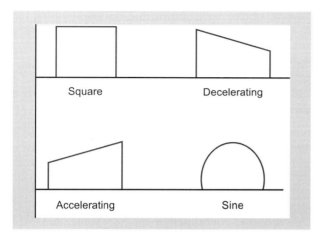

Fig. 3 Four different types of inspiratory flow patterns

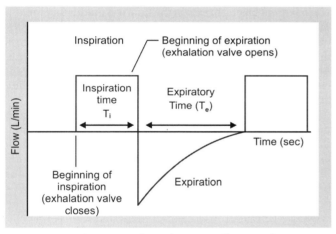

Fig. 4 Flow time scalar with constant flow waveform

Expiratory flow is always decelerating in a mechanical breath irrespective of the inspiratory flow pattern. **Figure 4** shows a complete mechanical breath with a square wave flow inspiratory pattern.

Changes in the mechanical properties of the lungs from atelectasis, edema or bronchoconstriction may cause high-inflation pressures (increasing the risk of barotrauma).

Pressure-targeted Mode

A predefined target pressure is set on the control panel of the ventilator. The ventilator generates flow to achieve the same pressure during the inspiration; the volume, however, is an independent variable which will depend on the impedance of the respiratory system.

The underlying reason for mechanical ventilation guides the selection of the mode of ventilation. Volume targeted ventilation should be used when strict control of V_T is required, e.g. ARDS.[8] Conversely, in patients with asthma and COPD strict control of airway pressure is desired so pressure targeted ventilation is preferred.

Control Mode or Controlled Mandatory Ventilation

Controlled mandatory ventilation (CMV) mode is appropriate for the patients who are either deeply sedated, paralyzed or have no spontaneous efforts of their own. The breaths delivered are time triggered. No matter how strong is the patient's breathing effort, the ventilator does not deliver gas flow unless it is time triggered. **Figures 5A and B** respectively show ventilator waveforms for pressure and VC-CMV. It is used when the aim is to provide complete rest to the patient or in cases such as chest trauma where paradoxical movements of chest due to flail segment impede the ventilation.

Assist Control Ventilation

It is a time triggered or patient triggered CMV mode. It is the appropriate mode of ventilation when we want to provide full support to the patient, but patient has spontaneous efforts.

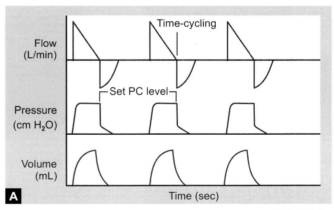

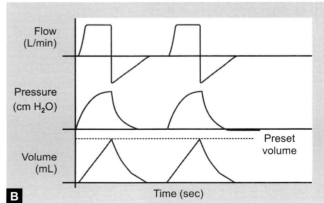

Figs 5A and B Control mode ventilation (A) Pressure control, and (B) Volume control
Abbreviation: PC, pressure control.

There are two types of breaths: (1) controlled and (2) assisted. Control breaths are time triggered, pressure or volume targeted and time cycled. Assisted breaths are patient triggered, volume or pressure targeted and time cycled. The sensitivity level is set in the ventilator and when the ventilator senses a spontaneous effort, mechanical breath is delivered to achieve the same target as the control breaths.

The major problem with this mode is that all the appropriately sensed efforts are converted to a mechanical breath, which may lead to hyperventilation and respiratory alkalosis when the patient's respiratory rate (RR) is high. Also because it involves assisted breaths there may be inappropriate sensing, if the trigger sensitivity is not correctly set leading to wasted efforts[9] or there may be a delayed response time of the ventilator which can cause a patient ventilator dysynchrony.

Assist control (AC) ventilation can be either a pressure controlled **(Fig. 6A)** or volume controlled **(Fig. 6B)**. In VC mode, setting of adequate gas flow is very important. If flow is less then patient will have flow hunger and dysynchrony will result. Patients may not stop breathing even when the flow ceases and this may cause dysynchrony. We may need to adjust the sensitivity.[10]

Several studies have shown that the decelerating ramp flow curve associated with PC mode may improve gas distribution and allows the patient to vary inspiratory gas flow during spontaneous breathing efforts.

Intermittent Mandatory Ventilation and Synchronized Intermittent Mandatory Ventilation

Intermittent mandatory ventilation (IMV) involves delivery of breaths (volume or pressure targeted) at set intervals (according to the set RR). However, the patient can breathe spontaneously between mandatory breaths at any desired baseline pressure without receiving a mandatory breath (contrast from AC mode).[11]

Synchronized intermittent mandatory ventilation (SIMV) is similar to IMV except that the mandatory breaths may be either patient triggered or time triggered **(Fig. 7)** IMV has an inherent drawback of stacking of breaths, which happens when patient takes a breath at the time of a mandatory breath. To overcome this, SIMV was developed in which ventilator waits for the patient to take a spontaneous breath. If it does not sense patient effort, then it delivers time-triggered breath. Advantage of IMV and SIMV over AC mode is that patient can breathe spontaneously to his own V_T, thus avoiding hyperventilation which may be seen in AC mode.[11]

Both IMV and SIMV have been used to wean patients from mechanical ventilation. As the mandatory rate is lowered, the patient gradually assumes a greater part of the work of breathing (WOB). However, IMV or SIMV can significantly increase WOB for spontaneous breaths.[12] The spontaneous breaths can be supported with pressure support [SIMV + pressure support ventilation (PSV)] if we want to reduce the WOB.

Both IMV and SIMV were used as a weaning mode, however, studies have shown that they do not fasten the weaning process rather can delay it.[13-15]

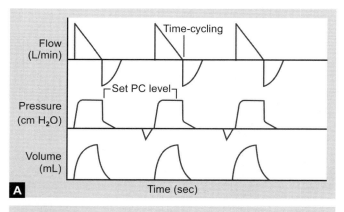
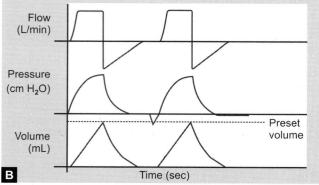

Figs 6A and B Assist control ventilation.
(A) Pressure control, and (B) Volume control
Abbreviation: PC, pressure control.

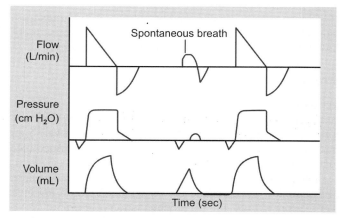

Fig. 7 Synchronized intermittent mandatory ventilation mode

Dual Modes of Ventilation

Newer ventilators offer many dual modes of ventilation. For the ER physician all of them are not important, however, we will discuss one of such modes in brief.

Pressure-regulated Volume Control

Problem with regular VC is high-airway pressures, which can cause barotrauma. Pressure-regulated VC was developed with purpose to deliver set V_Ts at minimum pressure level. It is a volume targeted, pressure limited and time-cycled mode. The ventilator automatically adjusts inspiratory PC level according to the changes in the properties of lung on a breath to breath basis.

However, it has inherent limitations. If patient demand and effort increases higher V_Ts are generated and the pressure support level is decreased. It means patient is getting less support when he actually requires more.[16]

Spontaneous Modes

Continuous Positive Airway Pressure

Ventilators can also provide continuous positive airway pressure (CPAP) for spontaneously breathing patients. It helps in preventing atelectasis and treating and preventing hypoxemia.

Pressure Support Ventilation

It is a patient triggered, pressure limited and flow-cycled ventilation **(Fig. 8)**. The ventilator provides a constant pressure during inspiration once it senses that the patient has made an inspiratory effort. Inspiratory pressure, PEEP, flow-cycle criteria and the sensitivity level are set. Rise time is the time taken to reach the target pressure. It can be changed according to the comfort of the patient. High rise time and inadequate flows can result in patient ventilator asynchrony.[17]

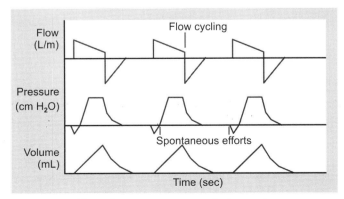

Fig. 8 Pressure support ventilation mode

Inspiratory flow in PSV ends when the ventilator senses that the flow has dropped to a certain level (flow cycling). Breathing through endotracheal tube increases the WOB.[18] PSV overcomes WOB for spontaneously breathing patients breathing through a ventilator circuit. Patients, who have a high respiratory drive and flow requirements may benefit by PSV compared to VC-CMV.[19] High pressure settings than required by patient and air leaks may cause patient-ventilator dysynchrony.[20]

INITIATION OF VENTILATION

Initially, a controlled or AC mode is selected to decrease the WOB and provide complete relaxation to the respiratory muscles. Later, mode can be changed to either a SIMV or a PSV.

Fraction of Inspired Oxygen

For patients with severe hypoxemia, the initial fraction of inspired oxygen (FiO_2) should be set at 100%. Arterial blood gas (ABG) should be done to see the partial pressure of oxygen, which should be targeted at 80–100 mm Hg for most patients, except those with COPD and ARDS where lower targets may be allowed. FiO_2 should be titrated and brought down to less than 50%, if feasible.

Respiratory Rate

It refers to the number of breaths per minute intended to maintain partial pressure of carbon dioxide (PCO_2) in normal range or patient's normal. It varies from 12 to 20 depending upon the clinical condition.

Minute Ventilation

In resting patients with healthy lungs and metabolic rates, minute ventilation (V_E) setting between 80 mL per kg and 100 mL/kg usually results in normocapnia. However, most of the patients presenting to ER have a different from normal metabolic rate. V_E varies directly with the metabolic rate. Metabolic rate is estimated on the basis of an individual's gender and body surface area (BSA).[21] BSA can be calculated using the DuBois BSA formula:

$$BSA = 0.007184 \times Ht^{0.725} \times W^{0.425}$$

Where BSA = body surface area in square meters, Ht = body height in centimeters and W = body weight in kilograms.

$$V_E = 4 \times BSA \text{ (Men)}$$
$$V_E = 3.5 \times BSA \text{ (Women)}$$

Minute ventilation requirements change in many pathological conditions. E.g. V_E increases by 5% for every °F above 99°F or 9% per °C above 37°C. Metabolic acidosis causes a 20% rise in V_E.

Tidal Volume

The normal spontaneous V_T for a healthy adult is about 5–7 mL/kg body weight. Earlier total body weight was used to derive the V_T. But now ideal or the predicted body weight (PBW) is used.[22,23]

Predicted body weight (in kg) may be derived as:

Men = 50 + 2.3 × (height in inches – 60)

Women = 45.5 + 2.3 × (height in inches – 60)

For patients presenting to ER with apparently normal lungs, such as patients with a drug overdose an initial V_T of 5–7 mL/kg and a rate of 10–20 breaths per minute are generally accepted. A V_T of more than 9–10 mL/kg is not recommended because of the risk of high pressures.

Pressure Control Setting

It should be selected to achieve the target V_T as mentioned above. Care should be taken that the pressure should not be too high so as to avoid barotrauma. It will vary according to the C of lung and chest wall and airway resistance. Those with compliant lungs and low-airway resistance will require less pressure to deliver the same V_T.

Duration of Inspiration to the Duration of Expiration Ratio

It refers to the ratio of the inspiratory to the expiratory time. Different ventilators have different settings. Some will allow to directly set I:E ratio, some however; will allow setting of inspiratory time and rate only and will decide I:E ratio from the set values. Usually I:E ratio is kept at 1:2, however, it may be required to change the I:E ratio in certain situations. It will be discussed under the section "ventilation in special conditions".

Total Cycle Time

It is the time of one cycle of inspiration and expiration. If RR is kept at 10 per minute, then one cycle of inspiration and expiration will be 6 seconds, i.e. total cycle time will be 6 seconds. Now either we can set I:E ratio as 1:2, which will make T_i as 2 seconds and T_E as 4 seconds. Some ventilators do not have I:E setting, but require setting T_i. Setting T_i as 2 seconds will set I:E ratio as 1:2.

Some ventilators use gas flow rate to decide the I:E ratio. Increasing the flow rate will cause T_i to decrease and T_E to increase. In the above example, T_i is 2 seconds. If the V_T set is 500 mL, then this 500 mL volume needs to be delivered to the patient in a time of 2 seconds, which will equals to a flow of 250 mL/second or 15 L/min. Flow rate affects RR and V_T of a spontaneously breathing patient.[24,25]

Positive End-expiratory Pressure

Positive end-expiratory pressure is defined as positive pressure at the end of exhalation during either spontaneous breathing or mechanical ventilation. **Figure 9** shows pressure time scalar in which the baseline pressure is elevated (PEEP).

Usually, clinicians set a minimum PEEP of 5 cm H_2O. The explanation behind this practice is that the glottis usually provides a physiological PEEP of around 5 cm H_2O in spontaneously breathing nonintubated patients. Intubation of trachea removes this PEEP. So, PEEP may be applied through the ventilator to prevent the atelectasis.[26] However, some patients may require higher PEEP, e.g. pulmonary edema and ARDS.

Trigger or Sensitivity

It can be set as pressure (1–5 cm H_2O) or flow (1–5 L/min). High trigger will mean that ventilator will ignore those spontaneous efforts of the patient, which produce a pressure or flow less than that which is set in ventilator. These spontaneous breaths will not be supported by the ventilator.

VENTILATION IN SPECIAL CONDITIONS

Bronchial Asthma

Severe bronchospasm causes longer time constant and severe inhomogeneity of time constant of lung units leading to air trapping. This is also called auto-PEEP.[27] In other words, there is insufficient time for complete inspired air to flow out of the lungs before the next inspiration occurs. This can cause increased intrathoracic pressure and decreased venous return resulting in hemodynamic collapse. So the target of ventilation in such patients should be to minimize air trapping and achieve hemodynamic stability. It can be

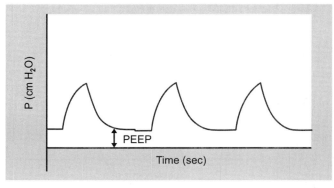

Fig. 9 Pressure–time scalar showing elevated baseline pressure
Abbreviation: PEEP, positive end-expiratory pressure.

achieved by providing long expiratory times, which can be achieved by the following settings:
- Frequency (f) = 8–10 breaths per minute
- V_T = 4–8 mL per kg
- T_I = Less than or equal to 1 second
- I:E ratio = 1:4–1:5
- Gas flow = 80–100 L/min
- PEEP 0–5 cm H_2O (in case severe asthma it should be kept at zero)
- Descending flow waveform pattern
- Airway plateau pressure (P_{plat}) less than 30 cm H_2O

Permissive hypercapnia refers to the strategy of accepting a higher PCO_2 while maintaining a pH more than 7.2. It aims to avoid air trapping.

If P_{plat} more than 30 cm H_2O and PCO_2 more than 90 mm Hg—deeper sedation and/or paralysis should be considered.

Chronic Obstructive Airway Disease

Pressure control-CMV may be ideal for such patients as it provides flow on demand to meet the patient's needs. Basic principle of ventilation is same as in asthma. Aim is to minimize auto-PEEP or air trapping, which occurs because of expiratory flow limitation.[28] Ventilator settings will be similar to those for asthma.

Controlled hypoventilation refers to the strategy of ventilation in which we aim a normal pH by targeting patient's baseline PCO_2.

When patients are spontaneously breathing and having trouble triggering breaths due to air trapping and auto-PEEP, setting the PEEP at about 75–80% of intrinsic PEEP may make triggering easier.[29,30]

Acute Respiratory Distress Syndrome

Acute respiratory distress syndrome patients can be one of the most difficult ones to intubate and ventilate in ER. Intubation has a high-risk of hypoxemia during the procedure and ventilating the lungs even after a successful intubation can be a nightmare.

Acute respiratory distress syndrome lungs are poorly compliant and need higher PEEP levels.[31,32] A lung-protective ventilation strategy gives a higher priority to the lung protection compared to the traditional goals of acid-base balance.[23] It minimizes mechanical overinflation of lung and lung inflammation or biotrauma. Open lung approach should be followed, which includes using maneuvers to open the collapsed lung, to maintain them in the same state without causing overdistension.[33]

Initiate ventilation with FiO_2 100%, RR—15–25/min, V_T 6–8 mL/kg of PBW and a PEEP of 10–15 cm H_2O. Total ventilation should be gradually brought down to 6 mL/kg. P_{plat} should be targeted to less than 30 cm H_2O. I:E ratio should be kept between 1:2 and 1:1.5.

Later, the PEEP may need to be titrated to find the optimum PEEP.[26] It is the PEEP level, which optimizes oxygenation while having the least detrimental effect on hemodynamics, oxygen delivery and airway pressures.[34,35] It has also been defined as the level of PEEP at which the static C is highest.[36] There are a number of strategies to find optimum PEEP. These methods most commonly consist of using a PEEP/FiO_2 table aimed at providing acceptable oxygenation,[26] titrating PEEP to reach a maximal C using stress index,[37] or a decremental PEEP approach.[38]

Recruitment maneuvers refer to a strategy of ventilation, which involves transient application higher transpulmonary pressures to open previously atelectatic alveoli. Several methods have been described, the most commonly used of which is a sustained inflation breath; e.g. CPAP of 40 cm H_2O for 40 seconds.[39] Another method is a stepwise increase in PEEP accompanied by low levels of PC ventilation.[40]

The best recruitment technique is still unknown and may be according to specific circumstance.[41]

It is worth remembering although P_{plat} target of less than 30 cm H_2O is accepted as a rule, but patients who are obese or have ascites or abdominal distension may need higher P_{plat}.[42]

Head Trauma

Head trauma patients may have an increased intracranial blood volume or elevated intracranial pressure (ICP). Such patients need intubation and mechanical ventilation for either poor sensorium or decreased respiratory drive. The aim is to provide sufficient ventilation to keep PCO_2 in normal range. Higher PCO_2 can cause cerebral vasodilatation leading to increase in ICP. However, higher intrathoracic pressure must be avoided as they may be transmitted to the brain causing elevation of ICP. So, PEEP should be judiciously used.

Pregnant Patient

Pregnancy results in a number of physiologic changes that have a direct bearing on the ventilatory strategy.

Important changes, which must be remembered, are:
- Increased metabolic rate
- Increased minute ventilation
- Respiratory alkalosis (PCO_2 about 30 mm Hg)
- Reduced chest wall C
- Mucosal edema and increased vascularity
- Increased intra-abdominal pressure

Therefore, in the pregnant mechanically ventilated patient, the minute volume setting should be adjusted to a PCO_2 target between 28 mm Hg and 32 mm Hg.[43] Higher peak airway pressures may be acceptable due to reduced chest wall C. Smaller diameter endotracheal tubes should be used. A rapid sequence intubation is mandatory in view of apparent full stomach and high risk of pulmonary aspiration.

Long-acting sedative agents should not be used, if delivery is imminent, as they may depress the fetus.

WHAT TO DO AFTER INITIATING VENTILATION?

- Constant vigilance is required after intubation and setting ventilator. Optimum delivery of breaths needs to be ensured
- Monitor vitals and oxygen saturation after intubation
- Monitor the parameters on the ventilator screen, e.g. if PC mode is used, see how much volume is being delivered to the patient. It may be grossly inadequate, if lung C is poor. In VC mode, peak airway pressure is influenced greatly by airway resistance and therefore is not reflective of end-inspiratory alveolar pressure. Alveolar pressure at end inspiration in VC mode is approximated by the P_{plat}, which can be measured with the ventilator at the end of inspiration by means of an inspiratory hold maneuver
- Check alarm limits in the ventilator. The ventilator may be cutting off the delivery of gases in inspiration, if the pressure limit gets exceeded (too low pressure limit)
- Do ABG after 15 minutes.[44] Adjust the parameters (if required) according to the ABG report
- Do a chest X-ray to check for endotracheal tube and nasogastric tube position and to rule out complications like tube malposition, lung collapse or pneumothorax, etc.
- After ensuring effective ventilation, the most important goal is to provide comfort to the patient. Initiate sedation infusion according to your institutional protocol
- Avoid neuromuscular blockers. However, they may be necessary in some cases like ARDS
- Periodic reevaluation of patient is needed. Initiate liaison with the ICU team for further management and shifting to ICU and anesthetist if patient is due to go to operating room or with radiology team, if an imaging procedure like computed tomography (CT) scan is planned.

TRANSPORTING INTUBATED PATIENTS

Patients need to be shifted to ICU after initial resuscitation. Some patients may be directly shifted to the operating room; some may require a radiologic procedure such as CT scan or magnetic resonance imaging (MRI) before shifting to ICU. Although transporting any critically ill patient involves risk, but patients on vasopressors, ARDS patients and those who have difficult airway have a much higher risk of adverse events.

Manual resuscitators are still used frequently in the transport of patients from ER. However, alteration in patient's respiratory status occurs frequently when manual resuscitators are used for transportation as compared to the transport ventilators.[45,46] So, a transport ventilator is recommended in such a case because it provides stable minute ventilation and also frees the caregiver to perform other tasks. Adverse events include but are not limited to incorrect measurement of vitals, arrhythmias, hypotension, hypertension, increased ICP, endotracheal tube blockage, loss of airway and cardiac arrest.

Following points should be remembered:
- There should be a written protocol and a dedicated transport team
- Transport ventilator should be preferred to a manual resuscitator
- Monitoring during transport should include cardiac monitor (including electrocardiogram, blood pressure monitoring, pulse oximetry and end tidal CO_2 monitoring) with defibrillating capacity. Other equipment should include airway management equipment, oxygen supplies, resuscitation drugs and intravenous fluids
- If patient is to be shifted to MRI suite, it must be ensured that the ventilator, gas hoses that plug into wall outlets and syringe pumps are MRI compatible.

COMPLICATIONS AND SIDE EFFECTS OF INTUBATION AND VENTILATION (TABLE 3)

Table 3 Complications and side effects of intubation and ventilation

Intubation	Mechanical ventilation
Hypoxemia during intubation	Hemodynamic collapse—decreased venous return
Failed intubation, esophageal intubation and unilateral intubation	Inability to ventilate—difficult to ventilate situations, e.g. severe exacerbations of asthma and COPD, ARDS
Injury to teeth	Air trapping and auto-PEEP
Hemodynamic response to intubation—hypertension and tachycardia	Pneumothorax
Hemodynamic collapse—secondary to sedatives and positive pressure ventilation	Atelectasis
Injury to trachea and vocal cords	Tube blockage and lung collapse
Bleeding	Accidental extubation
	Decreased renal blood flow

Abbreviations: COPD, chronic obstructive pulmonary disease; ARDS, acute respiratory distress syndrome; PEEP, positive end-expiratory pressure.

CONCLUSION

- Prompt evaluation of patients presenting to ER should identify those who may need intubation and mechanical ventilation. Ensure patient comfort and safety
- Constant vigilance is required after intubation and setting ventilator. Blood gas analysis should be performed to

confirm effective ventilation. Avoid fall in blood pressure and immediately treat, if occurs
- Sudden drastic change in measured ventilatory or hemodynamic parameters should prompt evaluation for life-threatening conditions and assessment of the ventilator settings.

REFERENCES

1. Bates JH, Rossi A, Milic-Emili J. Analysis of the behavior of the respiratory system with constant inspiratory flow. J Appl Physiol. 1985;58:1840-8.
2. Hubmayr RD, Gay PC, Tayyab M. Respiratory system mechanics in ventilated patients: techniques and indications. Mayo Clin Proc. 1987;62:358-68.
3. Chatburn RL, Volsko TA. Mechanical ventilators. In: Wilkins RL, Stoller JK, Kacmarek, RM (Eds). Egan's Fundamentals of Respiratory Care, 9th edition. St Louis: Mosby; 2009. pp. 965-1000.
4. Harrison RA. Monitoring respiratory mechanics. Crit Care Clin. 1995;11:151-67.
5. Sanborn WG. Monitoring respiratory mechanics during mechanical ventilation: where do the signals come from? Respir Care. 2005;50:28-52.
6. Aslanian P, El Atrous S, Isabey D, et al. Effects of flow triggering on breathing effort during partial ventilatory support. Am J Respir Crit Care Med. 1998;157:135-43.
7. Rau JJ, Shelledy DC. The effect of varying inspiratory flow waveforms on peak and mean airway pressures with a time-cycled volume ventilator: a bench study. Respir Care. 1991;36:347.
8. Brower R, Thompson BT. Tidal volume in acute respiratory distress syndrome—one size does not fit all. Crit Care Med. 2006;34:263-4; author reply 264-7.
9. Tobin MJ, Jubran A, Laghi F. Patient-ventilator interaction. Am J Respir Crit Care Med. 2001;163:1059-63.
10. Marini JJ, Rodriguez RM, Lamb V. The inspiratory workload of patient initiated mechanical ventilation. Am Rev Respir Dis. 1986;134:902-9.
11. Weisman IM, Rinaldo JE, Rogers RM, et al. Intermittent mandatory ventilation. Am Rev Respir Dis. 1983;127:641-7.
12. Mecklenburgh JS, Latto IP, Al-Obaidi TA, et al. Excessive work of breathing during intermittent mandatory ventilation. Br J Anaesth. 1986;58:1048-54.
13. Brochard L, Rauss A, Benito S, et al. Comparison of three methods of gradual withdrawal from ventilatory support during weaning from mechanical ventilation. Am J Respir Crit Care Med. 1994;150:896-903.
14. Esteban A, Frutos F, Tobin MJ, et al. A comparison of four methods of weaning patients from mechanical ventilation. Spanish Lung Failure Collaborative Group. N Engl J Med. 1995;332:345-50.
15. Trevisan CE, Vieira SR. Noninvasive mechanical ventilation may be useful in treating patients who fail weaning from invasive mechanical ventilation: a randomized clinical trial. Crit Care. 2008;12:R51.
16. Guldager H, Nielsen SL, Carl P, et al. A comparison of volume control and pressure-regulated volume control ventilation in acute respiratory failure. Crit Care. 1997;1:75-7.
17. Croci M, Pelosi P, Chiumello D, et al. Regulation of pressurization rate reduces inspiratory effort during pressure support ventilation: a bench study. Respir Care. 1996;41:880-4.
18. Kacmarek RM, McMahon K, Staneck K. Pressure support level required to overcome work of breathing imposed by endotracheal tubes at various peak inspiratory flow rates. Respir Care. 1998;33:933.
19. Ely EW, Baker AM, Dunagan DP, et al. Effect on the duration of mechanical ventilation of identifying patients capable of breathing spontaneously. N Engl J Med. 1996;335:1864-9.
20. Stroetz RW, Hubmayr RD. Patient-ventilator interactions. Monaldi Arch Chest Dis. 1998;53:331-6.
21. Harris JA, Benedict FG. A biometric study of human basal metabolism. Proc Natl Acad Sci USA. 1918;4:370-3.
22. Miller MR, Crapo R, Hankinson J, et al. General considerations for lung function testing. Eur Respir J. 2005;26:153-61.
23. The Acute Respiratory Distress Syndrome Network. Ventilation with lower tidal volumes as compared with traditional tidal volumes for acute lung injury and the acute respiratory distress syndrome. N Engl J Med. 2000;342:1301-8.
24. Georgopoulos D, Mitrouska I, Bshouty Z, et al. Effects of breathing route, temperature and volume of inspired gas, and airway anesthesia on the response of respiratory output to varying inspiratory flow. Am J Respir Crit Care Med. 1996;153:168-75.
25. Puddy A, Younes M. Effect of inspiratory flow rate on respiratory output in normal subjects. Am Rev Respir Dis. 1992;146:787-9.
26. Dammann JF, McAslan TC. PEEP: its use in young patients with apparently normal lungs. Crit Care Med. 1979;7:14-9.
27. Pepe PE, Marini JJ. Occult positive end-expiratory pressure in mechanically ventilated patients with air flow obstruction: the auto-PEEP effect. Am Rev Respir Dis. 1982;126:166-70.
28. Rossi A, Gottfried SB, Zocchi L, et al. Measurement of static compliance of the total respiratory system in patients with acute respiratory failure during mechanical ventilation. The effect of intrinsic positive end-expiratory pressure. Am Rev Respir Dis. 1985;131:672-7.
29. Gay PC, Rodarte JR, Hubmayr RD. The effects of positive expiratory pressure on isovolume flow and dynamic hyperinflation in patients receiving mechanical ventilation. Am Rev Respir Dis. 1989;139:621-6.
30. Ranieri VM, Giuliani R, Cinnella G, et al. Physiologic effects of positive end-expiratory pressure in patients with chronic obstructive pulmonary disease during acute ventilatory failure and controlled mechanical ventilation. Am Rev Respir Dis. 1993;147:5-13.
31. Gattinoni L, D'Andrea L, Pelosi P, et al. Regional effects and mechanism of positive end-expiratory pressure in early adult respiratory distress syndrome. JAMA. 1993;269:2122-7.
32. Gattinoni L, Pelosi P, Crotti S, et al. Effects of positive end-expiratory pressure on regional distribution of tidal volume and recruitment in adult respiratory distress syndrome. Am J Respir Crit Care Med. 1995;151:1807-14.
33. Lachmann B. Open up the lung and keep the lung open. Intensive Care Med. 1992;18:319-21.
34. Suter PM, Fairley HB, Isenberg MD. Optimum end-expiratory airway pressure in patients with acute pulmonary failure. N Engl J Med. 1975;292:284-9.
35. Peruzzi WT. The current status of PEEP. Respir Care. 1996;41:273-81.

36. Maggiore SM, Jonson B, Richard JC, et al. Alveolar derecruitment at decremental positive end-expiratory pressure levels in acute lung injury: comparison with the lower inflection point, oxygenation and compliance. Am J Respir Crit Care Med. 2001;164:795-801.
37. Grasso S, Stripoli T, De Michele M, et al. ARDSnet ventilatory protocol and alveolar hyperinflation: role of positive end-expiratory pressure. Am J Respir Crit Care Med. 2007;176:761-7.
38. Suarez-Sipmann F, Böhm SH, Tusman G, et al. Use of dynamic compliance for open lung positive end-expiratory pressure titration in an experimental study. Crit Care Med. 2007;35:214-21.
39. Brower RG, Lanken PN, MacIntyre N, et al. Higher versus lower positive end-expiratory pressures in patients with the acute respiratory distress syndrome. N Engl J Med. 2004;352:327-36.
40. Meade MO, Cook DJ Guyatt GH, Slutsky AS, et al. Ventilation strategy using low tidal volumes, recruitment maneuvers, and high positive end expiratory pressure for acute lung injury and acute respiratory distress syndrome. JAMA. 2008;299:637-45.
41. Pelosi P, Gama de Abreu M, Rocco PR. New and conventional strategies for lung recruitment in acute respiratory distress syndrome. Critical Care. 2010;14:210.
42. Gattinoni L, Chiumello D, Carlesso E, et al. Bench-to-bedside review: chest wall elastance in acute lung injury/acute respiratory distress syndrome patients. Crit Care. 2004;8:350-5.
43. Campbell LA, Klocke RA. Implications for the pregnant patient. Am J Respir Crit Care Med. 2001;163:1051-4.
44. Task Force on Guidelines, Society of Critical Care Medicine. Guidelines for standards of care for patients with acute respiratory failure on mechanical ventilatory support. Crit Care Med. 1991;19:275-8.
45. Nakamura T, Fujino Y, Uchiyama A, et al. Intrahospital transport of critically ill patients using ventilator with patient triggering function. Chest. 2003;123:159-64.
46. Austin PN, Campbell RS, Johanningman JA, et al. Transport ventilators. Respir Care Clin N Am. 2002;8:119-50.

CHAPTER 18

Use of Blood and Blood Products in Emergency

Aseem K Tiwari, Ravi C Dara, Dinesh Arora

INTRODUCTION

The transfusion of the blood components in emergencies, if not done rationally, can increase the morbidity and mortality of patients.[1] The immediate availability of blood components for life-threatening hemorrhages requires a rapid and focused approach, as excessive bleeding threatens the survival of patients. Early recognition of major blood loss and immediate effective interventions are vital to avoid hypovolemic shock and its consequences. One of the effective interventions is the rapid provision of blood components, for which effective communication between emergency team and blood bank is a must. Transfusion support is vital for any patient in hemorrhagic shock. The transfusion of the right component to the right patient in the right quantity and at the right time has been the guiding principle for resuscitating emergency/trauma patients. The emergency team and blood bank also needs disaster preparedness, presently, more than ever before.

The entire chapter has been dealt with in three major sections:
1. Responsibility of emergency and blood bank team.
2. Transfusion approach in emergency and massive transfusion protocol (MTP).
3. Use of specific blood components.

RESPONSIBILITY OF EMERGENCY AND BLOOD BANK TEAM

Responsibility of Emergency Team: Ordering Blood Component in an Emergency

Every hospital should have a protocol for ordering blood component in an emergency, which should be clear and simple so that everyone understands and follows them. Simplified protocol given by WHO in clinical use of blood[2] is as follows:

- Insert an intravenous (IV) cannula. Use it to take the blood sample for compatibility testing, set up an IV infusion of normal saline or a balanced salt solution (e.g. Ringer's lactate or Hartmann's solution). Send the blood sample to the blood bank as quickly as possible.
- Clearly label the blood sample tube and the blood request form. If the patient is unidentified, which may happen in a disaster-like situation or road traffic accident, use some form of emergency identification system (e.g. emergency admission number). Use the patient's name, only when you are sure that you have the correct information. If you are not sure then an identifier like "Unknown 1" can be used. Preferably two identifiers should be used; so along with "Unknown 1" you can use patient's hospital enrollment/registration number (for e.g. patient id: 12345).
- If you have to send another request for blood for the same patient within a short period, use the same identifiers which were used in the first request form and blood sample so the blood bank staffs know they are dealing with the same patient. In the interim, even if the real name is identified it should not be used until the patient has stabilized clinically.
- If there are several staff members working with emergency cases, one person should take charge of ordering blood components and communicating with the blood bank about the particular patient (s). This is especially important, if several injured patients are involved at the same time.
- Tell the blood bank how quickly the blood is needed for each patient. Communicate using words that have been previously agreed with the blood bank to explain how

urgently blood is required. For example we follow the terminology of immediate, urgent and routine. Immediate, urgent and routine denotes 5 minutes, 15 minutes and 30 minutes, respectively.
- Make sure that both you and the blood bank staff know:
  - Who is going to bring the blood to the patient (for example, general duty assistant at authors' institute)
  - Where the patient will be, e.g. emergency room, operating theater or delivery room.
- The blood bank may send group O (and possibly RhD negative) blood, especially, if there is any risk of errors in patient identification. During an acute emergency, this may be the safest way to avoid a serious mismatched transfusion.

Responsibility of Blood Bank: Issuing Blood in Emergency

In critical patients, the emergency physician may ask for group-specific uncross-matched or uncross-matched blood. In such situations, the request may contain a signed statement from the emergency medical team indicating that clinical status of patient is too critical to wait for completion of pretransfusion compatibility testing. However, signed statement is not necessary before an immediate/urgent transfusion and does not preclude blood bank to issue blood in emergency. Every hospital needs to have a written emergency protocol. The emergency protocols at authors' institute are discussed below.

Emergency Protocols

Blood bank should keep aside at least two O-negative units for any exigency. Turnaround time (TAT)-based approach is suggested, which matches the degree of urgency in transfusing blood components to a patient in an emergency setting. It has been divided in three categories: (1) immediate, (2) urgent, and (3) routine.
- *Immediate transfusion (TAT—5 minutes)*:
  - Issue uncross-matched group O red blood cells (RBCs) if the patient's blood group is unknown
  - Use D-negative blood, if the recipient's Rh status is unknown, especially, if the patient is female.
- *Urgent transfusion (TAT—15 minutes)*: Issue group specific uncross-matched, if the patient's blood group is known or can be typed.
- *Routine transfusion (TAT—30 minutes)*: Issue group-specific cross-match compatible blood.

When blood is requested in emergency, blood bank should take the following steps:
- Document on the unit as "uncross-matched" or "compatibility testing not completed" at the time of issue of unit in the immediate and urgent protocol.
- Complete the compatibility tests promptly, even after issue. If any incompatibility is detected during the completion of compatibility tests, the emergency medical team should be notified and blood transfusion should be stopped.
- O-negative units should be issued only in emergency situations where the recipient blood group is unknown at the time of transfusion, up to 2 units; thereafter group-specific blood unit to be issued (as the patient should have had their blood group tested by this time). This is important to conserve precious O-negative inventory.

Blood Check at Administration

Final administration check of the blood unit must be done by trained and competent emergency physician. All patients receiving transfusion must be positively identified by last name, first name, and unique identification number and must match the details on blood component label and document(s). All blood components should be administered using standard blood administration set with an integral mesh filter (170–200 µ).

TRANSFUSION APPROACH IN EMERGENCY AND MASSIVE TRANSFUSION PROTOCOL

Trauma patients generally present with varying grades of hemorrhage and shock. The approach with respect to blood component transfusion to such patients can only be understood, if we understand various classes of hemorrhage which have been classified as follows:
- *Class I hemorrhage*: Blood volume loss of up to 15%. The heart rate is minimally elevated or normal, and there is no change in blood pressure, pulse pressure, or respiratory rate.
- *Class II hemorrhage*: There is a 15–30% blood volume loss and is manifested clinically as tachycardia (heart rate of 100–120), tachypnea (respiratory rate of 20–24) and a decreased pulse pressure, although systolic blood pressure changes minimally, if at all. The skin may be cool and clammy, and capillary refill may be delayed.
- *Class III/IV hemorrhage*: Involves a 30–40% or more than 40% blood volume loss, resulting in a significant drop in blood pressure and changes in mental status.

While no treatment is necessary in Class I, Class II requires crystalloids, e.g. Ringer's lactate solution, which rapidly distributes between the intra- and extravascular spaces. Volume of crystalloid needed to restore intravascular volume is three times the estimated blood loss. Blood components are required only in Class III and Class IV hemorrhages. Earlier there was a traditional approach to give crystalloids and RBCs and transfuse first frozen plasma (FFP) only when more than 5–10 RBC units were transfused. However, this approach has given way to a newer approach described next.

Newer Approach—Transfusion for Severe Ongoing Hemorrhage (Class III/IV)

If the bleeding in trauma patients is unlikely or difficult to be controlled quickly, immediate transfusion of blood components in a 1:1:1 ratio of RBC, FFP and platelets should be considered. In simple terms, if the emergency team recognizes that the patient will require four or more units of RBCs in 1 hour (or more than 10 units in 12–24 hours), they should start transfusing six units of RBCs, six units of FFP and six units of random donor platelets (or one unit of single donor apheresis platelets as one unit of apheresis platelets is equivalent to six units of random donor platelets). Hypothermia must be controlled during transfusions with the help of inline warmers.

Studies supporting newer approach of 1:1:1 blood components transfusion are:

- A trial that randomly assigned 680 patients with major bleeding from severe trauma to receive transfusion of one versus two units of RBC for every unit of FFP and platelets (i.e. FFP to platelets to RBC of 1:1:1 versus 1:1:2) found slightly better outcomes with the 1:1:1 approach.[3] Patients assigned to 1:1:1 were more likely to have adequate hemostasis (86% vs. 78%) and had fewer exsanguination deaths at 24 hours (9% vs. 15%). Overall mortality at 1 and 30 days were not different between the groups, although there was a trend favoring 1:1:1 at both time points. Adverse events were also similar between the groups.[3]
- A retrospective study of 246 patients who presented to an Army combat support hospital in Iraq has produced some data to evaluate the merits of this regimen.[4] When patients who received massive transfusion were stratified by transfusion therapy regimen, patients who received a high ratio of FFP to RBCs (median of 1:1.4) had a survival rate of 81%, compared with 66% for those with an intermediate ratio (median 1:2.5) and 35% for those who received a low ratio of FFP to RBCs (median of 1:8).[4]
- In a retrospective study of 467 massively transfused trauma patients, 30-day survival was increased in patients transfused at a high FFP:RBC ratio (i.e. ≥1:2) as well as in those transfused at a high platelet:RBC ratio (i.e. ≥1:2).[5] The combination of high FFP and high platelet to RBC ratios was associated with decreased truncal hemorrhage and increased 6-hour, 24-hour, and 30-day survivals, with no change in deaths due to multiple organ failure.
- In a retrospective study of 694 massively transfused trauma patients who did not receive fresh whole blood, those receiving a high ratio of apheresis platelets (equivalent to six units of pooled platelets) per stored RBC unit (i.e. ratio ≥1:8) had a higher 24-hour survival (95%) compared with those receiving a medium (i.e. ratio 1:16–1:8, 87%) or a low ratio (i.e. <1:16, 64%).[6] On multivariate analysis, higher FFP:RBC ratios and higher apheresis platelets:RBC ratios were both independently associated with improved survival at both 24 hours and 30 days.

Massive Transfusion Protocol should be in place in every hospital and this protocol should be activated as soon as the emergency team recognizes the presence or likelihood of severe ongoing hemorrhage. One example of MTP followed at authors' institute adapted from publication in Journal of American College of Surgeons[7] is shown below **(Flow chart 1)**.

ROLE OF SPECIFIC BLOOD COMPONENTS

The decision to transfuse the blood components should not depend only on transfusion triggers, but should depend on clinical condition of patient, rate of ongoing bleeding, cardiopulmonary status and operative intervention. The ultimate goal of blood component transfusion is to restore volume and oxygen-carrying capacity. Role of whole blood and different blood components in emergency situation is described next.

Transfusion of Whole Blood

Whole blood has high levels of potassium, ammonia, and hydrogen ions and has no clotting factors. With the advent of blood component therapy, the use of whole blood has become obsolete. Although it provides volume expansion along with increased oxygen-carrying capacity, it may cause volume overload and dilutional coagulopathy in patients.

Transfusion of Red Cells

Red cell transfusion always remains an important unanswered question and often depends on clinical circumstances. In trauma patients, if hemodynamics does not improve after administration of 2–3 L of crystalloid, two units of RBCs should be transfused. Further transfusions will depend on response to the initial transfusion.

Antihuman globulin cross-matched compatible with antibody screen negative RBCs are best, but take considerable time. If the patient's condition warrants, emergency physician can transfuse immediately using type-O Rh-positive or type-O Rh-negative for males and type-O Rh-negative for girls and women of childbearing age, until group-specific uncross-matched or group-specific cross-matched blood is available.

- *ABO*—patients with blood type B or A may receive O RBC while type AB recipients can receive A or B RBCs. Patient should be switched back to original ABO type, if blood bank inventory permits, and the patient is stable with bleeding stopped. This is important as type B patient who received type O RBC do not get too much passively transferred anti-B from the donors.
- Rh-negative individual may be switched to Rh-positive RBCs—but should be avoided in women of childbearing potential. Can be done if an Rh-negative patient is likely to receive massive RBC transfusion that will deplete the existing ABO compatible, ABO inventory. Rh immunoglobulins (RhIgs) prophylaxis can be given

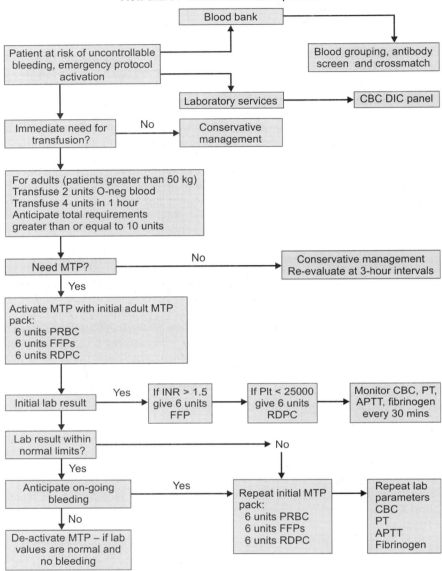

Flow chart 1 Massive transfusion protocol

Abbreviations: CBC, complete blood count; MTP, massive transfusion protocol; PRBC, packed red blood cell; FFPs, fresh-frozen plasmas; APTT, activated partial prothrombin time; RDPC, random donor platelets concentrate; PT, prothrombin time

to prevent anti-D formation in childbearing females following Rh incompatible transfusion.

Transfusion of Clotting Factors (First-frozen Plasma and Cryoprecipitate) and Platelets

Transfusion of IV crystalloid and red cells in hemorrhage increases the risk of coagulopathy due to dilution of clotting factors and platelets and also due to hypothermia. For bleeding patients (more than four units of packed RBCs transfused in the first few hours or chest tube continues to drain >200 mL of blood per hour) we suggest using 1:1:1 ratio approach of RBC, FFP and random donor platelets. This means 1 RBC:4 FFPs:6 RDP for an adult patient. If apheresis platelets are used; one unit would be equivalent to six units of random donor platelets.

When to transfuse cryoprecipitate will depend on assessment of fibrinogen levels. Fibrinogen concentration below 100 mg/dL is generally treated with 10 units of cryoprecipitate (each unit of cryoprecipitate raises the fibrinogen level by about 5 mg/dL).

First frozen plasma can be transfused irrespective of Rh status of blood component; for example, A-positive can be safely transfused to A-negative recipient. If ABO blood group compatible FFPs are not available, use "universal plasma", group AB plasma.

Thawed plasma can be kept at 4°C for 24 hours. This plasma has decreased levels of labile factors like FVIII and FV, but other factor levels are sufficient. It saves time in urgent transfusion settings.

Cryoprecipitate can be safely transfused across the ABO and Rh blood groups. Thawed plasma is a good alternative in emergency transfusion.

Platelets (random donor platelets) can be safely transfused across the ABO and Rh blood group. While in apheresis transfusing O platelets to non-O blood group recipient has to be done cautiously since they may contain high titer isoagglutinins. In such cases, it is a good idea to remove plasma to reduce transfer of isoagglutinins.

CONCLUSION

Inappropriate use of blood transfusion can increase the morbidity and mortality. So rational approach to be adopted for transfusion of blood and blood component in emergency. Rapid and focused approach is needed in case of life threatening hemorrhage. Rapid provision of blood product is one of the effective interventions. Transfusion of right blood component in right patient in right amount at right time is the key for resuscitation.

REFERENCES

1. Royal College of Obstetricians and Gynaecologist. Blood transfusion in obstetrics. Green-top guideline No. 47. London: RCOG; 2007.
2. World Health Organization, Geneva. (2001). Clinical use of blood. [online] Available from *http://www.who.int/blood-safety/clinical_use/en/Handbook_EN.pdf*. [Accessed October, 2016].
3. Holcomb JB, Tilley BC, Baraniuk S, et al. Transfusion of plasma, platelets, and red blood cells in a 1:1:1 vs a 1:1:2 ratio and mortality in patients with severe trauma: the PROPPR randomized clinical trial. JAMA. 2015;313:471-82.
4. Borgman MA, Spinella PC, Perkins JG, et al. The ratio of blood products transfused affects mortality in patients receiving massive transfusions at a combat support hospital. J Trauma. 2007;63:805-13.
5. Holcomb JB, Wade CE, Michalek JE, et al. Increased plasma and platelet to red blood cell ratios improves outcome in 466 massively transfused civilian trauma patients. Ann Surg. 2008;248:447-58.
6. Perkins JG, Cap AP, Spinella PC, et al. An evaluation of the impact of apheresis platelets used in the setting of massively transfused trauma patients. J Trauma. 2009;66:S77-84.
7. Riskin DJ, Tsai TC, Riskin L, et al. Massive transfusion protocols: The role of aggressive resuscitation versus product ratio in mortality reduction. J Am Coll Surg. 2009;209:198-205.

CHAPTER 19

Arterial Blood Gas Analysis

Sudha Kansal, Rajesh Chawla, Tarun S

INTRODUCTION

Arterial blood gas (ABG) analysis is a common and useful tool in intensive care patients. It gives information on oxygenation status and acid-base disorders. ABG measures the oxygen tension (PaO_2), oxyhemoglobin saturation (SaO_2), acidity (pH), carbon dioxide tension ($PaCO_2$), and bicarbonate (HCO_3) concentration in arterial blood. Some blood gas analyzers (CO oximeter) also measure the methemoglobin, carboxyhemoglobin, and hemoglobin levels. The newer available machines measure lactate and electrolytes too. ABG analysis provides immense information, which helps in management of the critically ill patients. A thorough understanding of acid-base balance is mandatory.

INDICATIONS

- To assess derangement of oxygenation, its severity and cause
- Assessment of acid-base disorder to identify primary disorder/disorders and plan its management
- To check response to the interventions
- Aids in adjustment of ventilator settings
- For detection of abnormal hemoglobins (carboxy and methemoglobin) and its severity.

ABSOLUTE CONTRAINDICATIONS[1]

- An abnormal modified Allen test
- Local infection or distorted anatomy at the puncture site
- Severe peripheral vascular disease of the artery selected for sampling
- Active Raynaud's syndrome.

Selection of Artery

- Radial artery (preferred)
- Femoral artery in case of shock, if radial artery is not palpable (beware of coagulopathy)
- Avoid brachial artery sampling due to poor collateral circulation and risk of limb ischemia.

Precautions while Taking Arterial Blood Gas Sample

- Avoid air bubbles (air contamination: spurious increase in PaO_2)
- Analyze within 30 minutes (blood cells consume O_2, produce CO_2, lower pH)
- If delay cool to 5°C, immediately
- Avoid excessive use of heparin (drop in $PCO_2 > PO_2$, pH usually remains unchanged).

DEFINITIONS OF ACID–BASE DISORDERS

- *Normal pH*—7.36–7.454
- *Acidemia*—fall in arterial pH
- *Alkalemia*—rise in arterial pH
- *Acidosis*—a process that acidifies body fluids (increased H^+ concentration) and if unopposed leads to fall in pH. This can be caused by a fall in the serum bicarbonate (HCO_3) concentration and/or an elevation in PCO_2
- *Alkalosis*—a process that alkalinizes body fluids (decreased H^+ concentration) and if unopposed leads to rise in pH. This can be caused by an elevation in the serum HCO_3 concentration and/or a fall in PCO_2.

NOMENCLATURE

- *Metabolic disorder*: Primary change in HCO_3 (increased in alkalosis and reduced in acidosis)
- *Respiratory disorder*: Primary change in H_2CO_3, i.e. CO_2 (increased in acidosis and reduced in alkalosis).
  Primary disorders not only change acid-base equilibrium directly but also set in motion secondary compensatory changes in the other member of the PCO_2-HCO_3^- pair. It requires normal lungs and kidneys.
- *Simple acid-base disorder*: The presence of a single primary disorder with the appropriate respiratory or renal compensation.
  Remember that compensation never returns the pH fully back to normal.
- *Mixed acid-base disorder*: It means simultaneous presence of more than one acid-base disorder. Mixed acid-base disorders can be suspected from the patient's history, from a lesser- or greater-than-expected compensatory respiratory or renal response, and from analysis of the serum electrolytes and anion gap. *Always correlate with history.*

Compensatory Respiratory and Renal Responses

The Henderson-Hasselbalch equation shows that the pH is determined by the ratio of the serum bicarbonate (HCO_3) concentration and the PCO_2 **(Table 1)**.[2]

$$pH = pK + log(HCO_3)/(H_2CO_3)$$
$$= kidney/lung$$
$$= (Metabolic/respiratory)$$
$$H^+ = 24 \times PCO_2/HCO_3 - (Validity\ check)\ Formula\ 1$$

In case of primary respiratory acid-base disorder, renal compensation occurs in two phases:
1. *Acute phase*: Small change in serum HCO_3 (in the same direction as the PCO_2 change), due to whole body buffering mechanisms. Renal compensation is minimal.
2. *Chronic phase*: Occurs over hours to days. Kidneys respond by producing larger changes in serum HCO_3 (again, in the same direction as the PCO_2). These HCO_3 changes mitigate the change in pH.

Respiratory compensation in metabolic acidosis or alkalosis is a rapid response. With metabolic acidosis, for example, the response begins within 30 minutes.[3]

The compensatory renal and respiratory responses are thought to be mediated, at least in part, by parallel pH changes within sensory and regulatory cells including renal tubule cells and cells in the respiratory center.[4] The magnitude of the compensatory response is proportional to the severity of the primary acid-base disturbance.

Thus, a high HCO_3 concentration may be due to metabolic alkalosis or compensation for chronic respiratory acidosis. Conversely, a low HCO_3 may be due to metabolic acidosis or compensation for chronic respiratory alkalosis.

Analogous issues apply to a high or low PCO_2.

Always interpret ABG in context of clinical history. It is preferable to have baseline PCO_2 and HCO_3 values, if available.

Blood pH and H⁺ ion Concentration

- pH and H^+ ion concentrations are inversely related
- Accurate estimation of proton concentration can be made from pH due to the nearly linear relationship
- At pH of 7.4—H^+ concentration is 40 nEq/L **(Table 2)**.

pH AND PARTIAL PRESSURE OF CARBON DIOXIDE RELATIONSHIP IN RESPIRATORY DISORDERS

$$\frac{\Delta H^+}{\Delta PaCO_2} < 0.3 \text{—Chronic} \quad \text{—Formula 2}$$

More than 0.8—acute
0.3–0.8—acute on chronic

EQUATIONS FOR ANALYSIS OF ACID–BASE DISORDERS—COMPENSATIONS

Metabolic Compensation of Respiratory Disorder—Remember 1,2,4,5

Respiratory acidosis—Formula 3:

$$\Delta HCO_3 = Change\ from\ 24;\ \Delta PCO_2 = Change\ from\ 40$$
$$Acute:\ \Delta HCO_3^- = 1/10\ (\Delta PCO_2)$$
$$Chronic:\ \Delta HCO_3^- = 4/10\ (\Delta PCO_2)$$

Add ΔHCO_3 to 24 (normal HCO_3). Match with HCO_3 on ABG. If two match, it is simple respiratory disorder. If calculated HCO_3 is more or less than on ABG, there is primary metabolic alkalosis and metabolic acidosis respectively also.

Table 1 Compensatory responses of acid–base disorder			
Disorder	Primary disturbance	Compensatory response	Mechanism of compensatory response
Metabolic acidosis	Decrease in HCO_3	Decrease in PCO_2	Hyperventilation
Metabolic alkalosis	Increase in HCO_3	Increase in PCO_2	Hypoventilation
Respiratory acidosis	Increase in PCO_2	Increase in HCO_3	Increased H^+ secretion
Respiratory alkalosis	Decrease in PCO_2	Decrease in HCO_3	Decreased H^+ secretion

Abbreviations: PCO_2, partial pressure of carbon dioxide; HCO_3, bicarbonate.

pH	H⁺ nEq/L	
7.70	20	For H⁺ concentration sequentially multiply 40 nEq/L with 0.8 between pH of 7.4 and 7.8
7.60	25	
7.50	32	
7.40	40	
7.30	50	For H⁺ concentration sequentially multiply 40 nEq/L with 1.25 between pH of 6.8 and 7.4
7.20	63	
7.10	79	
7.00	100	
6.90	126	

Table 2 Blood pH and hydrogen ion concentration value

Respiratory alkalosis—Formula 4:

$$\text{Acute: } \Delta HCO_3^- = 2/10\ (\Delta PCO_2)$$
$$\text{Chronic: } \Delta HCO_3^- = 5/10\ (\Delta PCO_2)$$

Subtract ΔHCO_3 from 24 (normal HCO_3). Match with HCO_3 on ABG. Similar interpretation as above.

Respiratory Compensations for Metabolic Disorders

Metabolic acidosis—Formula 5:

$$\text{Expected } PCO_2 = [(1.5\ HCO_3) + 8] + (-2)$$
$$\text{Match with ABG } PCO_2$$

Metabolic alkalosis—Formula 6:

$$\text{Expected } PCO_2 = [(0.7\ HCO_3) + 21] + (-2)$$

If ABG PCO_2 is more or less than calculated PCO_2, there is primary respiratory acidosis or alkalosis respectively also.

ANION GAP CONCEPT

- Organisms exist in a state of electroneutrality

$$\text{Anion gap} = Na^+ - (Cl^- + HCO_3^-)\text{—Formula 7}$$

- Normal $10 + (-2)$ mmol/L
- The "normal" anion gap in patients with hypoalbuminemia is about 2.5 mEq/L lower for each 1 g/dL decrease in the plasma albumin concentration from normal
- Corrected AG = Calculated AG + 2.5 [(alb) normal, i.e. 4 – (alb) measured]—*Formula 8*
- If the anion gap is elevated, calculate the osmolal gap in case of compatible situations.

Osmolal Gap

- *Osmolal gap = Measured osmolality—calculated osmolality—Formula 9*
- *S osmolal = $2(Na) + BUN/2.8 + glucose/18$—formula 10*
- Normal osmolal gap less than 15 mOsm/L.

Elevated Osmolal Gap

- Lactic acid and acetoacetate
- Methanol and ethylene glycol
- Alcohol and isopropyl alcohol
- Mannitol.

Hyperchloremic Nongap Acidosis

- Predominantly due to loss of HCO_3^-
- Check urine anion gap (UAG)—clue to site of loss; renal versus gastrointestinal
- *Urine anion gap = (Urine Na^+ + Urine K^+) – Urine Cl^-—formula 11*
- *Negative UAG—($UCl^- \gg UNa^+ + UK^+$) – GI loss of HCO_3^-*
- *Positive UAG—($UCl^- < UNa^+ + UK^+$) – Renal tubular acidosis*

If metabolic alkalosis—check spot urinary chloride:
- Urine Cl^- more than 20 mEq/L or more than 20 mEq/L.

INTERPRETATION OF ARTERIAL BLOOD GAS

Two aspects of analysis of ABG are:
1. Assessment of oxygenation.
2. Assessment of acid-base disturbances.
   Normal values of blood gas are given in **Table 3**.

Assessment of Oxygenation

1. It is equally or even more important to assess oxygenation while interpreting the ABG
2. PaO_2:
   - Less than 45 mm Hg—severe
   - 45–59 mm Hg: moderate
   - 60–79 mm Hg: mild

Always check alveolar PO_2 (PAO_2) – PaO_2 gradient (where PAO_2 is pressure of alveolar oxygen and PaO_2 is pressure of arterial oxygenation).

Equation for the calculation of PAO_2:

$$PAO_2 = (760 - 47) \times FiO_2 - (PCO_2/0.8)\text{—formula 12}$$
$$= 150 - (PCO_2/0.8)\text{ or room air}$$

Where 760—barometric pressure at sea level, 47—water vapor pressure, 0.8—respiratory quotient.
Check on room air, if possible.

$$(A - a)\ O_2\ \text{gradient} = PAO_2 - PaO_2$$
$$\text{Normal: 5–25 mm Hg}$$

SEVEN STEPS OF ANALYSIS OF ARTERIAL BLOOD GAS

Step 1

Perform validity check to assess the consistency of the ABG:
- $H^+ = 24 \times PCO_2/HCO_3$—*Formula 1*

Table 3 Normal values of blood gas

	Normal range	For calculation
pH	7.34–7.45	7.4
PCO_2	35–45	40
HCO_3	22–26	24
PO_2	≥80	≥95

Abbreviations: PCO_2, partial pressure of carbon dioxide; HCO_3, bicarbonate; PO_2, partial pressure of oxygen.

- Calculate H^+ from pH (*see* **Table 2**)
- Match the two. If both correlate then ABG is valid.

Step 2

To assess whether the patient is acidemic or alkalemic.

Action

Look at the pH. If less than 7.4 primary disorder is acidosis and if more than 7.4 it is alkalosis.

Step 3

Next step is to determine the overriding disturbance. Respiratory or metabolic.

Action

Check HCO_3 and PCO_2 on ABG. For interpretation (**Table 1**)

Step 4

If primary respiratory disturbance, calculate whether it is acute or chronic as the metabolic compensation will vary.

Action

Calculate $\Delta H^+/\Delta PCO_2$—Formula 2.

Step 5

If metabolic disturbance—check anion gap; if metabolic acidosis—correct anion gap to serum albumin.

Action

Measure Na^+, Cl^-, HCO_3^-, Albumin—Formula 7 and 8.

Step 6

Now determine whether compensatory mechanism is appropriate to know whether it is a simple or mixed disorder.

Action

Check formulas—*Formulas 3–6*.

Step 7

- In anion gap acidosis, calculate if there is a hidden disturbance, as two can coexist
- Check $\Delta AG/\Delta HCO_3$
- If $\Delta AG/\Delta(HCO_3^-)$ between 1.0 and 2.0—uncomplicated anion gap metabolic acidosis
- If $\Delta AG/\Delta(HCO_3^-)$ less than 1.0, then a concurrent nonanion gap metabolic acidosis is present
- If $\Delta AG/\Delta(HCO_3^-)$ more than 2.0, then a concurrent metabolic alkalosis is present.

Causes of Anion Gap Metabolic Acidosis

MUDPILERS
- M = Methanol
- U = Uremia
- D = Diabetic ketoacidosis/alcoholic ketoacidosis
- P = Paraldehyde
- I = Isoniazid
- L = Lactic acidosis
- E = Ethanol/ethylene glycol
- R = Rhabdomyolysis/renal failure
- S = Salicylates

Nonanion Gap Acidosis

HARDUPS
- H = Hyperalimentation
- A = Acetazolamide
- R = Renal tubular acidosis
- D = Diarrhea
- U = Ureteropelvic shunt
- P = Posthypocapnia
- S = Spironolactone.

Acute Respiratory Acidosis (Chronic Respiratory Acidosis = Chronic Obstructive Pulmonary Disease/Restrictive Lung Disease): Any Hypoventilation State

- Central nervous system (CNS) depression (drugs/cerebrovascular accident)
- Nerve damage beyond CNS:
  – High spinal cord injury
  – Phrenic palsy.
- Guillain-Barré syndrome
- Airway obstruction
- Pulmonary edema
- Hemo-/pneumothorax

- Myopathy and electrolyte disturbances—hypokalemia and hypophosphatemia
- Neuromuscular disorders—myasthenia gravis, Eaton-Lambert syndrome, aminoglycosides and colistin
- Chest wall deformity—Kyphoscoliosis and flail chest.

Metabolic Alkalosis

CLEVERPD
- C = Contraction
- L = Licorice*
- E = Endo: Conn's, Cushing's, Bartter's*
- V = Vomiting and NG aspirate
- E = Excess alkali*, electrolyte disturbance—hypokalemia* and hypomagnesemia
- R = Refeeding alkalosis*
- P = Posthypercapnia
- D = Diuretics

*Associated with high urine Cl levels.

Respiratory Alkalosis

CHAMPS
- C = CNS disease—meningitis, encephalitis and hemorrhage
- H = Hypoxia, hepatic failure and heart failure
- A = Anxiety
- M = Mechanical ventilators
- P = Progesterone, pneumonia, pulmonary embolism, and pregnancy
- S = Salicylates/sepsis

STRONG ION DIFFERENCE VERSUS TRADITIONAL APPROACH

The Stewart or strong ion approach to acid-base disturbances has gained acceptance among many intensivists because of perceived weaknesses of the traditional approach in the evaluation of patients with critical illnesses.[4,5]

As per Stewart approach, dissociation (and pH) is governed by laws of physical chemistry:
- *Law of conservation of mass*: Amount of substance in a solution remains constant unless added or removed or generated or destroyed by chemical reaction
- *Law of conservation of electric charge*: Sum of all cations always equal sum of all anions
- *Law of mass action*: Dissociation equilibrium of all incompletely dissociated substance must be satisfied at all times.

According to this approach HCO_3^- is a dependent variable. Three mathematically independent determinant of blood pH are:
1. Strong ion difference (SID) **(Fig. 1)**:
   - $SID = [(Na^-) + (K^+) + (Ca^{2+}) + (Mg^{2+})] - [(Cl^-)] = (HCO_3^-) + (A^-)$

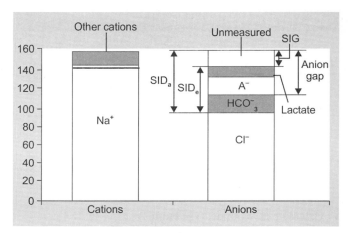

Fig. 1 Ion difference

- $SIDa = [(Na^+) + (K^+) + (Ca^{2+}) + (Mg^{2+})] - [(Cl^-)]$
- $SIDe = (HCO_3^-) + (A^-)$
  A^-—Total charges contributed by all nonbicarbonate buffers, primarily albumin, phosphate and in whole blood, hemoglobin
  – Normal SID is 40-42.
2. Total weak acid buffers (A TOT) = Total A^- and its weak acid $[(A^-) + (HA)]$.
3. Partial pressure of CO_2.

Strong ion gap (SIG) = SIDa – SIDe. It is due to unmeasured anions. It represents standard base excess (SBE).

Metabolic acidosis:
- Decrease in SID by addition of strong anions.

Metabolic alkalosis:
- Increase in SID by additions of strong cations (with weak anions).

Stewart approach is much more cumbersome and may be more prone to error, given its dependence upon multiple measurements of different variables. When measurements obtained from automated blood chemistry devices are used to calculate the SIG, the results can also vary substantially depending upon which device is used.[6] Therefore, the traditional approach in the analysis of all acid-base disturbances is preferred.

Moreover, if serum albumin concentration is considered in the traditional analysis of acid-base disturbances, Stewart approach is nonsuperior over the traditional Schwartz-Bartter approach to acid-base disturbances.[7,8]

CONCLUSION

Thus, analysis of ABG is an essential tool in management of critically ill patients. Always remember to assess oxygenation problem first. Next follow stepwise approach and correlate to clinical history while interpreting the ABG. ABG is a useful bedside tool in management of ICU patients.

REFERENCES

1. American Association for Respiratory Care. AARC clinical practice guideline. Sampling for arterial blood gas analysis. Respir Care. 1992;37:913-7.
2. Adrogué HJ, Madias NE. Secondary responses to altered acid-base status: the rules of engagement. J Am Soc Nephrol. 2010;21:920-3.
3. Wiederseiner JM, Muser J, Lutz T, et al. Acute metabolic acidosis: characterization and diagnosis of the disorder and the plasma potassium response. J Am Soc Nephrol. 2004;15:1589-96.
4. Rose BD, Post TW. Clinical Physiology of Acid-base and Electrolyte Disorders, 5th edition. New York City: McGraw-Hill; 2001. p. 542.
5. Carreira F, Anderson RJ. Assessing metabolic acidosis in the intensive care unit: does the method make a difference? Crit Care Med. 2004;32:1227-8.
6. Balasubramanyan N, Havens PL, Hoffman GM. Unmeasured anions identified by the Fencl-Stewart method predict mortality better than base excess, anion gap, and lactate in patients in the pediatric intensive care unit. Crit Care Med. 1999;27:1577-81.
7. Nguyen BV, Vincent JL, Hamm JB, et al. The reproducibility of Stewart parameters for acid-base diagnosis using two central laboratory analyzers. Anesth Analg. 2009;109:1517-23.
8. Rastegar A. Clinical utility of Stewart's method in diagnosis and management of acid-base disorders. Clin J Am Soc Nephrol. 2009;4:1267-74.

CHAPTER 20

Oxygen Therapy

Poulomi Chatterji, Bhawna Sharma

INTRODUCTION

Oxygen though ubiquitously present is actually a drug—it can be life-saving but can also be lethal in some cases. Oxygen is essential to cellular metabolism, unfortunately, it is difficult to assess cellular function. Certain organs are very dependent on oxygen like brain and heart, thus it is possible that even minor degrees of hypoxia can produce varying effects on coronary or cerebral circulation. Studies have shown a partial pressure of arterial oxygen (PaO_2) of 30 mm Hg is generally adequate to maintain cellular metabolism.[1-3]

INDICATIONS[1-7]

- Hypoxemic and hypercapnic respiratory failure
- Acute myocardial infarction
- Postoperative and perioperative states
- Acute asthma and exacerbation of chronic obstructive pulmonary disease (COPD)
- Conditions of tissue hypoxia with normal PaO_2 (normoxic hypoxia):
  – Anemic condition—supplemental oxygen may be used as a temporary measure
  – Carboxyhemoglobin—in these cases, PaO_2 may be characteristically normal, partial pressure of arterial carbon monoxide (PaCO) level has to be measured. If PaCO level is more than 40% indicates brain involvement, hence hyperbaric therapy, if available, is indicated
  – Sickle cell crisis—it is documented that deoxygenated states can cause sickling of cells, hence oxygen would be useful. However, oxygen toxicity should also be avoided in these conditions
- Respiratory distress
- Shock
- Hypotension
- To prevent postsurgical infections **(Table 1)**.

Table 1 Significance of differences of partial pressure of arterial oxygen and peripheral capillary oxygen saturation

PaO_2 values – SpO_2 values	Significance
97 mm Hg—100%	Normal young person
80 mm Hg—95%	Normal young person during sleep
70 mm Hg—93%	Lower limit of normal
60 mm Hg—90%	Respiratory failure
50 mm Hg—85%	Significant respiratory failure Patient needs admission
40 mm Hg—75%	Significant respiratory failure Normal venous blood values
30 mm Hg—60%	Unconscious

Abbreviations: PaO_2, partial pressure of arterial oxygen; SpO_2, peripheral capillary oxygen saturation.

TYPES OF HYPOXIA[4,7]

Types of hypoxia have been described in **Table 2**.

OXYGEN DEVICES

In a self-ventilating hypoxic patient, hypoxia is generally corrected by increasing the fraction of inspired oxygen (FiO_2). The actual concentration of oxygen delivered to the alveoli depends on the interaction between the oxygen delivery system and the patients breathing. In a hypoxic patient, inspiratory flow rates are high and respiratory pause is generally absent, thus a greater proportion of gas gets entrained in the apparatus. Hence, a substantially lower

Table 2 Types of hypoxia

Hypoxic hypoxia	Low PaO_2 caused by low-oxygen supply	• High altitude • Ventilatory failure—post-arrest, neuromuscular disease • Shunt Anatomical—R to L shunt Physiological—pneumonia, pneumothorax and ARDS
Anemic hypoxia	Arterial oxygen tension is normal but less availability due to low or physiological abnormal hemoglobin	Massive hemoptysis, carbon monoxide poisoning and methemoglobinemia
Stagnant hypoxia	Inadequate circulation causing insufficient oxygen tension	Left ventricular failure, pulmonary embolism and hypovolemia
Cytotoxic hypoxia	Normal transport of oxygen but inadequate cellular metabolism	Cyanide toxicity and arsenic toxicity

Abbreviations: PaO_2, partial pressure of arterial oxygen; ARDS, acute respiratory distress syndrome.

proportion of oxygen actually gets delivered to the alveolar level.[8-10]

Fraction of inspired oxygen delivered depends on the following described here.

Patient Factors[11,12]

Inspiratory flow rate:
- Tidal volume
- Respiratory rate
- Presence of a respiratory pause.

Device Factors

- Volume of the mask
- Tightness of fit
- Oxygen concentration
- Air vent size.

Types

Types of oxygen devices have been described in **Flow chart 1**.

Components:
- *Oxygen source and flow control*: Generally oxygen is supplied through cylinders, concentrators or central oxygen supply of the hospital. There is a valve device to control flow, rate often indicated by a flow meter
- *Connecting tubing*: The bore of the tube is important as narrower the bore, the lesser the amount of oxygen delivered.
- *Reservoir*: Reservoir is important as it ensures the oxygen supply for the next breathing effort, however, too large a reservoir has the problem of CO_2 rebreathing. In a nasal cannula, nasopharynx is the reservoir, the mask is the reservoir in a facemask, tent is the reservoir in an oxygen tent.
- *Expiratory device*: It is important to let out the expired air out in the environment, so that the air is not rebreathed. A facemask has holes in ask to let out the air. A continuous positive airway pressure (CPAP) system has holes in the expiratory limb.
- *Humidification*: It is important especially in high-flow systems; it may cause excess dryness and irritation. In that case, external humidifier or heat and moisture exchanger can be used. Other systems use natural humidification of nasopharynx.

Variable Oxygen Devices[11-15]

These supply oxygen at a variable rate depending on the patient's respiratory rate between 2 L/min and 15 L/min. These generally have a low reservoir capacity either being the nasopharynx or the volume of the mask. Depending on their reservoir capacity they have been divided into:
- *No capacity systems*: Nasal cannula and nasopharyngeal catheters
- *Low-capacity systems (capacity <100 mL)*: Simple and nebulizer facemask for children
- *Medium-capacity systems (capacity 100–250 mL)*: Simple and nebulizer mask for adults
- *High-capacity systems (capacity 250–1,500 mL)*: Facemask with reservoir bag
- *Very high-capacity systems (capacity >1,500 mL)*: Incubators and oxygen tents.

Nasal Prongs (Fig. 1)

Figure 1 shows nasal prongs and **Table 3** describes its working.

Facemask

For facemask, *see* **Figures 2 and 3**.

Types:
- Oxygen mask
- Reservoir facemask.

Simple mask: **Figure 2** shows simple facemask and **Table 4** describes the working of simple facemask.

Reservoir facemask:[16,17]
- High-oxygen, low-flow and variable performance device
- The reservoir empties during inspiration, and ambient air is entrained from vents

SECTION 2 Resuscitation and Critical Care in Emergency

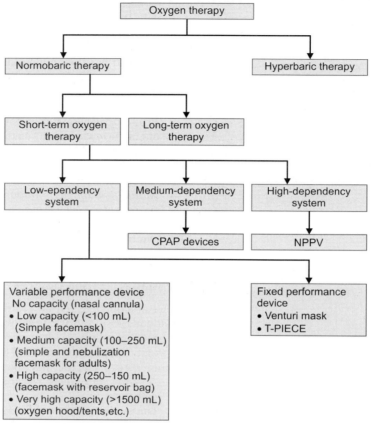

Flow chart 1 Oxygen therapy and oxygen devices

Abbreviations: CPAP, continuous positive airway pressure; NPPV, noninvasive positive pressure ventilation
Source: Adapted from ward's anesthetic equipment 6th edn.

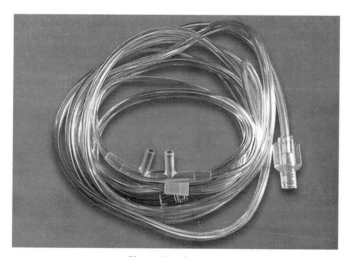

Fig. 1 Nasal prongs

- The mask with a reservoir bag must remain inflated during both inspiration and expiration. The patient inhales oxygen preferentially from the reservoir

- The rate of oxygen delivered depends on:
  – Mask fit
  – Capacity of reservoir bag
  – Oxygen flow rates
  – Patients inspiratory flow rate.

Types:
- Partial rebreathing
- Nonrebreathing.

Partial rebreathing mask:
- Simple mask with a reservoir bag
- Oxygen flow should always be supplied to maintain the reservoir to at least one-third to one-half on inspiration. The reservoir receives fresh gas exhaled gas approximately equal to the volume of the patient's anatomic dead space
- The flow of 6–10 L/min—the system provided FiO_2 of 40–70%.

Nonrebreathing mask:
- Do not permit mixing of exhaled gases with fresh gas supplied. The remaining exhaled air exits through vents. The presence of one-way valve ensures a fresh oxygen

CHAPTER 20 Oxygen Therapy

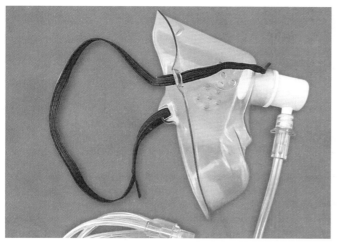

Fig. 2 Simple facemask

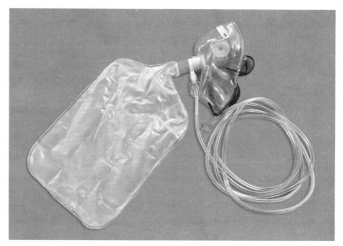

Fig. 3 Non-rebreathing mask

Table 3 Working of nasal prongs

Method	Amount of FiO$_2$	Precautions	Advantages	Disadvantages
Nasal prongs	Low flow—24–44% 1 L/min—24% 2–28% 3–32% 4–36% 5–40% 6–44%	To check whether both prongs are in patients nostrils In patient with chronic lung disease to deliver 2–3 L/min	• Patient able to talk and eat • Can be used in home setting • Well tolerated • Inexpensive	• May cause irritation to nasal mucosa • May cause epistaxis

Abbreviation: FiO$_2$, fraction of inspired oxygen.

Table 4 Working of simple facemask

Method	Amount of oxygen	Precautions	Advantages	Disadvantages
Simple facemask	Low flow (6–10 L/min) 35–50%	Frequently check placement of mask Check for claustrophobia CO$_2$ retention may occur unless flow rate <2 L/min or minute ventilation is high	Can provide increased oxygen demand for a limited period of time	Tight seal required Difficult to keep mask over mouth and nose Oxygen wasting Uncomfortable for patient while speaking or eating Problematic with RT in situ

Abbreviation: RT, ryles tube

supply with minimal dilution from the entrainment of room air. It provides a higher FiO$_2$ than partial rebreathing mask provided the mask fits correctly **(Fig. 3)**.
- Minimum flow rate required is 10 L/min
- Delivered FiO$_2$ of this system is 75–90% at flow rates of 12–15 L/min **(Table 5)**.

Fixed Performance Systems

Venturi Mask

Oxygen concentration is determined by the venturi principle—oxygen passing through a small orifice entrains air to a predictable dilution. The venturi principle depends

Table 5 Working of partial rebreathing or non-rebreathing mask

Method	FiO_2 delivered	Precaution	Advantages	Disadvantages
Partial rebreathing mask	75–80%	Reservoir bag should be two-thirds filled during inspiration Reservoir bag should be free of kinks	Patient can inhale room air through openings in mask, if oxygen supply briefly interrupted	Tight seal required (eating and talking is difficult)
Non-rebreathing mask	Flow rate—12–15% FiO_2—80–100%	Maintain flow rate so that reservoir bag collapses only slightly during inspiration Check valves are functioning properly	Delivers highest possible oxygen concentration Suitable for spontaneously breathing patient with severe hypoxemia	Not useful for long-term therapy Malfunction can cause CO_2 retention Feeling of suffocation Expensive

Abbreviation: FiO_2, fraction of inspired oxygen.

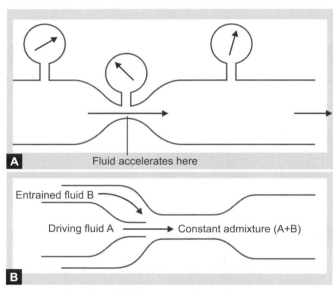

Figs 4A and B Venturi principle—the physics
Source: Adapted from Ward's anesthetic equipment, 6th edition. Amsterdam, Netherlands: Elsevier; 2012.

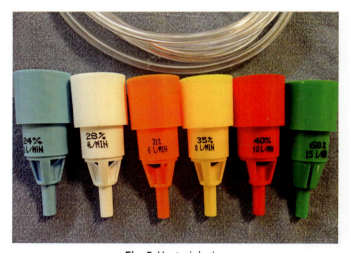

Fig. 5 Venturi device

on the Bernoulli's effect, when fluid flows through a narrow constriction, it accelerates, gaining kinetic energy from the surrounding potential energy, thus a negative pressure surrounding is created, this entrains the surrounding fluid through the constriction **(Figs 4A and B)**. The FiO_2 is adjusted by changing the venturi "valve" and setting the appropriate oxygen flow rate. The larger orifice results in the system behaving like a simple mask. However, a fixed delivery system is possible at a lower FiO_2, higher the FiO_2 required, lower the oxygen flow rate **(Fig. 5)**.

Venturi system is independent of the patient effort as the rate of oxygen flow is more than the patients inspiratory flow rate.

T-piece

- Provides accurate FiO_2
- Used on end of endotracheal (ET) tube when weaning from ventilator **(Fig. 6)**
- Provides good humidity. It fits securely over tracheostomy tube.

Medium-dependency Systems[18]

Continuous positive airway pressure mask with oxygen supply: The fresh gas flow in the system should be more than the total inspiratory rate of the patient that would ensure a positive pressure in the system **(Fig. 7)**.

High-dependency Systems

In addition to supplying oxygen, these can also be used for low-positive pressure ventilation (noninvasive positive-

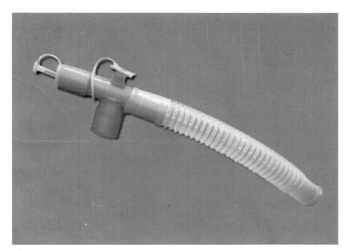

Fig. 6 T-piece with endotracheal tube connection

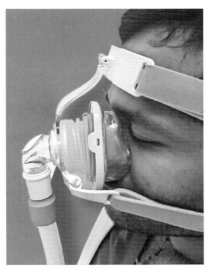

Fig. 7 Continuous positive airway pressure nasal mask

pressure ventilation) by means of facemask or nasal mask. These can be used to avoid intubation and during weaning.[18-22]

LONG-TERM OXYGEN THERAPY[23]

- Oxygen prescribed a low-flow rate at least 16 hours a day including night
- Long-term oxygen therapy (LTOT) improves sleep, survival and cognition
- Oxygen sources include—oxygen cylinder and oxygen concentrators
- Oxygen delivered through—nasal cannula, transtracheal catheters, etc.

Indications

- Patient with SaO_2 < 88%, PaO_2 < 55 mm Hg
- Patient with saturation of oxygen (SaO_2) between 88% and 90%, PaO_2 between 55 mm Hg and 60 mm Hg with:
  - Polycythemia
  - Cor pulmonale.

If LTOT is prescribed during an acute exacerbation—arterial blood gas (ABG) should be repeated in 30–90 days after discharge.

HYPERBARIC OXYGEN THERAPY[24-27]

- Implies oxygen delivery at increased ambient pressure generally at 2–3 atmospheres
- This increases the amount of oxygen dissolved in plasma from 2 mL/100 mL plasma to 2–6 mL/100 mL of plasma.

Indications

- Carbon monoxide poisoning
- Decompression sickness
- Thermal burns
- Treatment of gas gangrene
- Chronic refractory osteomyelitis
- Compartment syndrome.

WHICH OXYGEN DELIVERY SYSTEM TO USE?

- Level of FiO_2 used
- Patient comfort
- Indication of oxygenation
- Economical use of oxygen
- Minimum resistance of the system.[28,29]

GOALS OF OXYGEN THERAPY[29]

- Treatment of hypoxemia
- Decreased work of breathing
- Decreased myocardial oxygen demand.

MONITORING

For oxygen therapy monitoring **(Table 6)**.

OXYGEN TOXICITY[30,31]

Toxicity of oxygen caused by free radical injury due to superoxide, hydroxyl and oxygen singlet. At higher pressures, the protective natural scavenging mechanism of the body is lost. The toxicity is related to the FiO_2 of the air inspired. Generally, anything above 60% for more than 6 hours may be injurious. Studies have shown, if clinically allowed, can be tried for air breaks. Generally, normobaric therapy affects lungs, while hyperbaric therapy affects central nervous system, eyes in addition to lungs.[32]

Symptoms and Signs

- Nasal stuffiness
- Fatigability
- Substernal chest pain
- Nasal stuffiness and sore throat
- Headache

Table 6 Oxygen therapy monitoring

Patient severely hypoxemic, critically ill	Start at 15 L/min via reservoir facemask, once stabilized, can be tapered to maintain saturation between 94% and 98%. If at risk of type-2 respiratory failure to maintain SpO_2 between 88% and 92%
Patient moderately hypoxemic, seriously ill	Start O_2 via facemask at 6 L/min, if no improvement in condition, increase to up to 15 L/min via reservoir bag. SpO_2 to be maintained between 94% and 98%
COPD-like condition, at risk of type-2 respiratory failure	Venturi mask (at 4 L/min) preferred, to maintain SpO_2 between 88% and 92%. Should repeat ABG after 30–60 min to see the PaO_2 and $PaCO_2$ levels

Abbreviations: SpO_2, peripheral capillary oxygen saturation; COPD, chronic obstructive pulmonary disease; ABG, arterial blood gas; $PaCO_2$, partial pressures of carbon dioxide.
Source: Adapted from ERS guidelines on Oxygen therapy, 2013.

- Nausea and vomiting
- Radiological signs of atelectasis (adhesive atelectasis)—mimicking acute respiratory distress syndrome
- Hypoventilation.

Evaluation

- Pattern and breathing rate
- Pink color in nail beds, conjunctiva and lips
- Whether disorientation or difficulty in cognition present
- Regular ABG for PaO_2 and hemoglobin concentration.

Complications

- Absorption atelectasis
- Hypoventilation
- Bronchopulmonary dysplasia
- Retrolental fibroplasia
- Drying of mucous membranes (if humidifier not used)
- Fire-related hazards.

Weaning

- Patients with chronic lung disease may require oxygen for longer periods of time
- Weaning to be attempted once vitals like respiratory rate, pulse rate, SaO_2 and blood pressures are settled

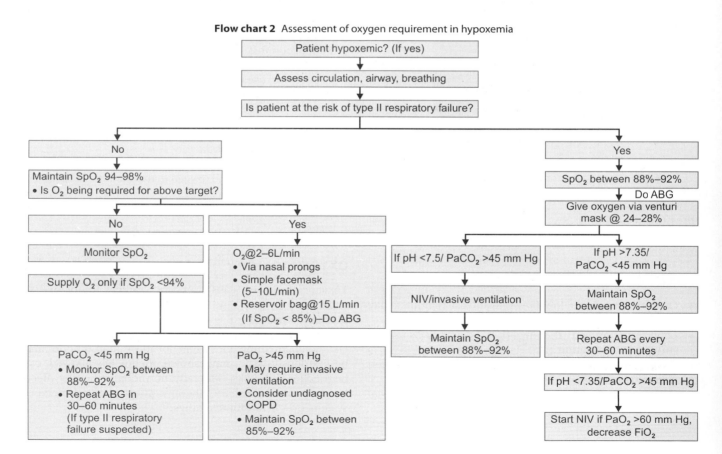

Flow chart 2 Assessment of oxygen requirement in hypoxemia

- The oxygen requirement should be assessed by reducing the FiO_2 and evaluating every 30 minutes using an arterial blood gas. However, pulse oximeter is preferred as is less invasive **(Flow chart 2)**.

SUMMARY

- Oxygen is a drug, hence, except for emergencies, should be prescribed
- Oxygen is the treatment of hypoxemia and not breathlessness
- The target saturation should always be prescribed in case of type-1 respiratory failure between 94% and 98%. In type-2 respiratory failure, between 88% and 92%
- Various devices are available for delivery of oxygen, indication of use, patient comfort, target saturation and efficient usage of oxygen to be considered while deciding the device
- Oxygen has its own sets of complications; hence, weaning should be attempted while patient has stable vitals.

REFERENCES

1. Ooi R, Joshi P, Soni N. An evaluation of oxygen delivery using nasal prongs. Anaesthesia. 1992;47:591-3.
2. Sim MA, Dean P, Kinsella J, et al. Performance of oxygen delivery devices when the breathing pattern of respiratory failure is simulated. Anaesthesia. 2008;63:938-40.
3. Groves N, Tobin A. High flow nasal oxygen generates positive airway pressure in adult volunteers. Aust Crit Care. 2007;20:126-31.
4. West JB. Respiratory Physiology. The Essentials, 6th edition. Philadelphia: Lippincott: Williams & Wilkins; 2000.
5. Hameed SM, Aird WC, Cohn SM. Oxygen delivery. Crit Care Med. 2003;31:S658-67.
6. Guyton AC. Textbook of Medical Physiology, 10th edition. Philadelphia: Saunders; 2000.
7. Boyd O. Optimisation of oxygenation and tissue perfusion in surgical patients. Intensive Crit Care Nurs. 2003;19:171-8.
8. Vermeij CG, Feenstra BW, Adrichem WJ, et al. Independent oxygen uptake and oxygen delivery in septic and postoperative patients. Chest. 1991;99:1438-43.
9. Gattinoni L, Brazzi L, Pelosi P, et al. A trial of goal-oriented hemodynamic therapy in critically ill patients. SvO_2 Collaborative Group. N Engl J Med. 1995;333:1025-32.
10. Hayes MA, Timmins AC, Yau EH, et al. Elevation of systemic oxygen delivery in the treatment of critically ill patients. N Engl J Med. 1994;330:1717-22.
11. Leach RM, Treacher DF. The pulmonary physician in critical care 2: Oxygen delivery and consumption in the critically ill. Thorax. 2002;57:170-7.
12. Wheeler AP, Bernard GR, Thompson BT, et al. National Heart, Lung, and Blood Institute Acute Respiratory Distress Syndrome (ARDS) Clinical Trials Network. Pulmonary-artery versus central venous catheter to guide treatment of acute lung injury. N Engl J Med. 2006;354:2213-24.
13. Cairo JM. Administering medical gasses: regulators, flowmeters, and controlling devices. In: Cairo JM, Pilbeam SP (Eds). Mosby's respiratory care equipment. St. Louis: Mosby; 1999. pp. 62-88.
14. Branson RD. The nuts and bolts of increasing arterial oxygenation: devices and techniques. Respir Care. 1993;38:672-86; discussion 87-9.
15. Breakell A, Townsend-Rose C. The clinical evaluation of the Respi-check mask: a new oxygen mask incorporating a breathing indicator. Emerg Med J. 2001;18:366-9.
16. Jones HA, Turner SL, Hughes JM. Performance of the large-reservoir oxygen mask (Ventimask). Lancet. 1984;1:1427-31.
17. Campbell DJ, Fairfield MC. The delivery of oxygen by a Venturi T-piece. Anaesthesia. 1996;51:558-60.
18. Nava S, Hill N. Noninvasive ventilation in acute respiratory failure. Lancet. 2009;374:250-9.
19. Duncan AW, Oh TE, Hillman DR. PEEP and CPAP. Anaesth Intensive Care. 1986;14:236-50.
20. Lindner KH, Lotz P, Ahnefeld FW. Continuous positive airway pressure effect on functional residual capacity, vital capacity and its subdivisions. Chest. 1987;92:66-70.
21. Brochard L, Mancebo J, Elliott MW. Noninvasive ventilation for acute respiratory failure. Eur Respir J. 2002;19:712-21.
22. Highcock MP, Morrish E, Jamieson S, et al. An overnight comparison of two ventilators used in the treatment of chronic respiratory failure. Eur Respir J. 2002;20:942-5.
23. O'Driscoll BR, Howard LS, Davison AG. BTS guideline for emergency oxygen use in adult patients. Thorax. 2008;63:vi1-68.
24. Guo S, Counte MA, Romeis JC. Hyperbaric oxygen technology: an overview of its applications, efficacy, and cost-effectiveness. Int J Technol Assess Health Care. 2003;19:339-46.
25. Weaver LK. Clinical practice. Carbon monoxide poisoning. N Engl J Med. 2009;360:1217-25.
26. Juurlink DN, Buckley NA, Stanbrook MB, et al. Hyperbaric oxygen for carbon monoxide poisoning. Cochrane Database Syst Rev. 2005;(1):CD002041.
27. Weaver LK, Valentine KJ, Hopkins RO. Carbon monoxide poisoning: risk factors for cognitive sequelae and the role of hyperbaric oxygen. Am J Respir Crit Care Med. 2007;176:491-7.
28. Iscoe S, Beasley R, Fisher JA. Supplementary oxygen for nonhypoxemic patients: O_2 much of a good thing? Crit Care. 2011;15:305.
29. Garcia de la Asuncion J, Belda FJ, Greif R, et al. Inspired supplemental oxygen reduces markers of oxidative stress during elective colon surgery. Br J Surg. 2007;94:475-7.
30. de Jonge E, Peelen L, Keijzers PJ, et al. Association between administered oxygen, arterial partial oxygen pressure and mortality in mechanically ventilated intensive care unit patients. Crit Care. 2008;12:R156.
31. Eastwood G, Bellomo R, Bailey M, et al. Arterial oxygen tension and mortality in mechanically ventilated patients. Intensive Care Med. 2012;38:91-8.
32. Bennett M. Randomised controlled trials. In: Fledmeier J (Eds). Hyperbaric Oxygen 2003—Indications and Results. The UHMS Hyperbaric Oxygen Therapy Committee Report. Durham NC: Undersea and Hyperbaric Medicine Society; 2003. pp. 1212-37.

CHAPTER 21

Acute Pain Management in Emergency Department

Sonam Kaushika, Devendra Richhariya, Manish Garg

INTRODUCTION

Pain is an unpleasant and emotional experience originating in real or potential damaged tissues. Pain is the most common and most undertreated condition in emergency department. In our experience, in most of the cases treatment of pain improves the patient satisfaction. Various drugs are available for treating acute pain in the various forms. The management of acute pain requires an experienced emergency physician who has good knowledge of the analgesics and anesthetics, contraindications, precautions, side effects, administration methods, and monitoring requirements.

PAIN CATEGORIES

Somatic pain: It is localized in the body tissues like nociceptive pain and neuropathic pain.

Psychogenic pain: It is a pain with no known physical cause.

Acute pain: It is a protective mechanism that alerts the individuals to harmful objects, sudden onset and relief after removal of its mediators that stimulate receptors, acute pain stimulates autonomic nervous system causes increased heart rate and respiratory rate, elevated blood pressure, pallor or flushing, dilated pupils, diaphoresis, increase in blood sugar, gastric acid secretion decrease in gastric motility. Acute pain also causes fear, anxiety, and general sense of unease.

Chronic pain: It develops gradually, persistent or intermittent chronic pain can produce depression and sleeping disorders.

MECHANISM INVOLVED IN NOCICEPTIVE PAIN

- *Nociceptors*: Ending of small unmyelinated or lightly myelinated afferent neurons
- *Stimulators*: Chemical, mechanical and thermal mild stimulation: positive, pleasurable sensation (e.g. tickling); strong stimulation: pain

These differences are a result of the frequency and amplitude of the afferent signal transmitted from the nerve endings to the central nervous system (CNS)
- *Location*: In muscles, tendons, epidermis, subcutaneous tissue, visceral organs; they are not evenly distributed in body (in skin more than in internal structures) **(Fig. 1)**.

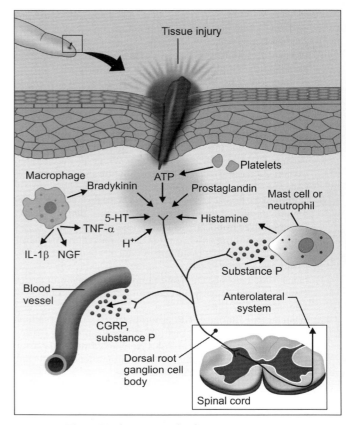

Fig. 1 Mechanism involved in nociceptive pain

Afferent Pathways

- From nociceptors → transmitted by small A-delta fibers and C-fibers to the spinal cord → form synapses with neurons in the dorsal horn (DH)
- From DH → transmitted to higher parts of the spinal cord and to the rest of the CNS by spinothalamic tracts

*The small unmyelinated C-neurons are responsible for the transmission of diffuse burning or aching sensations; the larger, myelinated A-delta fibers occurs much more quickly. A-fibers carry well-localized, sharp pain sensations.

Efferent Analgesic System

Inhibition of Pain Signals

Mechanisms: Pain afferents stimulate the neurons in gray matter surrounding the cerebral aqueduct in the midbrain results in activation of efferent (descendent) antinociceptive pathways from there the impulses are transmitted through the spinal cord to the DH; there they inhibit or block transmission of nociceptive signals at the level of DH **(Fig. 2)**.

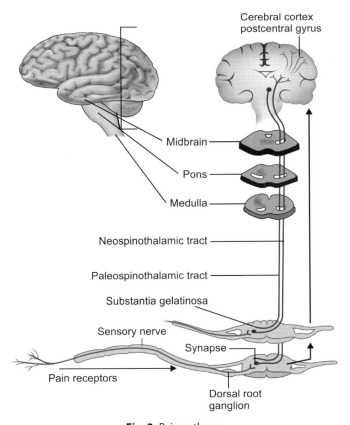

Fig. 2 Pain pathway

ASSESSMENT OF PAIN IN EMERGENCY DEPARTMENT

Objective

- Recognition of pain and measurement of its intensity.
- Treatment adapted to the intensity, the patient and the pathology.
- Systematic and regular reassessment permitting an appreciation of the efficiency of the treatment.

Evaluation

- Ask patients about their pain intensity, location, onset, duration, variation, and quality.
- The Clinical Effectiveness Committee standard of analgesia for moderate and severe pain should be given within 20 minutes of arrival in the emergency department and the effectiveness of analgesia should be re-evaluated within 30 minutes of receiving the first dose of analgesia in case of severe pain and 60 minutes in case of moderate pain.
- There are multiple assessment tools in use for assessment of pain **(Figs 3 and 4; Tables 1 and 2)**.

Pain as the Fifth Vital Sign and JCI Standards of Care

Joint Commission International (JCI) launched the "pain as the fifth vital sign" initiative, requiring a pain intensity rating (0–10) at all clinical encounters. There are four primary vital signs: body temperature, blood pressure, pulse, and respiratory rate.

Pain defined in JCI guidelines, as "whatever the experiencing person says it is, existing whenever she or he says it does". This definition emphasizes that pain is a subjective experience with no objective measures. It also stresses that the patient, not clinician, is the authority on the pain and that his or her self-report is the most reliable indicator of pain.

The JCI's pain standards make patient pain free during hospital stay.

INDICATIONS OF URGENT PAIN MANAGEMENT IN MEDICAL EMERGENCIES

- Acute subarachnoid headache
- Acute myocardial infarction

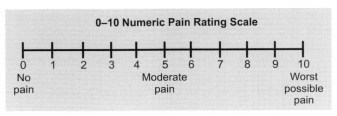

Fig. 3 Numeric pain rating scale (0–10) in adults

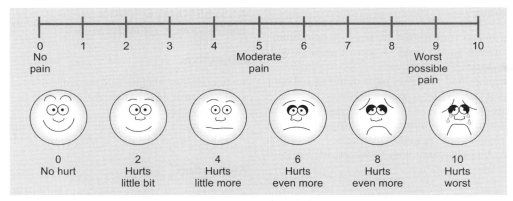

Fig. 4 Wong-Baker faces pain rating scale (age >7 years) in children

Table 1 Behavioral pain score in unconscious or comatose patients

Item	Description	Score
Facial expression	• Relaxed • Partially tightened (e.g., brow lowering) • Fully tightened (e.g., eyelid closing) • Grimacing	1 2 3 4
Upper limbs	• No movement • Partially bent • Fully bent with finger flexion • Permanently retracted	1 2 3 4
Compliance with mechanical ventilation	• Tolerating movement • Coughing but tolerating ventilation most of the time • Fighting ventilator • Unable to control ventilation	1 2 3 4

Table 2 Pediatric pain scale (FLACC) (age 0–7 years) in pediatric

Parameter	0	1	2
Face	No expression	Occasional grimace	Frequent to constant quivering chin
Legs	Normal position or relaxed	Uneasy restless, tense	Kicking or legs drawn up
Activity	Lying quiet	Squirming, shifting back and forth, tense	Arched, rigid or jerking
Cry	No cry	Moans or whimpers	Crying steadily
Consolability	Content, relaxed	Reassurance, hugging	Difficult to console

Score: 0, no pain: 1–3, mild pain; 4–7, moderate pain; 8–10, severe pain; *FLACC*: Face, legs, activity, cry, consolability

- Acute aortic dissection
- Acute pancreatitis
- Acute appendicitis
- Acute renal and ureteric colic due to calculus
- Ectopic pregnancy
- Anal fissure
- Trauma with head injuries, trunk and limb fractures, joint dislocations
- Electrical and thermal burns
- Acute rheumatoid arthritis in joints
- Analgesia during chest tube insertion, reducing fractures and dislocations.

POTENTIAL CAUSES FOR PAIN CONTROL FAILURE

- Failure to assess pain
- Failure to document pain
- Failure to implement pain guidelines
- Failure to meet patient expectation.

TREATMENT OF PAIN IN EMERGENCY DEPARTMENT

The implementation of analgesia is based on two steps:
1. *Step 1*: Pain relief as quickly as possible. It continues until the goal is not reached.
2. *Step 2*: Maintaining the pain relief with appropriate prescriptions **(Tables 3 and 4)**.

World Health Organization (WHO) three-step ladder for prescribing analgesics is well described in **Figure 5**.

When a non-opioid drug no longer adequately controls the pain, an opioid analgesic should be added. Opioid medications have strong potential of drug abuse in patients and medical personnel, so they are marked in schedule H, L and X of Drugs and Cosmetics Act **(Box 1)**.

Narcotic Drugs and Psychotropic Substances (NDPS; third amendment) rules, 2015 defined registered medical

CHAPTER 21 Acute Pain Management in Emergency Department

Table 3 Recommended dosing protocol

Medication (class)	Oral formulations	Recommended dosing protocol			Comments
		Starting dose	Usual dose	Maximum dose	
Nonopioid analgesics					
Acetaminophen	*Tablets*: 325, 500, 650 mg; 650 mg CR *Suspensions and solutions*: 160 mg/5 mL; 500 mg/15 mL	*Dose*: 1–2 tabs p.o. q6h p.r.n.	Adults: 325–650 mg q4–6h or 1000 mg 3–4 times per day	Do not exceed 4000 mg/day	No anti-inflammatory effect; rapid hepatotoxic effect if overdosed
Tramadol	*Tablets*: 50 mg *Extended-release*: 100, 200, 300 mg SR	Start dose at 25mg/day, titrating dose by 25 mg every 3 days, until reaching 25 mg q.i.d. The total daily dose may then be increased by 50 mg every 3 days as tolerated, to reach target dose of 50 mg q.i.d.	50–100 mg p.o. q4–6h p.r.n.: 100–300 mg q.d. for SR Immediate-release formulation: 50–100 mg q4–5h (not to exceed 400 mg/day)	400 mg/day	Maximum dose for SR form is 300 mg/day
Salicylates					
Aspirin	*Tablets*: 81, 162, 325, 500, 650, 975 mg	500 mg/day	325–650 mg p.o. q4h p.r.n.	4000 mg/day	Bleeding risk is the most significant concern
Diflunisal	*Tablet*: 500 mg	500 mg/day	500–1000 mg followed by 250–500 mg q8–12h	Maximum daily dose: 1.5 g	Approved for acute or long-term use for symptomatic treatment of (1) mild to moderate pain, (2) osteoarthritis, and (3) rheumatoid arthritis
Nonselective NSAIDs					
Ibuprofen	*Tablets*: 100, 200, 400, 600, 800 mg *Suspension*: 40 mg/mL; 100 mg/5 mL	600 mg/day	400–600 mg p.o. q4–6h p.r.n.	3200 mg/day	Use with caution in patients with history of peptic ulcer
Naproxen	*Tablets*: 250, 375, 500 mg *SR*: 375, 500 mg *Suspension*: 125 mg/5mL	500 mg/day	250–500 mg p.o. b.i.d.	1500 mg/day for 3–5 days	Maintenance dose is maximum 1000 mg/day for 6 months
Ketoprofen	*Tablets*: 12.5 mg *Capsules*: 25, 50, 75 mg *Extended-release*: 100, 150, 200 mg SR	50 mg/day	25–50 mg p.o. q6–8h	300 mg/day	Maximum dose for SR form is 200 mg/day
Meclofenamate sodium	*Tablets*: 50, 100 mg	50 mg/day	50–100 mg p.o. q4–6h	400 mg/day	Use lowest effective dose, shortest treatment duration: give with food and use with caution in patients with history of peptic ulcer
Piroxicam	*Capsules*: 10, 20 mg	10 mg/day	20 mg p.o. once daily	20 mg/day	May divide daily dose b.i.d.
Diclofenac	*Tablets*: 50 mg *Delayed-release*: 25, 50, 75, 100 mg SR	50 mg/day	50 mg p.o. b.i.d.–t.i.d.	150 mg/day	Alternative dose for SR form is 100 mg p.o daily
Nabumetone	*Tablets*: 500, 750 mg	500 mg/day	500–2000 mg once daily	2000 mg/day	May divide daily dose to b.i.d.

Abbreviations: CR, controlled release; SR, sustained release

Drug	Oral dose	IMI, SCI, IVI dose	Notes
Paracetamol	20 mg/kg initially, than 15 mg/kg every 4 h		Maximum 90 mg/kg/day (up to 4 g) for 2 days then 60 mg/kg/day
Ibuprofen	5–10 mg/kg every 8 h		Maximum 40 mg/kg/day up to 2 g/day
Naproxen	5 mg/kg every 12 h		Maximum 10–20 mg/kg/day up to 1 g/day
Diclofenac	1 mg/kg every 8 h 1 mg/kg every 12 h (rectally)		Maximum 3 mg/kg/day up to 150 mg/day
Codeine	0.5–1 mg/kg every 4 h	0.5–1 mg/kg every 3 h Not for IV use	Maximum 3 mg/kg/day
Morphine	0.2–0.3 mg/kg every 4 h	0.1–0.15 mg/kg every 3 h	
Tramadol	1–1.5 mg/kg every 6 h	1 mg/kg every 6 h	Maximum 6 mg/kg/day up to 400 mg/day

Abbreviations: IMI, intramuscular injection; SCI, subcutaneous injection; IVI, intravenous injection

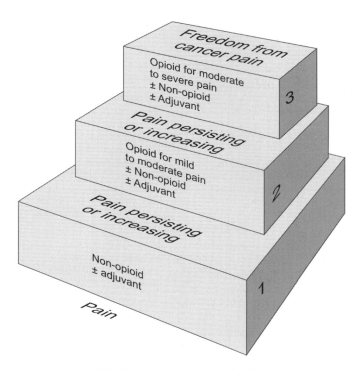

Fig. 5 Three-step analgesic ladder

Box 1 Scheduled* drugs in Indian gazette

Issued by Registered Pharmacist on written prescription of RMP (Registered Medical Practitioner) only:
- Schedule 'H' & schedule 'L' drugs—"H" for Hazardous & "L" for Lethal
- Narcotics & Opioids**—Morphine, Codeine, Fentanyl
- Sedatives–Pentobarbital & Barbiturates, Diazepam, Chlordiazepoxide, Lorazepam
- Schedule 'X' drugs–Ketamine-Conscious sedation (NDPS 2014 Amendment)
- Schedule 'Y' drugs- undertaking drug trials on new sedatives and analgesic drugs

* All scheduled drugs are classified in Drug and Cosmetics Act, 1945, recently updated in 2014
**Cultivation/production/manufacture, possession, sale, purchase, transport, storage, consumption or distribution of any of the following substances, except for medical and scientific purposes and as per the rules or orders and conditions of licences that may be issued, is illegal.

practitioner (RMP) trained in pain relief and medical institution like hospitals having emergency departments and pain clinics providing palliative care and pain relief in cancer patients.

Registered Medical Practitioner

Registered medical practitioner means any person registered as a medical practitioner under the Indian Medical Council Act, 1956 (102 of 1956) or under any law for the registration of medical practitioner for the time being in force, or registered as a dentist under the Dentists Act, 1948 (16 of 1948) or under any law for the registration of dentists for the time being in force and has undergone training in *pain relief* and palliative care for prescription of essential narcotic drugs for pain relief and palliative care or training care or training in opioid substitution therapy for prescription of essential narcotic drugs for treatment of opioid dependence.

A registered medical practitioner may possess essential narcotic drug, for use in his practice but not for sale or distribution, not more than the quantity mentioned in the **Table 5**.

Explanation: The expression "for use in his practice" covers only the actual direct administration of the drugs to a patient under the care of the registered medical practitioner

Table 5 Essential narcotic drug with prescribed quantity

Sl. No.	Name of the essential narcotic drug	Quantity
(1)	(2)	(3)
1.	Morphine and its salts and all preparations containing or more than 0.2% of Morphine	500 mg
2.	Methyl morphine (commonly known as codeine) and ethyl morphine and their salts (including dionine), all dilutions and preparations except those which are compounded with one or more other ingredients and containing not more than 100 mg of the drug per dosage unit and with a concentration of not more than 2.5% in undivided preparations and which have been established in therapeutic practice	2,000 mg
3.	Dihydroxycodeinone (commonly known as oxycodone and dihydroxycodeinone), its salts (such as Eucodal, Boncodal Dinarcon, Hydrolaudin, Nucodan, Percodan, Scophedal, Tebodol and the like), its esters and the salts of its ester and preparation, admixture, extracts or other substances containing any of these drug	250 mg
4.	Dihydrocodeinone (commonly known as hydrocodone), its salts (such as Dicodide, Codinovo, Diconone, Hycodan, Multacodin, Nyodide, Ydroced and the like) and its esters and salts of its ester, and preparation, admixture, extracts or other substances containing any of these drugs	320 mg
5.	1-phenethyl-4-N-propionyalnilino-piperdine (the international-nonproprietary name of which is fentanyl) and its salts and preparations, admixture, extracts or other substance containing any of these drugs	Two transdermal patches one each of 12.5 µg/hr and 25 µg/hr

in accordance with established medical standards and practices.

"Prescription" means a prescription given by a RMP for the supply of any of the essential narcotic and opioid drugs to a patient for medical use in accordance with these rules.

Registered medical practitioner and conditions relating to their prescriptions: No prescription for the supply of essential narcotic drugs shall be given by a registered medical practitioner otherwise than in accordance with the following conditions, namely:
- The prescription shall be in writing, dated and signed by the practitioner with his full name, address and registration number and shall specify the name and address of the person to whom the prescription is given and the total quantity of the essential narcotic drug to be supplied along with daily dose and period of consumption.
  Provided that where such drug to be supplied on the prescription is a patent or proprietary medicine, it shall be sufficient to state the quantity and strength of the medicine to be supplied.
- The prescription shall not be given for the use of prescriber himself.

MCI Code of Ethics for Doctors in Writing Narcotics, Opioids and Sedatives

Evasion of Legal Restrictions: The physician shall observe the laws of the country in regulating the practice of medicine and shall also not assist others to evade such laws. He could be cooperative in observance and enforcement of sanitary laws and regulation in the interest of public health. A physician should observe the provisions of the State Acts like Drugs and Cosmetics Act, 1940; Pharmacy Act, 1948; Narcotic Drugs and Psychotropic Substances Act, 1985; Medical Termination of Pregnancy Act, 1971; Transplantation of Human Organs Act, 1994; Mental Act, 1987; Environmental Protection Act, 1986; Prenatal Sex Determination Test Act, 1994; Drugs and Magic Remedies (Objectionable Advertisement) Act, 1954; Persons with Disabilities (Equal Opportunities and Full Participation) Act, 1995, and Bio-Medical Waste (Management and handling) Rules, 1988 and such other Acts, Rules, Regulations made by the Central or State Governments or local administrative bodies or any other relevant Act relating to the protection and promotion of public health.

In 2016, Gazette notification by Ministry of Health and Family Welfare (MOHFW) has banned over 344 medicines of fixed drug combinations found harmful to patients in research studies, which include analgesics combinations with other analgesics, narcotics, antacids, local anesthetics, anticoagulants, antibiotic, antidepressants, antipsychotics, antiallergics, antitussives, steroids, and sedatives.

Note: An emergency physician should be careful about prescribing banned drugs and drug combinations, otherwise he can be barred from practice by State Medical Council temporarily by giving warning notice, and doctor can be sued for negligence in care under Consumer Protection Act, in prescribing banned drugs, thus harming patients.

In India, currently, pain management is double-edged sword, if no pain relief to patient, then he complains against doctor to hospital administration. If doctor prescribes freely analgesics, especially narcotics, then NDPS officials raids the premises to scrutinize the narcotics register.

If doctor gives overdose of opioid analgesics, it can cause respiratory depression; nonsteroidal anti-inflammatory drugs (NSAIDs) analgesic overdose may causes renal failure in adults and hepatic failure in children, leading to allegations of malpractice and liable for hefty amounts of compensation to patient for damages and punishment, if patient dies due to overdose.

If doctor prescribes banned analgesic drug combinations, due to lack of awareness about recent notifications by Ministry of Health and Family Welfare (MOHFW), then doctor can be debarred from clinical practice by Medical Council of India (MCI).

Procedural Analgesia and Conscious Sedation in Pediatrics

An analgesic relieves pain, whereas sedatives relieve fear and anxiety. Some analgesics like narcotics have both sedative and analgesic properties, which made them useful in certain medical procedures like chest tube insertion, joint reduction in dislocations and reduction of fractures in trauma cases. Conscious sedation is induced by lesser dose of sedative, causing minimal depression in level of consciousness, wherein patient is awake but may have droopy eyes and slightly slurred speech. The patient should be able to respond to verbal command or physical stimulation and to maintain protective airway reflexes.

Conscious sedation by midazolam is used in pediatrics for conducting CT scan and X-ray in trauma and emergencies.

CONCLUSION

Pain is the most common presentation in emergency department. Pain management should be priority. Over the last decade various methods for assessment of pain and management strategies are developed. Adequate pain treatment in emergency improves the quality and patient satisfaction. Every emergency physician should be expert in Efficient and effective management of painful condition.

BIBLIOGRAPHY

1. Abdullah M. Ketamine. A new look at an old drug. M Abdullah. anaesthetics.ukzn.ac.za/.../Ketamine_a_new_look_at_an_old_drug_...(accessed on 12/21/11)
2. Bailey B, Bergeron S, Gravel J, et al. Efficacy and impact of intravenous morphine before surgical consultation in children with right lower quadrant pain suggestive of appendicitis: A Randomized Controlled Trial. Annals of Emergency Medicine. 2007;(50):371-8.
3. Ballantyne JC, Carr DB, Chalmers TC, et al. Postoperative patient-controlled analgesia: meta-analyses of initial randomized control trials. J Clin Anesth. 1993;5:182-93.
4. Bartfield JM, Flint RD, McErlean M, Broderick J. Nebulized fentanyl for relief of abdominal pain. Acad Emerg Med. 2003;10(3):215-8.
5. Baxter AD. Respiratory depression with patient-controlled analgesia. Can J Anaesth. 1994;41:87-90.
6. Bijur PE, Kenny MK, Gallagher EJ. Intravenous morphine at 0.1 mg/kg is not effective for controlling severe acute pain in the majority of patients. Annals of Emergency Medicine. 2005;46:362-7.
7. Bijur PE, Latimer CT, Gallagher EJ. Validation of a verbally administered numerical rating scale of acute pain for use in the emergency department. Academic Emergency Medicine. 2003;10:390-2.
8. Birnbaum A, Esses D, Bijur PE, Holden L, Gallagher EJ. Randomized double-blind placebo-controlled trial of two intravenous morphine dosages (0.10 mg/kg and 0.15 mg/kg) in emergency department patients with moderate to severe acute pain. Ann Emerg Med. 2007;49(4):445-53.
9. Blumstein HA, Moore D. Visual Analog Pain Scores do not define desire for analgesia in patients with acute pain. Academic Emergency Medicine. 2003;10:211-4.
10. Borland M, Jacobs I, King B, O'Brien D. A randomized controlled trial comparing intranasal fentanyl to intravenous morphine for managing acute pain in children in the emergency department. Ann Emerg Med. 2007;49(3):335-40. Epub 2006 Oct 25.
11. Bradshaw H, Woolridge D. Sickle cell crisis. In: Emergency Department Analgesia. Cambridge University Press, New York; 2008. pp. 365-79.
12. Bradshaw M, Sen A. Use of a prophylactic antiemetic with morphine in acute pain: randomised controlled trial. Emerg Med J. 2006;23(3):210-3.
13. Burton JH, Miner J. In: Emergency Sedation and Pain Management. Cambridge University Press. New York; 2008; pp. 49-53.
14. Campbell T, Hughes J, Girder S. Relationship of ethnicity, gender, and ambulatory blood pressure to pain sensitivity: effects of individualized pain rating scales. Journal of Pain. 2004;5:183-91.
15. Chang AK, Bijur PE, Campbell CM, Murphy MK, Gallagher EJ. Safety and efficacy of rapid titration using 1mg doses of intravenous hydromorphone in emergency department patients with acute severe pain: the "1+1" protocol. Ann Emerg Med. 2009;54(2):221-5. Epub 2008 Nov.
16. Chang AK, Bijur PE, Davitt M, Gallagher EJ. Randomized Clinical Trial Comparing a Patient-Driven Titration Protocol ofIntravenous Hydromorphone With Traditional Physician-Driven Management of Emergency Department Patients With Acute Severe Pain. Ann Emerg Med. 2009 Jun 27. [Epub ahead of print].
17. Chang AK, Bijur PE, Meyer RH, Kenny MK, Solorzano C, Gallagher EJ. Safety and efficacy of hydromorphone as an analgesic alternative to morphine in acute pain: a randomized clinical trial. Ann Emerg Med. 2006;48(2):164-72. Epub 2006 Apr 27.
18. Chang AK, Bijur PE, Napolitano A, Lupow J, Gallagher EJ. Two milligrams iv hydromorphone is efficacious for treating pain but is associated with oxygen desaturation. J Opioid Manag. 2009;5(2):75-80.
19. Clark RF, Wei EM, Anderson PO. Meperidine: therapeutic use and toxicity. J Emerg Med. 1995;13(6):797-802.
20. Coman M, Kelly AM. Safety of a nurse-managed, titrated analgesia protocol for the management of severe pain in the emergency department. Emerg Med (Fremantle). 1999;11:128-31.

21. Cordell WH, Wright SW, Wolfson AB, Timerding BL, Maneatis TJ, Lewis RH, Bynum L, Nelson DR. Comparison of intravenous ketorolac, meperidine, and both (balanced analgesia) for renal colic. Ann Emerg Med. 1996;28(2):151-8.
22. Curtis KM, Henriques HF, Fanciullo G. A Fentanyl- Based Pain Management Protocol Provides Early Analgesia For Adult Trauma Patients. The Journal of Trauma. 2007;63(4):819-26.
23. Curtis KM, Henriques HF, Fanciullo G. A Fentanyl-Based Pain Management Protocol Provides Early Analgesia For Adult Trauma Patients. The Journal of Trauma. 2007;63(4):819-26.
24. Ducharme J. Pain, Big Gain: Effective Pain Management. ACEP SA 2011, http://webapps.acep.org/sa/Syllabi/SU-78.pdf.
25. Eray O, Cete Y, Oktay C, Karsli B, Akça S, Cete N, Ersoy F. Intravenous single-dose tramadol versus meperidine for pain relief in renal colic. Eur J Anaesthesiol. 2002;19(5):368-70.
26. Evans E, Turley N, Robinson N, Clancy M. Randomised controlled trial of patient controlled analgesia compared with nurse delivered analgesia in an emergency department. Emerg Med J. 2005;22(1):25-9.
27. Ferrante FM, Covino BG. Patient-controlled analgesia: a historical perspective. In: Ferrante FM, Ostheimer GW, Covino BG, eds. Patient-controlled analgesia. Boston: Blackwell Scientific Publications. 1990. pp. 3-9.
28. Fosnocht DE, Swanson ER. Use of triage pain protocol in the ED. American Journal of Emergency Medicine. 2007;25(7):791-3.
29. Frakes MA, Lord WR, Kociszewski C, Wedel SK. Efficacy of fentanyl analgesia for trauma in critical care transport. American Journal of Emergency Medicine. 2006;24:286-9.
30. Friedman BW, Kapoor A, Friedman MS, Hochberg ML, Rowe BH. The relative efficacy of meperidine for the treatment of acute migraine: a meta-analysis of randomized controlled trials. Ann Emerg Med. 2008;52(6):705-13. Epub 2008 Jul 16.
31. Fry M, Holdgate A. Nurse-initiated intravenous morphine in the emergency department: efficacy, rate of adverse events and impact on time to analgesia. Emerg Med (Fremantle). 2002;14:249-54.
32. Fry M, Holdgate A. Nurse-intiated intravenous morphine in the emergency department: Efficacy, rate of adverse events and impact on time to analgesia. Emergency Medicine. 2002;14(3):249-54.
33. Fulda GJ, Giberson F, Fagraeus L. A prospective randomized trial of nebulized morphine compared with patient-controlled analgesia morphine in the management of acute thoracic pain. J Trauma. 2005; 59(2):383-8; discussion 389-90.
34. Furyk JS, Grabowski WJ, Black LH. Nebulized fentanyl versus intravenous morphine in children with suspected limb fractures in the emergency department: a randomized controlled trial. Emerg Med Australas. 2009;21(3):203-9.
35. Galinski, et al. Management of severe acute pain in emergency settings: ketamine reduces morphine consumption American Journal of Emergency Medicine. 2007;25(4)385-90.
36. Galinski M, Dolveck F, Borron SW, Tual L, et al. A randomized, double-blind study comparing morphine with fentanyl in prehospital analgesia. Am J Emerg Med. 2005;23(2):114-9.
37. Gonzalez, et al. Intermittent injection vs patient-controlled analgesia for sickle cell crisis pain: comparison in patients in the emergency department. Arch Intern Med. 1991;151(7):1373-8.
38. Grass JA. Patient-Controlled Analgesia. Anesth Analg. 2005;101:S44-S61.
39. Gurnani A, Sharma PK, Rautela RS, Bhattacharya A. Analgesia for acute musculoskeletal trauma: low-dose subcutaneous infusion of ketamine. Anaesth Intensive Care. 1996;24:32-6.
40. Gutstein HB, Akil H. Opioid Analgesics. In: Hardman JG, Limbrid LE, Gilman AG, ed. Goodman and Gilman's the pharmacological basis of therapeutics, 10th edn. New York: McGraw-Hill; 2001. p. 569-619.
41. Henderson SO, Swadron S, Newton E. Comparison of intravenous ketorolac and meperidine in the treatment of biliary colic. J Emerg Med. 2002;23(3):237-41
42. Hodgins MJ. Interpreting the meaning of pain severity scores. Pain Research Management. 2002;7(4): 192-8.
43. http://painconsortium.nih.gov/pain_scales/index.html (Accessed on 11/21/11)
44. http://www.ipcaz.org/pages/new.html (Accessed on 11/21/11).
45. Hwang U, Richardson LD, Sonya TO, Morrison RS. The effect of emergency department crowding on the management of pain in older adults with hip fracture. J Am Geriatr Soc. 2006;54: 270-5.
46. Javery KB, Ussery TW, Steger HG, Colclough GW. Comparison of morphine and morphine with ketamine for postoperative analgesia. Can J Anaesth. 1996;43:212-5.
47. Kanowitz A, Dunn TM, Kanowitz EM, et al. Safety and effectiveness of fentanyl administration in pre-hospital pain management. Prehospital Emergency Care. 2006;10(1):1-7.
48. Kaplan CP, Sison C, Platt SL. Does a Pain Scale improve pain assessment in the pediatric emergency department? Pediatric Emerg Care. 2008;24(9):605-8.
49. Kelly AM, Barnes C, Brumby C. Nurse initiated narcotic analgesia reduces time to analgesia for patients with acute pain in the emergency department. Canadian Journal of Emergency Medicine. 2005;7(3):149-54.
50. Lester L, Braude DA, Niles C, Crandall CS, et al. Low-dose ketamine for analgesia in the ED: a retrospective case series. Am J Emerg Med. 2010;28:820-76.
51. Lvovschi V, Auburn F, Bonnet P, et al. Intravenous morphine titration to treat severe pain in the ED. American Journal of Emergency Medicine. 2008;26:676-82.
52. Mahar PJ, Rana JA, Kennedy CS, Christopher NC. A randomized clinical trial of oral transmucosal fentanyl citrate versus intravenous morphine sulfate for initial control of pain in children with extremity injuries. Pediatr Emerg Care. 2007;23(8):544-8.
53. Michael, et al. Patient Controlled Analgesia for Hip Fractures in the Emergency Department: A Prospective Randomized Controlled Trial. Research Forum Abstract. Annals of Emergency Medicine. 2005. pp. 46(3).
54. Miner JR, Kletti C, Herold M, Hubbard D, Biros MH. Randomized clinical trial of nebulized fentanyl citrate versus iv fentanyl citrate in children presenting to the emergency department with acute pain. Acad Emerg Med. 2007;14(10):895-8.
55. Miner JR, Kletti C, Herold M, Hubbard D, Biros MH. Randomized clinical trial of nebulized fentanyl citrate versus i.v. fentanyl citrate in children presenting to the emergency department with acute pain. Acad Emerg Med. 2007;14(10):895-8.
56. Morton NS. Ketamine for procedural sedation and analgesia in pediatric emergency medicine: a UK perspective. Paediatr Anaesth. 2008;18:25-9.

57. O'Connor AB, Zwemer FL, Hays DP, Feng C. Intravenous opioid dosing and outcomes in emergency patients: a prospective cohort analysis. Am J Emerg Med. 2010;28(9):1041-50.
58. Paoloni R, Talbot-Stern J. Low incidence of nausea and vomiting with intravenous opiate analgesia in the ED. Am J Emerg Med. 2002;20(7):604-8.
59. Paris P, Yealy D. Pain Management. In: Marx JA, ed. Rosen's Emergency Medicine: Concepts and Clinical Practice. St. Louis, MO: Mosby; 2002. pp. 2555-77.
60. Pines JM, Hollander JE. Emergency Department Crowding is Associated with Poor care for patients with severe pain. Annals of Emergency Medicine. 2008;51(1):1-5.
61. Porrecca F, Ossipov MH. Nausea and vomiting side effects with opioid analgesics during treatment of chronic pain: mechanism, implications, and management options. Pain Medicine. 2009;10(4):654-62.
62. Silka PA, Roth MM, Moreno G, Merrill L, Geiderman JM. Pain scores improve analgesic administration patterns for trauma patients in the emergency department. Acad Emerg Med. 2004;11:264-70.
63. Strassels SA, McNicol E, Suleman R. Pharmacotherapy of pain in older adults. Clinics in Geriatric Medicine. 2008;24:275-98.
64. Talbot-Stern J, Paoloni R. Prophylactic metoclopramide is unnecessary with intravenous analgesia in the ED. Am J Emerg Med. 2000;18(6):653-7.
65. Thomas S, Benevelli W, Brown D, et al. Safety of fentanyl for analgesia in adults undergoing air medical transport from trauma scenes. Air Med J. 1996;15:57-9.
66. Thomas SH. Emergency Department Analgesia: An Evidence–Based Guide. Cambridge University Press. New York; 2008. pp. 47-9.
67. Thomas SH. Emergency Department Analgesia: An Evidence-Based Guide. Cambridge University Press. 2010
68. Todd KH, Ducharme J, Choiniere M, et al. PEMI Study Group. Pain in the emergency department: results of the pain and emergency medicine initiative (PEMI) multicenter study. J Pain. 2007;8:460-6.
69. Walder B, Schafer M, Henzi I, Tramer MR. Efficacy and safety of patient-controlled opioid analgesia for acute postoperative pain: a quantitative systematic review. Acta Anaesthesiol. Scand 2001;45:795-804.
70. Wong D, Baker C. Pain in children: comparison of assessment scales. Pediatric Nursing. 1998;14:901-7.
71. Yeoh BS, Taylor DM, Taylor SE. Education initiative improves the evidence-based use of metoclopramide following morphine administration in the emergency department. Emerg Med Australas. 2009;21(3):178-83.
72. Zimmer G. Acute pain management. In: Tintinalli J, Kelen G, Stapczynski J eds. Emergency Medicine: A Comprehensive Study Guide. New York, NY: NcGraw-Hill; 2004. pp. 257-64.

Section 3

Cardiac Emergencies

- **Chest Pain**
  Rohit Goel, Rashmi Xavier, Nagendra Singh Chouhan, Praveen Chandra
- **Palpitations**
  Shashank Chauhan, Ram NG, HR Tomar
- **Syncope**
  Brajesh Kumar Mishra
- **Acute Coronary Syndrome: Risk Stratification**
  Mayank Jain, Rajneesh Kapoor
- **Cardiogenic Shock**
  Devendra Richhariya, Vikas Mudgal, Madhukar Shahi
- **Heart Failure**
  Vijay Kumar Chopra
- **Bradyarrhythmias**
  Jamal Yusuf, Safal, Saibal Mukhopadhyay
- **Tachyarrhythmia**
  Jamal Yusuf, Prattay Guhasarkar, Saibal Mukhopadhyay
- **Temporary Pacing**
  Kartikeya Bhargava
- **Hypertensive Emergency**
  Ravi R Kasliwal, Kushagra Mahansaria
- **Aortic Dissection**
  Rachit Saxena, Manvendra Singh, Dinesh Chandra, Anil Bhan
- **Care of Patient on Anticoagulation**
  Vinayak Agarwal, Devendra Richhariya
- **Cardiac Biomarkers**
  Rahul Mehrotra
- **Electrocardiogram Interpretation in Emergency**
  Kartikeya Bhargava
- **Role of Echocardiography in Emergency Room**
  Mansi Kaushik, Manish Bansal, Ravi R Kasliwal
- **Coronary Computed Tomography in Emergency**
  Kulbir Ahlawat, Devendra Richhariya
- **Precardiac Surgery Evaluation**
  Bhanu Prakash Zawar, Yatin Mehta
- **Postcardiac Surgical Emergencies**
  Nishant Arora, Yatin Mehta

Chapter 22

Chest Pain

Rohit Goel, Rashmi Xavier, Nagendra Singh Chouhan, Praveen Chandra

INTRODUCTION

Acute chest pain is one of the most common reasons for emergency hospital visits accounting for approximately 8 million visits per annum in the United States. The main difficulty arises in differentiating the acute coronary syndrome (ACS) patients and other life-threatening causes of chest pain with other nonlife-threatening noncardiovascular causes of chest pain. It has been seen that the mortality rates increases by twofold in acute myocardial infarction patients which were discharged prematurely from the hospital as compared to those admitted. Also in patients with low-risk of complications, the cost of further investigations and hospital admission needs to be weighed apart from the small risk associated with the diagnostic procedures.

Recent advances in the medical field have improved the accuracy and efficiency in the evaluation of patients with chest pain. Development of new cardiac biomarkers (acute MI), radionuclide studies for low-risk patients, multislice CT scan for coronary artery disease (CAD), pulmonary embolism, aortic dissection has improved the management of these patients. Also the setting of chest pain units and pain pathways for evaluating the low-risk patients helps in the better outcome of the patients.

CAUSES OF CHEST PAIN

The causes of chest pain vary from life-threatening conditions needing urgent medical care to those that are relatively benign and nonlife-threatening **(Fig. 1 and Table 1)**.

Studies have shown that approximately one-third to one-half of patients have musculoskeletal chest pain, 10–20% have a gastrointestinal causes, 10% have stable angina, 5% have respiratory conditions, and approximately 2–4% have acute myocardial ischemia (including myocardial infarction).

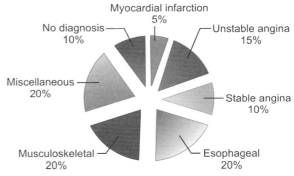

Fig. 1 Causes of chest pain

Table 1 Common causes of chest pain

Cardiac: Coronary artery disease, aortic valve disease, mitral valve disease, pericarditis, pulmonary hypertension and aortic stenosis *Pulmonary*: Pulmonary embolism, pneumothorax, pneumonia pleuritis *Vascular*: Aortic dissection, aortic aneurysm	*Musculoskeletol*: Costochondritis arthritis, muscular spasm *Gastrointestinal*: Ulcer disease, bowel diseases cholecystitis, pancreatitis, and hiatus hernia

Cardiac Causes

- *Myocardial ischemia*: Angina pectoris is defined as chest pain attributable to myocardial ischemia. Symptoms in chronic stable angina include heaviness, tightness, or constriction in the center or left side of the chest which gets precipitated on exertion and relieved by rest. Other associated symptoms include provocation with emotional stress or cold and radiating to the neck, jaw, and shoulder. Sometimes patient do not present with classical angina but, angina-like symptoms such as dyspnea, nausea and vomiting, diaphoresis, presyncope, or palpitations. These set of patients are mostly women, diabetics and elderly population.

Patients presenting with ACS (myocardial infarction and unstable angina) have anginal symptoms at rest, or new onset angina that is more frequent, prolonged in duration and occurs with less exertion. These patients should be referred to an emergency department and managed on a priority basis. Coronary heart disease (CHD) is the most common cause of myocardial ischemia. Other less common causes include coronary dissection, and vasospastic angina (Prinzmetal's angina) **(Tables 2 and 3)**.

- *Nonischemic causes of chest pain*:
  - *Aortic dissection*: This condition is rare but a true surgical emergency needing immediate care. Typical symptoms include acute onset of chest and back pain that is severe, sharp, and tearing in nature radiating anywhere to the chest or into the abdomen.
  - *Heart failure*: Patients with heart failure may present with chest discomfort, usually associated with dyspnea, orthopnea, cough and peripheral edema.
  - *Pericarditis*: Acute pericarditis refers to inflammation of the pericardium due to variety of causes. Patients often complain of pleuritic chest pain increasing on deep inspiration and relieved by sitting up and leaning forward. It is diagnosed based on history, physical examination, and electrocardiogram (ECG) findings. Etiologies include infections, drugs, autoimmune disorders, and malignancy.
  - *Stress cardiomyopathy*: Stress (takotsubo) cardiomyopathy or apical ballooning syndrome occurs in the setting of physical or emotional stress or critical illness. Its clinical presentation is similar to that of acute myocardial infarction and needs to be suspected in patients with no traditional risk factors for CAD and classical Echo findings.
  - *Mitral valve disease*: Patients with mitral stenosis uncommonly experience chest pain or heaviness. This is most often due to pulmonary arterial hypertension and right ventricular hypertrophy seen in these patients.

    Patients with mitral valve prolapse may also experience chest pain, is usually mild, but often troubling.

Pulmonary Causes

Life-threatening pulmonary causes of chest pain include pulmonary embolism and tension pneumothorax.

- *Pulmonary embolism*: The most common symptoms of pulmonary embolism include dyspnea, pleuritic chest pain, cough, sometimes hemoptysis. Often patients may have symptoms of deep venous thrombosis. Most common sign is sinus tachycardia. A high index of suspicion should be kept in mind while considering this diagnosis as it can be life-threatening if left undiagnosed. So past history of major surgery, malignancy, prolonged hospitalization and immobilization should be enquired into.
- *Pneumothorax*: Patients with spontaneous pneumothorax present with sudden onset of pleuritic chest pain and dyspnea. A diagnosis of tension pneumothorax is considered if the patient is hemodynamically unstable.

    Primary spontaneous pneumothorax is usually seen in young, tall, and thin individuals with no underlying lung disease. A secondary spontaneous pneumothorax occurs as a complication of underlying lung disease [e.g. chronic obstructive pulmonary disease (COPD)].
- *Pneumonia*: Patients may have chest pain, often pleuritic but associated with fever and productive cough.

Table 2 Features of myocardial ischemia and coronary occlusion

Pain: Severe, sudden onset, substernal, crushing, tightness, radiate to shoulder neck, back jaw, and arm may not be relieved by nitroglycerin	• Dyspnea • Syncope • Nausea • Vomiting • Extreme weakness • Diaphoresis • Increase in heart rate

Table 3 Differentiating features of cardiac and noncardiac chest pain

Characteristic	Ischemic cardiac chest pain	Noncardiac chest pain
Location	Central, diffuse	Peripheral, localized
Radiation	Jaw/neck/shoulder/arm (occasionally back)	Other or no radiation
Character	Tight, squeezing, choking	Sharp, stabbing, catching
Precipitation	Exertion and/or emotion	Spontaneous, provoked by posture, respiration or palpitation
Relieving factor	Rest, quick response to nitrates	Not relieved by rest, slow or no response to nitrates
Associated features	Breathlessness	Respiratory, gastrointestinal, locomotor or psychological

- *Malignancy*: Patients may complain of chest pain, typically on the same side as the primary tumor. Other symptoms include cough, hemoptysis, and dyspnea, and weight loss.
- *Pulmonary hypertension*: Patients with pulmonary hypertension may have chest pain on exertion in addition to exertional dyspnea and syncope.

Gastrointestinal Causes

- *Esophageal rupture/perforation*: Spontaneous rupture of esophagus (Boerhaave syndrome) may result from a sudden increase in intraesophageal pressure usually seen after vomiting.
- *Gastroesophageal reflux disease (GERD)*: It is the most common clinical condition mimicking angina pectoris. Sometimes patients may describe it as squeezing or burning pain, radiating to the back, neck, jaw, or arms. Pain can last for minutes to hours, and resolves spontaneously or with antacids. It may be seen after meals, during sleep.
- *Esophagitis*: Patients with esophagitis may present with sudden onset retrosternal chest pain. It may be associated with odynophagia. It can be due to candidiasis, cytomegalovirus (in HIV-AIDS), or radiation injury.
- *Others*: Hiatus hernias may cause chest pain in addition to symptoms of reflux. Esophageal motility disorders/esophageal spasm generally manifest with dysphagia, but sometimes patients may complain of chest pain.

Musculoskeletal Causes

Musculoskeletal causes are commonly seen in patients who present to the primary care physician with chest pain.
- *Isolated musculoskeletal chest pain syndrome*: Patients usually have local or regional chest wall tenderness without any other symptom. The most common causes are costochondritis and lower rib pain syndromes.
- *Rib pain*: Rib fractures are associated with pleuritic chest pain that is localized and reproducible with palpation. Patients often describe an associated injury/trauma, though some may occur without trauma. Other systemic disorders such as osteoporosis, metastasis, and infarction from sickle-cell anemia can also cause acute rib pain.

Psychiatric Causes

Chest pain is a common complaint in a wide variety of psychiatric disorders such as panic attack, depression, and somatization disorder. So a good clinical history and atypical symptoms in young individuals should raise a suspicion of underlying psychiatric illness.

However, patients with underlying psychiatric illness may have coexisting CAD; hence, a sound clinical judgment is needed.

Others

- *Substance abuse*: Cocaine abuse is commonly associated with myocardial ischemia. Other cardiac complications which can be seen include aortic dissection, coronary artery aneurysm, myocarditis and cardiomyopathy, and arrhythmias.

    Methamphetamine intoxication mimics cocaine and can cause similar cardiac complications.
- *Herpes zoster*: Sometimes chest pain may be the presenting symptom of herpes zoster, preceding the rash but is localized to a particular dermatome. Postherpetic neuralgia may also present with chest pain.
- *Domestic violence*: Patients may complain of chest pain or have chest pain in the setting of psychiatric conditions after suffering from intimate partner violence. In a community based population, chest pain was one of the many physical symptoms associated with domestic violence.

EVALUATION

A detailed clinical history, physical examination and relevant blood tests help in determining the probable cause of chest pain and the urgency of any intervention.

Unstable patients or patients with high suspicion of ACS or any other life-threatening condition (e.g. aortic dissection, pulmonary embolism, and Boerhaave syndrome) should be referred to the emergency department and managed on a priority basis **(Flow chart 1 and Table 4)**.

History

Patient presenting with chest pain should be evaluated with a detailed description of the pain and other associated symptoms.

Description

It often helps in differentiating cardiac from noncardiac chest pain. Symptoms associated with a relatively high risk of myocardial infarction include radiation to an upper

Flow chart 1 Step-by-step diagnostic approach

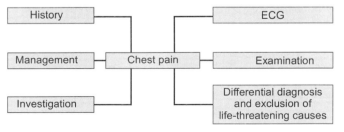

extremity, associated with diaphoresis or nausea and vomiting. However, no symptom alone or in combination helps in identifying patients in whom the diagnosis can be excluded safely.

Table 4 Differential diagnosis of chest pain

Potentially life-threatening causes	Common nonlife-threatening causes

• Acute coronary syndromes
  – Acute myocardial infarction
    - ST segment elevation MI
    - Non-ST segment elevation MI
  – Unstable angina
• Pulmonary embolism
• Aortic dissection
• Myocarditis (most common cause of sudden death in the young)
• Tension pneumothorax
• Acute chest syndrome (in sickle cell disease)
• Pericarditis
• Boerhaave's syndrome (perforated esophagus)
	• Gastrointestinal
	  – Biliary colic
	  – Gastroesophageal reflux
	  – Peptic ulcer disease
	• Pulmonary
	  – Pneumonia
	  – Pleurisy
	• Chest wall syndromes
	  – Musculoskeletal pain
	  – Costochondritis
	  – Thoracic radiculopathy
	  – Texidor's twinge (precordial catch syndrome)
	• Psychiatric
	  – Anxiety
	• Shingles

Quality

Chest pain can be pleuritic, positional, sharp or dull, ripping or tearing, or tender on palpation. It is also important to enquire whether the quality of the pain is similar to a previous episode if any. In a known case of CAD, pain similar to previous episodes is related to myocardial ischemia.
- A pleuritic chest pain gets worse on deep respiration. Causes include pericarditis, pulmonary embolism, pneumothorax, pleuritis, and pneumonia.
- Positional pain which improves on sitting and leaning forward suggests pericarditis.
- Ripping or tearing pain point toward aortic dissection.

Location and Radiation

Ischemic pain is often diffuse and poorly localized. Well-localized pain associated with finger tenderness is more likely to be musculoskeletal in nature.

Ischemic pain often radiates to the neck, throat, lower jaw, teeth, upper extremity, or shoulder **(Figs 2A to H)**.

Temporal Factors

Acute onset of chest pain suggests pneumothorax, aortic dissection, esophageal rupture/perforation, or pulmonary

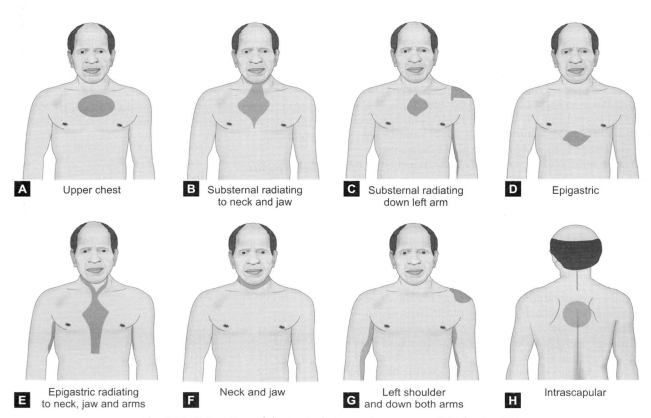

Figs 2A to H Locations of chest pain during angina or myocardial infarction (MI)

embolism. However, the onset of ischemic pain is more gradual (over a period of few minutes) and gradually increasing in intensity over time.

Chest discomfort that lasts only for seconds or is constant over weeks is unlikely to be ischemic in origin. Myocardial ischemic pain usually lasts not more than 20–30 minutes, though it may be prolonged in the setting of a myocardial infarction.

Exacerbating Factors

Chest discomfort on exertion is a classic symptom of angina. Sometimes esophageal pain can also present in a similar pattern. Other factors that may provoke ischemic pain include cold, emotional stress, meals, or sexual intercourse. Discomfort occurring with eating is suggestive of gastrointestinal etiology. Pain worsened on swallowing is likely to be esophageal in origin.

Relieving Factors

Pain that subsides with cessation of activity strongly suggests an ischemic origin. Pericarditis pain typically improves with sitting up and leaning forward.

Pain palliated by antacids or food is likely to be gastroesophageal in origin.

However, pain which responds to sublingual nitroglycerin is usually associated with cardiac etiology but may be due to esophageal spasm as well.

Other Associated Symptoms

Other associated symptoms may help in distinguishing the various etiologies of chest pain. However, sometimes even these symptoms may not reliably distinguish between cardiac and gastrointestinal origins of chest pain.
- *Cardiac symptoms*: Presyncope can be seen in patients with myocardial ischemia. However, it is also associated with other pathologies such as aortic dissection, a hemodynamically significant pulmonary embolus, or critical aortic stenosis.

  Palpitations are often the complaint in patients with ischemia due to ventricular ectopics or atrial fibrillation.
- *Pulmonary symptoms*: Exertional dyspnea may be considered an anginal equivalent, but it is also associated with other cardiac (e.g. aortic stenosis, atrial fibrillation) and pulmonary (e.g. asthma or chronic obstructive lung disease, pulmonary hypertension) causes of chest pain.

  Cough is associated with infection, neoplasm, pulmonary embolism, and gastroesophageal reflux disease (GERD).
- *Gastrointestinal symptoms*: GERD is associated with heartburn, regurgitation, and dysphagia. Belching, difficult or painful swallowing are suggestive of esophageal disease, although belching and indigestion may also be seen in patients with myocardial ischemia. Nausea and vomiting are often seen in the setting of myocardial ischemia in addition to gastrointestinal problems.
- *Musculoskeletal symptoms*: Occurrence of pain in the neck, thoracic spine, or shoulder may cause referred pain to the chest. Chronic widespread musculoskeletal pain is associated with fibromyalgia.
- *Systemic symptoms*: Presence of fever leads to infective or autoimmune etiologies for chest pain. Fatigue, weight loss, and other constitutional symptoms raise concerns for malignancy or rheumatologic etiologies.
- *Psychiatric symptoms*: Pain associated with panic may be due to panic disorder. Patients with depressed mood, decreased appetite, or sleep disturbances may have underlying depression.

Other Relevant Medical History

The clinical impression based on pain description and associated symptoms must be interpreted together with other aspects of the history.
- *Age*: Certain etiologies are more likely to occur at a particular age than others. For example, cardiovascular diseases (CVD) are more common in the elderly population even in the absence of traditional risk factors. Pneumonia is more common cause of chest pain in children.
- *Past medical history*: It is equally important in assessing the likelihood of various causes of chest pain. Diabetes, hypertension, smoking and dyslipidemia are traditional risk factors for CHD. Prolonged immobilization, recent surgery, and trauma all increase the probability of pulmonary embolism. Hence, knowledge about such risk factors provides important information regarding likelihood of a particular disease.

Physical Examination

- *Vital signs*: Presence of hemodynamic instability is an indication for immediate referral to the emergency department.

  Presence of hypoxemia points toward pulmonary or cardiac etiologies of chest pain whereas fever raises suspicion for infectious or autoimmune disease.

  In patients suspected of aortic dissection, blood pressure should be checked in both the arms and lower limbs.
- *Cardiac examination*: A complete examination should be performed to evaluate for rate, rhythm, murmurs, and extra heart sounds.

  In pericarditis one should examine in both supine and sitting and leaning forward position. This assesses for a pericardial rub which may only be present in the sitting position.

- *Pulmonary examination*: It should be done to evaluate for symmetrical breath sounds, wheezing, crackles, and any evidence of consolidation.
- *Musculoskeletal examination*: Chest pain reproducible with palpation may indicate musculoskeletal pain.

    Hyperesthesia associated with a rash is often due to herpes zoster. The presence of subcutaneous emphysema suggests Boerhaave syndrome or pneumothorax.
- *Abdominal examination*: A careful examination of the abdomen is required to assess for any referred pain, with attention to the right upper quadrant, epigastrium, and the abdominal aorta.

Electrocardiogram

An ECG should be obtained for all the patients with new onset of chest pain or any pain that is different from previous episodes of noncardiac pain. ECG is very helpful in the evaluation of patients with suspected myocardial ischemia as well as in making a diagnosis of many other etiologies.

Patients with ECG findings suggestive of ACS should be referred to the emergency room for further evaluation and management.

Those patients with a history suggestive of ACS but a normal ECG should have serial ECGs done and monitored in the emergency department. A normal ECG helps in ruling out ACS but findings must be interpreted in the context of the clinical history and physical examination.

Sometimes ECG also helps in making a diagnosis of nonischemic chest pain such as acute pericarditis (diffuse ST elevation with PR depression), pulmonary embolism [sinus tachycardia, right bundle branch block (RBBB), right axis deviation (RAD), and S1Q3T3 pattern]. So, in an emergency department, an ECG should be obtained in all the patients presenting with chest pain.

Other Studies

Laboratory tests and other studies such as chest radiograph, cardiac enzymes are determined on initial evaluation and varies depending upon the need. Many patients will not need any additional tests for their chest pain evaluation. When there is a possibility of ACS, cardiac enzymes (CK-MB and Trop-I) should be tested.

Chest X-ray if pneumonia, tension pneumothorax is the possibility. Two-dimensional (2D)-Echo for cardiac tamponade, aortic dissection, multislice CT for pulmonary embolism, and aortic dissection.

DIAGNOSTIC APPROACH

The following is a diagnostic approach toward patients presenting with chest pain in the emergency department with priority for life-threatening conditions.

Life-threatening conditions: Patients with life-threatening causes of chest pain should be referred immediately to the emergency department. These include patients with:
- Hemodynamic instability
- Sudden onset of chest pain and/or suspected life-threatening etiology such as pulmonary embolism, aortic dissection, esophageal rupture, and tension pneumothorax.
- Suspected ACS based on history (angina at rest, prolonged, or progressive) or ECG changes. Appropriate initial interventions should also be started such as 325 mg of aspirin tablet, sublingual nitroglycerin, and intravenous morphine.

EVALUATION OF CHEST PAIN OF CARDIAC ORIGIN

Evaluation of chest pain of cardiac origin is described in **Flow chart 2**.

EVALUATION OF CHEST PAIN OF VARIOUS CAUSES (FLOW CHART 3)

Evaluation for Stable Angina

Patients with symptoms consistent with stable angina should be evaluated for myocardial ischemia. The choice of diagnostic testing will depend upon the clinical setting, e.g. in patients with high suspicion for CHD, a stress test and/or myocardial perfusion scan should be done. Whereas in patients suspected for aortic stenosis or hypertrophic cardiomyopathy, an echocardiogram is more appropriate.

Also patients with multiple risk factors for CVD (e.g. diabetes, dyslipidemia, hypertension and/or tobacco use) or with atypical anginal symptoms (e.g. women, elderly, or diabetics), a noninvasive test can be performed if there is a strong clinical suspicion of myocardial ischemia.

Evaluation for Nonischemic Cardiac Etiologies

It depends upon the presenting signs or symptom which varies with the underlying etiology. For example, patients with pericarditis will have pleuritic chest pain and certain ECG findings.

Patients with acute decompensated heart failure will have associated dyspnea, orthopnea and peripheral edema.

Suspected Pulmonary Etiology

Patients with pulmonary causes for chest pain generally do not have symptoms consistent with classical angina. They have associated respiratory symptoms such as cough, sputum, and may be hypoxemic. A chest radiograph or any other chest imaging may be indicated depending upon the scenario.

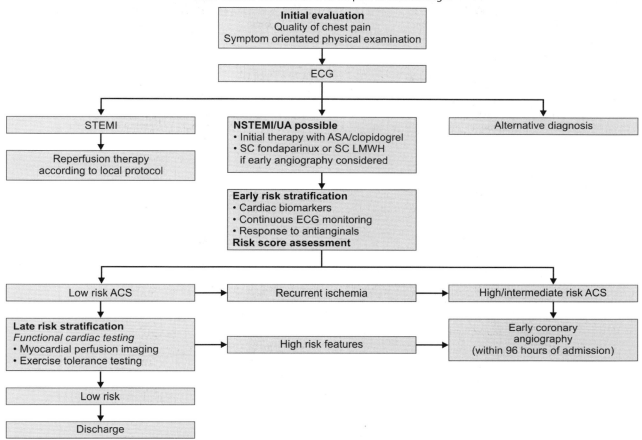

Flow chart 2 Evaluation of chest pain of cardiac origin

Suspected Gastrointestinal Etiology

Patients often complain of heartburn, regurgitation, pain with meals, and indigestion. However, some patients may also complain of angina like symptoms. These patients should be evaluated for myocardial ischemia, particularly if they have underlying risk factors for CVD, prior to evaluation/treatment for gastrointestinal pathology.

Patients with a normal cardiac evaluation and anginal-like chest pain often have GERD. GERD can be diagnosed based on clinical history and prompt response to therapy.

Suspected Musculoskeletal Etiology

If on evaluation there is point tenderness that is reproducible with palpation and there is no evidence of underlying systemic illness, further testing is not indicated. A trial of physiotherapy or nonsteroidal anti-inflammatory medication may help in confirming the diagnosis.

Suspected Psychiatric Etiology

If all other etiologies have been evaluated and ruled out (by history, physical examination, and/or testing) and the patient's history is consistent with psychiatric symptoms, he should be evaluated for psychiatric etiologies, particularly panic disorder. A therapeutic trial of cognitive behavioral therapy and/or antidepressant medication may be indicated.

Others

If all the other etiologies have been evaluated and ruled out or the history and physical examination are not consistent with the underlying etiologies, less common causes of chest pain such as herpes zoster and pain referred to the chest from other organs such as from the gallbladder, diaphragm, or from a disk herniation should be considered.

Patients with referred pain will often have associated symptoms or physical examination findings that support a particular diagnosis.

SUMMARY AND RECOMMENDATIONS

- The most common cause of chest pain in primary care practice is musculoskeletal pain and gastrointestinal conditions.

SECTION 3 Cardiac Emergencies

Flow chart 3 Evaluation of chest pain of various causes

```
Risk factors for cardiac disease?
• First episode of pain
• Pain radiating to arm or back
• Associated dizziness or collapse
• History of cardiac, clotting, connecting tissue or Kawasaki's disease
• Long standing diabetes mellitus
• Cocaine or other stimulant use
• Abnormal pulse or blood pressure
   │ Yes → ECG, CXR. If high risk, consider troponin +/− echo → Is there still a possibility of cardiac disease? → Yes → Discuss with cardiology
   │ No
   ▼
Risk factors for pulmonary embolus?
• Immobility or recent surgery
• Neoplasm
• Hypercoagulability
• Central venous catheter
• Pleuritic pain
• Hemoptysis
• Hypoxia
   │ Yes → CXR → CXR clear or minor abnormality? → Yes → Consider PE, ECG, V/Q scan, Discuss with respiratory unit
   │                                              → No
   │ No
   ▼
Respiratory symptoms or signs?
   │ Yes → CXR → Abnormal CXR → Yes → Pneumothorax, Pneumonia foreign body
   │                           → No → Exercise-induced asthma, Radiolucent foreign body, Hyperventilation
   │ No
   ▼
Pain related to eating? Abdominal tenderness?
   │ Yes → Consider gastrointestinal cause
   │ No
   ▼
Risk factors for serious psychiatric disease?
• Lowered affected or lack of motivation
• Hypervigilance
• Hyperventilation
• Social withdrawal
• Impairmental or function at school
• Drug and alcohol use
   │ Yes → Consider serious underlying psychological cause
   │ No
   ▼
Pain reproducible with movement or palpation?
   │ Yes → Consider musculoskeletal cause
   │ No
   ▼
Psychosomatic or undifferentiated chest pain?
   │ Yes → Reassure and then refer to LMO, general pediatrics or adolescent medicine
```

- Initial evaluation of chest pain starts with a detailed clinical history and physical examination. It helps in assessing the probability of various causes of chest pain and the need for further testing. ECG will be required in many patients suspected of myocardial ischemia.
- Patients with hemodynamic instability or life-threatening pathology [e.g. pulmonary embolism, aortic dissection, esophageal rupture, tension pneumothorax, acute coronary syndrome (ACS)] should be referred to the emergency department and managed on a priority basis.

Patients with suspected ACS due to classical history or ECG changes should be given 325 mg aspirin tablet to chew.
- Symptoms consistent with stable angina should be further evaluated for myocardial ischemia. The appropriate diagnostic test will depend on the most likely etiology.
- In patients with a negative work-up for myocardial ischemia or in whom clinical suspicion is low, further evaluation depends upon the most likely diagnosis that emerges from the initial evaluation.

BIBLIOGRAPHY

1. Adams JE III, Abendschein DR, Jaffe AS. Biochemical markers of myocardial injury: is MB creatine kinase the choice for the 1990s? Circulation. 1993;88:750-63.
2. American College of Emergency Physicians. Clinical policy for the initial approach to adults presenting with a chief complaint of chest pain, with no history of trauma. Ann Emerg Med. 1995;25:274-99.
3. Antman EM, Grudzien C, Sacks DB. Evaluation of a rapid bedside assay for detection of serum cardiac troponin T. JAMA. 1995;273:1279-82.
4. Antman EM, Tanasijevic MJ, Thompson B, et al. Cardiac-specific troponin I levels to predict the risk of mortality in patients with acute coronary syndromes. N Engl J Med. 1996;335:1342-9.
5. Braunwald E, Jones RH, Mark DB, et al. Unstable angina: diagnosis and management. Clinical practice guideline number 10. Rev. Rockville, Md.: Agency for Health Care Policy and Research, National Heart, Lung, and Blood Institute, May 1994. (AHCPR publication no. 94-0602.)
6. Colon PJ III, Mobarek SK, Milani RV, et al. Prognostic value of stress echocardiography in the evaluation of atypical chest pain patients without known coronary artery disease. Am J Cardiol. 1998;81:545-51.
7. Corey GA, Merenstein JH. Applying the acute ischemic heart disease predictive instrument. J Fam Pract. 1987;25:127-33.
8. Farkouh ME, Smars PA, Reeder GS, et al. A clinical trial of a chest pain observation unit for patients with unstable angina. N Engl J Med. 1998;339:1882-8.
9. Garber AM, Solomon NA. Cost-effectiveness of alternative test strategies for the diagnosis of coronary artery disease. Ann Intern Med. 1999;130:719-28.
10. Gaspoz JM, Lee TH, Cook EF, et al. Outcome of patients who were admitted to a new short-stay unit to "rule-out" myocardial infarction. Am J Cardiol. 1991;68:145-9.
11. Gaspoz JM, Lee TH, Weinstein MC, et al. Cost-effectiveness of a new short-stay unit to "rule out" acute myocardial infarction in low risk patients. J Am Coll Cardiol. 1994;24:1249-59.
12. Gibler WB, Runyon JP, Levy RC, et al. A rapid diagnostic and treatment center for patients with chest pain in the emergency department. Ann Emerg Med. 1995;25:1-8.
13. Goldman L, Cook EF, Brand DA, et al. A computer protocol to predict myocardial infarction in emergency department patients with chest pain. N Engl J Med. 1988;318:797-803.
14. Goldman L, Cook EF, Johnson PA, et al. Prediction of the need for intensive care in patients who come to emergency departments with acute chest pain. N Engl J Med. 1996;334:1498-504.
15. Goldman L, Weinberg M, Weisberg M, et al. A computer-derived protocol to aid in the diagnosis of emergency room patients with acute chest pain. N Engl J Med. 1982;307:588-96.
16. Gomez MA, Anderson JL, Karagounis LA, et al. An emergency department-based protocol for rapidly ruling out myocardial ischemia reduces hospital time and expense: results of a randomized study (ROMIO). J Am Coll Cardiol. 1996;28:25-33.
17. Goyal RK. Changing focus on unexplained esophageal chest pain. Ann Intern Med. 1996;124:1008-11.
18. Graff L, Joseph T, Andelman R, et al. American College of Emergency Physicians information paper: chest pain units in emergency departments—a report from the Short-Term Observation Services Section. Am J Cardiol. 1995;76:1036-9.
19. Hamm CW, Goldmann BU, Heeschen C, et al. Emergency room triage of patients with acute chest pain by means of rapid testing for cardiac troponin T or troponin I. N Engl J Med. 1997;337:1648-53.
20. Kontos M, Jesse RL, Anderson P, et al. Comparison of myocardial perfusion imaging and cardiac troponin I in patients admitted to the emergency department with chest pain. Circulation. 1999;99:2073-8.
21. Kuntz KM, Fleischmann KE, Hunink MG, et al. Cost-effectiveness of diagnostic strategies for patients with chest pain. Ann Intern Med. 1999;130:709-18.
22. Lee TH, Pearson SD, Johnson PA, et al. Failure of information as an intervention to modify clinical management: a time-series trial in patients with acute chest pain. Ann Intern Med. 1995;122:434-7.
23. Lee TH, Rouan GW, Weisberg MC, et al. Clinical characteristics and natural history of patients with acute myocardial infarction sent home from the emergency room. Am J Cardiol. 1987;60:219-24.
24. Lewis WR, Amsterdam EA, Turnipseed S, et al. Immediate exercise testing of low risk patients with known coronary artery disease presenting to the emergency department with chest pain. J Am Coll Cardiol. 1999;33:1843-7.
25. Lewis WR, Amsterdam EA. Utility and safety of immediate exercise testing of low-risk patients admitted to the hospital for suspected acute myocardial infarction. Am J Cardiol 1994;74:987-90.
26. Luscher MS, Thygesen K, Ravkilde J, et al. Applicability of cardiac troponin T and I for early risk stratification in unstable coronary artery disease. Circulation. 1997;96:2578-85.
27. National Heart Attack Alert Program Coordinating Committee 60 Minutes to Treatment Working Group. Emergency department: rapid identification and treatment of patients with acute myocardial infarction. Washington, DC: National Heart, Lung, and Blood Institute, September 1993. (NIH publication no. 93-3278.)
28. Newby LK, Christenson RH, Ohman EM, et al. Value of serial troponin T measures for early and late risk stratification in patients with acute coronary syndromes. Circulation. 1998;98:1853-9.
29. Nichol G, Walls R, Goldman L, et al. A critical pathway for management of patients with acute chest pain who are at low

risk for myocardial ischemia: recommendations and potential impact. Ann Intern Med. 1997;127:996-1005.
30. Panju AA, Hemmelgarn BR, Guyatt GH, et al. Is this patient having a myocardial infarction? JAMA. 1998;280:1256-63.
31. Pearson SD, Goldman L, Garcia TB, et al. Physician response to a prediction rule for the triage of emergency department patients with chest pain. J Gen Intern Med. 1994;9:241-7.
32. Polanczyk CA, Johnson PA, Cook EF, et al. A proposed strategy for utilization of creatine kinase-MB and troponin I in the evaluation of acute chest pain. Am J Cardiol 1999;83:1175-9.
33. Polanczyk CA, Johnson PA, Hartley LH, et al. Clinical correlates and prognostic significance of early negative exercise tolerance test in patients with acute chest pain seen in the hospital emergency department. Am J Cardiol. 1998;81:288-92.
34. Polanczyk CA, Lee TH, Cook EF, et al. Cardiac troponin I as a predictor of major cardiac events in emergency department patients with acute chest pain. J Am Coll Cardiol. 1998;32:8-14.
35. Pope JH, Aufderheide TP, Ruthazer R, et al. Missed diagnoses of acute cardiac ischemia in the emergency department. N Engl J Med. 2000;342:1163-70.
36. Pozen MW, D'Agostino RB, Selker HP, et al. A predictive instrument to improve coronary-care unit admission practices in acute ischemic heart disease: a prospective multicenter clinical trial. N Engl J Med. 1984;310:1273-8.
37. Pozen MW, D'Agostino RB, Mitchell JB, et al. The usefulness of a predictive instrument to reduce inappropriate admission to the coronary care unit. Ann Intern Med. 1980;92:238-42.
38. Prêtre R, Von Segesser LK. Aortic dissection. Lancet. 1997;349:1461-4.
39. Puleo PR, Meyer D, Wathen C, et al. Use of a rapid assay of subforms of creatine kinase MB to diagnose or rule out acute myocardial infarction. N Engl J Med. 1994;331:561-6.
40. Roberts RR, Zalenski RJ, Mensah EK, et al. Costs of an emergency department-based accelerated diagnostic protocol vs hospitalization in patients with chest pain: a randomized controlled trial. JAMA. 1997;278:1670-6.
41. Rusnak RA, Stair TO, Hansen K, et al. Litigation against the emergency physician: common features in cases of missed myocardial infarction. Ann Emerg Med. 1989;18:1029-34.
42. Ryan TJ, Antman EM, Brooks NH, et al. 1999 Update: ACC/AHA guidelines for the management of patients with acute myocardial infarction: executive summary and recommendations: a report of the American College of Cardiology/American Heart Association Task Force on Practice Guidelines (Committee on Management of Acute Myocardial Infarction). Circulation. 1999;100:1016-30.
43. Selker HP, Beshansky JR, Griffith JL, et al. Use of the acute cardiac ischemic time-insensitive predictive instrument (ACI-TIPI) to assist with triage of patients with chest pain or other symptoms suggestive of acute cardiac ischemia: a multicenter, controlled clinical trial. Ann Intern Med. 1998;129:845-55.
44. The Platelet Receptor Inhibition in Ischemic Syndrome Management in Patients Limited by Unstable Signs and Symptoms (PRISM-PLUS) Study Investigators. Inhibition of the platelet glycoprotein IIb/IIIa receptor with tirofiban in unstable angina and non-Q-wave myocardial infarction. N Engl J Med. 1998;338:1488-97. [Erratum, N Engl J Med 1998;339:415.]
45. Tosteson ANA, Goldman L, Udvarhelyi IS, et al. Cost-effectiveness of a coronary care unit versus an intermediate care unit for emergency department patients with chest pain. Circulation. 1996;94:143-50.
46. Weingarten SR, Riedinger MS, Conner L, et al. Practice guidelines and reminders to reduce duration of hospital stay for patients with chest pain: an interventional trial. Ann Intern Med. 1994;120:257-63.
47. Zimmerman J, Fromm R, Meyer D, et al. Diagnostic marker cooperative study for the diagnosis of myocardial infarction. Circulation. 1999;99:1671-7.

CHAPTER 23

Palpitations

Shashank Chauhan, Ram NG, HR Tomar

INTRODUCTION

Palpitations by definition are noticeably rapid, strong, regular or irregular sensation of heartbeat that could be because of a cardiac or a noncardiac cause. One may feel the palpitations in the chest, neck or throat. This feeling may or may not accompany other signs and symptoms of hemodynamic or neurological compromise.

ETIOLOGY

Most of the cases are triggered by a hyperadrenergic drive that causes a surge in the level of adrenaline in the circulation. This happens on overexertion, nervousness or when someone is anxious or excited. Food articles like caffeine, alcohol, excessive smoking, recreational drug abuse (cocaine, amphetamines, cannabis) can all bring on palpitations. Moreover, panic attacks too can trigger palpitations. Some medications like adrenergic agonists, thyroid medications can also trigger the same feeling of palpitations. Moreover, palpitations do occur in women during the menstrual cycle (luteal phase), pregnancy and around the menopausal period due to hormonal imbalance.

Apart from these relatively benign causes of palpitations presenting to emergency department (ED), emphasis should be made to identify and treat the more grievous and sometimes life-threatening palpitations in the ED, which turns out to be the true emergencies. Most patients with arrhythmias do not complain of palpitations. However, any arrhythmia including sinus tachycardia, atrial fibrillation, premature ventricular contractions or ventricular tachycardia can cause palpitations. These palpitations require a high precision and clinical acumen of an emergency physician and the cardiologist for successful reversion of cardiac arrhythmia, and thus saving a life.

DIFFERENTIAL DIAGNOSIS OF PALPITATIONS

Differential diagnosis includes:
- Arrhythmias
- Atrial fibrillation or flutter
- Bradycardia due to advance AV dissociation
- Sick sinus syndrome
- Multifocal atrial tachycardia
- Premature supraventricular or ventricular contractions
- Sinus tachycardia or arrhythmia
- Atrioventricular reentry tachycardia (AVRT) or AV nodal reentrant tachycardia (AVNRT).

Psychiatric Causes

Psychiatric causes are as follows:
- Anxiety disorders
- Panic attacks.

Drugs

Drugs include:
- Alcohol
- Caffeine
- Digitalis, phenothiazine, theophylline, beta-agonists
- Cocaine
- Tobacco.

Nonarrhythmic Cardiac Causes

Nonarrhythmic cardiac causes include:
- Atrial or ventricular septal defects
- Cardiomyopathy
- Congenital heart disease
- Congestive heart failure

- Mitral valve prolapse
- Pacemaker-mediated tachycardia
- Valvular diseases.

Extracardiac Causes

Extracardiac causes are:
- Anemia
- Electrolyte imbalance
- Fever
- Hyperthyroidism
- Hypoglycemia
- Pheochromocytoma
- Pulmonary disease.

Consensus or evidence-based guidelines for diagnosing and managing palpitations in the ED have not been developed. However, a recent cohort study of palpitation etiology in patients presenting to the ED claims to determine the etiology in 83% of patients. Of these 43% had palpitations caused by cardiac causes, 31% had palpitations caused by anxiety or panic disorders, 6% had palpitations due to the prescribed drugs or recreational drug abuse, 4% had palpitations caused by other noncardiac causes. No specific cause of the palpitations could be identified in 16% of patients. Psychiatric or emotional disturbances such as anxiety or somatization were found out to be the underlying problem for palpitations in many patients.

MANAGING PALPITATIONS

A 12-lead electrocardiogram (ECG) evaluation is appropriate in all patients who present with palpitations in the ED. In the event that the patient is having ongoing palpitation during the recording of ECG, the physicians may be able to confirm the diagnosis of arrhythmia on spot, and treat likewise. Many ECG findings warrant further cardiac investigation.

If the etiology of palpitations is not apparent after the history, physical examination and ECG are completed, consider ambulatory cardiac monitoring. The rule of thumb in managing palpitations due to arrhythmias is assessing the stability of the patient.

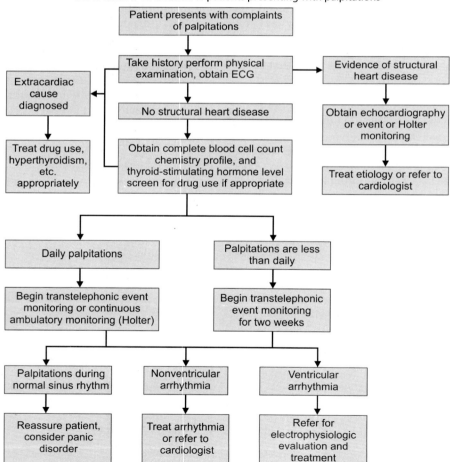

Flow chart 1 Evaluation of patients presenting with palpitations

If the patient is not compromised— no pain, no dyspnea, no hemodynamic or neurological compromise—you have some time. Take a short history and examination, get the patient monitored and acquire a 12-lead ECG and treat likewise.

If the patient is compromised—with pain, dyspnea, hemodynamic or neurological instability—*this is an emergency*. In such case, secure the airway if required, attach a defibrillator and treat as per the diagnosis.

MANAGEMENT PEARLS

Catecholamines release at times of intense emotional experience and sometimes with intense exercise may trigger ventricular or supraventricular tachycardias (SVTs). Similarly an increase in vagal tone after exercise occasionally can lead to episodes of atrial fibrillation. Some physicians may prematurely blame palpitations as anxiety. In one of the study done in the West, two-thirds of patients of SVTs were diagnosed with panic, stress or anxiety disorder, and one-half of the patients had unrecognized arrhythmia on the initial evaluation; this was particularly true among young females. Thus even in cases where panic disorder is suggested, ECG or Holter monitoring is important to pick the arrhythmia.

The **Flow chart 1** can be used in the evaluation of patients with palpitations.

Note: Careful risk stratification should be done to determine which patient requires admission and further investigations, and which patient can be safely discharged.

Not all patients presenting with palpitations in the ED are diagnosed there itself. For those in whom a specific diagnosis is not made, further workup will depend on the frequency and nature of symptoms. In such patients, referral for Holter ± echocardiography and subsequent cardiology follow-up should be advised.

The patients getting discharged from the ED should be given advice regarding future episodes of palpitations. Patients should be asked to refrain from stimulants such as caffeine, alcohol, etc. It is always beneficial to keep a record of such visits and the ECGs, as it aids in making the diagnosis. Patients of recurrent SVTs should be taught the vagal maneuvers to attempt to terminate the SVT episode till they reach to a hospital. This will improvise the quality care of patients and reduce the unwanted visits thus smoothening the patient flow in the ED.

BIBLIOGRAPHY

1. Barsky AJ. Palpitations, arrhythmias, and awareness of cardiac activity. Ann Intern Med. 2001;134(9 Pt 2):832-7.
2. Ehlers A, Mayou RA, Sprigings DC, et al. Pychological and perceptual factors associated with arrhythmias and benign palpitations. Psychosom Med. 2000;62(5):693-702.
3. Marx J, Walls R, Hockberger R. Rosen's emergency medicine: arrhythmias. Elsevier Health Sciences; 2013. p. 2808.
4. The Royal College of Emergency Medicine. (2015). Palpitations management in the ED. [online]. Available from *www.rcem.ac.uk*. [Accessed January, 2017].

CHAPTER 24

Syncope

Brajesh Kumar Mishra

INTRODUCTION

Syncope is a common, disabling, and often challenging symptom. It can cause fall and injury, and can be the warning sign before sudden cardiac death. *Syncope is defined as transient loss of consciousness (TLOC) due to transient global cerebral hypoperfusion,*[1] *it has three important features: (1) rapid onset, (2) short duration, and (3) complete recovery.* Differentiation of syncope from other causes of TLOC like seizure and "syncope mimics" (pseudoseizure, nonsyncopal TLOC and psychological disorder) is very important for emergency physician while evaluating such type of patient.

EPIDEMIOLOGY

Transient loss of consciousness events of suspected syncope are highly prevalent in the general population.[2] It affects about 50% of human being in their lifetime. First episode occurs generally around the age of 15 years, it is more common in female population, around age of 65 years. Syncope rises sharply as age increases. Syncope contributes to about 1% of total in hospital admission and 3% of emergency evaluation, although this is just tip of the iceberg because less than 50% of patients of syncope visit emergency department (ED) or consult their doctor.[3]

PATHOPHYSIOLOGY OR MECHANISM

Overall mechanism in syncope is transient cerebral hypoperfusion because of decreased cardiac output. Commonly, neurally mediated syncope occurs when ventricular filling is decreased by venous pooling that leads to a fall in cardiac output and blood pressure (BP). Activation of arterial baroreceptors results in rise in catecholamine levels, combined with reduced venous filling, and volume depleted ventricle. Activation of mechanoreceptors "C fibers" found in the atria, ventricles and pulmonary artery can result in "paradoxical" loss of peripheral sympathetic tone and an increase in vagal activity, which ultimately causes vasodilation and bradycardia leading to syncope or presyncope.

CLASSIFICATION

Syncope can be classified according to etiology or mechanism. Classification of syncope according to etiology modified by ESC guidelines versus classification according to mechanism modified by International Study on Syncope of Uncertain Etiology (ISSUE) classification is given in **Figure 1 and Table 1**.

There are two main objectives for evaluation of a patient with syncope in ED:
1. To identify the syncope so that an effective specific treatment strategy can be given
2. To assess the prognosis in view of death, severe adverse events, and syncope recurrence.

During ED evaluation the differential diagnosis of syncope is extensive, main focus remains on the treatment of underlying cause when this is obvious. However, the cause of syncope often remains unclear.

First challenge during evaluation of syncope is to differentiate it from seizure. Epilepsy, stroke, and head trauma, may present with TLOC and syncope-like situations. Taking careful history alone can narrow down the diagnosis. History of previous seizure, head injury, tongue bite, the presence of a tonic-clonic activity, abnormal posturing, incontinence of bowel or bladder, missed antiepileptic medication, and postictal confusion gives clue about seizure. While syncope associated with sweating or nausea and rapid return of orientation upon awakening

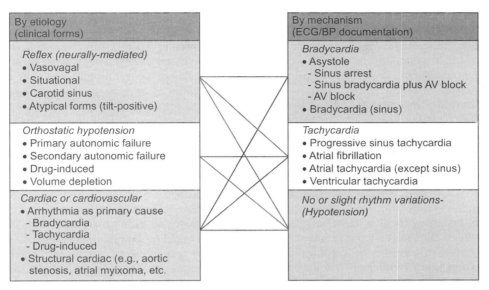

Fig. 1 Different types of syncope
Abbreviations: AV, atrioventricular; BP, blood pressure; ECG, electrocardiogram

Table 1 Classification of syncope	
Reflex syncope (neurally mediated)	• Vasovagal • Situational • Carotid sinus syncope • Atypical forms
Orthostatic hypotension	• Primary autonomic failure • Secondary autonomic failure • Drug-induced • Volume depletion
Cardiac arrhythmia	• Bradycardia • Tachycardia • Structural heart disease

It is very important to identify the life-threatening etiology like acute coronary syndrome (ACS), aortic dissection, leaking abdominal aortic aneurysm (AAA), subarachnoid hemorrhage (SAH), ruptured ectopic pregnancy and gastrointestinal (GI) bleed which may present as syncope in about 15% of cases. Missed diagnosis in these conditions can lead to medicolegal action in patients presenting as syncope. The physician evaluating a patient with TLOC should be alert for the possibility of this disease in addition to cardiovascular diagnosis of ominous significance.[4-10]

- *Cardiac syncope*: Cardiac causes which are associated with syncope include arrhythmia, ischemia, structural or valvular abnormalities (e.g. aortic stenosis), cardiac tamponade, and pacemaker malfunction. Brady and tachycardia is the second most common reason of syncope after reflex syncope.
- *Hemorrhage*: Large blood loss because of acute severe bleed can manifest as syncope. Important potential causes include: trauma, GI bleed, leaking aortic aneurysm, ruptured ovarian cyst, ectopic pregnancy rupture, and ruptured spleen.
- *Massive pulmonary embolism*: Hemodynamically significant pulmonary embolism (PE) is an uncommon but well-documented cause of syncope.[11]
- *Subarachnoid hemorrhage*: Patients presenting with syncope following a headache require evaluation for a possible SAH.

Common Conditions

- *Neurocardiogenic syncope*: Often referred to as vasovagal or vasodepressor syncope, neurocardiogenic syncope is the most common reason of syncope, accounting for 25–65% of cases.[12] In this condition, the cardiovascular reflexes mechanism that control the circulation become improper in response to a triggering factor, which results in vasodilation with or without bradycardia and a drop in BP leading to global cerebral hypoperfusion. Patients diagnosed with neurocardiogenic syncope have a benign course with no increase in mortality or morbidity.[13] Three types of responses are seen: (1) a cardioinhibitory response which is characterized by asystole, (2) a vasodepressor response presents as fall in BP, and (3) a mixed response with features of both. Significant bradycardia and/or hypotension accompany the acute loss of consciousness. Potential triggers are numerous and often determination of the underlying cause is made in the outpatient setting. Most patients with neurocardiogenic syncope experience a prodrome, which may include dizziness or lightheadedness, a sense of warmth, pallor, nausea or vomiting, abdominal pain, and diaphoresis, prior to their loss of consciousness. Examples include micturition or defecation syncope, situational syncope (e.g. while having blood drawn), or cough-mediated syncope.

- *Carotid sinus hypersensitivity*: It is a variant of neurocardiogenic syncope, resulting from pressure at the carotid sinus. External pressure to the neck can induce this reflex response. Common causes include shaving, a tight collar, and turning of the head.
- *Orthostasis*: Orthostatic syncope falls between 5 and 24% of syncope cases and can be defined by a fall in BP of 20 mm Hg or more, or a reflex tachycardia of more than 20 beats per minute. Orthostasis is most often caused by a loss of intravascular volume, from any number of causes, or by failure or instability of the autonomic nervous system. Nevertheless, clinicians should remain cautious because orthostasis can occur with cardiac syncope. Syncope from orthostatic hypotension is a diagnosis of exclusion in the ED, reserved for low-risk patients who have symptoms consistent with the diagnosis. Orthostatic hypotension can be an isolated disease (Bradbury-Eggleston syndrome) or can be a part of systemic disease like Parkinsonism or Shy-Drager syndrome. Postural orthostatic tachycardia syndrome (POTS) is characterized by symptoms of orthostatic intolerance because of milder form of chronic autonomic incompetence. Orthostatic vital signs are neither sensitive nor specific in assessing volume status or diagnosing syncope.[13-15] Many patients become symptomatic if their systolic BP drops below 90 mm Hg, but a large portion of the population who meets the definition of orthostasis do not have syncope. Elders, pregnant women, and patients taking drugs with vasodilating effects are predisposed to develop symptomatic orthostasis.
- *Medications*: The effects of medications account for 5–15% of syncopal events due to volume depletion or as a result in vasodilatation. Elderly patients are affected more due to the hypotensive effects of drugs because of renal sodium wasting, reduced baroreceptor sensitivity, decreased cerebral blood flow, and an impaired thirst mechanism that develops with aging. Medications often implicated include calcium channel blockers, beta-blockers, alpha-blockers, nitrates, antiarrhythmics, digoxin, diuretics (affecting volume status and electrolyte concentrations), erectile dysfunction medications, and medications affecting the QTc interval (e.g. antipsychotics and antiemetics).[16] Alcohol can also cause symptomatic orthostasis by impairing vasoconstriction.[17]

Other Conditions

- *Neurologic syncope*: True syncope is defined by an immediate, spontaneous return to baseline function following loss of consciousness, without new focal neurologic findings. Therefore, true neurologic causes leading to syncope are rare. Examples of neurologic syncope include: SAH, transient ischemic attack (TIA), subclavian steal syndrome, and migraine headache. Stroke and TIAs generally cause focal neurologic deficits that do not recover rapidly or completely.
- *Psychiatric syncope*: Anxiety and panic disorders can cause situational syncope. Emergency clinicians must be cautious when attributing syncope to psychiatric causes. Patients with hypoxia, inadequate cerebral perfusion, or other medical conditions may appear confused or anxious. Patients with psychiatric syncope are generally young, without cardiac disease, and complain of multiple episodes.[18]
- *Metabolic*: Metabolic causes of syncope include hypoxia, hypoglycemia, and hyperventilation. These comprises of less than 5% of cases of syncope.
- *Rare causes*: Rare causes of syncope include atrial myxoma, Takayasu's arteritis, systemic mastocytosis, and carcinoid. Anaphylaxis can involve syncope and loss of consciousness, and both patients and witnesses sometimes overlook or forget the more subtle, earlier symptoms, such as flushing, itching, hives, cough, bronchospasm, or abdominal cramping. In addition, these less dramatic symptoms may have resolved by the time the patient is evaluated.

Differentiation of syncope caused by neurally mediated hypotension, arrhythmias, seizures, and psychogenic causes has been described in **Table 2**.

MANAGEMENT

Evaluation and Investigation (Flow chart 1)

The utmost important parameters in evaluation of syncope are a careful history, physical examination, supine and upright BP, and a 12-lead ECG, followed by additional testing in selected patient subgroups, including carotid sinus massage, echocardiography, ECG monitoring, and tilt-table testing. A thorough history and clinical examination are by far the most important components of the evaluation of a patient with TLOC, which contribute to diagnosis in 25% of patients. During history special attention should be given to age and sex, surrounding circumstances, position, premonitory symptoms, index event witness, recovery, past medical history, medication, and family history. Based on this initial evaluation, patients can be divided into those with established syncope and those with nonsyncopal TLOC. Patients with syncope can be further classified into two groups: (1) those with a certain diagnosis and clear treatment plan and (2) those with an uncertain diagnosis. For the latter, attention should be on risk stratification of patients **(Flow chart 2)**. The patients who require hospitalization and/or an intensive timely outpatient cardiovascular evaluation should be identified. These patients may require exercise stress testing, cardiac catheterization, and electrophysiology

Table 2 Difference between syncope causes

	Neurogenic hypotension	Arrhythmias	Seizures	Psychogenic
Demographics and clinical setting	• Female > male sex • Younger age (<55 years) • More episodes (>2 standing, warm room emotional upset)	• Male > female sex • Older age (54 years) • Fewer episodes (<3) • During exertion or supine • Family history of sudden cardiac death	• Younger age (<45) • Any setting	• Female > male • Occurs in presence of others • Younger age (<40 years) • Many episodes even in a day • No identifiable triggers
Premonitory symptoms	• Longer duration (>5 sec) • Palpitations • Blurred vision • Nausea • Warmth • Diaphoresis • Lightheadedness	• Shorter duration (<6 sec) • Palpitations less common	• Sudden onset or brief aura (déjà vu, olfactory, gustatory, visual)	• Usually absent
Observation during event	• Pallor • Diaphoresis • Dilated pupils • Slow pulse, low BP • Incontinence may occur • Brief clonic movements may occur	• Blue, not pale • Incontinence can occur • Brief clonic movements can occur	• Blue face, no pallor • Frothing at the mouth • Prolonged syncope (duration >5 min) • Tongue biting • Horizontal eye deviation • Elevated pulse and BP • Incontinence more likely • Tonic-clonic movements if grand mal	• Normal color • Not diaphoretic • Eyes closed • Normal pulse and BP • No incontinence • Prolonged duration (minutes) is common
Residual symptoms	• Residual symptoms common • Prolonged fatigue common (>90%) • Oriented	• Residual symptoms uncommon (unless prolonged unconsciousness) • Oriented	• Residual symptoms common • Aching muscles • Disoriented • Fatigue • Headache • Slow recovery	• Residual symptoms uncommon • Oriented

(EP) testing. Conversely, patients who are presenting with only a single episode of syncope and are determined to be at low-risk for a cardiovascular event or death may require no further evaluation. Patients who fall between these two extremes can undergo further testing selected on the basis of results of the initial evaluation. There are subtle features in history and investigation which can assist clinicians in identifying high-risk patient with risk to life in comparison to low-risk patient who can be discharged safely **(Box 1)**.

INVESTIGATION

Laboratory Test

Blood tests are helpful in only less than 2% cases of syncope. Routine laboratory blood tests are helpful in identifying anemia and electrolyte abnormalities. Acute drop in hemoglobin can suggest bleeding. Arterial blood gas (ABG) test can reveal hypoxia suggestive of PE. Elevation of cardiac biomarkers may suggest ACS, PE, arrhythmia, and cardiac decompensation. Electrolyte imbalance contributing to TLOC can also be detected.

Electrocardiogram

The initial ECG can contribute to diagnosis in 5% of patients and suggests a probable diagnosis in another 5% of patients. ECG showing sinus bradycardia, sinus pauses, Mobitz type II atrioventricular (AV) block, high grade AV block or congenital heart block (CHB) suggests bradyarrhythmia as culprit. Right bundle branch block (RBBB), left bundle branch block (LBBB), and bifascicular block will require further evaluation. Extensive massive myocardial infarction can suggest ACS as a cause. PE may manifest as sinus tachycardia, RBBB and S1Q3T3 pattern. RBBB in V1–V3 with ST elevation may suggest Brugada syndrome, similarly Epsilon wave suggests arrhythmogenic right ventricular dysplasia (ARVD). Pre-excitation or Wolff-Parkinson-White (WPW) syndrome can also be detected with ECG. Abnormality of QT interval can lead to diagnosis of long or short QT interval. Ventricular

Flow chart 1 Diagnostic approach to the evaluation of patients with TLOC and syncope

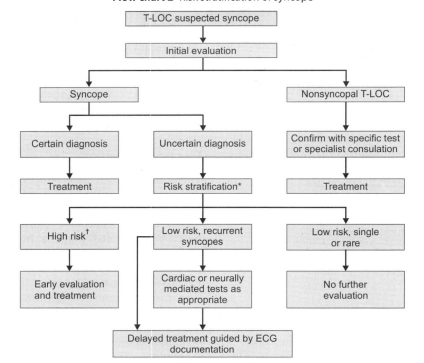

Abbreviations: SCD, sudden cardiac death; TLOC, transient loss of consciousness

Flow chart 2 Risk stratification of syncope

Abbreviation: TLOC, transient loss of consciousness.
*May require treatment laboratory investigations
†Risk for short-term serious events

Box 1 Important cardiac risk factors for syncope

- Severe structural heart disease (low heart function, previous heart attack, heart failure)
- Clinical or ECG suggestive of arrhythmia
- Syncope during physical exercise
- Palpitations during syncope
- Family history of sudden death
- Nonsustained VT
- Bifascicular block or QRS >120 msec
- Severe sinus bradycardia (<50 beats/min) in the absence of medications or physical training
- Pre-excitation
- Prolonged or very short QT interval
- Brugada ECG pattern (right bundle branch block with ST elevation in leads V1–V3)
- Arrhythmogenic right ventricular dysplasia ECG pattern (T wave inversion in leads V1–V3 with or without epsilon waves)
- ECG suggestive of hypertrophic dilated cardiomyopathy
- Clinical evidence or suspicion of a pulmonary embolus (clinical setting, sinus tachycardia, shortness of breath)
- Severe anemia

Table 3 Physiological changes as well as value and condition during head-up tilt test

Condition	Physiological change	Value
Vasovagal syncope	Delayed BP fall, bradycardia	Diagnostic if usual symptoms
Orthostatic hypotension	Immediate BP fall, no bradycardia	Diagnostic
Postural orthostatic tachycardia syndrome	Modest BP fall, tachycardia	Diagnostic if usual symptom
Psychogenic pseudo syncope	No physiological change (tachycardia)	Apparent loss of consciousness is diagnostic

tachycardia (VT) or nonsustained ventricular tachycardia (NSVT) can also confirm diagnosis. ECG monitoring can also be done with Holter, telemetry or loop recorder for better yield. Current guidelines recommend that an implantable event recorder should be tried when the mechanism of the syncope is unclear even after a complete evaluation.

Carotid Sinus Massage

This test is indicated in patient with syncope older than 40 years of age with unexplained reason, however, it is contraindicated in patient with history of recent stroke (within 3 months) or patient with carotid bruit. A pause of more than 3 seconds and fall in BP of more than 50 mm Hg is considered as criteria for hypersensitive carotid sinus syndrome.

Head-up Tilt Table Test

Tilt table test is done in patient with recurrent unexplained syncope when the cardiac evaluation and carotid sinus massage is noncontributory. This test demonstrates patient susceptibility for reflex syncope and is helpful in initiating treatment in these undiagnosed cases. It also helps in differentiating all the three types of neurogenic syncope: (1) cardioinhibitory, (2) vasodepressor, and (3) mixed response. It also helps in differentiation of orthostasis and reflex syncope, as well as psychogenic pseudoseizure and reflex syncope **(Table 3)**.

Ambulatory Blood Pressure

Ambulatory BP monitoring is an important test to diagnose syncope in elderly population because of recurrent hypotension due to autonomic failure.

Echocardiography

It is an important inexpensive noninvasive test. It confirms the cardiac diagnosis when there is suspicion of structural heart disease such as LV or RV dysfunction, valvular heart disease, pericardial effusion, cardiac tumor, myxomas, outflow tract obstruction, or hypertrophic cardiomyopathy (HCM). Yield of the test increases if there is history suggestive of cardiac diagnosis or abnormal ECG. The yield may go up to 27–40%.

Coronary Angiography or Computed Tomography Angiography and Electrophysiology Study

It is helpful in suspected ischemia or ischemia-related arrhythmia. EP study is helpful in establishing a diagnosis of sick sinus syndrome, carotid sinus hypersensitivity, heart block, supraventricular tachycardia (SVT), and VT. EP testing should be performed in patients when the initial evaluation suggests an arrhythmia as a cause of the syncope.

Dedicated syncope unit has shown better overall diagnosis and management of syncope patient. Initial evaluation gives a diagnosis in 21%, further workup reveals a diagnosis in 61% but in 18% diagnosis still remain uncertain.

TREATMENT

Treatment of a patient with syncope has three aims:
1. Prolong survival
2. Prevent traumatic injuries
3. Prevent recurrences.

The syncope treatment is based on the etiology and mechanism of the syncope. Current guidelines recommend that patients with syncope be hospitalized when there is known or suspected cardiac diagnosis, ECG suggestive of arrhythmic syncope, syncope with severe injury or during exercise, patients with a history of sudden unexplained death in family.

Single episodes of reflex syncope does not require any treatment, patients should be educated about common precipitating factors such as dehydration, prolonged

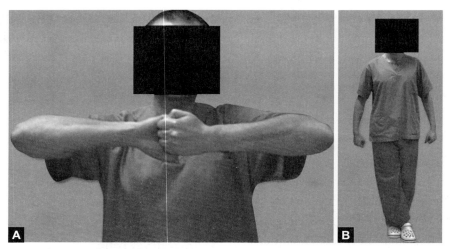

Figs 2A and B Counter-pressure maneuvers: (A) Arm tensing in left panel and (B) leg crossing in right panel

Table 4 Management of reflex syncope[1]		
Treatment	Class	LOE
Reassurance and education	I	C
Isometric physical counter-pressure maneuvers with a prodrome	I	B
Cardiac pacing should be considered in patients with dominant cardioinhibitory carotid sinus hyposensitivity	IIa	B
Cardiac pacing should be considered with frequent recurrent reflex syncope, age >40 years, and documented spontaneous cardioinhibitory response during monitoring of recurrent syncope	IIb	B
Midodrine may be indicated in patients with neurally mediated syncope refractory to conservative treatment approaches	IIb	B
Tilt training may be useful for education of patients, but long-term benefit depends on compliance	IIb	B
After alternative treatment has failed, cardiac pacing may be indicated in patients with a tilt-induced cardioinhibitory response; recurrent, frequent, unpredictable syncope; and age >40 years	IIb	C
Triggers of situations inducing syncope must be avoided as much as possible	III	C
Hypotensive drugs should be discontinued or modified	III	C
Cardiac pacing is not indicated in the absence of a documented cardioinhibitory reflex	III	C
Beta-blockers are not indicated	III	A

Abbreviation: LOE, level of evidence.
Source: Modified from Task Force for the Diagnosis and Management of Syncope, European Society of Cardiology (ESC), European Heart Rhythm Association (EHRA), et al. Guidelines for the diagnosis and management of syncope (version 2009): The Task Force for the Diagnosis and Management of Syncope of the European Society of Cardiology (ESC). Eur Heart J. 2009;30:2631-71.

standing, alcohol, and medications such as diuretics and vasodilators. Patients should also be taught to sit or lie down at the beginning of symptoms and to initiate physical counter-pressure maneuvers **(Figs 2A and B)**. One recent study reported that a standard education protocol decreased traumatic injuries and recurrences of syncope significantly. Expansion of volume by salt supplementation is also commonly recommended. Intake of approximately 500 mL of water immediately increases orthostatic tolerance to tilt in healthy subjects and may be of value as prophylaxis for syncope in blood donors.[19]

If syncope is refractory to nonpharmacological measures then drugs like alpha agonist midodrine, droxydopa and pyridostigmine can be considered for frequent hypotensive episodes.[20,21] Drugs with less proven efficacy like beta-blockers and fludrocortisone are also in use for reflex syncope **(Table 4)**.[22] Despite the widespread use of agents like midodrine and fludrocortisone, these drugs have proven to be ineffective in many prospective randomized clinical trials. Even though beta-blockers such as metoprolol, propranolol, and nadolol were previously considered by many to be first-line therapy, recent studies have reported contrary (not better than placebo).[23-27]

Orthostatic hypotension patient may be benefited by various nonpharmacological measures like tilt table training, increased salt intake, physical counter-pressure maneuvers, abdominal binder and compression stocking, midodrin and fludrocortisone are another alternative in these scenario.[28-31] Role of pacemakers in patients with neurally mediated syncope is debatable. Although the 2008 guidelines for device-based therapy state that pacemaker implantation has a IIb indication for the treatment of patients with highly symptomatic, neurally mediated syncope associated with bradycardia documented spontaneously or at the time of tilt-table testing.[32] Management of syncope because of specific clinical entity require the appropriate treatment for specific diagnosis, for example, a patient with syncope related to AV conduction block would require a pacemaker in most situations. However, a patient with syncope secondary to heart block on the background of an inferior wall myocardial infarction will not usually require a permanent pacemaker because the heart block usually resolves spontaneously after revascularization. Similarly, heart block resulting from neurally mediated syncope does not generally require pacemaker implantation. Management of a patient of WPW syndrome presenting with syncope typically involves catheter ablation. Management of a patient with syncope due to VT or in the setting of ischemic or nonischemic cardiomyopathy would probably include implantation of an implantable defibrillator. However, implantable cardioverter-defibrillator (ICD) implantation may not be required for patients with VT or ventricular fibrillation (VF) occurring within 48 hours of an acute myocardial infarction. For other types of syncope, treatment may involve cessation of a likely culprit drug, increased salt intake, education and counseling of the patient. In the case of syncope because of neurological or GI disease, respective super specialty must be involved.[33]

FUTURE PERSPECTIVE AND ADVANCEMENT

Syncope will be an important clinical problem in coming years because of increasing life expectancy and more frequent occurrence of cardiac disease in this subset. Over the next 5 years, additional studies will confirm the clinical and economic value of syncope evaluation units. This will lead to more widespread use of syncope evaluation units, much like chest pain emergency rooms which are now routinely used to evaluate patients with chest pain.[34] Clinical genetic testing is now available on a routine clinical basis for many of the inherited cardiac conditions that may be accompanied by syncope, including long-QT syndrome, ARVD, and hypertrophic cardiomyopathy (HCM). Therefore, it also seems likely that genetic testing will grow in diagnostic importance in the evaluation of patients with syncope.[35-40]

CONCLUSION

The evaluation and disposition of syncope in emergency department is not only complex but costly also. Many causes of syncope are benign but occasionally sign of life-threatening situation also. Some time patients of syncope remain undiagnosed after standard evaluation. Most of the studies about syncope focus on the risk stratification of the syncope on the basis of abnormal ECG, history of structural or arrhythmic heart disease, abnormal vital signs in emergency department, or combination of these features in elderly people. High risk syncope patient should be admitted and evaluated immediately. Since low risk patient are not" no risk" patient so they can appropriately followed up in regular interval.

REFERENCES

1. Task Force for the Diagnosis and Management of Syncope, European Society of Cardiology (ESC), European Heart Rhythm Association (EHRA), et al. Guidelines for the diagnosis and management of syncope (version 2009). Eur Heart J. 2009;30:2631-71.
2. Olde Nordkamp LR, van Dijk N, Ganzeboom KS, et al. Syncope prevalence in the ED compared to that in the general practice and population: a strong selection process. Am J Emerg Med. 2009;27:271-9.
3. Malasana G, Brignole M, Daccarett M, et al. The prevalence and cost of the faint and fall problem in the state of Utah. Pacing Clin Electrophysiol. 2011;34:278-83.
4. Linzer M, Yang EH, Estes NA, et al. Diagnosing syncope. Part 1: Value of history, physical examination, and electro-cardiography. Clinical Efficacy Assessment Project of the American College of Physicians. Ann Intern Med. 1997;126: 989-96.
5. Mattu A Syncope. (2009). (In) Head Emergencies. Audio series online. [online] Available from *www.audiodigest.org/pages/htmlos/3449.4.4231252564761264740/EM2609*. Audio-Digest Emergency Medicine. Volume 26, Issue 09. May 7, 2009. [Accessed January, 2017].
6. HCPUnet, Healthcare Cost and Utilization Project. Agency for Healthcare Research and Quality, Rockville, MD. [online] Available from *www.ahrq.gov/data/hcup/hcupnet.htm* [Accessed January, 2017].
7. Solbiati M, Casazza G, Dipaola F, et al. Syncope recurrence and mortality: a systematic review. Europace. 2015;17:300-8.
8. Kapoor WN, Karpf M, Wieand S, et al. A prospective evaluation and follow-up of patients with syncope. N Engl J Med. 1983;309:197-204.
9. Quinn JV, Stiell IG, McDermott DA, et al. Derivation of the San Francisco Syncope Rule to predict patients with short-term serious outcomes. Ann Emerg Med. 2004;43:224-32.
10. Middlekauff HR, Stevenson WG, Stevenson LW, et al. Syncope in advanced heart failure: high risk of sudden death regardless of origin of syncope. J Am Coll Cardiol. 1993;21:110-6.

11. Wolfe TR, Allen TL. Syncope as an emergency department presentation of pulmonary embolism. J Emerg Med. 1998;16:27-31.
12. Brignole M, Menozzi C, Bartoletti A, et al. A new management of syncope: prospective systematic guideline-based evaluation of patients referred urgently to general hospitals. Eur Heart J. 2006;27:76-82.
13. Soteriades ES, Evans JC, Larson MG, et al. Incidence and prognosis of syncope. N Engl J Med. 2002;347:878-85.
14. Baraff LJ, Schriger DL. Orthostatic vital signs: variation with age, specificity, and sensitivity in detecting a 450-mL blood loss. Am J Emerg Med. 1992;10:99-103.
15. Koziol-McLain J, Lowenstein SR, Fuller B. Orthostatic vital signs in emergency department patients. Ann Emerg Med. 1991;20:606-10.
16. Hanlon JT, Linzer M, MacMillan JP, et al. Syncope and presyncope associated with probable adverse drug reactions. Arch Intern Med. 1990;150:2309-12.
17. Narkiewicz K, Cooley RL, Somers VK. Alcohol potentiates orthostatic hypotension: implications for alcohol-related syncope. Circulation. 2000;101:398-402.
18. Kapoor WN, Fortunato M, Hanusa BH, et al. Psychiatric illnesses in patients with syncope. Am J Med. 1995;99:505-12.
19. Van dijk N, Quartieri F, Blanc JJ, et al. Effective of physical counter pressure maneuvers in preventing vasovagal syncope: the Physical Counterpressure Maneuver Trial (PC-Trial). J Am Coll Cardiol. 2006;48:1652-7.
20. Perez-Lugones A, Schweikert R, Pavia S, et al. Efficacy and safety of midodrine in patient with severe symptomatic patient with neurocardiogenic syncope: a randomized control study. J Cardiovasc Electrophysiol. 2001;12:935-8.
21. Samniah N, Sakaguchi S, Lurie KG, et al. Efficacy and safety of midodrine hydrochloride in patient with refractory vasovagal syncope. Am J Cardiol. 2001;88:A7, 80-3.
22. Sheldon R, Connolly S, Rose S, et al. Prevention of Syncope Trial (POST): A randomized, placebo controlled study of metoprolol in the prevention of vasovagal syncope. Circulation. 2006;113:1164-70.
23. Flevari P, Livanis EG, Theodorakis GN, et al. Vasovagal syncope. A prospective, randomized, crossover evaluation of the effect of propranolol, nadolol and placebo on syncope recurrence and patients' well-being. J Am Coll Cardiol. 2002;40:499-504.
24. Raviele A, Giada F, Menozzi D, et al. A randomized, double-blind, placebo-controlled study of permanent cardiac pacing for the treatment of recurrent tilt-induced vasovagal syncope. The Vasovagal Syncope and Pacing Trial (SYNPACE). Eur Heart J. 2004;25:17419.
25. Aydin MA, Mortensen K, Salukhe TV, et al. A standardized education protocol significantly reduces traumatic injuries and syncope recurrence: An observational study in 316 patients with vasovagal syncope. Europace. 2012;14:410-5.
26. Gurevitz O, Barsheshet A, Bar-Lev D, et al. Tilt training: Does it have a role in preventing vasovagal syncope? Pacing Clin Electrophsiol. 2007;30:1499-505.
27. Sheldon R, Connolly S, Rose S, et al. Prevention of Syncope Trial (POST): A randomized, placebo-controlled study of metoprolol in the prevention of vasovagal syncope. Circulation. 2006;113:1164-70.
28. Low PA, Gilden GL, Freeman R. Efficacy of midodrine vs placebo in neurogenic orthostatic hypotension, a randomized double blind multicenter study. Midodrine Study Group. JAMA. 1997;277:1046-51.
29. Van Leishout JJ, ten Harkel AD, Wieling W. Fludrocortisone and sleeping in head-up position limits the postural decrease in cardiac output in autonomic failure. Clin Auton Res. 2000;10:35-42.
30. Brignole M, Menozzi C, Moya A, et al. Pacemaker therapy in patients with neurally mediated syncope and documented asystole: Third International Study on Syncope of Uncertain Etiology (ISSUE-3): A randomized trial. Circulation. 2012;125:256671.
31. Palmisano P, Zaccaria M, Luzzi G, et al. Closed-loop cardiac pacing vs. conventional dual chamber pacing with specialized sensing and pacing algorithms for syncope prevention in patients with refractory vasovagal syncope: Results of a long-term follow-up. Europace. 2012;14:103843.
32. Epstein AE, DiMarco JP, Ellenbogen KA, et al. ACC/AHA/HRS 2008 guidelines for device-based therapy of cardiac rhythm abnormalities: A report of the American College of Cardiology/American Heart Association Task Force on Practice Guidelines (Writing Committee to Review the ACC/AHA/NASPE 2002 Guideline Update for Implantation of Cardiac Pacemakers and Antiarrhythmia Devices): Developed in collaboration with the American Association for Thoracic Surgery and Society of Thoracic Surgeons. Circulation. 2008;117:e350408.
33. Kanjwal K, Karabin B, Kanjwal Y, et al. Preliminary observations on the use of closed-loop cardiac pacing in patients with refractory neurocardiogenic syncope. J Interv Card Electrophysiol. 2010;27:69-73.
34. Douglas L Mann, Douglas P Zipes, Peter Libby, et al. Braunwald's Heart Disease: A Textbook of Cardiovascular Medicine, 10th edition. Philadelphia: Saunders; 2015.
35. Sun W, Zheng L, Qiao Y, et al. Catheter ablation as a treatment for vasovagal syncope: long-term outcome of endocardial autonomic modification of the left atrium. J Am Heart Assoc. 2016;5:e003471.
36. Kidd SK, Doughty C, Goldhaber SZ. Syncope (Fainting). Circulation. 2016;133:e600-2.
37. Ungar A, Del Rosso A, Giada F, et al. Early and late outcome of treated patients referred for syncope to emergency department. The EGSYS 2 follow-up study. Eur Heart J. 2010;31:2021-6.
38. Hindricks G, Pokushalov E, Urban L, et al. Performance of a new implantable cardiac monitor in detecting and quantifying atrial fibrillation. Results of the XPECT trial. Circ Arrhythm Electrophysiol. 2010;3:141-7.
39. Petkar S, Iddon P, Bell W, et al. REVISE (Reveal in the Investigation of Syncope and Epilepsy) study [abstract]. Eur Heart J. 2009;30(Suppl 1):15 [abstract: 245].
40. Krahn A, Andrade JG, Deyell MW. Selective appropriate diagnostic tools for evaluating the patient with syncope/collapse. Prog Cardiovasc Dis. 2013;55:402-9.

CHAPTER 25

Acute Coronary Syndrome: Risk Stratification

Mayank Jain, Rajneesh Kapoor

INTRODUCTION

Chest pain is a very common reason to attend the emergency department (ED). Acute coronary syndrome (ACS) is a frequent cause of chest pain and ACS is associated with both a short-term and a longer-term adverse prognosis. The diagnosis of an ACS in the ED should be followed by risk stratification and treatment. In this chapter, we focus on clinical guideline recommendations for risk stratification and the challenges relating to the implementation of these guidelines in every day clinical practice.

Acute coronary syndrome includes ST-elevation myocardial infarction (STEMI), non-ST elevation acute myocardial infarction (NSTEMI) or unstable angina (UA).

RISK STRATIFICATION AFTER ST-ELEVATION MYOCARDIAL INFARCTION

The process of risk stratification following STEMI occurs in several stages: initial findings, in-hospital course [coronary care unit (CCU), intermediate care unit], and at the time of hospital discharge. The tools used to form an integrated and dynamic assessment of the patient consist of baseline demographic information, serial electrocardiograms (ECGs) and serum and plasma cardiac biomarker measurements, hemodynamic monitoring data, a variety of noninvasive tests, and if performed, the findings at cardiac catheterization. These findings, integrated with the occurrence of in-hospital complications, can provide information regarding survival.

Initial Findings

Certain demographic and historical factors portend a worse prognosis in patients with STEMI. Five simple baseline parameters have been reported to account for more than 90% of the prognostic information for 30-day mortality. These characteristics are given in descending order of importance: age, systolic blood pressure, Killip classification **(Table 1)**, heart rate, and location of myocardial infarction (MI) **(Table 2)**.

A 12-lead ECG provides prognostic information about ACS. Mortality is greater in anterior wall STEMI than with inferior STEMI. Patients of inferior wall MI with right ventricle involvement as suggested by ST-segment elevation in V_4R, have greater mortality rate than inferior infarction without right ventricular involvement. Patients with multiple leads showing ST elevation have increased mortality rate, especially if their infarct is anterior in location. A patient with persistent advanced heart block (e.g. type II second-degree or third-degree AV block) or new intraventricular conduction abnormalities (bifascicular or trifascicular) in the course of STEMI have a worse prognosis.

Diabetes mellitus (DM), in particular, appears to confer a more than 40% increase in adjusted risk for death by 30 days. Surviving diabetic patients also experience a more

Table 1 30-day mortality based on hemodynamic (Killip) class

Killip class	Characteristics	Patients (%)	Mortality rate (%)
I	No evidence of CHF	85	5.1
II	Rales, ↑ JVD, or S3	13	13.6
III	Pulmonary edema	1	32.2
IV	Cardiogenic shock	1	57.8

Abbreviations: CHF, congestive heart failure; ↑JVD, increased jugular venous distention; S3, third heart sound.
Source: Adapted from Lee KL, Woodlief LH, Topol EJ, et al. Predictors of 30-day mortality in the era of reperfusion for acute myocardial infarction: results from an international trial of 41,021 patients. GUSTO-I Investigators. Circulation. 1995;91:1659-68.

Table 2 Acute myocardial infarction: Electrocardiogram subset and correlated infarct-related artery and mortality

Category	Anatomy of occlusion	ECG findings	30-day mortality rate (%)	1-year mortality rate (%)
1. Proximal LAD	Proximal to first septal perforator	ST ↑ V_1–V_6, I, aVL and fascicular or bundle branch block	19.6	25.6
2. Mid-LAD	Proximal to large diagonal but distal to first septal perforator	ST ↑ V_1–V_6, I, aVL	9.2	12.4
3. Distal LAD or diagonal	Distal to large diagonal or diagonal itself	ST ↑ V_1–V_4, I, aVL, V_5, V_6	6.8	10.2
4. Moderate-to-large inferior (posterior, lateral, right ventricular)	Proximal RCA or left circumflex	ST ↑ II, III, aVF, and any of the following: (a) V_1, V_3R, V_4R (b) V_5, V_6 (c) R > S in V_1, V_2	6.4	8.4
5. Small inferior	Distal RCA or left circumflex branch	ST ↑ II, III, aVF, only	4.5	6.7

Abbreviations: ECG, electrocardiogram; LAD, left anterior descending (coronary artery); ↑, increased; RCA, right coronary artery.
Note: Mortality rate based on GUSTO I cohort population in each of the 5 year categories, all receiving reperfusion therapy.
Source: Topol EJ, Van de Werf FJ. Acute myocardial infarction: early diagnosis and management. In: Topol EJ (Ed). Textbook of Cardiovascular Medicine. New York: Lippincott-Raven; 1998.

complicated post-MI course, including a greater incidence of postinfarction angina, infarct extension, and heart failure. These higher rates of complications probably relate to the extensive accelerated atherosclerosis and higher risk for thrombosis and heart failure associated with DM.

In addition, several validated clinical risk stratification tools may be used at initial evaluation to assess the short- and long-term risk for death after MI. In addition to the patient's age and historical factors such as diabetes and previous MI, clinical signs of heart failure, including tachycardia and hypotension, are common in many of these clinical risk assessment scores.

The *Thrombolysis in Myocardial Infarction (TIMI) risk score* incorporates eight variables obtained from the history, physical examination, and ECG **(Table 3 and Fig. 1)**. In patients treated with fibrinolysis, a TIMI score of 9 or greater predicts a 30-day mortality of approximately 35%. In patients with a TIMI score of 0 or 1, the 30-day mortality rate is less than 2%. The strongest predictor of poor prognosis is advanced age (where age >75 years receives 3 points and age 65–74 years receives 2 points). Other variables that predict a poor prognosis include hypotension, Killip class II-IV at presentation, tachycardia, history of diabetes or hypertension, anterior ST elevation [also complete left bundle branch block (LBBB)], low body weight and a time to treatment of more than 4 hours.

The *Global Registry of Acute Coronary Events (GRACE) score* is used to predict in-hospital mortality in patients with ACS. Risk is calculated based on Killip class, heart rate, systolic blood pressure, creatinine level, age, presence or absence of cardiac arrest at admission, presence or absence of cardiac biomarkers, and ST-segment deviation. Patients with a score of less than or equal to 60 have a less than or equal to 0.2% probability of in-hospital mortality, whereas patients with a score of more than or equal to 250 have a more than or equal to 52% probability of in-hospital mortality.

Based on Combined Abciximab REteplase Stent Study in Acute Myocardial Infarction (CARESS-in-AMI) and Trial of Routine ANgioplasty and Stenting after Fibrinolysis to Enhance Reperfusion in Acute Myocardial Infarction (TRANSFER-AMI) trials, the American College of

Table 3 TIMI risk model for prediction of short-term mortality in ST-segment elevation myocardial infarction patients

History	
Age 65–74 years	2 points
Age ≥75 years	3 points
Angina or DM/HTN	1 point
Physical examination	
HR >100 bpm	2 points
SBP <100 mm Hg	3 points
Killip class II-IV	2 points
Weight <67 kg	1 point
Presentation	
Anterior ST elevation or LBBB	1 point
Time to treatment >4 hour	1 point
TIMI risk score = total points (0–14)	

Abbreviations: DM/HTN; diabetes mellitus or hypertension; HR, heart rate; LBBB, left bundle branch block; SBP, systolic blood pressure; TIMI, thrombolysis in myocardial infarction.

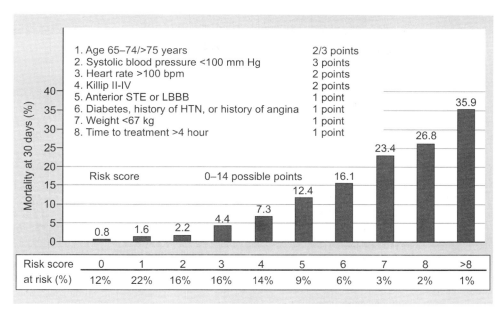

Fig. 1 Calculation of Thrombolysis in Myocardial Infarction (TIMI) risk score
Abbreviations: STE, ST-elevation; LBBB, left bundle branch block; HTN, hypertension
Source: Morrow DA, Antman EM, Charlesworth A, et al. TIMI risk score for ST-elevation myocardial infarction: a convenient, bedside, clinical score for risk assessment at presentation—an intravenous nPA for treatment of infarcting myocardium early II trial substudy. Circulation. 2000;102(17): 2031-7.

Cardiology/American Heart Association (ACC/AHA) now recommends abandoning the use of the terms "facilitated" and "rescue" and rather decide on transfer for percutaneous coronary intervention (PCI) based on the patient's level of risk. High-risk patients **(Table 4)** who receive fibrinolysis as the primary reperfusion strategy should be transferred to a PCI-capable facility as soon as possible. PCI can then be performed immediately or as needed. For low-risk patients, this management strategy is a class IIb recommendation.

Hospital Course

Hospital mortality from STEMI depends directly on the severity of left ventricular (LV) dysfunction. Risk stratification via physical findings, estimation of infarct size, and in appropriate patients, invasive hemodynamic monitoring provides an assessment of the likelihood of a complicated hospital course and may also identify important abnormalities, such as hemodynamically significant mitral regurgitation, that convey an adverse long-term prognosis **(Table 5)**. In particular, the development of heart failure after MI entails a higher risk for sudden cardiac death. Recurrent infarction and new stroke during hospitalization for STEMI also, not surprisingly, confer a higher risk for death.

Assessment at Hospital Discharge

After STEMI, patient's short- and long-term survival depends on the LV function, ischemic myocardium and serious ventricular arrhythmias **(Fig. 2)**.

RISK STRATIFICATION OF UNSTABLE ANGINA AND NON-ST-SEGMENT ELEVATION MYOCARDIAL INFARCTION

Introduction

The clinical presentation of non-ST-elevation acute coronary syndrome (NSTE-ACS) can be variable, ranging from progressive exertional angina to postinfarction angina. Because NSTEMI is distinguished from unstable angina (UA) by the presence of elevated serum levels of cardiac biomarkers, serial measurements in patients presenting with ACS should be performed. With improvements in the diagnosis and risk stratification of patients with UA and NSTEMI, therapeutic approaches to NSTE-ACS have continued to evolve.

Clinical Characteristics Indicative of High Risk

Symptoms may include an acceleration of ischemic symptoms within the preceding 48 hours, angina at rest (>20 minutes), congestive heart failure (S3 gallop, pulmonary edema and rales), known reduced LV function, hypotension, new or worsening mitral regurgitation murmur, age older than 75 years, diffuse ST-segment changes on an ECG (≥0.5–1 mm), and the presence of elevated serum cardiac biomarkers [typically creatine kinase-myocardial band (CK-MB), troponin T, or troponin I]. Patients at intermediate or low risk have angina of short duration, have no ischemic ST-segment changes on ECG, are negative for cardiac biomarkers, and are hemodynamically stable **(Table 6)**.

Table 4 ACC/AHA definitions of high-risk patients with acute myocardial infarction

Defined in CARESS-in-AMI
- STEMI patients with one or more of the following:
  - Extensive ST-segment elevation
  - Previous MI
  - New-onset LBBB
  - Killip class > II or EF≤35% for inferior MI
- Anterior MI with ≥2 mm or more ST elevation in two or more leads

Defined in TRANSFER-AMI
- More than or equal to 2 mm ST elevation in two anterior leads or ST elevation ≥1 mm in inferior leads with at least
  - SBP <100 Hg
  - HR >100 bpm
  - Killip class II-III
  - ≥2 mm ST-segment depression in anterior leads
  - ≥1 mm of ST elevation in right-sided lead V4 indicative of RV infarct

Abbreviations: EF, ejection fraction; HR, heart rate; LBBB, left bundle branch block; MI, myocardial infarction; RV, right ventricular; SBP, systolic blood pressure; STEMI, ST-segment elevation myocardial infarction; UFH, unfractionated heparin.
Source: Adapted from Kushner FG, Hand M, King SB, et al. 2009 focused updates: ACC/AHA guidelines for the management of patients with ST-elevation myocardial infarction (updating the 2004 guideline and 2007 focused update) and ACC/AHA/SCAI guidelines on percutaneous coronary intervention (updating the 2005 guideline and 2007 focused update). J Am Coll Cardiol. 2009;54:2205-41.

Table 5 Hemodynamic classifications of patients with acute myocardial infarction

A. Based on clinical examination		B. Based on invasive monitoring	
Class	Definition	Subset	Definition
I	Rales and S3 absent	I	Normal hemodynamics PCWP <18, CI >2.2
II	Crackles, S3 gallop, elevated jugular venous pressure	II	Pulmonary congestion PCWP <18, CI >2.2
III	Frank pulmonary edema	III	Peripheral hypoperfusion PCWP <18, CI >2.2
IV	Shock	IV	Pulmonary congestion and peripheral hypoperfusion PCWP <18, CI >2.2

Abbreviations: CI, cardiac index; PCWP, pulmonary capillary wedge pressure
Source: (A) Modified from Killip T, Kimball J. Treatment of myocardial infarction in a coronary care unit: a two year experience with 250 patients. Am J Cardiol. 1967;20:457-64. (B) From Forrester J, Diamond G, Chatterjee K, et al. Medical therapy of acute myocardial infarction by the application of hemodynamic subsets. N Engl J Med. 1976;295:1356-62.

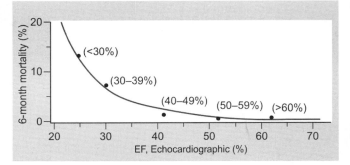

Fig. 2 Impact of left ventricular function on survival following MI. The curvilinear relationship between the left ventricular ejection fraction (EF) in patients treated in the reperfusion era is shown. In patients with a left ventricular EF below 40%, the rate of mortality markedly increases at 6 months
Source: Modified from Volpi A, De Vita C, Franzosi MG, et al. Determinants of 6-month mortality in survivors of myocardial infarction after thrombolysis. Results of the GISSI-2 database. The AdHoc Working Group of the Gruppo Italiano per lo Studio della Sopravvivenzanell'Infarto Miocardico (GISSI)-2 Database. Circulation. 1993;88:416.

Electrocardiogram

The initial ECG can help risk-stratify patients with UA. Ideally, this should be performed within 10 minutes of arrival to the ED. Patients with ST-segment deviation (i.e. ST-depression or transient ST-elevation) more than or equal to 0.5 mm or with pre-existing LBBB are at increased risk for death or MI at 1 year after presentation. ST-segment elevation more than or equal to 0.5 mm in lead aVR raises the possibility of left main or three-vessel coronary artery disease (CAD).

Non-ST-Elevation Acute Myocardial Infarction

Non-ST elevation acute myocardial infarction (NSTEMI) predicts a poorer prognosis among patients with NSTE-ACS. Multivariate predictors of NSTEMI in patients with ACS include prolonged chest pain (>60 minutes), ST-segment deviations (depression or transient elevation), and new or recent onset of angina (in the past month). Elevations in the levels of troponin I or troponin T, contractile proteins released from necrotic cardiac myocytes are independently predictive of morbidity and mortality among patients with UA. According to the European Society of Cardiology/American College of Cardiology (ESC/ACC), troponin elevations in this clinical setting are, by definition, NSTEMI. Risk stratification involves considering clinical characteristics and ECG findings to make early triage decisions.

Clinical Risk Classification Systems

Numerous scores have been derived to facilitate risk assessment and guide medical therapy in patients with NSTE-ACS. It is important to note that these scores can also be used to determine which patients may benefit most from

Table 6 Risk stratification of patients with unstable angina

High risk	Intermediate risk	Low risk
One of the following must be present:	No high-risk feature but must have one of the following:	No high-or intermediate-risk features present
Accelerating tempo of ischemic symptoms in preceding 48 hour	Prior MI, peripheral or cerebrovascular disease	
Prolonged ongoing rest pain (>20 min): Moderate or high likelihood of CAD	Prolonged rest pain (>20 min) that resolves	Increased frequency or duration of angina
Pulmonary edema: Most likely caused by ischemia	Rest angina (>20 min or relieved with rest or sublingual NTG)	Angina provoked by less exertion
Rest angina with dynamic ST changes ≥0.5 mm	Nocturnal angina	New-onset angina (within 2 weeks to 2 months)
New or worsening rales, S3, or MR murmur	New-onset, severe angina within 2 weeks with moderate or high likelihood of CAD	
Hypotension, bradycardia, tachycardia		
Bundle branch block, new or presumed new	T-wave changes	Normal or unchanged ECG
Sustained ventricular tachycardia	Pathologic Q waves or resting ST depression (<1 mm) in multiple lead groups	
Positive serum cardiac biomarkers	Slightly elevated CK-MB, troponin T, troponin I (e.g. troponin T 0.01 ng/mL but <0.1 ng/mL) Age older than 70 years	Normal cardiac markers

Abbreviations: CAD, coronary artery disease; CK-MB, creatine kinase myocardial band; ECG, electrocardiogram; MI myocardial infarction; MR, mitral regurgitation; NTG, nitroglycerin.

early invasive therapy as opposed to a more conservative approach.

The *Braunwald classification system* risk-stratifies patients with UA at presentation **(Table 7)**. Braunwald defined UA according to the characteristics of anginal pain and the underlying cause. Patients with increasing Braunwald class have been shown to have increasing risk of recurrent ischemia and death at 6 months.

The *TIMI UA risk score*, based on the TIMI IIB and ESSENCE (Efficacy and Safety of Subcutaneous Enoxaparin in Non-Q wave Coronary Events) trials, incorporates the combination of age, clinical characteristics, ECG changes, and cardiac markers for risk stratification **(Fig. 3)**. A higher risk score correlated with an increase in the incidence of death, new or recurrent MI, and recurrent ischemia requiring revascularization. This simple, rapid assessment of risk at initial evaluation identifies high-risk patients who can derive benefit from an early invasive strategy and more intensive antithrombotic therapy. This risk score also predicts the severity of angiographic findings, including the extent of CAD, thrombus burden, and flow impairment. An even simpler score, the TIMI risk index (age in decades × heart rate/systolic blood pressure), predicts mortality in patients with NSTEMI.

The *GRACE* prediction score, which incorporates nine clinical variables derived from the medical history and clinical findings on initial presentation and during hospitalization, can be used to estimate the in-hospital and 6-month outcomes for patients hospitalized with any form of ACS. Although perhaps more accurate, it is more complex than the TIMI risk score and is not easily calculated by hand.

Table 7 Braunwald classification of unstable angina

Class	Characteristics
I	*Exertional angina* New onset, severe, or accelerated Angina of <2 month duration More frequent angina Angina precipitated by less exertion No rest angina in last 2 months
II	*Rest angina, subacute* Rest angina within the last month but none within 48 hours of presentation
III	*Rest angina, acute* Rest angina within 48 hours of presentation
Clinical circumstances	
A	*Secondary unstable angina* Caused by a noncardiac condition, such as anemia, infection, thyrotoxicosis, or hypoxemia
B	*Primary unstable angina*
C	*Postinfarction unstable angina* Within 2 weeks of documented myocardial infarction

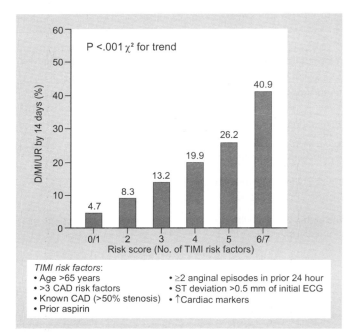

Fig. 3 TIMI risk score for NSTE-ACS. The number of risk factors present is counted
Source: Antman EM, Cohen M, Bernink PJ, et al. The TIMI risk score for unstable angina/non-ST elevation MI: a method for prognostication and therapeutic decision making. JAMA. 2000;284:835-42.

Table 8 GUSTO risk score	
Risk score	30-day mortality rate (%)
0–5	0.4
6–10	2.8
11–15	8.7
16–19	25.0
20–22	41.7
Scoring system	
Points are assigned based on the following criteria:	
Age (year)	Points
50–59	2
60–69	4
70–79	6
80+	8
Clinical history	
Prior heart failure	2
Prior stroke/TIA	2
Prior MI/revasc./chronic angina	1
Vitals and laboratory values	
Heart rate ≥90 beats/min	3
Elevated troponin and CK-MB	3
Creatinine >1.4 mg/dL	2
CAP (µg/L) >20	2
10–20	1
Anemia	1

Abbreviations: CK-MB, creatine kinase-myocardial band; CRP, C-reactive protein; GUSTO, Global Utilization of Strategies to Open Occluded Arteries; MI, myocardial infarction; revasc., revascularization; TIA, transient ischemic attack.

Other risk stratification scores based on the PURSUIT (Platelet Glycoprotein IIb/IIIa in Unstable Angina: Receptor Suppression Using Integrilin Therapy) and the GUSTO IV-ACS (Global Use of Strategies To Open Occluded Coronary Arteries IV-Acute Coronary Syndrome) trials **(Table 8)** have also been described. Together, these various clinical risk stratification systems help to identify high-risk patients likely to benefit most from more aggressive therapy.

Early Risk Stratification Recommendations

Patients who present with suspected ACS should be quickly assessed and should undergo early risk stratification for adverse cardiovascular events. This should include a history and physical examination focused on high-risk features of ACS [prolonged chest pain at rest, syncope, signs of congestive heart failure (CHF), etc.], an ECG, and laboratory biomarkers of cardiac injury, preferably troponin I or T.

A 12-lead ECG should be performed immediately upon arrival at the ED, with the standard being within 10 minutes of arrival for patients with symptoms suggestive of ACS.

Common ECG findings in UA/NSTEMI include ST-segment depression, transient ST-segment elevation, and T-wave inversion. However, approximately 20% of patients with an NSTEMI confirmed by cardiac enzymes have no ischemic ECG changes. Moreover, a "normal" ECG pattern is not sufficient to rule out ACS in patients with chest pain (>4% of patients presenting with chest pain and normal ECG patterns are diagnosed with UA). Persistent ST-segment elevation of more than 1 mm in two or more contiguous leads or new LBBB suggests acute STEMI and should be considered for emergency reperfusion therapy. As previously mentioned, ST-segment elevation more than 0.5 mm in lead aVR raises the possibility of left main or three-vessel CAD. T-wave inversions are the least specific of ECG changes in ACS. However, new, deep, symmetric T-wave inversions of more than 2 mm across the precordium in patients presenting with UA (Wellens' syndrome) often correspond to acute ischemia, usually related to a severe proximal left anterior descending artery stenosis. In this setting, revascularization often results in improved ventricular function and normalization of the ECG.

In patients in whom the initial ECG is not diagnostic but the anginal symptoms persist, serial ECGs should be performed in 15- to 30-minute intervals. This is done in order to detect the development of ST-segment depression or elevation. Posterior circulation ischemia or infarction should be suspected and the use of posterior ECG leads and echo imaging should be considered.

Biomarkers

Patients with chest discomfort possibly consistent with ACS should undergo measurement of biomarkers of myocardial injury.

Testing Strategy

The 2007 National Academy of Clinical Biochemistry (NACB) practice guidelines recommend measurement of biomarkers of cardiac injury in patients with symptoms that suggest ACS **(Box 1)**. Cardiac troponin I (cTnI) or cardiac troponin T (cTnT) with greater specificity recommended as the preferred first-line markers, but CK-MB (by mass assay) is an acceptable alternative. Another sample should be drawn 3–6 hours later, if initial set of markers is negative.

Troponins: Cardiac troponin I and T are contractile proteins found only in cardiac myocytes and are the preferred assays to document the presence of cardiac necrosis; clinical trials have used troponin levels for diagnosis and prognosis in ACS. Serum levels of troponins I and T typically rise within 3–12 hours after myocardial necrosis and remain elevated afterward for much longer than CK (10–14 days). Although troponins are more sensitive and specific for myocardial injury than CK and CK-MB, elevated troponin levels can be seen in other nonischemic cardiac conditions (advanced heart failure and acute pericarditis) and in the setting of renal insufficiency. In the setting of NSTE-ACS, troponins have important prognostic significance beyond that specified by clinical criteria, with elevated levels portending a worse prognosis. In the *GUSTO* IIb trial of patients with UA, the 30-day mortality rate for patients with an elevated troponin T level (>0.1 ng/mL) was 11.8%, compared with 3.9% for patients with normal troponin levels. Elevated troponin levels in the setting of NSTE-ACS have also been associated with increased likelihood of multivessel disease, high-risk culprit lesions, and intracoronary thrombus visible at the time of angiography.

Creatine kinase: Among the most commonly used biochemical markers for the evaluation of patients with suspected ACS are CK and the MB isoenzyme of CK, measured serially every 6–8 hours for the first 24 hours. Total CK levels peak at 12–24 hours after the onset of symptoms, and CK-MB levels peak at 10–18 hours after the onset of symptoms. The CK-MB isoenzyme is more specific and more sensitive than the total CK measurement for documenting myocardial necrosis. Although a low level of CK and CK-MB is usually found in normal patients, values above the upper limit of normal for a given laboratory suggest the presence

---

Box 1 National Academy of Clinical Biochemistry Recommendations for Use of Biochemical Markers for Risk Stratification in Acute Coronary Syndrome

Class I
1. Patients with suspected ACS should undergo early risk stratification based on integrated assessment of symptoms, physical examination findings, electrocardiography findings, and biomarkers (level or evidence: C).
2. A cardiac troponin is the perferred marker for risk stratification and, if available, should be measured in all patients with suspected ACS. In patients with a clinical syndrome consistent with ACS, a maximal (peak) concentration exceeding the 99the perentile of values for a reference control group should be considered indicative of increased risk for death and recurrent ischemic events (level of evidence: A).
3. Blood should be obtained for testing on arrival at the hospital, followed by serial sampling, with the timing of sampling based on clinical circumstances. For most patients, blood should be obtained for testing on arrival at the hospital and 6 to 9 hours later (level of evidence: B).

Class IIa
4. Measurement of high-sensitivity C-reactive protein (hsCRP) may be useful, in addition to a cardiac troponin, for risk assessment in patients with a clinical syndrome consistent with ACS. The benefits of therapy based on this strategy remain uncertain (level of evidence: A).
5. Measurement of B-type natriuretic peptide (BNP) or N-terminal pro-BNP (NT-proBNP) may be sudeful, in addition to a cardiac troponin, for risk assessment in patients with a clinical syndrome consistent with ACS. The benefits of therapy based on this strategy remain uncertain (level of evidence: A).

Class IIb
6. Measurement of markers of myocardial ischemia, in addition to cardiac troponin and an ECG, may aid in excluding ACS in patients with a low clinical probability of myocardial ischemia (level of evidence: C)
7. A multimarker strategy that includes measurement of two or more pathobiologically diverse biomarkers, in addition to a cardiac troponin, may aid in enhancing risk stratification in patients with a clinical syndrome consistent with ACS. BNP and hsCRP are the biomarkers best studied via this approach. The benefits of therapy base on this strategy remain uncertain (level of evidence: C).
8. Early repeated sampling of cardiac troponin (e.g. 2-4 hours after arrival) may be appropriate, if tied to therapeutic strategies (level of evidence: C).

Class III
Biomarkers of necrosis should not be used for routine screening of patients with a low clinical probability of ACS (level of evidence: C).

Source: From Morrow DA, Cannon CP, Jesse RL, et al. National Academy of Clinical Biochemistry Laboratory Medicine practice guidelines: Clinical characteristics and utilization of biochemical markers in acute coronary syndromes. Circulation. 2007;115:e356.

of myocardial necrosis. Many nonischemic conditions, such as pericarditis, skeletal muscle injury, and renal failure, can cause elevations of total CK levels or, less likely, an increase in CK-MB.

Recommendations for Immediate Management and Triage

The initial management of patients with suspected ACS is dependent on the predicted risk of adverse cardiovascular outcomes. Patients can be initially categorized as low, intermediate, or high risk depending on the historical and clinical findings. The use of risk stratification models such as the TIMI, GRACE, and PURSUIT risk scores can also assist in determining which patients are at increased risk. Patients with probable or possible ACS whose initial 12-lead ECG and cardiac biomarker levels are normal should be monitored on telemetry. Repeat ECGs and repeat cardiac biomarker measurements should be performed at scheduled intervals 6–8 hours apart.

In *low- and intermediate-risk patients* (Table 9) whose serial ECGs and cardiac biomarkers are normal, a conservative strategy may be considered and a cardiac stress test should be performed in the ED or monitoring facility. For low-risk patients, it is also appropriate to consider performing the stress test as an outpatient within 72 hours. The optimal time for testing may be determined at the discretion of the physician and in consideration of the patient's wishes. For such patients who are referred for outpatient stress testing, the initiation of antiplatelet and anti-ischemic pharmacotherapy should be strongly considered.

High-risk patients and low-risk patients who have a positive stress test with high-risk features should be admitted to the hospital for in-patient management. Patients with active ongoing ischemia or hemodynamic or electrical instability should be admitted to the intensive care unit.

Noninvasive Stress Testing

Stress testing has been thought to be contraindicated in the evaluation of patients with UA because of the concern for acute occlusion with increased cardiac workloads in the presence of unstable plaques. However, patients at low or even intermediate risk who remain pain free for at least 12–24 hours and without any symptoms of heart failure can safely undergo functional testing. Intermediate-risk patients include those with age older than 70 years; slightly elevated cardiac biomarkers (e.g. troponin T > 0.01 ng/mL but <0.1 ng/mL); T-wave changes; pathologic QS; minimal resting ST-depression (<1 mm) on ECG; rest angina or present with atypical symptoms; and prior history of MI, CABG, peripheral or cerebrovascular disease, or aspirin use.

Patients who have normal myocardial perfusion scan without fixed or reversible perfusion defects can be safely discharged from the hospital and followed up on an outpatient basis. However, cardiac catheterization should be considered for patients found to have high-risk features on stress testing because they are at increased risk for adverse ischemic

Table 9 Short-term risk for death or nonfatal myocardial ischemia in patients with unstable angina

Feature	High risk At least one of the following features must be present:	Intermediate risk No high-risk features but must have one of the following:	Low risk No high- or intermediate-risk features but may have any of the following:
History	Accelerating tempo of ischemic symptoms in the preceding 48 hours	Previous MI, peripheral or cerebrovascular disease, or CABG-previous ASA use	
Character of pain	Prolonged ongoing (> 20 min) pain at rest	• Prolonged (>20 min) rest angina, now resolved, with intermediate or high likehood or CAD • Rest angina (> 20 min) or relieved with rest or sublingual nitroglycerin • Nocturnal angina • New-onset or progressive CCS class III or IV angina in the past 2 weeks without prolonged (20 min) rest pain but with an intermediate or high likehood or CAD	• Increased angina frequency severity or duration • Angina provoked at a lower threshold • New-onset angina with onset 2 weeks to 2 months before initial evaluation
Clinical findings	• Pulmonary edema, most likely caused by ischemia • New or worsening MR murmur • S3 or new or worsening rales • Hypotension, bradycardia, tachycardia • Age >75 years	Age >70 years	

Contd...

Contd...

Feature	High risk At least one of the following features must be present:	Intermediate risk No high-risk features but must have one of the following:	Low risk No high- or intermediate-risk features but may have any of the following:
Electrocardiogram	• Angina at rest with transient ST-segment changes >0.05 mV • Bundle branch block, new or presumed new • Sustained ventricular tachycardia	• T-wave changes • Pathologic Q waves or resting ST-segment depression <0.1 mV in multiple lead groups (anterior, interior, lateral)	• Normal or unchaged ECG
Cardiac markers	Elevated cTnI, cTnT, or CK-MB	Slightly elevated cTnI, cTnT, or CK-MB	Normal

Abbreviations: ASA, acetylsalicylic acid; CABG, coronary artery bypass grafting; CCS, Canadian Cardiovascular Society; MR, mitral regurgitation.
Source: Anderson JL, Adams CD, Antman EM, et al. ACC/AHA 2007 guidelines for the management of patients with unstable angina/non-ST-elevation myocardial infarction: A report of the American College of Cardiology/American Heart Association Task Force on Practice Guidelines (Writing Committee to Revise the 2002 Guidelines for the Management of Patients With Unstable Angina/Non-ST-Elevation Myocardial Infarction): Developed in collaboration with the American College of Emergency Physicians, the Society for Cardiovascular Angiography and Interventions, and the Society of Thoracic Surgeons: Endorsed by the American Association of Cardiovascular and Pulmonary Rehabilitation and the Society for Academic Emergency Medicine. Circulation. 2007;116:e148-304.

Table 10 Initial management strategy in NSTE-ACS: Early invasive versus conservative (Selective invasive) approach

Early invasive	Conservative
• Hemodynamic instability • Arrhythmia instability • High-risk score (e.g. TIMI, GRACE, and PURSUIT) • Elevated troponin T or I • Refractory angina despite aggressive medical therapy • Prior PCI within 6 months or prior CABG • Signs or symptoms of congestive heart failure • New or worsening mitral regurgitation • Left ventricular function <40%	• Low risk score (e.g. TIMI, GRACE, and PURSUIT) • Physician or patient preference in low-to-intermediate risk patient

Abbreviations: CABG, coronary artery bypass grafting; GRACE, Global Registry of Acute Coronary Events; NSTE-ACS, non-ST-elevation-acute coronary syndrome; PCI, percutaneous coronary intervention; PURSUIT, Platelet Glycoprotein IIb/IIIa in Unstable Angina: Receptor Suppression Using Integrilin Therapy; TIMI, Thrombolysis in Myocardial Infarction.

events. If patients are unable to exercise, pharmacologic stress testing can be performed instead with dobutamine or a vasodilator such as adenosine or regadenoson.

Initial Conservative versus Initial Invasive Strategy

Two approaches to managing patients with NSTE-ACS have evolved. Based on a host of factors, including an overall assessment of patient risk, a decision to pursue either an early invasive strategy or an initial conservative strategy needs to be made early in the management of NSTE-ACS **(Table 10)**. Overall, patients selected to have early invasive therapy will have coronary angiography performed within 24 hours of admission, or sooner, depending on the clinical situation. Those patients elected to a conservative strategy are managed with optimal medical therapy and undergo angiography only in selected circumstances such as development of recurrent symptoms or objective evidence of ischemia while on appropriate medical therapy. Patients who have refractory angina despite medical therapy, hemodynamic instability, or electrical instability are recommended to undergo an early invasive strategy. For patients who are initially stabilized but are at high risk for adverse events, it is reasonable to undergo an early invasive strategy.

Initial Conservative Strategy

After receiving aspirin, patients who undergo an initial conservative strategy should receive an *anticoagulant* and be started on *clopidogrel therapy*. Enoxaparin and fondaparinux are the anticoagulants of choice; unfractionated heparin (UFH) is an acceptable alternative. Of note, if fondaparinux

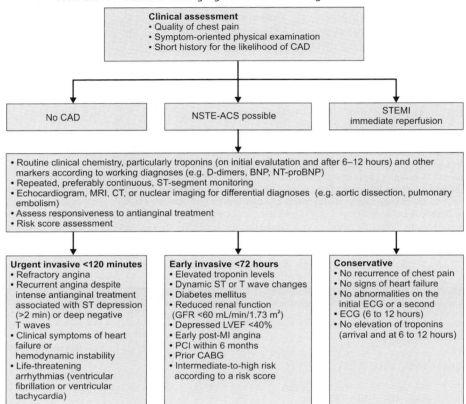

Flow chart 1 Decision-making algorithm for the management of NSTE-ACS

Abbreviations: BNP, B-type natriuretic peptide; CABG, coronary artery bypass grafting; CAD, coronary artery disease; CT, computed tomography; ECG, electrocardiogram; GFR, glomerular filtration rate; LVEF, left ventricular ejection fraction; MRI, magnetic resonance imaging; NT-proBNP, N-terminal pro b-type natriuretic peptide; NSTE-ACS, non-ST-elevation acute coronary syndrome; STEMI, ST-elevation myocardial infarction.
Source: From Bassand JP, Hamm CW. Diagnosis and treatment of non-ST-segment elevation acute coronary syndromes: European Society of Cardiology guidelines. Eur Heart J. 2011;32:369.

is used and an invasive strategy is ultimately employed, then another anticoagulant with factor IIa activity (UFH) must be coadministered to prevent catheterization-associated thrombosis.

Initial Invasive Strategy

After receiving aspirin, patients who undergo an initial invasive strategy should receive *anticoagulation with enoxaparin, UF, or bivalirudin*. Before proceeding with catheterization, it is recommended to administer a *second antiplatelet agent*. These agents include clopidogrel or ticagrelor. Prasugrel may also be utilized after angiographic definition. A glycoprotein IIb/IIIa inhibitor such as eptifibatide or tirofiban may be considered. Once angiography is performed, the appropriate subsequent therapy depends on the management plan **(Flow chart 1)**.

CONCLUSION

The optimal risk stratification of NSTE-ACS patients is a key priority in emergency medicine. Risk stratification based on prognostic scoring, such as GRACE, improves the selection of higher-risk patients for invasive management. However, the accuracy of diagnostic strategies is key to preventing inappropriate hospital admissions, minimizing avoidable morbidity and costs.

BIBLIOGRAPHY

1. Achar SA, Kundu S, Norcrohs WA. Diagnosis of Acute Coronary Syndrome. Am Fam Physician. 2005;72:119-26.
2. Antman EM, Cohen M, Bernink PJ, et al. The TIMI score for unstable angina/non ST elevation MI: a method for prognostication and therapeutic decision making. JAMA. 2000;284:835-42.
3. Bertrand ME, Simoons ML, Fox KA, et al. Management of Acute Coronary Syndromes in patients presenting without persistent ST-segment elevation. Eur Heart J. 2002;23:1809-40.
4. Boersma E, Pieper KS, Steyerberg EW, et al. Predictors of outcome in patients with acute coronary syndromes without persistent ST-segment elevation. Results from an international trial of 9461 patients. Circulation. 2000;101:2557-67.
5. Bramlage P, Messer C, Bitterlich N, et al. The effect of optical Medical therapy on 1-year mortality after acute myocardial infarction. Heart. 2010;96:804-9.
6. Braunwald E, Antman EM, Beasley JW, et al. ACC/AHA 2002 Guideline update for the management of patients with unstable angina and non ST-segment elevation myocardial infarction; a report of the American College of Cardiology/American Heart Association Task Force on Practice Guidelines (Committee on the Management of patients with Unstable Angina). Circulation. 2002;106:1883-90.
7. Bugiardini R. Risk stratification in acute coronary syndrome: focus on unstable angina/non ST-segment elevation myocardial infarction Heart. (Editorial). 2004;90:729-31.
8. Granger CB, Goldberg RJ, Dabbous O, et al. Predictors of hospital mortality in the Global Registry of Acute Coronary Events. Arch Intern Med. 2003;163:2345-53.
9. Kaur P, Rao TV, Shankar Subbiayan S, et al. Prevalence and distribution of cardiovascular risk factors in an urban industrial population in South India-A cross sectional study. JAPI. 2007;55:771-6.
10. Kennon S, Price CP, Mills PG, et al. Cumulative risk assessment in unstable angina: clinical, electrocardiographic, autonomic and biochemical markers. Heart. 2004;90:739-44.
11. Prabhakaran D, Shah P, Chaturvedi V, et al. Cardiovascular risk factor prevalence among men in a large industry of northern India. Nat Med J India. 2005;8:59-65.
12. Sabatine MS, Marrow DA, de Lemos JA, et al. Multimarker approach to risk stratification in non ST-segment elevation acute coronary syndromes. Simultaneous assessment of troponin I, Creactive protein, and B-type natriuretic peptide. Circulation. 2002;105:1760-3.
13. Syed Z, Scirica BM, Stultz CM, et al. Risk-Stratification following Acute Coronary Syndromes using a novel electrocardiographic technique to measure variability in morphology. Computers in Cardiology. 2008;35:13-6.
14. Yan AT, Yan RT, Tan Mary, et al. Risk scores for risk stratification in acute coronary syndromes: useful but simpler is not necessarily better. European Heart Journal. 2007;28:1072-8.
15. Yeolekar ME. Coronary artery disease in Asian Indians. Journal of Postgraduate Medicine. 1998;44:1,26-28.

CHAPTER 26

Cardiogenic Shock

Devendra Richhariya, Vikas Mudgal, Madhukar Shahi

INTRODUCTION

Shock is the final outcome of the circulatory collapse and inadequate supply of oxygenated blood to the tissues and the vital organs. Traditionally, shock is classified into four major types: (1) hypovolemic shock (excessive fluid loss from the body), (2) obstructive shock (blood flow obstruction in the large blood vessels conditions like pulmonary embolism, cardiac tamponade, and tension pneumothorax), (3) distributive shock (sepsis and anaphylactic reaction), and (4) cardiogenic shock caused by various conditions affecting the myocardium. Various characteristics of different types of shock are described in Chapter 14 (Overview of Shock). According to epidemiological data septic shock (distributive shock) is the most common shock followed by cardiogenic and hypovolemic shock **(Fig. 1)**.

Cardiogenic shock is the syndrome develops due to primary cardiac dysfunction resulting tissue and organ hypoperfusion with progressive multiorgan failure. Most common cause of cardiogenic shock is acute myocardial infarction (MI) particularly involving the anterior wall. Other causes include impairment of mechanical function of the heart, cardiomyopathies, and arrhythmias. Sometime establishing the etiology of cardiogenic shock is not easy. Invasive hemodynamic monitoring, specific biomarkers, and echocardiography are helpful in establishing the cause. Management of cardiogenic shock is always difficult and mortality in cardiogenic shock is still high about 50-70%. Since, MI is common cause of cardiogenic shock, early recognition, utilization of advanced revascularization therapy, and circulatory support help in reducing the mortality and improves the survival also.

DEFINITION

Cardiogenic shock is defined by the presence of specific clinical and hemodynamic criteria. Cardiogenic shock can easily be diagnosed by easy to assess clinical criteria. This is possible that hypotension may not present in early stage of compensated shock where normotension is maintained by high systemic vascular resistance compensating for low cardiac index **(Table 1)**. Group of people who are prone to cardiogenic shock is shown in **Box 1**.

ETIOLOGY

Knowledge of etiology is important for management of cardiogenic shock. Etiology of cardiogenic shock is classified as conditions affecting the myocardium, mechanical cause, and arrhythmic causes. Out of which most common is MI affecting the myocardium. Complications of MI like acute mitral regurgitation, ventricular septal defect, and cardiac tamponade due to cardiac free wall rupture also result in cardiogenic shock. Other important causes of cardiogenic shock are right ventricular failure, myocarditis, valvular heart

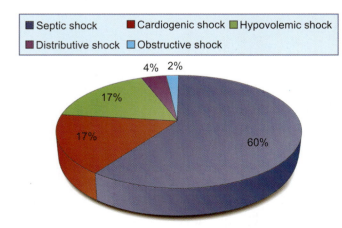

Fig. 1 Percentage of various types of shock in clinical practice

Table 1 Definition of cardiogenic shock

Clinical criteria	Hemodynamic criteria
Systolic blood pressure <90 mm Hg for more than 30 minutes or requirement of vasopressor to maintain BP >90 mm Hg. Clinical features of tissue and organ hypoperfusion like altered mental status, cold and clammy skin decreased urine output, raised serum lactate	Low cardiac output state with cardiac index <1.8 L/min/m^2 or <2–2.2 L/min/m^2 (on pharmacological or mechanical support) with elevated pulmonary capillary wedge pressure 15 mm Hg. Elevated indices of cardiac preload LVEDP >18 mm Hg and RVEDP >10–15 mm Hg

Abbreviations: LVEDP, left ventricular end diastolic pressure; RVEDP, right ventricular end-diastolic pressure.

Box 1 Risk factors for cardiogenic shock

- Older age
- Female sex
- Anterior wall MI
- Hypertension
- Diabetes mellitus
- Multivessel coronary artery disease
- History of MI
- STEMI with LBBB
- History of heart failure

Abbreviations: MI, myocardial infarction; STEMI, ST-segment elevation myocardial infarction; LBBB, left bundle branch block.

Table 2 Etiology of cardiogenic shock

Myocardial causes	• Myocardial infarction (MI) left or right infarction • Cardiomyopathy • Myocarditis • Toxins and cytotoxic drugs • Medication (calcium channel blocker, beta-blockers, digoxin, antiarrhythmic drugs, and antidepressant) • Ventricular hypertrophy
Mechanical causes	• Valvular heart disease • Mechanical complications of MI (papillary muscle dysfunction, ventricular septal rupture, and cardiac free wall rupture) • Hypertrophic cardiomyopathy • Outflow tract obstruction • Atrial thrombus and atrial tumor • Aortic dissection • Cardiac trauma (myocardial contusion)
Arrhythmic causes	• Supraventricular or ventricular arrhythmia • Bradyarrhythmias

disease, arrhythmias, and advanced stage cardiomyopathies **(Table 2)**.

Figure 2 showing myocardial infarction-related complications as a cause cardiogenic shock.

PATHOPHYSIOLOGY

Cardiogenic shock occurs when about 40% of left ventricle is damaged predominantly due to ischemia. Right ventricular infarction is also recognized as the cause of cardiogenic shock in few cases. Thrombotic occlusion of artery supplying the major part of the heart is underlying pathology of the cardiogenic shock. Coronary occlusion induces depression of myocardial contractility. Reduction in myocardial contractility produces the low cardiac index and hypotension. Low cardiac index and hypotension cause severe tissue hypoperfusion which is measured by the raised serum lactate. Initially compensatory vasoconstriction occurs in which normotensive state is maintained. If this preshock stage is not recognized early and not treated well, this condition progresses to severe or refractory cardiogenic shock **(Flow chart 1)**. Inflammatory derangement capillary leakage and microcirculatory derangement also contribute to development of severe or refractory shock. According to various studies older age group, low left ventricular ejection fraction (LVEF), low cardiac index, low systolic BP, requirement of vasopressor and mechanical support, and high serum lactate level are associated with high mortality rates in cardiogenic shock.

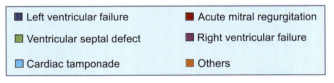

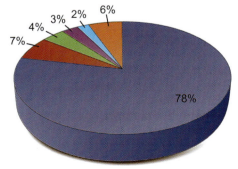

Fig. 2 Distribution of myocardial infarction-related complications as a cause of cardiogenic shock

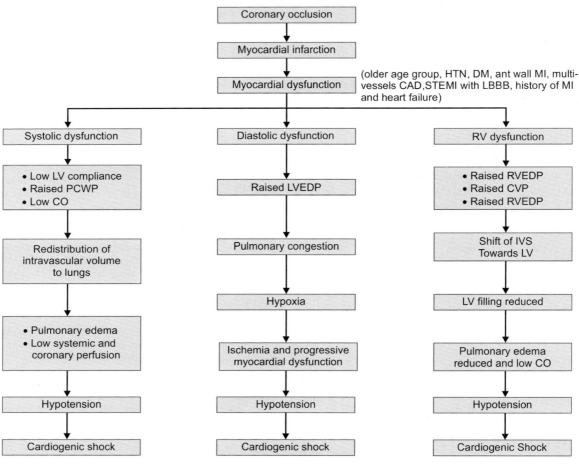

Flow chart 1 Pathophysiology of cardiogenic shock

Abbreviations: MI, myocardial infarction; HTN, hypertension; LV, left ventricular; LVEDP, left ventricular end-diastolic pressure; RVEDP, right ventricular end-diastolic pressure; CVP, central venous pressure; CO, cardiac output; PCWP, pulmonary capillary wedge pressure; IVS interventricular septum.

DIAGNOSIS

Cardiogenic shock develops gradually as preshock stage (patient at risk of cardiogenic shock), mild shock (responsive to low dose inotropic support), severe shock [responsive to high dose inotropic support or intra-aortic balloon pump (IABP)], and refractory shock (when mechanical support is required). Diagnosing the cardiogenic shock in early stage is challenging and vital as reversibility almost impossible in advanced and refractory stage. Various clinical features and hemodynamics are suggestive of cardiogenic shock **(Table 3)**.

This is also important to establish the type of shock for appropriate management. Emergency physician should know the differentiating features of hypovolemic, distributive, and cardiogenic shock **(Table 4)**.

Table 3 Diagnosis of cardiogenic shock on the basis of clinical and hemodynamic features	
Clinical features	Hemodynamic features
• Signs of hypoperfusion like cool moist skin, pale or cyanosis, slow speech, low sensory perception lethargy confusion • Oliguria or anuria	• Systolic BP <90 mm Hg for more than 30 minutes • Requirement of vasopressors to maintain the systolic BP >90 mm Hg • Low cardiac index (<2.2 L/min/m^2) • Raised pulmonary wedge pressure (>15 mm Hg)

Various supporting tests like biochemical test, hemodynamic monitoring, and echocardiography are also helpful in this regards. Bedside echocardiography is the key investigations along with electrocardiogram (ECG)

Table 4 Hemodynamic features of various types of shock

	Hypovolemic shock	Distributive shock	Cardiogenic shock
Pulmonary wedge pressure	Low	Low or normal	Raised
Cardiac output	Low	Raised	Low
SVR	Raised	Low	Raised
Mixed venous O$_2$ saturation	Low	Raised	Low

Abbreviation: SVR, systemic vascular resistance.

Table 5 Differentiating features of LVMI and RVMI

	LVMI	RVMI
Clinical features	Pulmonary congestion S3, S4 new MR	Clear lung fields right sided S3 new TR, hypotension with distended neck veins
ECG	ST-elevation in standard leads	ST-elevation in V4R
Hemodynamics	Raised pulmonary wedge pressure	RAP >10 mm Hg RAP/PAWP >0.8
Specific management	Fluid restriction Preload and after load reduction Reperfusion therapy Inotropes	Fluid resuscitation Avoid preload reduction Reperfusion therapy Inotropes

Abbreviations: LVMI, left ventricular myocardial infarction; RVMI, right ventricular myocardial infarction, MR, mitral regurgitation; TR, tricuspid regurgitation; ECG, electrocardiogram; RAP, right atrial pressure; PAWP, pulmonary arterial wedge pressure.

and biochemical test for acute coronary syndrome as MI is important cause of cardiogenic shock. Important cardiac parameters like global systolic function, pressers, pericardial fluid, and inferior vena cava can be assessed by the bedside echocardiography. Pulmonary artery catheterization (PAC) is helpful in providing the information about left or right ventricular filling pressures, systemic and pulmonary vascular resistance, right ventricular ejection fraction, and oxygen saturation. Monitoring of mixed venous oxygen saturation (SvO$_2$) is not only useful for diagnostic purpose but also helpful in reducing the mortality when SvO$_2$ is maintained within therapeutic target during initial hours of shock treatment.

It is also important to distinguish between the left ventricular myocardial infarction (LVMI) and the right ventricular myocardial infarction (RVMI) as the cause of cardiogenic shock with the help of clinical features, ECG, and the hemodynamic features because mortality risk for cardiogenic shock is due to primary right ventricular dysfunction nearly as high as left ventricular dysfunction. Differentiating features between LVMI and RVMI are shown in **Table 5**.

MANAGEMENT

Management of cardiogenic shock should be started early to normalize hemodynamic parameter and to prevent the further damage of organ and deterioration of the

Box 2 Therapeutic target for hemodynamic parameters.
Mean arterial pressure >60 mm Hg

- Pulmonary wedge pressure <18 mm Hg
- Central venous pressure 8–12 mm Hg
- Urine output >0.5 mL/h/kg
- Arterial blood pH 7.3–7.5
- Central venous O$_2$ saturation (SvO$_2$) >70%

patient. Immediate management of shock includes fluid therapy, vasoactive therapy, and ventilator therapy along with correction of electrolyte imbalance. Along with the symptomatic treatment therapy should be directed at the underlying cause. Most cases of cardiogenic shock are due to MI, prompt reperfusion therapy should be instituted. Revascularization therapy [percutaneous transluminal coronary angioplasty (PTCA) or coronary artery bypass grafting (CABG)] reduces the hospitalization, long-term mortality, and MI-related mechanical complication. Management of the cardiogenic shock should target to maintain hemodynamic parameter within therapeutic range **(Box 2)**. Maintaining the hemodynamic parameters within therapeutic range is suggestive of adequate management strategies and positive outcome.

Management of cardiogenic shock is multiphasic, and **Table 6** showing various modalities of treatment used in cardiogenic shock.

Table 6 Modalities of treatment in cardiogenic shock

Intensive care unit support	Revascularization support	Mechanical support	Special situation

• Fluid administration
• Vasoactive agents*
  (vasopressor and inotrope)
• Ventilator support
• PA catheter
	• Thrombolysis
	• PCI
	• CABG
		• IABP
		• ECMO
		• Percutaneous left ventricular assist device (LVAD), e.g. tandem heart, impella
			• RVMI with shock
			• Surgical repair of mechanical complication
			  (acute MR, free wall rupture)

Abbreviations: IABP, intra-aortic balloon pump; RVMI, right ventricular myocardial infarction; PCI, percutaneous coronary intervention; ECMO, extracorporeal membrane oxygenation; CABG, coronary artery bypass grafting; MR, mitral regurgitation; PA, pulmonary artery.
*Vasoactive agents (vasopressor and inotrope) are described in chapter 13.

INTENSIVE CARE UNIT SUPPORT

Fluid Administration

First step of management is assessment of intravascular fluid status and fluid responsiveness. Fluid therapy should be used cautiously under the guidance of invasive monitoring and maintenance of target CVP. Generally, 250–500 mL of crystalloid fluid is given over 30 minutes.

Vasopressor Support

Vasopressor agents are added to the ongoing therapy when hypotension persists despite fluid therapy. For maintaining the mean arterial pressure (MAP) (>60 mm Hg) vasopressor agents are required to maintain adequate coronary and tissue perfusion.
- *Noradrenaline*: Primarily is vasoconstrictor and weak inotrope. Noradrenaline is vasopressor of choice in cardiogenic shock, helpful in increasing the coronary blood flow. Dose of noradrenaline is 0.02–1 µg/kg/min.
- *Vasopressin*: Primarily a vasoconstrictor usually added to the noradrenaline when requirement to noradrenaline exceeds 0.4 µg/kg/min.
- *Phenylephrine*: Pure vasoconstrictor and used when hypotension is associated with tachycardia.

Inotrope Support

Inotrope support maintains the adequate MAP related to stabilization of cardiogenic shock. MAP relating mostly to central hemodynamics but does not correlate peripheral tissue perfusion. There is compensatory peripheral vasoconstriction mechanism due to which compromised tissue perfusion occurs. Inotropes are indicated when features of tissue hypoperfusion persists despite adequate fluid and target MAO.
- *Dobutamine*: It is an inotrope of choice in cardiogenic shock; started with the dose of 2–20 µg/kg/min when systolic BP is above 90 mm Hg. It improves the peripheral perfusion but produce hypotension and tachyarrhythmia due to mild systemic vasodilatory and positive chronotropic effect.
- *Milrinone*: The main use of milrinone is in decreasing the RV load in advanced nonischemic cardiomyopathies. Milrinone provides inotropic with less chronotropic and less arrhythmic effects.
- Dopamine and adrenaline are less commonly used in cardiogenic shock due to their arrhythmic and undesirable hemodynamic results.

Ventilator Support

Mechanical ventilation improves patient comfort, reduces stress, fatigue and correct acidosis, hypoxia, and improves tissue perfusion.

Intensive care support is summarized as VIP mnemonic, i.e. *V* (ventilation), *I* (infuse-fluid therapy), *P* (pump-vasoactive drugs).

Pulmonary Artery Catheterization

Pulmonary artery catheter insertion may be helpful in monitoring of patient with cardiogenic shock. It gives information about hemodynamic parameters like right and left ventricular filling pressures, systemic and pulmonary vascular resistance, right ventricular ejection fraction, and mixed venous oxygen (SvO_2) saturation and thermodilution-derived cardiac out. PAC is associated with various periprocedural complications so should be performed by expert. Appropriate interpretation of data of PAC is helpful in differentiating the different types of shock and to guide appropriate management.

Revascularization Support

Myocardial infarction is the important cause of cardiogenic shock. Early revascularization [percutaneous coronary intervention (PCI) or CABG] is the lifesaving intervention in cardiogenic shock management. Urgent coronary angiography with support of IABP and PTCA or CABG is recommended in patient with cardiogenic shock due to left ventricular failure complicating acute MI or new left bundle branch block (LBBB) MI **(Flow chart 2)**.

Flow chart 2 Revascularization support in cardiogenic shock

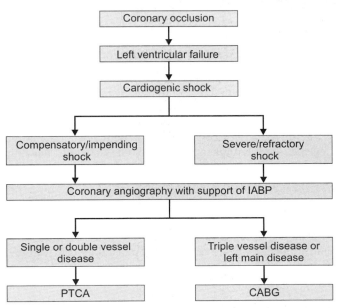

Abbreviations: IABP, intra-aortic balloon pump; PTCA, percutaneous transluminal coronary angioplasty; CABG, coronary artery bypass grafting.

Fibrinolytic Therapy

Fibrinolytic therapy is started if presentation of early or compensatory stage of cardiogenic shock with ST segment elevation myocardial infarction (STEMI) to hospital is less than 3 hours, no contraindications to therapy, and PCI intervention facility is not available. Concurrent use of IABP is also beneficial.

Currently available fibrinolytic agents are alteplase, reteplase, tenecteplase, urokinase, prourokinase anistreplase, streptokinase. Intravenous doses of fibrinolytic agents in acute MI are as follows:

Streptokinase: 1.5 million IU (infused over 1 hour in 45 mL NaCl).

Alteplase: 15 mg loading dose followed by 50 mg* over 30 min and 35 mg** over next 1 hour (total duration of infusion 90 min) and concurrent use of heparin

Reteplase: Given as double bolus by 10 U+10 U (no infusion), 10 U bolus over 2 min wait for 30 min and repeat 10 U over 2 min and concurrent use of heparin.

Tenecteplase: 30–50 mg single weight based bolus over 5–10 sec and concurrent use of heparin.

---

*0.75 mg/kg not to exceed 50 mg over 30 min.
**0.50 mg/kg and not to exceed 35 mg over next 1 hour.

Percutaneous Transluminal Coronary Angioplasty

Various studies shows decrease in mortality rates if successful reperfusion done in cardiogenic shock complicating acute MI.

Coronary Artery Bypass Grafting

Patient with cardiogenic shock with triple vessel disease or left main coronary artery disease, CABG provides favorable outcome.

Mechanical Support

Mechanical support is ultimate approach to improve hemodynamic parameters. Nowadays a number of devices are available with different mechanism of action and effectiveness. These devices provide cardiac chambers (right left biventricular) support. IABP, extracorporeal membrane oxygenation (ECMO), and percutaneous left ventricular assist device (LVAD) are available for mechanical support. These devices are indicated when all ICU measures fail to provide adequate tissue and organ perfusion and risk of multiorgan failure develops. IABP is commonly used to improve hemodynamic parameters. 30-days mortality was not reduced by use of IABP in cardiogenic shock complicating MI according to IABP-SHOCK II trials. No reduction of short-term mortality is noted by use of IABP and Impella pump and Tandem Heart device are not found superior to IABP according to few randomized studies. Thus, further improvement in mechanical device is required which provides not only hemodynamic stabilization but also improves patient outcome.

Intra-aortic Balloon Pump

Several physiological parameters are improved with the use of IABP. IABP provides reduction in myocardial oxygen demand, pulmonary wedge pressure, LV afterload along with improvement in coronary blood flow, and cardiac output. Various indications are shown in **Table 7**. IABP is associated with various complications like arterial wall trauma, limb ischemia, thrombus dislodgement, thrombocytopenia, red blood cell hemolysis, hemorrhage, balloon rupture or leak, and infection. Hemodynamic effect of IABP depends on the balloon volume, heart rate and rhythm, and systemic vascular resistance. **Table 8** showing how to select balloon size in specific patient and their characteristics. Ideal balloon function in 1:3 sequence where every third ventricular beat is augmented by IABP. If heart rate is above 140 beats/min, switch to 1:2 sequence until rate slow. Be aware of presence of pulse in left arm, indicate tip of balloon not obstructing

Table 7	IABP is indicated in various conditions apart from cardiogenic shock
Medical	• Cardiogenic shock • Acute anterior wall MI • Complications of MI like acute MR and VSR • High-risk angioplasty • Ventricular arrhythmia secondary to ischemia
Surgical	• High-risk cardiac patient • Bridge to CABG and heart transplant • Postoperative low cardiac output • Weaning from bypass open heart surgery
Others	• Drug-induced heart failure • Myocardial contusion aortic stenosis
IABP contraindicated in acute aortic dissection, aortic regurgitation chronic end-stage heart disease, irreversible brain damage	

Abbreviations: IABP, intra-aortic balloon pump; MI, myocardial infarction; MR, mitral regurgitation; VSR, ventricular septal rupture; CABG, coronary artery bypass grafting.

subclavian orifice and subclavian flow is not occluding. For optimal hemodynamics balloon should be deflated just before LV ejection (at QRS complex) **(Fig. 3)**.

Extracorporeal Membrane Oxygenation (Fig. 4)

It consists of blood pump, the heat exchanger, and the oxygenator. Indicated in severe hypercapnia with pH <7.20, PaO_2:FiO_2 <50–1,000 mm Hg, alveolar-arterial oxygen gradient >600 mm Hg, and transpulmonary shunt >30%.

Main challenges in ECMO are patient selection, system logistic, and complication like limb ischemia bleeding complications. Currently ECMO is used as bridge therapy to heart transplantation.

Percutaneous Left Ventricular Assist Device

Currently available percutaneous LVADs are Tandem Heart and Impella. They are inserted percutaneously through femoral artery and provide pulsatile support via pump.

Table 8 Selection of balloon size			
Height of patient	<5'	5'–5'4"	5'4"–6'
Balloon volume	25 mL	34 mL	40 mL
Length	165 mm	221 mm	258 mm
Diameter	15 mm	15 mm	15 mm
Catheter size	7.5F	7.5F	7.5F

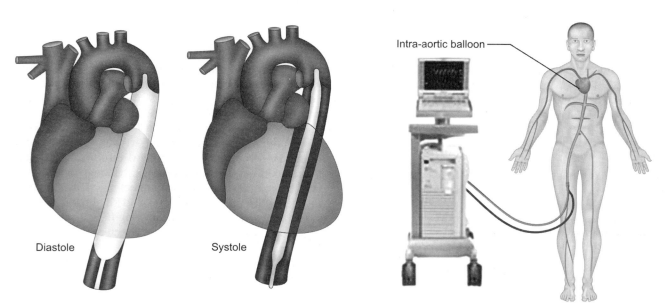

Fig. 3 Intra-aortic balloon pump (IABP): balloon inflated in diastole with closure of aortic valve. Balloon remains inflated till ventricular systole Inflation of balloon displaces the blood toward aorta and coronaries and promotes coronary perfusion and blood flow. Collapse of balloon decreases the left ventricular (LV) work by reducing the resistance of LV ejection.

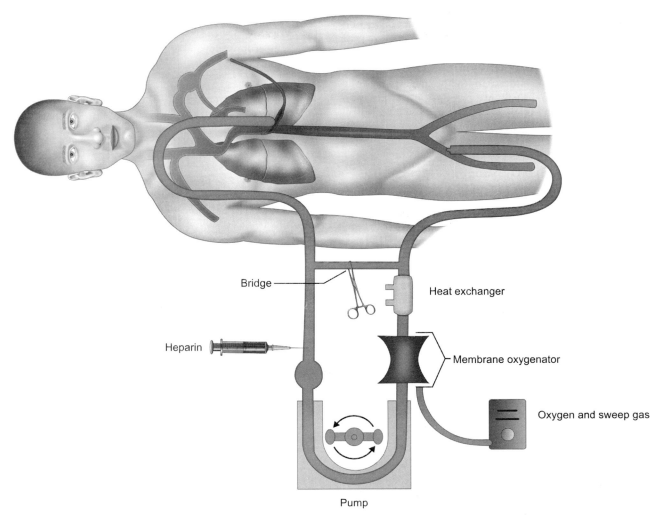

Fig. 4 Extracorporeal membrane oxygenator

LVADs provide higher cardiac index, higher MAP, and lower pulmonary wedge pressure. There is no 30-day survival benefit by using LVAD. They are used in refractory cardiogenic shock as bridging strategies to heart transplantation.

SPECIAL SITUATION

Right Ventricular Myocardial Infarction with Shock

Right ventricular MI is suspected in all patients with inferior wall MI with shock. RVMI is mostly associated with inferior and posterior wall MI and mortality is also high. Clinical triad of raised jugular venous pressure, clear lung fields in presence of inferior or posterior wall MI (ST-elevation in V3R and V4R) suggestive of RVMI. Echocardiography also helpful in diagnosis. Therapeutic approach is quite different from left ventricular failure. Maintain right ventricular preload with intravenous fluid, avoid use of nitrates and diuretics, and maintain A-V synchrony with the help of pacing in case of high degree of heart block. Use of pharmacological circulatory support, revascularization support, and mechanical support is the mainstay of therapy.

Mechanical Complication of Acute MI (Acute Mitral Regurgitation, Papillary Muscle Rupture, Ventricular Septal Rupture, and Free Wall Rupture)

Acute mitral regurgitation is usually associated with inferior wall MI and ischemia of posterior papillary muscle. Acute mitral regurgitation develops within 2–7 days after the MI and clinically present as pulmonary edema hypotension and cardiogenic shock. Echocardiography is extremely useful. All therapeutic measures should be implemented as described above. However, definitive therapy is surgical valve repair or replacement.

Patient with ventricular septal rupture present with severe or refractory cardiogenic shock. Characteristics, pansystolic murmur and parasternal thrill, are present on examination and echocardiography is diagnostic modality of choice. Early use of circulatory and mechanical support followed by surgical repair is definitive therapy.

Reversible Myocardial Dysfunction (Myocarditis, Sepsis Induced-myocardia Dysfunction)

Few reversible causes of myocardial dysfunctions are sepsis-induced myocardial dysfunction, inflammatory myocarditis, and myocardial dysfunction after cardiopulmonary bypass. Inflammatory cytokines (tumor necrosis factor and IL1) play an important role in sepsis and myocarditis. Combination of inotropic support and IABP is required for days to week to allow sufficient time for recovery. If these measures fail mechanical support with LVAD can be considered.

CONCLUSION

Cardiogenic shock develops due to multiple causes like MI, cardiomyopathies, and myocarditis. Restoration of effective tissue perfusion and cellular metabolism are the ultimate goals for the prescribed therapy. Early circulatory support and revascularization is the mainstay of treatment and also improves the survival in cardiogenic shock complication in acute MI.

BIBLIOGRAPHY

1. Abrams D, Combes A, Brodie D. Extracorporeal membrane oxygenation in cardiopulmonary disease in adults. J Am Coll Cardiol. 2014;63(25 Pt A):2769-78.
2. Aissaoui N, Puymirat E, Tabone X, et al. Improved outcome of cardiogenic shock at the acute stage of myocardial infarction: A report from the USIK 1995, USIC 2000, and FAST-MI French Nationwide Registries. Eur Heart J. 2012;33:2535-43.
3. Ammirati E, Oliva F, Cannata A, et al. Current indications for heart transplantation and left ventricular assist device: A practical point of view. Eur J Intern Med. 2014;25:422-9.
4. Arlt M, Philipp A, Voelkel S, et al. Hand-held minimised extracorporeal membrane oxygenation: A new bridge to recovery in patients with out-of-centre cardiogenic shock. Eur J Cardiothoracic Surg. 2011;40(3):689-94.
5. Bednarczyk JM, White CW, Ducas RA, et al. Resuscitative extracorporeal membrane oxygenation for in hospital cardiac arrest: a Canadian observational experience. Resuscitation. 2014;30:2014.
6. Belletti A, Castro ML, Silvetti S, et al. The effect of inotropes and vasopressors on mortality: a meta-analysis of randomized clinical trials. Br J Anaesth. 2015;115:656-75.
7. Cheng JM, Den Uil, Hoeks C, et al. Percutaneous left ventricular assist devices vs. intra-aortic balloon pump counterpulsation for treatment of cardiogenic shock: A meta-analysis of controlled trials. Eur Heart J. 2009l;30:2102-8.
8. De Backer D, Biston P, Devriendt J, et al. SOAP II Investigators. Comparison of dopamine and norepinephrine in the treatment of shock. N Engl J Med. 2010;362(9):779-89.
9. De Backer D, Hollenberg S, Boerma C, et al. How to evaluate the microcirculation: report of a round table conference. Crit Care. 2007;11(5):R101.
10. Delaney AP, Dan A, McCaffrey J, et al. The role of albumin as a resuscitation fluid for patients with sepsis: A systematic review and meta-analysis. Crit Care Med. 2011;39:386-91.
11. Feldman D, Pamboukian SV, Teuteberg JJ, et al. The 2013 International Society for Heart and Lung Transplantation Guidelines for mechanical circulatory support: Executive summary. J Heart Lung Transplant. 2013;32:157-87.
12. Felker GM, Benza RL, Chandler AB, et al. Heart failure etiology and response to milrinone in decompensated heart failure. J Am Coll Cardiol. 2003;41:997-1003.
13. Fincke R, Hochman JS, Lowe AM, et al. Cardiac power is the strongest hemodynamic correlate of mortality in cardiogenic shock: A report from the SHOCK trial registry. J Am Coll Cardiol. 2004;44:340-8.
14. Fuhrmann JT, Schmeisser A, Schulze MR, et al. Levosimendan is superior to enoximone in refractory cardiogenic shock complicating acute myocardial infarction. Crit Care Med. 2008;36:2257-66.
15. Guenther S, Theiss HD, Fischer M, et al. Percutaneous extracorporeal life support for patients in therapy refractory cardiogenic shock: Initial results of an interdisciplinary team. Interact. Cardiovasc Thorac Surg. 2014;18:283-91.
16. Harvey S, Harrison DA, Singer M, et al. Assessment of the clinical effectiveness of pulmonary artery catheters in management of patients in intensive care (PAC-Man): a randomised controlled trial. 2005;366(9484):472-7.
17. Hochman JS, Sleeper LA, Webb JG, et al. Early revascularization and long-term survival in cardiogenic shock complicating acute myocardial infarction. JAMA. 2006;295:2511-5.
18. Jansen TC, van Bommel J, Schoonderbeek FJ, et al. Early Lactate-Guided Therapy in Intensive Care Unit Patients. Am J Respir Crit Care Med. 2010;182:752-61.
19. Jeffries PR, Whelan SK. Cardiogenic shock: current management. Crit Care Nurs Q. 1988;11:48-56.
20. Jeger RV, Lowe AM, Buller CE, et al. Hemodynamic parameters are prognostically important in cardiogenic shock but similar following early revascularization or initial medical stabilization: a report from the SHOCK Trial Chest. 2007;132:1794-803.
21. Jeger RV, Urban P, Harkness SM, et al. Early revascularization is beneficial across all ages and a wide spectrum of cardiogenic shock severity: A pooled analysis of trials. Acute Card Care. 2001;13:14-20.
22. Kagawa E, Dote K, Kato M, et al. Should we emergently revascularize occluded coronaries for cardiac arrest?: rapid-response extracorporeal membrane oxygenation and intra-arrest percutaneous coronary intervention. Circulation. 2012;126(13):1605-13.
23. Kar B, Gregoric ID, Basra SS, et al. The percutaneous ventricular assist device in severe refractory cardiogenic shock. J Am Coll Cardiol. 2001;57:688-96.
24. Kolh P, Windecker S, Alfonso F, et al. 2014 ESC/EACTS Guidelines on myocardial revascularization: The Task Force on Myocardial Revascularization of the European Society of

Cardiology (ESC) and the European Association for Cardio-Thoracic Surgery (EACTS). Developed with the special contribution of the European Association of Percutaneous Cardiovascular Interventions (EAPCI). Eur J Cardiothorac Surg. 2014;46(4):517-92.
25. Lim N, Dubois MJ, De Backer D, et al. Do all nonsurvivors of cardiogenic shock die with a low cardiac index? Chest. 2003;124(5):1885-91.
26. Maharaj R, Metaxa V. Levosimendan and mortality after coronary revascularisation: a meta-analysis of randomised controlled trials. Crit Care. 2011;15:R140.
27. McMurray JJ, Adamopoulos S, Anker SD, et al. ESC Guidelines for the diagnosis and treatment of acute and chronic heart failure 2012: The Task Force for the Diagnosis and Treatment of Acute and Chronic Heart Failure 2012 of the European Society of Cardiology. Developed in collaboration with the Heart Failure Association (HFA) of the ESC. Eur Heart J. 2012;33:1787-847.
28. National Institute for Health and Clinical Excellence (NICE) interventional procedure guidance 482. Extracorporeal membrane oxygenation (ECMO) for acute heart failure in adults. 2014.
29. Pages ON, Aubert S, Combes A, et al. Paracorporeal pulsatile biventricular assist device versus extracorporeal membrane oxygenation-extracorporeal life support in adult fulminant myocarditis. J Thorac Cardiovasc Surg. 2009;137:194-7.
30. Prondzinsky R, Lemm H, Swyter M, et al. Intra-aortic balloon counterpulsation in patients with acute myocardial infarction complicated by cardiogenic shock: The prospective, randomized IABP SHOCK Trial for attenuation of multiorgan dysfunction syndrome. Crit Care Med. 2010;38(1):152-60.
31. Reynolds HR, Hochman JS. Cardiogenic shock: current concepts and improving outcomes. Circulation. 2008;117:686-97.
32. Rivers E, Nguyen B, Havstad, S, et al. Early Goal-Directed Therapy in the Treatment of Severe Sepsis and Septic Shock. N Engl J Med. 2001;345:1368-77.
33. Russell JA, Walley KR, Gordon AC, et al. Interaction of vasopressin infusion, corticosteroid treatment, and mortality of septic shock. Crit Care Med. 2009;37:811-18.
34. Sakamoto S, Taniguchi N, Nakajima S, et al. Extracorporeal life support for cardiogenic shock or cardiac arrest due to acute coronary syndrome. Ann Thorac Surg. 2012;94:1-7.
35. Scheidt S, Wilner G, Mueller H, et al. Intra-aortic balloon counterpulsation in cardiogenic shock. N Engl J Med. 1973; 288:979-84.
36. Sheu JJ, Tsai TH, Lee FJ, et al. Early extracorporeal membrane oxygenator-assisted primary percutaneous coronary intervention improved 30-day clinical outcomes in patients with ST-segment elevation myocardial infarction complicated with profound cardiogenic shock. Crit. Care Med. 2010;38:1810-7.
37. Soar J, Deakin C, Lockey A, et al. Adult advanced life support. Summary of changes in advanced life support since 2010 Guidelines. Resusc Counc UK (2015).
38. Steg PG, James SK, Atar D, et al. Task Force on the management of ST-segment elevation acute myocardial infarction of the European Society of Cardiology (ESC)1. ESC Guidelines for the management of acute myocardial infarction in patients presenting with ST-segment elevation. Eur Heart J. 2012;33(20):2569-619.
39. Stegman BM, Newby LK, Hochman JS, et al. Post-myocardial infarction cardiogenic shock is a systemic illness in need of systemic treatment. J Am Coll Cardiol. 20012;59(7):644-47.
40. Stub D, Bernard S, Pellegrino V, et al. Refractory cardiac arrest treated with mechanical CPR, hypothermia, ECMO and early reperfusion (the CHEER trial). Article in press. Resuscitation. 1-7 (2015).
41. Thiele H, Zeymer U, Neumann FJ, et al. Intra-aortic balloon counterpulsation in acute myocardial infarction complicated by cardiogenic shock (IABP-SHOCK II): final 12 months results of a randomised, open-label trial. Lancet. 2013;382:1638-45.
42. Thiele H, Zeymer U, Neumann FJ, et al. Intra-aortic balloon support for myocardial infarction with cardiogenic shock. N Engl J Med. 2012;367:1287-96.
43. Torgersen C, Schmittinger CA, Wagner S, et al. Hemodynamic variables and mortality in cardiogenic shock: a retrospective cohort study. Crit Care. 2009;13:R157.
44. Vincent JL, De Backer D. Circulatory Shock. N Engl J Med. 2013;18369:1726-34.
45. Vincent JL, Rhodes A, Perel A, et al. Clinical review: Update on hemodynamic monitoring–a consensus of 16. Crit Care. 2011;15:229.
46. Yancy CW, Jessup M, Bozkurt B, et al. ACCF/AHA Practice Guideline 2013 ACCF/AHA Guideline for the Management of Heart Failure A Report of the American College of Cardiology Foundation/American Heart Association Task Force on Practice Guidelines. J Am Coll Cardiol. 2013;62(16):e147-239.

CHAPTER 27

Heart Failure

Vijay Kumar Chopra

INTRODUCTION

Acute heart failure is one of the most common causes of emergency admissions in our country and the incidence is steadily rising. Increasing prevalence of coronary artery disease (CAD), greater survival after myocardial infarction (MI) due to coronary care units (CCUs) and rising incidence of diabetes mellitus (DM) in our country are some of the important factors. Of late, there has been a greater awareness of heart failure with preserved ejection fraction where left ventricular ejection fraction (LVEF) is over 40%. The most common causes of acute heart failure is exacerbation of chronic heart failure (CHF). However, other important causes are accelerated hypertension, acute myocardial infarction, valvular disease, myocarditis, and renal failure.

INITIAL CLINICAL ASSESSMENT

For patients with preexisting CHF, one should identify the precipitating factors and the status of fluid overload and perfusion.[1] For patients with known CAD new onset ischemia is an important cause. Other common exacerbating factors are tachyarrhythmia, thyroid disease, anemia, infection, chronic kidney disease, chronic pulmonary disease, and pulmonary emboli.[2] Excessive fluid and salt intake and coadministration of certain drugs is known to worsen heart failure and should also be enquired into *the four hemodynamic profiles*. The key components of acute heart failure are elevation of filling pressure and reduction of cardiac output, which do not necessary occur together as shown in **Figure 1**.[1] The most common manifestation is generally profile B with congestion and adequate perfusion **(Box 1)**. A good history and a thorough physical examination can yield important information. Orthopnea, nocturnal cough, and progressive effort intolerance are indicative of elevated filling pressure in this setting. Raised jugular venous

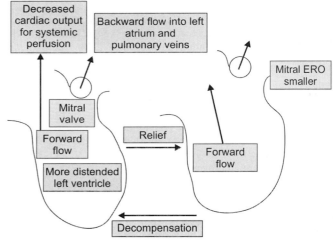

Fig. 1 Key components of acute heart failure
Abbreviation: ERO, effective regurgitant orifice

Box 1 Evidence of congestion

- Orthopnea
- Elevated jugular venous pressure
- Rales (rarely)
- Hepatomegaly
- Ascites
- Edema (more common in older patients)
- Valsalva square wave

pressure (JVP), hepatomegaly, and bilateral crepitation are usually present but not always. Electrocardiogram, chest X-Ray, elevated natriuretic peptides, and echocardiography are the most important initial investigations. In the absence of pulmonary edema, arterial desaturation may or may not be present.

Patients with heart failure and low ejection fraction may also decompensate with profile C "cold and wet" but rarely with profile "cold and dry".

Hemodynamic profiles of patients hospitalized for heart failure include profile A, B, C, and L. Most patients can be classified as having one of these four profiles in a 2-minute bedside assessment, although in practice some patients may qualify for both profile B and profile C **(Fig. 2)**. This classification helps guide consideration of initial therapy and prognosis. The clinical criteria for congestion (columns) concern dryness and wetness, the clinical evidence of perfusion (rows) concern coldness or warmth **(Box 2)**. For the "cold and dry" category, the label "L" is used instead of "D" to avoid the implication that heart failure invariably progresses.

Cardiac output is frequently reduced from normal but reaches critical levels only with patients with cardiogenic shock. Clinical estimation of perfusion can be made by temperature of extremities, examination of pulses and sensorium and presence of cyanosis. In heart failure with preserved ejection fraction decompensation is usually characterized by profile B. In these patients, severe compromise of resting cardiac output and perfusion generally does not occur unless a patient has severe restrictive, infiltrative or hypertrophic disease with very small left ventricular cavity or severe mitral regurgitation.

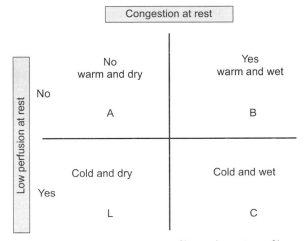

Fig. 2 Two minute assessment of hemodynamic profile

Box 2 Congestion at rest

- Evidence of low perfusion
- Narrow auscultated pulse pressure
- Cool extremities
- May be sleepy and obtunded
- Suspect from ACEI/ARB hypotension
- Progressive oliguria

Abbreviations: ACEI, angiotensin-converting enzyme inhibitors; ARB, angiotensin receptor blocker.

Management

An initial assessment of hemodynamic profile of the patient as assessed by symptoms and physical examination is crucial in deciding the line of management. For patients with normal resting hemodynamic profile, therapy is directed toward the relief of congestion with intravenous (IV) diuretics. The use of inotropes to increase contractility has generally been shown to be deleterious, unless organ perfusion is critically compromised and renal hypoperfusion limits reduction of filling pressures. In patients with acute heart failure with previous CHF, filling pressure can often be lowered to 15–16 mm Hg from baseline levels of over 30 mm Hg at admission.[3] As the filling pressures are reduced, cardiac output usually increases.[3] This is due to multiple factors including increase in contractility from decreased myocardial oxygen consumption and improved gradient for myocardial perfusion. Improvement in ejection due to decreased systemic vascular resistance and reduction in mitral regurgitation are also important factors.[4] Echocardiography is extremely useful for following the progress and may reveal reduction in mitral regurgitant fraction as clinical improvement occurs. There is also a greater renin-angiotensin sympathetic system activation, which is initially adaptive but later contributes to symptoms and prognosis.[5]

Profile A

For patients, who appear to be in Profile A "warm and dry" without clinical evidence of increased filling pressure or hypoperfusion on clinical examination, the diagnosis of heart failure may not explain the presenting symptoms and one should look for other causes such as pulmonary or hepatic disease.

Profile B "Warm and Wet"

This is the most common cause of admission for acute heart failure and the priority here is reduction of filling pressure. The filling pressure in these patients may be increased due to volume overload, systemic vasoconstriction or both. Most patients will require IV diuretics for fluid removal. Where vasoconstriction or severe hypertension is present, vasodilators are the first line of therapy along with diuretics. In some patients, positive pressure mask may be needed. IV loop diuretic either by bolus or by infusion are generally effective and sometime may be needed to combine with oral metolazone, if not effective alone.[6]

Use of adjunctive therapies beyond diuretics has not been shown to improve outcomes in these patients. IV inotropes generally worsen the prognosis and have been associated with increased arrhythmias, more ischemic events and more adverse events after discharge from hospital.[7] Nitroglycerin and nitroprusside may accelerate early symptomatic improvement, but have not proved to change outcomes during hospitalization or after discharge and can result in hypotension.[8] Endothelin antagonists have not been proven to be useful.[9] Vasopressin antagonists are effective in increasing serum-sodium levels in setting of hyponatremia and fluid overload and are associated with increased diuresis due to free water clearance. They also require careful monitoring of sodium levels to avoid hypernatremia. However, no long-term benefit has been shown.[10]

Cardiorenal Syndrome

An important cause of inadequate clinical response is cardiorenal syndrome, which occurs in about 25% of patients hospitalized with heart failure and is equally common among patients with low and preserved ejection fraction.[11] Its manifestation includes—renal dysfunction at the time of admission, failure to respond to high-dose diuretics, worsening renal function during diuresis despite persistent volume overload and progressive uremia after euvolemic state has been achieved. This syndrome is associated with longer hospital stay, and higher postdischarge mortality. It is most likely to occur in patients with severe right ventricular dysfunction, prolonged volume overload and chronically elevated right atrial pressures.[12]

In Profile B patients with very high blood pressure, systematic vascular resistance is elevated and is often accompanied by low-pulse pressure. In this situation, diuresis can result in renal dysfunction without symptomatic relief. However, if both blood pressure and cardiac output are low, severe vasoconstriction may be difficult to diagnose without hemodynamic monitoring.

Some patients have persistent hypotension with diuretics or vasodilators despite apparently normal cardiac output as judged by good pulse pressure and warm extremities. This indicates excessive vasodilation, which can be due to intrinsic liver disease in which circulating vasodilator substances have been implicated.

Profile C "Wet and Cold"

Less than 5% of patients present with true cardiogenic shock in which system perfusion is low, organ function is jeopardized and serum lactates are high.[1] They need urgent attention and perfusion needs to be optimized before congestion can be treated. Sometimes reduction of filling pressure with diuretics can improve cardiac output, but at times there is a dilemma whether the initial choice should be a vasodilator or an inotrope. When systematic resistance is very high, IV vasodilators can simultaneously increase cardiac output and reduce filling pressures.[13] If effective, this strategy is preferable. However, cardiac output can be increased by inotropes with some vasodilatory effects such as low-dose dobutamine and milrinone. However, they increase ischemic events and exacerbate subendocardial injury, which may worsen long-term outcomes.[14] The dose therefore should be kept as low as possible while watching for atrial fibrillation and tachyarrhythmias. After the desired goal of initial and volume they should be tapered as soon as possible.

Profile L "Dry and Cold"

Patients rarely present with this profile[15] and therefore any such patient should be carefully checked for occult profile C. If truly, the filling pressure is decreased cautious trial of fluid repletion, preferably by oral route without diuretics is better. However, there are several caveats to this. Unless postural hypotension is present, this approach may not improve clinical status and may lead to congestion. IV inotropes provide only temporary improvement. Vasodilators may increase resting cardiac output but lead to symptomatic hypotension. In the presence of tachycardia, beta blockers may be cautiously started and uptitrated very gradually.[16]

Direct Hemodynamic Monitoring

In patients with cardiogenic shock, hemodynamic monitoring may provide valuable information and guide titration of pressor agents and the need for mechanical circulatory support. Pulmonary artery catheterization can be done at the bedside and should be undertaken, if patients fail to respond to or deteriorate during usual therapy. Hemodynamic monitoring is strongly recommended to help re-evaluate optimization of filling pressures and systematic vascular resistance while oral agents are adjusted during weaning from inotropic infusions in patients who appear to be dependent on them. It is not recommended as a routine practice, if a patient is responding to the usual treatment. In carefully selected patient, a good beside echocardiography can yield useful information regarding cardiac hemodynamics and can be used repeatedly.

SPECIFIC AGENTS USED DURING HOSPITALIZATION

Diuretics, IV vasodilators, and IV inotropes are the major drugs used during acute management of decompensated heart failure.

Diuretics

Loop diuretics are generally considered as the first-line therapy. They are effective and well tolerated. Rapid IV administration of Frusemide may rarely cause ototoxicity. A common problem is under dosing with these drugs. When glomerular filtration rate (GFR) is reduced, higher doses must be used because they are secreted in the proximal tubule and act from the luminal side on the loop of Henle. Thiazides and spironolactone are weaker diuretics and may be ineffective when GFR is below 40 mL.

In patients with more advanced heart failure, distal tubule reabsorption may limit the efficacy of loop diuretics. In this situation, a combination of metolazone and loop diuretics is very effective. However, potassium levels needs to be watched for carefully with this combination as hypokalemia may occur and can precipitate ventricular arrhythmias. Muscle aches are common with brisk diuresis. Most patients with heart failure receive potassium-sparing angiotensin-converting enzyme (ACE) inhibitors and frequently spironolactone also. In patients with diabetes and renal dysfunction hyperkalemia can result in this situation. Potassium-rich fruits and salt substitutes containing potassium are often given to these patients and can further aggravate hyperkalemia. Metabolic alkalosis, increased uric acid, hyponatremia and neurohormonal activation are the other side effect of potent diuretics and need to be watched for.

In certain patients, when IV diuretics have suboptimal effect, IV infusions of loop diuretics have been shown in some studies to be of help.[17] Ultrafiltration and other form of dialysis may be useful in patients with inadequate diuresis and are very useful in patients who have difficulty achieving diuresis with conventional medications.

Intravenous Vasodilators

After diuretics, IV vasodilators are the most useful medicine for acute management of heart failure. They reduce filling pressures, increase cardiac output and reduce mitral regurgitation, resulting in immediate improvement of symptoms. When used carefully, they generally do not increase heart rate or result in arrhythmias unless there is severe hypotension.

Nitroglycerin

This is one of the safest and most widely used agents in acute heart failure for both acute ischemia and heart failure due to ischemia or vasoconstriction. The individual responses are highly variable and thus require careful monitoring. Headache and tachycardia may occur in some patients.[18]

Nitroprusside

This was the first vasodilator to be used in heart failure[19] and is very effective in patients with severe hypertension with increased systemic vascular resistance. The onset and offset of action is very rapid with a half-life of approximately 2 minutes. Once filling pressures are nearly normal, further vasodilator may not be necessary. Its major limitation is gastrointestinal and central nervous system side effects from cyanide toxicity, which are more likely to occur with impaired hepatic perfusion or hepatic dysfunction and in patients receiving large doses for more than 48 hours. Reduction and cessation of nitroprusside is generally enough to treat this complication.

Nesiritide

It is a recombinant form of B-type natriuretic peptide and lowers filling pressures and improves symptoms in decompensated heart failure.[20] Blood pressure needs to be monitored because it has a longer half-life of 18 minutes. Bradycardia and headache may occur occasionally. It potentiates the effect of concomitant diuretics. This effect may persist after infusion is stopped. It has been shown to be effective for decreasing filling pressures and relieving symptoms.

Angiotensin Receptor and Neprilysin Inhibitor

A recent welcome addition is a new drug called angiotensin receptor and neprilysin inhibitor (ARNI). This is an oral drug which upon ingestion breaks down into valsartan [angiotensin receptor blocker (ARB)] and sacubitril, which inhibits neprilysin. Neprilysin is a natural enzyme which results in breakdown of natriuretic peptides. Thus, the administration of this drug results in elevated levels of natriuretic peptides due to inhibition of their breakdown and ARB valsartan. In recent trials, this drug has shown dramatic results in reducing mortality and morbidity in CHF and currently a trial is under way to assess its efficacy in acute heart failure.

Intravenous Inotropic Agents

Though widely used inotropic agents pose their own problems. They are associated with more tachyarrhythmias and ischemic events.[21] Also, the efficacy of diuretics and tolerability of ACE inhibitors may be overestimated in the presence of inotropic stimulation. This may prolong hospitalization or increase the chances of early rehospitalization. The appropriate use of inotropic agents therefore is in a situation when they provide benefits not offered by initial therapies. They should be used until the cause of hypotension and deranged hemodynamic profile has been elucidated till diuresis become effective in patients with refractory heart failure and till renal, lung or liver functions have improved significantly.[22] Tapering of inotropes at time, become difficult due to hypotension and in this situation temporary or permanent discontinuation of beta-blockers and ACE inhibitors in severely compromised patients may help. Despite all these limitations they are still extremely useful, especially in situations where despite adequate therapy congestion or hypotension is persistent.

The change in distribution of stroke volume as ventricular loading conditions are improved, so that more of the total stroke volume is ejected forward and less flows backward into the left atrium. The mitral effective regurgitant orifice is significantly reduced after therapy.

Dobutamine

This is the most commonly used inotropic agent. It stimulates beta-adrenergic receptor with little effect on alpha-adrenergic receptors, so that contractility is increased with peripheral and pulmonary vasodilation. Cardiac output is increased, filling pressures are reduced and diuresis is potentiated. However, it causes tachycardia, especially in patients with atrial fibrillation and also results in increased ventricular arrhythmias and ischemia. When indicated, the lowest dose possible should be used. Increase in diuresis and improvement in renal function can be seen at 1–2 µg/kg/min. Treatment for more severe hypoperfusion requires higher doses and tachyphylaxis is generally seen. Maximum doses are usually 10–15 µg/kg/min. Occasionally, its prolonged administration is accompanied by increased eosinophil count, skin rash, and eosinophilic myocarditis.

Dopamine

Dopamine stimulates beta receptors, alpha receptors and dopaminergic receptors that cause vasodilation in renal and peripheral vasculature. At doses up to 5 µg/kg/min, it is predominantly vasodilatory. After 5 µg/kg/min, alpha receptor stimulation dominates, resulting is vasoconstriction. Dopamine also causes release of norepinephrine, resulting in independent stimulation of alpha and beta receptors. In low doses, its beneficial effects are clinically similar to dobutamine with similar adverse effects. It is usually indicated in rapidly changing situations in which modest inotropy and vasodilation may be adequate, but further increase in pressure is required. In this situation, one can start with 4 µg/kg/min and wean off when a dose of 3 µg/kg/min is reached. There is no significant advantage of combining dobutamine and dopamine for enhanced renal function in heart failure and it increases the risk of arrhythmias and ischemia.

Milrinone

Milrinone increases cyclic adenosine monophosphate by inhibiting its breakdown rather than increasing its production through stimulation of beta receptor. It acts synergistically with beta agent stimulating to achieve further increase in cardiac output than either agent alone. These are more effective than beta-adrenergic agent, when beta-blockers have already been given. The degree to which cardiac output increases and systemic resistance decreases is variable and therefore some patients may exhibit predominant vasodilator. Thus, there is a significant incidence of hypotension with milrinone unlike dobutamine. It results in lesser tachycardia than dopamine and dobutamine, but has a similar incidence of arrhythmias and ischemia. It has a longer half-life of 6 hours unlike dopamine and dobutamine, which are in minutes. It is generally started as an infusion at a dose of 0.5 µg/kg/min and titrated up to a maximum of 75 µg/kg/min. It is excreted renally and therefore in renal dysfunction dose adjustment is needed. Its prolonged use can increase its half-life up to 18 hours. Therefore, after discontinuing its infusion at least 48 hours of observation is required.

Epinephrine and Norepinephrine

These are full beta-receptor agonists, which increase contractility, heart rate, and peripheral resistance while promoting arrhythmias and ischemia. They can provide significant additional short-term inotropic and blood pressure support over minutes to hours before other therapies. Kidney failure, hepatic failure, and gangrene can result from the use of these agents. When fatal hypotension is imminent, they are used at a starting dose of 0.1 µg/min. This can be preceded by a static dose of 0.25 mg of epinephrine to maintain survival for a brief period. Boluses of calcium may be helpful particularly in the presence of conditions that may lower serum calcium such as transfusions, dialysis, and cardiopulmonary bypass. They are highly arrhythmogenic and may exaggerate ongoing myocardial necrosis.

Vasopressin

It is used to potentiate the use of catecholamines in patients who remain severely hypotensive despite high-dose pressor support. It can be used for hours to days in doses of 0.52–1 U/min. When added to norepinephrine, it can result in about 30 mm Hg increase in systolic blood pressure. It is sometimes associated with profound water diuresis. As with other vasoconstrictors, it can result in ischemic injury and necrosis of organs and limbs.

ESCALATING SUPPORT

In a small minority of patients with rapid deteriorating hemodynamics, which threatens their survival a quick, aggressive support for stabilization or for definitive intervention is required. The goal in these cases is stabilization of patient to a point at which definitive intervention or surgical therapy can be offered or spontaneous recovery occurs. The evidence of this situation usually includes more than one of the following:

- Systolic blood pressure below 75 mm Hg
- Cardiac index below 1.5–1.8 L/min/m^2
- It is important to identify these patients quickly. The evidence of rapid deterioration consists of one or more of the following:
  - Systemic acidosis with positive lactate levels anuria
  - Obtundation and shock with rise of transaminase level to thousands of U/L
  - Altered sensorium.

Dopamine is the most common first-line drug administered in this situation, but if the situation does not improve within minutes, escalation would include more intense inotropic support with epinephrine at escalating doses. Vasopressin is frequently added as well, as discussed previously. For the patients with otherwise robust health, consultation regarding surgical options should be obtained immediately. The role for the intra-aortic balloon pump for intermediate stabilization has been well established for cardiogenic shock caused by acute myocardial infarction. The pump is usually inserted while other therapies are under way by the bedside or in the cardiac catheterization suite. When it can be performed expeditiously, balloon pump insertion seems reasonable for other cases of cardiogenic shock with underlying CAD. For cardiogenic shock of other causes, its role is less clear, and plans for insertion should not detract from progress to more definitive intervention. Some experts advocate its use for stabilization of medical therapy and anesthesia regardless of cause, whereas others believe that it offers little benefit for patients without epicardial CAD and moreover, increases the risk of vascular and infectious complications.

Extracorporeal membrane oxygenator and left ventricular assist devices are available in some specialized centers used judiciously, they are lifesaving as a bridge to recovery, surgery or heart transplant.

Survivals of patients presenting with acute heart failure have improved dramatically since 1980, the medical advances reflect understanding of the role of neurohormonal stimulation and antagonism, the physiology and evaluation of congestion leading to decompensation, and the indications for devices to avert sudden death and enhance synchrony. Most therapies investigated for acute decompensation have been unsuccessful attempts to encompass the broad population of hospitalized patients. Clinicians remain optimistic that more specific neurohormonal or metabolic profiling will identify a subset of patients who would benefit from specific antagonists or metabolic manipulation. Therapy tailored to individual targets seems more promising than the blind application of all approved therapies until cumulative intolerance. However, the majority of new therapies is more likely to achieve long-term effects when initiated electively during clinical stability than during decompensation.

Quality-of-life and survival after heart failure have improved significantly for last three decades. This has largely been due to understanding of the basic pathophysiology specially the role of neurohormonal activation, definitive interventional therapies, and support devices. New drugs on the horizon, especially ARNI, appear to be very promising and may yet be the most significant advance in pharmacotherapy after ACE inhibitors. The readmission rate often acute heart failure is still disturbingly high. This may be due to failure to uptitrate the doses and inadequate counseling regarding lifestyle modification. It is important to quickly triage these patients on presentation to the emergency ward to decide who requires more aggressive approach to their disease. Such patients should be offered high-technology solution to reduce mortality and morbidity.

CONCLUSION

Heart failure is common clinical syndrome in emergency department characterized by dyspnea fatigue and features of fluid overload. Patient with heart failure has high morbidity and mortality. Initial evaluation of heart failure by history physical examination ECG and echocardiography. Systolic and diastolic heart failure can be diagnosed by echocardiography. Premature death occurs in patient with heart failure due lack of awareness about heart failure. Early recognition of symptoms and immediate medical attention improve the outcome for patient with heart failure.

REFERENCES

1. Jessup M. Abraham WT, Casey DE, et al. 2009 focused update: ACCF/AHA Guidelines for the Diagnosis and Management of Heart Failure in Adults: a report of the American College of Cardiology Foundation/American Heart Association Task Force on Practice Guidelines: developed in collaboration with the International Society for Heart and Lung Transplantation. Circulation. 2009;119:1977-2016.
2. Fonarow GC, Abraham WT, Albert NM, et al. Factors identified as precipitating hospital admissions for heart failure and clinical outcomes: findings from OPTIMIZE-HF. Arch Intern Med. 2008;166:847-54.
3. Stevenson LW, Bruken RC, Belil D, et al. Afterload reduction with vasodilators and diuretics decreases mitral regurgitation during upright exercise in advanced heart failure. J Am Coll Cardiol. 1990;15:174-80.
4. Palardy M, Stevenson LW, Tasissa G, et al. Reduction in mitral regurgitation during therapy guided by measured filling pressures in the ESCAPE trial. Circ Heart Fail. 2009;2:181-8.
5. Kaye DM, Lambert GW, Lefkovits J, et al. Neurochemical evidence of cardiac sympathetic activation and increased central nervous system norepinephrine turnover in severe congestive heart failure. J Am Coll Cardiol. 1994;23:570-8.
6. Channer KS, McLean KA, Lawson-Matthew P, et al. Combination diuretic treatment in severe heart failure: a randomized controlled trial. Br Heart J. 1994;71:146-50.
7. Elkayam U, Tasissa G, Binanay C, et al. Use and impact of inotropes and vasodilator therapy in hospitalized patients with severe heart failure. Am Heart J. 2007;153:98-104.
8. Publication Committee for the VMAC Investigators (Vasodilatation in the Management of Acute CHF). Intravenous nesiritide vs nitroglycerin for treatment of decompensated congestive heart failure: a randomized controlled trial. JAMA. 2002;287:1531-40.
9. McMurray JJ, Teerlink JR, Cotter G, et al. Effects of tezosentan on symptoms and clinical outcomes in patients with acute heart failure: The VERITAS randomized controlled trials. JAMA. 2007;298:2009-19.
10. Pang PS, Konstam MA, Krasa HB, et al. Effects of tolvaptan on dyspnoea relief from the EVEREST trials. Eur Heart J. 2009;30:2233-40.
11. Krumholzm HM, Chen YT, Vaccarino V, et al. Importance of venous congestion of worsening renal function in patients >

or = 65 years of age with heart failure. Am J Cardiol. 2000;85: 1110-3.
12. Mullens W. Abrahams Z, Francis GS, et al. Importance of venous congestion for worsening of renal function in advanced decompensated heart failure. J Am Coll Cardiol. 2009;53:589-96.
13. Stevenson LW, Dracup KA, Tillisch JH. Efficacy of medical therapy tailored for severe congestive heart failure in patients transferred for urgent cardiac transplantation. Am J Cardiol. 1989;63:461-4.
14. Dickstein K, Cohen-Solal A, Filippatos G, et al. ESC Guidelines for the diagnosis and treatment of Acute and Chronic Heart Failure 2008: the task Force for the Diagnosis and Treatment of Acute and Chronic Heart Failure 2008 of the European Society of Cardiology. Developed in collaboration with the Heart Failure Association of the ESC (HFA) and endorsed by the European Society of Intensive Care Medicine (ESICM). Eur Heart J. 2008;29:2388-442.
15. Nohria A. Tsang SW, Fang JC, et al. Clinical assessment identifies hemodynamic profiles that predict outcomes in patients admitted with heart failure. J AM Coll Cardiol. 2003;41:1797-804.
16. Stevenson LW. Heart Failure: A companion to Braunwald's Heart Disease. 2012. p 639.
17. Dormans TP, van Meyel JJ, Gerlag PG, et al. Diuretic efficacy of high dose furosemide in severe heart failure: bolus injection versus continuous infusion. J Am Coll Cardiol. 1996;28: 376-82.
18. Publication Committee for the VMAC Investigators (Vasodilatation in the Management of Acute CHF). Intravenous nesiritide vs nitroglycerin for the treatment of decompensated congestive heart failure: a randomized controlled trial. JAMA. 2002;287:1531-40.
19. Guiha NH, Cohn JN, Mikulic E, et al. Treatment of refractory heart failure with infusion of nitroprusside. N Engl J Med. 1994;291:587-92.
20. Colucci WS, Elkayam U, Horton DP, et al. Intravenous nesiritide, a natriuretic peptide, in the treatment of decompensated congestive heart failure. Nesiritide Study group. N Engl J Med. 2000;343:246-53.
21. Gheorghiade M, Gattis WA, Klein L. OPTIME in CHF trial: rethinking the use of inotropes in the management of worsening chronic heart failure resulting in hospitalization. Eur J Heart Fail. 2003;5:9-12.
22. Stevenson LW. Clinical use of inotropic therapy for heart failure: looking backward or forward? Part I: inotropic infusions during hospitalization. Circulation. 2003;109;367-72.

CHAPTER 28

Bradyarrhythmias

Jamal Yusuf, Safal, Saibal Mukhopadhyay

INTRODUCTION

Heart rate (corresponding to ventricular rate) below 60/minute in an adult is referred to as bradyarrhythmia or bradycardia.[1] While accurate prevalence data for symptomatic bradyarrhythmias is not available, a rough inference can be made from data regarding number of permanent pacemaker implants; the figures for Europe being 938 per million inhabitants in 2011.[2] Data regarding natural history is mainly derived from very old studies performed at the beginning of the pacemaker era, but suffice to say that while pacemaker implant is clearly lifesaving in cases of advanced atrioventricular (AV) block, its role may be limited to symptom management and prevention of falls in patients with sinus node dysfunction; nevertheless over a quarter of permanent pacemakers in the UK are implanted for sinus node dysfunction.[3-9]

ETIOLOGY

Bradycardia could be due to either intrinsic or extrinsic causes or a combination of the two. The most important intrinsic cause is age-related degenerative disease. Other intrinsic causes include ischemia affecting sinus node or conduction tissue, infiltrative diseases (e.g. sarcoidosis and amyloidosis), collagen vascular diseases (e.g. systemic lupus erythematosus), congenital heart diseases affecting sinus node or conduction system [(e.g. congenitally corrected transposition of the great arteries (ccTGA)], infections (e.g. diphtheritic myocarditis), genetic cardiomyopathies, primary genetic conduction disorders, post-cardiac surgery and post-catheter ablation.[10]

Extrinsic causes include vagotonia due to physical conditioning or in vasovagal reflex or carotid sinus hypersensitivity. Rate-limiting drugs (e.g. beta-blockers), dyselectrolytemia (e.g. hyperkalemia), metabolic derangements (e.g. hypothyroidism), and raised intracranial pressure are some other extrinsic causes that need to be kept in mind while evaluating a case of bradycardia; the clinical and electrocardiogram (ECG) manifestation of each of these is unique enough to provide a hint to the alert mind and help guide further testing.

SYMPTOMS

Symptoms of bradycardia may be subtle and persistent due to a chronic low-output state (easy fatigability, poor functional capacity, exertional dyspnea, cognitive impairment and dizziness) or episodic and dramatic in intermittent bradycardias (syncope or presyncope associated with traumatic falls).

CLASSIFICATION

The most useful classification of bradyarrhythmias is based on the site of abnormality in impulse generation and/or propagation. Broadly, there are two groups:
1. Abnormalities of sinus node and intra-atrial conduction (includes abnormalities in impulse generation as well as conduction).
2. Abnormalities at level of AV node and below (includes abnormalities in impulse conduction only).

Abnormalities of Sinus Node and Intra-atrial Conduction (Includes Abnormalities in Impulse Generation as well as Conduction)

Sinus Bradycardia

In an adult, sinus bradycardia is diagnosed when there are less than 60 P-waves per minute on the ECG (or P-P interval of more than 1 second), with a regular P-P interval, every

P-wave being followed by a QRS interval, PR interval between 0.12 and 0.2 seconds and a normal P-wave axis (upright in leads I and II, inverted in aVR). When the P-wave axis is consistently abnormal (beyond 0–75 degrees), it generally indicates that there is sinus arrest and an alternative atrial pacemaker has taken over (atrial rhythm rather than sinus bradycardia).

Persistent sinus bradycardia is frequently physiological (e.g. in well-conditioned athletes) or may be due to the effect of rate-limiting drugs like beta-blockers. Conditions causing parasympathetic stimulation may lead to transient sinus bradycardia (as during a vasovagal episode). Symptomatic sinus bradycardia when a part of sick sinus syndrome may require a permanent pacemaker implant.

Sinus Pause

A sudden drop in the P-wave frequency indicates a sinus pause. This is to be differentiated from both, a sinus exit block and sinus arrhythmia. While sinus arrhythmia results in a gradual and cyclical change in P-P interval (frequently related to the respiratory cycle), sinus pauses are abrupt and non-cyclical. On the other hand, a type II second-degree sinoatrial (SA) exit block leads to an abrupt increase in the P-P interval, which is an exact multiple of the normal P-P interval; however with superimposed sinus arrhythmia, the differentiation between type II second-degree SA exit block and a sinus pause may be difficult on the surface ECG. Practically, though, this differentiation is not of much significance as the management of both would be on similar lines.

Sinoatrial Exit Block

Sinoatrial exit block refers to the delay in or inability of formed impulse to conduct to the right atrium. As the P-wave is generated on the surface ECG due to atrial depolarization, whether the impulse is not generated or whether it is generated but not conducted to the atrium, both manifest as dropped P-waves. SA exit block includes:

- *First-degree SA exit block*: This is due to delayed conduction of the generated impulse to the right atrium; as no P-wave is dropped it cannot be diagnosed from the surface ECG.
- *Type I second-degree SA exit block (Wenckebach)*: This is due to progressive delay in impulse transmission to the atrium, finally resulting in a dropped impulse. It manifests on the surface ECG as progressive shortening of the P-P interval culminating in a dropped P-wave, with the P-P interval preceding the dropped beat being the shortest. It is frequently mistaken for sinus arrhythmia.
- *Type II second-degree SA exit block*: This is manifested as abrupt increase in P-P interval, due to sudden blocked P-wave with the increased P-P interval being an exact multiple of normal P-P interval. As discussed earlier, this may at times be difficult to differentiate from a sinus pause on the surface ECG.
- *Complete (type III) SA exit block*: None of the generated impulses is conducted to the atrium, resulting in complete absence of normal P-waves. An atrial or junctional pacemaker may take over, providing an atrial escape rhythm (with abnormal P-waves, as discussed in the section on sinus bradycardia) or a junctional escape rhythm (with no visible P-waves).

Sinus Arrest

This is due to non-generation of the sinus impulse, leading to complete absence of normal P-waves. It is indistinguishable from type III SA exit block on the surface ECG; the two can only be distinguished with a sinus node electrode during electrophysiologic evaluation.

Hypersensitive carotid sinus syndrome: The cardioinhibitory type of hypersensitive carotid sinus syndrome is characterized by sinus arrest or complete SA exit block during carotid sinus stimulation, leading to a ventricular pause exceeding 3 seconds; less commonly the ventricular pause may be due to AV block. Patients with symptomatic ventricular pauses exceeding 3 seconds or documented asymptomatic pauses exceeding 6 seconds on prolonged monitoring, with little or no prodromal symptoms, leading to frequent syncope and falls, are most likely to benefit from a permanent pacemaker.[11] A dual-chamber pacemaker with a rate-drop algorithm and rate hysteresis is appropriate in this situation.[11,12]

Sick sinus syndrome: Sick sinus syndrome refers to a combination of various sinus node abnormalities (pathological sinus bradycardia, prolonged sinus pauses, SA exit block and sinus arrest); more than one of these may be seen at different times. The bradycardia-tachycardia syndrome, characterized by alternation of paroxysms of rapid regular or irregular atrial tachyarrhythmias with periods of slow atrial and ventricular rates, is also a part of this spectrum. The anatomic basis of sick sinus syndrome may involve total or subtotal destruction of sinus node, areas of nodal-atrial discontinuity, inflammatory or degenerative changes in nerves and ganglia around the node, and pathologic changes in the atrial wall; occlusion of sinus node artery may have a role. Symptomatic patients of sick sinus syndrome are candidates for permanent pacemaker implant, with dual-chamber pacing likely superior to ventricular-only pacing with regard to incidence of atrial fibrillation (AF) and pacemaker syndrome.[13,14] Atrial-only pacing is usually avoided for fear of pacing failure, in case patient goes on to develop AV conduction defect in future. Also, a recent trial has shown an increased incidence of paroxysmal AF as well as pacemaker reoperation with atrial-only pacing vis-à-vis dual-chamber pacing.[15] Tachycardia-bradycardia syndrome patients require a combination of pacemaker for the bradycardia and pharmacotherapy for tachycardia control.

Abnormalities at Level of AV Node and below (Includes Abnormalities in Impulse Conduction Only)

First-degree AV Block

Every atrial impulse is conducted to the ventricle, although with a delay, evident on the surface ECG as a prolongation of the PR interval beyond 0.2 seconds. PR intervals as long as 1 second have been noted, and may even exceed the P-P interval, a phenomenon known as skipped P-waves. First-degree AV block may occur due to conduction delay in the AV node (A-H interval), in the His-Purkinje system (H-V interval), or at both sites. Uncommonly, equally delayed conduction over both bundle branches can produce PR prolongation without significant QRS widening. Occasionally, intra-atrial conduction delay can also prolong the PR interval. Practically, first-degree AV block with a normal QRS is most likely due to delay at AV node; with a wide QRS, delay could be at the AV node or the His-Purkinje system or both. While first-degree AV block by itself is considered benign, select patients with marked PR prolongation (beyond 300 milliseconds) and persistent symptoms owing to shortening of left ventricular filling time and diastolic mitral regurgitation, may be considered for DDD pacing **(Fig. 1)**.[16,17]

Mobitz Type I Second-degree AV Block (Wenckebach)

This is characterized by serial prolongation of the PR interval till a P-wave is blocked completely. The increment in PR interval is maximum in the second beat of the Wenckebach group and each subsequent increment is progressively smaller. While a classic Wenckebach phenomenon is easy to recognize, certain caveats must be kept in mind **(Fig. 2)**. For one, a pure 2:1 AV block can be either type 1 or type 2; if the QRS is normal, the block is more likely to be type 1—a careful search for transition to 3:2 block at some stage (with PR prolongation in the second cycle) may be useful. Secondly, type 1 AV block with a high ratio of conducted beats (e.g. 8:7) may give an impression of having a constant PR interval due to the small increments in consecutive beats; here comparing the PR interval just before and just after the dropped beat readily reveals the variation in PR interval. Prognosis-wise, a type 1 AV block is more likely to be suprahisian, especially when accompanied with a narrow QRS and have a relatively benign course **(Fig. 3)**.

Mobitz Type II Second-degree AV Block

In Mobitz type II block, some P-waves are blocked abruptly, but PR interval of the conducted beats is constant. Type II AV block is more likely to be infranodal, worsening with atropine, exercise or isoproterenol and improving with carotid sinus massage. Infranodal blocks are more likely to progress to complete AV block as compared to blocks at level of AV node; and may present with Stokes-Adams attacks. Most cases require a permanent pacemaker implant once reversible causes are ruled out; a dual-chamber pacemaker that maintains AV synchrony is an appropriate choice **(Fig. 4)**.

Third-degree (Complete) AV Block

Complete AV block is a type of complete AV dissociation, where none of the P-waves is conducted to the ventricles; both atria and ventricles are controlled by independent pacemakers. Symptoms are predominantly governed by the stability and rate of escape rhythm. For blocks at the level of AV node (usually congenital), the escape focus is generally within or close to the His bundle—this focus is relatively more stable and can provide ventricular rates up to 60/minute. Acquired complete heart block is, however, frequently infra-

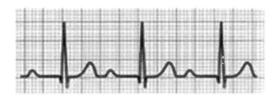

Fig. 1 First-degree AV block

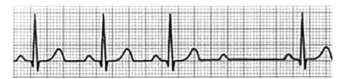

Fig. 3 Second-degree AV block (2:1 block)

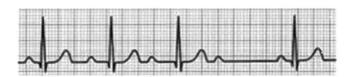

Fig. 2 Second-degree AV block (Mobitz I or Wenckebach)

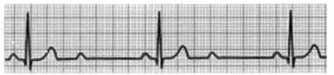

Fig. 4 Second-degree AV block (Mobitz II)

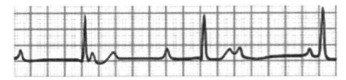

Fig. 5 Third-degree AV block with junctional escape

hisian, due to trifascicular involvement, and the distal escape foci can rarely provide rates beyond 40/minute. Acquired complete AV block, unless reversible, almost invariably requires permanent pacing; even where reversible causes are suspected temporary pacing support needs to be provided. Congenital complete AV block may however be observed, without any intervention, if it is asymptomatic and the patient consistently has an escape rate above 50/minute with normal QRS duration and normal left ventricular function (LVF); whenever symptoms or high risk features appear permanent pacing is indicated **(Fig. 5)**.[18-24]

MANAGEMENT

The most tricky aspect in the management of brady-arrhythmias is not implanting a pacemaker (which is possibly the simplest aspect); rather it is reaching an accurate diagnosis and then deciding whether or not to treat the condition in a given patient.

While persistent bradycardia is easy to diagnose from the resting ECG, the diagnosis of intermittent bradycardia can be elusive and the diagnostic modality needs to be chosen as per the patient's symptom frequency. When the symptoms occur on a daily basis; 24-hour Holter monitoring is likely to have a good yield. However, extended Holter or external loop recorder may be required for less frequent (e.g. weekly) symptoms and an implantable loop recorder may be required for occasional symptoms (frequency less than once a month).[25,26] A carotid sinus massage (in absence of contraindications) may prove useful in patients above 40 years of age, when carotid sinus hypersensitivity is suspected.[27] While evaluating a patient for symptoms of intermittent bradycardia (e.g. syncope) other causes with similar presentation must also be ruled out (e.g. tachyarrhythmias, severe aortic stenosis, etc.).

Once a diagnosis of bradyarrhythmia is established, the next step is correlating it with the patient's symptoms. This is because benefit of treatment is much better established when bradycardia is shown to reproduce the symptoms in a given patient; otherwise there always lies the possibility that the bradycardia is an incidental finding and the symptoms are due to a different etiology. However, the same is easier said than done; and frequently patients are implanted a permanent pacemaker based on reasonable level of suspicion even when recorded bradyarrhythmic events have not reproduced the symptoms. In this scenario, it is worthwhile to have a lower threshold for treatment of advanced AV blocks vis-à-vis sinus node dysfunction.

Once a decision to treat a persistent or recurrent bradyarrhythmia (not attributable to reversible causes) is taken, drug therapy has no role; the choice is only of the type of pacemaker to be implanted. The choice of pacemaker device and specific algorithms (for conditions like carotid sinus hypersensitivity) have already been discussed in the relevant sections. Suffice to say that as of date, with the exception of patients with permanent AF, dual-chamber pacing is preferable to single-chamber pacing; cost constrains however must be taken into account.

REFERENCES

1. Olgin J, Zipes DP. Specific arrhythmias: diagnosis and treatment. In: Mann DL, Zipes DP, Libby P, Bonow RO (Eds). Braunwald's Heart Disease: A Textbook of Cardiovascular Medicine, 10th edition. Philadelphia, PA: Elsevier Saunders; 2014.
2. Eucomed. (2013). Medical Technology—key facts and figures. [online] Available from *http://archive.eucomed.org/medical-technology/facts-figures* [Accessed November 2016].
3. Edhag O. Long-term cardiac pacing. Experience of fixed-rate pacing with an endocardial electrode in 260 patients. Acta Med Scand Suppl. 1969;502:9-110.
4. Edhag O, Swahn A. Prognosis of patients with complete heart block or arrhythmic syncope who were not treated with artificial pacemakers. A long-term follow-up study of 101 patients. Acta Med Scand. 1976;200(6):457-63.
5. Friedberg CK, Donoso E, Stein WG. Nonsurgical acquired heart block. Ann N Y Acad Sci. 1964;111:835-47.
6. Johansson BW. Complete heart block. A clinical, hemodynamic and pharmacological study in patients with and without an artificial pacemaker. Acta Med Scand Suppl. 1966;451:1-127.
7. Michaelsson M, Jonzon A, Riesenfeld T. Isolated congenital complete atrioventricular block in adult life: a prospective study. Circulation. 1995;92(3):442-9.
8. Shaw DB, Holman RR, Gowers JI. Survival in sinoatrial disorder (sick-sinus syndrome). Br Med J. 1980;280:139-41.
9. Sutton R, Kenny RA. The natural history of sick sinus syndrome. Pacing Clin Electrophysiol. 1986;9(6Pt 2):1110-4.
10. Brignole M, Auricchio A, Baron-Esquivias G, et al. 2013 ESC Guidelines on cardiac pacing and cardiac resynchronization therapy: the Task Force on cardiac pacing and resynchronization therapy of the European Society of Cardiology (ESC). Developed in collaboration with the European Heart Rhythm Association (EHRA). Eur Heart J. 2013;34(29):2281-329.
11. Brignole M, Menozzi C, Moya A, et al. Pacemaker therapy in patients with neurally mediated syncope and documented asystole: Third International Study on Syncope of Uncertain Etiology (ISSUE-3): a randomized trial. Circulation. 2012;125(21):2566-71.
12. Brignole M, Sutton R, Menozzi C, et al. Early application of an implantable loop recorder allows effective specific therapy in patients with recurrent suspected neurally mediated syncope. Eur Heart J. 2006;27(9):1085-92.
13. Healey JS, Toff WD, Lamas GA, et al. Cardiovascular outcomes with atrial-based pacing compared with ventricular pacing:

14. Castelnuovo E, Stein K, Pitt M, et al. The effectiveness and cost-effectiveness of dual-chamber pacemakers compared with single-chamber pacemakers for bradycardia due to atrioventricular block or sick sinus syndrome: systematic review and economic evaluation. Health Technol Assess. 2005;9(43):iii, xi-xiii, 1-246.
15. Nielsen JC, Thomsen PE, Hojberg S, et al. A comparison of single-lead atrial pacing with dual-chamber pacing in sick sinus syndrome. Eur Heart J. 2011;32(6):686-96.
16. Barold SS. Indications for permanent cardiac pacing in first-degree AV block: class I, II, or III? Pacing Clin Electrophysiol. 1996;19(5):747-51.
17. Carroz P, Delay D, Girod G. Pseudo-pacemaker syndrome in a young woman with first-degree atrioventricular block. Europace. 2010;12(4):594-6.
18. Jaeggi ET, Hamilton RM, Silverman ED, et al. Outcome of children with fetal, neonatal or childhood diagnosis of isolated congenital atrioventricular block. A single institution's experience of 30 years. J Am Coll Cardiol. 2002;39(1):130-7.
19. Michaelsson M, Engle MA. Congenital complete heart block: an international study of the natural history. Cardiovasc Clin. 1972;4(3):85-101.
20. Villain E, Coastedoat-Chalumeau N, Marijon E, et al. Presentation and prognosis of complete atrioventricular block in childhood, according to maternal antibody status. J Am Coll Cardiol. 2006;48(8):1682-7.
21. Breur JM, Udink Ten Cate FE, Kapusta L, et al. Pacemaker therapy in isolated congenital complete atrioventricular block. Pacing Clin Electrophysiol. 2002;25(12):1685-91.
22. Karpawich PP, Gillette PC, Garson A Jr, et al. Congenital complete atrioventricular block: clinical and electrophysiologic predictors of need for pacemaker insertion. Am J Cardiol. 1981;48(6):1098-102.
23. Beaufort-Krol GC, Schasfoort-van Leeuwen MJ, Stienstra Y, et al. Longitudinal echocardiographic follow-up in children with congenital complete atrioventricular block. Pacing Clin Electrophysiol. 2007;30(11):1339-43.
24. Dewey RC, Capeless MA, Levy AM. Use of ambulatory electrocardiographic monitoring to identify high-risk patients with congenital complete heart block. N Engl J Med. 1987;316:835-9.
25. Edvardsson N, Frykman V, van Mechelen R, et al. Use of an implantable loop recorder to increase the diagnostic yield in unexplained syncope: results from the PICTURE registry. Europace. 2011;13(2):262-9.
26. Furukawa T, Maggi R, Bertolone C, et al. Additional diagnostic value of very prolonged observation by implantable loop recorder in patients with unexplained syncope. J Cardiovasc Electrophysiol. 2012;23(1):67-71.
27. Task Force for the Diagnosis and Management of Syncope; European Society of Cardiology (ESC); European Heart Rhythm Association (EHRA); Heart Failure Association (HFA); Heart Rhythm Society (HRS); Moya A, Sutton R, Ammirati F, et al. Guidelines for the diagnosis and management of syncope (version 2009). Eur Heart J. 2009;30(21):2631-71.

CHAPTER 29

Tachyarrhythmia

Jamal Yusuf, Prattay Guhasarkar, Saibal Mukhopadhyay

INTRODUCTION

Tachyarrhythmia is defined as abnormal heart rhythms with a ventricular rate of 100 or more beats per minute, are frequently symptomatic and often result in patients seeking care at the emergency department. Signs and symptoms related to the tachyarrhythmia may include shock, hypotension, heart failure, shortness of breath, chest pain, acute myocardial infarction, palpitations and/or decreased level of consciousness. Tachyarrhythmias are broadly characterized as supraventricular tachycardia (SVT), defined as a tachycardia in which the driving circuit or focus originates, at least in part, in tissue above the level of the ventricle [i.e. sinus node, atria, atrioventricular (AV) node, or His bundle] and ventricular tachycardia (VT), defined as a tachycardia in which the driving circuit or focus solely originates in ventricular tissue or Purkinje fibers.[1] Because of differences in prognosis and management, the distinction between SVT and VT is critical early in the acute management of a tachyarrhythmia. In general (with the exception of idiopathic VT), VT often carries a much graver prognosis, usually implies the presence of significant heart disease, results in more profound hemodynamic compromise and therefore requires immediate attention and measures to revert to sinus rhythm. On the other hand, SVT is usually not lethal and often does not result in hemodynamic collapse; therefore, more conservative measures can be applied initially to convert to sinus rhythm.[1]

ELECTROCARDIOGRAPHIC FEATURES

The electrocardiogram (ECG) is the most important tool in arrhythmia analysis. An electrophysiological study is more definitive, however is not available at every center. Initially, a 12-lead ECG and a long continuous recording with use of the lead that shows distinct P waves (usually leads II, III, aVF, V1 or aVR) is recorded and analyzed. The ECG obtained during an episode of arrhythmia may be diagnostic by itself, obviating the need for further diagnostic testing. **Flow chart 1** depicts an algorithm for diagnosis of specific tachyarrhythmias from the 12-lead ECG. The following important questions are to be asked in order, while analyzing an ECG with a tachyarrhythmia.[2]

QRS Duration

In general, if the QRS is narrow (duration less than 120 msec, referred to as narrow-complex tachycardias) during the tachycardia, the ventricle is being activated via the normal His-Purkinje system and thus the origin of the tachycardia is supraventricular. A wide QRS (duration exceeding 120 msec) during tachycardia suggests VT or a SVT in specific scenarios. SVT with a concurrent bundle branch block (BBB) or intraventricular conduction defect can produce wide-complex tachycardias despite a supraventricular origin. A narrow-complex tachycardia almost always makes the diagnosis of SVT, but a wide-complex tachycardia can be supraventricular or ventricular. Fusion or capture beats and AV dissociation are diagnostic of VT but are often not present or are difficult to detect.

Regularity of Rhythm

An irregularly irregular rhythm points toward atrial fibrillation (AF). A regular or a regularly irregular rhythm can be seen in either SVTs or VTs.

Characteristic of P Waves

- P wave morphology, association with QRS complexes, atrial rate, PR and RP intervals and the response of the P waves to carotid sinus massage or adenosine further

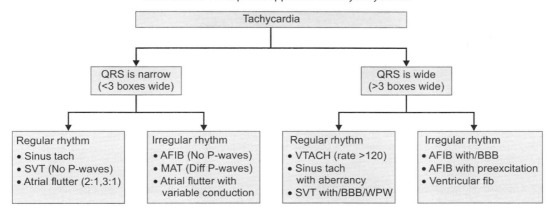

Flow chart 1 A simplified approach to tachyarrhythmias

Abbreviations: Tach, tachycardia; SVT, supraventricular tachycardia; AFIB, atrial fibrillation; MAT, multifocal atrial tachycardia; VTACH, ventricular tachycardia; BBB, bundle branch block; WPW, Wolff-Parkinson-White syndrome.

helps to narrow down the differential diagnosis of the tachyarrhythmia.
- Once these questions have been addressed, one needs to assess the significance of the arrhythmia in view of the clinical setting. Should it be treated, and if so, how? A practical overview of various arrhythmias will be presented here.

SUPRAVENTRICULAR TACHYCARDIAS

An SVT is a paroxysmal tachycardia arising above the level of His bundle. It is a commonly encountered tachycardia in emergency department. Sinus tachycardia and paroxysmal supraventricular tachycardia (PSVT) are mostly without complication and are easily manageable. Atrial flutter and AF are serious tachycardias.[3] Patient with multifocal atrial tachycardia (MAT) usually have underlying pulmonary or cardiac disease. PSVT are classified on the basis of the specific conduction pathway involved—atrioventricular reentrant tachycardia (AVRT) and atrioventricular nodal reentrant tachycardia (AVNRT).

Clinical Presentation

Common complaints by patient are:
- Increased heart beats
- Anxious feeling
- Dizziness
- Chest heaviness or discomfort
- Pulsatile feeling in neck
- Breathlessness.

Supraventricular tachycardia is usually seen in structurally normal heart and precipitating factors are excessive intake of coffee, alcohol, or thyroid dysfunction.

Approach to a Patient with Supraventricular Tachycardia[1]

- A detailed patient's history and physical examination is important to rule out structural heart disease
- Duration and frequency of episodes
- Possible trigger factors (caffeine, exercise, etc.)
- History of heart and lung disease
- SVTs are sudden in onset and offset
- Sinus tachycardia accelerates and decelerates gradually[1] (**Table 1**).

Electrocardiographic Features

Supraventricular tachycardias present with narrow complex tachycardia with QRS duration of less than 120 msec. Few cases of SVT can have a QRS duration of greater than 120 msec (**Flow chart 2**).

Two-dimensional echocardiography is helpful to rule out structural heart disease. Laboratory investigations like serum electrolytes, thyroid profile can be done and electrophysiological study (EPS) is done to identify the exact mechanism of arrhythmia and catheter ablation is reserved for patients with drug resistant SVT, SVT associated with syncope, wide QRS tachycardia, and individual who do not wish to take long-term medications.

Atrioventricular Nodal Reentrant Tachycardia

Atrioventricular nodal reentrant tachycardia has a rate between 150 bpm and 230 bpm. The R-R interval is regular and a retrograde P wave may be present. The retrograde P wave may be difficult to distinguish in the standard ECG trace. PSVT may produce aberrant conduction and a widened QRS.

Table 1 Differentiating features of tachycardia				
Tachycardia	Age	Underlying conditions	Presentation	Baseline ECG
Paroxysmal SVT	All ages	Structurally normal heart	Fast onset and offset palpitation	Preexcitation common in AVRT
Atrial fibrillation, atrial flutter, multifocal atrial tachycardia	>50 years	HTN, IHD, RHD and pulmonary disease	Abrupt onset and offset irregular palpitaion	LVH and repolarization abnormalities
Sinus tachycardia	10–30 years	Normal heart	Progressive onset and slow termination	Normal

Abbreviations: ECG, electrocardiogram; SVT, supraventricular tachycardia; AVRT, atrioventricular reentrant tachycardia; LVH, left ventricular hypertrophy; IHD, ischemic heart disease; RHD, rheumatic heart disease; HTN, hypertension.

Flow chart 2 Approach to narrow complex tachyarrhythmia

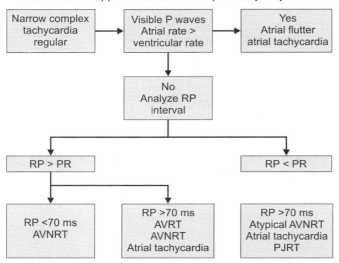

Abbreviations: AVRT, atrioventricular reentrant tachycardia; AVNRT atrioventricular nodal reentrant tachycardia; PJRT, permanent junctional reciprocating tachycardia.

The reentrant pathway is functionally permitted by a fast and slow pathway that exists within the AV node.

Atrioventricular Reentrant Tachycardia

Atrioventricular reentrant tachycardia is due to a concealed AV bypass tract which creates the reentrant circuit. The AV bypass tract usually allows retrograde conduction only.

Sinus Node and Intra-atrial Reentrant Tachycardias

Intra-atrial reentrant tachycardias are commonly seen in postcardiac surgery patients caused by re-entry in sinus node and atria, respectively.

Wolff-Parkinson-White Syndrome (WPW)

Activation of ventricular muscle by impulses originating in atria and conducted by bypass tracts causes preexcitation. Many forms of aberrant connections are possible.

The patients present with episodic SVT, specific ECG abnormalities can be elicited that consist of:[2]
- PR interval less than 120 msec
- Delta wave: Slurring of the initial part of QRS complex
- QRS duration greater than 120 msec.

Association of WPW is seen with mitral valve prolapse syndrome (MVPS), ischemic heart diseases (IHD), hypertrophic cardiomyopathy (HCM), sick sinus syndrome, Ebstein's anomaly, and rheumatic fever.

Treatment of Supraventricular Tachycardia

Vagal Maneuver

Carotid sinus massage stimulates baroreceptors triggering a reflexive increase in the activity of the vagus nerve and sympathetic withdrawal. Both of this causes a slowing conduction through the AV node, thus helping in blocking reentry.[4] A physical examination to rule out a carotid bruit is necessary. Resuscitation equipment should be ready to attach the monitor for continuous ECG monitoring. Pressure is applied in a firm circular manner at the level of the cricoid cartilage for about 5 seconds. Repeat the procedure on the opposite side if the tachyarrhythmia persists.

Drug Therapy

Drug therapy and long-term management of SVT[5] have been described in **Tables 2 and 3**.

Catheter Ablation

Catheter ablation has very high success rates greater than 95% and recurrence rates are few about less than 5% in patients with accessory pathways. Complications of catheter ablation include perforation, bleeding, AV fistula, venous thrombosis, pulmonary embolism, myocardial perforation, valve damage, systemic embolism and rarely death.

VENTRICULAR TACHYCARDIAS

Ventricular tachycardias are the common cause for sudden cardiac deaths. They are aberrant cardiac rhythms from

Table 2 Drug therapy for immediate control of SVT

Drugs	Doses	Side Effects
SVT without preexcitation		
Adenosine	Give 6 mg rapid intravenous followed by fluid bolus; if no response within 1–2 minutes, give 12 mg more	Facial flushing, chest pain, and hypotension; transient asystole bronchospasm, atrial fibrillation and ventricular fibrillation
Verapamil	5 mg every 3–5 minutes, to maximum 15 mg	Hypotension, heart block and negative inotropic effect
Diltiazem	0.25 mg/kg of body weight over a 2-minutes period; if no response, additional dose of 0.35 mg/kg over a 2-minutes period; maintenance infusion of 5–15 mg/h	Hypotension, heart block and negative inotropic effect
Metoprolol	5 mg over a 2-minute period; up to 3 doses in 15 minutes	Hypotension, heart block, bradycardia and bronchospasm
SVT with preexcitaion or WPW with atrial fibrillation		
Procainamide	30 mg/min continuous infusion to a maximal dose of 17 mg/kg (maintenance infusion of 2–4 mg/min)	Hypotension, widening of QRS complex and torsades de pointes
Flecainide	2 mg/kg over a 10-minute period	Negative inotropic effect, conducting atrial flutter and widening of QRS
Ibutilide	If ≥60 kg: 1 mg over a 10-minute period, If<60 kg: 0.01 mg/kg over a 10-minute period. Repeat once if no response after 10 minute.	Prolongation of QT interval and torsades de pointes

Abbreviations: SVT, supraventricular tachycardia; WPW, Wolff-Parkinson-White syndrome

Table 3 Drugs for long-term management of SVT

Drugs	Doses	Side effects	Contraindication
Beta-blockers • Metaprolol • Atenolol	50–200 mg daily 80–240 mg daily	Hypotension and heart block	Asthma, CHF
Calcium channel blockers • Diltiazem • Verapamil	180–360 mg daily 120–480 mg daily	Hypotension and heart block	CHF
Digoxin	0.125–0.375 mg daily	Digitalis toxicity	Preexcitation
First-line drugs			
Flecainide	100–300 mg daily	VT enhanced, AV nodal conduction and interaction with digoxin	Ischemic and structural heart disease
Propafenone	450–900 mg daily		
Second-line drugs			
Amiodarone	200 mg daily	Skin discoloration, thyroid dysfunction, GI, pulmonary corneal deposit, optic neuritis, tremor	
Sotalol	160–320 mg daily	Hypotension, heart block and bradycardia	

Abbreviations: SVT, supraventricular tachycardia; CHF, congestive heart failure; VT, ventricular tachycardia; AV, atrioventricular.

single premature ventricular complexes (PVC) to sustained monomorphic VT, polymorphic VT, and ventricular fibrillation (VF). Ischemic and dilated cardiomyopathies are the common cause for ventricular tachycardia. Patient should be investigated for the presence of underlying structural heart disease as the prognosis depends on it.

Clinical Approach to a Patient with Wide Complex Tachycardia

The QRS greater than 120 msec in ECG are called wide complex tachycardia and are common in clinical practice.[6] Wide QRS complex are seen in VT, SVT with aberrancy or

BBB and SVT with antegrade conduction over an accessory pathway (preexcited tachycardia). Drug toxicities and electrolyte imbalances are also present as QRS.

Medical history and physical examination are very important and helpful in diagnosis. A history of angina, myocardial infarction, or congestive cardiac failure is strong indicators for the presence of VT. Young patients are more likely to have idiopathic VT. Hemodynamic tolerance for the arrhythmia is a poor guide to diagnosis as both SVT and VT can present with hemodynamic collapse. On the contrary, idiopathic VTs may be well tolerated hemodynamically.

Clinical examination of the patient can help in differentiating and categorizing these patients. Clinical signs of AV dissociation include cannon A waves in the jugular venous pulse, variability in the intensity of the first heart sound and variability in arterial blood pressure. Vagal maneuvers that result in termination of tachycardia indicate the presence of SVT. However, these tests are not very reliable as a few VTs can also terminate with vagal maneuvers.

Electrocardiographic Features

Various electrocardiographic features suggestive of VT[7] are as follows **(Table 4)**:
- AV dissociation
- Fusion or capture beats
- QRS width [left bundle branch block (LBBB) >160 msec, right bundle branch block (RBBB) >140 msec]
- Extreme left axis
- Concordance in all precordial leads
- LBBB morphology with right axis deviation.

Monomorphic Ventricular Tachycardia

Various structural heart diseases are known to predispose to monomorphic VT. The scars present in the myocardium act as substrates for reentry. Large ventricular scars seem to predispose more frequent VTs. The most common substrate for VT is ventricular scarring related to IHD, which is present in approximately 60% of patients.[8] Patients with dilated cardiomyopathies, arrhythmogenic right ventricular cardiomyopathy (ARVC), prior cardiac surgery (particularly for correction of congenital anomalies or valve surgery), sarcoidosis or hypertrophic cardiomyopathy can also have ventricular scarring and VT.

Polymorphic Ventricular Tachycardia

Polymorphic VT is defined by a changing QRS morphology from beat to beat. The term literally means "twisting of points". It is commonly a sustained arrhythmia often requiring emergency cardioversion. It can be self-limiting in some patients. Evaluation of the underlying substrate for polymorphic VT is important. Acute ischemia is common cause of polymorphic VT in most cases. Other conditions associated with polymorphic VT are long QT syndrome and Brugada syndrome. Coronary angiography is important investigation to exclude ischemia. Correction of electrolyte is a very important step. Special consideration should be given to hypokalemia and hypomagnesemia. Stabilization of heart failure is also important. Amiodarone is also effective in controlling episodes of polymorphic VT.

Acute Management

The initial management of a patient with sustained monomorphic VT caused by underlying structural heart disease is determined by the nature of the symptoms and the patient's hemodynamic state.[9] Patients presenting with hemodynamic instability, myocardial ischemia and pulmonary edema should be promptly electrically cardioverted. Reversible causes of VT, such as electrolyte imbalances, acute ischemia, hypoxia, and drug toxicities, should be corrected.[10]

In patients who are hemodynamically stable, pharmacological reversion of VT can be attempted. Lidocaine is the first-line agent and is very useful in the setting of myocardial ischemia. In other settings, especially in patients with slow and stable VT not related to ischemia, the efficacy of lidocaine is limited. Intravenous procainamide is a better choice in such patients. Procainamide has the ability to rapidly slow and terminates VT in the nonischemic setting. Use of procainamide is limited by hypotension, which occurs in approximately 20% of these individuals. Overall it is acutely

Table 4 Features in favor of SVT and VT	
Features in favor of supraventricular tachycardia (SVT)	Features in favor of ventricular tachycardia (VT)
• Initiation with a premature P wave • Tachycardia complexes identical to those in resting rhythm • "Long-short" sequence preceding initiation • Changes in the P-P interval preceding changes in the R-R interval • QRS contours consistent with aberrant conduction (V1, V6) • Slowing or termination with vagal maneuvers • Onset of the QRS to its peak (positive or negative) <50 msec • Fusion beats, capture beats QRS duration ≤0.14 sec	• Initiation with a premature QRS complex • Tachycardia beats identical to premature ventricular contractions (PVCs) during sinus rhythm • "Short-long" sequence preceding initiation • Changes in the R-R interval preceding changes in the P-P interval • QRS contours inconsistent with aberrant conduction (V1, V6) • Atrioventricular (AV) dissociation or other non-1:1 AV relationship • Onset of the QRS to its peak (positive or negative) ≥50 msec • QRS duration >0.14 sec left axis deviation (especially 90° to180°)

effective in 75% patients. Amiodarone is also useful, but its onset of action is slower than lidocaine or procainamide. If used, it should be loaded with an intravenous dose and still the results of acute termination studies have been variable. However, at many centers amiodarone is preferred as it is less likely to produce hypotension and prolonged QTc predisposing to torsades de pointes.

Secondary Prevention

Recurrence of VT is frequent problem. Medical therapy can also be beneficial in the secondary prevention of VT.[11] Mexiletine can be used as a second-line therapeutic agent for recurrent ventricular arrhythmias, particularly in combination with other antiarrhythmic medications, although adverse effects can limit its use. Catheter ablation is an option in patients who have recurrent VT or shocks inspite of optimal medical therapy or who have unacceptable side effects with medical therapy. Catheter ablation can also be lifesaving in patients with incessant VT. Catheter ablation is also beneficial in controlling recurrent VT in patients with dilated cardiomyopathies and arrhythmogenic right ventricular dysplasia (ARVD). Implantable cardioverter defibrillators (ICDs) effectively treat ventricular arrhythmias. But ICDs provide inappropriate shocks and can produce a huge psychological impact as well as increase mortality.

REFERENCES

1. Orejarena LA, Vidaillet H Jr, DeStefano F, et al. Paroxysmal supraventricular tachycardia in the general population. J Am Coll Cardiol. 1998;31(1):150-7.
2. Josephson ME, Wellens HJ. Differential diagnosis of supraventricular tachycardia. Cardiol Clin. 1990;8(3):411-42.
3. Bhandari AK, Anderson JL, Gilbert EM, et al. Correlation of symptoms with occurrence of paroxysmal supraventricular tachycardia or atrial fibrillation: a transtelephonic monitoring study. The Flecainide Supraventricular Tachycardia Study Group. Am Heart J. 1992;124(2):381-6.
4. Blomstrom-Lundqvist C, Scheinman MM, Aliot EM, et al. ACC/AHA/ESC guidelines for the management of patients with supraventricular arrhythmias executive summary: a report of the American College of Cardiology/American Heart Association Task Force on Practice Guidelines and the European Society of Cardiology Committee for Practice Guidelines (Writing Committee to Develop Guidelines for the Management of Patients with Supraventricular Arrhythmias). Circulation. 2003;108(15):1871-909.
5. Winniford MD, Fulton KL, Hillis LD. Long-term therapy of paroxysmal supraventricular tachycardia: a randomized, double-blind comparison of digoxin, propranolol and verapamil. Am J Cardiol. 1984;54(8):1138-9.
6. Akhtar M, Shenasa M, Jazayeri M, et al. Wide QRS complex tachycardia. Reappraisal of a common clinical problem. Ann Intern Med. 1988;109(11):905-12.
7. Baerman JM, Morady F, DiCarlo LA Jr, et al. Differentiation of ventricular tachycardia from supraventricular tachycardia with aberration: value of the clinical history. Ann. Emerg Med. 1987;16(1):40-3.
8. Garratt CJ, Griffith MJ, Young G, et al. Value of physical signs in the diagnosis of ventricular tachycardia. Circulation. 1994;90(6):3103-7.
9. Zipes DP, Camm AJ, Borggrefe M, et al. ACC/AHA/ESC 2006 Guidelines for Management of Patients with Ventricular Arrhythmias and the Prevention of Sudden Cardiac Death: a report of the American College of Cardiology/American Heart Association Task Force and the European Society of Cardiology Committee for Practice Guidelines (writing committee to develop Guidelines for Management of Patients with Ventricular Arrhythmias and the Prevention of Sudden Cardiac Death): developed in collaboration with the European Heart Rhythm Association and the Heart Rhythm Society. Circulation. 2006;114(10):e385-484.
10. Lemery R, Brugada P, Bella PD, et al. Nonischemic ventricular tachycardia. Clinical course and long-term follow-up in patients without clinically overt heart disease. Circulation. 1989;79(5):990-9.
11. Ohe T, Aihara N, Kamakura S, et al. Long-term outcome of verapamil-sensitive sustained left ventricular tachycardia in patients without structural heart disease. J Am Coll Cardiol. 1995;25(1):54-8.

CHAPTER 30

Temporary Pacing

Kartikeya Bhargava

INTRODUCTION

Temporary pacing refers to electrical stimulation of cardiac chambers (usually ventricle, occasionally atrium) as a part of the treatment of bradyarrhythmia or tachyarrhythmia. The underlying arrhythmia may be transient, intermittent or persistent and the temporary pacing aims to establish adequate hemodynamics till the arrhythmia resolves completely or definitive therapy usually in the form of permanent pacing is performed. Though, most commonly, temporary pacing is performed as a life-saving emergency measure in a patient with symptomatic bradycardia till a permanent pacemaker is implanted; there are many more indications of temporary pacing that will be discussed later.

TYPES OF TEMPORARY PACING

Temporary pacing is performed most commonly in the ventricles in order to provide adequate ventricular rate in patients with symptomatic atrioventricular (AV) block; but can also be performed in the atrium in patients with symptomatic bradycardia due to sinus node dysfunction or in patients with intact AV conduction and frequent supraventricular or ventricular tachyarrhythmias so as to prevent occurrence of the arrhythmias (ventricular fibrillation or polymorphic ventricular tachycardia) or overdrive treat the arrhythmia (supraventricular tachycardia) if it occurs. *Dual-chamber AV sequential* temporary pacing is often performed through epicardial wires in postoperative patients, though it can be performed transvenously to improve hemodynamic performance in certain patients with AV block such as those with acute inferior and right ventricular myocardial infarction (MI).

Temporary pacing can also be classified according to the route of electrical stimulation as follows:
- *Transvenous pacing*: The pacing lead (**Fig. 1**) is inserted in the right ventricle (or atrium) through a transvenous route from access via either femoral, internal jugular or subclavian vein. It can be fluoroscopically guided or performed blindly in the emergency or intensive care unit (ICU).
- *Transcutaneous external pacing*: The pacing is performed noninvasively via transcutaneous adhesive patches placed on the chest wall in anteroposterior or anterolateral configuration connected to an external defibrillator with pacing capability. This means of stimulation is painful and used only when transvenous pacing is not immediately available and can be instituted in the emergency often as a bridge to transvenous pacing.
- *Epicardial pacing*: The pacing is performed usually in the postoperative period through temporary epicardial fine pacing wire electrodes implanted during cardiac surgery.

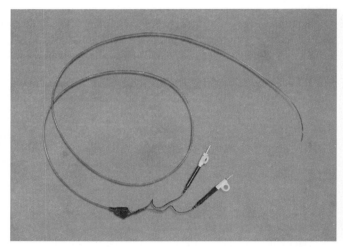

Fig. 1 Transvenous temporary pacing lead. The lead has two electrodes (distal tip and the proximal ring) at its tip and two connecting pins, distal and proximal at the other end where it connects with the pulse generator via a connecting cable

The wires are usually removed before discharge from the hospital and hence this means is not available to the emergency physician.
- *Transesophageal pacing*: The pacing is performed through a flexible pacing electrode placed in the mid-esophagus (for atrial pacing) or the fundus of the stomach (for ventricular pacing). This approach is better tolerated in a conscious patient than transcutaneous pacing as it is painless but is not frequently used clinically.

INDICATIONS OF TEMPORARY PACING

Most commonly temporary pacing is performed as an emergency procedure in patients with symptomatic and/or life-threatening bradycardia, although many elective indications of temporary pacing also exist **(Box 1)**. In general, emergency temporary pacing is reserved for patients with bradycardia who have recurrent syncope occurring at rest (mostly AV block), or hemodynamically instability due to bradycardia or ventricular tachyarrhythmias. The patients with sinus node dysfunction are usually not symptomatic at rest and if pacing is indicated, they can directly undergo permanent pacing. Temporary transvenous pacing poses the risks of not only infection but also damage to venous access sites that may potentially be needed for permanent pacing; and hence should be avoided if possible without compromising patient's safety.

Among patients with acute MI, one needs to be more proactive and aggressive with temporary pacing in those with anterior MI. Sinus bradycardia and AV block associated with acute inferior MI are usually hemodynamically well tolerated, responsive to drugs and fluids, not life-threatening and infrequently need temporary pacing. AV block in most patients with acute inferior MI recovers spontaneously with time and permanent pacing is only rarely necessary. On the other hand, bradyarrhythmias or new intraventricular conduction disturbances associated with acute anterior MI can result in unpredictable and sudden hemodynamic deterioration and warrant temporary pacing although, many of them may not require permanent pacing.

Elective temporary pacing is usually required to cover for any pacing support in catheterization lab or surgical procedures in patients with high risk of AV block or bradycardia.

TEMPORARY PACING PROCEDURE

Transvenous Pacing

The temporary pacing is best performed under fluoroscopic visualization in catheterization laboratory, however, it is often performed blindly at the bedside as an emergency procedure, especially if catheterization laboratory facility is not available. Though, many routes of venous access, each

Box 1 Indications of temporary cardiac pacing

Emergency indications:
- Complete or second degree (Mobitz II or advanced or high grade) AV block with recurrent syncope at rest as a bridge to permanent pacing
- Ventricular tachyarrhythmias related to bradycardia
- Bradyarrhythmias in acute MI:
    - Ventricular asystole
    - Symptomatic or hemodynamically significant bradycardia unresponsive to atropine: Sinus bradycardia or second degree type 1 AV block
    - Complete AV block associated with hypotension, or wide QRS escape rhythm or ventricular arrhythmias
    - Mobitz type II AV block
    - Intraventricular conduction defects at high risk of unpredictable complete AV block or asystole even with absence of symptomatic bradycardia, e.g. new or indeterminate bifascicular block with prolonged PR interval, bilateral bundle-branch block, alternating bundle-branch block
- Recurrent polymorphic ventricular tachycardia with or without QT prolongation, not adequately controlled by drugs
- Recurrent monomorphic ventricular tachycardia or supraventricular tachycardia not controlled with drugs in order to overdrive treat the arrhythmia

Elective indications:
- Catheterization laboratory procedures with potential for requirement of temporary pacing support
    - Pacemaker pulse generator replacement in patients with complete AV block or pacing dependence
    - Permanent pacemaker system explantation usually for infection
    - Immediately prior to permanent pacemaker or CRT-device implantation in patients with AV block or left bundle-branch block
    - Alcohol septal ablation for hypertrophic cardiomyopathy
    - Rotablation of coronary stenosis especially right coronary artery
    - Transcatheter aortic valve implantation
- Noncardiac surgery under general anesthesia in patients with high risk of AV block
- *Cardiac surgery*: Epicardial pacing wires are routinely placed for any perioperative pacing requirement

Abbreviations: AV, atrioventricular; CRT, cardiac resynchronization therapy; MI, myocardial infarction.

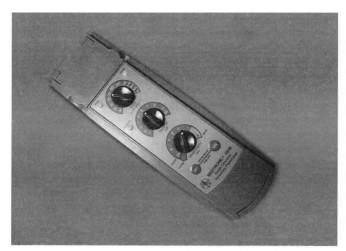

Fig. 2 Temporary pacing pulse generator. This is a single chamber pulse generator and has three knobs for adjusting pacing rate, output and sensitivity; light indicators for pace, sense and low battery; switches to turn on or off; a port for connecting the connecting cable and a battery that can be replaced. The model shown also has capability of delivering rapid pacing (beyond 180/min) mainly used for rapid atrial pacing to terminate supraventricular tachycardia or atrial flutter

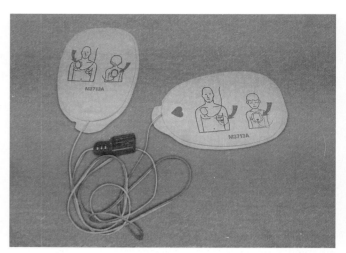

Fig. 3 Transcutaneous patches for pacing and defibrillation. The two patches are attached to the right anterior and left lateral (or posterior) chest wall as shown and are connected to the external defibrillator using the attached connecting cable

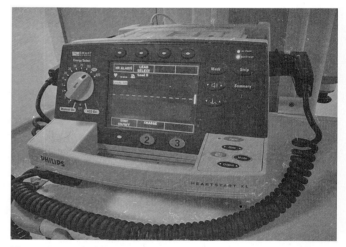

Fig. 4 External defibrillator. The external defibrillator can deliver transcutaneous temporary pacing through patches shown in Figure 3. The rate and output of pacing can be adjusted as per the patients need, tolerability and capture threshold

with its advantages and disadvantages are available, the femoral vein (in catheterization lab) and the right internal jugular vein (bedside) are the most suitable and most commonly used approaches. In general, the subclavian veins especially the left should be avoided for temporary pacing since these may be needed in future for permanent pacemaker implantation.

The procedure entails placement of a venous sheath using Seldinger's technique taking all aseptic precautions in a sterile environment, positioning of the temporary pacing lead (**Fig. 1**) in the right ventricle (or atrium) preferably under fluoroscopy, connecting the lead to an external pulse generator (**Fig. 2**), ensuring adequacy of electrical pacing parameters and finally securing the lead with sutures to the skin to avoid its displacement. Some experience is needed to negotiate the lead from the right atrium across the tricuspid valve in the right ventricle and echocardiography can sometimes be very useful in guiding the lead placement in absence of fluoroscopy at the bedside.

Transcutaneous Pacing

The external transcutaneous pacing can be easily performed without much learning curve using transcutaneous defibrillation patches (**Fig. 3**) and an external defibrillator (**Fig. 4**) with pacing capability. The patches can be placed preferably in anteroposterior configuration on the chest but an anterolateral configuration can be used in an emergency situation. Though, this means of pacing is painful and often requires the patient to be sedated; it can be very useful due to universal availability in emergency wards and coronary care units and ease of use. Moreover, this is often very useful to transfer a patient from a small nursing home to a facility with catheterization laboratory.

COMPLICATIONS OF TEMPORARY PACING

As with any invasive procedure, transvenous temporary pacing can also lead to complications in 14–20% of patients, the frequency of which increases with the duration of pacing.

> **Box 2** Complications of temporary transvenous pacing
>
> *Venous access-related complications:*
> - Hematoma and bleeding at puncture site, femoral pseudoaneurysm
> - Venous thrombosis and pulmonary embolism
> - Pneumothorax (internal jugular or subclavian puncture) or hemothorax
> - Infection at local puncture site
>
> *Lead placement-related complications:*
> - Catheter knotting
> - Tricuspid valve injury
> - Myocardial perforation and cardiac tamponade
> - Air embolism
>
> *Pacing lead-related and electrical issues:*
> - Lead dislodgement or disconnection
> - Cardiac perforation and tamponade
> - Extracardiac (phrenic nerve) stimulation
> - Increase pacing threshold
> - *Ventricular arrhythmias*: Ectopics and tachycardia due to mechanical effect of the lead or inappropriate pacing due to improper sensing

The complications may be related to the venous access, mechanical effects of the pacing lead or to the electrical issues **(Box 2)**.

POST-PROCEDURE CARE

Care of the patient after temporary transvenous pacing in the emergency and ICUs is very important to prevent complications and recognize them promptly if they occur. The salient points are mentioned here.

- *Post-procedure and periodic chest X-ray and electrocardiogram (ECG)*: A chest X-ray should be performed to ascertain the position of the pacing lead and also look for any pneumothorax or hemothorax. Similarly, an ECG should be performed post-procedure and repeated if needed to assess adequate sensing and pacing. If there are any doubts, an echocardiogram should be performed to look for lead position and presence of pericardial effusion.
- *Continuous ECG monitoring*: The patients with temporary pacemaker should have continuous ECG monitoring in order to promptly recognize any loss of pacing or occurrence of ventricular arrhythmias.
- *Checking electrical parameters, system integrity and pulse-generator battery*: At least once daily checking of sensing and pacing parameters, lead connections and need for battery change should be performed and adequacy of parameters programmed should be ensured. The pacing output should be programmed to at least three times the pacing threshold. The underlying rhythm should also be checked by gradually reducing the pacing rate to below intrinsic rate to assess the continued need for temporary pacing. Lack of pacing and asystole often occurs due to loose connections or rise in pacing threshold.
- *Care of the access site*: An occlusive dressing with antibiotic or antiseptic ointment should be performed at the site of puncture and sheath access to prevent infection. The dressing should be changed if soiled and once daily. If the sheath is in place, it should be flushed periodically with heparinized saline to prevent thrombosis.
- *Prevention of infection*: Prophylactic antibiotics that cover *Staphylococcus* should be used especially if a femoral route has been chosen for temporary pacing. If the temporary pacing is to be used for a prolonged period (>7 days) or any sign of local infection is seen, the pacing site and lead should be changed to prevent systemic infection.

CONCLUSION

Temporary cardiac pacing involves electrical stimulation of the heart usually the ventricles in order to treat bradyarrhythmias and sometimes tachyarrhythmias and is commonly performed transvenously using a pacing lead and pulse generator. It should be used judiciously and only when necessary for an appropriate length of time in order to avoid its complications. Choice of the approach, the access site, and the duration of pacing needs to be individualized based on the patient's requirements and routine post-procedure care taken to prevent complications from this procedure.

CHAPTER 31

Hypertensive Emergency

Ravi R Kasliwal, Kushagra Mahansaria

INTRODUCTION

In the year 2000, more than one-quarter of the world's adult population, nearly 1 billion people were estimated to have hypertension. It is expected to rise to 1.5 billion by the year 2025.[1] Hypertension is one of the major risk factors that contribute to the development of cardiovascular diseases (CVDs).[1,2] Many evidence-based guidelines have addressed the burden of hypertension, providing recommendations for the outpatient management of chronic hypertension.[3-9] In contrast, only a few studies in the past have addressed the epidemiology of acute hypertension.

A retrospective cohort study from 2005–2007 defined acute hypertension as a systolic blood pressure more than or equal to 180 mm Hg, which occurred in approximately 14% of all patients presenting to the emergency.[10] Moreover, acute hypertensive episodes affect nearly 1% of all patients having chronic essential hypertension.[11-13]

We know that chronic hypertension is an established risk factor for many diseases affecting the cardiovascular, cerebrovascular, and renal systems. In contrast, the abrupt increase in blood pressure (BP) during episodes of hypertensive emergencies can cause acute end-organ damage with significant morbidity. Prompt treatment plays a vital role in limiting morbidity and mortality.[14,15] Accelerated hypertension is among the most misunderstood diseases seen in clinical practice and is often mismanaged by a reflex need to rapidly decrease the blood pressure without giving proper thought behind the pathophysiological mechanisms leading to the acute rise in BP. Knowledge of current principles and available therapies is of utmost importance in the management of this growing problem in India.

CLASSIFICATION

The stages of hypertension as recommended in the most recent report of the Joint National Committee on Prevention, Detection, Evaluation and Treatment of High Blood Pressure (JNC-7, 2003)[3] have been summarized in **Table 1**. The 5th report of JNC published in 1993 proposed to classify hypertensive crisis as either *hypertensive emergencies* or *hypertensive urgencies*.[16]

Table 1 Stages of hypertension [Joint National Committee on Prevention, Detection, Evaluation and Treatment of High Blood Pressure (JNC 7)]

Stage	Systolic blood pressure (SBP) (mm Hg)	Diastolic blood pressure (DBP) (mm Hg)
Normal	<120	<80
Prehypertension	121–139	80–89
Stage 1	140–159	90–99
Stage 2	≥160	≥100

This classification remains useful today. Severe elevations in BP were classified as either hypertensive emergencies or as hypertensive urgencies depending on the presence or absence of end-organ damage (cardiovascular, cerebrovascular or renal). When an acute elevation in blood pressure is accompanied by encephalopathy or acute nephropathy, the term *malignant hypertension* has been used.[17] This term has been discontinued and falls under the classification of hypertensive emergencies. A systolic blood pressure (SBP) more than 190 mm Hg and/or diastolic blood pressure (DBP) more than 100 mm Hg on two consecutive readings following surgery is referred to as *postoperative hypertension*.[18,19]

This classification is essential to formulate a treatment plan. In hypertensive urgency, blood pressure should be reduced within 24–48 hours. In contrast, in hypertensive emergency (including postoperative hypertension),[20] blood pressure should be lowered immediately to target levels as per the presentation (summarized in **Table 2**) in order to prevent end-organ damage.

Table 2 Target blood pressure (BP) goals for specific emergencies

Condition	Target BP goal
Hypertensive encephalopathy	Mean arterial pressure (MAP) lowered by maximum 20% or to diastolic blood pressure (DBP) 100–110 mm Hg within first hour then gradual reduction in BP to normal range over 48–72 h
Ischemic stroke	MAP lowered no more than 15%–20%, DBP not less than 100–110 mm Hg in first 24 h (thrombolytic protocols in stroke may allow slightly more aggressive management)
Intracerebral hemorrhage	MAP lowered by 20%–25%
Hypertensive retinopathy	MAP lowered by 20%–25%
Left ventricular failure	MAP to 60–100 mm Hg
Aortic dissection	Systolic blood pressure (SBP) 100–120 mm Hg
Acute renal insufficiency	MAP lowered by 20%–25%
Pregnancy-induced hypertension	SBP 130–150 mm Hg, DBP 80–100 mm Hg

Table 3 Secondary causes of hypertensive crisis

Cause	Example
Renal parenchymal	Chronic pyelonephritis, primary glomerulonephritis, etc.
Renovascular	Atherosclerosis, fibromuscular dysplasia, polyarteritis nodosa
Systemic disorders	Systemic lupus erythematosus (SLE), systemic sclerosis, vasculitides
Endocrine	Pheochromocytoma, Cushing's syndrome, Conn's syndrome
Drugs	Cocaine, amphetamines, cyclosporine, clonidine withdrawal, phencyclidine, etc.
Other	Coarctation of aorta

EPIDEMIOLOGY

Of the estimated 1 billion people living with essential hypertension, around 30% are undiagnosed.[1] Of these 1 billion, only a quarter have adequate blood pressure control.[21] Increasing age, male gender, and ethnicity adversely affect both the incidence and prevalence of hypertension.[7,8,22–25] Similarly, the epidemiology of hypertensive crises resembles the distribution of essential hypertension, being much higher among male gender, older population and certain ethnic groups like people of Latin-American and African-American descent.[14,26] Risk factors for exacerbation of episodes of hypertensive emergencies include inadequate blood pressure control in hypertensive patients. This may be complicated by lack of accessibility to a physician and nonadherence to treatment.[13,25,27,28] Illicit drug use is a growing problem in both developed and developing countries and has been found to be another risk factor that might be easily overlooked. These factors have led to an increase in the incidence of hypertensive crisis despite the development of increasingly effective antihypertensive treatments.[29] A detailed history is the key to finding a cause in most patinets.[30]

PATHOGENESIS

The pathogenesis of hypertensive crises is poorly understood. In most cases, there appears to be a triggering factor that causes acute rise in BP on patients with preexisting hypertension. Most likely, an abrupt rise in systemic vascular resistance mediated by humoral vasoconstrictors leads to initiation of the crisis.[31,32] The resulting increase in BP causes mechanical stress and endothelial cell damage causing increased vascular permeability, platelet activation, fibrin deposition, and activation of the coagulation cascade. Further elevations in BP worsen endothelial injury and cause fibrinoid necrosis of the arterioles.[31,32] This results in ischemia, releasing more vasoactive mediators. The renin-angiotensin-aldosterone system gets activated, leading to further vasoconstriction and production of proinflammatory cytokines.[33,34] A vicious cycle generates causing hypoperfusion of end-organs, ischemia, and dysfunction that manifest as a hypertensive emergency.[33,34]

Although in most cases accelerated hypertension complicates underlying essential hypertension, it can also develop *de novo* or can complicate secondary hypertension. The secondary causes of hypertensive crisis are summarized in **Table 3**.[31,35,36]

CLINICAL PRESENTATION

The clinical presentation depends on the end-organ affected. These are summarized in **Box 1**.[15]

The signs and symptoms therefore vary from patient-to-patient depending upon the end organ involved. The most frequent presenting signs in patients with hypertensive emergencies are chest pain, dyspnea, and neurologic deficits.[13] Usually, organ dysfunction is uncommon with a DBP less than 130 mm Hg (except in children and pregnant women).[21] It is also important to note that the rate of increase of BP is a more important predictor of organ dysfunction compared to absolute level of BP.[37] **Box 2**[38] lists common clinical characteristics of hypertensive emergency.

ASSESSMENT

Initial Assessment

Early triage is critical for timely and appropriate therapy.[39] History taking should inquire about the duration of

Box 1 Clinical outcomes of hypertensive emergency

- Cerebral infarction
- Hypertensive encephalopathy
- Acute aortic dissection
- Acute myocardial infarction, acute coronary syndrome
- Pulmonary edema with respiratory failure
- Preeclampsia, eclampsia, HELLP syndrome
- Acute renal failure
- Microangiopathic hemolytic anemia
- Antepartum hemorrhage

Abbreviation: HELLP, hemolysis, elevated liver enzymes, and low platelet count.

Box 2 Clinical characteristics of hypertensive emergencies

- *Blood pressure (in mm Hg)*: Systolic >220; Diastolic >140
- *Fundoscopy*: Exudates, hemorrhages, papilledema
- *Neurological*: Altered sensorium, headache, visual field defects, seizures, coma, focal deficits
- *Cardiac*: Congestive heart failure, dyspnea, angina
- *Renal*: Oliguria, proteinuria, azotemia
- *Gastrointestinal*: Nausea, vomiting, abdominal pain

hypertension, BP control, prescription and nonprescription drugs, compliance to antihypertensive medications, and use of recreational drugs. Sympatholytic medications such as clonidine are notorious for causing severe rebound hypertension. Cocaine and phencyclidine are sympathomimetics that cause severe increases in blood pressure.

Knowledge of preexisting comorbidities is an important part of the initial evaluation and guides further management. A family history of sudden death, premature cardiac disease, or endocrine disorders should prompt the clinician to consider pheochromocytoma, multiple endocrine neoplasm, and hyperthyroidism as possible causes of episodic blood pressure increase and tachycardia in a young healthy patient. The most vital part of the history is assessment of signs and symptoms associated with the patient's chief complaint and targeted evaluation of end organs looking for specific manifestations, such as headache, seizures, weakness, or sensory loss, chest pain, dyspnea, edema, and decreased urine output. The presence of symptoms alone does not confirm a hypertensive emergency, but it suggests that an organ might be affected, requiring further assessment.

Physical Examination

The physical examination should focus on identifying presence or absence of end-organ dysfunction. For example, an altered sensorium along with associated fundoscopic features may be suggestive of hypertensive encephalopathy.[40,41] A sudden onset of a severe headache (usually described by the patient as the "worst headache of their life") indicates subarachnoid hemorrhage.

The basis of cardiac evaluation rests on prompt identification of features of acute coronary syndrome (ACS) including acute myocardial infarction (MI) and angina. Atypical symptoms especially in the diabetic patients should also be investigated appropriately.[14,42] Aortic dissection should be suspected in patients presenting with sudden onset of severe chest pain, mediastinal widening, and unequal pulses. A contrast computed tomography (CT) or magnetic resonance imaging (MRI) confirms diagnosis.[43,44]

Initial Laboratory Studies

A complete blood count with smear, renal function test including electrolytes, urinalysis and electrocardiograph (ECG) should be obtained in all patients. Electrolyte abnormalities such as hypokalemia and hypomagnesemia increase the risk of cardiac arrhythmias including ventricular tachycardia/fibrillation. A chest X-ray should be routinely ordered in patients complaining of chest pain or dyspnea. A CT head should be considered in patients presenting with symptoms of neurologic dysfunction.[40,45]

INITIAL THERAPEUTIC APPROACH

The therapeutic approach should be to refrain from a rapid reduction in BP as this approach has been found to be associated with considerable morbidity.[46-48] In patients presenting with hypertensive urgencies, oral medications are used to gradually lower the blood pressure over a period of 24–48 hours. The target BP goals in hypertensive emergencies is summarized in **Table 2**.[49] Rapid and controlled BP reduction to target goals should be achieved in order to prevent organ damage.[46-48] Care should be taken to not lower blood pressure rapidly and to normal levels.[50-52]

PHARMACOLOGICAL THERAPY FOR HYPERTENSIVE CRISIS

Hypertensive Urgencies

In case of hypertensive urgencies, the choice of oral antihypertensive agents is summarized in **Table 4**.[38]

- *Captopril* is a well-tolerated angiotensin-converting enzyme inhibitor (ACEI) that effectively reduces blood pressure in hypertensive urgencies.[53] Responsiveness to captopril can be enhanced by the addition of a loop diuretic.
- *Clonidine* is a centrally acting α-agonist. It causes drowsiness and may be a poor choice when monitoring of mental status is important.
- *Labetalol* is a combined α- and β-blocker.[54,55] Like any β-blocker it should be avoided in patients with airway disease, symptomatic bradycardia, congestive heart failure (CHF) or those with higher than a 1st degree heart block.

Table 4 Oral antihypertensive agents for hypertensive urgencies

Agent	Dose	Onset of action	Duration of action	Precautions
Captopril	25 mg	15–30 min	2–6 h	Can cause renal failure in bilateral renal artery stenosis
Clonidine	0.1–0.2 mg, can be repeated hourly to a total dose of 0.6 mg	30–60 min	8–16 h	Drowsiness, dry mouth
Labetalol	200–400 mg, repeated every 2–3 h	0.5–2 h	2–12 h	Bronchoconstriction, heart block, orthostatic hypotension
Prazosin	1–2 mg, repeated hourly as needed	1–2 h	8–12 h	First dose syncope, palpitation, orthostatic hypotension

- *Prazosin* is an α-blocker that can have limited benefit in the management of pheochromocytoma.

Hypertensive Emergencies

Clinical presentation guides the choice of antihypertensive agents in hypertensive emergencies. The various agents that are used today in clinical practice are summarized in **Table 5**.[24,56-58]

Sodium nitroprusside is an arterial and venous vasodilator that decreases both afterload and preload.[59] It increases intracranial pressure while decreasing cerebral blood flow making it unsuitable for use in patients presenting with associated neurological symptoms.[60] It is also rapidly degraded by light, requiring special handling and making it cumbersome to use and store. One of the major concerns is the metabolism of sodium nitroprusside into cyanogen and thiocyanate. Due to this, cyanide toxicity has been reported in patients, sometimes leading to sudden cardiac arrest. It should be used with caution in patients with impaired hepatic, renal and cardiac function.[61]

Nitroglycerin is a potent venodilator but can reduce afterload at high doses. It also dilates collateral coronary vessels and may be of particular use in patients presenting with concurrent coronary ischemia or in post-CABG.[62] However, tolerance to IV nitroglycerin maybe observed within 24–48 hours of infusion, which can cause hypotension and reflex tachycardia.

Nicardipine, a second-generation intravenous dihydropyridine calcium antagonist, has been growing in popularity in the management of a high percentage of hypertensive emergencies. In a large multicenter trial, nicardipine was found to be as effective as nitroprusside,[63] with an added benefit of reducing both cerebral and cardiac ischemia.[64]

Clevidipine is a newer, ultra-short-acting, third-generation dihydropyridine calcium antagonist. It inhibits calcium influx through L-type channels, thereby causing vascular smooth muscle relaxation of small arteries and decreasing peripheral vascular resistance.[65,66] Several trials have shown clevidipine to be very effective in the control of postoperative hypertension.[67,68]

Fenoldopam is a short-acting dopamine agonist. It activates dopamine receptors on the renal tubules, inhibiting sodium reabsorption and resulting in diuresis. It also improves creatinine clearance especially in patients with renal dysfunction.[69,70] Due to these properties, fenoldopam may be the drug of choice in these patients.[71]

Hydralazine is a direct-acting vasodilator. It improves blood flow across the uterine vessels. Therefore, it was used in the management of eclampsia and preeclampsia. However, it can cause a rapid fall in BP that can last up to 12 hours.[72] Due to unpredictability of its antihypertensive effects and difficulty in titration, it has very limited use.

Enalaprilat, the active form of enalapril, is an ACEI. ACEIs may have an important role countering the pathogenic role of angiotensin II.[31] Enalaprilat is particularly useful in patients presenting with CHF and is contraindicated in pregnancy.

Esmolol is an ultra-short-acting cardioselective β-blocker that can be used safely in patients with acute myocardial infarction. Studies have found esmolol to be safe even in patients who have relative contraindication β-blocker therapy.[73]

Labetalol is a combined α$_1$-blocker and a nonselective β-blocker possessing intrinsic sympathomimetic activity and having an α: β blocking ratio of 1:7, labetalol has little or no effect on heart rate.[74,75] It reduces the systemic vascular resistance while maintaining cerebral, renal, and coronary blood flows.[75] Being lipid insoluble, labetalol is ideal for use in eclampsia/preeclampsia because little placental transfer occurs.[76]

Phentolamine is an α-blocker and had found importance in the management of acute hypertension secondary to pheochromocytoma.[77] However, since nitroprusside and labetalol are more easily titrated, phentolamine is rarely used today.

CONCLUSION

The incidence and prevalence of people living with hypertension is growing in India every day. As a result, the number of hospital visits in our country due to hypertensive

Table 5 Pharmacological agents used in hypertensive emergencies

Drug	Dose	Onset of action	Duration of action	Adverse effects	Indications
Sodium nitroprusside	0.25–10 µg/kg/min IV infusion	Few seconds	1–2 min	Nausea, vomiting, cyanide toxicity	Most hypertensive emergencies; use cautiously in patients with high intracranial pressure or azotemia
Nitroglycerin	5–100 µg/min IV infusion	1–5 min	5–30 min	Headache vomiting, methemoglobinemia caution in right ventricular infarct	Cardiac ischemia, flash pulmonary edema; use cautiously in right ventricular infarction or with recent use of phosphodiesterase inhibitors
Nicardipine	5–15 mg/h IV infusion	5–10 min	15–30 min, may last several hours	Tachycardia, headache, flushing, local phlebitis	Most hypertensive emergencies; *Caution*: Causes coronary steal in cardiac ischemia
Fenoldopam	0.1–0.3 µg/kg/min IV infusion	5–10 min	30 min	Tachycardia, headache, nausea, flushing	Best for renal hypertensive emergencies
Enalaprilat	1.25–5 mg IV every 6 h	15–30 min	6–12 h	Significant fall in BP in high renin states	Acute left ventricular failure, flash pulmonary edema; avoid in acute myocardial infarction (MI)
Hydralazine	10–20 mg 10–40 mg IM	10–20 min IV 20–30 min IM	1–4 h IV 4–6 h IM	Tachycardia, flushing, headache, vomiting, worsening angina	Eclampsia; *Caution*: Gives erratic response
Clevidipine	1–2 mg/h then titrate to maximum 16 mg/h IV infusion	2–4 min	5–15 min	Headache, nausea, vomiting, hypotension, rebound hypertension, reflex tachycardia	Postoperative hypertension, hypertensive emergency in renal dysfunction or acute heart failure
Esmolol	250–500 µg/kg/min IV bolus, then 50–100 µg/kg/min IV infusion; repeat bolus after 5 min or increase infusion to 300 µg/kg/min	1–2 min	10–30 min	Nausea, hypotension, bronchoconstriction, heart failure, 1st degree heart block	Aortic dissection, perioperative hypertension
Labetalol	20–80 mg IV bolus every 10 min; or 0.5–2 mg/min IV infusion	5–10 min	3–6 h	Vomiting, dizziness, nausea, orthostatic hypotension, bronchoconstriction, heart block	Most hypertensive emergencies, ideal for preeclampsia; *Caution*: With acute heart failure
Phentolamine	5–15 mg IV bolus	1–2 min	10–30 min	Tachycardia, flushing, headache	Pheochromocytoma and other conditions with catecholamine excess

emergencies also are on the rise. It is imperative for the emergency physicians and other medical personnel working in the emergency department to have a proper understanding of the pathophysiology and presentation of hypertensive crises and distinguish urgency from an emergency. Prompt treatment based on correct diagnosis can prevent severe end-organ morbidity. As such, the treating physicians should also know the various treatments available and their dosing including adverse effects. These are again summarized in **Table 6**[23,38,49,57,58,78] for the benefit of the reader.

Many medications are available to treat hypertensive emergencies but none is universally recognized as being superior to the others. The appropriate therapeutic approach is specific to patients depending on their clinical presentation. With appropriate identification and management, hypertensive crises can be halted and reversed.

Table 6 Choice of pharmacological agent in hypertensive emergency according to presentation

Condition	Preferred drugs	Drugs to avoid
Acute pulmonary edema/heart failure	Fenoldopam/nitroprusside + nitroglycerin (up to 60 μg/min) + loop diuretic	Hydralazine, β-blockers
Myocardial ischemia and infarction	Labetalol/esmolol + nitroglycerin (up to 200 μg/min) ± Nicardipine/fenoldopam if BP uncontrolled or poorly controlled	Hydralazine, minoxidil, diazoxide, nitroprusside
Hypertensive encephalopathy	Labetalol/nicardipine/fenoldopam	β-blockers, methyldopa, clonidine, diazoxide, hydralazine, nitroglycerin
Acute aortic dissection	Labetalol or nicardipine + esmolol or nitroprusside + esmolol/ IV metoprolol	Hydralazine, minoxidil
Preeclampsia, eclampsia	Labetalol/nicardipine	Diuretics, angiotensin-converting enzyme inhibitors (ACEIs)
Acute renal failure, Microangiopathic anemia	Fenoldopam/nicardipine	
Intracerebral hemorrhage	Nimodipine (oral)/nicardipine/ labetalol/ nitroprusside/enalaprilat	β-blockers, methyldopa, clonidine, diazoxide, hydralazine, nitroglycerin
Hyperadrenergic states/sympathetic overdrive	Phentolamine/nitroprusside/labetalol/nicardipine/verapamil. Alternatively, fenoldopam ± a benzodiazepine (in cocaine overdose)	β-blockers (in cocaine overdose)

REFERENCES

1. Kearney PM, Whelton M, Reynolds K, et al. Global burden of hypertension: analysis of worldwide data. Lancet. 2005;365(9455):217-23.
2. Mills KT, Bundy JD, Kelly TN, et al. Global Burden and Control of Hypertension in 2010: Analysis of Population-Based Studies from 89 Countries. Circulation. 2015;131(Suppl 1):A32.
3. Chobanian AV, Bakris GL, Black HR, et al. The seventh report of the joint national committee on prevention, detection, evaluation, and treatment of high blood pressure: the JNC 7 report. JAMA. 2003;289(19):2560-71.
4. Dasgupta K, Quinn RR, Zarnke KB, et al. The 2014 Canadian Hypertension Education Program recommendations for blood pressure measurement, diagnosis, assessment of risk, prevention, and treatment of hypertension. Can J Cardiol. 2014;30(5):485-501.
5. James PA, Oparil S, Carter BL, et al. 2014 evidence-based guideline for the management of high blood pressure in adults: report from the panel members appointed to the Eighth Joint National Committee (JNC 8). JAMA. 2014;311(5):507-20.
6. Mancia G, Fagard R, Narkiewicz K, et al. 2013 ESH/ESC guidelines for the management of arterial hypertension: the Task Force for the Management of Arterial Hypertension of the European Society of Hypertension (ESH) and of the European Society of Cardiology (ESC). Blood Press. 2013;22(4):193-278.
7. Whitworth JA; World Health Organization, International Society of Hypertension Writing Group. 2003 World Health Organization (WHO)/International Society of Hypertension (ISH) statement on management of hypertension. J Hypertens. 2003;21(11):1983-92.
8. Prevention of cardiovascular disease. World Health Organization; 2007.
9. Weber MA, Schiffrin EL, White WB, et al. Clinical practice guidelines for the management of hypertension in the community. J Clin Hypertens. 2014;16(1):14-26.
10. Shorr AF, Zilberberg MD, Sun X, et al. Severe acute hypertension among inpatients admitted from the emergency department. J Hosp Med. 2012;7(3):203-10.
11. Kuppasani K, Reddi AS. Emergency or urgency? Effective management of hypertensive crises. JAAPA. 2010;23(8):44-9.
12. Owens WB. Blood pressure control in acute cerebrovascular disease. J Clin Hypertens. 2011;13(3):205-11.
13. Zampaglione B, Pascale C, Marchisio M, et al. Hypertensive urgencies and emergencies prevalence and clinical presentation. Hypertension. 1996;27(1):144-7.
14. Bennett NM, Shea S. Hypertensive emergency: case criteria, sociodemographic profile, and previous care of 100 cases. Am J Public Health. 1988;78(6):636-40.
15. Varon J, Fromm Jr RE. Hypertensive crises. The need for urgent management. Postgrad Med. 1996;99(1):189-91, 195-6, 199-200, passim.
16. The fifth report of the Joint National Committee on detection, evaluation, and treatment of high blood pressure. Arch Intern Med. 1993;153(2):154-83.
17. Carey RM, Cutler J, Friedewald W, et al. The 1984 report of the joint national committee on detection, evaluation, and treatment of high blood pressure. Arch Intern Med. 1984;144(5):1045-57.
18. Gal TJ, Cooperman LH. Hypertension in the immediate postoperative period. Br J Anaesth. 1975;47(1):70-4.
19. Halpern NA, Goldberg M, Neely C, et al. Postoperative hypertension: A multicenter, prospective, randomized comparison between intravenous nicardipine and sodium nitroprusside. Crit Care Med. 1992;20(12):1637-43.

20. Goldman L, Caldera D. Risks of general anesthesia and elective operation in the hypertensive patient. Anesthesiology. 1979;50(4):285-92.
21. Varon J, Marik PE. The diagnosis and management of hypertensive crises. Chest. 2000;118(1):214-27.
22. Dannenberg AL, Garrison RJ, Kannel WB. Incidence of hypertension in the Framingham Study. Am J Public Health. 1988;78(6):676-9.
23. Pak KJ, Hu T, Fee C, et al. Acute hypertension: a systematic review and appraisal of guidelines. Ochsner J. 2014;14(4):655-63.
24. Varon J, Marik PE. Clinical review: The management of hypertensive crises. Crit Care. 2003;7(5):374-84.
25. Vaughan CJ, Delanty N. Hypertensive emergencies. Lancet. 2000;356(9227):411-7.
26. Kaplan NM. Treatment of hypertensive emergencies and urgencies. Heart Dis Stroke. 1992;1(6):373-8.
27. Lip GY, Beevers M, Potter JF, et al. Malignant hypertension in the elderly. QJM. 1995;88(9):641-7.
28. Smith CB, Flower LW, Reinhardt CE. Control of hypertensive emergencies. Postgrad Med. 1991;89(5):111-9.
29. Kozak LJ, DeFrances CJ, Hall MJ. National hospital discharge survey: 2004 annual summary with detailed diagnosis and procedure data. Vital Health Stat 13. 2006(162):1-209.
30. Shea S, Misra D, Ehrlich MH, et al. Predisposing factors for severe, uncontrolled hypertension in an inner-city minority population. N Engl J Med. 1992;327(11):776-81.
31. Ault MJ, Ellrodt AG. Pathophysiological events leading to the end-organ effects of acute hypertension. Am J Emerg Med. 1985;3(6):10-5.
32. Wallach R, Karp RB, Reves J, et al. Pathogenesis of paroxysmal hypertension developing during and after coronary bypass surgery: a study of hemodynamic and humoral factors. Am J Cardiol. 1980;46(4):559-65.
33. Funakoshi Y, Ichiki T, Ito K, et al. Induction of interleukin-6 expression by angiotensin II in rat vascular smooth muscle cells. Hypertension. 1999;34(1):118-25.
34. Han Y, Runge MS, Brasier AR. Angiotensin II induces interleukin-6 transcription in vascular smooth muscle cells through pleiotropic activation of nuclear factor-κB transcription factors. Circ Res. 1999;84(6):695-703.
35. Milne F, James S, Veriava Y. Malignant hypertension and its renal complications in black South Africans. S Afr Med J. 1989;76(4):164-7.
36. Yu SH, Whitworth JA, Kincaid-Smith PS. Malignant hypertension: aetiology and outcome in 83 patients. Clin Exp Hypertens A. 1986;8(7):1211-30.
37. Rey É, LeLorier J, Burgess E, et al. Report of the Canadian Hypertension Society Consensus Conference: 3. Pharmacologic treatment of hypertensive disorders in pregnancy. Can Med Assoc J. 1997;157(9):1245-54.
38. Vidt DG. Emergency room management of hypertensive urgencies and emergencies. J Clin Hypertens. 2001;3(3):158-64.
39. Jackson RE. Hypertension in the emergency department. Emerg Med Clin North Am. 1988;6(2):173-96.
40. Garcia Jr JY, Vidt DG. Current management of hypertensive emergencies. Drugs. 1987;34(2):263-78.
41. Hickler RB. Hypertensive emergency: a useful diagnostic category. Am J Public Health. 1988;78(6):623-4.
42. Fromm RE, Varon J, Gibbs LR. Congestive heart failure and pulmonary edema for the emergency physician. J Emerg Med. 1995;13(1):71-87.
43. Khan IA, Nair CK. Clinical, diagnostic, and management perspectives of aortic dissection. Chest. 2002;122(1):311-28.
44. Kouchoukos NT, Dougenis D. Surgery of the thoracic aorta. N Engl J Med. 1997;336(26):1876-89.
45. Vidt DG. Current concepts in treatment of hypertensive emergencies. Am Heart J. 1986;111(1):220-5.
46. Bannan LT, Beevers D, Wright N. ABC of blood pressure reduction. Emergency reduction, hypertension in pregnancy, and hypertension in the elderly. Br Med J. 1980;281(6248):1120-2.
47. Bertel O, Marx BE, Conen D. Effects of antihypertensive treatment on cerebral perfusion. Am J Med. 1987;82(3):29-36.
48. Reed WG, Anderson RJ. Effects of rapid blood pressure reduction on cerebral blood flow. Am Heart J. 1986;111(1):226-8.
49. Johnson W, Nguyen ML, Patel R. Hypertension crisis in the emergency department. Cardiol Clin. 2012;30(4):533-43.
50. Ferguson RK, Vlasses PH. Hypertensive emergencies and urgencies. JAMA. 1986;255(12):1607-13.
51. Gifford RW Jr. Management of hypertensive crises. JAMA. 1991;266(6):829-35.
52. Rahn KH. How should we treat a hypertensive emergency? Am J Cardiol. 1989;63(6):C48-50.
53. Biollaz J, Waeber B, Brunner HR. Hypertensive crisis treated with orally administered captopril. Eur J Clin Pharmacol. 1983;25(2):145-9.
54. Catapano MS, Marx JA. Management of urgent hypertension: A comparison of oral treatment regimens in the emergency department. J Emerg Med. 1986;4(5):361-8.
55. Ghose R. Acute management of severe hypertension with oral labetalol. Br J Clin Pharmacol. 1979;8(S2):189S-93S.
56. Marik PE, Varon J. Hypertensive crises: challenges and management. Chest. 2007;131(6):1949-62.
57. Adebayo O, Rogers RL. Hypertensive emergencies in the emergency department. Emerg Med Clin North Am. 2015;33(3):539-51.
58. Chuda RR, Castillo SM, Poddutoori P. Hypertensive crises. Hosp Med Clin. 2014;3(1):e111-27.
59. Friederich JA, Butterworth JF. Sodium nitroprusside: twenty years and counting. Anesth Analg. 1995;81(1):152-62.
60. Hartmann A, Buttinger C, Rommel T, et al. Alteration of intracranial pressure, cerebral blood flow, autoregulation and carbondioxide-reactivity by hypotensive agents in baboons with intracranial hypertension. Neurochirurgia. 1989;32(02):37-43.
61. Nightingale S. New Labeling For Sodium-Nitroprusside Emphasizes Risk Of Cyanide Toxicity. Amer Medical Assoc 515 N State ST, Chicago, IL 60610; 1991.
62. Flaherty JT, Magee PA, Gardner TL, et al. Comparison of intravenous nitroglycerin and sodium nitroprusside for treatment of acute hypertension developing after coronary artery bypass surgery. Circulation. 1982;65(6):1072-7.
63. Halpern NA, Sladen RN, Goldberg JS, et al. Nicardipine infusion for postoperative hypertension after surgery of the head and neck. Crit Care Med. 1990;18(9):950-5.
64. Schillinger D. Nifedipine in hypertensive emergencies: a prospective study. J Emerg Med. 1987;5(6):463-73.

65. Rodríguez G, Varon J. Clevidipine: a unique agent for the critical care practitioner. Crit Care Shock. 2006;9(2):37-41.
66. Bailey JM, Lu W, Levy JH, et al. Clevidipine in adult cardiac surgical patients: a dose-finding study. Anesthesiology. 2002;96(5):1086-94.
67. Kieler-Jensen N, Jolin-Mellgård Å, Nordlander M, et al. Coronary and systemic hemodynamic effects of clevidipine, an ultra-short-acting calcium antagonist, for treatment of hypertension after coronary artery surgery. Acta Anaesthesiol Scand. 2000;44(2):186-93.
68. Powroznyk A, Vuylsteke A, Naughton C, et al. Comparison of clevidipine with sodium nitroprusside in the control of blood pressure after coronary artery surgery. Eur J Anaesthesiol. 2003;20(09):697-703.
69. Shusterman NH, Elliott WJ, White WB. Fenoldopam, but not nitroprusside, improves renal function in severely hypertensive patients with impaired renal function. Am J Med. 1993;95(2):161-8.
70. White WB, Halley SE. Comparative renal effects of intravenous administration of fenoldopam mesylate and sodium nitroprusside in patients with severe hypertension. Arch Intern Med. 1989;149(4):870-4.
71. Reisin E, Huth MM, Nguyen BP, et al. Intravenous fenoldopam versus sodium nitroprusside in patients with severe hypertension. Hypertension. 1990;15(2 Suppl):I59-62.
72. Shepherd AM, Ludden TM, McNay JL, et al. Hydralazine kinetics after single and repeated oral doses. Clin Pharmacol Ther. 1980;28(6):804-11.
73. Mooss AN, Hilleman DE, Mohiuddin SM, et al. Safety of esmolol in patients with acute myocardial infarction treated with thrombolytic therapy who had relative contraindications to beta-blocker therapy. Ann Pharmacother. 1994;28(6):701-3.
74. Lund-Johansen P, Omvik P. Acute and chronic hemodynamic effects of drugs with different actions on adrenergic receptors: a comparison between alpha blockers and different types of beta blockers with and without vasodilating effect. Cardiovasc Drug Ther. 1991;5(3):605.
75. Pearce CJ, Wallin JD. Labetalol and other agents that block both alpha-and beta-adrenergic receptors. Cleve Clin J Med. 1994;61(1):59-69.
76. Rosei EA, Trust P, Brown J, et al. Intravenous labetalol in severe hypertension. Lancet. 1975;2(7944):1093-4.
77. Ziegler MG. Advances in the acute therapy of hypertension. Crit Care Med. 1992;20(12):1630-1.
78. Baumann BM, Cline DM, Pimenta E. Treatment of hypertension in the emergency department. J Am Soc Hypertens. 2011;5(5):366-77.

CHAPTER 32

Aortic Dissection

Rachit Saxena, Manvendra Singh, Dinesh Chandra, Anil Bhan

INTRODUCTION

There is no cardiovascular pathology which is more life-threatening than an acute aortic dissection to the extent that the nearest comparison which can be made is only to a volcano waiting to erupt. If untreated it has an extremely high mortality of about 1% per hour during the first 48 hours and hence lies the importance of its early identification and urgent surgical intervention. The aim of this chapter is to describe the entity of aortic dissection and help the emergency physician team to clinically differentiate acute aortic dissection from other sinister causes of chest pain especially acute myocardial infarction (AMI), the management of which is absolutely opposite.

DEFINITION

The wall of the aorta is made up of three layers namely, tunica interna (endothelium), tunica media (smooth muscle cells and connective tissue) and tunica externa (collagen fibers). The three layers together give tremendous tensile strength to the aorta to bear the continuous stress of the cardiac output. Acute aortic dissection is an entity wherein there is a breach in the continuity of the tunica intima thereby resulting in formation of another lumen called the false lumen within the layer of tunica media (**Fig. 1**). The blood now flows both within the actual lumen of the aorta as well as within the layers of the aortic wall. Therefore, the tensile strength of the disintegrated aortic wall is greatly reduced and there is very high risk of free aortic wall rupture resulting in exsanguinating hemorrhage. This condition differs from aortic aneurysm wherein there is increase in the luminal diameter of the aorta but the structural integrity of the aortic wall is well maintained.

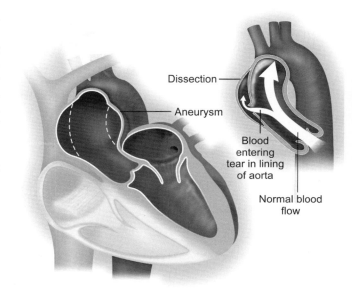

Fig. 1 The first picture shows dilatation of the aorta but with all layers intact whereas the second picture shows an intimal tear leading to formation of a false lumen

CLASSIFICATION

Anatomically, there are two classification systems for aortic dissection (**Fig. 2**):
1. *DeBakey classification*: It is based upon the location of intimal tear and the extent of dissection.
    - *DeBakey type A*: When the intimal tear is in the ascending aorta but the false lumen extends into the arch and often beyond it.

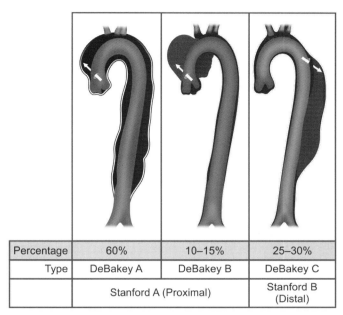

Fig. 2 Classification of aortic dissection (the arrowheads show the proximal intimal tear)

- *DeBakey type B*: When the intimal tear is in the ascending aorta and the false lumen is limited only to the ascending aorta.
- *DeBakey type C*: When the intimal tear is in the descending thoracic aorta and the false lumen extends distally.
2. *Stanford classification*: It is based solely on the location of intimal tear and is more commonly used as it is more pertinent in planning the management strategy:
   - *Stanford type A*: When the intimal tear is located in the ascending aorta or the arch of aorta.
   - *Stanford type B*: When the intimal tear is located in the descending thoracic aorta.

Aortic dissection can also be classified on the basis of duration of symptoms which help to decide the urgency with which intervention should be sought:
- *Acute aortic dissection*: Duration of symptoms less than 2 weeks. It requires urgent intervention.
- *Subacute aortic dissection*: Duration of symptoms from 2–4 weeks.
- *Chronic dissection*: Duration of symptoms more than 4 weeks and intervention can be planned electively.

PATHOPHYSIOLOGY

Aortic dissection can occur in a variety of clinical settings:
- *Connective tissue disorders*: In patients with connective tissue disorders, e.g., Marfan syndrome, Ehlers-Danlos syndrome, the aortic wall has inherent structural weakness due to pathological arrangement of the smooth muscle cells in the arterial wall. Therefore due to the continuous hemodynamic stress in these patients the aortic wall is predisposed to intimal tear and formation of false lumen within the tunica media of the aortic wall.
- *Bicuspid aortic valve*: Patients with a structural bicuspid aortic valve have inherent pathological distribution of smooth muscle cells in the tunica media. This structural abnormality exists even if the bicuspid aortic valve is functionally normal.
- *Aortic valvular heart disease*: The proximal aorta in patients with aortic valve regurgitation or stenosis is under constant hemodynamic stress and if the valve is unaddressed for a long time the proximal aorta is liable to aneurismal dilatation which further increases the stress and weakens the aortic wall leading to intimal tear progressing to aortic dissection.
- *Atherosclerotic aneurysm*: This usually occurs in elderly patients with atherosclerotic aortic wall with uncontrolled hypertension which results in a continuous stress to the aortic wall leading to aneurysmal dilation and ultimately culminating into aortic dissection.
- *Trauma*: Blunt thoracic injury, sudden deceleration injury, and seat belt injury can lead to intimal tears at the aortic isthmus because this is the most fixed part of the aorta. Traumatic dissections are usually associated with chest polytrauma and hemothorax and it is important to differentiate whether the hemothorax is because of chest wall trauma or it is a result of aortic dissection and contained rupture of the aorta.
- *Inflammatory disease of the aorta (aortoarteritis)*: Relatively uncommon but aortoarteritis can manifest with aortic dissection.
- *Post-cardiac surgery*: Again an uncommon cause of aortic dissection usually secondary to clamping of the aorta or dissection arising from aortic suture line or aortic cannulation site.

CLINICAL IMPLICATIONS

Aortic Rupture

The tensile strength of the aortic wall is severely compromised and therefore there is very high risk of fatal aortic wall rupture leading to exsanguination hemorrhage either in the pleural cavity or the pericardial cavity. If there is a communication with the tracheobronchial tree as in cases of long standing aortic aneurysm, it can manifest as massive hemoptysis.

Aortic Valve Regurgitation

Proximal extension of the dissection flap into the aortic root leads to loss of suspension of the aortic valve cusps leading acute severe aortic valve regurgitation **(Fig. 3)**.

Coronary Insufficiency

Extension of the dissection flap into the coronary ostia more commonly the right coronary ostium can lead to myocardial infarction **(Fig. 3)**. Patient may present with all clinical signs and symptoms of inferior wall myocardial infarction if the blood flow to the right coronary ostium is jeopardized.

Cerebral Malperfusion

Dissection flap may compromise the blood flow to any of the carotid arteries and the patient may present with features of complete spectrum of neurological deficit ranging from transient ischemic attack to dense hemiplegia or brain death.

Visceral Malperfusion

The abdominal viscera may have malperfusion leading to mesenteric ischemia which if unattended can lead to massive bowel gangrene.

Limb Ischemia

Limb ischemia compromised flow to any of the limbs can lead to critical limb ischemia progressing to gangrene.

CLINICAL FEATURES

In order to clinically differentiate aortic dissection from other non-aortic pathologies it is important to critically examine patient's habitus, clinical signs, and symptoms.

Patient Profile

- *Connective tissue disorder*: A patient with connective tissue disorder, e.g. Marfan's syndrome, is easily identified by the body habitus and the various skeletal abnormalities **(Fig. 4)**.
- Elderly patient with history of hypertension and dyslipidemia.

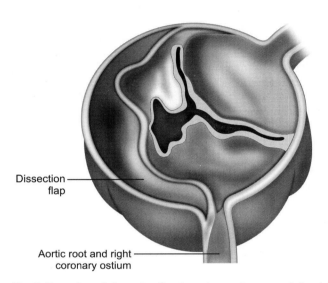

Fig. 3 Extension of dissection flap into the aortic root and the right coronary ostium. The aortic valve cusps have been avulsed from their attachment with the aortic wall thereby leading to severe aortic regurgitation

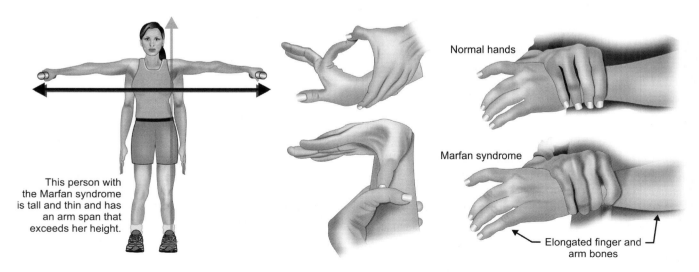

Fig. 4 Marfan's patient is tall and thin and arm span is more than the height. There is extreme laxity in the movement of the thumb and fingers. The fingers are long and the arm circumference is less

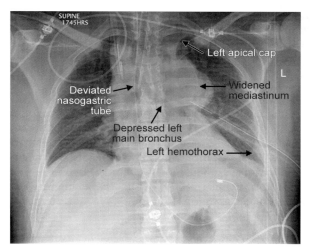

Fig. 5 Chest roentgenogram in a polytrauma patient with left hemothorax (left intercostal tube in situ) with widened mediastinum suggestive of traumatic aortic dissection

- *Polytrauma patient*: In a patient with history sudden deceleration injury with chest roentgenogram suggestive of widened mediastinum should be suspected to have traumatic aortic dissection **(Fig. 5)**.

SYMPTOMS

Pain

History of chest pain is the most common symptom. It is of utmost importance for an emergency physician to differentiate it from chest pain resulting from myocardial infarction. Chest pain in acute aortic dissection is usually sudden onset, localized, severe, sharp, tearing with radiation to interscapular area. Patients with acute type B dissection usually complain of a similar type of back pain or flank pain. Whereas a patient of AMI usually has diffuse precordial heaviness as if a huge weight has been placed on his chest with radiation to left arm or ipsilateral jaw. Unlike acute aortic dissection, patients with AMI may give history of previous episodes of precordial discomfort.

Dyspnea

Patients with acute type A dissection can have acute onset dyspnea of varying severity secondary to acute aortic regurgitation, coronary insufficiency or cardiac tamponade. Patients with acute type B dissection can have dyspnea secondary to massive hemothorax due to leak from the dissected aorta.

Neurological Symptoms

Neurological symptoms can be very variable from mild confusion and irritability secondary to cerebral hypoperfusion to dense neurological deficits like hemiparesis or hemiplegia or even coma. This type of neurological deficits (hemiplegia) is usually not seen in AMI.

Hypertensive Crisis

It is secondary to renal malperfusion.

Abdominal Pain

Abdominal pain can be secondary to progression of dissection flap in the abdominal aorta or a manifestation of mesenteric ischemia. Patients with mesenteric ischemia are "toxic looking" in hypovolemic shock and have all clinical signs of acute abdomen. The prognosis of mesenteric ischemia is extremely poor.

Acute Limb Ischemia

Many a times limb ischemia is the only clinical manifestation of aortic dissection and is secondary false lumen obstructing the flow of blood into the femoral artery.

Asymptomatic

Although uncommon but sometimes patient might not have any symptom at all and these patients are usually elderly.

CLINICAL SIGNS (TABLE 1)

General Physical Examination

There is a wide range of presentation ranging from an absolutely asymptomatic individual to one who is confused, agitated or with varying degree of mental deficits.

Blood Pressure

Hypertension

Hypertensive response could be a part of preexisting hypertension or sympathetic response to pain or systolic hypertension consequent to severe aortic regurgitation. This can be a feature of AMI as well as acute aortic dissection.

Hypotension

Hypotension again can be a feature of AMI as well as acute aortic dissection. In AMI the cause is myocardial dysfunction whereas in aortic dissection the cause is hemopericardium and cardiac tamponade.

Wide Pulse Pressure

It is due to severe aortic regurgitation and is typical of acute aortic dissection.

Table 1 Clinical differentiation of acute aortic dissection versus acute myocardial infarction

	Aortic dissection	Acute myocardial infarction
History	Connective tissue disorder Marfans syndrome	Angina pectoris
Pain: Character	Sharp, excruciating	Heaviness, crushing
Pain: Localization/radiation	Well localized Typical propagation pattern	Vague chest pain-radiating left upper limb
Examination: Blood pressure differential (arms)	Present	Absent
Pulse differentials (limbs, carotids)	Present	Absent
Aortic regurgitation	Wide pulse pressure Mumur	Absent
Pericardial effusion	Muffled heart sounds	Absent
Malperfusion	Pain/paresthesia limbs Pain abdomen	Absent

Pulse Differential

Interarm differential of more than 20 mm Hg is significant and is a characteristic feature of aortic dissection.

Jugular Venous Pressure

Jugular venous pressure (JVP) can be raised in aortic dissection.

Auscultation

Muffled heart sounds is typical of aortic dissection. Cardiac murmur of aortic regurgitation is typical of aortic dissection.

INVESTIGATIONS

The aims of investigating in a suspected aortic dissection patient are:
- Confirm diagnosis
- Ascending aorta involved or not (type A or type B)
- Site of proximal intimal tear
- Extent of dissection
- Diameter of aorta
- Involvement of coronary ostia, arch vessels, and visceral arteries
- Pericardial effusion
- Left ventricular function
- Valve function (especially aortic valve regurgitation).

Chest Roentgenogram

A routine chest X-ray posteroanterior view has a low sensitivity (67%) and specificity to show any abnormal finding. In about 12–20% cases the chest X-ray may be absolute normal. Findings suggestive of aortic dissection are:
- *Mediastinal widening*: In aortic dissection due to the presence of false lumen the combined aortic diameter is increased which manifests as widened mediastinum on chest roentgenogram (**Fig. 6**).
- *Calcium sign*: In the elderly many a times the aortic intima has calcific deposits which are seen at the outer margin of the aorta on chest roentgenogram. In presence of aortic dissection this calcific intima gets deviated medially due to propagation of the false lumen (**Fig. 7**).
- Tracheal deviation.
- Pleural effusion.

Electrocardiogram

In a patient with severe chest pain but a normal electrocardiogram (ECG), always keep a possibility of aortic dissection in mind. About 1–2% patients with acute aortic dissection can actually have ST elevation myocardial infarction due to the involvement of coronary artery [right coronary artery (RCA) > left coronary artery (LCA)]. If thrombolytic therapy is mistakenly administered to these patients there is a risk of 70% mortality.

Transthoracic Echocardiography

A transthoracic echocardiography (TTE) can provide us the following details:
- Presence of dissection flap
- Site of entry point
- Aortic arch vessel occlusion
- Dilatation of aorta

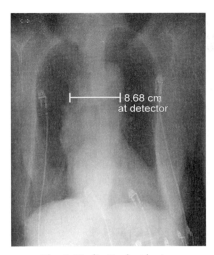

Fig. 6 Mediastinal widening

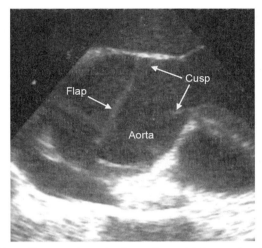

Fig. 8 Transesophageal echocardiographic image showing presence of an intimal flap in the ascending aorta

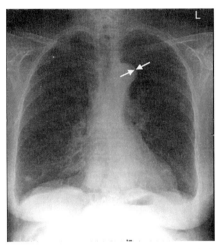

Fig. 7 The intimal calcification gets displaced medially (arrows)

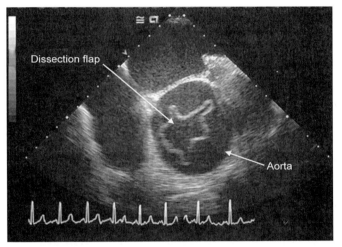

Fig. 9 Transesophageal echocardiographic image showing a circumferential intimal flap in the ascending aorta diagnostic of aortic dissection

- Aortic valve regurgitation, other valve status
- Pleural or pericardial effusion.

Disadvantages of TTE

- Low sensitivity and specificity (59% and 83%).
- Difficulty due to technical problems, narrow intercostal spaces, obesity and emphysematous chest.

Transesophageal Echocardiography

Transesophageal echocardiography (TEE) can be performed rapidly and is relatively noninvasive and can provide better details as compared to TTE (**Figs 8 and 9**).
- Pericardial effusion
- Pericardial tamponade

- Aortic regurgitation or other valve status.
- Involvement of proximal coronary artery
- Left ventricular (LV) function/RWMA (regional wall motion abnormalities).

Computed Tomography

Contrast enhanced tomography is perhaps the most relevant investigation modality to fulfill most of the aims of investigation mentioned above except that it fails to provide a functional assessment of the heart and valves. It is rapid, minimally invasive and less operator-dependent. 3D reconstruction can visualize entire course of dissection. It can identify entry point, dissection membrane, true and the false lumen, extent of dissection, arch involvement and perfusion of major aortic branches (**Figs 10 to 12**). It delineates the

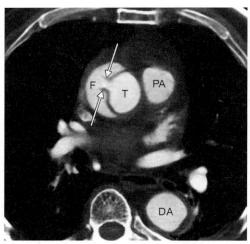

Fig. 10 Computed tomography angiographic cross-section showing aortic dissection. The arrowheads show the proximal intimal tear which is the entry point for dissection. The intima has separated from the aortic wall leading to a false lumen (F) and a true lumen (T)
Abbreviations: PA, pulmonary artery; DA, descending thoracic aorta.

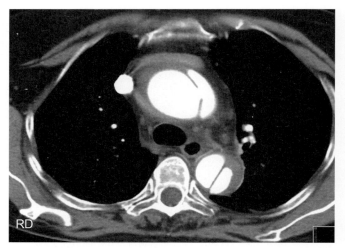

Fig. 12 Computed tomography angiographic cross-section showing dissection flap in both the ascending as well as the descending thoracic aorta with proximal intimal tear in the ascending aorta

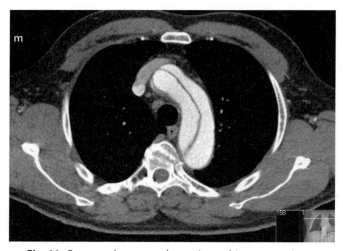

Fig. 11 Computed tomography angiographic cross-section at T4 level showing dissection flap in the arch of aorta

coronary artery anatomy. Its sensitivity is around 82–100% and specificity around 90–100%. The disadvantages are:
- Dissection obscured by complete thrombosis of false lumen
- May not identify proximal intimal tear
- Aortic regurgitation
- Use of contrast
- Movement of patient creates inferior quality of the scan.

Magnetic Resonance Imaging

Magnetic resonance imaging (MRI) has some advantages over other imaging modalities like:
- Localize proximal intimal tear, extent of dissection
- Identifies arch vessels involvement
- Severity of aortic regurgitation or flow patterns in true lumen and false lumen
- Can evaluate LV functions
- No contrast material or no radiation hazard
- Sensitivity and specificity in the range of 95–100%.

But the major draw back of an MRI is the time it takes to acquire the images which is a major concern when the patient is sick and needs immediate surgical intervention. MRI can be considered to be a better imaging modality for follow-up of these patients **(Fig. 13)**.

Aortography

This is of historical interest and the findings suggestive of dissection are **(Fig. 14)**:
- Double lumen or intimal flap
- Compressed true aortic lumen
- Aortic regurgitation
- Occlusion of branch vessels.

Disadvantages
- Invasive procedure
- Harmful effect of contrast material
- Iatrogenic propagation of dissection.

DIAGNOSTIC STRATEGY (FLOW CHART 1)

Diagnostic strategy includes:
- High index of suspicion
- Suspect aortic dissection if:
  - Young patient with connective tissue disorder (Marfan's syndrome)
  - Old patient less than 60 years with history of hypertension

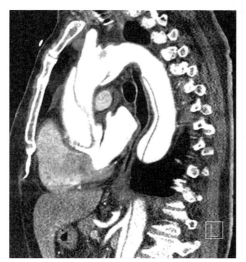

Fig. 13 Magnetic resonance imaging sagittal section showing dissection flap extending from the root of aorta across the arch of aorta and extending into the descending thoracic aorta

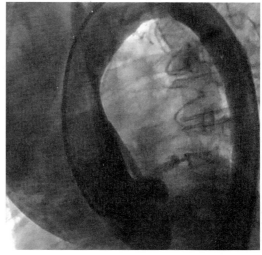

Fig. 14 Aortography showing a large (poorly opacified) false lumen and a much small (densely opacified) true lumen

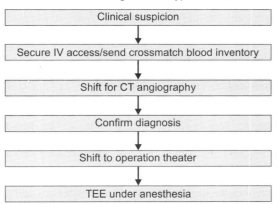

Flow chart 1 Management of type A dissection

Abbreviations: CT, computed tomography; TEE, transesophageal echocardiography

- Unexplained syncope
- *Pain*: Severe, excruciating, well localized pain with history of typical radiation pattern
- Unexplained stroke
- Acute congestive heart failure
- Pulse differential
- Evidence of malperfusion—lower limb ischemia:
  - Mesenteric ischemia
  - Renal ischemia.

AIMS OF TREATMENT

- Prevent death
- Prevent irreversible end-organ damage
- Surgical repair of ascending aorta precedes percutaneous or vascular surgical interventions addressing peripheral vascular complications.

EXCEPTIONS

- Irreversible stroke
- Advanced debilitating systemic illness
- More than 80 years with multiple major complications
- New onset hemiplegia—not an absolute contraindication
- Paraplegia—chances of spinal cord deficit improvement are low.

MANAGEMENT OF TYPE A AORTIC DISSECTION

Acute type A aortic dissection is always to be managed surgically. The procedure involves replacement of the entire dissected ascending aorta and at least the undersurface of the aortic arch. The aortic valve has to be replaced simultaneously if it is morphologically diseased but if the aortic valve per se is normal it can be repaired.

MANAGEMENT OF TYPE B AORTIC DISSECTION

The optimal treatment strategy for type B dissection is still debated. Medical treatment prevents death in majority of case and the operative mortality of type B dissection is high. The long-term outcome of surgically and medically managed patients is similar. Hence, a "complication specific" approach for type B dissection is preferred.

The medical management is called as the anti-impulse therapy which was proposed by Wheat and associates in 1965.

It is based on the observation that factors responsible for progression of aortic dissection are change in pressure over time (dP/dT). Neither high blood pressure nor high blood flow alone governs the rate of progression. The backbone of the anti-impulse therapy is a combination of vasodilator therapy along with the sympathetic control by β-blockade.

- *Target*: Mean arterial pressure = 60–75 mm Hg
  - Systolic pressure = 100–110 mm Hg
  - Heart rate = 60–80 bpm
- *Eliminate pain*: Morphine
- *Beta blockade*:
  - *Esmolol*: 500 μg/kg IV bolus; 50 μg/kg/min infusion (max 200 μg/kg/min)
  - *Propranolol*: 1 mg every 5 minutes to achieve target heart rate (HR) (max 10 mg)
- *Sodium nitroprusside (SNP)*: 20 μg/min (max 800 μg/min)
- *Refractory hypertension*: Angiotensin-converting enzyme *inhibitor* (ACEI)—enalapril.

Indication for intervention in type B aortic dissection:
- Persistent pain
- Refractory arterial hypertension
- Progression or expansion of dissection
- Aortic rupture or impending rupture
- Impaired distal organ perfusion
- Sizable localized false aneurysm
- Young with connective tissue disorder—Marfan syndrome without complications.

Surgical Management of Type B Aortic Dissection

Surgical intervention for type B aortic dissection includes replacement of the entire descending thoracic aorta along with the diseased segment of the abdominal aorta with reimplantation of the mesenteric vessels.

CONCLUSION

Diagnosing the aortic dissection in emergency department is a challenge. Chest pain and associated clinical features and investigation do not always diagnose this condition. Understanding the potential risk factors of aortic dissection, typical and atypical presentation, high index of suspicion, advanced imaging technique reliably includes or excludes the condition. After diagnosing the condition, the management of pain, heart rate and blood pressure and hemodynamic stability is important.

BIBLIOGRAPHY

1. Ando M, Okita Y, Tagusari O, et al. A surgically treated case of Takayasu's arteritis complicated by aortic dissections localized in the ascending and abdominal aorta. J Vasc Surg. 2000;31:1042-5.
2. Ankel F. Aortic dissection. In: Marx JA, Hockberger RS, Walls RM, et al, editors. Rosen's emergency medicine: concepts and clinical practice. 7th edition. Philadelphia: Mosby Elsevier Publishing; 2010. p. 1088–92. Chapter 83.
3. Babatasi G, Massetti M, Bhoyroo S, et al. Pregnancy with aortic dissection in Ehler-Danlos syndrome. Staged replacement of the total aorta (10-year follow up). Eur J Cardiothorac Surg. 1997;12:671-4.
4. Beach C, Manthey D. Painless acute aortic dissection presenting as left lower extremity numbness. Am J Emerg Med. 1998;16:49-51.
5. Bushnell J, Brown J. Clinical assessment for acute thoracic aortic dissection. Ann Emerg Med. 2005;46:90-2.
6. Chen K, Varon J, Wenker OC, et al. Acute thoracic aortic dissection: the basics. J Emerg Med. 1997;15:859-67.
7. Chew HC, Lim SH. Aortic dissection presenting with atrial fibrillation. Am J Emerg Med. 2006;24:379-80.
8. Choi JB, Yang HW, Oh SK, et al. Rupture of ascending aorta secondary to tuberculous aortitis. Ann Thorac Surg. 2003;75:1965-7.
9. Daily PO, Trueblood HW, Stinson EB, et al. Management of acute aortic dissections. Ann Thorac Surg. 1970;10(3):237-47.
10. DeBakey ME, McCollum CH, Crawford ES, et al. Dissection and dissecting aneurysms of the aorta: 20-year follow-up of 527 patients treated surgically. Surgery. 1982;92:1118.
11. Demiroyoguran NS, Karcioglu O, Topacoglu H, et al. Painless aortic dissection with bilateral carotid involvement presenting with vertigo as the chief complaint. Emerg Med J. 2006;23:e15.
12. Den Uil CA, Caliskan K, Bekkers JA. Intractable supraventricular tachycardia as first presentation of thoracic aortic dissection: case report. Int J Cardiol. 2010;144:e5-7.
13. Fisher A, Holroyd BR. Cocaine-associated dissection of the thoracic aorta. J Emerg Med. 1992;10:723-7.
14. Gallagher EJ. Clinical utility of likelihood ratios. Ann Emerg Med. 1998;31:391-7.
15. Greenwood WR, Robinson MD. Painless dissection of the thoracic aorta. Am J Emerg Med. 1986;4:330-3.
16. Haffner JW, Parrish SE, Hubler JR, et al. Risk factor documentation for life-threatening disease in the US emergency department patients [abstract 209]. Ann Emerg Med. 2006;48:S65.
17. Hagan PG, Neinaber CA, Isselbacher EM, et al. The International Registry of Acute Aortic Dissection (IRAD)– new insights into an old disease. JAMA. 2000;283:897-903.
18. Hiratzka LF, Bakris GL, Beckman JA, et al. 2010 ACCF/AHA/AATS/ACR/ASA/ SCA/SCAI/SIR/STS/SVM guidelines for the diagnosis and management of patients with thoracic aortic disease. Circulation. 2010;121:e266-369.
19. Hsu YC, Lin CC. Paraparesis as the major initial presentation of aortic dissection: report of four cases. Acta Neurol Taiwan. 2004;13:192-7.
20. Huang SM, Du F, Wang CY, et al. Aortic dissection presenting as isolated lower extremity pain in a young man. Am J Emerg. Med. 2010;28:1061.e1-3.
21. Joo JB, Cummings AJ. Acute thoracoabdominal aortic dissection presenting as painless, transient paralysis of the lower extremities: a case report. J Emerg Med. 2000;19:333-7.
22. Karascostas D, Anthomelides G, Ioannides P, et al. Acute paraplegia in painless aortic dissection. Rich imaging with poor outcomes. Spinal Cord. 2010;48:87-9.
23. Kim TE, Smith DD. Thoracic aortic dissection in an 18-year-old woman with no risk factors. J Emerg Med. 2010;38:e14-44.

24. Kimura N, Yamaguchi A, Noguchi K, et al. Type B aortic dissection associated with *Salmonella* infection. Gen Thorac Cardiovasc Surg. 2007;55:212-6.
25. Klompas M. Does this patient have an acute thoracic aortic dissection? JAMA. 2002;287:2262-72.
26. Knaut AL, Cleveland JC. Aortic emergencies. Emerg Med Clin North Am. 2003;21:817-45.
27. Lakhi NA, Jones J. Takayasu's arteritis in pregnancy complicated by peripartum aortic dissection. Arch Gynecol Obstet. 2010;282:103-6.
28. Larson EW, Edwards WD. Risk factors for aortic dissection: a necropsy study of 161 patients. Am J Cardiol. 1984;53:849-55.
29. Lee CC, Chang WT, Fang CC, et al. Sudden death caused by dissecting thoracic aortic aneurysm in a patient with autosomal dominant polycystic kidney disease. Resuscitation. 2004;63:93-6.
30. Liu JF, Ge QM, Chen M, et al. Painless type B aortic dissection presenting as acute congestive heart failure. Am J Emerg Med. 2010;28:646.e5-7.
31. Liu WP, Ng KC. Acute thoracic aortic dissection presenting as sore throat: report of a case. Yale J Biol Med. 2004;77:53-8.
32. Madu EC, Shala B, Baugh D. Crack-cocaine-associated aortic dissection in early pregnancy-a case report. Angiology. 1999;50:163-8.
33. McDermott JC, Schuster MR, Crummy AB, et al. Crack and aortic dissection. Wis Med J. 1993;92:453-5.
34. Meron G, Kurkciyan I, Sterz F, et al. Non-traumatic aortic dissection or rupture as a cause of cardiac arrest: presentation and outcome. Resuscitation. 2004;60:143-50.
35. Nadour W, Goldwasser B, Beiderman RW, et al. Silent aortic dissection presenting as transient locked-in syndrome. Tex Heart Inst J. 2008;35:359-61.
36. Palmiere C, Burkhardt S, Staub C, et al. Thoracic aortic dissection associated with cocaine abuse. Forensic Sci Int. 2004;141:137-42.
37. Perron AD, Gibbs M. Thoracic aortic dissection secondary to crack cocaine ingestion. Am J Emerg Med. 1997;15:507-9.
38. Ragucci MV, Thistle HG. Weight lifting and type II aortic dissection. A case report. J Sports Med Phys Fitness. 2004;44:424-7.
39. Risk identification for all physicians – thoracic aortic dissections: "tearing" apart the data. CMPA bulletin R10812E 2008. Available at: https://www.cmpa-acpm.ca/ cmpapd04/ docs/resource_files/risk_id/2008/com_ri0812-e.cfm. AccessedOctober 8, 2008.
40. Rogers RL, McCormack R. Aortic disasters. Emerg Med Clin North Am. 2004;22:887-908.
41. Schorr JS, Horowitz MD, Livingstone AS. Recreational weight lifting and aortic dissection: case report. J Vasc Surg. 1993;17:774-6.
42. Shihata M, Preforius V, MacArthur R. Repair of an acute type A aortic dissection combined with an emergency cesarean section in a pregnant woman. Interact Cardiovasc Thorac Surg. 2008;7:938-40.
43. Stout CL, Scott EC, Stokes GK, et al. Successful repair of a ruptured Stanford type B aortic dissection during pregnancy. J Vasc Surg. 2010;51:990-2.
44. Sung PS, Fang CW, Chen CH. Acute aortic dissection mimicking basilar artery occlusion in a patient presenting with sudden coma. J Clin Neurosci. 2010;17:952-3.
45. Suzuki T, Mehta RH, Ince H, et al. Clinical profiles and outcomes of acute type B aortic dissection in the current era: lessons from the International Registry of Acute Aortic Dissection (IRAD). Circulation 2003;108(Suppl 1):11312-7.
46. Thoracic aortic dissection: Medicolegal difficulties. CMPA Bulletin IS0768-E 2008. Available at: https://www.cmpa-acpm.ca/cmpapd04/docs/resource_files/infosheets/2007/com_is0768-e.cfm. Accessed March 11, 2011.
47. Von Koloditsch Y, Schwartz AG, Nienaber CA. Clinical prediction of acute aortic dissection. Arch Intern Med. 2000;160:2977-82.
48. Vuckovic SA. An usual presentation of ascending aortic arch dissection. J Emerg Med. 2000;19:149-52. Acute Aortic Dissection 325
49. Woo K, Schneider JI. High-risk chief complaints I: chest pain – the big three. Emerg Med Clin North Am. 2009;27:685-712.
50. Young J, Herd AM. Painless acute aortic dissection and rupture presenting as syncope. J Emerg Med. 2002;22:171-4.

CHAPTER 33

Care of Patient on Anticoagulation

Vinayak Agarwal, Devendra Richhariya

INTRODUCTION

Anticoagulants prevent blood from clotting at a normal rate of coagulation and are taken by patients, who suffer from deep venous thrombosis, stroke, myocardial infarction, cardiac valve replacement, or atrial fibrillation. Oral anticoagulant is prescribed to prevent blood clot formation on and around the mechanical valve. Patient on anticoagulation should be under physician supervision. When anticoagulation not started in adequate dose, formation of blood clot may occur, and can produce a stroke. Over anticoagulation can cause bleeding, both externally and internally. The therapeutic international normalized ratio (INR) value range is 1.0–3.5. Anticoagulant therapy is helpful in following situations:
- Atrial fibrillation
- Coronary artery disease
- Myocardial infarction
- Hypercoagulable states
- Deep vein thrombosis
- Pulmonary embolism
- Ischemic stroke
- Restenosis from stents.

TYPES OF ANTICOAGULANTS

Coumarins

Coumarins are oral anticoagulants and vitamin K antagonists. Warfarin (Coumadin) is important member in this class. Full anticoagulant effect develops in 48–72 hours. Heparin is used with warfarin if immediate effects are required. Acenocoumarol (Acitrom) is similar to warfarin but with longer half-life and lesser interactions. It is available as 1, 2 and 4 mg tablets. Most commonly warfarin started with loading dose of 10 mg, and 5 mg on first 3 days. Warfarin may be started with low-molecular weight heparin (LMWH) or unfractionated heparin (UFH) and should be overlapped for 4–5 days. Recommended INR range is according to indication. Major side effect of warfarin is bleeding tendency, and bleeding risk increases as INR increases. Age is also major risk factor for bleeding and warfarin has teratogenic effect and cause peripartum bleeding in pregnancy so generally contraindicated in pregnancy. Warfarin should be avoided during pregnancy unless absolutely indicated, like women with mechanical heart valves.

New Oral Anticoagulants

These are inhibitors of factor IIa and factor Xa. Efficacy of new oral anticoagulants (NOACs) is similar to warfarin in preventing stroke. Patients who are prescribed NOACs are freed from regular blood tests.

ADVANTAGES

- Quick onset of action, so no need to start overlap therapy with heparin
- Short half-life, over anticoagulation can be controlled easily
- Few drugs and food interaction.

DISADVANTAGES

- High cost, so poor compliance
- No monitoring is possible if needed
- No specific antidote
- Serious bleeding in renal dysfunction patients and elderly.

MEDICINES THAT INCREASE THE RISK OF BLEEDING IN PATIENTS ON ORAL ANTICOAGULANTS

- *Medicines with antiplatelet action*: Aspirin, clopidogrel, dipyridamole, nonsteroidal anti-inflammatory drugs, prasugrel, and ticagrelor.
- *Medicines that increase serotonin and reduce platelet aggregation*: Selective serotonin reuptake inhibitors (SSRIs) and serotonin-noradrenaline reuptake inhibitors.
- *Medicines that can cause thrombocytopenia*: Disease modifying antirheumatic drugs (DMARDs).
- *Medicines that increase acid secretion*: Aminophylline and theophylline.
- *Local gastrointestinal irritation*: Bisphosphonates, corticosteroids, potassium chloride, and tetracyclines.

HEPARIN AND LOW MOLECULAR WEIGHT HEPARIN

Standard heparin combined with antithrombin III (enhance its activity) inhibits factor Xa activity thus rate-limiting step of prothrombin → thrombin

- Traditionally, if patient required a parenteral anticoagulation then standard heparin was the choice but due to life-threatening bleeding and thrombocytopenia low molecular weight heparin (LMWH) approved since 1987.
- LMWH is more highly processed product derived from standard heparin by fractionated method mainly inhibit Xa activity and does not require monitoring of the activated partial thromboplastin time (APTT) coagulation parameter (it has more predictable plasma levels) and side effects are few, e.g. fraxiparine, enoxaparin, and fondaparinux.

MONITORING ANTICOAGULATION THERAPY: TARGET INR

- For prosthetic heart valve: INR 2.5–3.5
- All other conditions including deep vein thrombosis, pulmonary thromboembolism, and atrial fibrillation: INR 2–3
- Higher INR is beneficial in patient with recurrent thromboembolic event while on anticoagulation
- Check INR four times per week, initially in the first week of therapy then two times per week for next 2–3 weeks as fluctuation are more common
- If INR stable, check INR once a week or once a fortnight
- Very stable INR once a month
- If any signs of external or internal bleeding like bruising, epistaxis, hematuria, hemoptysis, hematemesis and melena appears, then patients should report to emergency department or they involved in a major trauma or suffer profuse or prolonged bleeding (>15 minutes)
- If patient develops following symptoms, they should report to emergency department:
  - New onset shortness of breath and postvalve surgery feature may suggestive of valve thrombosis
  - Stroke and sharp pain in limbs or cold limbs, if clot reaches to brain it produce stroke if reaches to limb it produce severe pain
  - Fever and anemia after valve replacement may indicate infection.

BLOOD TESTS USED IN EMERGENCY DEPARTMENT TO MONITOR ANTICOAGULANTS

- Warfarin and acitrom by getting prothrombin time (PT) and INR
- Heparin: by getting partial thromboplastin time (PTT) and APTT.

MANAGEMENT OF OVER ANTICOAGULATION

- Vitamin K is used as an antidote to coumarins anticoagulants (warfarin and acitrom)—for stopping bleeding by correcting high PT and INR
- In case of over anticoagulation INR greater than 4 without bleeding, skipping one or more dose is sufficient to achieve the therapeutic range. Oral 1 mg or 0.5 mg intravenous vitamin K can be added for faster correction and reduces the risk of minor hemorrhages. Avoid subcutaneous injection of vitamin K due to variable absorption
- In case of over anticoagulation with major bleeding, hospitalize the patient, vitamin K alone is not sufficient because its full effect occurs after 12–24 hours, infusion of fresh frozen plasma (FFP) or coagulation factor concentrate is also required. Recheck INR after 6–8 hours then daily for next 3 days
- In case of bleeding patient with normal INR suspect any other pathology may require temporary lowering of INR
- Protamine is used as antidote to heparin—correct deranged APTT.

EDUCATION TO PATIENT ABOUT ANTICOAGULATION

Patient must:
- Check the strength of tablet before taking
- Take the drug at same time daily
- Regularly check PT or INR as advised by physician, regular follow-up
- Inform doctor or report to emergency department if INR is higher than target INR of bleeding
- Young females on anticoagulation should take extra care
- Always plan and supervise pregnancy, regular checkup during pregnancy, and consider hospital delivery only.

CONCLUSION

The benefits of anticoagulation are well documented in various conditions like mitral valve disese, prosthetic heart valve, atrial fibrillation. Dose and duration of anticoagulant should be titrated according to the indication. INR should be maintained within therapeutic range. Patient should be educated about importance of monitoring of INR. overanticoagulation is managed by vitamin K. Vitamin K is safe and reduces the incidence of bleeding.

BIBLIOGRAPHY

1. AIIMS guidelines on anticoagulation. *http://www.aiims.edu/en/departments-and-centers/specialty-centers.html?id=407.*
2. Ansell J, Hirsh J, Poller L, Bussey H, Jacobson A, Hylek E. The pharmacology and management of the vitamin K antagonists: the Seventh ACCP Conference on Antithrombotic and Thrombolytic Therapy. Chest. 2004;126(3 Suppl):204S-233S.
3. Baglin TP, Cousins D, Keeling DM, Perry DJ, Watson HG. Safety indicators for inpatient and outpatient oral anticoagulant care: [corrected] Recommendations from the British Committee for Standards in Haematology and National Patient Safety Agency. Br J Haematol. 2007;136:26-9.
4. Douketis JD, Spyropoulos AC, Spencer AS, Mayr M, Jaffer KJ, Eckman MH, Dunn AS, Kunz R. Perioperative management of antithrombotic therapy: American College of Chest Physicians Evidence-Based Clinical Practice Guidelines, 9th edn. Chest. 2012;141:326S-50S.
5. Garcia DA, Baglin TP, Weitz JI, Samama MM. Parenteral anticoagulants: American College of Chest Physicians Evidence-Based Clinical Practice Guidelines, 9th edn. Chest; 2012. p. 141.
6. Gopalakrishnan S. Oral Anticoagulants: Current Indian Scenario. *http://www.apiindia.org/medicine_update_2013/chap90.pdf.*
7. Kaluski E, Maher J, Gerula CM. New oral anticoagulants: good but not good enough. JACC. 2012;60:1434.
8. Keeling D, Baglin T, Taite C, et al. Guidelines on oral anticoagulation with warfarin – fourth edition. British Journal of Haematology doi:10.1111/j.1365-2141. Pengo V, Cucchini U, Denas G, Erba N, Guazzaloca G, La RL, De M, Testa V, S, Frontoni R; 2011
9. Moser M, Bode C. Anticoagulation in atrial fibrillation – a new era has begun. Hamostaseologie. 2012;32:37-9.
10. Prisco D, Nante G, Iliceto S. Standardized low-molecular-weight heparin bridging regimen in outpatients on oral anticoagulants undergoing invasive procedure or surgery: an inception cohort management study. Circulation. 2009;119:2920-7.
11. Schulman S, Crowther MA. How I treat with anticoagulants in 2012: new and old anticoagulants, and when and how to switch. Blood. 2012;119:3016-23.
12. Singer DE, Albers GW, Dalen JE, Fang MC, Go AS, Halperin JL, Lip GY, Manning WJ. Antithrombotic therapy in atrial fibrillation: American College of Chest Physicians Evidence-Based Clinical Practice Guidelines, 8th edn. Chest. 2008; 133:546S-92S.
13. Suzuki S, Yamashita T, Kato T, et al. Incidence of major bleeding complication of warfarin therapy in Japanese patients with atrial fibrillation. Circ J. 2007;71:761-5.
14. Tzeis S, Andrikopoulos G. Novel anticoagulants for atrial fibrillation: a critical appraisal. Angiology. 2012;63:164-70.
15. Veitch AM, Baglin TP, Gershlick AH, Harnden SM, Tighe R, Cairns S. Guidelines for the management of anticoagulant and antiplatelet therapy in patients undergoing endoscopic procedures. Gut. 2008;57:1322-9.
16. Woods K, Douketis JD, Kathirgamanathan K, Yi Q, Crowther MA. Low-dose oral vitamin K to normalize the international normalized ratio prior to surgery in patients who require temporary interruption of warfarin. J Thromb Thrombolysis. 2007;24:93-7.

CHAPTER 34

Cardiac Biomarkers

Rahul Mehrotra

INTRODUCTION

In the practice of medicine, any measurable characteristic that is indicative of the presence of a particular disease state can be called as the biomarker of the disease. A biomarker may be a physical characteristic, a chemical substance or a biological process. Biomarkers have found a great role in the practice of medicine and are routinely used for detection of subclinical disease, differentiation of acute from chronic disease, assessment of severity, risk stratification, selecting the treatment modality, monitoring the progression of disease and response to therapy. The increased use of biomarkers for all these purposes has resulted in overall improved patient care. Cardiac markers are biomarkers measured to evaluate heart function. They are often discussed in the context of myocardial infarction, but other conditions can lead to an elevation in cardiac marker level.

Most of the early markers identified were enzymes, and as a result, the term "cardiac enzymes" is sometimes used. However, not all of the markers currently used are enzymes. For example, in cardiac troponin is a myocardial protein and not a cardiac enzyme.

Biomarkers are also routinely used in cardiology and have a critical role to play in cardiac emergencies like acute coronary syndrome (ACS) where the treatment approach is changed altogether depending upon the detection of elevated markers of cardiac injury in blood. Besides, they are also useful in triaging the patients presenting with chest pain or breathlessness who may not have ACS but may in fact be having acute pulmonary embolism (PE) with deep vein thrombosis (DVT), heart failure (HF) or have no cardiovascular disease at all. Biomarkers are very useful in the setting of the emergency room where there is a need of rapid triage, early diagnosis and institution of life saving treatment with little chance of error since the symptoms and signs of these diseases may not always be present, may be confusing and are usually not specific. For example, a completely normal electrocardiogram (ECG) does not exclude the possibility of ACS.[1]

Also, the patients cannot be kept in triage for long owing to space crunch in most busy centers and a timely decision to safely discharge the patients has to be taken. Any error in this can be very dangerous, not only for the patient, but also for the doctors and the institution in the current era.

One of the largest numbers of medicolegal litigations against doctors has been for patients with chest pain who were sent home from the emergency room, who later developed ACS.[2]

It has thus become imperative to do this balancing act in the emergency room and cardiac biomarkers are the key players in this.

In this chapter, we review the common cardiac biomarkers in the blood and their use in the emergency department.

THE IDEAL CARDIAC BIOMARKER

As discussed above, biomarkers can have several roles and it is an ideal situation if a single biomarker provides multiple informations which are pivotal to the management in the emergency. An ideal cardiac biomarker is thus expected to have most of the attributes, like early detection in blood, highly specific for cardiac injury, be low cost and have a sensitive assay to detect it **(Box 1)**. Clearly no such ideal cardiac biomarker exists[3,4] and usually a multimarker strategy (discussed later) is practiced depending on the clinical scenario, for optimal outcomes. In the subsequent sections, we discuss the common cardiac emergencies along with the role of appropriate blood biomarkers.

Box 1 Attributes of an ideal biomarker

- Found in high concentration in the heart and not found in other tissues even in pathological states
- Have low molecular weight so released early in the blood, ideally before myocardial necrosis
- Should peak early and remain elevated for several days
- The level in blood should be proportional to the size of myocardial injury and be indicative of risk
- Should trigger effective therapy
- There should be a sensitive assay available to detect it
- Should have low cost and be widely available

ACUTE CORONARY SYNDROME

Acute coronary syndrome is one of the most common cardiac emergencies with devastating consequences. It results from the rupture or erosion of an atherosclerotic plaque leading to formation of coronary thrombus. The working diagnosis of ACS is made based on the presence of typical symptoms, which is further characterized by ECG changes. The final diagnosis, however, is based on the detection of elevated cardiac specific biomarker (preferably cardiac specific troponin).

Based on these findings, ACS is subclassified into one of the three clinical syndromes—ST segment elevation myocardial infarction (STEMI), non-ST segment elevation myocardial infarction (NSTEMI) or unstable angina **(Flow chart 1)**. As clear from the names of these, ECG plays an important role in the working diagnosis of these entities but a key role is played by the cardiac biomarker—now almost exclusively cardiac specific troponin.[5]

Elevated cardiac specific troponin is much more specific for cardiac tissue, is very sensitive for myocardial necrosis, and has a useful temporal profile as compared to other cardiac enzymes used previously [like creatine kinase (CK) and CK-MB]. It has also been shown to relate directly with infarct size and thus act as a prognostic marker also. Therefore, it is the preferred biomarker recommended for use in myocardial infarction (MI) and the new definition of MI is based solely on the level of troponin. It is recommended that any patient coming to the emergency with suspected MI should have troponin done immediately and another value 3–6 hours later.[6] Rather than only absolute elevated values, temporal rise and fall is very important for diagnosis of MI. Although troponin is quite specific to cardiac injury, it cannot differentiate ischemic injury (in MI) from other types of myocardial injury (like in sepsis, acidosis, and trauma).[7] As such elevations of troponin can be seen in a variety of clinical conditions and disease states but the clinical scenario and time trend of the values should be carefully looked at in these situations to arrive at a diagnosis of MI.

This approach of using troponin only for diagnosis of MI has resulted in diagnosis of more episodes of myocardial infarctions correctly owing to its sensitivity and specificity,

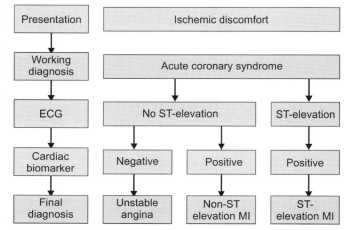

Flow chart 1 Algorithm for diagnosis of acute coronary syndrome

Abbreviations: ECG, electrocardiogram; MI, myocardial infarction.

but also has been shown to be more cost-effective than doing both, troponin and CK-MB.

Myoglobin is also a cardiac biomarker which is detectable quite early in blood following acute MI (within 2 hours). However, it is not specific for cardiac injury and is also not widely available. However, it can be used sometimes as part of a multimarker strategy for diagnosis of acute MI (see later). CK-MB similarly is sometimes utilized since it remains elevated till much later after acute MI. Cardiac specific troponins (I or T) however remain the preferred biomarkers for diagnosis for ACS.

DEEP VEIN THROMBOSIS AND PULMONARY EMBOLISM

Acute pulmonary embolism (PE) is associated with high mortality and morbidity. Besides, there are no specific sign or symptoms of PE. As such, it is also known as the "great mimic". The clinical presentation may resemble acute myocardial infarction, dissection of aorta, acute HF, acute asthma or even syncope. It is very important to diagnose and institute appropriate treatment for PE in the emergency department. DVT is a related entity equally important to diagnose.

D-dimer is the only biomarker which is used in the scenario of DVT and PE.

Endogenous fibrinolysis breaks down the fibrin rich clot to D-dimers. The detection of elevated circulating D-dimer by enzyme-linked immunosorbent assay (ELISA) is therefore an indicator of clot formation and endogenous fibrinolysis due to any reason. It is a sensitive indicator of DVT and PE but is not specific for DVT or PE. Elevated D-dimer can be seen in any systemic illness like sepsis, MI, cancer or even postoperatively up to months. However, it has a great negative predictive value. It is most useful thus in ruling out acute PE or DVT in appropriate clinical setting. For example, in a patient presenting to emergency, suspected of having acute PE, with no other systemic illness, a negative D-dimer virtually rules out DVT/PE and no further testing is required for this purpose. In case of an elevated value in this scenario, further testing in the form of ultrasound of leg veins or CT angiography of chest is required to diagnose PE. However, it has a limited role in the admitted patient with multiple comorbidities or in a patient with recent history of trauma, surgery or any systemic illness, owing to its nonspecificity. D-dimer can also be used as part of multimarker strategy where there is a need to rule out other conditions like MI or acute HF which may have similar presentation (as discussed later).

The use of D-dimer is thus very useful in the emergency for triage of patients who require costly and potentially harmful testing (like CT scanning) and potentially life-saving treatment, by optimizing the resource utilization in busy emergency room settings.

CARDIAC BIOMARKERS IN HEART FAILURE

B-type natriuretic peptide (BNP) and N-terminal pro-B-type natriuretic peptide (NT pro-BNP) are polypeptides secreted mainly by the ventricles of the heart in response to excessive stretching of heart muscle cells (cardiomyocytes). They have vasodilator and natriuretic properties and are also released from blood vessels and kidneys. Circulating BNP and NT pro-BNP are measured by immunoassay and elevated levels are shown to be indicative of HF (left as well as right, acute as well as chronic). Systematic studies have shown that elevated natriuretic peptides, released as a response to myocardial stretch, can be used as indicators of elevated myocardial load. They have been found to be a useful triage tool for diagnosis, prognosis, and monitoring response to treatment in patients with acute decompensated HF.[8] In a study, the negative predictive value was 96% for BNP below 50 pg/mL and the positive predictive value was 83% for a cutoff value of 100 pg/mL, relative to clinical assessment by cardiologists.[9] BNP and NT pro-BNP have been recommended for use in acute decompensated HF scenario by the guidelines from HF association of America and from the UK.

It has now been shown that BNP and NT pro-BNP are elevated in chronic HF with preserved ejection fraction (HFpEF). The European Society of Cardiology guidelines of 2016 have incorporated this approach in the diagnosis of HFpEF and cutoffs have been proposed.[10] There is no difference between BNP and NT-pro BNP when used as markers of HF but different cutoff values are to be used for each of these (>35 pg/mL for BNP; >125 pg/mL for NT pro-BNP). Elevated BNP and NT-pro BNP are also predictors of prognosis and can be used as markers of response to treatment. As discussed above, they are not specific for HF and elevated values can be found in diverse situations like pulmonary hypertension, acute MI, severe sepsis, renal disease, etc.

MULTIMARKER STRATEGY

In the emergency setting, it is often necessary to differentiate diverse clinical conditions, having similar clinical presentation but markedly different treatment and prognosis. There is thus a need to test for the possibility of multiple clinical conditions rapidly and accurately in order to diagnose and institute appropriate therapy at the earliest. It clearly implies that use of biomarkers one by one would be detrimental in this scenario. In view of this need, several biomarkers are used together according to the clinical scenario and several point-of-care kits incorporating these multiple markers have also been made available. For example, in a patient who presents with acute onset dyspnea where it is necessary to differentiate between acute PE and acute MI, the use of D-dimer, along with troponin could be useful. Also, multiple biomarkers could be used to provide additional information related to prognosis and timing of the index event. For example, in a patient with ischemic chest pain of very short duration will require the use of troponin along with myoglobin while in a patient with typical ECG changes but a history of ischemic chest discomfort 2–3 weeks before will require the use of troponin and CPK-MB in view of the temporal profile of these markers.

The disadvantage of this approach is increased cost and sometimes leading to inappropriate management. Besides, these have not been recommended as a preferred strategy and exercising clinical judgment in choosing the appropriate biomarkers, in a given clinical situation, is recommended.

SUMMARY AND FUTURE PERSPECTIVE

Cardiac biomarkers are an indispensable tool for diagnosis, prognosis and risk stratification in the emergency department. The use of biomarkers results in optimizing scarce resources in busy emergency departments. Judicious use of biomarkers results in rapid triage, institution of appropriate therapy in a timely manner and is also very useful in preventing mishaps on account of missing out on critical diagnosis. Some of the cardiac biomarkers like troponin and natriuretic peptides also contribute to prediction of future risk and thus, in devising of aggressive approach for sicker patients. A multimarker approach is sometimes used as a point-of-care device but it requires more experience and refinement before it can be widely recommended. There are several biomarkers being studied for their higher sensitivity, specificity, and prognostic value in different clinical conditions. A very sensitive troponin assay is being developed for early detection and risk stratification in MI. Similarly markers of inflammation [high-sensitivity C-reactive protein (hsCRP)] are being evaluated for defining their role in the scenario in ACS. Numerous other biomarkers (metalloproteinases) are being evaluated for different stages of atherosclerosis and we are likely to see greater use of low cost, easy to use biomarkers with superior diagnostic and prognostic accuracy in the emergency room.

REFERENCES

1. Kumar A, Cannon CP. Acute coronary Syndromes: Diagnosis and Management, part I. Mayo Clin Proc. 2009;84:917.
2. Katz DA, Williams GC, Brown RL, Aufderheide TP, Bogner M, Rahko PS, et al. Emergency physician's fear of malpractice in evaluation of patients with possible acute cardiac ischemia. Ann Emerg Med. 2005;46(6):525-33.
3. Morrow DA, de Lemos JA. Benchmarks for the assessment of novel cardiovascular biomarkers. Circulation. 2007;115(8):949-52.
4. Vasan RS. Biomarkers of cardiovascular disease: molecular basis and practical considerations. Circulation. 2006;113(19):2335-62.
5. Thygesen K, Alpert JS, Jaffe AS, Simoons ML, Chaitman BR, White HD, et al. Third universal definition of myocardial infarction. J Am Coll Cardiol. 2012;60(16):1581-98.
6. Rusnak RA, Stair TO, Hansen K, Fastow JS. Litigation against the emergency physician: Common features in cases of missed myocardial infarction. Ann Emerg Med. 1989;18(10):1029-34.
7. D'Antono B, Dupris G, Arsenault A, Burelle D. Silent ischemia: Silent after all? Can J Cardiol. 2008;24(4):285-91.
8. Lindenfeld J, Albert NM, Boehmer JP, Collins SP, Ezekowitz JA, Givertz MM, et al. Heart Failure Society of America. HFSA 2010 Comprehensive Heart Failure Practice Guideline. J Card Fail. 2010;16(6):e1-194.
9. Braverman AC. Acute aortic dissection: clinician update. Circulation. 2010;122:184-8.
10. Ponikowski P, Voors AA, Anker SD, Bueno H, Cleland JG, Coats AJ, et al. 2016 ESC Guidelines for the diagnosis and treatment of acute and chronic heart failure: The task force for the diagnosis and treatment of acute and chronic heart failure of the European Society of Cardiology (ESC) developed with the special contribution of the heart Failure Association (HFA) of the ESC. Eur J Heart Fail. 2016;18(8):891-975.

CHAPTER 35

Electrocardiogram Interpretation in Emergency

Kartikeya Bhargava

INTRODUCTION

The electrocardiogram (ECG) is often the first investigation in any patient presenting with symptoms related to cardiovascular disease. Rather, it is seen as an extension of a good history and physical examination in view of its almost universal availability. Emergency physicians are usually the first ones and often the only ones to analyze the electrocardiogram performed in a patient presenting in an emergency department. Hence, it is imperative that they should have proficiency in reading and analysis of ECGs so as to arrive at a diagnosis rapidly and take appropriate clinical decisions regarding treatment. This chapter is not supposed to be a comprehensive review of ECG diagnosis, rather it tries to summarize ECG findings to assist interpretation in a typical patient presenting in the emergency department with symptoms of cardiovascular disorders, such as chest or epigastric pain, palpitations, syncope or presyncope, breathlessness, etc. The findings on ECG in certain systemic or noncardiac conditions that can assist in the clinical diagnosis and therapy are also mentioned. The various groups of cardiovascular conditions in which ECG is of diagnostic value are listed in **Box 1**.

A systematic approach to read and analyze the ECG is essential to arrive at an accurate diagnosis and the steps (not necessarily in the order given) that can be used in this approach are mentioned in **Box 2**. However, it is important to realize that in an emergency, especially if the patient is hemodynamically unstable, a rapid diagnosis may be needed based on the most significant finding correlated with patient's symptoms and a stepwise approach can be deferred to a later time.

The following sections discuss various ECG patterns grouped according to the ECG findings that may be seen in patients presenting in the emergency department. The description of each finding and its clinical correlation

Box 1 Cardiovascular conditions where electrocardiogram (ECG) is likely to be useful

- Arrhythmias:
  Bradyarrhythmia and tachyarrhythmias, Wolff-Parkinson-White (WPW) syndrome, long QT syndrome, and others
- Acute coronary syndrome (ACS):
  ST-elevation myocardial infarction (STEMI), non-ST-elevation myocardial infarction (NSTEMI), and noncoronary causes of ST-elevation
- Miscellaneous nonarrhythmic cardiac emergencies:
  – Aortic dissection
  – Acute pulmonary embolism
  – Acute pericarditis
- Electrocardiogram in systemic conditions presenting in emergency:
  – Electrolyte imbalance: Hypokalemia, hyperkalemia, hypocalcemia, and hypercalcemia
  – Hemorrhagic stroke
  – Pericardial effusion
  – Myxedema
  – Cor pulmonale due to chronic obstructive airway disease (COAD)
  – Drug effects and toxicities

with the cardiovascular disorder is not comprehensively presented but can be found elsewhere in this book.

CARDIAC ARRHYTHMIAS

One of the most common uses of ECG is a diagnosis of an abnormal rhythm. The arrhythmias include disorders with abnormally fast rhythm (tachyarrhythmia) or abnormally slow rhythm (bradyarrhythmia). Sometimes, though an abnormal rhythm may not be present at the time of presentation, but an abnormal finding during sinus rhythm ECG may point to a specific rhythm disorder during the time of symptoms. For

> **Box 2** Steps in systematic analysis of electrocardiogram (ECG)
>
> 1. Rate and rhythm
> 2. Relationship between P waves and QRS complexes, PR interval
> 3. *QRS duration, morphology and amplitude*: Presence of bundle branch block or intraventricular conduction defect, ventricular preexcitation; pathological Q-waves; left or right ventricular enlargement or hypertrophy, fragmentation and notches
> 4. *ST-segment and T wave abnormalities*: ST segment elevation or depression; early repolarization pattern; T wave inversion, flattening, tall and pointed patterns, etc.
> 5. QRS axis in the frontal plane and fascicular blocks
> 6. *P wave morphology*: Site of atrial origin, left or right atrial enlargement or hypertrophy patterns
> 7. *Intervals*: PR interval, QT interval, PP and RR intervals
> 8. *Miscellaneous*: Paced ECG interpretation, disease specific diagnostic patterns—acute pulmonary embolism, arrhythmogenic right ventricular dysplasia, electrolyte imbalance, etc.

example, presence of ventricular preexcitation during sinus rhythm may suggest episodes of supraventricular tachycardia (SVT) in a patient with palpitations. Similarly, presence of left bundle branch block (LBBB) in a patient with history of syncope may suggest intermittent complete atrioventricular (AV) block.

Tachyarrhythmias

Any rhythm with a rate more than 100 beats/min qualifies to be called as tachycardia. These can be classified based on the QRS duration and regularity of the ventricular rhythm as shown in **Flow chart 1**. The patients with tachyarrhythmias usually present with complaints of palpitations, presyncope or syncope, breathlessness and/or chest discomfort. Though, the details regarding the diagnosis of these are beyond the scope of this chapter, a few comments are outlined next for the aid of emergency physician.

Sinus Tachycardia

Sinus tachycardia is identified by gradual onset (history), normal or reduced PR interval and a P wave morphology suggestive of sinus node origin (negative in lead aVR, positive in leads I, II, III, aVF and biphasic in lead V1). It is usually secondary to some other underlying cause that can be physiological (anxiety, fever and pregnancy) or pathological (pulmonary embolism and myocardial ischemia, etc.).

Paroxysmal Supraventricular Tachycardia

Paroxysmal SVT (PSVT) starts abruptly and presents with symptoms of palpitations. It shows regular RR intervals with

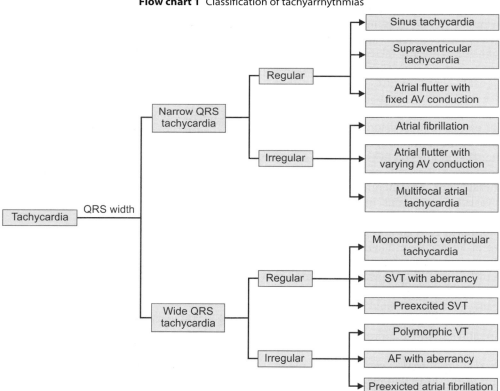

Flow chart 1 Classification of tachyarrhythmias

Abbreviations: AV, atrioventricular; AF, atrial fibrillation; SVT, supraventricular tachycardia; VT, ventricular tachycardia

CHAPTER 35 Electrocardiogram Interpretation in Emergency

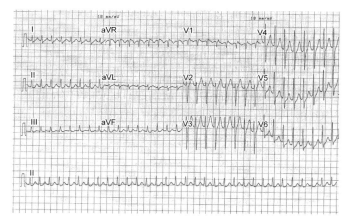

Fig. 1 Paroxysmal supraventricular tachycardia (PSVT) due to atrioventricular nodal re-entrant tachycardia (AVNRT). A regular narrow QRS tachycardia with QRS morphology that is normal is diagnostic of PSVT. Note the lead V1 shows a small positive deflection similar to r' after the S waves that suggest presence of P waves occurring just at the end of the QRS complex. These P waves may also be visible as small negative deflections in leads II, III, and aVF immediately at the end of QRS. This location of P waves during PSVT indicates a diagnosis of AVNRT—the most common mechanism of PSVT

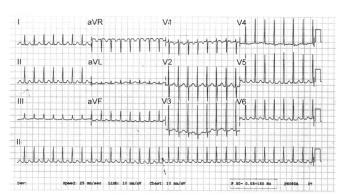

Fig. 2 Paroxysmal supraventricular tachycardia (PSVT) due to atrioventricular reciprocating tachycardia (AVRT). Another example of regular narrow QRS tachycardia where the P waves are seen in the ST segment. The most common mechanism of this pattern is AVRT wherein the re-entrant circuit involves antegrade conduction over the normal atrioventricular (AV) node-His-Purkinje system and retrograde conduction over an accessory pathway. A similar pattern of ECG can also occur in a focal atrial tachycardia, however, that is much less common

rate varying from 140 beats/min to 220 beats/min. The various subtypes of PSVT **(Figs 1 to 3)** can also be inferred from the ECG based on the location of the P waves in the cardiac cycle, however, since the acute treatment of different subforms of the PSVTs is more or less same, their identification is not of paramount importance in the emergency. The QRS complexes during SVT are usually narrow, however, preexisting bundle branch block (BBB) or transient aberrant conduction can result in wide QRS complexes during SVT.

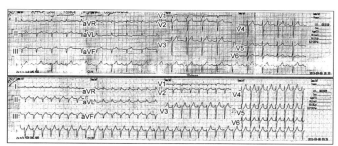

Fig. 3 Electrocardiograms (ECGs) of sinus rhythm (top panel) and paroxysmal supraventricular tachycardia (PSVT) (bottom panel) showing identical QRS morphology. Note that in both panels, the 12-lead ECG is displayed at half voltage (5 mm/mV) resulting in small QRS amplitude. The rhythm strip in both panels displays lead II at standard 10 mm/mV voltage. The sinus rhythm ECG was recorded immediately after termination of PSVT with injection of metoprolol that also explains prolonged PR interval during sinus rhythm. The P waves are not visible during the regular narrow QRS PSVT suggesting AVNRT as the likely diagnosis

The clue lies in the fact that the QRS morphology is typical of either right or LBBB in SVT with aberrancy.

Atrial Flutter

Atrial flutter can be recognized by rapid atrial rate (220–350/min, usually 300/min) with P waves of single morphology occurring in a saw-tooth pattern without any isoelectric line between them. The ventricular rate and rhythm depends on the AV conduction pattern and can be rapid or controlled and regular or irregular.

Atrial Fibrillation

Atrial fibrillation presents with rapid irregular ventricular rhythm with P waves that are either not visible or exist as small, nonuniform undulations (fibrillatory waves). The QRS complexes are usually narrow but can be wide if there is aberrant intraventricular conduction (transient BBB), preexisting BBB **(Fig. 4)** or ventricular preexcitation. The clue to recognition of atrial fibrillation is markedly irregular RR intervals.

Monomorphic Ventricular Tachycardia

Monomorphic ventricular tachycardia (MMVT) presents as a regular wide QRS tachycardia. It is the most common cause of wide QRS tachycardia in clinical setting and its diagnosis is even more likely if the patient has structural heart disease or prior myocardial infarction (MI) **(Figs 5 to 7)**. The ECG pointers to a diagnosis of MMVT as against the other differential diagnosis of SVT with aberrancy include AV dissociation, fusion and capture beats, wider QRS [>140 ms with right bundle branch block (RBBB) type and >160 ms with LBBB type], precordial concordance **(Fig. 5)**, and northwest axis of the QRS in the frontal plane. Though,

Preexcited Supraventricular Tachycardia

Any SVT can present as a wide QRS complex tachycardia in patients with ventricular preexcitation or WPW syndrome. The QRS morphology does not resemble that during sinus rhythm or typical BBB but suggests the location of commonly found accessory pathways. The sinus rhythm ECG (of prior times or recorded after termination of SVT) shows typical preexcitation pattern with short PR interval, delta waves and wide QRS complexes.

Polymorphic Ventricular Tachycardia

Polymorphic VT presents as an irregular tachycardia with wide QRS complexes with marked variation in the morphology of the QRS complexes from beat-to-beat. If the tachycardia is sustained, the patient is usually hemodynamically unstable. It can exist in the presence of normal QT interval, but is more common with QT interval prolongation, when it is known as "torsades de pointes" due to appearance on the ECG as if the QRS complexes are twisting around a point or line.

Bradyarrhythmias

The normal heart rate in an adult person at rest varies from 60 to 100 beats per minute. Any rhythm where the heart rate is less than 60 beats/min is known as bradyarrhythmia. Atrioventricular (AV) block of second or higher degree even with a ventricular rate more than 60 beats/min is classified as bradyarrhythmia. These rhythm disorders can occur due to either sinus node dysfunction (disorder of impulse formation or conduction) or AV block (disorder of impulse conduction). The patients with bradyarrhythmia usually present with complaints of syncope or presyncope, weakness or fatigue and/or breathlessness on exertion. Though, commonly these rhythm disorders occur as a result of degenerative diseases of the electrical system, at times reversible causes like drugs, electrolyte imbalance or acute myocardial ischemia or infarction (**Fig. 8**) may be the causative mechanism.

- Sinus node dysfunction can present as sinus pauses, sinus arrest with junctional or ventricular escape beats and rhythm, sinus bradycardia or sinoatrial exit block (**Fig. 9**). Other ECG manifestations that may be found in patients with so called sick sinus syndrome include AV block, BBB, atrial fibrillation, and episodes of bradycardia alternating with tachycardia (tachy-brady syndrome).
- Atrioventricular block presents as delay in conduction (prolonged PR interval, first degree AV block) or block of some (second degree, **Fig. 10**) or all (third degree or complete AV block, **Fig. 11**) atrial impulses to the ventricles. The need for temporary and permanent pacemaker implantation depends on the presence and severity of symptoms, presence of reversible causes, ventricular rate, QRS width and underlying heart disease.

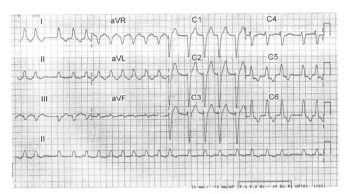

Fig. 4 Atrial fibrillation with aberrant conduction. Irregular wide QRS complex tachycardia with predominantly negative QRS complexes in lead V1 (LBBB type) with no identifiable P waves indicating a diagnosis of atrial fibrillation (AF). The typical LBBB morphology of the QRS suggests aberrant intraventricular conduction rather than ventricular tachycardia. Also, marked irregularity of RR intervals clinches the diagnosis of AF

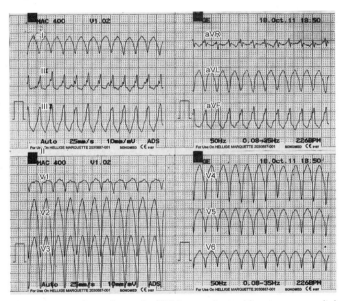

Fig. 5 Ventricular tachycardia (VT) in a patient with prior myocardial infarction (MI). A regular wide QRS tachycardia with predominantly negative QRS complexes in V1 [left bundle branch block (LBBB) type] is displayed. The clues to the diagnosis of VT include history of prior MI, atrioventricular dissociation (best seen in V1), negative concordance of QRS in the precordial leads, axis-morphology discordant pattern (LBBB morphology with right axis deviation of QRS in the frontal plane) and QRS morphology not resembling typical LBBB

many algorithms exist to help in differentiation of MMVT from SVT with aberrancy; the history of prior infarction, QRS morphology not resembling typical LBBB or RBBB and QRS morphology different from baseline indicate a diagnosis of ventricular tachycardia (VT).

CHAPTER 35 Electrocardiogram Interpretation in Emergency 277

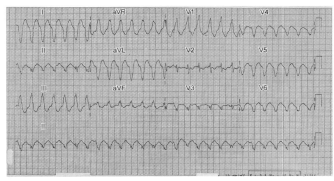

Fig. 6 Ventricular tachycardia (VT) in a patient with idiopathic dilated cardiomyopathy. A regular wide QRS tachycardia with predominantly positive QRS in lead V1 [right bundle branch block (RBBB) type] is shown. The clues to the diagnosis of VT include AV dissociation (best seen in rhythm strip of lead II), markedly wide QRS complexes, Q waves in lead V6 and QRS morphology not resembling typical RBBB among many others. Note that the QRS looks deceptively narrow in lead V2 and an erroneous diagnosis of supraventricular tachycardia can be made if this lead is chosen as the only monitoring lead and a 12-lead ECG is not recorded

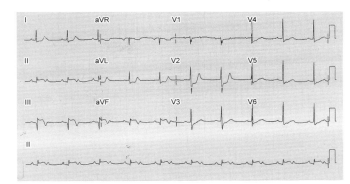

Fig. 8 Acute inferior-posterior myocardial infarction (MI). Sinus rhythm with 2 to 1 atrioventricular block with narrow QRS complexes in the conducted beats is seen. The leads II, III, and aVF show ST segment elevation with prominent Q waves indicating acute evolving inferior wall MI. Notice that large R wave in lead V2 with marked ST depression suggests presence of concomitant posterior wall MI. ST segment elevation that is greater in lead III than in lead II indicate involvement of the right coronary artery and presence of AV block suggests a proximal location of the culprit lesion

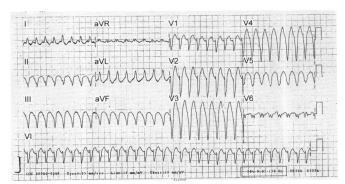

Fig. 7 Ventricular tachycardia (VT) in a patient with arrhythmogenic right ventricular dysplasia (ARVD). A regular wide QRS tachycardia with LBBB type pattern and left axis of the QRS in the frontal plane is shown. The presence of atrioventricular (AV) dissociation (seen best in rhythm strip of lead V1) and negative precordial concordance clinches the diagnosis of VT. Note that during LBBB type VTs, left axis deviation of QRS complex is suggestive of ARVD as the underlying diagnosis, whereas a right axis deviation is more common with idiopathic outflow tract VTs

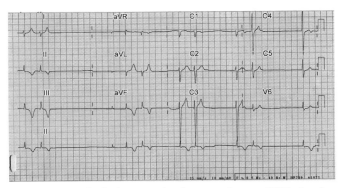

Fig. 9 Sinus node dysfunction. An electrocardiogram (ECG) showing sinus pauses and junctional escape beats and rhythm in a patient with sinus node dysfunction is displayed. Also, note that marked T wave inversion in inferior leads that could be either due to underlying heart disease (e.g. myocardial ischemia) or due to cardiac memory as a result of prior persistent ventricular escape rhythm. Also present in this tracing is possibly left posterior fascicular block (right axis deviation of QRS; qR pattern in leads II, III, and aVF; and rS pattern in leads I and aVL)

ST-SEGMENT DEVIATION

The ST-segment is the deflection from the end of QRS complex to the onset of T wave and is normally isoelectric. Deviation of the ST segment upward (ST elevation) or downward (ST depression) in various ECG leads is an important sign of many heart diseases, the most important of which is coronary artery disease. In fact, presence or absence of ST-segment elevation is a means of classifying acute MI into STEMI or NSTEMI.

Few important points are provided below in reference to ST-segment deviation and its utility in the emergency.
- The ECG leads can be grouped according to the region of the ventricle (mainly the left) that they overlie. These are known as contiguous leads and include:
  - *Inferior wall*: Leads II, III and aVF
  - *Anterior wall*: Leads V1 to V6
  - *Anterolateral wall*: V4 to V6, I and aVL
  - *Anteroseptal wall*: V1 to V3, aVR

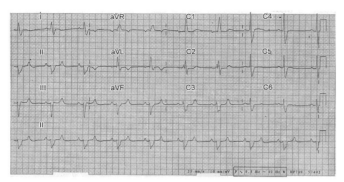

Fig. 10 Two to one atrioventricular (AV) block. Sinus tachycardia with 2 to 1 AV block with RBBB and LAFB in the conducted beats is seen. Notice that there are two P waves for each QRS complex, and the PR intervals of the conducted beats are constant as are PP and RR intervals. A wide QRS complex in the conducted beat (RBBB in this case) suggests Infra-Hisian location of the AV block and need for permanent pacemaker implantation even in the absence of bradycardia related symptoms

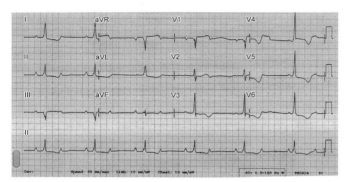

Fig. 11 Complete atrioventricular (AV) block. Sinus rhythm with complete AV block and a slower wide QRS (ventricular) escape rhythm is seen. Note that the P waves occur at a much faster rate, and have no association with the QRS complexes (AV dissociation). The clue to the presence of AV dissociation is varying apparent PR intervals in the presence of constant RR and PP intervals

- *Right ventricle*: Right-sided precordial leads V1 to V6
- *Posterior wall*: Leads V7 to V9.
- The ST elevation of 1 mm (0.1 mV) or greater in two or more contiguous leads in a patient with chest discomfort is indicative of STEMI **(Figs 8 and 12)**. A prompt recognition of STEMI suggests the need of emergency reperfusion therapy in the form of either primary angioplasty or thrombolysis.
- The ST elevation and depression both are suggestive of myocardial ischemia. ST elevation has localizing value but ST depression does not. Hence, ST elevation in leads II, III and aVF indicates acute inferior wall MI. ST depression in these leads may indicate myocardial ischemia but not necessarily in inferior wall of the left ventricle.

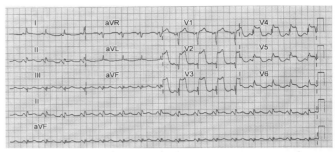

Fig. 12 Acute anterior wall myocardial infarction (MI). Marked ST elevation is seen in precordial leads V2 to V6 indicating acute anterior wall MI and involved of left anterior descending (LAD) coronary artery. Notice, that the inferior leads also show ST-segment elevation. This pattern suggests that the site of culprit lesion in the LAD artery is distal to the origin of the septal and diagonal branches. Hence, ECG not only helps in diagnosis but indicates the culprit vessel and localizes the site of lesion

Box 3 Noninfarction causes of ST-segment elevation

- Acute pericarditis
- Coronary artery spasm
- Left ventricular aneurysm
- Left bundle branch block
- Left ventricular hypertrophy
- Early repolarization syndrome
- Hypertrophic cardiomyopathy
- Acute pulmonary embolism

- Serial changes in ECGs taken over time have more importance than fixed changes.
- The ECG not only has value in diagnosis of MI but also helps in localization of infarct, culprit artery localization, estimation of infarct size, timing of infarction, risk stratification, and prognostication.
- Various other causes of ST elevation apart from STEMI exist and should be considered if diagnosis of MI is doubtful. These are listed in **Box 3**.
- The ST-segment depression indicates myocardial ischemia especially if it is greater than 1 mm, present in two or more contiguous leads, of horizontal or downsloping (rather than upsloping) nature or if associated with marked T wave changes.
- The ST-segment depression of less than 1 mm especially if present in the absence of typical chest discomfort is commonly nonspecific and is seen in a variety of clinical conditions.

T WAVE CHANGES

The T wave represents part of the recovery period of the ventricles (repolarization). The T wave is normally upright in leads I, II, and V4 to V6; inverted in aVR; usually upright in aVF

Box 4 T wave abnormalities

- T wave inversion associated with ST segment deviation and/or abnormal Q waves: Myocardial ischemia or infarction, digitalis effect or toxicity **(Fig. 13)**
- Diffuse deep T wave inversion (usually nonspecific and seen in variety of conditions): Myocardial ischemia, evolving MI, apical or hypertrophic cardiomyopathy, cardiac memory, electrolyte imbalance, and cerebrovascular accidents
- Asymmetric T inversion in lateral precordial leads: Left ventricular hypertrophy
- Asymmetric T inversion in right precordial leads: Right ventricular hypertrophy and acute pulmonary embolism
- Peaked T waves in precordial leads: Hyperkalemia
- Peaked T waves in V1 and V2 with positive QRS complexes: Posterior wall myocardial infarction

Table 1 ECG criteria of bundle branch blocks and fascicular blocks

Left bundle branch block	Right bundle branch block

• QRS duration >120 ms
• Wide notched R waves in V5, V6, I and aVL
• Small or absent initial r wave in right precordial leads V1 and V2 followed by deep S waves
• Absent septal waves in left-sided leads—V6 and lead I
• Prolonged intrinsicoid deflection (>60 ms) in V5 and V6
	• QRS duration >120 ms
	• Wide notched R waves (rsr', rsR' or rSR') patterns in right precordial leads—V1 and V2
	• Wide and deep S waves in left precordial leads—V5 and V6
	• Bifascicular block
	  – RBBB and LAFB
	  – RBBB and LPFB

Left anterior fascicular block	Right anterior fascicular block
• Left axis deviation (QRS axis in the frontal plane −45 to −90°) • rS pattern in leads II, III, and aVF • qR pattern in lead aVL • QRS duration <120 ms	• Right axis deviation (QRS axis in frontal plane >120°) • qR pattern in leads II, III and aVF • rS pattern in leads I and aVL • QRS duration <120 ms

Abbreviations: ECG, electrocardiogram; RBBB, right bundle branch block; LAFB, left anterior fascicular block; LPFB, left posterior fascicular block.

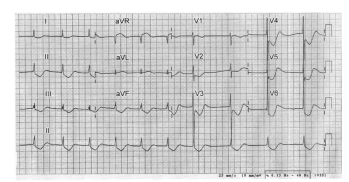

Fig. 13 Digitalis toxicity. This is an ECG of a patient with permanent AF and digitalis toxicity. The P waves are absent and the ventricular rhythm is irregular with narrow QRS complexes. Importantly there is marked ST-segment depression with T wave inversion in most leads. Note, that the J point (end of QRS) is also markedly depressed in leads V3 to V6 that differentiates it from digitalis effect wherein the ST depression and T wave inversion is present without J point depression. Note is also made of large amplitude R waves in V5 and V6 due to underlying left ventricular hypertrophy

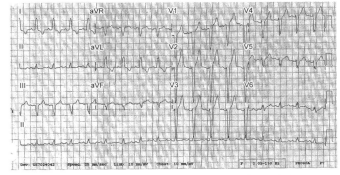

Fig. 14 Left bundle branch block (LBBB). Sinus tachycardia is present with wide QRS complexes that have predominantly negative QRS in lead V1, notching in V4 to V6, absent (very small) r in lead V1 and absent q waves in leads V6, I and aVL. These are typical features of LBBB

and can be variable in III, aVL, and V1. The T wave changes can often be nonspecific and should always be interpreted along with the ST-segment abnormalities and clinical setting. The common T wave abnormalities are described in **Box 4**.

QRS MORPHOLOGY, AMPLITUDE AND DURATION AND AXIS PATTERNS

The normal coordinated simultaneous activation of both right and left ventricle is responsible for normal QRS complex that is narrow (QRS duration <100 ms), has normal axis in the frontal plane and has normal amplitude in various leads (in absence of normal left and right ventricular thickness).

Delay or block in conduction in left or the right bundle branches results in sequential activation of the ventricles with resultant right or LBBB pattern. The block in conduction of the left anterior and posterior fascicles **(Fig. 9)** does not result in QRS widening but causes change in the QRS axis in the frontal plane. The diagnostic criteria for left and right BBB and fascicular blocks are summarized in **Table 1**. A diagnosis of BBB especially LBBB **(Fig. 14)** or bifascicular block in a patient presenting with history of syncope or presyncope may suggest intermittent complete AV block as the cause and requirement of additional evaluation and possible pacemaker implantation. All physicians should have an imprint of typical LBBB and RBBB patterns inscribed in their minds for an accurate diagnosis of many arrhythmias.

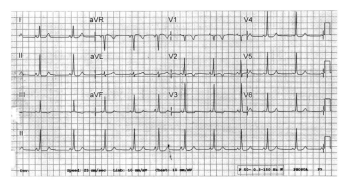

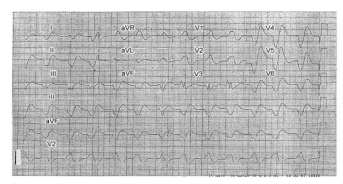

Fig. 15 Wolff-Parkinson-White (WPW) syndrome. Sinus rhythm with short PR interval, delta waves and wide QRS complexes are present indicating ventricular preexcitation due to an accessory pathway. The negative delta and QRS in lead V1 suggests a right sided pathway. The presence of symptoms or documented arrhythmias related to accessory pathways in a patient with ventricular preexcitation makes a diagnosis of WPW syndrome. Note is made of marked irregularity in sinus rhythm that is as a result of sinus arrhythmia due to respiratory variation

Fig. 16 Hyperkalemia. A regular rhythm with markedly wide and bizarre QRS complexes that are not preceded by P waves—sinoventricular rhythm. The T waves start immediately after the end of QRS complexes with almost absent ST-segment. These are ECG features of severe hyperkalemia

Similarly, presence of an antegradely conducting accessory pathway (WPW syndrome, **Figure 15**) results in preexcitation of the ventricle in which it is inserted resulting in sequential activation of ventricles. The QRS complex in this situation of ventricular preexcitation occurs as a result of fusion of activation of ventricles by the accessory pathway and the normal AV node—His-Purkinje system and is wide with an initial delta wave. Recognition of WPW syndrome or ventricular preexcitation during sinus rhythm in a patient with episodic palpitations may indicate PSVT as a cause of palpitation.

MISCELLANEOUS ELECTROCARDIOGRAM FINDINGS IN EMERGENCY

Many other findings in the ECG may be present that may provide an important clue to the diagnosis in the emergency setting. These include:
- *Wide QRS complexes with absent P waves*: Hyperkalemia (**Fig. 16**)
- *Low voltage ECG*: Pericardial effusion, hypothyroidism, thick chest wall, obesity, emphysema, and incorrect standardization
- *Electrical alternans*: Cardiac tamponade
- *Prolonged QT interval*: Congenital long QT syndrome, drug inducted QT prolongation, hypocalcemia, and hypomagnesemia
- *Osborn wave*: Abnormal wave seen at the end of QRS and seen classically in hypothermia.

CONCLUSION

The ECG plays an important role in the initial diagnostic evaluation of all patients presenting with symptoms related to cardiovascular disorders or at times systemic illnesses in the emergency. Emergency physicians cannot afford to miss the finding of ST-segment elevation, the hallmark of diagnosis of acute MI as it may result in disastrous consequences. Studies have shown that emergency physicians are usually good and accurate at diagnosing MI from the ECG, but are not up to the mark in diagnosis of cardiac arrhythmias. A systemic approach to ECG interpretation as outlined in this chapter can be useful to arrive at a quick and accurate diagnosis in most patients presenting in the emergency.

CHAPTER 36

Role of Echocardiography in Emergency Room

Mansi Kaushik, Manish Bansal, Ravi R Kasliwal

INTRODUCTION

Prompt diagnosis and rapid institution of appropriate therapeutic measures are the most important goals in the management of patients presenting to the emergency room (ER). Given the time-sensitive and critical nature of the illnesses leading to ER presentation, the diagnosis must be established quickly, which limits the scope of the investigative workup available for the initial evaluation of these patients. Therefore, in most patients, a focused clinical assessment combined with bedside diagnostic tools, such as X-ray, electrocardiogram (ECG), and laboratory investigations, need to form the basis for initial triaging. However, since a cardiac etiology may underlie almost every clinical presentation resulting in ER admission, some form of cardiac evaluation is invariably required in many of these patients. Echocardiography has emerged as a highly useful diagnostic modality for this purpose. Its portability, safety, easy availability, and ability to provide comprehensive information about cardiac structure and function within a short period of time make it ideally suited for use in the ER setting. Because of these attributes, echocardiography has now become almost an extension of clinical examination. Previous studies have shown that addition of a screening echocardiogram significantly improves the diagnostic accuracy of physical examination and reduces unwarranted downstream diagnostic and therapeutic referrals.[1-4]

In this review, we discuss the role of echocardiography in the initial evaluation and management of patients presenting to ER with various clinical presentations.

PATIENTS PRESENTING WITH ACUTE CHEST PAIN

Chest pain is one of the most common reasons for ER visits. A number of cardiac and noncardiac conditions can cause chest pain, such as acute coronary syndrome (ACS), aortic dissection, pulmonary embolism, acute pericarditis, lower respiratory tract infection, acute cholecystitis, acute pancreatitis, costochondritis, etc. Echocardiography plays an important role as a first-line diagnostic modality in the differential diagnosis of these conditions and plays a pivotal role in the overall management of patients presenting with ACS.[5-8]

Acute Coronary Syndrome

The term ACS encompasses a wide spectrum of clinical presentations ranging from unstable angina, non-ST elevation myocardial infarction (NSTEMI) and ST elevation myocardial infarction (STEMI) to even sudden cardiac death. The diagnosis of ACS is traditionally based on clinical presentation, ECG changes, and the abnormalities in the cardiac biomarkers.[9] However, many patients with ACS present with nondiagnostic ECGs and cardiac biomarkers typically take 6–8 hours to become abnormal. Given these constraints, echocardiography can be a useful tool for establishing the diagnosis of ACS and has a class I indication for this purpose.[10]

In the ischemic cascade, abnormalities of left ventricular (LV) systolic and diastolic function develop very early, much before the appearance of ECG changes. Accordingly, the presence of new regional wall motion abnormalities (RWMA) on echocardiography will strongly support a diagnosis of ACS in a patient with typical chest pain but nondiagnostic baseline ECG. However, echocardiography may not be much helpful for diagnosing ACS in a patient with known coronary artery disease (CAD) when the extent of preexisting RWMA is not known.

For the purpose of initial diagnosis of ACS, a positive echocardiogram should meet one of the following criteria:
- Abnormal wall motion of two or more contiguous segments visible in two different views, or

- Global LV hypokinesia with an ejection fraction (EF) of less than 40%.[11]

In patients who do not have any evidence of LV systolic dysfunction and also have normal cardiac biomarkers, stress echocardiography (either dobutamine or exercise) can be performed to rule out significant CAD prior to discharge from the ER. Such approach has more than or equal to 90% sensitivity and specificity for identifying subjects at risk for having cardiac events.[12]

Abnormalities of LV diastolic function appear even before the development of RWMA and therefore have even greater sensitivity for detection of myocardial ischemia. However, these abnormalities are too nonspecific to be used routinely for this purpose. Their utility currently lies mainly in the assessment of intracardiac hemodynamics and guiding management, rather than in the initial diagnosis of ACS. However, the diastolic phase abnormalities may have diagnostic value on strain imaging as discussed next.

Apart from establishing the diagnosis of ACS, echocardiography also permits recognition of the underlying culprit vessel, assessment of the extent of myocardial damage and its hemodynamic consequences, and helps in detection of mechanical complications of myocardial infarction (MI), if any (discussed further in subsequent sections).

In CAD, LV RWMA usually follow the distribution of coronary vascular territory. Therefore, the pattern of regional myocardial involvement during ACS helps in identification of the underlying culprit artery **(Fig. 1)**. This information not only has diagnostic utility, but also helps in determining the choice of treatment modality and the urgency with which such treatment needs to be instituted.

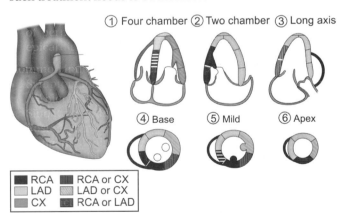

Fig. 1 The typical distribution of coronary vascular supply
Abbreviations: LAD, left anterior descending; LCX, left circumflex; RCA, right coronary artery.
Source: Adapted from Lang RM, Bierig M, Devereux RB, et al. Recommendations for chamber quantification: a report from the American Society of Echocardiography's Guidelines and Standards Committee and the Chamber Quantification Writing Group, developed in conjunction with the European Association of Echocardiography, a branch of the European Society of Cardiology. J Am Soc Echocardiogr. 2005;18:1440-63.

The extent of myocardial damage can be determined by estimating either wall motion score index (WMSI) or more commonly, LVEF. For estimation of WMSI, segmental wall motion of each LV myocardial segment is scored as 1 = normal, 2 = hypokinetic, 3 = akinetic, and 4 = dyskinetic or aneurysmal, in a 16 segment model. The score for each segment is then added and the total score is divided by the number of segments analyzed to obtain WMSI. WMSI provides a semiquantitative estimate of overall LV systolic function with higher WMSI signifying greater amount of myocardial damage and thus, worse LV systolic function.[13,14]

In clinical practice, however, LVEF is the most commonly used measure of LV systolic function. In patients with ACS, LVEF has immense diagnostic, prognostic and therapeutic value and is central to almost every therapeutic decision-making, not just during the acute stage, but during the entire course of illness.

Estimation of LVEF by echocardiography is simple and easy to perform. Modified biplane Simpson's technique is the recommended method for this purpose.[15] This method requires tracing of endocardial border of the LV in apical four-chamber and two-chamber views in both end-diastolic and end-systolic frames. The automated software onboard the echocardiography machine performs the calculations required to estimate LV volumes and EF. Alternately, LVEF can also be estimated visually by eyeballing, which, in fact, is the most common method used in real-life clinical practice. With experienced echocardiographers, LVEF estimation by eyeballing has been shown to have high degree of accuracy.[16] More recently, three-dimensional (3D) echocardiography has also become available and has been shown to be more accurate than two-dimensional (2D) echocardiography for estimation of LV volumes and EF.[13,17,18]

Role of Adjunctive Techniques

As discussed earlier, the diagnostic evaluation of CAD by echocardiography traditionally relies on segmental wall motion analysis, either at rest or during stress. While this approach has been extensively validated over the years, it has certain limitations. Most important of these are inability to detect subtle changes in myocardial contractile function and the lack of information about myocardial perfusion. Strain imaging and myocardial contrast echocardiography (MCE) overcome these limitations and their incorporation during conventional echocardiography has been shown to have incremental value in the evaluation of chest pain patients in the ER.

Strain imaging is a sensitive modality for detection of myocardial contractile dysfunction. The currently used speckle tracking echocardiography (STE) permits comprehensive assessment of myocardial deformation in different directions, which has important diagnostic implications in the evaluation of CAD[19,20] **(Fig. 2)**. As longitudinal deformation of LV is determined predominantly

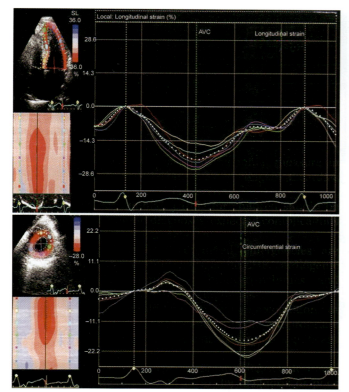

Fig. 2 Speckle tracking echocardiography-based measurement of left ventricular longitudinal and circumferential strain

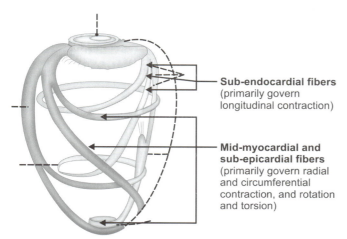

Fig. 3 Arrangement of muscle fibers in the left ventricular myocardium and their contributions in causing myocardial deformation

by subendocardial myocardial fibers, longitudinal strain (LS) is the first one to get affected with the onset of myocardial ischemia **(Fig. 3)**. In contrast, circumferential deformation which is determined primarily by the subepicardial fibers gets involved much later when the myocardial injury has become transmural. This unique structural-functional relationship

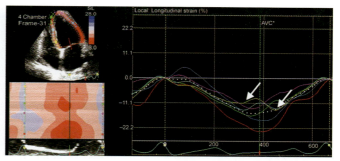

Fig. 4 Reduced systolic longitudinal strain with post-systolic shortening (arrows) in basal septum (yellow trace)

of LV myocardial contractile apparatus can be exploited for the purpose of early detection of myocardial ischemia, for differentiating subendocardial injury from transmural injury and for predicting myocardial viability.[20]

Subendocardial myocardial fiber dysfunction can be detected by strain imaging either as reduced systolic LS, increased post-systolic strain (PSS), and/or as delayed decay of peak LS during diastole **(Fig. 4)**. These strain abnormalities can be used for diagnosing CAD and may have incremental value over wall motion analysis.[21] Furthermore, increased PSS and impaired diastolic decay of strain may persist for a reasonable period of time after acute myocardial ischemia and can serve as ischemic myocardial memory.[22,23]

When impairment of LS is not accompanied by concomitant reduction in circumferential strain (CS), it usually indicates nontransmural injury whereas concomitant reduction of both LS and CS indicates transmural infarct. Thus, assessment of CS can be helpful not only in diagnosing ACS,[21] but more importantly, in identifying total coronary occlusions[24] and in predicting late LV remodeling and overall clinical outcomes[20] **(Figs 5A to D)**. Furthermore, CS can also help in differentiating STEMI from acute myocarditis which may have similar clinical presentations. As myocarditis preferentially affects epicardial and mid-myocardial layers, it causes more marked impairment of CS, unlike ischemia which generally results in greater impairment of LS. Accordingly, in patients with preserved LVEF, impaired global CS (less negative than –19.3%) has been shown to differentiate acute myocarditis from STEMI with sensitivity 72% and specificity 74%.[25]

Unlike strain imaging, MCE provides information about myocardial perfusion and thus bridges the gap between echocardiography and nuclear imaging. Because of its ability to assess myocardial perfusion, MCE has been shown to have high sensitivity for detection of subendocardial ischemia and can be useful in triaging the patients presenting with suspected ACS. In a study involving 400 patients presenting to ER with chest pain but normal ECG and biomarkers, dipyridamole-atropine stress echocardiography with MCE had significantly higher accuracy (sensitivity and specificity 97% and 74%, respectively) for diagnosing as compared to

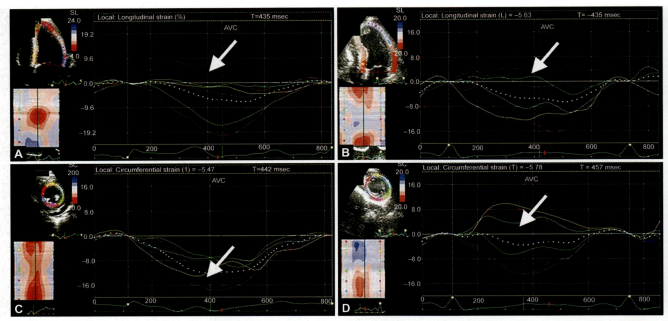

Figs 5A to D Differential involvement of left ventricular longitudinal and circumferential strain in patients with subendocardial and transmural infarcts. (A) Longitudinal strain is impaired but (B) circumferential strain is preserved in basal segments in a patient with subendocardial infarct; (C and D) Both longitudinal and circumferential strains are impaired in apical segments in a patient with transmural infarct

wall motion analysis alone (sensitivity and specificity 63% and 91%, respectively).[26]

Aortic Dissection

Acute aortic dissection is a potentially fatal disease which presents as acute severe chest pain often radiating to interscapular region. Although chest pain in aortic dissection generally has typical character, it has often been misdiagnosed as ACS because of low index of suspicion and also because of occurrence of nonspecific ECG changes in aortic dissection. Sometimes, aortic dissection may result in a true STEMI also, due to occlusion of a coronary artery ostium by the dissection flap. Since, the management of ACS is completely opposite of that of acute aortic dissection, accurate distinction between the two conditions is of paramount importance.

The patient profile, pattern of chest pain, and the presence of unequal peripheral pulses provide important clues to the underlying diagnosis of aortic dissection, which can then be confirmed with the help of imaging. Echocardiography is an excellent modality for initial evaluation of patients with aortic dissection, particularly those with proximal aortic dissection **(Figs 6A to D)**. Transthoracic echocardiography (TTE) has 77–80% sensitivity and 93–96% specificity for diagnosing proximal aortic dissection, whereas the same for transesophageal echocardiography (TEE) are 98% and 95%, respectively.[27,28] The sensitivity of TTE for detecting distal aortic dissection is much lower, but TEE can generally diagnose most of the dissections involving descending thoracic aorta. The diagnosis of aortic dissection on echocardiography is based on detection of an undulating intimal flap within the aortic lumen that separates the true and false channels and has motion independent of that of the aortic wall. The flap should be identified in more than one view. TEE can demonstrate intimal tear in the vast majority of cases and also permits recognition of true and false lumina. The false lumen is often larger and has less blood flow than the true lumen. Partial thrombosis of the false lumen is seen frequently and total thrombosis is an occasional finding. Doppler study can also be used for differentiating true lumen from the false lumen. Apart from diagnosing aortic dissection, echocardiography is also helpful in detecting its potential complications such as hemopericardium, coronary involvement, and aortic insufficiency.

Pulmonary Embolism

Pulmonary embolism is a less common but potentially lethal cause of chest pain. It more often presents as shortness of breath or as hemodynamic collapse. Chest pain usually occurs when emboli are relatively small resulting in peripheral pulmonary infarction.

The imaging modality of choice for diagnosing acute pulmonary embolism is computed tomographic pulmonary angiography (CTPA).[29] However, echocardiography provides useful initial clues toward the possibility of under-

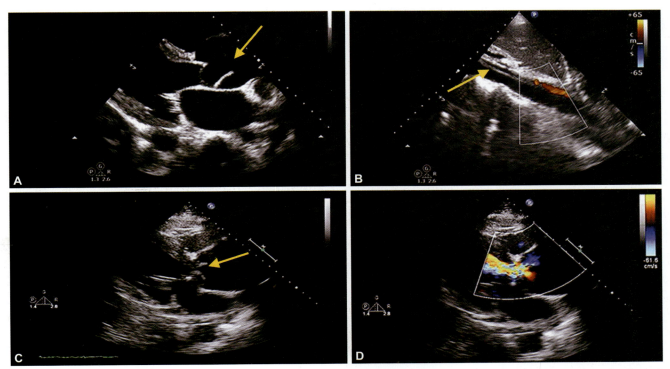

Figs 6A to D Two examples of acute aortic dissection. (A) Intimal flap (arrow) is seen in the aortic root; (B) In the same patient, the dissection flap (arrow) is seen extending into the abdominal aorta also; (C and D) Intimal flap (C, arrow) in another patient is prolapsing through the aortic valve causing severe aortic regurgitation

lying pulmonary embolism, permits assessment of the hemodynamic significance of the embolism—an important determinant of the treatment strategy and in some cases may also reveal thrombi in main pulmonary artery and its branches, right atrium (RA) and/or right ventricle (RV) **(Figs 7A and B)**.

Echocardiographic features corroborative of pulmonary embolism include dilatation of pulmonary artery with evidence of increased RV afterload in the form of RV dilatation/dysfunction, D-shaped LV cavity caused by leftward shift of the interventricular septum and Doppler evidence of pulmonary hypertension with or without evidence of increased RA pressure. RV systolic dysfunction in pulmonary embolism often has a typical regional pattern, affecting mainly the free wall with sparing of RV apex. This is known as McConnell's sign and is highly specific for pulmonary embolism but has low sensitivity.[30,31] As such, echocardiography itself has low sensitivity to rule out pulmonary embolism.[29] Therefore, while an abnormal echocardiogram can help confirm the diagnosis of pulmonary embolism, particularly in a hemodynamically compromised patient in whom CTPA may not be feasible, it should not be the only modality to rule out the diagnosis or to risk stratify patients with stable hemodynamics. Additionally, emergency physicians should also be vigilant about other causes of RV pressure/volume overload, such as obstructive airway disease, idiopathic pulmonary hypertension, right ventricular myocardial infarction (RVMI), primary tricuspid regurgitation (TR), etc. when diagnosing pulmonary embolism based on echocardiography alone.

DYSPNEA/SHORTNESS OF BREATH

Acute onset dyspnea can be due to cardiac or noncardiac conditions. Echocardiography is very helpful in distinguishing between the two and in providing detailed description of the underlying cardiac pathology when such a condition is found. Dyspnea is therefore a class I indication for performing echocardiography.

There are a number of cardiac conditions that can result in acute dyspnea. The common ones include:
- Predominant LV systolic dysfunction—due to MI, dilated cardiomyopathy, stress cardiomyopathy, etc.
- Predominant LV diastolic dysfunction—due to long-standing hypertension, hypertrophic cardiomyopathy, restrictive cardiomyopathy, aortic stenosis, etc.
- Valvular heart diseases—mitral stenosis, mitral regurgitation (MR), aortic stenosis, aortic regurgitation, prosthetic heart valve (PHV) malfunction, etc.

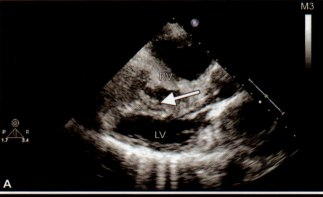
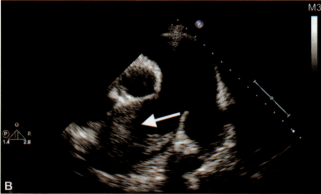

Figs 7A and B A patient with massive pulmonary embolism. (A) Right ventricle is grossly dilated and the interventricular septum (arrow) is deviated toward the left ventricle; (B) Markedly dilated main pulmonary artery with complete occlusion of right pulmonary artery with thrombus (arrow)
Abbreviations: LV, left ventricle; RV, right ventricle.

- Pericardial diseases, such as cardiac tamponade, constrictive pericarditis, etc.
- Cardiac tumors such as LA myxoma, etc.
- Pulmonary embolism, idiopathic pulmonary hypertension, etc.

In all the above conditions, echocardiography is able to demonstrate the underlying structural abnormality in detail. In addition, it also permits comprehensive assessment of intracardiac hemodynamics which helps in determining the role of these abnormalities in causation of dyspnea and in planning appropriate treatment strategy.

Predominant LV diastolic dysfunction has recently emerged as an important cause of dyspnea. It is estimated that almost half of all patients presenting with heart failure have normal or near normal LVEF with LV diastolic dysfunction being the dominant abnormality.[32] This entity is termed as "heart failure with preserved EF" or HFpEF. Assessment of LV diastolic function is central to the recognition of this entity and echocardiography is the most commonly utilized modality for this purpose. Using echocardiography, LV diastolic function is assessed by integrating information

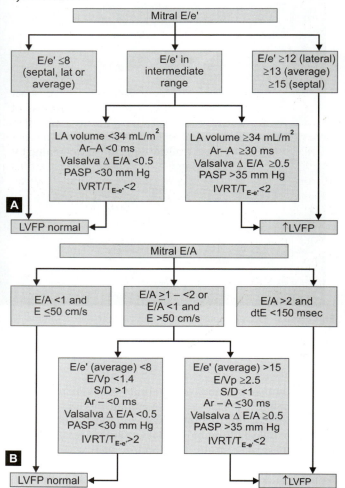

Flow chart 1 Algorithm for echocardiographic assessment of left ventricular diastolic function and estimation of left ventricular filling pressure in presence of normal (A) or reduced (B) left ventricular systolic function

Abbreviations: A, mitral inflow late diastolic velocity; Ar, atrial reversal wave in pulmonary vein flow; D, pulmonary vein flow diastolic velocity; dtE, deceleration time of mitral inflow early diastolic velocity; E, mitral inflow early diastolic velocity; e'- mitral annular early diastolic velocity; IVRT, isovolumic relaxation time; LA, left atrium; LVFP, left ventricular filling pressure; PASP, pulmonary artery systolic pressure; S, pulmonary vein flow systolic velocity; $T_{E-e'}$, time interval between the onset of mitral E and e' velocities, measured from the onset of QRS complex on ECG; Vp, mitral inflow propagation velocity.
Source: Adapted from Nagueh SF, Appleton CP, Gillebert TC, et al. Recommendations for the evaluation of left ventricular diastolic function by echocardiography. J Am Soc Echocardiogr. 2009;22:107-33.

derived from interrogation of mitral inflow pattern, mitral annular motion, pulmonary vein flow pattern, etc. The American Society of Echocardiography has recommended algorithms for stepwise assessment of LV diastolic function and LV filling pressure in different patient populations[33] **(Flow chart 1)**.

Estimation of LV filling pressure is of paramount importance even in patients with frank LV systolic dysfunction. In these patients, elevated LV filling pressure is not only an adverse prognostic marker,[34] it has major therapeutic implications as well. The need for diuretics, intravenous fluids, inotropes, vasodilators, etc.; timing of introduction of beta-blockers; timing of coronary intervention; ambulation and mobilization of patients after acute MI, etc. are all influenced by the status of LV filling pressure.

Among valvular lesions, mitral stenosis is the most common condition that presents with acute shortness of breath. Development of atrial fibrillation is the usual culprit in these patients. In contrast, acute shortness of breath in other valvular heart diseases generally occurs due to worsening LV systolic dysfunction, development of infective endocarditis (IE) or traumatic disruption of valvular apparatus. Aortic stenosis may result in acute dyspnea even in absence of LV systolic dysfunction because of LV hypertrophy with consequent LV diastolic dysfunction. PHV malfunction can occur because of valve thrombosis, structural degeneration, progressively worsening pannus formation or IE.

HYPOTENSION AND HEMODYNAMIC INSTABILITY

Hypotension and shock are commonly encountered in the ER. They can be cardiogenic in origin or may result from noncardiac causes, such as hemorrhage, hypovolemia or sepsis. As shock requires aggressive early intervention in order to prevent end organ damage due to inadequate tissue perfusion, distinguishing cardiogenic shock from shock of other etiologies is extremely important. The major advantage of echocardiography is that it can quickly determine whether the shock is cardiogenic or noncardiogenic,[8,35] apart from also providing plenty of hemodynamic information that is useful irrespective of the type of shock. A brief 2D echocardiographic examination itself can help in excluding common cardiac causes of hypotension such as:
- Extensive MI with severe LV systolic dysfunction
- Right ventricular infarction
- Mechanical complication of MI
- Nonischemic severe LV systolic dysfunction
- Pericardial effusion with tamponade
- Massive pulmonary embolism, etc.

Even in patients with noncardiogenic shock, echocardiography often provides useful clues to the underlying etiology. For example, in patients with hypovolemic shock, echocardiography often reveals a small underfilled and hyperdynamic LV, which is a reliable indicator of intravascular volume depletion. Similarly, a collapsed inferior vena cava (IVC) in a patient with unexplained shock indicates an urgent ultrasound evaluation of the peritoneal cavity to look for abdominal hemorrhage.[36]

A more formal assessment of hemodynamics can also be performed by echocardiography, which helps in characterization of the type of shock. LV filling pressure can be estimated as described above, whereas RV filling pressure (same as mean RA pressure or central venous pressure) is derived from IVC size and collapsibility[37] **(Table 1)**. Mean and systolic pulmonary pressures can be estimated from pulmonary regurgitation and TR jets. For systemic cardiac output, LV stroke volume is calculated first which is then multiplied with heart rate. LV stroke volume is usually calculated by multiplying 2D-derived LV outflow tract (LVOT) area with Doppler-derived LVOT velocity time integral.[38] Alternately, it can also be calculated by subtracting LV end-systolic volume from LV end-diastolic volume derived using the modified Simpson's method. By combining all this data, systemic vascular resistance (SVR) can be calculated as:

SVR (Wood units) = [Mean aortic pressure (mm Hg) − mean RA pressure (mm Hg)]/systemic cardiac output (L/min)

In the above equation, mean systemic blood pressure is used as a surrogate for mean aortic pressure whereas the other two values are obtained from echocardiography.

Once systemic cardiac output, LV filling pressure, pulmonary pressures, and central venous pressure are available, it is quite easy to determine the underlying mechanism of shock, i.e. hypovolemic, cardiogenic, septic or a combination of these.

Right Ventricular Myocardial Infarction

Right ventricular myocardial infarction occurs in almost 50% of all cases of inferior wall MI, but hemodynamically significant RVMI is less common.[39] Recognition of RVMI in patients with inferior wall MI is important because not only RVMI is associated with worse prognosis;[40-42] the management of the two conditions is also vastly different.[40,42,43] Echocardiography plays a vital role in the diagnosis of RVMI. In these patients, it usually reveals a dilated RV with regional RV hypokinesia/akinesia. TR is common due to dilatation of the tricuspid annulus. Tissue Doppler imaging may provide additional information. A study revealed that a tricuspid annular peak systolic velocity less than 12 cm/sec had a sensitivity of 81%, specificity of 82%, and negative predictive value of 92% for diagnosing RVMI in patients presenting with acute inferior wall MI.[44]

Table 1 Estimating mean right atrial pressure from inferior vena cava size and collapsibility

Inferior vena cava diameter	Collapse on sniff	Mean right atrial pressure (mm Hg)
<2.1 cm	>50%	3 (range 0–5)
>2.1 cm	<50%	15 (range 10–20)
Indeterminate cases		8 (range 5–10)

Mechanical Complications of Myocardial Infarction

Acute MI can result in several mechanical complications that are among the few most catastrophic cardiac conditions and are associated with very high mortality rates despite best treatment. Early recognition is extremely crucial for improving outcome of these conditions and echocardiography is the most useful modality for this purpose.[43,45-48]

Common mechanical complications of MI include ventricular septal rupture (VSR), chordal or papillary muscle rupture leading to acute MR, contained free wall rupture with pseudoaneurysm formation, and complete free wall rupture[43] **(Figs 8A to C)**.

Post-MI VSR occurs in roughly 1–3% of all STEMI, mainly during the early phase of acute infarction. In case of anterior wall MI, the defect is usually located in the distal part of the septum whereas inferior wall MI results in basal septal rupture. 2D echocardiography may reveal a discrete defect, or there may be multiple channels traversing through the necrotic myocardium. The diagnosis of large discrete defect can be easily made by TTE but small defects may not be visible. TEE is required when TTE is suboptimal and there is high clinical suspicion.

Papillary muscle necrosis and rupture occurs in roughly 1% of all cases of STEMI. It is more common after inferior wall MI and can result from even a modest size infarct. Rupture usually involves the posteromedial papillary muscle as it has single blood supply. Echocardiography is useful in delineating the exact anatomic defect and in assessment of MR severity. However, conventional parameters of MR severity may not be applicable in this setting due to small regurgitant volume with nondilated LA and LV.[49] Accordingly, a chordal or papillary muscle rupture should always be suspected when there is an eccentric jet of MR with a relatively normal-sized LA in a patient of acute MI.

Rupture of the free wall of the LV occurs in about 1% of the patients with MI. It mainly occurs in patients with a transmural MI involving the inferolateral wall. When there is complete free wall rupture, it usually results in immediate cardiac tamponade and sudden death. However, when the defect is small, the patients may sometimes escape immediate death. In such cases, echocardiography will reveal pericardial collection of variable magnitude with features of cardiac tamponade. However, it is often difficult to visualize the actual defect as the defect may appear just like a "slit" in the myocardium and the location of the pericardial collection also does not always correlate with the site of rupture.[50]

A pseudoaneurysm is the contained rupture of LV free wall, but rarely it may also form as a result of VSR. Majority of pseudoaneurysms are seen in inferoposterior or inferolateral regions. It is important to distinguish a pseudoaneurysm from a true aneurysm as the former has high risk of spontaneous rupture whereas a true aneurysm seldom ruptures spontaneously. In a true aneurysm, there is continuity of the endocardium in the area of dilatation and the wall of the aneurysm is formed by the stretched but intact LV myocardium. In contrast, in a pseudoaneurysm there is breach of endocardial continuity and the wall of the sac is composed of pericardium with little or no myocardial tissue. In addition, the size of communication relative to the size of the aneurysm may also help in making this distinction. The ratio of the diameter of entry to the maximum diameter of the pseudoaneurysm is usually less than 0.5, whereas it is much larger in a true aneurysm. However, this feature has only 60% sensitivity.[51]

Cardiac Tamponade

Cardiac tamponade should be suspected in every patient presenting with acute breathlessness with hypotension. Immediate pericardiocentesis is lifesaving in such patients and an echocardiogram is very helpful in making the diagnosis.

On echocardiography, pericardial effusion is seen as an echo-free space between pericardium and the heart. The characteristic finding in cardiac tamponade with large effusion is a "swinging heart" appearance. The 2D echocardiographic and Doppler signs that indicate increased intrapericardial pressure and presence of tamponade in patients with large pericardial effusion include early diastolic RV collapse, late diastolic RA inversion, abnormal ventricular

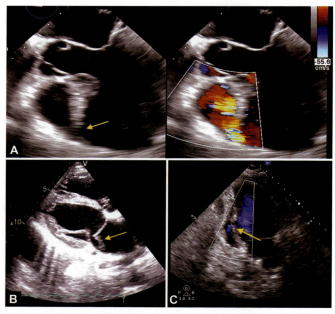

Figs 8A to C Examples of mechanical complications of myocardial infarction. (A) There is apical ventricular septal rupture (arrow) with left-to-right shunt through the defect; (B) One of the papillary muscles has got ruptured and is seen attached to the anterior mitral leaflet and prolapsing into the left atrium. The anterior mitral leaflet itself is flail; (C) Contained rupture of the inferior wall. Blood flows through the defect (arrow) into a small pseudoaneurysm

septal motion, characteristic respiratory variation in mitral and tricuspid inflow velocities, and dilated and noncollapsing IVC.[52]

Apart from establishing the diagnosis, echocardiography is also helpful in guiding pericardiocentesis by demonstrating the maximum site of fluid accumulation, suggesting the best trajectory for needle insertion, helping confirm the intrapericardial position of the needle tip, and finally by assessing the immediate post-procedure outcome.[53,54]

ECHOCARDIOGRAPHY IN STROKE PATIENTS

Cardiogenic embolus is an important cause of stroke, accounting for approximately 20% of all ischemic strokes.[55] Therefore, cardiac evaluation is required in all stroke patients who present with clinical features suggestive of cardioembolism (i.e. young age, presence of atrial fibrillation, known valvular heart disease, etc.).

A variety of cardiac conditions can lead to systemic embolism. The common sources of cardioembolism include **(Figs 9A to F)**:

- Left atrial/LA appendage (LAA) thrombus
- Left ventricular thrombus
- Vegetations (infective/noninfective)
- Cardiac tumors
- Prosthetic heart valve thrombi
- Paradoxical embolism through patent foramen ovale (PFO)/atrial septal defect (ASD)
- *Miscellaneous*:
  – Mitral annular calcification
  – Sclerotic aortic valve
  – Mitral valve prolapse, etc.

Left Atrial/Left Atrial Appendage Thrombus

Left atrial/LAA thrombi account for more than 45% of cardiogenic thromboembolic events. They are most often associated with atrial fibrillation or rheumatic mitral stenosis. TEE is the modality of choice for detection of LA/LAA thrombi and has nearly 100% sensitivity for this purpose. In comparison, the sensitivity of TTE for detection of LA/LAA thrombi is only 39–63%.[56] However, both TTE and TEE can easily detect spontaneous echo contrast within LA, which is a precursor to thrombus formation and has strong association with the risk of systemic embolism.[57]

Systemic emboli are frequently seen among patients with dilated cardiomyopathy as well. Though LV thrombi are supposed to be the source of emboli in these patients, LA thrombi are four times more frequent than LV thrombi.[58]

Left Ventricular Thrombus

Left ventricular thrombus is mainly seen in patients with recent MI, LV aneurysm or dilated cardiomyopathy. Thrombi most often occur in the apical region of LV, in the presence

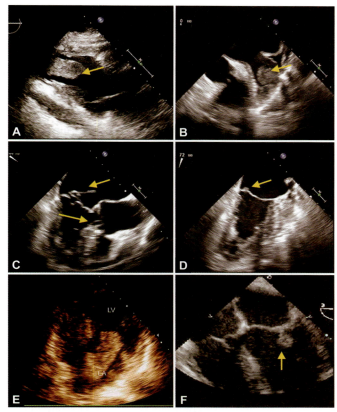

Figs 9A to F Common causes of cardioembolic stroke. (A) Large left ventricular apical clot (arrow) in a patient with anterior wall myocardial infarction; (B) Left atrial appendage clot (arrow); (C) Vegetations (arrows) attached to both mitral and aortic valve leaflets; (D) Sessile vegetation (arrow) on the atrial surface of the mitral leaflet in a patient with nonbacterial thrombotic endocarditis; (E) Large left atrial myxoma (arrow) prolapsing into the left ventricular cavity through the mitral orifice; (F) Papillary fibroelastoma (arrow) attached to the mitral leaflet

of regional akinesis or dyskinesis. TTE in combination with ultrasound contrast is a good modality for detection of LV thrombi and TEE is usually not required. Echocardiography also helps in assessing the risk of embolism. A large sized, mobile thrombus hanging in the LV cavity is associated with high risk of embolism. Similarly, hyperkinetic segments adjacent to the thrombus and an echo-lucent center (suggesting actively growing thrombus) also indicate high risk of embolization.

Valvular Sources of Systemic Embolism

Systemic embolism is a common complication in patients with PHVs, particularly mechanical PHVs. The risk is much higher in patients with subtherapeutic anticoagulation level. Although echocardiography is the modality of choice for evaluation of PHV related thrombi, acoustic shadowing due to valve structure often proves a limiting factor. TEE provides much better visualization as compared to TTE, particularly in case of mitral PHVs.

Infective endocarditis is another common cause of valve related embolic events. Echocardiography is useful in detecting the underlying heart disease responsible for IE, identifying vegetations, and diagnosing complications of IE. A vegetation is an irregularly shaped, often flagellar, echogenic, mobile mass, usually attached to the valve leaflets but may also be attached to chordae, chamber walls or any intracardiac implant such as pacemaker lead, indwelling catheter or PHV sewing ring. Vegetations may be sessile or pedunculated. Large vegetations (>10 mm size) with high mobility and multiple sites of involvement are at higher risk of embolization. For detection of vegetations and abscesses, TEE is more sensitive than TTE with overall sensitivity 90–100% as compared to only 40–63% for the latter.[59] In a comparative study involving 66 cases of suspected IE, TEE had a sensitivity of 94% compared with 44% for TTE, but both had high specificity approaching 100%.[60]

Vegetations can also form in absence of IE. This is known as nonbacterial thrombotic endocarditis (NBTE) and is usually seen in patients with connective tissue disorders, malignancies, etc. Vegetations in NBTE are most commonly found on the mitral valve and usually on the atrial side of the leaflets. Unlike IE, these vegetations are generally sessile and not more than 5–10 mm in size.

Finally, calcific specks or fragments of valve tissue can also embolize rarely in patients with mitral annular calcification, aortic sclerosis, etc.

Cardiac Tumors

Cardiac tumors that are commonly associated with systemic embolization are LA myxoma and papillary fibroelastomas. A young patient in sinus rhythm presenting with embolic stroke should raise the suspicion of cardiac tumor or IE.

Left atrial myxomas are most often attached to the interatrial septum, in the region of fossa ovalis. They are usually pedunculated and have a nonhomogeneous "cluster of grapes" appearance with areas of echolucency and calcification. LA myxomas can often be confused with LA thrombus and need to be differentiated from the latter. Unlike LA myxoma, an LA thrombus has an amorphous echogenic appearance, is usually sessile and is commonly located in the posterior portion of the LA.[61,62]

Papillary fibroelastomas most often arise from aortic or mitral valve.[61] These tumors are small in size (generally 0.5–2.0 cm in diameter) and have distinct appearance. They are irregular and frond-like in shape, pedunculated, mobile and attached to the downstream side of the valve. Mobility makes them prone to embolization. Because of the attachment on the valve, fibroelastomas are often mistaken for vegetations. However, the lack of any evidence of infection and their appearance should help in differentiating fibroelastomas from vegetations.

Paradoxical Embolism

In patients with ASD or PFO, blood flow is predominantly in left-to-right direction. However, there can be a transient reversal of the shunt when RA pressure exceeds LA pressure as occurs during coughing or straining. During these brief periods of shunt reversal, a thrombus from the venous system may travel to the left side of the heart, resulting in systemic embolism.

While it is easier to diagnose ASD by echocardiography, diagnosis of a PFO may be challenging. Injecting agitated saline contrast along with Valsalva maneuver or coughing can help uncover intermittent right-to-left interatrial shunting. TEE with saline contrast is superior to TTE with contrast for the diagnosis of PFO.[63] A PFO is considered potentially significant for causing stroke when more than 10 microbubbles appear in the LA within three cardiac cycles.

SYNCOPE

Syncope is defined as "sudden temporary loss of consciousness associated with a loss of postural tone and spontaneous recovery not requiring electrical and chemical cardioversion". It is a clinical diagnosis and a detailed history and good physical examination should be able to suggest the diagnosis in the vast majority of the cases. However, echocardiography is often required to rule out underlying structural heart disease. Various structural heart diseases that can result in syncope include:
- Acute MI
- Ischemic or nonischemic LV systolic dysfunction (usually due to ventricular tachyarrhythmias)
- Severe aortic stenosis—valvular, subvalvular, or supravalvular
- Hypertrophic obstructive cardiomyopathy
- Large atrial myxoma
- Cardiac tamponade
- Aortic dissection
- Massive pulmonary embolism
- Severe pulmonary hypertension
- Severe pulmonary stenosis, etc.

Echocardiography aids in the accurate diagnosis of the underlying structural heart disease when present. However, it should be remembered that echocardiography should not be a routine diagnostic tool for evaluation of syncope, unless the underlying cause is unexplained by history and physical examination or when the patient has significant cardiac history or has an abnormal ECG.[64]

FEVER OF UNKNOWN ORIGIN

Echocardiography is generally not required in the evaluation of most patients with fever. However, when patients with cardiac conditions predisposing to IE present with fever, echocardiography is routine indicated. In addition, it is also needed to rule out IE in some patients with no underlying heart disease when no other cause for fever is found despite extensive evaluation.

CONCLUSION

Noninvasive nature, portability and instantaneous diagnostic capability render echocardiography a highly suited diagnostic modality for use in the ER. It offers vital information for early diagnosis, provides extensive anatomic and hemodynamic information and is also very useful in guiding therapeutic procedures. However, echocardiography is an operator-dependent technique and this becomes even more relevant in ER setting where diagnosis needs to be established quickly and the acoustic window may not always be good. Therefore, proper training of the users and following standardized imaging protocols are essential to maintain optimum diagnostic accuracy of this technique.

REFERENCES

1. Bansal M, Singh S, Maheshwari P, et al. Value of interactive scanning for improving the outcome of new-learners in transcontinental tele-echocardiography (Vision-in-Tele-Echo) study. J Am Soc Echocardiogr. 2015;28(1):75-87.
2. Cardim N, Fernandez Golfin C, Ferreira D, et al. Usefulness of a new miniaturized echocardiographic system in outpatient cardiology consultations as an extension of physical examination. J Am Soc Echocardiogr. 2011;24(2):117-24.
3. Mjolstad OC, Dalen H, Graven T, et al. Routinely adding ultrasound examinations by pocket-sized ultrasound devices improves inpatient diagnostics in a medical department. Eur J Intern Med. 2012;23(2):185-91.
4. Skjetne K, Graven T, Haugen BO, et al. Diagnostic influence of cardiovascular screening by pocket-size ultrasound in a cardiac unit. Eur J Echocardiogr. 2011;12(10):737-43.
5. Frenkel O, Riguzzi C, Nagdev A. Identification of high-risk patients with acute coronary syndrome using point-of-care echocardiography in the ED. Am J Emerg Med. 2014;32(6):670-2.
6. Arntfield RT, Millington SJ. Point of care cardiac ultrasound applications in the emergency department and intensive care unit–a review. Curr Cardiol Rev. 2012;8:98-108.
7. Shah BN, Ahmadvazir S, Pabla JS, et al. The role of urgent transthoracic echocardiography in the evaluation of patients presenting with acute chest pain. Eur J Emerg Med. 2012;19:277-83.
8. Labovitz AJ, Noble VE, Bierig M, et al. Focused cardiac ultrasound in the emergent setting: a consensus statement of the American Society of Echocardiography and American College of Emergency Physicians. J Am Soc Echocardiogr. 2010;23(12):1225-30.
9. Thygesen K, Alpert JS, White HD. Universal definition of myocardial infarction. J Am Coll Cardiol. 2007;50:2173-95.
10. Douglas PS, Khandheria B, Stainback RF, et al. ACCF/ASE/ACEP/ASNC/SCAI/SCCT/SCMR 2007 appropriateness criteria for transthoracic and transesophageal echocardiography: a report of the American College of Cardiology Foundation Quality Strategic Directions Committee Appropriateness Criteria Working Group, American Society of Echocardiography, American College of Emergency Physicians, American Society of Nuclear Cardiology, Society for Cardiovascular Angiography and Interventions, Society of Cardiovascular Computed Tomography, and the Society for Cardiovascular Magnetic Resonance endorsed by the American College of Chest Physicians and the Society of Critical Care Medicine. J Am Coll Cardiol. 2007;50(2):187-204.
11. Volpi A, De Vita C, Franzosi MG, et al. Determinants of 6-month mortality in survivors of myocardial infarction after thrombolysis. Results of the GISSI-2 data base. The Ad hoc Working Group of the Gruppo Italiano per lo Studio della Sopravvivenza nell'Infarto Miocardico (GISSI)-2 Data Base. Circulation. 1993;88:416-29.
12. Shah BN, Balaji G, Alhajiri A, et al. Incremental diagnostic and prognostic value of contemporary stress echocardiography in a chest pain unit: Mortality and morbidity outcomes from a real-world setting. Circ Cardiovasc Imaging. 2013;6:202-9.
13. Lang RM, Bierig M, Devereux RB, et al. Recommendations for chamber quantification: a report from the American Society of Echocardiography's Guidelines and Standards Committee and the Chamber Quantification Writing Group, developed in conjunction with the European Association of Echocardiography, a branch of the European Society of Cardiology. J Am Soc Echocardiogr. 2005;18:1440-63.
14. Armstrong WF, Ryan T. Echocardiography and coronary artery disease. In: Armstrong WF, Ryan T (Eds). Feigenbaum's Echocardiography. Philadelphia, USA: Lippincott Williams and Wilkins; 2010. pp. 427-72.
15. Lang RM, Badano LP, Mor-Avi V, et al. Recommendations for cardiac chamber quantification by echocardiography in adults: an update from the American Society of Echocardiography and the European Association of Cardiovascular Imaging. J Am Soc Echocardiogr. 2015;28:1-39. e14.
16. Gudmundsson P, Rydberg E, Winter R, et al. Visually estimated left ventricular ejection fraction by echocardiography is closely correlated with formal quantitative methods. Int J Cardiol. 2005;101:209-12.
17. Jenkins C, Moir S, Chan J, et al. Left ventricular volume measurement with echocardiography: a comparison of left ventricular opacification, three-dimensional echocardiography, or both with magnetic resonance imaging. Eur Heart J. 2009;30:98-106.
18. Dorosz JL, Lezotte DC, Weitzenkamp DA, et al. Performance of 3-dimensional echocardiography in measuring left ventricular volumes and ejection fraction: a systematic review and meta-analysis. J Am Coll Cardiol. 2012;59:1799-808.
19. Geyer H, Caracciolo G, Abe H, et al. Assessment of myocardial mechanics using speckle tracking echocardiography: fundamentals and clinical applications. J Am Soc Echocardiogr. 2010;23:351-69. quiz 453-5.
20. Bansal M, Sengupta PP. Longitudinal and circumferential strain in patients with regional LV dysfunction. Curr Cardiol Rep. 2013;15:339.

21. Sarvari SI, Haugaa KH, Zahid W, et al. Layer-specific quantification of myocardial deformation by strain echocardiography may reveal significant CAD in patients with non–ST-segment elevation acute coronary syndrome. JACC Cardiovasc Imaging. 2013;6:535-44.
22. Asanuma T, Fukuta Y, Masuda K, et al. Assessment of myocardial ischemic memory using speckle tracking echocardiography. JACC Cardiovasc Imaging. 2012;5:1-11.
23. Ishii K, Imai M, Suyama T, et al. Exercise-induced post-ischemic left ventricular delayed relaxation or diastolic stunning: is it a reliable marker in detecting coronary artery disease? J Am Coll Cardiol. 2009;53:698-705.
24. Grenne B, Eek C, Sjøli B, et al. Acute coronary occlusion in non-ST-elevation acute coronary syndrome: outcome and early identification by strain echocardiography. Heart. 2010;96:1550-6.
25. Hsiao JF, Koshino Y, Bonnichsen CR, et al. Differentiating acute myocarditis from acute myocardial infarction: diagnostic value of LV deformation by 2-D speckle tracking echocardiography. J Am Coll Cardiol. 2011;57:E309.
26. Gaibazzi N, Reverberi C, Squeri A, et al. Contrast stress echocardiography for the diagnosis of coronary artery disease in patients with chest pain but without acute coronary syndrome: incremental value of myocardial perfusion. J Am Soc Echocardiogr. 2009;22:404-10.
27. Hiratzka LF, Bakris GL, Beckman JA, et al. 2010 ACCF/AHA/AATS/ACR/ASA/SCA/SCAI/SIR/STS/SVM guidelines for the diagnosis and management of patients with Thoracic Aortic Disease: a report of the American College of Cardiology Foundation/American Heart Association Task Force on Practice Guidelines, American Association for Thoracic Surgery, American College of Radiology, American Stroke Association, Society of Cardiovascular Anesthesiologists, Society for Cardiovascular Angiography and Interventions, Society of Interventional Radiology, Society of Thoracic Surgeons, and Society for Vascular Medicine. J Am Coll Cardiol. 2010;55:e27-e129.
28. Evangelista A, Flachskampf FA, Erbel R, et al. Echocardiography in aortic diseases: EAE recommendations for clinical practice. Eur J Echocardiogr. 2010;11:645-58.
29. Konstantinides SV, Torbicki A, Agnelli G, et al. 2014 ESC guidelines on the diagnosis and management of acute pulmonary embolism. Eur Heart J. 2014;35:3033-69.
30. McConnell MV, Solomon SD, Rayan ME, et al. Regional right ventricular dysfunction detected by echocardiography in acute pulmonary embolism. Am J Cardiol. 1996;78:469-73.
31. Sosland RP, Gupta K. Images in cardiovascular medicine: McConnell's Sign. Circulation. 2008;118:e517-8.
32. Yancy CW, Jessup M, Bozkurt B, et al. 2013 ACCF/AHA guideline for the management of heart failure: a report of the American College of Cardiology Foundation/American Heart Association Task Force on Practice Guidelines. J Am Coll Cardiol. 2013;62:e147-239.
33. Nagueh SF, Appleton CP, Gillebert TC, et al. Recommendations for the evaluation of left ventricular diastolic function by echocardiography. J Am Soc Echocardiogr. 2009;22:107-33.
34. Iwahashi N, Kimura K, Kosuge M, et al. E/e' two weeks after onset is a powerful predictor of cardiac death and heart failure in patients with a first-time ST elevation acute myocardial infarction. J Am Soc Echocardiogr. 2012;25:1290-8.
35. Ferrada P, Evans D, Wolfe L, et al. Findings of a randomized controlled trial using limited transthoracic echocardiogram (LTTE) as a hemodynamic monitoring tool in the trauma bay. J Trauma Acute Care Surg. 2014;76:31-7; discussion 37-8.
36. Lyon M, Blaivas M, Brannam L. Sonographic measurement of the inferior vena cava as a marker of blood loss. Am J Emerg Med. 2005;23:45-50.
37. Rudski LG, Lai WW, Afilalo J, et al. Guidelines for the echocardiographic assessment of the right heart in adults: a report from the American Society of Echocardiography endorsed by the European Association of Echocardiography, a registered branch of the European Society of Cardiology, and the Canadian Society of Echocardiography. J Am Soc Echocardiogr. 2010;23:685-713; quiz 786-8.
38. Quinones MA, Otto CM, Stoddard M, et al. Doppler Quantification Task Force of the Nomenclature and Standards Committee of the American Society of Echocardiography. Recommendations for quantification of Doppler echocardiography: a report from the Doppler Quantification Task Force of the Nomenclature and Standards Committee of the American Society of Echocardiography. J Am Soc Echocardiogr. 2002;15:167-84.
39. Goldstein JA. Pathophysiology and management of right heart ischemia. J Am Coll Cardiol. 2002;40:841-53.
40. Kakouros N, Cokkinos DV. Right ventricular myocardial infarction: pathophysiology, diagnosis, and management. Postgrad Med J. 2010;86:719-28.
41. Ondrus T, Kanovsky J, Novotny T, et al. Right ventricular myocardial infarction: from pathophysiology to prognosis. Exp Clin Cardiol. 2013;18:27-30.
42. O'Rourke RA, Dell'Italia LJ. Diagnosis and management of right ventricular myocardial infarction. Curr Probl Cardiol. 2004;29:6-47.
43. Antman EM, Morrow DA. ST-segment elevation myocardial infarction: management. In: Bonow RO, Mann DL, Zipes DP, Libby P (Eds). Braunwald's Heart Disease: A Textbook of Cardiovascular Medicine. Missouri: Saunders; 2012. pp. 1111-70.
44. Ozdemir K, Altunkeser BB, Icli A, et al. New parameters in identification of right ventricular myocardial infarction and proximal right coronary artery lesion. Chest. 2003;124:219-26.
45. Deshmukh HG, Khosla S, Jefferson KK. Direct visualization of left ventricular free wall rupture by transesophageal echocardiography in acute myocardial infarction. Am Heart J. 1993;126:475-7.
46. Hanlon JT, Conrad AK, Combs DT, et al. Echocardiographic recognition of partial papillary muscle rupture. J Am Soc Echocardiogr. 1993;6:101-3.
47. Ballal RS, Sanyal RS, Nanda NC, et al. Usefulness of transesophageal echocardiography in the diagnosis of ventricular septal rupture secondary to acute myocardial infarction. Am J Cardiol. 1993;71:367-70.
48. Panidis IP, Mintz GS, Goel I, et al. Acquired ventricular septal defect after myocardial infarction: detection by combined two-dimensional and Doppler echocardiography. Am Heart J. 1986;111:427-9.
49. Zoghbi WA, Enriquez-Sarano M, Foster E, et al. Recommendations for evaluation of the severity of native valvular regurgitation with two-dimensional and Doppler echocardiography. J Am Soc Echocardiogr. 2003;16:777-802.

50. Purcaro A, Costantini C, Ciampani N, et al. Diagnostic criteria and management of subacute ventricular free wall rupture complicating acute myocardial infarction. Am J Cardiol. 1997;80:397-405.
51. Yeo TC, Malouf JF, Oh JK, et al. Clinical profile and outcome in 52 patients with cardiac pseudoaneurysm. Ann Intern Med. 1998;128:299-305.
52. Klein AL, Abbara S, Agler DA, et al. American Society of Echocardiography clinical recommendations for multimodality cardiovascular imaging of patients with pericardial disease: endorsed by the Society for Cardiovascular Magnetic Resonance and Society of Cardiovascular Computed Tomography. J Am Soc Echocardiogr. 2013;26:965-1012.
53. Callahan JA, Seward JB, Nishimura RA, et al. Two-dimensional echocardiographically guided pericardiocentesis: experience in 117 consecutive patients. Am J Cardiol. 1985;55:476-9.
54. Tsang TS, Enriquez-Sarano M, Freeman WK, et al. Consecutive 1127 therapeutic echocardiographically guided pericardiocenteses: clinical profile, practice patterns, and outcomes spanning 21 years. Mayo Clin Proc. 2002;77:429-36.
55. Cardiogenic brain embolism. The second report of the Cerebral Embolism Task Force. Arch Neurol. 1989;46:727-43.
56. Schweizer P, Bardos P, Erbel R, et al. Detection of left atrial thrombi by echocardiography. Br Heart J. 1981;45:148-56.
57. Kasliwal RR, Mittal S, Kanojia A, et al. A study of spontaneous echo contrast in patients with rheumatic mitral stenosis and normal sinus rhythm: an Indian perspective. Br Heart J. 1995;74:296-9.
58. Vigna C, Russo A, De Rito V, et al. Frequency of left atrial thrombi by transesophageal echocardiography in idiopathic and in ischemic dilated cardiomyopathy. Am J Cardiol. 1992;70:1500-1.
59. Evangelista A, Gonzalez-Alujas MT. Echocardiography in infective endocarditis. Heart. 2004;90:614-7.
60. Shively BK, Gurule FT, Roldan CA, et al. Diagnostic value of transesophageal compared with transthoracic echocardiography in infective endocarditis. J Am Coll Cardiol. 1991;18:391-7.
61. Peters PJ, Reinhardt S. The echocardiographic evaluation of intracardiac masses: a review. J Am Soc Echocardiogr. 2006;19:230-40.
62. Auger D, Pressacco J, Marcotte F, et al. Cardiac masses: an integrative approach using echocardiography and other imaging modalities. Heart. 2011;97:1101-9.
63. Schneider B, Zienkiewicz T, Jansen V, et al. Diagnosis of patent foramen ovale by transesophageal echocardiography and correlation with autopsy findings. Am J Cardiol. 1996;77:1202-9.
64. Chang NL, Shah P, Bajaj S, et al. Diagnostic yield of echocardiography in syncope patients with normal ECG. Cardiol Res Pract. 2016;2016:1251637.

CHAPTER 37

Coronary Computed Tomography in Emergency

Kulbir Ahlawat, Devendra Richhariya

INTRODUCTION

We all know that chest pain and related symptoms like chest discomfort with squeezing pressure and burning sensation in epigastric precordial or pericardial area are the most common presentation in emergency department (ED). About 60–85% of patients with chest pain presenting to ED do not have acute coronary syndrome (ACS). Presentation of patients with chest pain is increasing in ED and emergency physician are very careful while discharging these patient from emergency because mortality in wrongly discharge patient is about 25%. Meanwhile, observing all patients in emergency for a longer period of time is neither logical nor economical. Initial triaging is to identify the patient with low-risk chest pain and discharge them safely, but this is also true that traditional cardiovascular risk factors and clinical scores are not enough to discharge the patient safely because even in low-risk patients adverse events are about 1–2%. This is a challenge for an emergency physician to accurately and efficiently diagnose the myocardial infarction (MI) and also noncardiac fatal causes of acute chest pain like aortic dissection and pulmonary embolism (PE) at the same time. Electrocardiogram (ECG) and cardiac enzyme are traditional methods used as first diagnostic tool for chest pain evaluation and in some institute exercise treadmill, stress echo, and myocardial perfusion imaging are also performed for risk stratification and to look for functional ischemia; these tests carry false positive and false negative results. At the same time, a package of tests exerts logistic burden on emergency medical services and on patients. So early imaging is necessary for risk stratification. Coronary computed tomography (CT) is an advanced cardiac noninvasive imaging modality with excellent diagnostic accuracy for the detection of coronary artery disease and a safe efficient and cost effective tool. Coronary CT angiography (CTA) has been shown to be a highly sensitive test for the detection of coronary artery disease (CAD) with negative predictive values approaching 97–99%. Triple rule out (TRO) CT examines coronary, pulmonary and thoracic aorta in a single test and is helpful in diagnosing the fatal causes of acute chest pain like acute PE and aortic dissection. Coronary CT is an attractive modality for rapid triaging of chest pain, reduces the hospitalization, and is cost effective without compromising the safety and quality of care.

INDICATIONS OF CORONARY COMPUTED TOMOGRAPHY ANGIOGRAPHY (CT ANGIOGRAPHY OF HEART)

Following are the indications for coronary CTA:
- Coronary CTA is useful in patients with nonacute symptoms representing an ischemic equivalent and low or intermediate group of CAD.
- It is also appropriate in patients who have low or intermediate probability of CAD and normal, nondiagnostic, or uninterpretable ECG or cardiac biomarkers.
- Cardiac CT is excellent for detection and quantification of calcified portions of coronary plaque and for differentiation of calcified, mixed, and noncalcified plaques.
- Coronary CTA is an appropriate first test in patients who are unable to exercise due to osteoarthritis, and who have either a low or intermediate probability of CAD.
- Coronary CTA has promise as a novel imaging modality in the acute setting because it is readily available, rapid and requires minimal additional expertise to perform the imaging.
- Coronary CTA is a useful screening tool for the assessment of coronary arteries for obstructive disease in young- and middle-aged patients presenting for noncoronary cardiac surgery such as valve repair, resection of cardiac masses, and aortic surgery.

CHAPTER 37 Coronary Computed Tomography in Emergency

Table 1 Acute chest pain suspicion of acute coronary syndrome

High risk	Intermediate risk	Strong suspicion of CAD/PE/aortic dissection	Very low-risk
Positive ECG and cardiac enzyme	Inconclusive ECG cardiac enzyme no known CAD → CTA	Triple rule out CT	Outpatient follow-up
Standard protocol for management of acute coronary syndrome and invasive coronary angiography	If abnormal, perform invasive coronary angiography. If normal → discharge	Triple rule out if positive, management according to diagnosis	Ambulatory follow-up

Abbreviations: CAD, coronary artery disease; CTA, CT angiography; PE, pulmonary embolism.

- Coronary CTA is a safe test with newly diagnosed heart failure. The objective is to exclude CAD as a cause of heart failure.
- Coronary CTA gives accurate assessment of in-stent restenosis in post-percutaneous transluminal coronary angioplasty (PTCA) patients coming in ED with nonacute chest pain.
- Coronary CTA is indicated for symptomatic patients with prior coronary artery bypass grafting (CABG) to evaluate for graft patency, graft thrombosis, malposition, aneurysms, and pseudoaneurysms.
- Cardiac CT can be used to differentiate between a subacute and an old MI. An acute myocardial infarct will appear as a hypoperfused, akinetic area of myocardium with normal wall thickness. In old MI, patients usually develop wall thinning in relation to normal, adjacent myocardium. In some instances, fatty metaplasia or calcification may be seen in CTA in old MI.
- Cardiac CT is a reasonable choice as the first modality in assessing all of the congenital anomalies in a single study, e.g. patients with suspected Turner's syndrome may have multiple congenital anomalies, including a bicuspid aortic valve, coarctation of the aorta, elongation of the transverse aortic arch, atrial or ventricular septal defect, and partial anomalous pulmonary venous return. All anomalies can be screened in a single study of CTA.
- Prior to invasive procedures, cardiac CT is useful for pulmonary vein mapping, coronary vein mapping, and for localizing bypass grafts and other retrosternal anatomy.
- Computed tomography angiography is useful for evaluating the right ventricular morphology and function, including in cases of suspected arrhythmogenic right ventricular dysplasia (ARVD).
- It is useful for evaluating native or prosthetic cardiac valves in the setting of valvular dysfunction and for evaluating cardiac masses.
- Finally, cardiac CT is an appropriate test for evaluation of the pericardium.

Coronary Computed Tomography in Emergency Department

Early implementation of CTA in the ED, for the evaluation of low to intermediate risk chest pain associated with reduced

Table 2 Inclusion and exclusion criteria for coronary computed tomography

Inclusion criteria	Exclusion criteria
• Chest pain • Low to intermediate risk • TIMI score 0–2 • Normal ECG and cardiac enzyme • Inconclusive cardiac enzyme • Admission to rule out CAD	• Atrial fibrillation • Known CAD • History of PTCA • Deranged creatinine • Beta-blocker or contrast allergy • Obesity weight >150 kg

Abbreviations: CAD, coronary artery disease; PTCA, percutaneous transluminal coronary angioplasty.

length of stay and a safe alternative to standard ED evaluation, rules out CAD by direct visualization of the coronary arteries (**Tables 1 and 2**).

Possible algorithm for coronary CT-based protocol for chest pain evaluation in ED shown in **Flow chart 1**.

CONTRAINDICATIONS FOR CORONARY CT IN THE ED

Following are the contraindications to CT:
- Inability to remain still, breath-hold, or follow instructions
- Renal insufficiency
- Cardiac arrhythmias
- Beta-blockers are given to patients undergoing CTA to bring the heart rate down so as to allow gating. If a patient has a contraindication to beta-blockade, such as asthma.
- Anaphylactic reaction to intravenous iodinated contrast agents is considered an absolute contraindication, though less severe allergic reactions may be acceptable if the patient has been adequately premedicated, usually with a combination of intravenous or oral diphenhydramine and corticosteroids.

PREPARATION FOR CORONARY CT

- Patient undergoes coronary CT while in ED or after completing observation protocol.
- Troponin and creatinine test are performed simultaneously. Coronary CT is performed only after creatinine result. Usually the troponin results are repeated while patient are in observation unit.

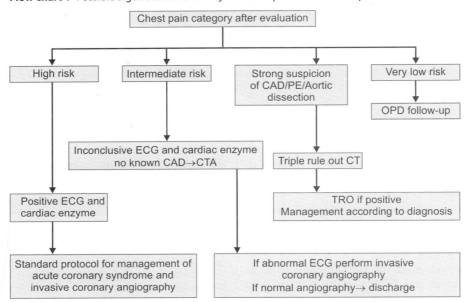

Flow chart 1 Possible algorithm for coronary CT-based protocol for chest pain evaluation in ED

- Patient with heart rate (HR) more than 70 beats/min beta-blocker should be given to achieve the heart rate less than 65 beats/min. Calcium channel blockers are alternative to beta-blockers.
- Contrast is calculated on the basis of weight of the patient and given as the bolus technique.
- Radiology technician or attending physician instructs the patient about breath holding.
- Image acquisition during single breath hold.
- Patient should not move during the image acquisition.
- Patient may feel warm sensation during contrast injection.
- Heart rate reducing medication and fast scan (64–320 cross section per rotation) help in acquiring the images with no artifact.
- Low radiation exposure with lower tube voltage technique and with advanced CT scan.

INTERPRETATION AND REPORTING OF CORONARY CT (FIGS 1A TO C)

Interpretation and reporting of CTA is done by radiologist with special training in cardiac imaging and CTA. Degree of stenosis is observed and measured by electronic calipers. Narrowing of left main, left anterior descending, right coronary artery, circumflex and their branches are expressed and reported in percentage: mild stenosis (<50% luminal narrowing); moderate stenosis (50–69% luminal narrowing); severe stenosis (>70% luminal narrowing) **(Tables 3 and 4)**.

Value of calcium scoring in ACS evaluation of patient in ED is debatable. Large calcium deposits in coronaries make interpretation of images difficult. Calcification in coronary

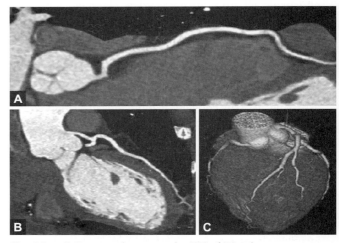

Figs 1A to C Computed tomography (CT) of (A) right coronary artery and (B) left anterior descending artery, and (C) volume-rendered three-dimensional reconstruction show absence of coronary plaque or stenosis. A negative CT coronary with good image quality has a very high negative predictive value and may spare the patient a diagnostic invasive angiogram

Table 3 Possible triaging scale on the basis of coronary CT report

0	Negative CT finding
1	Mild (<49% stenosis)
2	Moderate (50–69% stenosis)
3	Severe (>70% stenosis)

Table 4 Coronary CT as decision making tool: Degree of stenosis and recommendation for management

0–25%	26–49%	50–69%	>70%
• Patient can be discharged safely • Follow-up in OPD	• Patient can be discharged • OPD follow-up for preventive measures	• Possible CAD • Further evaluation needed before discharge	• Possible CAD • Hospitalization and evaluation

arteries is a marker of atherosclerosis and may be considered for long-term management of cardiac risk in outpatient but not for acute setting in ED.

FACTORS AFFECTING THE QUALITY OF CORONARY CT IMAGES

Fast heart rate: Image quality will be poor if heart rate more than 65/min. Patients with high heart rate are unsuitable for CT coronary.

Atrial fibrillation: Ectopy or ECG artifacts result in degradation of image quality.

Extensive coronary calcification: Obscures the coronary lumen making analysis of segments or even entire arteries difficult.

Pre-existing CAD: Patient with history of CAD usually have extensive coronary calcifications and/or coronary stents produce metal artifacts, and prior coronary bypass grafting with extensively calcified native vessels and small caliber distal coronary arteries also make interpretation of images difficult.

Obesity (body mass index over 40 kg/m^2): Increases radiation scatter within the patient's body and consequently degrades image quality.

ADVANTAGES OF CORONARY CT IN EMERGENCY DEPARTMENT

Following are the advantages of coronary CT in ED:
- It acts as a surrogate for catheterization laboratory angiography
- Provide better understanding of disease
- CT is safe, efficient, costs effective, reduces ED visits and hospitalization
- ED physicians and patients believe the results
- Higher satisfaction rates
- Improve chest pain triaging.

"TRIPLE RULE OUT" PROTOCOL

Acute chest pain is the most common presentation in ED. In view of wide spectrum causes of acute chest pain, not all life-threatening causes are of cardiac origin. Emergency physician should consider other noncardiac causes of chest pain like PE

Box 1 Triple rule out protocol

Triple rule out protocol is helpful in diagnosis of following conditions:

• *Acute aortic syndrome*: Including aortic dissection, aneurysm, penetrating aortic ulcer, intramural hematoma • Pulmonary embolism • Acute coronary syndrome	• Pneumothorax • Pleurisy • Pneumonia • Mesothelioma

and acute aortic syndrome, which are less common than ACS but immediately life-threatening. Apart from initial triaging, other investigation like D-dimer are used for diagnosis but nonspecific and elevated in other conditions also. Whenever there is high clinical suspicion, multidetector row CT (MDCT) is used to examine three vascular territories simultaneously pulmonary aorta and coronary arteries **(Box 1)**. "Triple rule out" CT protocol is associated with higher radiation dose. Coronary CT imaging with TRO protocol is the modality of choice for suspected PE and aortic pathology such as aortic dissection and aneurysm. Triple rule out protocol covers the whole chest and is helpful in assessment of vascular as well as nonvascular pathologies of the entire chest.

Patient Selection

Triple rule out CT protocol is recommended in acute chest pain patients with inconclusive cardiac enzyme and ECG and combine suspicion of acute PE and ACS, acute PE and aortic dissection.

Patients with elevated cardiac enzyme, ECG changes of ACS, pregnancy, previous contrast reaction, and nephropathy should be excluded.

CONCLUSION

Computed tomography angiography has been shown to be a safe and efficient way to determine which patients have no significant CAD. CTA is a valuable asset to clinical decision-making, in that it allows for the discharge of many patients who would otherwise be admitted for further observation and testing. CTA is not without its limitations, but as technology improves, so will the detail of images, which will improve the diagnostic capabilities of the modality. Triple rule out protocol not only diagnoses ACS but also noncardiac life-threatening emergencies like acute pulmonary embolism and acute aortic dissection.

BIBLIOGRAPHY

1. Achenbach S. Cardiac CT: State of the art for the detection of coronary arterial stenosis. J Cardiovasc Comput Tomogr. 2007;1(1):3-20.
2. Achenbach S, Marwan M, Ropers D, et al. Coronary computed tomography angiography with a consistent dose below 1 mSv using prospectively electrocardiogram-triggered high-pitch spiral acquisition. Eur Heart J. 2010;31:340-6.
3. Arbab-Zadeh AA, Miller JM, Rochitte CE, et al. Diagnostic accuracy of computed tomography coronary angiography according to pre-test probability of coronary artery disease and severity of coronary arterial calcification—The CORE-64 International Multicenter Study. J Am Coll Cardiol. 2012;59:379-87.
4. CT coronary angiography for risk stratification in the emergency department. [online] available from *http://www.ihe-online.com/feature-articles/ct-coronary-angiography-for-risk-stratification-in-the-emergency-department/* [Accessed February, 2017].
5. Deseive S, Pugliese F, Meave A, et al. Image quality and radiation dose of a prospectively electrocardiography-triggered high-pitch data acquisition strategy for coronary CT angiography: the multicenter, randomized PROTECTION IV study. J Cardiovasc Comput Tomogr. 2015;9:278-85.
6. Goldstein JA, Chinnaiyan KM, Abidov A, et al. The CT-STAT (Coronary computed tomographic angiography for systematic triage of acute chest pain patients to treatment) trial. J Am Coll Cardiol. 2011;58:1414-22.
7. Hoffmann U, Bamberg F, Chae CU, et al. Coronary computed tomography angiography for early triage of patients with acute chest pain—The ROMICAT (Rule out myocardial infarction using computer assisted tomography) Trial. J Am Coll Cardiol. 2009;53:1642-50.
8. Hoffmann U, Truong QA, Fleg JL, et al. Design of the rule out myocardial ischemia/infarction using computer assisted tomography: a multicenter randomized comparative effectiveness trial of cardiac computed tomography versus alternative triage strategies in patients with acute chest pain in the emergency department. Am Heart J. 2012;163:330-8, 338.e1.
9. Hoffmann U, Truong QA, Schoenfeld DA, et al. Coronary CT angiography versus standard evaluation in acute chest pain. N Engl J Med. 2012;367:299-308.
10. Kamimura M, Moroi M, Isobe M, et al. Role of coronary CT angiography in asymptomatic patients with type 2 diabetes mellitus. Int Heart J. 2012;53:23-28.
11. Litt H. Application of Coronary CT in the Emergency Department. [online] Available from *http://www.nasci.org/Portals/4/Meetings/RSSACardiacCTA2013/ED-CT-litt.pdf* [Accessed February, 2017].
12. Litt HI, Gatsonis C, Snyder B, et al. CT angiography for safe discharge of patients with possible acute coronary syndromes. N Engl J Med. 2012;366:1393-403.
13. Raff GL, Chinnaiyan KM. The role of coronary CT angiography in triage of patients with acute chest pain. Rev Esp Cardiol. 2009;62(9):961-5.
14. Truong QA, Schulman-Marcus J, Zakroysky P, et al. Coronary CT angiography versus standard emergency department evaluation for acute chest pain and diabetic patients: is there benefit with early coronary CT angiography. 2016. Results of the Randomized Comparative Effectiveness ROMICAT II Trial. J Am Heart Assoc. 2016;5(3):e003137. Published on behalf of the American Heart Association, Inc., by Wiley Blackwell.
15. Truong QA, Hayden D, Woodard PK, et al. Sex differences in the effectiveness of early coronary computed tomographic angiography compared with standard emergency department evaluation for acute chest pain: the rule-out myocardial infarction with Computer-Assisted Tomography (ROMICAT)-II Trial. Circulation. 2013;127:2494-2502.

CHAPTER 38

Precardiac Surgery Evaluation

Bhanu Prakash Zawar, Yatin Mehta

INTRODUCTION

Cardiac surgical patient are investigated extensively before surgery. However, evidence from studies using intraoperative transesophageal echocardiography suggest that as many as 5% of patients have additional undocumented pathology (e.g. valvular heart disease, patent foramen ovale).[1,2] Therefore, thorough preoperative evaluation is essential to identify the risk factors, assess the risk of surgery, optimize medical condition if necessary and take written informed consent, if necessary.

HISTORY

In majority of cases, the diagnosis would have already been established. So, preoperative assessment invariably begins with a review of the patient's medical record. The presence of risk factors known to be associated with increased perioperative mortality and morbidity like age greater than 60 years, arterial and pulmonary hypertension, body mass index (BMI) less than 20 or greater than 35 kg/m², congestive heart failure, peripheral vascular disease, diabetes mellitus, renal insufficiency, acute coronary syndromes, chronic pulmonary obstructive disease, neurological disease, and previous cardiac surgery should be sought. Drug history is very important. Patient on medications like steroids, bronchodilators, antihypertensive, anticoagulants, antiplatelets, antibiotics, antidiabetics, immunosuppressants, etc. should be noted. Some medications may need discontinuation before cardiac surgery like anticoagulant, potent antiplatelets, oral antidiabetics, angiotensin-converting enzyme (ACE) inhibitors, etc. If the patient is on anticoagulation warfarin should be stopped 3–7 days before surgery and international normalized ratio (INR) should be generally less than 1.5 for surgery. Heparin should be discontinued 6 hours before cardiac surgery. History of allergy to any drug or food should be noted, especially fish allergy as there are higher chances of protamine reaction in these patient. Signs and symptoms of cardiorespiratory disease (e.g. angina, dyspnea, orthopnea, impaired exercise tolerance, (pre)syncope) should be actively looked for. The severity of symptoms and effort tolerance should be documented using conventional indices; for example, the Canadian Cardiovascular Society angina score,[3] the New York Heart Association (NYHA) classification[4] of functional capacity,[4] and the Duke activity status index.[5] A short systematic examination should be conducted to exclude any gastrointestinal, renal, hepatic, neurological, metabolic or hematological disease. A symptom suggestive of gastroesophageal reflux necessitates the use of strategies to reduce the risk of regurgitation and pulmonary aspiration during anesthesia. Furthermore, a history suggestive of upper gastrointestinal tract pathology, such as hiatus hernia, may contraindicate the use of transesophageal echocardiography intraoperatively.

PHYSICAL EXAMINATION

Physical examination should be focused on the cardiovascular and respiratory systems. Examination should include heart rate, blood pressure measurement in supine and sitting position, respiratory rate; characterization of the heart rhythm, gentle palpation of the carotid, femoral and peripheral arteries, and auscultation of the precordium, carotid arteries and lung fields. Allen's test although not specific but should be performed to confirm the presence of an adequate collateral (ulnar) circulation in patient who are likely to undergo radial artery cannulation. Assessment of dentition, mouth opening and cervical mobility should be done to predict difficult airway.

INVESTIGATIONS

A blood count, coagulation profile, blood group, serum electrolytes, urea, creatinine and liver function test, a 12-lead electrocardiogram (ECG), and a left heart catheter should be regarded as routine preoperative investigations in virtually all cardiac surgical patients. A plain posteroanterior chest skiagram provides information about heart size, pulmonary vasculature, lung size, trachea, signs of cardiac failure and bony cage of the chest. Left heart catheterization typically comprises coronary angiography (useful in coronary artery patients), aortography, left ventriculography (ventricular function), and manometry. This provides information about the sites and severity of coronary artery stenosis, mitral and aortic valve function, and left ventricular (LV) morphology and function. ECG is done to detect arrhythmias, conduction changes, myocardial injury, and myocardial infarction. Exercise stress testing is a noninvasive test. It is useful in patient with chest pain of unknown etiology, and for quantification and prognosis in patients with known coronary artery disease (CAD). Currently many treadmill protocols are available of which Bruce protocol is most familiar. Pharmacological stress testing, e.g. dobutamine stress echocardiography is suitable for patient who are unable to exercise adequately. Transthoracic echocardiography is frequently used to define cardiac anatomy and assess ventricular and valvular function. Regional wall motion abnormality can be seen and it is helpful in deciding optimum preoperative management and perioperative monitoring and care. Additional investigations such as respiratory function tests, arterial blood gas analysis, carotid ultrasonography and angiography, creatinine clearance and evaluation of a permanent pacemaker or cardio-defibrillator[6] should be conducted, as appropriate.

RISK ASSESSMENT AND STRATIFICATION

Cardiac surgeries still have a certain risk of death and serious complications despite of advances in surgical techniques, anesthesia, and critical cardiac care. It is essential that the cardiac anesthesiologist understands how risk is assessed and that the patient and his or her relatives are adequately informed about the risk of surgery. In the late 1980s, Parsonnet and colleagues[7] identified 14 independent risk factors for death after cardiac surgery. The so-called Parsonnet score was adopted by many centers worldwide and is still in use today. The European System for Cardiac Operative Risk Evaluation (EuroSCORE)[8] was developed in the late 1990s, across 128 centers in eight European states in 19,030 patients undergoing cardiac surgery. Based on the EuroSCORE, the patients were categorized as, patients with low risk (EuroSCORE 0–2), moderate risk (EuroSCORE 3–5), and high risk (EuroSCORE greater than 6) of in-hospital mortality following cardiac surgery. The model has not been validated till date in India and Australia. The study involved assessment of 17 risk factors identified in EuroSCORE model. The additive EuroSCORE can be satisfactorily applied to low- and moderate-risk Indian patients but is less accurate for high-risk Indian patients undergoing cardiac surgery.[9] For high-risk patients, the logistic EuroSCORE[10] provides a more accurate prediction than the simple additive score.

CONCLUSION

Inpatient undergoing cardiac surgery extensive cardiac evaluation, preoperative cardiac risk assessment, and stratification are the part of routine workup. The main goal is to provide risk adjusted mortality rates for the preoperative patient and adequate patient and family counseling. Various complex or simplified models are available and can serve as a tool for risk assessment and stratification for perioperative mortality and morbidity.

REFERENCES

1. Benson MJ, Cahalan MK. Cost-benefit analysis of transesophageal echocardiography in cardiac surgery. Echocardiography 1995;12(2):171-83.
2. Fanshawe M, Ellis C, Habib S, et al. A retrospective analysis of the costs and benefits related to alterations in cardiac surgery from routine intraoperative transesophageal echocardiography. Anesth Analg. 2002;95(4):824-7.
3. Campeau L. Letter: Grading of angina pectoris. Circulation. 1976;54(3):522-3.
4. Fleisher LA, Fleischmann KE, Auerbach AD, et al. 2014 ACC/AHA guideline on perioperative cardiovascular evaluation and management of patients undergoing noncardiac surgery: a report of the American College of Cardiology/American Heart Association Task Force on Practice Guidelines. J Am Coll Cardiol; 2014.
5. Hlatky MA, Boineau RE, Higginbotham MB, et al. A brief self-administered questionnaire to determine functional capacity (the Duke Activity Status Index). Am J Cardiol. 1989;64(10): 651-4.
6. Diprose P, Pierce JMT. Anaesthesia for patients with pacemakers and similar devices. Contin Educ Anaesth Crit Care Pain. 2001;1:166-70.
7. Parsonnet V, Dean D, Bernstein AD. A method of uniform stratification of risk for evaluating the results of surgery in acquired adult heart disease. Circulation. 1989;79(6):I3-12.
8. Nashef SA, Roques F, Michel P, et al. European system for cardiac operative risk evaluation (EuroSCORE). Eur J Cardiothorac Surg. 1999;16(1):9-13.
9. Malik M, Chauhan S, Mali V. Is EuroSCORE applicable to Indian patients undergoing cardiac surgery? Ann of Card Anaesth. 2010;13(3):241-5.
10. Roques F, Michel P, Goldstone AR, et al. The logistic EuroSCORE. Eur Heart J. 2003;24(9):881-2.

CHAPTER 39

Postcardiac Surgical Emergencies

Nishant Arora, Yatin Mehta

INTRODUCTION

Cardiac surgery is an evolving surgical specialty which had significant morbidity and mortality in past, but with streamlining of the specialty by protocols for every aspect of cardiac surgery the morbidity and mortality both have come down significantly in the last few decades.

Quality surgical as well as anesthetic care with utmost attention to every detail can further improve the outcomes.

POSTCARDIAC SURGICAL EMERGENCIES

Pathophysiology

Postcardiac surgical emergencies arise as:
- *Immediate*:
  - It can be as a result of paravalvular aortic or mitral regurgitation postvalve replacement or unintentional damage to coronaries while doing the valve repair or replacement. (The most notorious in this is the accidently involvement of left circumflex artery in mitral valve surgery).
  - Bleeding
  - Arrhythmias.
- *Early* as a direct effect of the kind of surgery done and its success, anticoagulants (i.e. heparin) and their reversal agent (i.e. protamine) used, excessive bleeding and early collection of blood around the heart.
  - Acute coronary syndrome (ACS) following surgery
  - Bleeding requiring re-exploration
  - Early tamponade—collection of blood around heart requiring re-exploration of the chest
  - Tension pneumothorax
  - Atrial fibrillation (AF) and other dysrhythmias
  - Stroke
  - Acute kidney injury (AKI)
  - Acute decompensated congestive heart failure or low cardiac output syndrome (LCOS)
  - Respiratory failure.
- *Delayed* because of partial or complete failure of surgery done, e.g. graft getting compromised post, coronary artery bypass graft (CABG) surgery or delayed tamponade.
  - ACS
  - Paravalvular aortic regurgitation (AR) or mitral regurgitation (MR)
  - Delayed tamponade
  - AKI
  - ADCHF
  - Respiratory failure.

IMMEDIATE POSTOPERATIVE COMPLICATIONS

Immediate Paravalvular Aortic Regurgitation or Mitral Regurgitation

If this is diagnosed immediately after coming off cardiopulmonary bypass (CPB) by transesophageal echocardiography (TEE).

Treatment

It requires going back on CPB and placing the valve in appropriate manner as to treat the paravalvular AR/MR.

However if it happens to be a delayed complication (delayed diagnosis or delayed presentation), it can also be treated in cardiac catheterization laboratory by device closure of the regurgitation.

Late Paravalvular Aortic Regurgitation or Mitral Regurgitation

Most of the paravalvular leaks are hemodynamically insignificant. However, large ones lead to heart failure, intravascular hemolysis and increased risk of infectious endocarditis. Hemolysis is also common in small paravalvular leaks. Redo surgeries are associated with very high risk which leads to development of transcatheter closure devices. These techniques are less invasive and of immense use in high-risk patients.

Diagnosis

Diagnosis is aided by continuing sign and symptoms of heart failure in postoperative period (or even later) with evidence of hemolysis like falling hematocrit, rising bilirubin, elevated lactate dehydrogenase (LDH) activity, changed reticulocyte counts, etc. The diagnosis is confirmed by echocardiography.

Treatment

It is either surgical or using the transcatheter closure devices. Reoperation is the choice of procedure when paravalvular leaks are associated with significant dysfunction or mechanical instability of the prosthetic valve or associated with infective endocarditis.

Transcatheter device closure is reserved for small paravalvular leaks.

Excessive Bleeding in a Postcardiac Surgery Patient

Excessive Bleeding

Considering the complexity of cardiac surgery, the inflammatory cascade generated by CPB machine and circuit, bleeding will remain an issue which requires due attention. But with the institutional protocols being in place for the kind of patients who will need to be reexplored for bleeding, the decision-making is not difficult.

What is Significant Bleeding?

Various criteria have been used to define excessive bleeding:
- As a rough guide, it is the chest tube and mediastinal tube drainage of more than 200 mL/h for 4 h, greater than 1,000 mL(s) in total, or a sudden drainage of 400 mL(s).
- Any sudden and significant increase in drainage is considered as a genuine reason to reexplore the mediastinum and chest because it signifies a disruption of surgical anastomosis or a slippage of clips or bleeding from aortic cannulation site.
- In pediatric cardiac surgeries, it is significant if the chest tube drainage and mediastinal tube drainage is more than 10 mL/kg in the first hour after the surgery or a total of more than 20 mL/kg over the first 3 hours after surgery.
- At times, postoperatively cardiac surgery patients bleed more. In such cases, early diagnosis and intervention helps in preventing impairment of hemodynamics, anemia, impairment of hemostasis, tamponade, and reduction of innate coagulation factors.
- Use of heparin and thrombolytic agents in preoperative period may leads to deranged hemostasis and increased risk of bleeding. Also the use of CPB leads to platelet destruction, dilutional coagulopathy, and activation of inflammatory and coagulation cascades. However, these are not the only factors leading to increased bleeding after any cardiac surgery.

Manage postoperative bleeding according to **Flow chart 1**.

Prophylaxis and Treatment Modalities

- Stop platelet inhibiting drugs in advance if possible (especially clopidogrel for 5-7 days)
- Avoid hypertension after aortotomy
- Rule out surgical cause and achieve hemostasis with reasonable speed (delaying closure also increases propensity to bleed)
- Limit fluids, dilution aids hemorrhage
- *Chest radiograph*: To get an idea of collection
- *Neutralize heparin*: More protamine is suggested in a dose of 0.5-1 mg/kg if activated clotting time (ACT) is more than 150 seconds or the activated partial thromboplastin time (aPTT) is more than 1.5 times control
- Warm the patient to above 36°C as hypothermia is known to increase bleeding tendencies
- Apply positive end-expiratory pressure (PEEP) of 5-10 cm H_2O. Although it has not a proven role, but it is still used with the theoretical rationale of a tamponade effect on the bleeders and oozing
- Desmopressin in the dose of 0.2-0.4 ug/kg intravenously is suggested when bleeding time is prolonged with expected platelet defect
- Epsilon aminocaproic acid in a bolus dose of 50 mg/kg, followed by 25 mg/kg/h is used as antifibrinolytic prophylaxis
- Similarly tranexamic acid in a bolus dose of 10 mg/kg, followed by 1 mg/kg/h can be used as antifibrinolytic prophylaxis
- Platelet transfusion in pediatrics is weight guided as a dose of 1 U/10 kg when platelet count is less than 100,000/mm^3. However in adults, platelet transfusion is not weight guided
- Fresh frozen plasma (FFP) in a dose of 15 mL/kg are transfused when the partial thromboplastin (PT) or aPTT is more than 1.5 times control
- Cryoprecipitate in dose of 1 U/4 kg when the fibrinogen levels are less than 1 g/L or 100 mg/dL
- Recombinant factor VIIa with a risk of graft occlusion in CABGs.

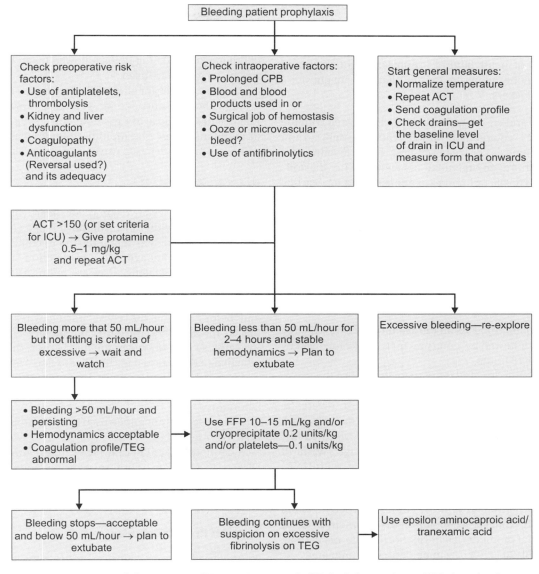

Flow chart 1 Management of excessive bleeding in postoperative period

Abbreviations: ACT, activated clotting time; ICU, intensive care unit; FFP, fresh-frozen plasma; TEG, thromboelastography; CPB, cardiopulmonary bypass; OR, operating room.

Acceptable Limit

Bleeding below 50 mL/h for 2 hours is acceptable to consider the patient for extubation.

Arrhythmias

Arrhythmias are one of the most common complications in the postoperative period after cardiac surgery.

Tachyarrhythmias

Postsurgically, most common arrhythmia seen is AF; commonly seen is stable AF, so does not require direct current shock as an emergent maneuver. Normally, amiodarone is given first as a slow bolus and followed by infusion.

Atrial fibrillation: After cardiac surgeries, AF is not a rare entity and occurs in nearly 30–40% of patients. While the cause is poorly understood, AF has a strong association with increased mortality and morbidity in terms of stroke and prolonged hospital stay.

The factors linked to the occurrence of AF are age, male sex, prior episode of AF, surgeries related to mitral valve, and a history of heart failure. Prophylaxis and treatment modalities can be achieved by amiodarone, magnesium, and/or beta-blockers.

Etiology: Fluid and electrolyte imbalance associated with the use of diuretics, enlargement of left atrium or right atrium because of stenosis or regurgitation of atrioventricular valves, left atrium enlargement associated with diastolic dysfunction, hypoxia, pulmonary embolism, and myocardial infarction.

Management of AF is rate control and if possible convert rhythm to sinus rhythm or rate control with anticoagulants.

Amiodarone is relatively less depressant to the heart than other antiarrhythmic drugs. It is used in the dose of 150–300 mg intravenously to manage acute postoperative AF. Its use is therefore justified in patients with poor left ventricular function than other antiarrhythmic drugs.

Regimen for amiodarone: As an intravenous infusion, 150 mg in 10 minutes, followed by 1 mg/min for 6 hours, followed by 0.5 mg/min for 18 hours.

Atrial fibrillation longing more than 48 justifies the use of echocardiography; preferably TEE to rule out left atrial clots. TEE should be done before any intervention to revert the rhythm. Use of thromboembolic prophylaxis in such cases is warranted. In those with risk factors like previous stroke, heart failure, diabetes mellitus, advanced age, warfarin is used with a target international normalized ratio (INR) between 2 and 3.

Ventricular fibrillation: It is most commonly occurs while coming off CPB, which is acceptable at that moment (it is not a surprise at that moment). Defibrillation by internal cardiac defibrillation 10–20 J (1–4 J/kg in pediatrics) is sufficient.

However, if it occurs late in the course like in postcardiac surgical intensive care unit (ICU), it is treated as any witnessed arrest with ventricular fibrillation and treated on the same lines. The only difference is that there can be internal cardiac massage after opening the chest if the need so arises. The dose for external defibrillation is 150–200 J biphasic.

Ventricular Tachycardia

Stable or unstable ventricular tachycardia (VT): Stable VT may be given a trial of medical treatment, however if unstable the treatment is again defibrillation.

Other arrhythmias are not very common in postcardiac surgery barring pediatric surgery where they may occur.

Prophylaxis and Management

Prophylaxis for arrhythmias: Though not proven with certainty to have a predictable antiarrhythmic, anti-ischemic effect, magnesium in the dose of 2 g slow intravenous dose and lignocaine 100 mg bolus followed by an infusion at the rate of 2 mg/min are used.

A universal drug for all kind of arrhythmias is amiodarone. Though there is no scientific evidence to support its use, magnesium in a dose of 2 g is frequently given prior to CABG in many institutes. The multidisciplinary team will have to come to a rationale based use of such drugs as a prophylaxis.

Bradycardias

Bradycardia, especially complete heart block, is most commonly seen either in aortic valve replacement (AVR) on adults or in ventricular septal repairs in children because of the unintended damage to the conduction system. For the same reason, the pacing wires are left in AVR for 72 hours and for nearly 48 hours in CABG or mitral valve replacement.

At the completion of the open heart procedure or CABG and before closing the chest, pacing wires are normally placed epicardially at the end of the surgery as a prophylactic measure, so that whenever the need arises, the wires can be attached to the external pacemaker to tide over the crisis.

Later, if the patient is pacing dependent, the patient may be given a permanent pacemaker in the cardiac catheterization laboratory.

The most common mode used in the postoperative period is DDD.

A cautionary note here is never to leave the patient with DOO or VOO because it is just a sensing mode.

EARLY POSTOPERATIVE COMPLICATIONS

Tension Pneumothorax

Normally in the immediate postsurgical time, this emergency is not seen because mediastinal and chest tubes are in place (unless the tubes are blocked with blood or kinked); however, it may occur on the side where the chest tube is not placed. It may also occur later in postoperative period when the chest tube is removed.

Most of the times, if it is tension pneumothorax it is diagnosed clinically and confirmed on chest X-ray (CXR) or while putting the chest drain on mere clinical suspicion.

If the hemodynamics suddenly gets deranged, differential diagnosis of tension pneumothorax should be kept in mind along with other causes. Check the chest tube or any blockade with blood, or crimping. And if found so, then release the blockade or crimping. If it does not get resolved, then place wide bore angiocaths in the anterolateral part of chest above

T4 level. Consider placing intercostal drain on ipsilateral side (with pneumothorax).

Pericardial Tamponade

Cardiac tamponade is a common but largely unrecognized cause of the low cardiac output syndrome after cardiac surgery. It happens when the heart gets compressed by blood and/or clots and/or fluid accumulating in the mediastinum.

Hemodynamic derangement due to tamponade is seen in nearly 3–6% of the patients requiring massive/multiple blood/blood products for bleeding after surgery.

Postoperative pericardial tamponade is called acute when it is within 24 hours of surgery. Delayed pericardial tamponade on the contrary develops after 10–14 days after surgery. Delayed tamponade is known to occur in patients on preoperative anticoagulants.

Reduced filling of the heart because of tamponade causes hemodynamic collapse. As the collection or tamponade increases, pressure inside heart increases in order to compensate. However, if the pressure because of tamponade is more than pressure because of filling inside the heart, diastolic collapse of ventricle (right ventricle first) happens leading to severe deterioration of hemodynamics. Reduced venous return leads to reduced filling (lesser end-diastolic volume) which in turn leads to reduced end-systolic volume. This explains the low-cardiac output syndrome in pericardial tamponade.

When the tamponade increases acutely or is severe because of the sheer volume of tamponade, the filling of the ventricle (especially right) occurs only during atrial systole.

Low-cardiac output causes increased sympathetic discharge to compensate by constricting veins to increase return to heart. Increased heart rate because of increased sympathetic discharge also compensates partially for the low-cardiac output syndrome.

Low-cardiac output, reduced atrial natriuretic factor (because of decreased atrial size and because of tamponade) and increased adrenergic discharge in turn lead to reduced urine output.

The tamponade that happens postoperatively is very different from tamponade arising of medical reasons (which happen slowly and is therefore well tolerated) because postoperative pericardial tamponade can be regional as well global, clotted and unclotted, pericardium open and communicating with the pleural cavity.

In a slowly increasing pericardial collection (especially medical), compensatory changes occurring over a period do not allow hemodynamic collapse even in presence of a major collection in the pericardial cavity (more than 1,000 mL).

Many surgeons leave the pericardial cavity open and in communication with pleural cavity, so, at times it may be well tolerated even with large volumes. If clotted however, and compressing on a particular chamber, it may produce severe symptoms, much in contrast to the volume, e.g. a localized clot behind atrium does not allow to fill and hence deranged hemodynamics.

The signs and symptoms in postsurgical tamponade may not be as seen in classical tamponade.

When to Consider?

If in a patient who had been bleeding significantly in postoperative period, and his bleeding appears to have reduced but the hemodynamic collapse still occurs then it is wise to think about tamponade.

Treatment includes intravenous fluids and inotropes but not those alone; getting a second opinion from a senior, bedside echocardiography and a CXR are very important in diagnosis. A very high degree of suspicion should be kept for this diagnosis.

If the hemodynamic suddenly deteriorates, it is advisable to open the chest and not wait for the diagnosis.

Diagnosis of tamponade is considered in a postcardiac surgery patient whose hemodynamics deteriorate along with (or without) a classical triad of lower blood pressure, increased heart rate and increased filling pressures, and/or low-cardiac output. However, it may also present as slowly increased requirement of inotropes and vasopressors.

The classic findings of elevated central venous pressure or equalization of intracavity pressures (in all chambers of heart) may or may not occur. Similar clinical picture is seen in postoperative biventricular failure. Intermittent positive pressure ventilation (IPPV) deteriorates it further because of excessive additional pressure on the heart leading to further reduction of filling. Increased pulse pressure variation and stroke volume variation with IPPV when seen with increased central venous pressure and reduced cardiac output should be sufficient to ring the bell toward tamponade.

With a widened cardiac shadow in CXR, significant pericardial collection on echocardiography, reduced drainage, and deranged hemodynamics—the patient is a candidate for urgent exploration of the chest for relieving tamponade.

Similarly, if you have a patient who is not maintaining hemodynamics despite two inotropes, and good amount of intravenous fluids, you must consider tamponade.

Management of Early Postoperative Complication

- *ECG*: Dampened QRS with tachycardia and electrical alternans
- *CXR*: Mediastinal widening; associated pleural effusion may be seen
- *Echocardiographic signs of tamponade*:
  - *Two-dimensional echocardiography*: Systolic collapse of right atrium and left atrium (atrial diastole) and diastolic collapse of right ventricular (RV) [left ventricular (LV) collapse does not occur, but occasionally it may occur] along with fluid all around

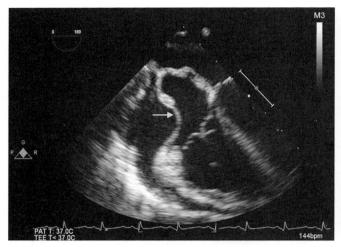

Fig. 1 Systolic collapse of right atrium in pericardial tamponade

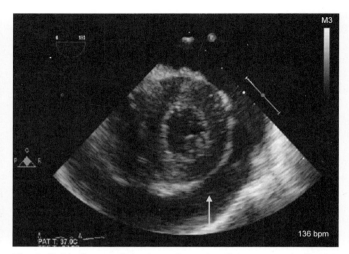

Fig. 3 Fluid all around the heart in pericardial tamponade (fluid is even around the anterior most part of heart indicating that it is severe)

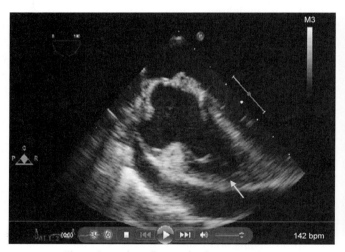

Fig. 2 Diastolic collapse of right ventricular in pericardial tamponade

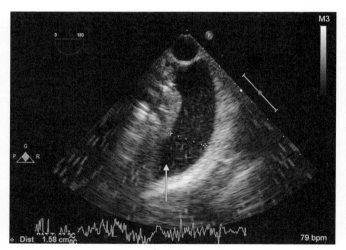

Fig. 4 Associated pleural collection in a case of pericardial tamponade (tiger claw sign depicting the left pleural collection: claw tip on left side)

the heart. However, these may not necessarily be seen in a postcardiac surgery patient **(Figs 1 to 4)**.

However, if the fluid is present all around the heart, more the fluid moves anterior, more is the severity.

Clotted blood may make TTE less sensitive for diagnosis, because the pericardial and ventricular wall delineation becomes difficult. Mechanical ventilation also makes TTE difficult. TEE is preferred if possible.

Note here that unclotted blood is echolucent whereas clotted blood is echodense and looks like myocardium.

Grading of severity of tamponade on two-dimensional echocardiography:
- *Mild*: Less than 0.5 cm at its maximum
- *Moderate*: 0.5–2 cm at its maximum
- *Severe*: More than 2 cm at its maximum.

However, the pericardial tamponade that occurs after surgery does not follow this index of severity. Rather, even a small amount of clotted blood behind right atrium may cause severe hemodynamic compromise by decreasing the inflow.

Management

The exploration of chest for removing clots and relieving tamponade is the definitive treatment. It may happen that the tamponade is acute and severe, in that case it may need to be explored as an emergency in postcardiac surgery unit only.

If tamponade occurs later than 2 weeks, it is justified to proceed with pericardiocentesis.

While the preparations are made to explore the chest, it is advisable to go liberal with intravenous fluids (IV) and increasing inotropic doses. Both these measures manage to improve cardiac output till definitive measures are taken.

Ventilation should be managed with lowest tidal volume and PEEP which allows acceptable gas exchange as the mechanical ventilation causes increased pressure on the already compromised heart and its venous return.

Sedation should be used with utmost caution as the innate sympathetic discharge may be compromised which is required to maintain hemodynamics.

Acute Coronary Syndrome Following Cardiac Surgery

Myocardial ischemia in postoperative period is not as uncommon as thought. It occurs in nearly 30–45% of patients who underwent CABG. It is detectable in the form of electrocardiogram (EKG) and echocardiographic changes in the form of regional wall motion abnormalities (RWMAs). Significant RWMAs are associated with worse outcomes.

Causes

Though there is revascularization of the heart but during the procedure itself, plaques can rupture; later in postoperative period grafts can clot or the lie of the grafts may make them prone to kinking and occlusion, air bubbles (especially in the immediate postoperative period while coming off CPB), stunning, tachycardia, excessive use of inotropes all can lead to acute myocardial infarction.

During valvular repair, coronary artery may get occluded accidentally and may lead to hemodynamic instability, most of the times immediately going back on CPB if recognized then and correcting the cause. The notorious amongst these is the left circumflex artery getting included while doing mitral valve repair or replacement.

The handling of the tissues during cardiac surgery leads to troponin I levels getting elevated even without myocardial infarction. The acceptable limit of troponin levels in postoperative period is 10 times the normal. However, if it exceeds 20 times the normal, it probably indicates ischemia and is associated with increased morbidity and mortality in postoperative period.

Postoperative ischemia is probably caused by the arterial grafts (left internal mammary artery graft and radial graft) or the native diseased vessels going in spasm. The reason for spasm is the endothelial dysfunction because of handling during surgery and preexisting atherosclerosis. Apart from the endothelial dysfunction, it can be due to the usage of vasoconstrictors, calcium, preoperative withdrawal of calcium channel blockers, probably thromboxane released by platelets causing the spasm.

The treatment for the vasospasm of the arterial grafts and native vessels is the use of glyceryl trinitrate (GTN) and/or calcium channel blockers (diltiazem) and/or phosphodiesterase inhibitors.

Some institutes have the policy for prophylactic use of GTN or calcium channel blockers for preventing vasospasm. Use of dilators for the purpose of vasospasm is fraught with the risk of low perfusion pressure for the coronaries itself and the increased need for volume.

Intra-aortic balloon counterpulsation (IABC) can be a great help in alleviating the crisis both by increasing flow to coronaries by diastolic pressure augmentation (inflation of balloon during diastole) and reduced afterload (deflation of balloon in systole), thereby reducing cardiac work and increasing oxygen supply to heart.

Intractable Hypotension or Vasoplegia

It is also commonly seen during postoperative period because of the CPB and because of the drugs like angiotensin converting enzyme inhibitors being used in preoperative period. It requires vasoconstrictors and if not corrected with that, one may have to proceed with the use of methylene blue.

It may not be amenable to even intravascular volume and vasoconstrictors like selective alpha-agonists or vasopressin. Administration of vasoconstrictors must be guided by objective assessment of cardiac function on pulmonary artery catheters/echocardiography/other monitoring, because optimization of blood pressure by vasoconstrictors may make us miss a LCOS state.

Gastrointestinal Emergencies

These require emergent surgical or medical care that are rare after cardiac surgery but these do occur in nearly 1% of patients undergoing cardiac surgery.

The most common complication among these is upper gastrointestinal bleeding from duodenal or gastric ulceration or varices. For this reason, the stress ulcer prophylaxis is important.

Mesenteric Ischemia

It is another dreaded complication that has a very high mortality. It may occur because of hypoperfusion that may happen during CPB or because of embolization to the splanchnic vessels during aortic manipulation. The embolization can be treated in catheterization laboratory by interventional radiologist if a removable thrombus is localized. Mortality remains high.

Stroke and Other Neurological or Neurosurgical Complications

What happens during surgery presents in the postoperative period as stroke/cognitive defects/focal deficits?

Neurosurgical Complications

The complications like subdural hematoma (SDH)/extradural hematoma (EDH) may happen inside operation theater and present in postoperative period. SDH may happen because of a heparinized patient (for putting in CPB) having poor venous drainage from brain (venous cannula malpositions). EDH also happens partially because of heparinization (for CPB) having undiagnosed cerebral aneurysms or very high blood pressure during the perioperative period.

Not all patients with the SDH or EDH require neurosurgical intervention for drainage. Only those with significant midline shifts on computed tomography (CT) scan need to be operated as emergency. Transferring these patients to CT suites is very tedious and risky because they may be on life support systems like ventilatory and inotropic support, although with the advent of portable CT at bedside, it has become easier.

Neurological Complications

What happens during surgery presents in the postoperative period as stroke/cognitive defects/focal deficits?

Stroke or cognitive defects: So, the treatment of perioperative stroke is actually preventive. The reason being that by the time it presents in the postoperative period as a deficit, the irreversible damage is already done.

Neurologic events happening in the postoperative period have a strong association with increased mortality, increased length of stay in ICU and hospital, and reduced lifespan. Neurological complication not only includes stroke but cognitive dysfunction, visual deficits, coma as well. In fact, cognitive dysfunction has an incidence of nearly 80% in the perioperative period. All these lead to a poor quality of life, even though the cardiac issue may be resolved.

Still therapies are tried with mixed benefits both in digital subtraction angiography (DSA) catheterization laboratory and as a neurosurgical procedure.

The incidence of these neurological emergencies, postcardiac surgery is not very high but its occurrence is ominous. With the improved preventive and therapeutic techniques there is improved survival rate and lifespan. Because of rising population in general and geriatric population surviving more, the requirement of cardiac surgeries is increasing.

Neurological injuries are more common after heart surgery in the geriatric age group. Though the mortality rate because of cardiac surgeries have gone down, but the rate of neurological complications have remained nearly the same. The neurological injuries in the perioperative period leads to nearly 20% increased mortality in comparison to those without neurological dysfunction. The morbidity also increases in the population with neurological deficits in the perioperative period. The mechanism of neurological injuries is cerebral embolism and hypoperfusion because of low perfusion pressure, inflammatory mediators because of CPB, preexisting neurological deficits or problems.

Hemodynamic Instability

Periods of hemodynamic instabilities are more than numbered while undergoing cardiac surgeries especially CABG that too in geriatric patients who may have compromised circulation to the brain. The fall in mean arterial pressure by 10 mm Hg or more during cardiac surgery is associated with a three times risk for stroke and more for cognitive deficits.

Diabetes mellitus (poorly controlled DM) and age (with increasing age) are associated more with neurological episodes especially with poorer outcomes.

Once cerebral injury is diagnosed, the main measures to be taken in the ICU are:
- Glucose control
- Prevention of hypertension
- Prevention of seizures
- Maintenance of normoxia and normocarbia
- Prevention of raised intracranial pressure.

AKI or Cardiac Surgery-associated AKI (CSA-AKI)

Cardiac surgery-associated-AKI as the name indicates is AKI associated with cardiac surgery. It has a huge impact on the quality of life in perioperative period and even in later life after surgery. The etiology of this complication is governed by multiple factors especially related to perioperative management and use of pharmacological agents.

Significant implications for short- and long-term outcomes are:
- Increased infections
- Increased stay in hospital and increased ICU stay
- Later, dependency on dialysis
- Greater mortality.

Risk Factors of CSA-AKI

- Advanced age
- Female gender
- Severe left ventricle dysfunction
- Congestive heart failure (CHF)
- Diabetes mellitus (DM)
- Peripheral vascular disease
- Chronic obstructive pulmonary disease (COPD)
- Valve surgery
- Emergency surgery
- Prolonged CPB time
- Excessive and prolonged hemodilution on CPB
- Combined procedures and severe left ventricular (LV) dysfunction
- Use of IABP
- Preoperatively elevated serum creatinine (SCr).

It is seen in up to 30% of subjects after CPB. Fortunately, only up to 5% require dialysis, but in that 5%, the mortality rate is very high. AKI is the strongest independent risk factor for death after CPB.

The risk is least in CABG alone, but increases exponentially for valve replacement and is greatest after combined procedures.

Unfortunately, this complication and its effect on mortality have not reduced despite better understanding of pathophysiology, pharmacotherapeutics, and the advances in renal replacement therapy (RRT).

Diagnosis

The AKI is a complex diagnosis. Many diagnostic criteria have been applied for the AKI (for example, percentage change in serum creatinine, requirement for hemodialysis).

There are two classifications, which need special mention:
1. The risk injury failure loss end-stage kidney disease (RIFLE) classification (glomerular filtration rate, creatinine and urine output).
2. Acute kidney injury network (AKIN) classification (creatinine and urine output).

Even these well-validated criteria based classifications are not completely reliable as these do not guide about the actual site of kidney injury whether tubular or glomerular. Also, both these depend more on change in serum creatinine.

Society of thoracic surgeons (STS) bedside risk tool and many other such models are used to predict the kidney dysfunction or need for dialysis in advance.

Newer biomarkers are also being studied to help in the early detection of AKI. Early detection of AKI leads to early institution of RRT and better outcomes.

Serum Creatinine

It is not sensitive and not consistent in diagnosis. It has a significant time lag in the diagnosis of AKI as well as its recovery. Multiple factors apart from AKI govern the increase and decrease of serum creatinine. Also, it does not guide about the nature of kidney injury whether ischemic or prerenal.

Other newer markers, which were found to have a better association with AKI, are NGAL (neutrophil gelatinase-associated lipocalin), KIM-1 (kidney injury molecule-1), IL-18 (interleukin-18), and L-FABP (liver-type fatty acid binding protein).

The risk of AKI requiring dialysis: 10–20% with baseline creatinine of 2.0–4.0 mg/dL and 25%, if more than 4.0 mg/dL

Perioperative Management of AKI-CPB

Perioperative management of AKI-CPB is described in **Flow chart 2**.

Goals:
- To maintain and replete intravascular volume
- Optimizing cardiac output or treating left ventricular failure
- Avoid nephrotoxic agents whenever possible
- Discontinue angiotensin converting enzyme inhibitors (ACEIs) or angiotensin II receptor blockers (ARBs) though its benefit is doubtful; in fact in diabetic nephropathy, it has been shown to be beneficial
- Maintaining adequate tissue perfusion primary goal
- Reasonable glycemic control and outcomes (<180 mg/dL, avoid fluctuations)
- Nesiritide or recombinant atrial natriuretic peptide has shown good results but larger trials are needed
- Avoid anemia (especially on CPB) but at the same time avoid excessive transfusion, because anemia decreases the renal DO_2, increases oxidative stress, and impaired hemostasis and transfused stored RBCs decrease tissue DO_2, is pro-inflammatory, increases oxidative stress, activates leukocytes and coagulation cascade
- Fenoldopam (D1 receptor agonist) also has shown positive results in smaller trials. Preoperative RRT as a prophylaxis in preoperative period for optimization is another option
- Be meticulous in closing and hemostasis as any reexploration is an added insult and the combination of

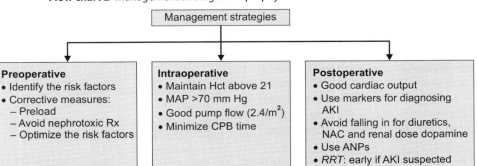

Flow chart 2 Management strategies for prophylaxis and treatment of CSA-AKI

Abbreviations: Hct, hematocrit; MAP, mean arterial pressure; CPB, cardiopulmonary bypass; NAC, N-acetylcysteine; RRT, renal replacement therapy; CSA-AKI, cardiac surgery-associated acute kidney injury; ANP, atrial natriuretic peptide.

insults including associated anemia and blood transfusion contribute to AKI
- Optimizing cardiac surgical procedure and CPB parameters

Alternate Strategies in Management of CPB

Pediatrics

Ultrafiltration (UF) has been studied a lot for its benefit for AKI. It is safe and reduces perioperative morbidity. The optimal use of UF is combined use of conventional ultrafiltration and modified ultrafiltration. More studies in larger trials are required for using ultrafiltration in a better way. There is still no consensus on best timing of initiation of RRT.

What Fluids to Use?

A good preload is important for prevention of AKI, but we are unclear as to what fluids are better for kidney. Recent studies have shown that PlasmaLyte is better than saline in reducing the risk of AKI in perioperative period. The chloride restriction reduces AKI as well as the need for renal replacement therapy.

The chloride is detrimental because of its thromboxane release, renal vasoconstrictive effect, and decreased GFR. Dexmedetomidine may also be beneficial.

Decompensated Heart Failure

In postcardiac surgery, decompensated heart failure may be encountered more often.

The causes may be preoperative left ventricular dysfunction, poor myocardial protection during CPB, prolonged CPB and cross-clamp time; chronic regurgitant lesions with left ventricular dysfunction, graft failure, involvement of coronaries in valve surgery.

It is one of the most common conditions requiring active management in the perioperative period. Postoperatively, decompensated heart failure is seen as an early occurrence of classical signs and symptoms of heart failure secondary to suboptimal heart function, often in those with preexisting heart failure. However, it does not mean that the ADCHF is an entity not seen in previously healthy subjects. It means that the clinicians should have a high index of suspicion for this condition in the perioperative period and the required skill in managing it.

Management of ADCHF in the perioperative period is very demanding and requires the in-depth knowledge of the pathophysiology behind ADCHF in perioperative period.

The myocardial stunning causes injury to heart which happens during CPB and it sometimes takes quite a long time to recover. During this time of recovery, we need to support heart by pharmacological means and support devices.

Pharmacological means: The intended purpose behind the pharmacological means is to support or improve the contractility while reducing the afterload or SVR at the same time.

The choice between the inotropes rests between drugs like adrenaline (0.05–0.2 µg/kg/min), milrinone (0.3–0.7 µg/kg/min), dopamine (5–20 µg/kg/min), (not much preferred because of the arrhythmogenic nature and the unwanted tachycardia), dobutamine (5–20 µg/kg/min). While all these drugs increase the contractility, only milrinone and dobutamine decrease the systemic vascular resistance (SVR) as well and that way seem more suitable.

The disadvantage with milrinone is that it cannot be used for a longer period as it produces thrombocytopenia, and that it reduces the SVR exponentially, at times so severe as to require a vasopressor to counter the effect and hence nullifying the purpose.

The devices that help the heart tide over the crisis are suitably called assist devices. The most common amongst these is the IABC which improves the coronary flow during diastole by getting inflated during diastole and reducing the afterload in systole by getting deflated during systole.

Use of IABC has been discussed earlier.

Postoperative Respiratory Failure

Postcardiac surgery respiratory failure is seen as ventilator dependency and may or may not be a direct complication of the cardiac surgery. The reason being, it may be a preexisting COPD or asthma leading to a type 2 respiratory failures (RFs), i.e. lack of drive leading to CO_2 retention and accompanying hypoxemia. In this case, however, the hypoxemia is very responsive to simple measures like increasing fraction of inspired oxygen (FiO_2) by a minimal proportion.

As a direct complication of the cardiac surgery, it occurs as type 1 RF which means a failure of exchange of gases, because of decompensated ADCHF or preexisting or new onset chest infection may not even respond to a FiO_2 of 100% if not accompanied by other measures. So, type 1 RF requires not just raising the FiO_2 but also raising the PEEP, antibiotics, chest physiotherapy, frequent suctioning, and other supportive measures.

Both these two classic types of RFs have distinctly different abnormalities in the mechanics of breathing, but they share the mechanisms finally leading to RF dysfunction, fatigue and hence ventilator dependence.

Types of Respiratory Failure

Type I RF: Severe hypoxemia which is nonresponsive to oxygen because of shunting of the pulmonary blood flow without oxygen pickup.

Type II RF: Increased partial pressure of CO_2 and accompanying hypoxemia caused by hypoventilation reason being the loss of drive at the respiratory center in central nervous system and/or suboptimal neuromuscular function and/or excess of dead space (COPD).

Type III RF: Reduced functional residual capacity (obesity/diaphragmatic muscular relaxation/effect of anesthesia) when combined with rising closing volume (especially in geriatric population) produces atelectasis and in turn leading to respiratory failure (resembling type I/type II or both).

Type IV RF: Circulatory failure or shock leading to RF. Its characteristic is that it is responsive to the treatment of shock.

Treatment

Treatment of any type of RF includes these key elements other than the chest supportive measures:
- Improvement of cardiac function
- Achieving improved oxygen carrying capacity by improving hemoglobin
- Improving arterial saturation
- Reducing oxygen requirement.
  The end point of each therapy is individualized.

Early freedom from ventilator dependency is done by prompt identification and correction of multiple factors which had been the cause of increased work load and/or compromised neuromuscular functions.

Aggressive early resuscitation is very important to avoid the vicious cycle of ventilator dependence. Acute management in such patients follow airway, breathing and chest compression (ABC) of resuscitation and not chest compression, airway and breathing (CAB) of the recent guidelines of cardiopulmonary resuscitation (CPR), because here the concern is RF. This means these patients need airway, ventilator management, and optimal management of circulation.

However, at the same time, open-minded approach is kept for prompt diagnosis and treatment plan for the cause of such condition early in course. It is guided not just by the clinical examination and laboratory evaluation but also supplemented by the results of focused intensive care interventions.

Reducing oxygen demand and improving delivery of oxygen: With its acceptable risks, tracheal intubation or noninvasive ventilation (NIV) ensures delivery of the high FiO_2. Also, it reduces the oxygen demand. Under normal circumstances, the work of breathing is very low, but in patients with acute hypoxemic RF (type I) and its associated tachypnea and lung stiffness, oxygen demand of the respiratory muscles alone can approach 100 mL/min. Increased work of breathing may result in high oxygen demand in other patients with other causes of restriction such as morbid obesity.

Optimizing cardiac output and hematocrit: Patients with LCOS because of preexisting heart disease may not tolerate large infusion of packed red blood cells (PRBCs). At the same time, it is a well-known fact that tissue hypoxia is made worse by concurrent anemia. In these kind of situations, a slow transfusion of packed cells may prevent anaerobic metabolism at a time, especially when cardiac output cannot be increased to adequate levels.

Management is also dependent on the type of RF:

The treatment for hypercapnia (type II RF) is different from the treatment for hypoxemia [type I acute hypercapnic respiratory failure (AHRF)]

Type I AHRF, where cyanosis, tachypnea, and refractory hypoxemia lead to early identification of airspace flooding by physical and radiologic examinations, it includes cardiogenic or permeability pulmonary edema, pneumonia, and lung hemorrhage, each having specific etiologies and therapy.

Therapy for patients with AHRF includes: (1) High FiO_2, e.g. high flow nasal oxygen cannula, (2) ventilator management so as to have minimal respiratory work, (3) low tidal volume strategy, (4) PEEP enough to have more than 90% saturation at minimal FiO_2, and (5) cardiovascular management to reduce airspace edema with an adequate cardiac output and oxygen transport to the peripheral tissues.

Management of type II RF or ventilatory failure: It needs attention to preventing atelectasis and correcting hypoperfusion until the abnormal neurologic condition resolves; bronchodilator therapy and ventilator settings to minimize intrinsic PEEP until the airways resistance is reduced sufficiently for the respiratory muscles to achieve adequate ventilation to be weaned off the ventilator. Initially, NIV may be tried but if not effective, invasive mechanical ventilation is done.

Perioperative Respiratory Failure

Occurs in patients in the perioperative period who are unusually susceptible to atelectasis, obesity, ascites, etc. surgery leading to splinting of thorax which reduces the end-expired lung volume and functional residual capacity (FRC) below the increased closing volume leading to progressive collapsed lung. Features can be of type I RF, or type II RF, or both. Treatment should be aimed at preventing lung collapse.

Approach to Management

Approach to management of perioperative respiratory failure has common modalities for both type I and type II RF:
- Changing position every 1–2 hours
- Chest physiotherapy and endotracheal suction
- 30°–45° head up tilt reduces the abdominal splinting effect
- NIV returns the end-expired lung volume to a position above the patient's closing volume

- Treatment of incisional pain (e.g. epidural anesthesia)
- Discontinuation of smoking at least 6 weeks prior to surgery makes a lot of difference and should be adhered to.

Hypoperfusion States Cause Type IV Respiratory Failure

Occurs in patients who have been intubated and stabilized with ventilatory support during resuscitation from a hypoperfusion state, type IV RF is most commonly due to cardiogenic, hypovolemic, or septic shock without associated pulmonary problems. Liberation from the ventilator of the patient with type IV RF is simple. When shock is corrected, the patient resumes spontaneous breathing and is extubated.

Respiratory muscle exercise for the recovered muscles and rest for the muscles which are fatigued go hand in hand for the weaning from ventilator in any respiratory failure.

CONCLUSION

To conclude, it is very optimistic to know and say that amongst all other surgical fields, the outcomes of cardiac surgery have become excellent, reason being it is driven by very strict protocols. Also, the postcardiac surgical emergencies are getting rarer because of advanced monitoring of vital parameters. In the coming times, point of care monitoring for excessive bleeding and the liberal use of TEE for any hemodynamic instability in postoperative period will actually reduce the two common complications, i.e. bleeding and tamponade apart from other complications getting diagnosed early like paravalvular regurgitation.

Mortality is already less; future lies in reducing the morbidity.

BIBLIOGRAPHY

1. Andropoulos DB, Brady KM, Easley RB, et al. Neuroprotection in Pediatric Cardiac surgery: What is On the horizon? Prog Pediatr Cardiol. 2010;29(2):113-222.
2. Grogan K, Stearns J, Hogue CW. Brain Protection in Cardiac Surgery. Anesthesiol Clin. 2008;26(3):521-38.
3. Hogue CW Jr, Palin CA, Arrowsmith JE. Cardiopulmonary bypass management and neurologic outcomes: an evidence-based appraisal of current practices. Anesth Analg. 2006;103(1):21-37.
4. Jesse Hall, John Kress, Gregory Schmidt (Eds). Principles of Critical Care, 4th edition. New York, NY: McGraw-Hill; 2015.
5. Joel A Kaplan, David L Reich, Steven N Konstadt (Eds). Kaplan's Cardiac Anesthesia: The Echo Era, 6th edition. Elsevier Health Sciences; 2011.
6. Joel L Kaplan (Ed). Miller's Anesthesia, 8th edition. Saunders; 2011.
7. Loepke AW, Priestley MA, Schultz SE, et al. Desflurane improves neurologic outcome after low-flow cardiopulmonary bypass in newborn pigs. Anesthesiology. 2002;97(6):1521-7.
8. Maiese K, Li F, Chong ZZ. New avenues of exploration for erythropoietin. JAMA. 2005;293(1): 90-5.
9. McAuliffe JJ, Loepke AW, Miles L, et al. Desflurane, isoflurane, and sevoflurane provide limited neuroprotection against neonatal hypoxia-ischemia in a delayed preconditioning paradigm. Anesthesiology. 2009;111(3):533-46.
10. McCullough JN, Zhang N, Reich DL, et al. Cerebral metabolic suppression during hypothermic circulatory arrest in humans. Ann Thorac Surg. 1999;67(6):1895-9.
11. McPherson RJ, Juul SE. Recent trends in erythropoietin-mediated neuroprotection. Int J Dev Neurosci. 2008;26(1):103-11.
12. Naureckas ET, Wood LH. The pathophysiology and differential diagnosis of acute respiratory failure. In: Hall JB, Schmidt GA, Kress JP, (Eds). Principles of Critical Care, 4th edition. New York, NY: McGraw-Hill; 2015.

SECTION 4

Respiratory Emergencies

- **Hemoptysis**
  Poulomi Chatterji, Bhawna Sharma

- **Acute Respiratory Failure**
  Chitra Mehta, Yatin Mehta

- **Acute Exacerbation of Asthma and Chronic Obstructive Pulmonary Disease**
  Ashish Kumar Prakash, Bornali Datta, Anand Jaiswal

- **Pneumonia**
  Ashish Kumar Prakash, Bornali Datta, Anand Jaiswal

- **Pneumothorax and Insertion of Chest Tube**
  Shaiwal Khandelwal, Ali Zamir Khan

- **Pulmonary Embolism**
  Saleh Fares, Omar Ghazanfar

CHAPTER 40

Hemoptysis

Poulomi Chatterji, Bhawna Sharma

INTRODUCTION

Hemoptysis is the expectoration of blood in sputum. The location may be upper respiratory tract, vocal cords, tracheobronchial tree or lung parenchyma.[1] Identification of location is important for proper management of the symptom. In most cases hemoptysis is self-limiting, but may be life-threatening. The difficulty in management of hemoptysis lies in the fact that it is difficult to predict which episode may be a massive one. Thus timely intervention is important.[2]

MASSIVE HEMOPTYSIS

There is no fixed definition. Various studies have quoted varying amounts—ranging from 100 mL to 600 mL over 24 hours. Most intensivists define massive hemoptysis as either more than or equal to 500 mL over 24 hours or 100 mL/hour. The cause of death may either be asphyxiation due to airway flooding by blood or aspiration.[1] Irrespective of the source of bleed, the bad prognostic factors are:
- Rate of bleed (most important)
- Amount of bleed
- Underlying condition of the lung
- Amount of blood aspirated in the lung.

Causes[3-6]

- *Pseudohemoptysis*:
  - Upper respiratory bleed
  - Hematemesis
- *Trauma*:
  - Penetrating chest trauma
  - Iatrogenic
  - Blunt chest trauma
- *Infective*:
  - Tuberculosis (active or healed—most common cause in India)
  - Bronchiectasis
  - Mycetoma and invasive mucormycosis
  - Pneumonia
  - Lung abscess
  - Parasitic (e.g. *Paragonimus*)
- *Neoplasm*:
  - Lung cancer
  - Bronchial adenoma
  - Metastasis to airway or lung parenchyma
- *Iatrogenic*:
  - Bronchoscopy
  - Airway stent
  - Aortobronchial fistula due to aortic graft or stent
  - Transthoracic needle aspiration
  - Pulmonary arterial catheterization
  - Erosion of tracheal tube to innominate artery
- *Cardiovascular*:
  - Arteriovenous malformation
  - Pulmonary infarction
  - Congenital heart disease
  - Mitral stenosis
  - Heart failure
  - Tricuspid endocarditis
- *Coagulopathies*:
  - Thrombocytopenia
  - Thrombasthenia
  - Disseminated intravascular coagulation
  - Iatrogenic
- *Others*:
  - Anticoagulants or antiplatelet agents
  - Dropsy

- Cocaine
- Nitrogen dioxide toxicity
- Bevacizumab therapy
- Anti-glomerular basement membrane disease (Goodpasture syndrome)
- Idiopathic hemosiderosis
- Granulomatosis with polyangiitis (Wegener's granulomatosis)
- Catamenial hemoptysis.

PULMONARY CIRCULATION

Lungs have dual blood supply:
1. Pulmonary artery
2. Bronchial artery.

Pulmonary Artery

Primarily involved in gas exchange process, arises from right ventricle. It is a low resistance system and a high volume system. It accounts for more than 99% of blood supply and less than 10% of causes of hemoptysis. Beyond terminal bronchioles it anastomosis with bronchial circulation for gas exchange.[6]

Bronchial Artery

It serves as a nutritional source of circulation. It arises from the systemic vascular bed. There are one or two arteries per lung commonly arising from aorta and at times from intercostal arteries. It is a high pressure (systemic pressure) system. In diseased lungs it often becomes tortuous and anastomosis with the pulmonary veins also get exaggerated (e.g. Rasmussen's aneurysm). Thus bleeding from bronchial artery rupture is more profuse than pulmonary artery rupture.[7]

EVALUATION (FLOW CHART 1)

As the patient presents to the emergency, one should try to answer the following questions:
- Rate of bleed and amount of bleeding
- Underlying pulmonary reserve
- Etiologic diagnosis
- Site of bleed.[8]

The given below questions can be asked.[3-5]

Present Episode

- Amount of blood coughed out
- Nature of expectoration—purulent or mucoid
- Is the episode recurrent?
- Any other site of bleed—nose, rectum, and gums
- Is it associated with breathlessness, rash or loss of weight and fever?

RISK FACTORS

- Is the patient smoker? If yes then pack years, whether current or past.
- Is there a known bleeding disorder?
- Is the patient taking any medication—antiplatelet, anticoagulant and aspirin?
- History of tuberculosis or exposure to the same?
- Was there history of thoracic stenting, recent hospitalization, deep vein thrombosis or any other suspected pulmonary, renal or cardiac disease?

FAMILY HISTORY

- Similar episode in family—in addition history of gastrointestinal bleed, and epistaxis.
- History of pulmonary embolism in family.

PHYSICAL EXAMINATION

- Is the patient dyspneic (using accessory muscles of respiration, tachypnic or cyanotic)
- Is the patient clubbed (suggestive of bronchiectasis and lung cancer)?
- Is there blood in the nose?
- Are there telangiectasias in the lips, tongue, or oral cavity?
- Are there skin rashes suggestive of vasculitis, systemic lupus erythematosus, infective endocarditis or fat embolism?
- Are there any adventitious sounds on auscultation (crepitations and bronchial breath sounds)?
- Is there a P2 component or murmur of tricuspid regurgitation suggestive of pulmonary hypertension?
- Is there a bruit suggestive of pulmonary arteriovenous malformation?
- Is there a heart murmur suggestive of mitral stenosis, mitral regurgitation, or septic emboli?
- Is there calf muscle tenderness suggestive of deep vein thrombosis?
- Saddle nose deformity with septal perforation and rhinitis suggestive of Wegener's granulomatosis.

INVESTIGATIONS

Investigations should be targeted for:
- Cause of bleed
- Starting treatment.

Laboratory Investigations

Blood investigations like complete blood count, platelet count, liver and renal function tests, coagulation profile, blood grouping and crossmatching studies should be done. Arterial blood gas analysis should be done to analyze the gas exchange abnormalities due to hemoptysis. Chest X-ray, urine analysis, antiglomerular antibodies should be analyzed if vasculitis is suspected. Sputum should be analyzed if infectious etiology is suspected. Sputum can also be analyzed for if malignant etiology is suspected.

Chest X-ray is useful in identifying lung mass, cavitary lesion or vasculitic lesion **(Fig. 1)**.[7]

Multidetector computed tomography (MDCT) is useful in identifying the site of bleed and also the etiology of bleed, especially the bronchial circulation.

Computed Tomography

It is useful in determination of site of bleed and parenchymal lesions like pulmonary tuberculosis, bronchogenic carcinoma, aspergilloma and airway lesions like bronchiectasis **(Figs 2 to 4)**. Contrast enhanced films are preferred as these would show structures like arteriovenous malformations, aneurysms. However, if a patient is too unstable to be moved in for a computed tomography scan, bronchoscopy should be performed first.[9-11]

Bronchoscopy

Bronchoscopy is the first-line investigation in a patient with massive hemoptysis. Rigid bronchoscopy should be the ideal tool. It not only helps in localizing the source of bleed but also helps in therapeutic measures better due to a larger working channel and better airway protection. However, it requires general anesthesia and cannot help to visualize beyond trachea and main bronchi.

Flexible bronchoscopy is good as a bedside procedure, can help to localize lesions up to the segmental level especially the central ones. However, the working channel being narrow poses a difficulty in airway protection, suctioning especially in massive hemoptysis. Thus in an ideal situation, combined use of both would be most useful **(Fig. 5)**.[12-15]

INITIAL RESUSCITATION

Airway

- Maintenance of airway is the first priority in management.
- Single lumen endotracheal tube is the first choice for intubation as it enables for suctioning and fiber-optic bronchoscopy.
- Double lumen endotracheal tube is useful to isolate and ventilate lung but only if bleeding site is isolated.

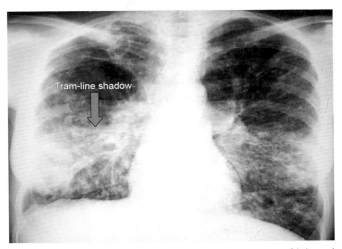

Fig. 1 Chest X-ray posteroanterior (PA) view suggestive of bilateral lower and middle zones tram-line shadows, cystic shadows suggestive of bronchiectasis

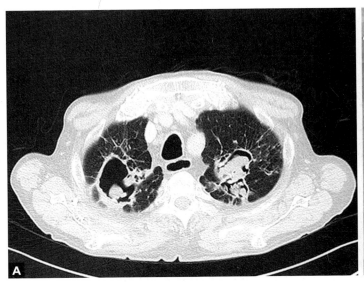
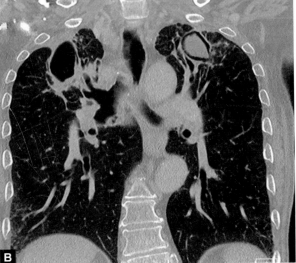

Figs 2A and B Bilateral upper lobar cavities with aspergilloma with bronchiectatic changes. Patient had presented with hemoptysis

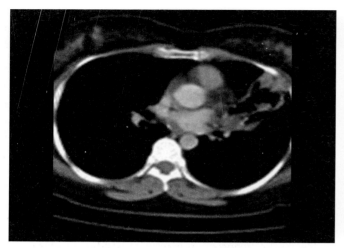

Fig. 3 Left upper lobe bronchiectasis, with mucous plugging (partial). This patient also presented with massive hemoptysis

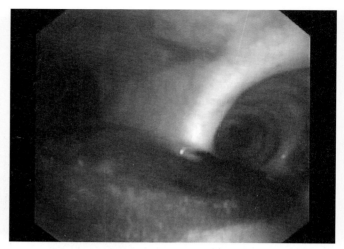

Fig. 5 Bronchoscopy showing bleeding from left main bronchus and spilling into right main bronchus

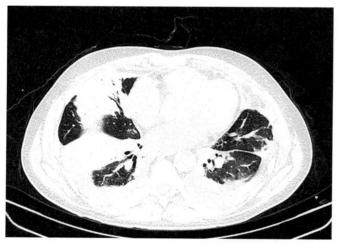

Fig. 4 Bilateral consolidation—patient presented with moderate hemoptysis

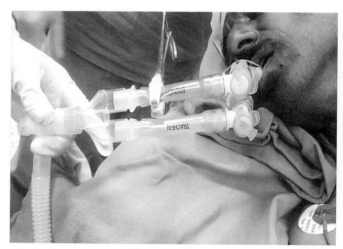

Fig. 6 Double-lumen endobronchial tube—blue colored part is the bronchial tube and transparent one is the tracheal tube

However, it requires expertise and not available in all centers. Moreover the lumen gets easily blocked by clots (Fig. 6).

Breathing

Massive amount of bleed in the airway causes difficulty in gas exchange. Saturation has to be maintained and above 95%, supplemental oxygen may be required. To prevent blood trickling to contralateral lung, patient to be positioned in lateral decubitus position on the bleeding side.

Circulation

At least two large bore intravenous lines should be inserted, fluid resuscitation should be started. Samples for grouping and crossmatching should be sent. If hemoptysis continues, O+ blood should be transfused.

LOCALIZATION OF SITE

History and physical examination is useful in localization of lesion in around 50% of cases.

Bronchoscopy is the first investigation of choice. Bronchoscopy done early during massive hemoptysis increases the likelihood of localization. However during bouts of massive hemoptysis, fiber-optic bronchoscope usage becomes difficult given its narrow working channel.

TOPICAL BRONCHOSCOPIC THERAPY

- Bronchoscopic irrigation with iced solution using 50 mL aliquots is useful in hemoptysis. The mechanism of action may be due to ice-induced local vasoconstriction.
- Use of epinephrine (1:20,000) is often useful in bleeding induced by endobronchial or transbronchial lung biopsy, however, its use in massive hemoptysis is not proved.
- Bronchoscopy induced topical hemostatic therapy.

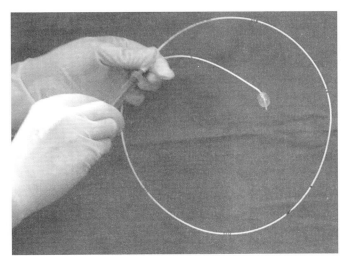

Fig. 7 Fogarty's catheter with inflated balloon before insertion

- Balloon tamponade using 4 Fr 100 cm long Fogarty's catheter which on inflation can stop bleeding up to the subsegmental bronchi. The balloon can be kept inflated for 48 hours. If no bleeding in next 6–8 hours of observation, it can be removed. Balloon tamponade is useful as a temporary measure preempting surgery or embolization **(Fig. 7)**.
- Tamponade therapy using oxidized regenerated cellulose (ORC) mesh has been found to be useful.[12-15]

MEDICAL TREATMENT

Medical management consists of maintenance of an adequate airway and to adopt measures to control bleeding. Patients are advised for rest and to take lateral decubitus with the affected side down. Cough suppressant and anxiolytics are usually advised, but should be weighed cautiously because they causes drowsiness and loss of cough reflex. If coagulopathy or thrombocytopenia is present, should be corrected with vitamin K, fresh frozen plasma and platelet transfusions. Generally, anemia is absent in acute hemoptysis, however, if symptomatic with other sources of bleeding, blood transfusions should be planned. In case of tubercular etiology, antitubercular therapy should be started. Broad-spectrum antibiotics should be prescribed to control bacterial inflammation in conditions like pneumonia or bronchiectasis.[2]

BRONCHIAL ARTERY EMBOLIZATION[21]

Arteriography should be opted for when hemoptysis is not controlled by therapeutic measures with bronchoscopy. Nonbronchial systemic collateral system feeding the axillary, subclavian arteries may also feed parenchymal cavities and arteriography identifies them. Embolotherapy is done with materials like polyvinyl alcohol, gelatin sponges, steel coils, etc. Recurrent hemoptysis may warrant arteriography of the pulmonary vessels. Rate of success in hemoptysis control varies in different studies ranging from 73% to 90% ranging from a period of follow-up of 1 to 60 months.[16]

Complications depend on the experience of interventionist. Rate of complications vary from 5% to 15%. Spinal cord damage is reported when embolization is done in a branch supplying spinal cord (anterior spinal artery).

Recurrent hemoptysis is seen in patients with multiple collaterals, especially in chronic lung disease (posttubercular lesion) and mycetoma. In that case, embolization may be used as a temporary measure before surgery.[16-20]

SURGERY[7,20-22]

The surgery indicated is a thoracotomy—may be video-assisted (VATS)—a lobectomy or pneumonectomy.

Indications

- Conservative measures like bronchoscopic tamponade or bronchial arterial embolization have failed.
- When there is contraindication for bronchial artery embolization (dye allergy and spinal artery arising from bronchial artery).
- Definitive therapy in patients (e.g. mycetoma) when patient is stable.
- Specific indications like:
  - Tracheoinominate fistula
  - Arteriovenous malformation
  - Chest injuries—penetrating
  - Aortic aneurysm
  - Hydatid cyst.

Contraindications

- Bilateral or diffuse disease
- Presence of pulmonary hypertension
- Severe hypoxemia and CO_2 retention
- Inoperable lung cancer.

The main complications post-surgery include:
- Persistent air leak from stump
- Infection of the stump
- In case spread of blood to opposite lung—pneumonia and sepsis. However, with the success of bronchoscopic tamponade and bronchial artery embolization, emergency surgeries have become uncommon.

CONCLUSION

Massive hemoptysis has a worse outcome when underlying lung is diseased, rate of bleed is high and bleeding volume is massive. However, timely interventions especially choosing proper candidates for interventions have significantly improved outcomes.

Flow chart 1 Evaluation and management of hemoptysis

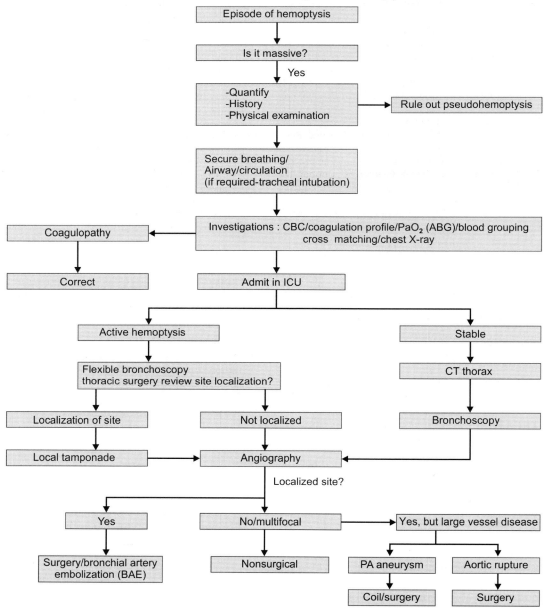

CLINICAL PEARLS

- Hemoptysis is a condition that warrants evaluation.
- Massive hemoptysis is potentially life-threatening condition and patients should be admitted in intensive care unit.
- History and clinical evaluation is helpful in assessing site of bleed.
- Laboratory investigations like coagulation profile, hemoglobin, etc. should be sent on an urgent basis.
- Radiological investigations like chest X-ray and MDCT thorax are indicated.
- Bronchoscopy especially flexible one is the first-line investigation, tamponade measures may be unsuccessful in massive cases, however, it is useful in localizing site.
- Bronchial artery embolization is successful in stopping bleeding in about 74–90% of cases.
- Surgery is the definitive management in some cases.

REFERENCES

1. Jean-Baptiste E. Clinical assessment and management of massive hemoptysis. Crit Care Med. 2000;28(5):1642-7.
2. Santiago S, Tobias J, Williams AJ. A reappraisal of the causes of hemoptysis. Arch Intern Med. 1991;151(12):2449-51.

3. Hirshberg B, Biran I, Glazer M, et al. Hemoptysis: etiology, evaluation, and outcome in a tertiary referral hospital. Chest. 1997;112(2):440-4.
4. Johnston H, Reisz G. Changing spectrum of hemoptysis. Underlying causes in 148 patients undergoing diagnostic flexible fiberoptic bronchoscopy. Arch Intern Med. 1989;149(7):1666-8.
5. Prasad R, Garg R, Singhal S, et al. Lessons from patients with hemoptysis attending a chest clinic in India. Ann Thorac Med. 2009;4(1):10-2.
6. Soares Pires F, Teixeira N, Coelho F, et al. Hemoptysis—etiology, evaluation and treatment in a university hospital. Rev Port Pneumol. 2011;17(1):7-14.
7. Wiggle DA, Waddell TK. Investigations and management of massive hemoptysis. In: Alexander GP, Pearson FG, Cooper JD (Eds). Pearson's Thoracic and Esophageal Surgery. London: Churchill Livingstone; 2008.
8. Amrhein TJ, Kim C, Smith TP, et al. Bronchial artery arising from the left vertebral artery: case report and review of the literature. J Clin Imaging Sci. 2011;1:62.
9. Cahill BC, Ingbar DH. Massive hemoptysis. Assessment and management. Clin Chest Med. 1994;15(1):147-67.
10. Conlan AA, Hurwitz SS, Krige L, et al. Massive hemoptysis. Review of 123 cases. J Thorac Cardiovasc Surg. 1983;85(1):120-4.
11. Revel MP, Fournier LS, Hennebicque AS, et al. Can CT replace bronchoscopy in the detection of the site and cause of bleeding in patients with large or massive hemoptysis? AJR Am J Roentgenol. 2002;179(5):1217-24.
12. Khalil A, Soussan M, Mangiapan G, et al. Utility of high-resolution chest CT scan in the emergency management of haemoptysis in the intensive care unit: severity, localization and aetiology. Br J Radiol. 2007;80(949):21-5.
13. Ketai LH, Mohammed TL, Kirsch J, et al. ACR appropriateness criteria hemoptysis. J Thorac Imaging. 2014;29(3):W19-22.
14. Lee YJ, Lee SM, Park JS, et al. The clinical implications of bronchoscopy in hemoptysis patients with no explainable lesions in computed tomography. Respir Med. 2012;106(3):413-9.
15. Set PA, Flower CD, Smith IE, et al. Hemoptysis: comparative study of the role of CT and fiberoptic bronchoscopy. Radiology. 1993;189(3):677-80.
16. O'Neil KM, Lazarus AA. Hemoptysis. Indications for bronchoscopy. Arch Intern Med. 1991;151(1):171-4.
17. Tak S, Ahluwalia G, Sharma SK, et al. Haemoptysis in patients with a normal chest radiograph: bronchoscopy-CT correlation. Australas Radiol. 1999;43(4):451-5.
18. Woo S, Yoon CJ, Chung JW, et al. Bronchial artery embolization to control hemoptysis: comparison of N-butyl-2-cyanoacrylate and polyvinyl alcohol particles. Radiology. 2013;269(2):594-602.
19. Menchini L, Remy-Jardin M, Faivre JB, et al. Cryptogenic haemoptysis in smokers: angiography and results of embolisation in 35 patients. Eur Respir J. 2009;34(5):1031-9.
20. Wong ML, Szkup P, Hopley MJ. Percutaneous embolotherapy for life-threatening hemoptysis. Chest. 2002;121(1):95-102.
21. Cremaschi P, Nascimbene C, Vitulo P, et al. Therapeutic embolization of bronchial artery: a successful treatment in 209 cases of relapse hemoptysis. Angiology. 1993;44(4):295-9.
22. Sellke FW, del Nido PJ, Swanson SJ. Sabiston and Spencer Surgery of the chest, 8th edition. Philadelphia: Saunders Elsevier; 2010.

CHAPTER 41

Acute Respiratory Failure

Chitra Mehta, Yatin Mehta

INTRODUCTION

Acute respiratory failure (ARF) is a commonly encountered condition in intensive care unit (ICU) and emergency department (ED). It may be the primary disease, or may be a complication of other conditions like cardiac failure or acute renal insufficiency.

DEFINITION

Acute respiratory failure occurs when the respiratory system fails to meet the oxidative, ventilatory, and metabolic demands of the body. There is a failure of gas exchange mechanisms in maintaining adequate oxygen delivery to the tissues, and/or adequate removal of carbon dioxide (CO_2) from the body.

EPIDEMIOLOGY

Acute respiratory failure is a major cause of morbidity and mortality in ICU setting. Both are found to increase in geriatric age group, and in presence of comorbidities. Hospital mortality has been found to be 30–40% in patients requiring ventilatory support. Mortality also varies according to the etiology. For acute respiratory distress syndrome (ARDS) it is about 40–45% and for acute exacerbation of chronic obstructive pulmonary disease (COPD) it is around 30%.

CLASSIFICATION

Acute respiratory failure has been divided into four types primarily:
1. Type I (hypoxemic) respiratory failure
2. Type II (hypercapnic) respiratory failure
3. Type III (perioperative) respiratory failure
4. Type IV (shock related) respiratory failure.

Type I (Hypoxemic) Respiratory Failure

It is characterized by the arterial oxygen tension (PaO_2) below 60 mm Hg (8.00 kPa) with normal or low arterial CO_2 tension ($PaCO_2$). This is the most common form of respiratory failure.

Type II (Hypercapnic) Respiratory Failure

It is characterized by $PaCO_2$ of more than 45 mm Hg, often accompanied by hypoxemia that gets easily corrected with supplemental oxygen.

Type III (Perioperative) Respiratory Failure

It specifically occurs in postoperative patients, most commonly secondary to atelectasis related to low functional residual capacity in the setting of altered chest wall, and/or abdominal wall compliance. Both type I and type II respiratory failures can occur during this period.

Type IV (Shock Related) Respiratory Failure

This refers to hypoperfusion-induced respiratory failure. It commonly occurs in a hemodynamically unstable patient during the process of resuscitation.

It is also important to differentiate between acute, chronic, and acute on chronic respiratory failures. This is particularly important in type II respiratory failure. Acute hypercapnic respiratory failure develops rapidly over minutes to days with inadequate compensation. This results in pH less than 7.3. On the other hand, chronic hypercapnic respiratory failure develops gradually over days to months, allowing adequate time for renal compensation to take place. So there is a near normal pH with raised serum bicarbonate levels. Elevated $PaCO_2$ with partial compensation, resulting in pH less than 7.35, characterizes acute on chronic ventilatory failure. Other signs like polycythemia and cor pulmonale may also help in identifying them. Acute and chronic differentiation may be relevant to type I respiratory failure as well. This is important in patients with interstitial lung diseases and in patients residing at high altitude areas.

Some people consider definition of hypoxemic respiratory failure too simplistic, as it gives no idea about the tissue oxygenation and overlooks the major determinants of oxygen delivery—cardiac output and hemoglobin level.[1-3]

PATHOPHYSIOLOGY

Efficacy of the lung is evaluated by its oxygenation and ventilation capacity. PaO_2 reflects oxygenation and $PaCO_2$ reflects ventilation. Alveolar-arterial oxygen gradient ($AaDO_2$) aids in evaluating oxygenation. It also helps in understanding the pathophysiological mechanisms. $AaDO_2$ can be determined with the help of alveolar gas equation:

$$PAO_2 = FiO_2 \times (P_{atm} - P_{H_2O}) - PaCO_2/R \quad (1)$$

Where,
PAO_2 = Alveolar PO_2
FiO_2 = Fraction of inspired oxygen
P_{atm} = Barometric pressure, 760 mm Hg at sea level
P_{H_2O} = Pressure of water vapor at standard temperature, normally 23 mm Hg
$PaCO_2$ = Arterial PCO_2
R = Respiratory quotient (R = 0.8)
The normal value of $AaDO_2$ increases with age and FiO_2.
$PaCO_2$ is a function of CO_2 production and alveolar ventilation, as can be seen in following relationship:

$$PaCO_2 = VCO_2 \times k/V_A \quad (2)$$

Where,
$PaCO_2$ = Partial pressure of CO_2 in arterial blood
VCO_2 = CO_2 production
V_A = Alveolar ventilation
K = Constant (0.863)

$$V_A = V_T - V_D \quad (3)$$

Where,
V_T = Tidal volume
V_D = Dead space volume

So $PaCO_2$ will rise if there is an increased CO_2 production, fall in tidal volume, or an increase in dead space volume.[4,5]

Respiratory failure may occur as a result of malfunction of any of respiratory components like airways, parenchyma, chest wall, respiratory muscles (intercostal + diaphragm), central and peripheral nervous systems.

Hypoxemic Respiratory Failure

Pathophysiological mechanisms responsible for type I failure are:
- Low FiO_2
- Ventilation/perfusion mismatch (V/Q)
- Shunt
- Diffusion abnormalities
- Hypoventilation
- Venous admixture (low mixed venous oxygen).

Low FiO_2 as a cause of hypoxemia is of importance at high altitude where barometric pressure is low. In clinical practice, one can suspect this, if there is sudden desaturation of a patient receiving supplemental oxygen. Interruption or disconnection of oxygen supply should be ruled out in this condition.

Diffusion abnormalities become clinically relevant only if there is a significant decrease in blood transit time in the pulmonary capillary bed and if there are coexistent V/Q abnormalities.

For all practical purposes V/Q mismatch and shunt mechanisms are the dominant causes of hypoxemia. Both result in an elevated $AaDO_2$.

V/Q mismatch: It is the most common mechanism resulting in hypoxemia. Ideal gas exchange can only exist if V/Q ratio is 1. Normal V/Q ratio is 0.8. A relative decrease in ventilation reduces the ratio, which impairs oxygenation and ventilation. If this ratio becomes near zero, it represents a shunt mechanism. A relative decrease in perfusion results in ratio more than 1, representing increased dead space. Clinically this becomes important only if the abnormality is quite severe. Response to supplemental oxygen can help in differentiating between V/Q mismatch and shunt.

Shunt: It is the right to left shunting of deoxygenated blood, which is responsible for causing hypoxemia. The deoxygenated blood bypasses the gas exchange area, and mixes with the oxygenated blood coming from other ventilated alveoli resulting in fall in oxygen content. This may occur in presence of anatomical right to left shunts (like atrial septal defect), or may occur in presence of physiological shunting when the V/Q ratio approaches 0 (like collapse, ARDS). Under normal circumstances also the anatomical shunts are present. This is secondary to admixture of blood from pulmonary circulation with bronchial and Thebesian circulations. It amounts to about 2-3% of shunt. Both anatomical and physiological shunts show poor response to supplemental oxygen.

In addition to above mechanisms, it has been observed that tissue hypoperfusion exacerbates the degree of hypoxia caused by other diseases. This is due to excess oxygen extraction at tissue level, resulting in low mixed venous oxygen saturation. Hypoxia can also occur if there is an increase in abnormal hemoglobins like carboxy or methemoglobin. In this situation, PaO_2 may remain normal but oxygen saturation falls resulting in low arterial oxygen content.[6,7] Various causes of type I respiratory failure are illustrated in **Box 1**.

Box 1 Causes of type I respiratory failure

- *Low FiO$_2$*: High altitude
- *Airways*: Chronic obstructive pulmonary disease (COPD), asthma, postintubation laryngeal edema, mucus plugging, bronchiectasis, and vocal cord paralysis
- *Lung parenchyma*: Pulmonary edema, acute respiratory distress syndrome (ARDS), pulmonary hemorrhage, lung contusion, pneumonia, alveolar proteinosis, hypersensitivity pneumonitis, transfusion-related lung injury, lung resection, aspiration, and radiation injury
- *Interstitium*: Pulmonary fibrosis, viral or atypical pneumonia
- *Pulmonary vasculature*: Pulmonary veno-occlusive disease, pulmonary embolism, intracardiac or intrapulmonary shunt
- *Pleural*: Pneumothorax and pleural effusion
- *Chest wall*: Kyphoscoliosis, thoracoplasty, massive obesity, chest wall trauma—flail chest and burns

Box 2 Causes of type II respiratory failure

- *Respiratory drive (reduced)*: Ondine's curse, drug overdose, obesity hypoventilation syndrome, traumatic brain injuries, carotid body resection, and metabolic alkalosis
- *Neural transmission (reduced)*
- *Spinal cord*: Cervical spine injury and tumor
- *Anterior horn cells*: Poliomyelitis, amyotrophic lateral sclerosis
- *Peripheral nerves*: Phrenic nerve injury, Guillain-Barré syndrome, critical illness polyneuropathy, Lyme disease, beriberi, and diphtheria
- *Neuromuscular junction*: Neuromuscular blocking agents, tick paralysis, organophosphorus poisoning, botulism, tetanus, myasthenia gravis, and Lambert-Eaton syndrome
- *Respiratory muscles*: Muscular dystrophy, polymyositis, malnutrition, dyselectrolytemia, and hypothyroidism
- *Chest wall*: Kyphoscoliosis, thoracoplasty, fibrothorax, flail chest, ankylosing spondylitis, and asphyxiating thoracic dystrophy

Hypercapnic Respiratory Failure

This type results when there is an imbalance between ventilatory demand and ventilatory capacity. Excessive increase in load, or a drastic fall in capacity may precipitate it. It may also occur when there is coexistent increased load and reduced capacity, though each may be of moderate severity. Pure hypoventilation as a sole cause can be identified by presence of normal AaDO$_2$. Hypercapnia can also occur as a part of hypoxic failure if the gas exchange derangements are quite severe.[8-10] Causes of hypercapnic respiratory failure are shown in **Box 2**.

CLINICAL PRESENTATION

Patients with respiratory failure have a varying clinical presentation. Dyspnea is the hallmark of respiratory failure. Neurological symptoms may also be present. Various clinical presentations are shown in **Table 1**.

DIAGNOSTIC APPROACH

Given the vast differential diagnosis of acute respiratory failure, it is imperative to obtain an extensive history from the patient. History of fever with chills indicates underlying infection. Sudden onset shortness of breath or chest pain may point toward pulmonary embolism, pneumothorax or myocardial infarction (if left sided chest pain). Increased cough and sputum in a smoker suggests acute exacerbation of COPD. Cardiogenic pulmonary edema is associated with chest pain, paroxysmal nocturnal dyspnea or orthopnea. Presence of sensorimotor abnormalities may suggest neuromuscular respiratory failure. Additional exposure history may help in diagnosing inhalational injury, aspiration, transfusion-related lung injury, hypersensitivity pneumonitis, pneumoconiosis, etc. A focused physical examination of cardiopulmonary system is also necessary.

Table 1 Clinical manifestations

Hypoxia	Hypercapnia
Central or peripheral cyanosis	Coma
Tachycardia or bradycardia	Asterixis
Hypertension or hypotension	Headache
Tachypnea accessory muscle use	Somnolence
Diaphoresis	Abdominal paradox (diaphragmatic fatigue)
Altered mentation	Warm extremities with bounding pulses
Anxiety	Myoclonic jerks
Confusion	Papilledema
Lactic acidosis	Slurred speech
Seizures	Signs of airway obstruction

All patients must have basic investigations including arterial blood gas analysis, chest radiography, electrocardiogram, and routine blood chemistry. A normal AaDO$_2$ gradient indicates hypoventilation as the only cause for respiratory failure. Abnormal hemoglobins can also be picked up in arterial blood gas analyzer with co-oximetry facility. Oxygen requirement gives an idea about the severity of the disease. A chest X-ray may help in making the correct diagnosis. A clear chest X-ray in presence of hypoxia and hypo- or normocapnia points toward pulmonary embolism, shock or anatomical shunts. A clear chest X-ray in presence of hypercapnia would indicate COPD, asthma, drug overdose or neuromuscular pathology. Localized shadow may indicate pneumonia or an infarct. Diffuse infiltrates suggest pulmonary edema, atypical pneumonia, pulmonary hemorrhage or pulmonary fibrosis. ARDS, which is a common cause of type I respiratory failure, has been redefined **(Table 2)**.[11-13]

Table 2	Berlin definition 2012 of ARDS
Timing	Within 1 week of known clinical insult or new or worsening respiratory symptoms
Chest imaging	Bilateral opacities on chest radiograph or chest computed tomographic scan
Origin of edema	Respiratory failure not fully explained by cardiac failure or fluid overload
Oxygenation	
Mild	PaO_2/FiO_2 ratio 200–300 mm Hg with PEEP or CPAP $>/= 5$ cm H_2O
Moderate	PaO_2/FiO_2 ratio 101–200 mm Hg with PEEP $>/= 5$ cm H_2O
Severe	PaO_2/FiO_2 ratio $</= 100$ mm Hg with PEEP $>/= 5$ cm H_2O

Abbreviations: ARDS, acute respiratory distress syndrome; PEEP, positive end-expiratory pressure; CPAP, continuous positive airway pressure.

Some special investigations may be required to substantiate the diagnosis like computed tomography of chest, echocardiography, serum chemistry like thyroid profile, calcium, magnesium, phosphorus levels, sputum and blood cultures, urinalysis, and cardiac biomarkers like troponins. Diagnostic pleural tap should be done if pleural effusion is present. In presence of severe hypoxemia, therapeutic decisions may have to be taken even if the data is incomplete. Decisions can later be revised when additional information is available. In recent times, bedside cardiothoracic ultrasound has been found to be a useful complimentary diagnostic tool.

MANAGEMENT

The management of respiratory failure is directed towards its cause, its clinical impact, and patient's underlying status. Primary aims of treatment are: (1) to ensure adequate oxygenation, (2) to improve respiratory acidosis, (3) to improve cardiac output if reduced, (4) to treat the primary condition and (5) to avoid predictable complications. It is essential to do the airway, breathing and circulation assessment right at the time of presentation.

When encountered in the ED, timely decision for hospitalization should be taken. Clinical features indicating the need for ICU admission are as follows:
- Severe breathlessness
- Poor/deteriorating general condition
- Altered mentation
- Significant comorbidities
- Cyanosis
- Acute onset
- Not able to speak full sentences
- Severe acidosis
- High oxygen requirement
- Hypotension.

Supplemental Oxygen

A reasonable goal is to achieve PaO_2 of 65–70 mm Hg with oxygen saturation of more than 90%. Various devices are used to deliver oxygen. They are divided into low- or high-flow systems, or open or closed systems. This depends upon their capacity to deliver oxygen at sufficient flow rates so as to meet the patient's flow demands. In a low flow system, lower the oxygen flow, and higher the patients flow requirements, higher the probability of entraining room air leading to lower FiO_2. Examples of low-flow systems are nasal cannula or facemask. Examples of high-flow devices are venturi masks, facemasks with reservoir bag, and resuscitation bag-mask-valve unit. Venturi mask is a fixed performance device ensuring delivery of precise oxygen concentrations from 24% to 60%. These are extremely useful in COPD patients where oxygen saturation has to be carefully titrated so as not to blunt the hypoxic drive of the patients.

Initial choice of the device is dependent on the severity of hypoxemia. A higher FiO_2 of 0.5–1.0 can be achieved with a nonrebreathing facemask with reservoir bag. For FiO_2 requirement of more than 0.7, early institution of mechanical ventilation should be considered, especially in the presence of hemodynamic instability.[14,15]

The level of acidosis, which needs to be treated, remains debatable. Recently it has been advocated that pH of more than 7.15 does not require bicarbonate therapy. However, in presence of coexistent cardiac arrhythmias, shock or decreased level of consciousness, secondary to no other obvious cause, pH may need to be increased to around 7.25. In addition to above, optimization of cardiac output and adequate hemoglobin concentration are essential in managing compromised oxygenation state. Intravenous fluids should be infused in a targeted and controlled manner. This is to prevent positive fluid balance, which is a predictor of poor outcome in ICU.

Continuous Positive Airway Pressure

Continuous positive airway pressure (CPAP) therapy maintains a CPAP throughout the respiratory cycle, and is similar to positive end-expiratory pressure (PEEP) of mechanical ventilation (MV). It has been found useful in alleviating hypoxemia by recruiting collapsed alveoli. It has been found beneficial in acute cardiogenic pulmonary edema, postsurgical respiratory failure and in chest trauma patients. It can be provided either by a facemask or nasal mask or helmet as an interface.

Noninvasive Ventilation

It is defined as a process of delivering positive pressure ventilation through a noninvasive interface (nasal mask, facemask). It can be delivered through either the modern ventilators, or portable noninvasive ventilation (NIV) devices. It has been found to be useful in acute exacerbation of COPD, immunocompromised patient with respiratory failure, acute cardiogenic pulmonary edema, postextubation support, and postoperative respiratory failure. Both NIV and CPAP have proven clinical benefit in above situations. They, however, have been found to have no impact on outcome in patients with ARDS or pneumonia. In fact, therapeutic trial with either of them in these two conditions, may actually cause unnecessary delay in intubation. NIV has been found to obviate the need for intubation in more than 50% of properly selected patients.[16-20]

Contraindications to NIV use are:
- Inability to protect airway, or clear secretions
- Cardiac or respiratory arrest
- Facial surgery or trauma
- Recent upper airway or esophageal surgery
- High risk of aspiration
- Anticipation of prolonged ventilatory support
- Obtundation except hypercapnic encephalopathy
- APACHE II Score greater than 34
- Initial pH less than 7.1
- Excessive secretions
- Upper airway obstruction
- Nonrespiratory organ failure—upper gastrointestinal bleeding and hemodynamic instability
- Facial burns
- Nonacceptance of NIV
- Excessive air leak around the interface.

Mechanical Ventilation

Initiation of MV is a clinically based bedside decision. Broad indications for MV are:
- Inadequate oxygenation by noninvasive means
- Increased $PaCO_2$ resulting in obtundation and respiratory muscle fatigue
- Increased work of breathing
- Inability to clear secretions
- High-risk of aspiration
- Decreased level of consciousness (GCS <8)
- Bulbar dysfunction
- Severe respiratory acidosis.

Current initial recommendations for ventilator strategies are:
- FiO_2 = 1.0
- Tidal volume = 8–10 mL/kg
- PEEP = 5
- Mode = Volume control.

This can later be modified to following settings:
- Low tidal volume strategy (<6 mL/kg)
- Peak airway pressure less than 35 cm of H_2O
- Permissive hypercapnia
- Higher levels of PEEP (5–15 cm H_2O)
- Early use of ventilator modes allowing spontaneous respiratory efforts.

Additional approaches for improving pulmonary gas exchange are recruitment maneuvers, prone positioning, high frequency ventilation, inverse ratio ventilation, inhaled nitric oxide, and extracorporeal membrane oxygenation (ECMO), or extracorporeal CO_2 removal ($ECCO_2R$). None of the above approaches except prone positioning and extracorporeal gas exchange therapy have been found to have unequivocal benefit.[21-25]

High-flow Oxygen Therapy

It is a technique where heated and humidified oxygen is delivered at high-flow rates (up to 50 lpm) through a specially designed nasal cannula. It can provide FiO_2 of 30–100%. This modality has been found to be associated with an enhanced patient comfort and decreased work of breathing. It acts primarily by generating a low level of PEEP and by reducing the physiological dead space. Its use is now being advocated prior to use of NIV in patients with ARF. It can also be safely used if NIV is contraindicated.[26,27]

All the abovementioned therapies provide only temporary benefit if the underlying disease is not treated simultaneously.

Definitive Therapy

Appropriate empirical antimicrobial agents should be initiated at first suspicion of underlying pneumonia. Bronchodilators and steroids should be prescribed in presence of asthma or COPD. Adequate humidification and mucolytics should be used for avoiding secretions from becoming tenacious. Diuretics should be started when pulmonary edema or fluid overload are suspected. Intercostal drains should be inserted for pneumothoraces or pleural effusions. Chest physiotherapy should be started timely and early mobilization of the patients should be done. Type III or postoperative respiratory failure presents usually to the ICU. It has to be managed on similar lines. Various strategies have been suggested to prevent its development like preoperative optimization of chronic lung diseases, early initiation of lung expansion maneuvers (incentive spirometry and deep breathing exercises), adequate analgesia, and use of CPAP where appropriate.

CONCLUSION

Acute respiratory failure is one of the most common conditions encountered in general emergency practices. Timely decision of admission to ICU is a prerequisite to successful treatment. ARF can have wide clinical manifestations ranging from sympathetic overactivity to encephalopathy with somnolence. All patients must have arterial blood gas analysis and chest radiography at the earliest. Supplemental oxygen and assisted ventilation should be initiated while waiting for the ICU shift.

REFERENCES

1. Kaynar AM. Respiratory failure treatment and management. [online] Available from *http://emedicine.medscape.com/article/167981-treatment* [Accessed November, 2016].
2. Pinson R. Revisiting respiratory failure. [online] Available from *www.acphospitalist.org/archives/2013/10/coding.htm* [Accessed November, 2016].
3. Schraufnagel D. Breathing in America: Diseases, Progress, and Hope. New York: American Thoracic Society; 2010.
4. Pinson R. Revisiting respiratory failure. [online] Available from *www.acphospitalist.org/archives/2013/11/coding.htm* [Accessed November, 2016].
5. Baruch M, Messer B. Criteria for intensive care unit admission and severity of illness. Surgery (Oxford). 2015;33(4):158-64.
6. Lee WL, Slutsky AS. Acute hypoxemic respiratory failure and ARDS. In: Broaddus VC, Mason RJ, Ernst JD, et al (Eds). Murray and Nadel's Textbook of Respiratory Medicine, 6th edition. Amsterdam: Elsevier; 2015. p. 2104.
7. Dakin J, Griffiths M. The pulmonary physician in critical care 1: pulmonary investigations for acute respiratory failure. Thorax. 2002;57:79-85.
8. Hill NS. Acute ventilator failure. In: Broaddus VC, Mason RJ, Ernst JD, et al. (Eds). Murray and Nadel's Textbook of Respiratory Medicine, 6th edition. Amsterdam: Elsevier; 2015. p. 2138.
9. Roussos C, Koutsoukou A. Respiratory failure. Eur Respir J Suppl. 2003;47:3s-14s.
10. Burns KE, Adhikari NK, Keenan SP, et al. Noninvasive positive pressure ventilation as a weaning strategy for intubated adults with respiratory failure. Cochrane Database Syst Rev. 2010;(8):CD004127.
11. ARDS Definition Task Force, Ranieri VM, Rubenfeld GD, et al. Acute respiratory distress syndrome: the Berlin Definition. JAMA. 2012;307(23):2526-33.
12. Karmpaliotis D, Kirtane AJ, Ruisi CP, et al. Diagnostic and prognostic utility of brain natriuretic peptide in subjects admitted to the ICU with hypoxic respiratory failure due to noncardiogenic and cardiogenic pulmonary edema. Chest. 2007;131(4):964-71.
13. Pepe PE, Potkin RT, Reus DH, et al. Clinical predictors of the adult respiratory distress syndrome. Am J Surg. 1982;144(1):124-30.
14. Wilson JG, Matthay MA. Mechanical ventilation in acute hypoxemic respiratory failure: a review of new strategies for the practicing hospitalist. J Hosp Med. 2014;9(7):469-75.
15. MacIntyre N, Huang YC. Acute exacerbations and respiratory failure in chronic obstructive pulmonary disease. Proc Am Thorac Soc. 2008;5(4):530-5.
16. Hill NS, Brennan J, Garpestad E, et al. Noninvasive ventilation in acute respiratory failure. Crit Care Med. 2007;35(10):2402-7.
17. Ray P, Birolleau S, Lefort Y, et al. Acute respiratory failure in the elderly: etiology, emergency diagnosis and prognosis. Crit Care. 2006;10(3):R82.
18. Calfee CS, Matthay MA. Nonventilatory treatments for acute lung injury and ARDS. Chest. 2007;131(3):913-20.
19. Zilberberg MD, Epstein SK. Acute lung injury in the medical ICU: comorbid conditions, age, etiology, and hospital outcome. Am J Respir Crit Care Med. 1998;157(4 Pt 1):1159-64.
20. Nava S, Hill NS. Noninvasive ventilation in acute respiratory failure. Lancet. 2009;374(9685):250-9.
21. Matthay MA, Ware LB, Zimmerman GA. The acute respiratory distress syndrome. J Clin Invest. 2012;122(8):2731-40.
22. Briel M, Meade M, Mercat A, et al. Higher vs lower positive end-expiratory pressure in patients with acute lung injury and acute respiratory distress syndrome: systematic review and meta-analysis. JAMA. 2010;303(9):865-73.
23. Bach JR, Gonçalves MR, Hamdani I, et al. Extubation of patients with neuromuscular weakness: a new management paradigm. Chest. 2010;137(5):1033-9.
24. Gehlbach BK, Hall JB. Respiratory failure and mechanical ventilation. In: Porter RS, (Ed). The Merck Manual, 19th edition. West Point, PA: Merck Sharp & Dohme Corp.; 2011.
25. The National Heart, Lung, and Blood Institute Acute Respiratory Distress Syndrome (ARDS) Clinical Trials Network; In: Wheeler AP, Bernard GR, Thompson BT, et al. Pulmonary-artery versus central venous catheter to guide treatment of acute lung injury. N Engl J Med. 2006;354(21):2213-24.
26. Roca O, Hernández G, Díaz-Lobato S, et al. Current evidence for the effectiveness of heated and humidified high flow nasal cannula supportive therapy in adult patients with respiratory failure. Critical Care. 2016;20(1):109.
27. Spoletini G, Alotaibi M, Blasi F, et al. Heated Humidified High-Flow Nasal Oxygen in Adults: Mechanisms of Action and Clinical Implications. Chest. 2015;148(1):253-61.

CHAPTER 42

Acute Exacerbation of Asthma and Chronic Obstructive Pulmonary Disease

Ashish Kumar Prakash, Bornali Datta, Anand Jaiswal

BRONCHIAL ASTHMA[1]

Bronchial asthma (BA) is a chronic respiratory illness which is because of hyperresponsive airways and is mainly characterized by symptoms of wheezing, dyspnea, chest tightness cough, and by variable expiratory airflow limitation. The most important aspect of asthma is that it is very much reversible and variable. Though various phenotypes of asthma like allergic, nonallergic, late onset, with fixed airflow, and obesity[2,3] have been identified but genetic influence and family history still remains very important. Asthma predominantly involves the larger airways. It affects 1–18% of populations in different countries. In India, the estimated prevalence of asthma is 2.05% among those aged older than 15 years, and a total burden of 18 million asthmatics.[4] The Global Initiative for Asthma (GINA) has defined asthma as *"Asthma is a heterogeneous disease, usually characterized by chronic airway inflammation. It is defined by the history of respiratory symptoms such as wheeze, shortness of breath, chest tightness and cough that vary over time and in intensity, together with variable expiratory airflow limitation"*.

CHRONIC OBSTRUCTIVE PULMONARY DISEASE[5]

Chronic obstructive sleep disease, i.e. chronic obstructive pulmonary disease (COPD), is a well-known clinical entity, and acute exacerbation of COPD is commonly encountered in emergency department (ED) **(Flow chart 1)**. It is high burden disease and is mostly because of aging and smoking, though the environmental smoke and other causes are also there. This is the third most common cause of death in United States of America.[5] In India, history of cooking with burning of biomass fuel, i.e. *chulha* smoke, is one of the causes of COPD. In India, the prevalence of chronic bronchitis is 3.49% in males and 2.7% in females.[4] COPD is a spectrum of lung abnormality which is physiologically characterized by persistent airflow obstruction. It involves both the lung parenchyma causing destruction of it which is histologically termed as emphysema and airway inflammation leading to chronic bronchitis.

The global initiative of COPD which forms the guideline for the management of COPD has defined COPD as[5] *"Chronic obstructive pulmonary disease (COPD) is a common,*

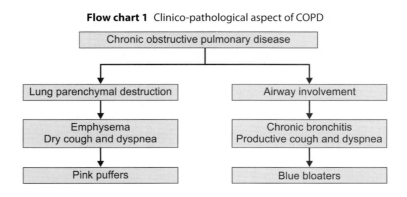

Flow chart 1 Clinico-pathological aspect of COPD

preventable and treatable disease that is characterized by persistent respiratory symptoms and airflow limitation that is due to airway and/or alveolar abnormalities usually caused by significant exposure to noxious particles or gases".

Chronic obstructive pulmonary disease develops because of multifactorial etiology and the risk factors include both genetic and environmental factors. Pathological changes are observed in almost every part of lung like central airways, small airways, and alveolar space. There are various proposed pathogenesis of COPD which includes proteinase-antiproteinase hypothesis, systemic inflammation, immunological mechanisms, oxidant-antioxidant balance, apoptosis, and ineffective repair. Apart from symptoms of cough and dyspnea, spirometry has also a diagnostic role; the postbronchodilator forced expiratory volume in 1 sec (FEV_1) to forced vital capacity (FVC) ratio less than 0.70. The patients of COPD have accelerated decline in FEV_1.

ACUTE EXACERBATION OF COPD AND ACUTE ASTHMA IN EMERGENCY

The acute exacerbation of COPD and asthma **(Table 1)** are the most common respiratory illness which require visit to the ED. Asthma and COPD are chronic lung diseases that can be differentiated traditionally by the presence or absence of reversibility, though not always helpful. For emergency setup, both airway diseases can be dealt as same entity.

Table 1 Exacerbations of acute asthma and chronic obstructive pulmonary disease

Acute asthma[1]	Acute exacerbation chronic obstructive pulmonary disease[5]
Exacerbations of asthma are episodes characterized by a progressive increase in symptoms of shortness of breath, cough, wheezing or chest tightness, and progressive decrease in lung function, i.e. they represent a change from the patient's usual status that is sufficient to require a change in treatment.	Chronic obstructive pulmonary disease exacerbations are defined as an acute worsening of respiratory symptoms that result in additional therapy.

Pathophysiology

Though the clinical manifestation of both the disease is very similar but there is no histopathological correlation. They have got different involvement at cellular level as cited in **Table 2**, which is very important from the management point of view. Chronic asthma sometimes behaves like COPD and there is now a clinical entity called asthma COPD overlap syndrome (ACOS). The pathogenesis may be similar to some extent and the Dutch hypothesis though disproved, has also shown that chronic asthma behaves like COPD.

Clinical Evaluation

Breathing difficulty is the most common manifestation with which the patients come to ED. It requires several steps for the risk stratification of patients presenting with shortness of breath (SOB). There should be methodological approach by the doctors present in ED. A proper history as well as a quick determination of the best management is mandatory.

History taking should include:
- Family history of asthma
- Smoking history
- Any cardiac disease
- Fever/sputum/hemoptysis/chest pain
- Previous intubation and intensive care unit (ICU) admission
- Chronic use of oral corticosteroid and medication compliance
- Use of short-acting beta-2 agonist (SABA), nocturnal awakening, and night symptoms.

After taking brief history, patient needs to be evaluated for severity of symptoms and clinical examination done. We can get cyanosis, nasal flaring, use of accessory muscles of respiration leading to intercostal or supraclavicular indrawing, tachycardia, tachypnea, hypotension, and altered level of consciousness. On auscultation, bilateral rhonchi are present mostly and may be associated with audible wheeze. In case of very severe illness, we may get silent chest on auscultation. We have to look for absence of unilateral breath sound. Crackles unilateral or bilateral can be auscultated **(Table 3)**.

The differential diagnoses for acute dyspnea are given in **Box 1**.[6]

Table 2 Different involvement of asthma and chronic obstructive pulmonary disease at cellular level

Inflammation	Asthma	Chronic obstructive pulmonary disease
Cells	Mast cells, eosinophil, $CD4^+$ T-cells, macrophages+	Neutrophils, $CD8^+$ T-cells, macrophages+++
Mediators	LTD4, histamine, IL-4, IL-5, ROS^+	LTB4, IL-8, TNF-α, ROS^{+++}
Effects	All airways, little fibrosis	Peripheral airway, lung destruction, fibrosis, squamous metaplasia
Response to steroids	+++	–

Table 3: Different breath sounds, their quality and associated conditions on examination

Breath sound (BS)	Quality	Associated conditions
Wheeze or rhonchi	Whistling/sibilant, musical	Caused by narrowing of airways, such as in asthma, chronic obstructive pulmonary disease, foreign body
Stridor	Whistling/sibilant, musical	Epiglottitis, foreign body, laryngeal edema, croup
Crackles	Cracking/clicking/rattling	Pneumonia, pulmonary edema, interstitial lung disease, heart failure
Hamman's sign (or mediastinal crunch)	Crunching, rasping	Pneumomediastinum, pneumopericardium
Silent chest/B/L decreased BS	Decreased or no breath sound	Acute severe asthma. B/L emphysema or bullous lung
Unilateral decreased BS	Breath sound decreased or absent on one side	Pleural effusion (dull percussion note), pneumothorax (hyperresonant percussion note)

Box 1: Differential diagnosis for acute dyspnea

Head and neck	Cardiac	Miscellaneous
• Angioedema • Anaphylaxis • Pharyngeal infection • Deep neck infection • Foreign body • Neck trauma	• ACS • Decompensated heart failure • Pulmonary edema (flash) • High output failure • Cardiomyopathy • Arrhythmia • Valvular dysfunction • Cardiac tamponade	• Hyperventilation • Anxiety • Pneumomediastinum • Lung tumor • Massive pleural effusion • Intra-abdominal process • Ascites • Pregnancy • Massive obesity
Pulmonary	**Toxic/metabolic**	**Neurological**
• COPD exacerbation • BA exacerbation • Pulmonary embolism • Pneumothorax • Pneumonia • ARDS • Lung contusion or injury • Hemorrhage	• Organophosphate • Salicylate • CO poisoning • Toxic ingestion • DKA • Sepsis • Anemia	• Stroke • Neuromuscular ds
		Chest wall
		• Rib fracture • Flail chest

Abbreviations: ACS, acute coronary syndrome; ARDS, acute respiratory distress syndrome; BA, bronchial asthma; CO, carbon monoxide; COPD, chronic obstructive pulmonary disease; DKA, diabetic ketoacidosis.

The baseline (routine) investigations which need to be done urgently are as follows:
- *Vital signs*: Heart rate (HR), blood pressure (BP), SaO$_2$ and consciousness level [Glasgow Coma Scale (GCS) scoring]
- Chest X-ray, electrocardiogram (ECG), blood gas monitoring (BGM) [arterial blood gas (ABG)], peak expiratory flow rate (PEF) and end-tidal CO$_2$ (EtCO$_2$)
- Total leukocytes counts with differential, renal function test (RFT), liver function test (LFT), C-reactive protein (CRP), procalcitonin (ProCal).

The assessment of severity can be done based on GINA guidelines **(Flow chart 2)**.[1]

Investigations

- *Laboratory investigations*: There is no specific laboratory test to clearly identify the asthma and acute exacerbation of chronic obstructive pulmonary disease (AECOPD) as the etiology of dyspnea. The test are helpful in identification of infective cause of exacerbation. The total leukocyte counts with differential count may show high neutrophil counts in bacterial infective exacerbations. Renal function test and liver function test (RFT and LFT) should also be done. Increased CRP and ProCal can be suggestive of infective exacerbations.[7,8] Though these may not be

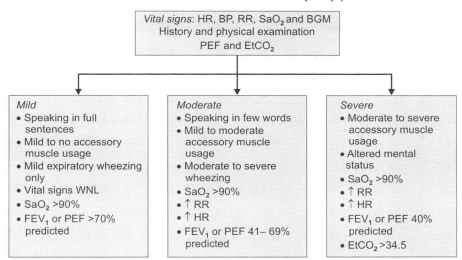

Flow chart 2 Clinical assessment of severity of dyspnea

Abbreviations: BP, blood pressure; BGM, blood gas monitoring; $EtCO_2$, end-tidal CO_2; FEV_1, forced expiratory volume in 1 sec; HR, heart rate; PEF, peak expiratory flow rate; RR, respiratory rate; SaO_2, arterial oxygen saturation; WNL, within normal limits.

accurate in settings of viral, fungal infections or may be falsely high in case of renal failure patients.[9] N-terminal pro b-type natriuretic peptide (NT-pro BNP)[10] and cardiac enzymes (Tropin-I/T, CPK-MB) may be raised indicating possible cardiac etiology. D-dimer although used for its negative predictive value, can be advised if pulmonary thromboembolism is suspected.

- *Radiology*: Chest X-ray is almost mandatory for patients with acute dyspnea. It is not a very specific test but is very much sensitive in detecting lung or cardiac causes of dyspnea. Pneumothorax, pneumonia or patchy consolidation or interstitial pattern can be seen on chest X-ray. Signs of heart failure like batwing appearance, cardiomegaly, bilateral shadows, and Kerly B lines may be seen. If chest X-ray is not informative, then we may have to ask for chest computed tomography (CT) or CT-pulmonary angiography. Two-dimensional (2D)-echocardiography and venous Doppler are also advised based on chest X-ray findings. Ultrasound of chest is also useful for detection of pleural pathology.
- *Electrocardiogram*: ECG is an essential component in evaluating patients for acute dyspnea. Increased mortality has been linked to adverse cardiovascular events.[11] ECG is very sensitive in detecting cardiac events like acute coronary syndrome (ACS) and arrhythmias. We can also get ECG changes in pulmonary embolism (S1Q3T3). The ECG changes is COPD because of clockwise rotation of heart, right atrial and ventricular hypertrophy, and P-wave verticalization due to flattening of the diaphragm leading to downward displacement of heart. The ECG changes are as follows:
  – S waves in leads I, II, and III
  – R/S ratio less than 1 in leads V5 or V6, and
  – The lead I sign—isoelectric P-wave, QRS amplitude less than 1.5 mm, and T-wave amplitude less than 0.5 mm in lead I.
- *Blood gas monitoring*: Arterial blood gas is a routine practice in emergency for patients of asthma and COPD. Though peripheral capillary oxygen saturation (SpO_2) is very sensitive and noninvasive, ABG is more accurate for hypercarbia and hypoxemia status. Sometimes the venous sample may also demonstrate about the CO_2 retention and can be used as surrogate to avoid the painful procedure of arterial puncture.[12-16]
- *Ultrasonography*: Ultrasonography (USG) is a very specific investigation and can be used if available in emergency to differentiate between cardiac or respiratory causes. It has been found to be very accurate in diagnosing COPD or asthma exacerbation.[17,18] The protocols which have been used are lung USG in critically ill (LUCI), bedside lung sonography in emergency (BLUE).
- *Microbiology*: Sputum Gram stain and cultures are advised for all admitted patients. In emergency, first goal is to stabilize the patient then send samples. Sputum for acid-fast bacilli (AFB) should be obtained for nonresponders as per Revised National Tuberculosis Control Programme (RNTCP) guidelines. We can use sputum as well as other respiratory samples like bronchial washings and endotracheal secretions for microbiological sampling.

Treatment

According to Global Initiative for Chronic Obstructive Lung Disease (GOLD) 2017 the acute exacerbation is classified as mild, moderate and severe and the management varies accordingly **(Flow chart 3)**.

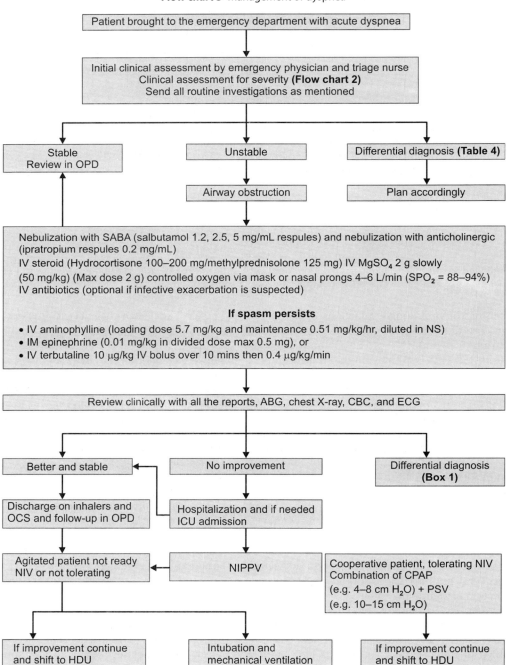

Flow chart 3 Management of dyspnea

Abbreviations: ABG, arterial blood gas; CBC, complete blood count; CPAP, continuous positive airway pressure; ECG, electrocardiogram; HDU, high dependency unit; NIV, noninvasive ventilation; NIPPV, noninvasive positive pressure ventilation; OCS, corticosteroids; PSV, pressure support ventilation; SABA, short-acting beta-2 agonist.

Mild	Short-acting bronchodilators (SABDs)
Moderate	SABDs + antibiotics and/or oral corticosteroids
Severe	Emergency visit and hospitalization, patients may be in respiratory failure

The drugs which are most commonly used for airway managements are as follows:
- *Beta-2 agonists*:
  - *Short-acting beta-2 agonists*: Salbutamol, salmeterol, levosalbutamol, terbutaline, and fenoterol
  - *Long-acting beta-2 agonists (LABA)*: Formoterol, salmeterol, indacaterol, olodaterol, and arformoterol
- *Anticholinergics*:
  - *Short-acting anticholinergics (SAMA)*: Ipratropium, oxitropium
  - *Long-acting anticholinergics (LAMA)*: Tiotropium, aclidinium, glycopyrronium, and umeclidinium
- Combination short-acting beta-2 agonists + anticholinergic
- Combination long-acting beta-2 agonist + anticholinergic
- *Methylxanthines*: Aminophyllines and theophylline
- *Inhaled corticosteroids (ICSs)*: Beclomethasone, budesonide, fluticasone, mometasone, and ciclesonide
- Combination long-acting beta-2 agonists + corticosteroids
- *Systemic corticosteroids (OCS or IV)*: Hydrocortisone, methylprednisolone, and prednisolone
- *Phosphodiesterase-4 inhibitors (PDE)*: Roflumilast
- *Leukotriene receptor antagonists*: Montelukast and zafirlukast.

To remember management, ABC is the main arm for treatment in acute exacerbation, which consists of antibiotics, bronchodilators and corticosteroids.
- *Antibiotics*: Based on local bacterial resistance and stewardship guidelines, antibiotics can be started for patients with history of producing purulent sputum. Change in amount, color, and consistency of sputum leads toward infective exacerbations, and antibiotics should be started. Initial empiric treatment should consist of an aminopenicillin, a macrolide or a tetracycline. If *Pseudomonas* or *Enterobacteriaceae* is suspected, combination therapy with antipseudomonal antibiotics like piperacillin or tazobactam or imipenem or meropenem plus amikacin or levofloxacin can be given.
- *Inhaled bronchodilators*: In emergency setup, it is the most important aspect of therapy for acute bronchospasm. We have various modes of delivery for inhaled bronchodilators. Both nebulizers as well as hand-held inhalers can be used in exacerbations. If patient is acidotic nebulizers preferably should be given by compressed air rather than oxygen (to avoid CO_2 narcosis). In ED, nebulization with either single or dual bronchodilators like salbutamol with ipratropium bromide can be given. Nebulized salbutamol can be given back to back till resolution of bronchospasm.
- *Inhaled or systemic corticosteroids*: Inhaled as well as systemic corticosteroids are regularly used for acute spasm. It is also considered first-line in the emergency management of the acute asthma and AECOPD. ICSs like beclomethasone 50–400 μg; budesonide 100, 200, 400 μg; fluticasone 50–500 μg through nebulization or hand-held devices can be used. Systemic corticosteroids are the mainstay of therapy for acute severe spasm in both asthma and COPD. Both the oral and the parenteral route have same bioavailability. If patient can take oral, parenteral treatment are reserved for patients who cannot take oral medication as there is no major difference between oral and IV with regards to relapse rate, treatment failure or mortality. Patients during hospitalization can be given oral/IV steroids and once stable should be discharged on oral corticosteroids for 7–14 days. The equivalent dose is 20 mg hydrocortisone, approximately 5 mg prednisolone, approximately 4 mg methylprednisolone, and approximately 0.75 mg dexamethasone.

The mode of delivery is mostly in inhaled form, may be through metered-dose inhalers, dry powder inhalers or nebulization which have their own pros and cons **(Table 4)**.[19]
- *Theophylline*: If bronchospasm persists and the patient is still breathless in spite of adequate steroids and inhaled bronchodilators, we can add parenteral aminophylline after excluding cardiac cause. Because of its high toxicity and drug interaction (with common used drugs like ciprofloxacin, clarithromycin, allopurinol, phenytoin), it should be maintained within therapeutic range 10–20 μg/mL.
- *Other drugs*: Intravenous magnesium sulfate though not supported by GOLD or GINA guidelines can be given as it has been found to reduce hospital admissions when other drugs had failed to reduce symptoms.[20] Kidney functions if normal, it can be given slow IV over 20 minutes. Parenteral terbutaline and intramuscular epinephrine can also be given in centers with experience of using the drugs. Heliox (mixture of 80% helium and 20% oxygen) can also be considered as an adjuvant in the management of severe asthma. For the penetration of drugs like bronchodilator, anticholinergic, and anti-inflammatory agents, the lower density of helium serves as a better transport modality than room air or oxygen-driven nebulizers.
- *Oxygen therapy*: In case of severe respiratory distress and bronchospasm, respiratory failure which is more common with AECOPD (both type1 and 2) can be seen. Hypoxia may be with hypercapnia (CO_2 narcosis), which is basically type 2 respiratory failure, is found commonly in advance stage COPD and is rare in acute asthma. In asthmatic attack, the patients are hyperventilating so hypocapnia or normocapnia are common. Oxygen therapy is recommended in both type 1 and 2 respiratory

Table 4 Pros and cons of metered-dose inhalers, dry powder inhalers, and nebulization

	Advantages	Disadvantages
Pressurized metered-dose inhalers (pMDI)	• Compact and portable • Multidose • Quick treatment time • Drug in sealed canister • Inexpensive	• High oropharyngeal deposition • Difficulty in hand mouth coordination • Propellant may cause "Cold Freon" effect and affect climate change
Dry powder inhaler (DPI)	• Compact and portable • Quick treatment time • Breath-actuated function removes need for coordination	• Need adequate inhalation flow to dispense • High oropharyngeal deposition • Humidity can cause drug degradation • Patients may be intolerant to additives, e.g. lactose
Nebulizers	• Large doses of drug can be given • Can be used with relaxed tidal breathing • Suitable for young, old and acutely ill patients • Many drug solutions can be aerosolized	• Bulky cumbersome and expensive • Wasted drug in nebulizer reservoir • Variations in aerosol output performance between models • Time-consuming • Need for power source • Regular cleaning and maintenance

failure to relieve severe respiratory distress and prevent tissue hypoxia. Oxygen therapy in case of COPD should be judiciously used to prevent CO_2 retention and respiratory acidosis. SPO_2 to be maintained between 88–94%. Pulse oximetry must be used to continuously monitor oxygen saturation. BGM is very useful in guiding the oxygen therapy and gives information about CO_2 status. The various delivery devices for oxygen comprises of nasal cannula, venturi mask, nonrebreather mask, reservoir cannula, and transtracheal catheter.

- *Admission to intensive care unit/critical care unit*: If the patient's condition further deteriorates (persistent respiratory distress, inability to maintain oxygen level above 90%, persistent hypercapnia, abnormal ABG, PaO_2 < 60 mm Hg and/or $PaCO_2$ > 60 mm Hg, alteration of mental status, acute confusion and drowsiness) even after above said measures then he can be shifted to ICU and noninvasive positive pressure ventilation (NIPPV) should be tried.
- *Noninvasive ventilation*: For patients with respiratory failure, assisted mode of ventilation must be given first trial through noninvasive mode and if patients does not tolerates it or is noncooperative then invasive mode of ventilation is applied after endotracheal intubation. Noninvasive ventilation (NIV) assists the patient in taking a breath and helps to maintain adequate oxygen. NIPPV is most popular mode of providing NIV in combination with continuous positive airway pressure (CPAP) with pressure support ventilation (PSV). It is the treatment of choice for persistent hypercapnic ventilator failure. NIV has proven role in AECOPD.[21-23] However, use of NIV in acute severe asthma has no clear benefit for reduced intubation or mortality.
- *Mechanical ventilation*: Intubation can be considered in patients with the following:
  - *NIV failure*: Worsening of ABG and/or pH in 1–2 hours; lack of improvement in ABG and or pH after 4 hours.
  - Severe acidosis (pH < 7.25) and hypercapnia ($PaCO_2$ > 60 mm Hg).
  - Tachypnea more than 35 breaths/minute.
  - *Other complications*: Metabolic abnormalities, sepsis, pneumonia, pulmonary embolism, barotrauma, and massive pleural effusion.

CONCLUSION

- For acute exacerbations, asthma and COPD are clinically similar.
- Proper clinical evaluation and exclusion of differential diagnosis is very important.
- *ABC*: Antibiotics, bronchodilator and corticosteroids are first-line treatment.
- Hypoxia with or without hypercapnia (type 1 and 2 respiratory failure) is more common with AECOPD.
- Controlled oxygen and NIPPV has important role in patients with type 1 and 2 respiratory failure.

REFERENCES

1. Reddel HK, Bateman ED, Becker A, et al. A summary of the new GINA strategy: a roadmap to asthma control. Eur Respir J. 2015;46(3):622-39.
2. Bel EH. Clinical phenotypes of asthma. Curr Opin Pulm Med. 2004;10:44-50.
3. Moore WC, Meyers DA, Wenzel SE, et al. Identification of asthma phenotypes using cluster analysis in the Severe Asthma Research Program. Am J Respir Crit Care Med. 2010;181:315-23.
4. Jindal SK, Aggarwal AN, Gupta D, et al. Indian study on epidemiology of asthma, respiratory symptoms and chronic bronchitis in adults (INSEARCH). Int J Tuberc Lung Dis. 2012;16:1270-7.

5. Global Initiative for Chronic Obstructive Lung Disease. (2017). GOLD 2017 Global Strategy for the Diagnosis, Management and Prevention of COPD. [online] Available from *http://goldcopd.org/gold-2017-global-strategy-diagnosis-management-prevention-copd/*.
6. Morgan WC, Hodge HL. Diagnostic evaluation of dyspnea. Am Fam Physician. 1998;57(4):711-6.
7. Schuetz P, Müller B, Christ-Crain M, et al. Procalcitonin to initiate or discontinue antibiotics in acute respiratory tract infections. Cochrane Database Syst Rev. 2012:CD007498.
8. Soler N, Esperatti M, Ewig S, et al. Sputum purulence-guided antibiotic use in hospitalised patients with exacerbations of COPD. Eur Respir J. 2012;40:1344-53.
9. Grace E, Turner RM. Use of procalcitonin in patients with various degrees of chronic kidney disease including renal replacement therapy. Clin Infect Dis. 2014;59(12):1761-7.
10. Wang TJ, Larson MG, Levy D, et al. Plasma natriuretic peptide levels and the risk of cardiovascular events and death. N Engl J Med. 2004;350:655-63.
11. Murray CJ, Atkinson C, Bhalla K, et al. The State of US health, 1990-2010: burden of diseases, injuries, and risk factors. JAMA. 2013;310:591-608.
12. Kelly AM, Kerr D, Middleton P. Validation of venous pCO_2 to screen for arterial hypercarbia in patients with chronic obstructive airways disease. J Emerg Med. 2005;28:377-9.
13. Kelly AM, Kyle E, McAlpine R. Venous pCO_2 and pH can be used to screen for significant hypercarbia in emergency patients with acute respiratory disease. J Emerg Med. 2002;22:15-9.
14. Sur E. COPD: is it all in the vein? Thorax. 2013;68(Suppl 3):P182.
15. McCanny P, Bennett K, Staunton P, et al. Venous vs arterial blood gases in the assessment of patients presenting with an exacerbation of chronic obstructive pulmonary disease. Am J Emerg Med. 2012;30:896-900.
16. Lim BL, Kelly AM. A meta-analysis on the utility of peripheral venous blood gas analysis in exacerbations of chronic obstructive pulmonary disease in the emergency department. Eur J Emerg Med. 2010;17:246-8.
17. Gallard E, Redonnet JP, Bourcier JE, et al. Diagnostic performance of cardiopulmonary ultrasound performed by the emergency physician in the management of acute dyspnea. Am J Emerg Med. 2015;33(3):352-8.
18. Silva S, Biendel C, Ruiz J, et al. Usefulness of cardiothoracic chest ultrasound in the management of acute respiratory failure in critical care practice. Chest. 2013;144(3):859-65.
19. Usmani OS, Branes PJ. Fishman Textbook of Pulmonary Medicine, 5th edition. pp. 1561, Table 46-5. Kew KM, Kirtchuk L, Michell CI. Intravenous magnesium sulfate for treating adults with acute asthma in the emergency department. Cochrane Database Syst Rev. 2014;(5):CD010909.
20. Lightowler JV, Wedzicha JA, Elliot MW, et al. Noninvasive positive pressure ventilation to treat respiratory failure resulting from exacerbations of chronic obstructive pulmonary disease: Cochrane systematic review and meta-analysis. BMJ. 2003;326(7382):185.
21. Rossi A, Appendini L, Roca J. Physiological aspects of noninvasive positive pressure ventilation. Eur Respir Mon. 2001;16:1-10.
22. Diaz O, Iglesia R, Ferrer M, et al. Effects of noninvasive ventilation on pulmonary gas exchange and hemodynamics during acute hypercapnic exacerbations of chronic obstructive pulmonary disease. Am J Respir Crit Care Med. 1997;156(6):1840-5.
23. Lim WJ, Mohammed Akram R, Carson KV, et al. Noninvasive positive and pressure ventilation for treatment of respiratory failure due to severe acute exacerbations of asthma. Cochrane Database Syst Rev. 2012;(12):CD004360.

Pneumonia

Ashish Kumar Prakash, Bornali Datta, Anand Jaiswal

INTRODUCTION

In our medical science we have studied thousands of diseases which can be broadly classified as:
- Infection
- Autoimmune
- Malignancy.

The most important thing that we have learnt in our practice is that among all the diseases, infection is a wholly treatable and preventable disease with the best outcome and none or minimal sequelae. Pneumonia is defined as lung infection by a microbiological agent. The spectrum of lung infection varies from:

LRTI—Lobar Consolidation—Multilobar Consolidation—ARDS-Sepsis-MODS

The word "pneumonia" almost always refers to a syndrome which is due to acute infection usually bacterial (may also be other microorganism), characterized by clinical and/or radiographic signs of consolidation of a part or parts of one or both lungs.[1]

Pneumonitis is sometimes used as a synonym for pneumonia, particularly when inflammation of lung has noninfectious etiology like chemical, radiation or interstitial **(Table 1)**.

PNEUMONIA IN EMERGENCY

To discuss totality pneumonia in it is beyond the scope of this book. Here we will provide a glimpse of acute pneumonia in adults. The most common cause of pneumonia with acute presentation are viruses, *Pneumococcus* and *Mycoplasma*. In India apart from those we can also get *Staphylococcus aureus, Klebsiella pneumoniae, Haemophilus influenzae, Legionella pneumophila* or others as a causative agent for community acquired pneumonia.[2]

Table 1 Classification of pneumonia[1]

Basis	Types
Anatomical location	- Lobar - Multilobar - Segmental - Subsegmental - Bronchopneumonia
Etiological (microbiological)	- Bacterial - Viral - Fungal - Parasitic - Chemical (e.g. Lipoid) - Physical (ionizing)
Empiricists	- Community-acquired pneumonia (CAP) - Hospital-acquired pneumonia (HAP) or nosocomial pneumonia - Ventilator-associated pneumonia (VAP) - Aspiration pneumonia - Immunocompromised host pneumonia
Behaviorists	- Easy pneumonia (responds to early treatment) - Difficult pneumonia (fails to do so)

CLINICAL EVALUATION

For typical pneumonia, cough, fever and chest pain are the common presentation with which the patients come to the emergency department. Cough may be with expectoration whitish to greenish; rarely patients can have hemoptysis. Mucopurulent sputum is mostly found with bacterial pneumonia. Patients may present only with high grade sudden onset of fever which is continuous, but many a times patients have already taken antipyretics for that. Chest pain can be pleuritic or dull aching in nature. Atypical presentation may also occur like poor oral uptake, nausea, vomiting, diarrhea, and change of mental status or disorientation. This is more common in elderly patients.

Table 2 Acute pneumonia in adult		
Pathophysiologic changes	Symptoms	Investigations
• Obstruction of bronchioles • Decrease gas exchange • Increase exudates	• Cough • Fever • Chills • Tachycardia • Tachypnea • Dyspnea • Pleural pain • Malaise • Respiratory distress • Decrease breath sound	• Chest X-ray • Sputum culture • ABG (arterial blood gas)

On general physical examination the patients are febrile with tachycardia and tachypnea. Sometimes relative bradycardia is also found in atypical pneumonia with *Mycoplasma, Legionella, Chlamydophila psittaci,* or *Francisella tularensis,* and *Mycoplasma pneumoniae* (**Table 2**).[3]

There are a few signs which can indicate serious illness or severe pneumonia like cyanosis, nasal flaring, use of accessory muscles of respiration leading to intercostal or supraclavicular in drawing, respiratory rate more than 30/min, heart rate more than 125/min, hypotension and altered level of consciousness.[4] While examining the respiratory system proper we may get decreased movement and tachypnea on inspection. On auscultation crackles are most common findings in pneumonia. If there is consolidation we can get classical signs like dull percussion note, tactile fremitus on palpation and bronchial breath sound as well as vocal fremitus, whispering pectoriloquy, bronchophony and egophony on auscultation.[5]

DIAGNOSTIC APPROACH

Radiology

Chest X-ray is always advisable for patients with clinical suspicion of pneumonia. We most commonly see the patchy consolidation mainly confined to the lobes with air bronchogram or interstitial infiltrates as nonhomogeneous opacity and or cavity. If chest X-ray is not informative, then we may have to ask for chest computed tomography (CT) to rule out mass, effusion, cavity, etc. Computed tomography, i.e. CT chest, is only advisable in case of nonresolving pneumonia or clinical worsening. Ultrasound of chest is also useful for detection of pleural effusion or pneumonia with parapneumonic effusion.

Microbiology

Sputum Gram's stain and cultures are advice for all admitted patients. The sputum Gram's stain is very useful for directing the choice of initial therapy but needs to be performed on a good quality sample and by a skilled microbiologist. Sputum for acid-fast bacilli should be obtained for nonresponders as per Revised National Tuberculosis Control Program guidelines. US Food and Drug Administration has also approved some newer test that include polymerase chain reaction (PCR), (multiplex PCR), for detecting atypical organism like *Chlamydia pneumoniae* and *M. pneumoniae* as well as 14 respiratory tract viruses. We can use it for sputum as well as for other respiratory samples like bronchial washings and endotracheal secretions. These tests are rapid, sensitive, and specific.[6]

Hematological

Total and differential leukocyte count (TLC and DLC) is of great value in dealing with pneumonia patients. In bacterial pneumonia, it is usually raised with neutrophilic predominance. It is also used for monitoring treatment response. Other important hematological test apart from routine liver and renal function test are C-reactive protein (CRP), erythrocyte sedimentation rate (ESR), and serum procalcitonin. CRP and ESR has good prognostic role and serum procalcitonin is of diagnostic value for bacterial pneumonia. Procalcitonin guidance for antibiotic had a great impact and it was found that there was reduction in antibiotic exposure without an increase in mortality or treatment failure.[7] Apart from these tests, urinary pneumococcal antigen and blood cultures are also of good diagnostic utility. Blood culture is only recommended for hospitalized patients and not for patients who need treatment on outpatient department (OPD) basis.

TREATMENT OF PNEUMONIA

The initial approach to the pneumonia patient by a clinician either in emergency or in OPD is to access the severity, send the investigations (radiology and microbiology as discussed), and start the empirical treatment. As per Indian guidelines the approach for pneumonia is depicted in **Flow chart 1**. To assess the severity of pneumonia there are

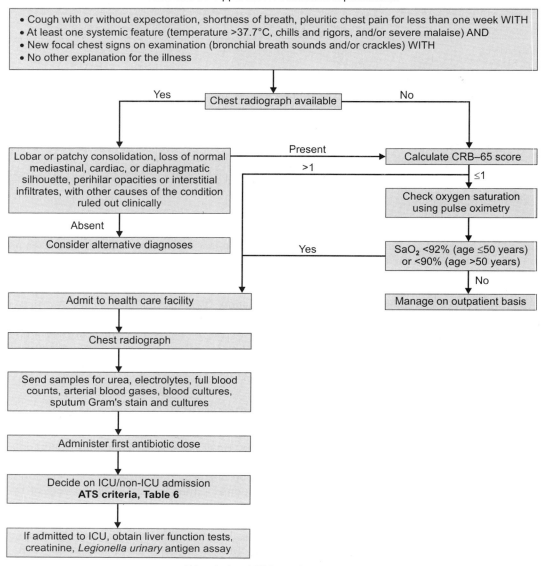

Flow chart 1 Approach for evaluation of pneumonia[2]

Abbreviation: ICU, intensive care unit.

various scoring systems (CURB-65, CRB-65, SMART-COP, SMRT-CO, ATS-IDSA criteria) which can help us to decide regarding admission [intensive care unit (ICU) or ward] and OPD management.[2] The most commonly used is CURB-65 [**c**onfusion, **u**rea >7 mmol/L, **r**espiratory rate >30 breaths/min, **b**lood pressure (systolic <90 mm Hg or diastolic <60 mm Hg), age >**65** years].

INITIAL EMPIRIC ANTIMICROBIAL THERAPY FOR CAP[4]

The initial empiric antimicrobial therapy for community-acquired pneumonia (CAP) is given in **Box 1**.

After empiric therapy we have to follow-up the patients and if there is no response to the therapy within after 48–72 hours they should be re-evaluated. Once the culture report is available, the pathogen targeted therapy, if not started earlier, can be started. The other supportive care needs to addressed are:
- Antipyretics
- Clear the airway
- Oxygen therapy if needed
- Adequate hydration and nutrition
- Evaluate for ICU care
- Need to be seen for requirement of ventilator (noninvasive or invasive).

Box 1 Initial empiric antimicrobial therapy for community-acquired pneumonia[4]

- OPD
  - Previously healthy and no recent antibiotic therapy:
    - Macrolide
    - Doxycycline
  - Presence of comorbidities:
    - Like CHF, COPD, DM, cancer or use of antibiotics within the past 3 months
    - Fluoroquinolone
    - A beta-lactam plus a macrolide
- IPD
  - Non-ICU
    - A respiratory fluoroquinolone
    - A macrolide plus beta-lactam
  - ICU
    - *Pseudomonas* not suspected:
      - A beta-lactam plus either azithromycin or a fluoroquinolone
    - *Pseudomonas* not suspected but patient allergic to beta-lactam:
      - A fluoroquinolone and aztreonam
    - *Pseudomonas* suspected:
      - An antipneumococcal, antipseudomonal beta-lactam(piperacillin-tazobactam, cefepime, imipenem, or meropenem plus ciprofloxacin or levofloxacin 750 mg; or the above beta-lactam plus aminoglycoside and azithromycin or the above beta-lactam plus an aminoglycoside and an antipneumococcal fluoroquinolone (in penicillin-allergic patients use aztreonam instead of the beta-lactam)
      - If methicillin-resistant *S. aureus* is suspected add vancomycin, or linezolid
      - India being a tuberculosis prevalent country fluoroquinolones are not recommended for empiric treatment

Abbreviations: CHF, congestive heart failure; COPD, chronic obstructive pulmonary disease; DM, diabetes mellitus; OPD, outpatient department; IPD, inpatient department.

SUMMARY

Pneumonia is the inflammation of the lung caused infection by bacteria viruses and other organisms and one of the common as well as potentially serious diseases seen in emergency department. To recognize the diagnosis, risk stratification, severity of illness, initiate early and appropriate empiric treatment including antibiotics and admission in right place are the challenges for the emergency physician in emergency department. Systematic approach is adopted to manage these patients as pneumonia is associated with 15% of the mortality in hospitalized patient.

REFERENCES

1. Seaton D. Pneumonia. In: Seaton A, Seaton D, Leitch GA (Eds). Crofton and Douglas's Respiratory Diseases; 5th edition. Oxford: Blackwell Science Ltd.; 2000. p. 356.
2. Gupta D, Agarwal R, Aggarwal AN, et al. Guidelines for diagnosis and management of community- and hospital-acquired pneumonia in adults: Joint ICS/NCCP(I) recommendations. Lung India. 2012;29(Suppl 2):S27-62.
3. Torres A, Menéndez R, Wunderink RG. Bacterial pneumonia and lung abscess. In: Broaddus VC, Mason RJ, Ernst JD, King Jr TE, Lazarus SC, Murray JF (Eds). Murray & Nadel's Textbook of Respiratory Medicine, 6th edition. Amsterdam; Elsevier; 2015. p. 557.
4. Mandell LA, Wunderink RG, Anzueto A, et al. Infectious Diseases Society of America/American Thoracic Society consensus guidelines on management of community-acquired pneumonia in adults. Clin Infect Dis. 2007;44 (Suppl 2):S27-72.
5. Vakil RJ, Golwalla AF. Physical Diagnosis: A Textbook of Symptoms and Physical Signs, 5th edition. Amsterdam: Elsevier; 1992.
6. Oosterheert JJ, van Loon AM, Schuurman R, et al. Impact of rapid detection of viral and atypical bacterial pathogens by real-time polymerase chain reaction for patients with lower respiratory tract infection. Clin Infect Dis. 2005;41(10):1438-44.
7. Schuetz P, Müller B, Christ-Crain M, et al. Procalcitonin to initiate or discontinue antibiotics in acute respiratory tract infections. Cochrane Database Syst Rev. 2012:CD007498.

CHAPTER 44

Pneumothorax and Insertion of Chest Tube

Shaiwal Khandelwal, Ali Zamir Khan

INTRODUCTION

A pneumothorax is defined as the accumulation of air in the pleural space with secondary collapse of the surrounding lung. It must be distinguished from bulla or air cysts within the lung. Pneumothoraces can be divided into spontaneous pneumothorax and traumatic pneumothorax. Spontaneous pneumothorax is subclassified as either primary spontaneous pneumothorax (PSP) or secondary spontaneous pneumothorax (SSP). Primary spontaneous pneumothorax occurs without a precipitating event in a person with no clinical evidence of lung disease. Many of these individuals have occult lung disease with subpleural blebs on computed tomography (CT) scans. Complication of underlying lung disease, most often chronic obstructive pulmonary disease (COPD), gives rise to secondary spontaneous pneumothorax. Blunt (nonpenetrating) or penetrating trauma disrupting the lung, bronchus, or esophagus causes traumatic (or nonspontaneous) pneumothorax. A subcategory of traumatic pneumothorax is iatrogenic pneumothorax, which occurs as a consequence of diagnostic or therapeutic maneuvers (i.e. thoracentesis, insertion of a central venous catheter, surgery, or mechanical ventilation).

CLASSIFICATION AND ETIOLOGY

Classification and etiology of pneumothorax have been described in **Table 1**.

PATHOPHYSIOLOGY

The pleural space has negative pressure during the entire respiratory cycle. This negative pressure is due to elastic recoil capacity of lung (collapsing nature) and the tendency of chest wall to expand. The negative pressure at the apex is more than the base, and this pressure difference keep the alveoli more distended in this region. Whenever a communication develops between an alveolus and the pleural space, air will move from the alveolus into the pleural space (due to negative pressure difference) until there is equalization of pressure or the communication is sealed. As a consequence pneumothorax enlarges and lung becomes smaller resulting in reduction of vital capacity of the lung and partial pressure of oxygen. Total lung capacity, functional residual capacity, and diffusing capacity are also reduced.

The reduction in arterial PaO_2 appears to be caused by low ventilation perfusion (V/Q) ratios, anatomic shunts, and occasionally, alveolar hypoventilation. If perfusion to the collapsed lung is preserved, there is an increase in pulmonary shunt and substantial hypoxemia. If perfusion to the collapsed lung is reduced by hypoxic vasoconstriction, hypoxemia may be minimal. In general, pneumothoraces occupying less than 25% of the hemithorax are not usually associated with significant shunts. Under normal circumstances, despite the degree of pneumothorax, hypoxemia tends to abate within 24 hours, presumably because of redistribution of pulmonary blood flow.

In tension pneumothorax, (mechanical ventilation, resuscitation, and trauma) the intrapleural pressure is more than the atmospheric pressure during entire expiration and inspiration. The collapsed lung produces hypoxia and reduced venous return due to compression of atria decreases the cardiac output and resulting in hypotension.

CLINICAL FEATURES

The clinical presentation depends on degree of lung collapse and underlying lung pathology.

Patient of pneumothorax may be asymptomatic or may be critically ill. Clinical manifestations are unreliable indicators of the size of the pneumothorax. The patients

Table 1 Classification and etiology of pneumothorax			
Primary spontaneous	*Secondary spontaneous*	*Traumatic*	*Iatrogenic*
• No underlying lung disease	Underlying lung disease	Due to blunt and traumatic chest injuries	Due to diagnostic and therapeutic procedure
• Subpleural bullae formation → smoking causes elastic fiber dysfunction → influx of neutrophils and macrophages, inflammation induced → obstruction of small airway → rise in alveolar pressure and air leak into lung interstitium.	• COPD • Asthma • Cystic fibrosis • Interstitial lung diseases • Connective tissue disease • *Carcinoma catamenial*: Female 30–40 years history of pelvic endometriosis, thoracic endometriosis related to menstruation	• Fall from height • Dashboard injury • Steering wheel injury • Road traffic accident	• Transthoracic needle aspiration or biopsy • Thoracentesis • Closed pleural biopsy • Transbronchial biopsy • Subclavian or jugular vein catheterization • Mechanical ventilation • Cardiopulmonary resuscitation • Nasogastric tube placement • Tracheostomy • Liver biopsy

Abbreviation: COPD, chronic obstructive pulmonary disease.

may present with chest pain, dyspnea, cyanosis, sweating, and tachycardia. Clinical examination may reveal pulsus paradoxus, respiratory distress, and tracheal deviation (to opposite side). There may be hyperresonance on percussion and auscultation may reveal ipsilateral decreased or absent breath sounds. Presence of chest pain and respiratory distress accompanied by tachycardia, tachypnea, and hypotension indicates tension pneumothorax. Rarely there may be cyanosis and altered level of consciousness.

In emergency department clinical evaluation should be the main determinant of the management strategy.

IMAGING MODALITIES

Imaging modalities used to identify pneumothorax are:
- *Chest X-ray*: Standard erect posteroanterior (PA) view, expiratory films, supine, and lateral X-rays
- CT scan.

Chest X-ray

Chest X-ray is used to detect:
- Absence of lung marking
- Mediastinal shift
- Presence of small pleural effusion
- Deep sulcus sign in occult pneumothorax.

CT Scanning

Not useful in routine cases but helpful in detection of small pneumothorax and size estimation, surgical emphysema and bullous lung disease and for identifying misplaced chest drain or additional lung pathology.

Size of pneumothorax: The differentiation of a "large" from a "small" pneumothorax can be done by the presence of a visible rim of greater than 2 cm between the lung margin and the chest wall (at the level of the hilum) and is easily measured with the picture archiving communication systems (PACS). Accurate pneumothorax size calculations are best achieved by CT scanning.

TREATMENT OF PNEUMOTHORAX

Primary Spontaneous Pneumothorax

Small Pneumothorax

In small pneumothorax:
- Provide oxygen and observation in emergency department
- Repeat chest X-ray after 24 hours, if no further increase in size then no further management only follow-up in outpatient department (OPD).

Large Pneumothorax

It needs:
- Hospitalization
- Chest tube insertion, if expansion of lung and no air leak
- Remove chest tube and repeat chest X-ray after 24 hours, if stable then no further management
- If large pneumothorax or air leak then surgical intervention needed.

Secondary Spontaneous Pneumothorax

Small or Large Pneumothorax

It needs:
- Hospitalization
- Oxygen inhalation
- Chest tube insertion
- *Surgery*: In patients with persistent air leak, recurrent pneumothorax and spontaneous hemothorax with professions like pilots, divers, etc.

- *Chemical pleurodesis*: Only be used if a patient is either unwilling or unable to undergo surgery. Rate of success is low with chemical pleurodesis.

CHEST DRAIN INSERTION

Chest drains are inserted into the pleural or mediastinal spaces to remove abnormal collections of air, blood, pus or fluid and in many acute and chronic conditions especially when respiratory function is compromised. The procedure is usually performed by surgeons and chest physicians, but every emergency physician should be well versed with the technique of insertion of chest drain.

Indications

Following are the indications of chest drain insertion:
- Pneumothorax:
  - In any ventilated patient
  - Tension pneumothorax
  - Persistent or recurrent pneumothorax
  - Large secondary pneumothorax
- Malignant pleural effusion
- Empyema and complicated pleural effusion
- Traumatic hemopneumothorax
- Postchest surgery.

Contraindications

It includes:
- Coagulopathy
- Dense lung adhesions
- Diaphragmatic hernia.

Preparation

- Identify the correct patient and side of insertion
- Review the radiology and indication for procedure
- Explain the procedure and obtain informed consent
- Arrange for equipment
- Secure intravenous line
- Mild sedation may be required if patient is apprehensive
- Monitoring of vitals and oxygen saturation during the procedure.

Equipment Required

- Sterile gown and gloves
- Sterile drapes
- Suture set
- Sterile gauze swabs
- Syringes and needles of various sizes
- Local anesthetic
- Scalpel and blade (no. 11)
- Betadine
- Local anesthetic—lignocaine 1 or 2%
- Suture—silk no. 1 on cutting needle
- Instrument for blunt dissection (e.g. curved clamp)
- Chest drain
- Connecting tubing
- Closed drainage system (including sterile water for underwater seal)
- Dressing material (Tegaderm).

Selection of Chest Tube of Appropriate Size

- *Spontaneous uncomplicated pneumothorax*: 16-22 Fr (small bore)
- *Unstable patient, bronchopleural fistula or mechanical ventilation*: 24-28 Fr
- *Complicated pneumothorax or hemothorax (trauma)*: 32 Fr (large bore) or larger
- *Pediatric*: 4 X endotracheal (ET) tube size
  - ET tube size = age/4 + 4
- *For Seldinger technique of insertion*: 14 Fr.

Position of Patient

Patient should be in:
- Supine position with arm abducted and placed by the side of the patient (preferred position)
- Upright position leaning over pillow or cardiac table if patient is breathless and cannot lie supine
- Lateral decubitus.

Procedure

Chest drains are usually inserted in the triangle of safety, which is defined anteriorly by the fold of pectoralis major, posteriorly by the fold of latissimus dorsi, and inferiorly by a line drawn downwards from nipple, which usually corresponds to 5th or 6th intercostal space in the midaxillary line **(Fig. 1)**.

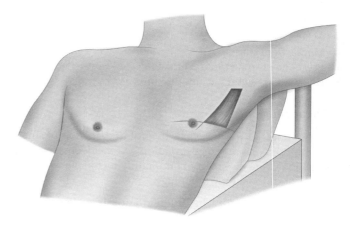

Fig. 1 Procedure for insertion of chest drain

Clean a large area appropriately with betadine and drape with sterile sheets. Aspirate and identify if air or fluid/blood can be aspirated. In case of loculated collections ultrasonography is helpful to identify the site of insertion of drain. In cases of severe cardiomegaly and distorted thoracic anatomy, blind insertion of a chest tube through the "triangle of safety" is not safe. If air or fluid is not found, the insertion site should be changed.

Infiltration of skin, subcutaneous tissue, chest wall muscles, and pleura is performed using generous amount of diluted local anesthetic. Up to 7 mg/kg of locally injected 1% lidocaine with epinephrine (1:100,000) can be used (up to 5 mg/kg if not using epinephrine).

Skin incision is made parallel to the intercostal space (size 1–2 cm) at the marked site.

Blunt dissection of subcutaneous tissues is done with a blunt artery forceps up to intercostal muscles. Insert the finger to explore the tract created and feel for the intercostal space.

Enter the pleural cavity using a blunt artery forceps (guarded by fingers) at the upper border of the lower rib (this avoids injury to the neurovascular bundle running at the lower border of each rib). One may encounter gush of air coming out (pneumothorax) or blood (hemothorax) or pleural fluid (effusion).

Keep the blades of the artery forceps open so as to create the tract for chest drain. Insert the finger through the wound into the intercostal space to feel inside the pleural cavity and rule out underlying dense lung adhesions. This maneuver also allows the surgeon to feel for the tract which facilitates in the insertion of chest tube.

The chest tube is held by blunt artery forceps just proximal to its tip and is inserted into the pleural cavity. Drain is directed toward apex in case of pneumothorax and toward base in case of fluids and then pushed into the pleural cavity for appropriate length. Successful drainage of pleural cavity can be achieved even if the tube is not placed at the ideal position. Drain manipulation and reposition should not be performed until the drain is functioning and draining the pleural cavity.

The drain is then connected to closed underwater seal drainage system. Look for the bubbling of air or column swing in the tubing. This confirms the presence of functioning tube in the pleural cavity.

Fix the drain with the help of vertical mattress suture taken near the drain. The whole length of string is wrapped around the drain tightly and then tied (the same suture would be utilized to close the wound after drain removal). Extra stitch may be applied to avoid peri drain leakage. Dressing is applied and drapes are removed.

Check for any kink or leakage in the tubing. Provide adequate length of the tubing and avoid loop of tube on the floor.

Postprocedure Drain Care

Not more than 1 L of fluid should be allowed to drain in case of massive pleural effusion, to avoid re-expansion pulmonary edema. The drain should be clamped and fluid drained intermittently (500 mL every few hours by releasing the clamp).

Chest X-ray must be done following the procedure to ensure the correct position of the drain. All holes of the drain should be inside the pleural cavity.

The dressing should remain clean and dry, change if it gets soaked or spoiled.

Adequate analgesia should be given to promote chest physiotherapy.

The underwater seal bottle should be kept below the level of chest.

Universal sterile precautions should be taken while changing the underwater seal bottle and should be done by a trained person.

Chest drains should never be clamped especially in patients with pneumothorax (clamping of drains in patients with air leaks can cause tension pneumothorax).

Daily drainage chart should be maintained and hourly drainage should be recorded in patients of hemothorax.

Drain Removal

Indications

Following are the indications of drain removal:
- Chest X-ray shows complete lung expansion (resolution of pneumothorax or hemothorax or pleural effusion)
- No air leak (ask the patient to cough and look for air bubbling at the underwater seal)
- Daily drainage should be less than 200 mL per day (should not be blood)
- Use an assistant while removing drains. Maintain asepsis. Clean the wound and tubing with betadine
- Cut the distal end of the suture and untie
- Explain the procedure to the patient and ask the patient to do inspiration and expiration on instruction. Ask the assistant to hold the ends of suture. Ask the patient to hold the breath at the peak of expiration and pull the drain out while the assistant pull the ends of suture to tighten the knot thereby sealing the wound as soon as the drain is pulled out. Ask the patient to resume breathing as the knot is tied. Extra stitch may be applied to secure an air tight closure. Sterile dressing is applied
- Check the integrity of the removed drain (especially for pigtail catheters)
- Chest X-ray is done 2 hours after drain removal to rule out pneumothorax symptomatic large pneumothorax need drain reinsertion otherwise observation with serial chest X-rays is required for small asymptomatic pneumothorax which resolves spontaneously.

- For drain reinsertion always make a separate incision. Never use the previous drain site for drain reinsertion even if the drain is inadvertently pulled out.

CONCLUSION

Pneumothorax can occur in various clinical settings, classified as primary and secondary pneumothorax. Small primary spontaneous pneumothorax often require no intervention, while a secondary spontaneous pneumothorax almost always requires drainage because of the high-risk of recurrence and complications. In an emergency situation, one should believe more on clinical findings rather than waiting for X-ray, and immediate treatment is required.

BIBLIOGRAPHY

1. Conces DJ Jr, Tarver RD, Gray WC, et al. Treatment of pneumothoraces utilizing small caliber chest tubes. Chest. 1988;94(1):55-7.
2. Melton LJ III, Hepper NG, Offord KP. Incidence of spontaneous pneumothorax in Olmsted County, Minnesota: 1950 to 1974. Am Rev Respir Dis. 1979;120(6):1379-82.
3. Northfield TC. Oxygen therapy for spontaneous pneumothorax. Br Med J. 1971;4(5779):86-8.
4. Ohata M, Suzuki H. Pathogenesis of spontaneous pneumothorax. With special reference to the ultrastructure of emphysematous bullae. Chest. 1980;77(6):771-6.
5. Ruckley CV, McCormack RJ. The management of spontaneous pneumothorax. Thorax. 1966;21(2):139-44.
6. Sahn SA, Heffner JE. Spontaneous pneumothorax. N Engl J Med. 2000;342(12):868-74.
7. Schramel FM, Postmus PE, Vanderschueren RG. Current aspects of spontaneous pneumothorax. Eur Respir J. 1997;10(6):1372-9.
8. Seremetis MG. The management of spontaneous pneumothorax. Chest. 1970;57(1):65-8.
9. Weissberg D, Refaely Y. Pneumothorax: experience with 1,199 patients. Chest. 2000;117(5):1279-85.
10. Withers JN, Fishback ME, Kiehl PV, et al. Spontaneous pneumothorax. Am J Surg. 1964;108:772-6.

CHAPTER 45

Pulmonary Embolism

Saleh Fares, Omar Ghazanfar

INTRODUCTION

Pulmonary embolism (PE) is described as the occlusion of the main arteries or one of its smaller branches of the pulmonary circulation.[1] There are various presentation of PE, it may present as incidental finding or as a clinically unimportant thromboembolism or grave presentation as massive PE and sudden death. Systematic approach is required in emergency department for diagnosis and management of PE also involvement of various medical, surgical, and radiology specialties. Confirmed diagnosis and effective treatment decreases the recurrence rate of PE and PE-related mortality except in cases where PE is associated with hemodynamic instability.

PATHOPHYSIOLOGY OF PULMONARY EMBOLISM

Pulmonary embolism and deep venous thrombosis are the part of same pathological process.

Pulmonary embolism is commonly caused by migration of a thrombus from other anatomical locations in the body and is often precipitated by a deep vein thrombosis (DVT) in the lower limb. This is a process referred to as venous thromboembolism (VTE). This is by far the most common cause of PE. A smaller proportion of PEs can be as a result of air, fat, talc or amniotic fluid. Other pathological conditions such as malignancy or prolonged immobilization increase the risk of PE. Various risk factors are illustrated in **Box 1**.

Pulmonary embolism results in obstruction of blood flow through the lungs and increases right ventricular pressure and leads to the presenting symptoms.

Risk factor for PEs is due to a triad of causes called the Virchow's triad and often more than one may be present in a patient. This comprises of three main components which include alteration in blood flow, vessel wall pathology, and hypercoagulability states.

Box 1 Risk factors for pulmonary embolism

- Elderly group
- History of venous thrombosis
- Previous surgery
- Immobilization for prolonged periods
- Stroke
- Heart failure
- Malignancies
- Obesity
- Pregnancy
- Hormone replacement therapy
- Genetic factors protein C, S antithrombin III deficiency antiphospholipid antibody syndrome (APLA)

The **Table 1** illustrates the various components of the Virchow's triad.[2]

The pathophysiology of PE most commonly involves the migration of a thrombus from deep veins in the lower limbs which travels through the venous circulation and results in occlusion of the major or minor vessels in the pulmonary circulation.

This pathway is illustrated in **Figure 1**.

CLINICAL SIGNS AND SYMPTOMS

The signs and symptoms can be across a broad spectrum and depend on the size and location of the occlusion. Smaller emboli tend to occur in the peripheral lung circulation and classically result in lung infarctions and tend to cause chest pain more commonly but not dyspnea, hypoxia or hemodynamic compromise. Larger PEs occlude major pulmonary vasculature and, typically cause dyspnea, hypoxia, hypotension, tachycardia, and syncope but due to not resulting in lung infarction classically do not cause chest pain. The typical presentation with pleuritic pain, dyspnea,

Table 1 Virchow's triad		
Alteration in blood flow	Vessel wall	Hypercoagulability states
Immobilization	Vascular surgery	Contraception (estrogen)
Surgery	Vascular catheterizations	*Genetic* Factor V, protein s, protein c, prothrombin mutation, antithrombin deficiency, hyperhomocysteinemia
Limb injury		
Pregnancy		
Obesity		
Malignancy		

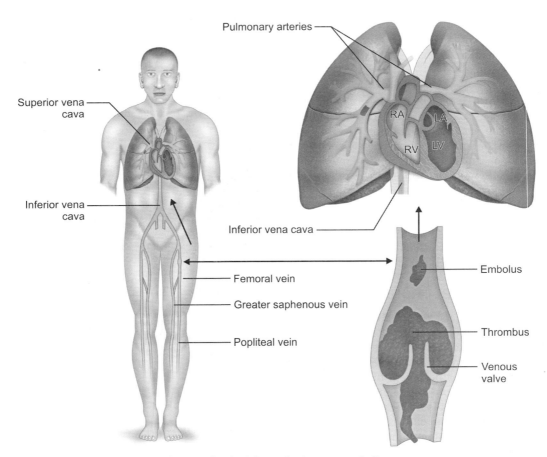

Fig. 1 Pathophysiology of pulmonary embolism
Abbreviations: RA, right atrium; LA, left atrium; RV, right ventricle; LV, left ventricle.

and tachycardia is often caused by a large emboli resulting in both major and minor vessel occlusions. It is for this reason that PEs can be difficult to detect, as smaller PEs cause chest pain alone and large PEs can be painless and mimic other cardiac conditions. It is therefore imperative that PEs are considered as a differential diagnosis especially because 15% of all sudden death are attributed to PEs.

Table 2[2] provides a detailed summary.

Table 2 Clinical signs and symptoms of pulmonary embolism	
Clinical symptoms	Physical signs
Dyspnea	No clinical findings
Pleuritic chest pain	Pleural friction rub
Cough with hemoptysis	Exudative pleural effusion
Cyanosis in severe cases	Left-sided parasternal heave
Cardiovascular collapse	Loud second heart sound
Sudden death	Raised JVP, low-grade pyrexia

Abbreviation: JVP, jugular venous pressure.

Box 2 The Wells score[3]

- Clinically suspected DVT: 3 points
- Alternative diagnosis is less likely than PE: 3 points
- Tachycardia (>100): 1.5 points
- Immobilization (>3 days)/surgery in the previous 4 weeks: 1.5 points
- History of previous DVT/PE: 1.5 points
- Hemoptysis: 1.0 points
- Malignancy (with treatment within 6 months) or palliative: 1.0 points

Abbreviations: DVT, deep venous thrombosis; PE, pulmonary embolism.

SCORING SYSTEMS FOR RISK STRATIFYING PULMONARY EMBOLISMS

The Wells score is given in **Box 2**.

Interpretation of Wells Score

Traditional interpretation includes:
- *Score greater than 6*: High (probability 59% based on data)
- *Score 2.0–6.0*: Moderate (probability 29% based on data)
- *Score less than 2.0*: Low (probability 15% based on data)

Alternative interpretation includes:
- *Score greater than 4*: PE likely. Consider diagnostic imaging
- *Score 4 or less*: PE unlikely. Consider D-Dimer to rule out PE.

Differential diagnosis of PE is given in **Box 3**.

MANAGEMENT (INVESTIGATIONS AND TREATMENT)

Blood Test

There is no specific blood investigation for the diagnosis of PE. In patients with low to moderate suspicion of a PE, a normal D-Dimer can be enough to rule out the possibility, it should be however noted that although the D-Dimer test is highly sensitive but, it is not specific and can be raised in several other conditions. When a PE is suspected it may be necessary to exclude other important causes of secondary PE. CBC, ESR, clotting profile, renal and liver function test.[3,4]

Diagnostic Imaging

There are several different imaging modalities used for the diagnosis of pulmonary embolism and include:
- *CT pulmonary angiogram*: Gold standard investigation
- Ventilation/perfusion scintigraphy (V/Q scan)
- Ultrasound Doppler of the lower extremities
- Chest X-ray: May show large pulmonary infarctions

Box 3 Differential diagnosis of pulmonary embolism

- Myocardial infarction
- Aortic dissection
- Acute exacerbation of asthma and COPD
- Pneumonia
- Pulmonary edema
- Pneumothorax
- Rib fractures
- Costochondritis

Abbreviation: COPD, chronic obstructive pulmonary disease.

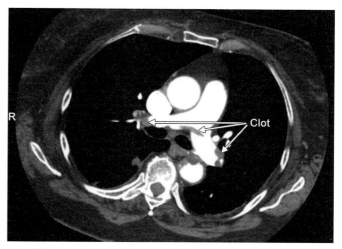

Fig. 2 CT scan showing clots in the pulmonary circulation

- MRI scan
- Spiral CT.[3,4]

In **Figure 2**, CT scan showing clots in the pulmonary circulation.

Electrocardiogram Findings

The classic signs are a large S wave in lead I, a large Q wave in lead III, and an inverted T wave lead III (S1Q3T3), but can also be present in patients who do not have the condition. Sinus tachycardia may also be present but can be present in

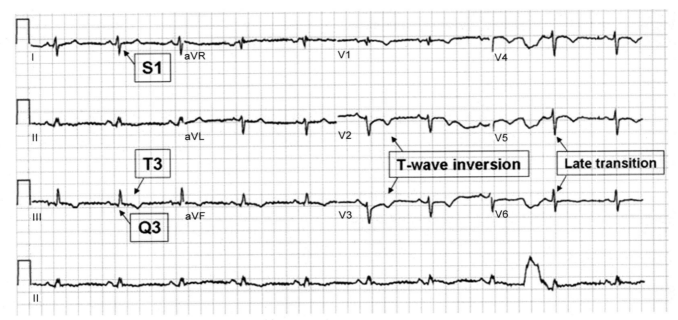

Fig. 3 Electrocardiogram findings in pulmonary embolism

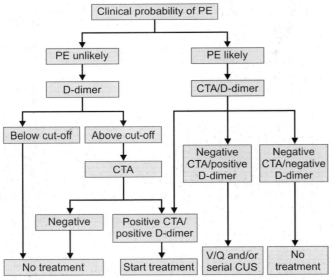

Flow chart 1 Diagnosis of pulmonary embolism

Abbreviations: CTA, computed tomography angiography; CUS, compression ultrasonography; PE, pulmonary embolism; V/Q, ventilation or perfusion.

a wide variety of other pathologies. The important thing to note is that very often patients with PE have entirely normal electrocardiogram **(Fig. 3)**.

Diagnosis of PE is well described in **Flow chart 1**.

Treatment Modalities

Immediate management is along the lines of the advanced cardiovascular life support (ACLS) guidelines to include airway, breathing, and circulation (ABC). This may include both respiratory support with high flow oxygen and/or intravenous fluids if there is hemodynamic instability. Anticoagulant therapy is the mainstay of treatment. Low-molecular-weight heparin (LMWH) or fondaparinux or unfractionated heparin is given initially, which is followed by warfarin, acenocoumarol or phenprocoumon therapy on discharge.

In PE, international normalized ratios (INRs) between 2.0 and 3.0 should be maintained with warfarin. Recurrent PE in patient on warfarin treatment, dose adjustment should be done to bring the INR range to 2.5–3.5. In patients with a malignancy, LMWH is preferred over warfarin. LMWH is also considered for pregnant women and can start at 6 weeks after delivery to avoid the teratogenic effects of warfarin. Usually warfarin therapy is given for 3–6 months in cases of PE, but in recurrent DVTs and PEs anticoagulant therapy is given lifelong.

Indication for Immediate Thrombolysis[3-6]

Immediate thrombolysis is clearly beneficial for patient with massive PE. Massive PE is associated with hemodynamic instability like hypotension and/or shock systolic blood pressure <90 mm Hg. Thrombolysis can be lifesaving.

Intervention radiologists are not increasingly using catheter-guided thrombolysis although this practice is yet not widespread.

Procedural Techniques

Inferior Vena Cava Filter

Inferior vena cava filters are only used if there is a contraindication for anticoagulant therapy. It is also sometimes used in patients to develop PEs despite anticoagulation.

Surgery

Surgical thrombectomy is very rarely used in current day practice in acute PEs although chronic PE leading to pulmonary hypertension is sometimes treated with pulmonary thromboendarterectomy.

Prognosis

Mortality from untreated PEs is said to be around 26% **(Box 4)**.

Advances in Treatment

There have been several new and novel ways of treating PEs. These include ultrasound-assisted thrombolysis, rheolytic embolectomy, rotational embolectomy, suction embolectomy, and thrombus fragmentation. As research goes on, it is expected that more advanced ways of treating pulmonary embolisms will come to the medical forefront.[7]

Prevention

Prevention of PE is of great importance because PE is difficult to diagnose due to its wide spectrum of presentation and treatment is not always successful.

Preventable measures should be applied in according to risk of PE measures which includes LMWH, lower limb antithrombosis stocking (compression stocking), pneumatic compression.

CONCLUSION

Nowadays, we have better understanding about risk factors of PE and advancement of diagnostic tools is helpful in early diagnosis of PE.[8] Management of PE needs multispecialty involvement. In spite of advancement in diagnostic and treatment modalities of PE, the recurrence rate and mortality rate are high. So prevention is of great importance and specific therapy is less important than risk stratification and prophylaxis of PE in hospitalized patient.

> **Box 4** Factors associated with poor outcome
>
> - Hypotension
> - Cardiogenic shock
> - Syncope
> - Evidence of right heart dysfunction
> - History of COPD and chronic heart failure
> - ECG changes including S1Q3T3
> - Risk of a fatal pulmonary embolism increases if anticoagulation is stopped
>
> *Abbreviation*: COPD, chronic obstructive pulmonary disease.

REFERENCES

1. Wikipedia. Pulmonary embolism. [online] Wikipedia website. Available from *https://en.wikipedia.org/wiki/Pulmonary_embolism.* [Accessed February, 2016].
2. NIH. How is pulmonary embolism diagnosed? [online] NIH website. Available from *http://www.nhlbi.nih.gov/health/health-topics/topics/pe/diagnosis.* [Accessed February, 2016].
3. Todd K, Simpson CS, Redfearn DP, et al. ECG for the diagnosis of pulmonary embolism when conventional imaging cannot be utilized: a case report and review of the literature. Indian Pacing Electrophysiol J. 2009;9(5):268-75.
4. Medscape. Pulmonary embolism. [online] medscape website. Available from *http://emedicine.medscape.com/article/300901-overview.* [Accessed February, 2016].
5. MDCalc. Pulmonary embolism severity index (PESI). [online] MDCalc website Available from *http://www.mdcalc.com/pulmonary-embolism-severity-index-pesi/.* [Accessed February, 2016].
6. Mayoclinic. Pulmonary embolism. [online] Mayoclinic website. Available from *http://www.mayoclinic.org/diseases-conditions/pulmonary-embolism/basics/prevention/con-20022849.* [Accessed February, 2016].
7. Tapson VF. Treatment, prognosis, and follow-up of acute pulmonary embolism in adults. [online] UptoDate website. Available from *http://www.uptodate.com/contents/overview-of-the-treatment-prognosis-and-follow-up-of-acute-pulmonary-embolism-in-adults.* [Accessed February, 2016].
8. Rahimtoola A, Bergin JD. Acute pulmonary embolism: an update on diagnosis and management. Curr Probl Cardiol. 2005;30(2):61-114.

SECTION 5

Neurological Emergencies

- **Vertigo**
  Kalpesh Sanariya, Abdul Muniem

- **Acute Headache**
  Devendra Richhariya, Rajeev Goyal

- **Acute Confusional State**
  Devendra Richhariya, Rajeev Goyal

- **Acute Stroke**
  Arun Garg, Devendra Richhariya

- **Status Epilepticus and Refractory Status Epilepticus**
  Atma Ram Bansal, Yeeshu Singh

CHAPTER 46

Vertigo

Kalpesh Sanariya, Abdul Muniem

INTRODUCTION

Dizziness is a common and vague symptom presenting in a variety of conditions to the emergency physician. The diagnosis is frequently challenging and in certain cases difficult to make with certainty based on history and examination alone. Because patient use the term to refer to a variety of different sensations, including feeling of faintness, spinning and other illusions of imbalance, motion and anxiety, it is frequently difficult to extract the exact information that patient want to convey. Dizziness is a broad term that includes light headedness, presyncope, disequilibrium and vertigo.[1]

Light headedness is the most frequently complained form of dizziness. It is nonspecific and the patient may describe it as giddiness or unsteadiness. Important history in light headedness is that there is never a history of fall. There are various causes of light headedness like low hemoglobin, head trauma, low blood sugar, hypotension and psychological causes like anxiety and depression **(Table 1)**.

Presyncope is described as a sensation of faintness or just going to loss of consciousness. It is usually felt when patient assumes upright position from lying or sitting position. Patient is usually asymptomatic in supine position. Causes of presyncope include postural hypotension which can be due to cardiac causes like ischemic heart disease, arrhythmia, dilated cardiomyopathy or due to drugs like antihypertensive, diuretics, and antiarrhythmics. Autonomic dysfunction from diabetes, sarcoidosis, autoimmune disorders or malignancy can also lead to presyncopal episodes. Cerebral hypoperfusion as in case of carotid atherosclerotic disease can also be a cause.

Disequilibrium means sensation of imbalance while walking without any rotatory sensations of head or surrounding. Patient complaints of unsteadiness while walking in the absence of spinning or fall of fear. It is usually seen in elderly people. Sensory peripheral neuropathy, vestibular dysfunction, decreased visual acuity as well as posterior column dysfunction are the main contributory factors in the elderly. There is no role of vestibular suppressants in this condition. Use of walking stick and vestibular rehabilitation can help the patient to maintain balance while walking.

Vertigo can simply be defined as a hallucination or sensation of spinning of self or surrounding. Vestibular system is responsible for keeping informed the central nervous system (CNS) of the primary position of the head in space, its relation to the pull of the gravity and direction of the head movements. Vertigo can be peripheral (the end organ or the peripheral nerve) or central (the brain stem or its connections to the cerebellum or cerebral cortex) in origin depends on level of the lesion.

Table 1	Types of dizziness	
Type	Definition	Percentage
Vertigo	Hallucinatory sensation of rotation of self or surrounding	40–60%
Disequilibrium	Imbalance while walking without any rotatory sensations	<15%
Presyncope	Sensation of faintness or just going to loss of consciousness	<15%
Lightheadedness	Nonspecific symptom, giddiness or heaviness in head	Up to 10%

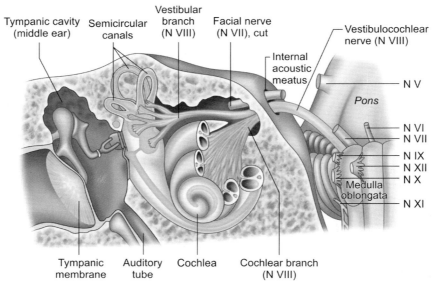

Fig. 1 Inner ear and its connections

Before going for evaluation of a case of vertigo a brief understanding of anatomy and physiology of the vestibular system will be helpful.

There are two components of vestibulocochlear nerve: (1) vestibular and (2) cochlear. Function of the cochlear nerve is hearing and vestibular nerve subserves equilibration, coordination, and orientation in space. Vestibular apparatus has three semicircular canals, which detects angular movements of the head and otolithic apparatus (utricle and saccule) which detects linear acceleration of the body (**Fig. 1**). Vestibular nuclei are connected with the following structures:

- Ocular motor nerve nuclei via medial longitudinal fasciculus which mediate vestibulo-ocular reflex (VOR) which maintain visual stability during head movements.
- To the cerebellum primarily to the flocculus and nodulus which help in modulation of the VOR.
- To the spinal cord via lateral and ventral vestibulospinal pathways which helps in maintenance of postural stability.
- To the cerebral cortex via thalamus which provide conscious awareness of the head position and movements in space.

Vertigo may occur either physiological stimulation or pathological lesion in any of these connections (**Fig. 2**).[2]

APPROACH TO THE PATIENT WITH ACUTE VERTIGO

History

When a patient presents with sudden onset giddiness to the emergency room, the most important clue to reach to the

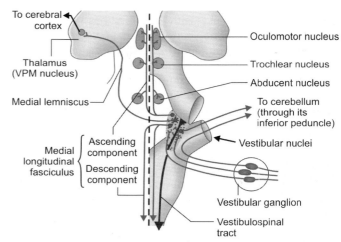

Fig. 2 Connections of the vestibular nucleus

diagnosis is history given by the patient. But as the symptom is often difficult to explain, he or she may not be able to convey right information to the examiner or sometimes the patient may be symptomatic or anxious that exacting proper history is often difficult. In that case physician will have to ask for related question to reach to a correct diagnosis.

Duration of the vertigo is the most important in determining the cause of vertigo. Vertigo lasting for seconds occurs in benign paroxysmal positional vertigo (BPPV), perilymphatic fistula and sometimes in migraine also. Vertigo in BPPV is triggered by change in position of the head while in perilymphatic fistula by loud sound. Vertigo lasting for minutes occurs in migraine, Meniere's disease, and transient ischemic attacks (TIAs). While long duration vertigo is usually seen in labyrinthitis, vestibular neuritis and central causes like stroke, multiple sclerosis or psychogenic origin.

Patient should be asked regarding whether the vertigo is better with eye open or closed. Vertigo that decreases with visual fixation is more likely to have vestibular component, while vertigo of central origin does not lessen with visual fixation.

Effect of the body position also gives important information for certain disease like vertigo in BPPV is typically reproduced by change in position of the head while in orthostatic hypotension patient feels vertiginous or dizzy on assuming the upright position.

Asking to the patient about other otological symptoms like tinnitus and hearing loss also guide to the certain diagnosis. There is history of fluctuating hearing loss of low frequency and tinnitus with aural fullness in Meniere's disease. The vertigo is frequently associated with nausea and vomiting. Labyrinthitis results in sudden onset hearing loss and/or tinnitus with vertigo lasting for hours. Vertigo in vestibular neuritis is usually not associated with hearing loss or tinnitus, an important feature that differentiate it from the acute labyrinthitis. Acute otitis media can present with acute onset vertigo with ear ache, discharge and fever. Otological manifestation of Wegener's granulomatosis includes vertigo, lower motor facial palsy, chronic otitis media, and sensorineural deafness.

History regarding the preceding illness like upper respiratory tract infection (URTI) before the onset of vertigo favors vestibular neuritis or labyrinthitis while patients with history of trauma or barotraumas may have perilymphatic fistula.

Patient should also be asked regarding other symptoms of CNS involvement like diplopia, dysarthria, ataxia and clumsiness of the extremities which favor central causes of vertigo. Symptoms of cardiovascular system like chest pain, dyspnea and palpitation point toward cardiac cause. History regarding psychiatric symptoms should also be asked in case of long duration of nonspecific isolated vertigo.

Other important history include history of trauma or surgery, history of other medical illness, drug history, history of neoplastic disease, and family history should be evaluated.[3]

Examination

Because vertigo could be a manifestation of a variety of neurological disorders, the neurological examination is important in evaluation of these patients.

Examination for nystagmus: The presence of nystagmus may indicate peripheral or central pathology. Central lesion will produce vertical, bidirectional or pure rotatory nystagmus, while peripheral lesion vertigo never produces pure vertical or pure rotational nystagmus. Abnormal saccades and smooth pursuit may also indicate central pathology. Eye examination with Frenzel glasses which use +30 diopter lenses to blur patient's vision and to remove visual fixation helps to uncover vestibular nystagmus. **Table 2** shows difference between the central and peripheral vertigo.

Dynamic Visual Acuity

It is a helpful test in detecting vestibular function. In this test visual acuity is measured when the head is still and when head is rotated back and forth by the examiner at about 1–2 per seconds. When there is fall in visual acuity

Table 2 Features of central versus peripheral vertigo

Signs/symptoms	Peripheral vertigo	Central vertigo
Onset	Acute	Subacute or slow
Direction	Torsional or horizontal, never vertical, direction is same in all gazes	Mostly vertical, may be in other direction, direction may change with change of gaze
Direction of spin	Toward fast phase (away from lesion)	Variable
Visual fixation	Inhibit nystagmus and vertigo	No inhibition
Severity of vertigo	Marked	Often mild
Vomiting and nausea	Severe	Usually mild
Deafness and tinnitus	Usually present	Usually not present
CNS symptoms	Usually absent	Usually present
Instability	Mild to moderate	Severe, unable to stand
Fatigability	Yes	No
Duration	Short duration, decrease over days	Persists
Causes	BPPV, labyrinthitis, vestibular neuritis	Vascular, demyelinating, neoplasm

Abbreviations: CNS, central nervous system; BPPV, benign paroxysmal positional vertigo.

during movements of the head more than one line on a near card or Snellen's chart is suggestive of bilateral vestibular involvement.[4]

Head Impulse Test

This test is particularly useful to differentiate between peripheral from central vertigo. The examiner sits in front of the patient. While patient focused on the examiner's nose, his head is suddenly rotated about 5–10° to one side and response is noted. In patients with normal VOR and normal vestibular function, there is movement of both the eyes in direction opposite to that of head movement and eye remain fixed on the examiner's nose. Testing is then repeated on the other side. In patients with impaired VOR like labyrinthitis or vestibular neuritis (peripheral causes of vertigo) there is initial movement of the eyes in the direction of the head and then there is corrective saccade which brings the patient's eye back to the examiner's nose **(Fig. 3)**.[2]

Romberg Test

In this test patient is asked to stand with feet together, eye closed, and arms outstretched. The ability of the patient to maintain balance is checked. The test could be abnormal in peripheral or central lesions. Ataxia due to central pathology is usually more severe. Patient with cerebellar infarction usually cannot stand without support, even with open eyes, whereas patient with acute vestibular neuritis or labyrinthitis can.

The Dix-Hallpike Test

The Dix-Hallpike test helps in the confirmation of BPPV. Purpose of this test is to stimulate various semicircular canals in different head positions and precipitate vertigo. To stimulate posterior semicircular canal, head is turned 45° to one side and wait for 20–30 seconds. Now supporting the neck, patient is quickly made to lie down with the head about 20° down from the edge of the bed and wait for 30 seconds. If posterior semicircular canal is involved than this maneuver will precipitate nystagmus and vertigo after latency of about 5 seconds. Direction of the nystagmus will be up and fast phase will be toward the ground. If on testing one side there is no nystagmus, then the test is repeated on the other side. On repeated testing, nystagmus will gradually decreases and then disappear **(Fig. 4)**.

Supine Roll Test

This test is performed when Dix-Hallpike test is negative and suspicion of BPPV is high. The patient is asked to lie supine with head in neutral position. In this position, the head is then moved to 90° to one side and look for vertigo and nystagmus. After allowing vertigo and nystagmus to settle down by bringing the head in neutral position, the test is

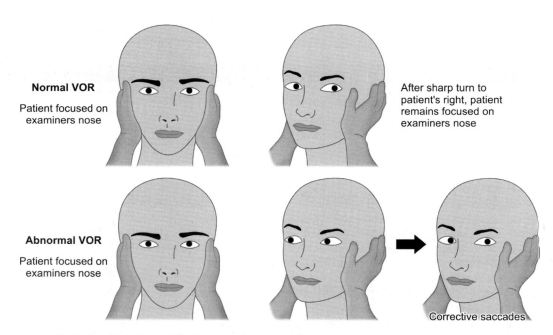

Fig. 3 Head-impulse test (HIT) in normal person and in patient with deficient vestibular function
Abbreviation: VOR, vestibulo-ocular reflex.

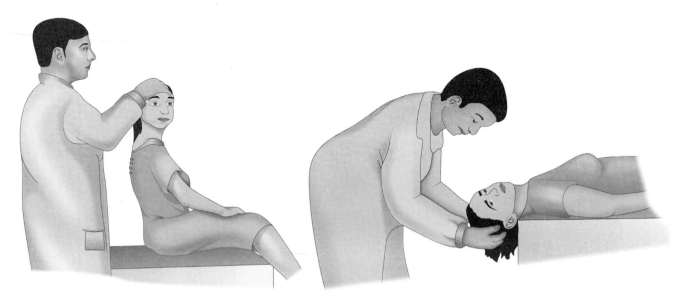

Fig. 4 Dix-Hallpike test

then repeated to other side. This maneuver is for testing of horizontal semicircular canal.

Central Nervous System Examination

Involvement of the other cranial nerves (CNs) should be looked for, like 9th and 10th CN in lateral medullary syndrome. 5th, 7th, and 8th CN could be involved in lesion at cerebellopontine angle. Other neurological symptoms like diplopia, dysarthria, ataxia, and clumsiness of the extremities should be specifically asked for which indicate involvement of the brain stem, cerebellum or its connections.

Cardiovascular System Examination

A quick look on the pulse for any irregularity, carotid bruits, lying and standing blood pressure should be sought.[3]

Investigations

There are list of investigations which can be performed in a patient presenting with acute vertigo. Proper history and examination can help to avoid unnecessary work up. Hearing loss could be accessed with pure tone audiogram which could be found in labyrinthitis and Meniere's disease. Urgent MRI of the brain should be done in patients suspected of having cerebellar stroke. It should also be requested in all patients with acute vertigo who have multiple risk factors for stroke. CT angiography of the head and neck vessels should be performed if posterior circulation TIAs are suspected. Electronystagmography (ENG) and caloric testing can be useful in cases of diagnostic uncertainty to establish unilateral or bilateral vestibular loss. Meniere's disease may be diagnosed with the help of electrocochleography.

Work up of cardiac condition by ECG, 2D echo, and Holter monitoring can be of value in detecting cardiac cause of vertigo. HUTT (head-up tilt test) should be performed in cases of orthostatic hypotension resulting in repeated dizziness episodes.[3]

Treatment

Treatment of acute vertigo depends on the cause of it. Vestibular suppressants are useful in acute stage to give symptomatic relief to the patient in cases if peripheral vertigo. Antihistaminics like cinnarizine, meclizine, dimenhydrinate, and promethazine are most frequently used medications. Diuretics and low sodium diet is helpful in Meniere's disease. Antimigrainous drugs are specifically useful in vestibular migraine. Steroids and antiviral agents are to be of value in vestibular neuritis. For the cases of BPPV, repositioning Epley's maneuver is therapeutic in significant number of cases.

Epley's Maneuver

This maneuver is done to correct vertigo when Dix-Hallpike test is positive. When there is vertigo and nystagmus while doing Dix-Hallpike maneuver, kept the same position maintained for about 60–90 seconds. The head is then rotated to 90° to the opposite side and wait for another 1–2 minutes. Patient is then asked to rotate toward the direction of the head for about 90° so that head will be facing toward the ground. Now patient may feel vertigo again. Wait for about

358 SECTION 5 Neurological Emergencies

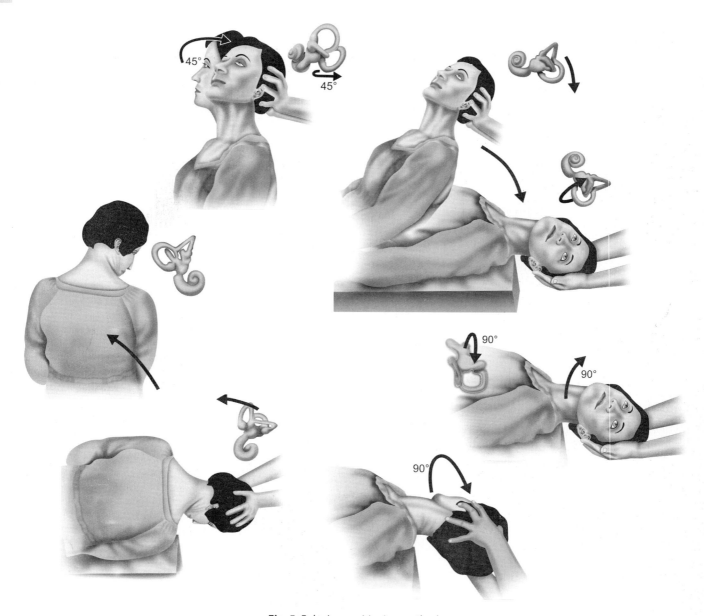

Fig. 5 Epley's repositioning method

1 minute. Now maintaining this position patient is asked to made upright position. Patient is instructed to avoid position and movements which precipitate vertigo. Patients with recurrent episodes of disabling vertigo, may be asked to learn vestibular rehabilitative exercise which can be performed at home **(Fig. 5)**.

A simplified algorithm showing easy approach toward patients with acute vertigo is shown in **Flow chart 1**.[5]

Flow chart 1 Approach toward patients with acute vertigo

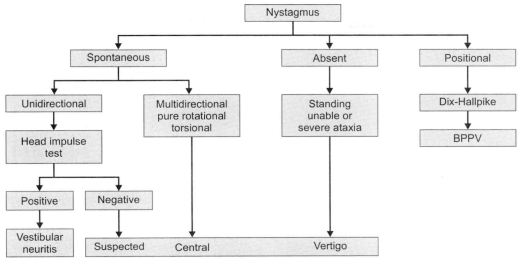

Abbreviation: BPPV, benign paroxysmal positional vertigo.

CONCLUSION

Vertigo is one of the common presenting complaints in emergency department. Mostly the causes are benign but vertigo may indicate some neurological condition also. Systematic evaluation and analysis is required to diagnose the condition correctly.

REFERENCES

1. Lee AT. Diagnosing the cause of vertigo: a practical approach. Hong Kong Med J. 2012;18(4):327-32.
2. Mehndiratta MM, Kumar R. Vertigo—A Clinical Approach. Medicine Update. 2010;20:12-22.
3. Godlee F. Put patients first and give the money back. BMJ. 2015;351:h5489.
4. Walker MF, Daroff RB. Dizziness and vertigo. In: Longo DL, Fauci AS, Kasper DL, Hauser SL, Jameson JL, Loscalzo J (Eds). Harrison's Principles of Internal Medicine, 18th edition. New York: McGraw Hill Professional; 2012.
5. Vanni S, Pecci R, Casati C, et al. STANDING, a four-step bedside algorithm for differential diagnosis of acute vertigo in Emergency Department. Acta Otorhinolaryngol Ital. 2014;34(6):419-26.

CHAPTER 47

Acute Headache

Devendra Richhariya, Rajeev Goyal

INTRODUCTION

Headache is one of the common symptoms presents in emergency department (ED). About 2–5% of patients in various EDs are due to headache; apart from these most of the patient with headache do not visit ED also. Important aspect of management of headache in emergency is identification of life-threatening causes of headache like subarachnoid hemorrhage (SAH) and meningitis and early initiation of the treatment in these life-threatening causes. It is frequent scenario that patient with acute headache immediately sent to nearest computed tomography (CT) scan center by general physician in view of attendant anxiety and in hope that this will identify some cause. But, this will delay in receiving the appropriate treatment while taking care full history alone and differentiate the fatal (need further investigation and immediate intervention) from nonfatal causes (need only reassurance and discharge). In other words, approach should be to classify the patient into two groups: primary headache like migraine tension or cluster and secondary headache like SAH, cerebrovascular accident (CVA), meningitis, temporal arteritis, carotid dissection, sinus thrombosis **(Flow chart 1)**. Educating the patient about probable causes and various treatment options are really helpful in headache management in emergency department.

OBJECTIVES FOR EMERGENCY PHYSICIAN IN ACUTE HEADACHE PATIENTS

Objectives for emergency physician in acute headache patients include:
- Identify secondary headache causes
- Rule out life-threatening causes
- Pain management
- Investigate

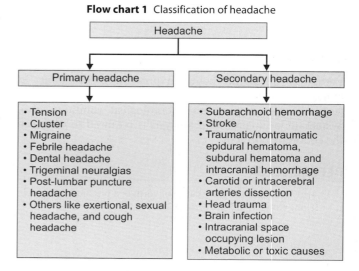

Flow chart 1 Classification of headache

- Manage appropriately
- Follow-up in primary headache patient.

PRIMARY HEADACHE

Pathophysiology

Brain parenchyma has no nerve innervations and pain sensation is referred from cranial vessels, which are only innervated areas in central nervous system, and neural events result in dilatation of blood vessels.

Migraine is not primarily a vascular event but associated with cranial blood vessels, trigeminal innervations of blood vessels, and reflex connection of trigeminal system with parasympathetic outflow.

Tension Headache

It is a most common type of headache presentation in ED. Tight or compression type sensation usually bilateral nonpulsatile type associated with stress and occurs daily not aggravated by exertion. Compliant of feeling constant pressure or weight on shoulders neck and head. Headache starts gradually but increase in severity at the end of the day. Once the secondary headache is excluded, tension headache can be treated with nonsteroidal anti-inflammatory drugs (NSAID), chlorpromazine, metoclopramide, and sumatriptan

Treatment of Tension Headache

Treatment for tension headache includes:
- Reassurance
- Anxiety and depression assessment
- If severe depression suicidal or refractory to treatment then psychiatrist consultation is needed
- *Minor tranquilizers*: Tricyclic antidepressant
- Treatment with diazepam, chlordiazepoxide, and aspirin is helpful
- *Alprazolam*: Antianxiety and antidepressant action.

Cluster Headache

As compared to migraine and tension headache, cluster headache is uncommon. Cluster headache is usually unilateral, short duration, and associated with parasympathetic autonomic features like lacrimation rhinorrhea, warm and redness of face. Headache is so severe that it awakens the patient from sleep. Objective of treatment in ED is to control the pain and abort the cluster headache. Start oxygen inhalation by facemask at the rate of 7–10 L/min for 15 minutes. Subcutaneous sumatriptan 6 mg is helpful in aborting the cluster headache attack. Subcutaneous sumatriptan is fast acting drug. Antiemetics should also be given to cluster headache patient. As recurrence is common after discharge from ED so adequate maintenance therapy should be prescribed to the patient.

Treatment of Cluster Headache

- Subcutaneous injection of sumatriptan 6 mg, abort cluster headache within 15 minute
- Inhalation of 100% oxygen
- Ergotamine 1 mg at bed time, total weekly dose not more than 14 mg
- Lithium 600–900 mg in chronic form
- Prophylactic drugs are prednisone, lithium, methysergide, ergotamine, and verapamil.

Migraine

Migraine is common headache disorder after tension headache. Migraine is typically unilateral recurrent throbbing associated with nausea, photophobia, and phonophobia either associated with aura (focal neurological symptoms) or without aura **(Table 1)**.

Table 1 Preventive and abortive medications for migraine

Preventive medications for migraine	
Propranolol	40–120 mg bd
Metaprolol	100–200 mg/day
Amitriptyline	25–75 mg hs
Valproate	400–600 mg bd
Flunarizine	5–15 mg/day
Serotonin antagonist • Pizotifen • Methysergide	0.3–3 mg/day 1–6 mg/day

Abortive medication for migraine		
Analgesics	Nonsteroidal anti-inflammatory drugs	Antiemetics
• Aspirin 500–650 mg • Paracetamol 500 mg • Propoxyphene 65 mg • Codeine 60 mg	• Ibuprofen 200–300 mg • Diclofenac 50–100 mg • Naproxen 500–700 mg • Flurbiprofen 50–100 mg	• Metoclopramide 5–10 mg • Chlorpromazine 10–25 mg • Promethazine 50–100 mg • Diphenhydrinate 50 mg

Management of Acute Attack of Migraine in Emergency Department

Analgesics and NSAIDs: Many patients of migraine respond to simple treatment drug should be given as early as symptoms are detected. Antiemetics should be given to facilitate the absorption of primary drugs.

Ergot derivatives:
- Ergot derivatives are low cost medication and with vasoconstriction effect
- Main adverse effects are nausea, vomiting, angina, cramps, numbness, and tingling
- Contraindicated in hepatic or renal failure, coronary artery disease, peripheral vascular disease, pregnancy, and hypertension.

Triptans

- Efficacy and safety is established by well-designed trials. Triptans are 5-HT1B/1D receptor antagonist
- Adverse effects are skin reaction, dizziness, hypertension, and chest discomfort
- Contraindicated in angina and coronary artery disease
- Sumatriptan, naratriptan, rizatriptan, zolmitriptan, and almotriptan are in use
- *Parenteral sumatriptan*: 6 mg of subcutaneous sumatriptan are highly effective in acute attack.

SECONDARY HEADACHE

Symptoms and causes of secondary headache are described in **Table 2**.

APPROACH TO ACUTE HEADACHE IN EMERGENCY DEPARTMENT

History Taking in Relation with Headache

- Sudden or gradual onset
- Exertional (cough sexual activity) or nonexertional
- Aggravating factors like supine position, bending forward (raised intracranial pressure), and closed setting (carbon monoxide poisoning)
- Location of pain occipital area with dizziness, ataxia, dysarthria, and dysphagia (posterior circulation stroke)
- Radiation of pain toward neck may be associated with meningitis, dissection, and SAH
- *Severity*: Maximum pain within minutes, SAH, venous sinus thrombosis, and intracranial hemorrhage.
- Any change of pattern in headache
- *Associated symptoms*: Nausea, vomiting, confusion, and altered behavior
- Syncope, seizure, change in vision, jaw pain, numbness, and weakness
- Any previous history of headache, CT head, hypertension, diabetes, and malignancy
- Pregnancy or postpartum status
- Medication history, anticoagulants, analgesics, and contraceptive pills
- Family history of SAH or migraine.

Examination

- Alertness/orientation/mental status
- Vitals signs hypertension, bradycardia, and fever
- Palpation of temporal artery and jaw movement

Table 2 Symptoms and causes of secondary headache	
Presenting symptoms in emergency	Most likely cause of headache
Severe sudden onset headache, altered mental status, history of hypertension, smoking, subarachnoid hemorrhage (SAH), cerebral aneurysm, arteriovenous malformation or trauma and coagulopathy	SAH/intracerebral hemorrhage/subdural hematoma
Fever, neck stiffness, altered behavior, seizures, photophobia, history of ear infection, brain surgery, trauma and immunocompromised status	Central nervous system infections or meningitis
Jaw pain, changes in vision, polymyalgia, and gradual onset of severe throbbing pain	Temporal arteritis
Dizziness, fatigue, weakness, nausea, vomiting, confusion, syncope, headache in winters, and dull frontotemporal pain	Carbon monoxide poisoning
Sudden moderate to severe pain around eye, unilateral vision change and redness	Acute glaucoma
Neck pain, vertigo history of trauma, stroke symptoms, Horner syndrome, and upper extremities weakness	Cervical artery dissection
Associated with nausea, vomiting, seizures, ocular nerve palsies, chemosis, proptosis, papilledema, pregnancy, postpartum, hypercoagulable, and oral contraceptive use	Venous sinus thrombosis
Chronic progressive headaches, papilledema, and history of malignancy	Intracerebral tumor/space occupying lesion/increased intracranial pressure /idiopathic intracranial hypertension
Headache associated with vertigo, vomiting, ataxia, and dysmetria	Cerebellar infarction

- Neurological examination, cranial nerve examination, meningeal signs and fundus examination.

ALARMING SIGNS AND SYMPTOMS IN ACUTE HEADACHE

These are:
- *First or worst headache*: Acute onset of headache particularly in elderly
- Progressively worsen headache
- Headache associated with fever, nausea, and vomiting
- Headache associated with papilledema, neck stiffness, and altered mental state
- Headache with syncope and seizure
- Immunocompromised status, HIV, and malignancy
- Pregnancy and postpartum status
- Headache after neurosurgery and shunt
- For all these patient neuroimaging should be considered.

NEUROIMAGING IN ACUTE HEADACHE

Choice of neuroimaging depends on the differential diagnosis. CT scan of head is choice of investigation in patient of acute headache presenting in emergency department.

CT scan contrast or noncontrast: For trauma and rule out SAH space occupying lesion in brain.

MRI/MR venography brain: For venous thrombosis aneurysm.

LABORATORY INVESTIGATIONS

- Lumbar puncture and cerebrospinal fluid (CSF) examination, meningitis, and SAH
- *Intraocular pressure*: Glaucoma
- *Carboxyhemoglobin*: Carbon monoxide
- *Erythrocyte sedimentation rate (ESR)*: Temporal arteritis.

DISPOSITION

If secondary cause of headache is identified after detailed examination and neuroimaging, patient should be admitted and manage appropriately. If workup is normal, patient should be discharged and follow-up with neurologist.

CONCLUSION

- Taking careful and specific history plays important part in evaluation of acute headache in emergency department.
- Identifying the alarming signs and symptoms while evaluating the headache indicate the high possibility of intracranial pathology and also provide strong indications to evaluate further with the help of CSF examination, or neuroimaging like CT scan head or both.
- Pain management is important irrespective of the cause.

BIBLIOGRAPHY

1. De Bruijn SFTM, Stam J, Kappelle LJ. Thunderclap headache as the first symptom of cerebral venous sinus thrombosis. Lancet. 1996;348(9042):1623-5.
2. Edmeads J. Emergency management of headache. Headache. 1988;28(10):675-9.
3. Fridriksson S, Hillman J, Landtblom AM, et al. Education of referring doctors about sudden onset headache in subarachnoid haemorrhage. A prospective study. Acta Neurol Scand. 2001;103(4):238-42.
4. Linn FH, Wijdicks EF, van der Graaf Y, et al. Prospective study of sentinel headache in aneurysmal subarachnoid haemorrhage. Lancet. 1994;344(8922):590-3.
5. Salomone JA 3rd, Thomas RW, Althoff JR, et al. An evaluation of the role of the ED in the management of migraine headaches. Am J Emerg Med. 1994;12(2):134-7.
6. Torelli P, Campana V, Cervellin G, Manzoni GC, et al. Management of primary headaches in adult Emergency Departments: a literature review, the Parma ED experience and a therapy flow chart proposal. Neurol Sci. 2010;31(5):545-53.
7. van Gijn J, van Dongen KJ, Vermeulen M, et al. Perimesencephalic haemorrhage: a nonaneurysmal and benign form of subarachnoid haemorrhage. Neurology. 1985;35(4):493-7.
8. van Gijn. Pitfalls in the diagnosis of sudden headache. Proc R Coll Physicians Edinburgh. 1999;29:21-31.
9. Ward TN, Levin M, Phillips JM. Evaluation and management of headache in the emergency department. Med Clin North Am. 2001;85(4):971-85.

CHAPTER 48

Acute Confusional State

Devendra Richhariya, Rajeev Goyal

INTRODUCTION

Acute confusional state is common and challenging presentation for emergency department physician. Acute confusional state is present in all age groups and in about 5-12% of total emergency patient. Acute confusional state is a generalized term used to describe altered mental state, delirium, acute brain failure, psychiatric disorder; it is difficult to define the acute confusional state when associated with disturbance in consciousness, attention, thought, perception, awareness, memory, and psychomotor behavior. Acute confusional state starts with irritability and disturbance in sleep cycle, bizarre behavior, and hyperalertness confusion. Most of the time family members are the first one who notice the confusion. Elderly people with comorbidities are common population that develops acute confusional state. Acute confusional state develops rapidly over days to week. In its hypoactive form patient present with lethargic condition while in hyperactive form patient will be agitated, restless, and anxious, in mixed variety fluctuation of symptoms occurs. Morbidity and mortality are high, if this condition remains untreated or missed in emergency department either due to subclinical nature of the disease or due to work load and also raises serious issue related to quality of the care. Patient with hypoactive symptoms like lethargy and elderly people are prone for "missed diagnosis" in emergency department. Patient with acute confusional state are vulnerable and may not cooperate with the staff so emergency physician should focus on maintaining airway, breathing, circulation, vitals and normal blood sugar level. This chapter discusses the risk factors, etiology, and approach to manage the acute confusional state **(Flow chart 1)**.

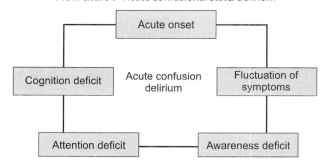

Flow chart 1 Acute confusional state/delirium

RISK FACTORS FOR ACUTE CONFUSIONAL STATE/DELIRIUM

Following are the risk factors for acute confusional state:
- Elderly male
- Multiple comorbidities
- Advance form of comorbidities
- Previous episode of delirium
- Advance dementia
- Chronic kidney disease
- End-stage liver disease
- Postoperative status like recent hip fracture
- Conditions like burn, hypoalbuminemia, dehydration, malnutrition, infection, and acquired immunodeficiency syndrome (AIDS)
- Multiple medications and dependence like benzodiazepine
- Alcohol abuse or withdrawal

- Socially neglected stressful people, visual or hearing problem, poor mobility, and terminally ill
- Prolong intensive care unit admission.

ETIOLOGY OF ACUTE CONFUSIONAL STATE/DELIRIUM

- *Systemic*: Infections including—urinary tract infection, malaria, pneumonia, sepsis, inadequate pain management, trauma (head injury), dehydration, hypothermia, and hyperthermia.
- *Metabolic*: Hypoxia, hyponatremia, hypoglycemia, hyperglycemia, renal, hepatic, thyroid dysfunction, thiamine, B12, and nicotine deficiency.
- *Central nervous system*: Stroke—ischemic or hemorrhagic, subarachnoid hemorrhage, subdural and epidural hematoma, meningitis, encephalitis, seizure, and postictal state, migraine, space occupying lesion, brain tumor, and brain abscess.
- *Cardiorespiratory system*: Acute myocardial infarction, heart failure, cardiogenic shock, and respiratory failure.
- *Medication*: Benzodiazepine, morphine, steroid, antiepileptics, antiparkinsonism, and anticholinergics.
- *Toxic substance*: Alcohol intoxication or withdrawal, substance misuse or withdrawal, and carbon monoxide poisoning.
- *Others*: Postoperative state, urinary retention bladder, catheterization, and physical retrain.

LIFE-THREATENING CAUSES OF ACUTE CONFUSIONAL STATE/DELIRIUM

- Hypoxia
- Hypoglycemia
- Stroke
- Hypertensive encephalopathy
- Wernicke's encephalopathy
- Meningitis or encephalitis
- Status epilepticus
- Poisoning.

CLINICAL PRESENTATION OF ACUTE CONFUSIONAL STATE/DELIRIUM IN EMERGENCY DEPARTMENT

- Acute or subacute onset with fluctuation of symptoms
- Clouding of consciousness
- Reduced level of alertness and arousal
- Deficit in attention, awareness, and concentration
- Disorientation for time and place
- Short-term memory deficit
- Altered sleep pattern (day time sleeping)
- Hallucination and illusion
- Agitation
- Asterixis
- Unsteady gait and tremors.

PATHOPHYSIOLOGY: ACUTE CONFUSIONAL STATE/DELIRIUM

Pathophysiology of delirium is shown in **Figure 1**.

DIFFERENTIAL DIAGNOSIS

It is very important for the emergency physician to identify the life-threatening cause of acute confusional state or delirium and manage urgently. Another important concern is to differentiate it from psychiatric illnesses as most of the causes of acute confusional state or delirium are reversible, if identify and treated urgently. One should not be confused with the presence of history of psychiatric illness because many medical conditions exacerbate the underlying psychiatric illness and make the situation more complex and here effective management depends on the high index of suspicion (**Table 1**).

Taking history of these patients is difficult as patients are often confused and disoriented. In most of the patients history alone give the diagnostic clues so emergency physician should obtain the information through previous medical records, family members, and friends. History of fever, headache, suicidal tendency, fall or trauma, alcohol use or any substance, and abuse should be recorded. Elderly are more vulnerable for acute confusional state or delirium so emphasis should be given on their medication chart and recent changes done in medication doses.

Important drugs that cause delirium need screening are benzodiazepines, opiates, antidepressants, muscle relaxant, anticholinergics, and sympathomimetics (**Table 2**).

Anticholinergic group of medication, narcotics, and benzodiazepines are the drugs which commonly precipitate delirium especially in elderly group of population. Promethazine, diphenhydramine, hydroxyzine, lomotil, meclizine, amitriptyline, and doxepin are the drugs with anticholinergic properties and generally prescribed to elderly. Generally elderly population with comorbidities are on multiple drugs regimens so while evaluating the delirium in emergency department it is mandatory to check the medication list regarding recent addition of any culprit medication and dose modification.

WORKUP FOR ACUTE CONFUSIONAL STATE/DELIRIUM IN EMERGENCY DEPARTMENT

Immediate Steps

Put the patient on monitoring device so that vital signs are recorded immediately. Airway breathing, and circulation can be assessed, and Ringer's lactate can be started if poisoning is suspected for circulatory support. Abnormal vital signs

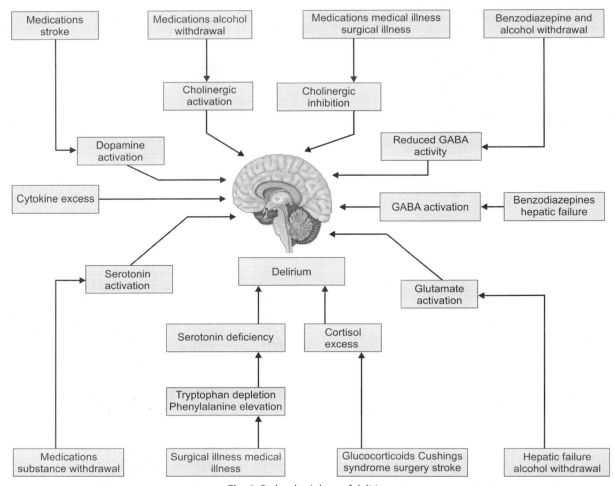

Fig. 1 Pathophysiology of delirium
Source: Flacker JM. J Gerontol Biol Sci. 1999;54:B239-46.

Table 1 Differentiating features between acute confusional state and other psychiatric illness		
Features	Acute confusional state	Other psychiatric illness
Onset	Acute	Subacute/chronic
Course	Fluctuating	Progressive/chronic
Duration	Hours to week	Month to years
Vitals	Abnormal	Normal
Attention	Abnormal	Normal
Orientation	Abnormal	Normal
Awareness	Abnormal	Normal
Reversibility	In most of cases	Usually not

in nonagitated patient are dangerous sign and indicate systemic illness. Use the point-of-care testing to identify the life-threatening cause immediately like random blood sugar, blood gases, and electrocardiogram (ECG).

Physical Examination

- Head, eyes, ears, nose, and throat examination
- Neck examination for stiffness

Table 2 Effects and clinical features of drugs causing delirium

Medications or toxidromes and their systemic effects		
Drugs	Effect	Clinical features
Alcohol benzodiazepines	Central nervous system (CNS) depression	Decrease motor activity and hypotension
Alcohol benzodiazepines Withdrawal	Agitation and excitation Hallucination	Sweating, tachycardia, and mydriasis
Opiates	Sedation	Hyperventilation and miosis
Opiates withdrawal	Anxiety	Nausea, vomiting, and tachycardia
Cholinergic	CNS depression	Salivation, lacrimation, urination, bradycardia, miosis are muscarinic effects Hypertension, tachycardia, and fasciculations are nicotinic effects
Anticholinergics	Agitation and coma	Tachycardia, flushed and dry skin, dry mucus membranes, hyperthermia, decreased bowel sounds, urinary retention, and mydriasis
Sympathomimetics	Agitation, seizures, and coma	Hypertension, tachycardia, hyperthermia, diaphoresis, hyperpnea, and mydriasis

- Cardiovascular and respiratory examination for any murmurs or abnormal lung sounds
- Abdominal and genitourinary examination
- *Neurological examination*: Glasgow coma scale (GCS) score, and asterixis can be seen in hepatic encephalopathy.

ACUTE CONFUSIONAL STATE/DELIRIUM ASSESSMENT TOOLS

There are several tools available for assessment of confusion in emergency department:
- *AVPU*: Simplest scale which stands for alertness, response to verbal, painful stimuli and unresponsiveness. There is no assessment of "response to painful stimuli" so limited usefulness this scale
- GCS was described 40 years ago and most familiar among physicians
- Richmond agitation sedation scale (RASS)
- *Confusion assessment method (CAM)*: First described by Inouye and colleagues in 1990 based on the *Diagnostic and Statistical Manual of Mental Disorders Revised 3rd edition* (DSM-III-R) criteria, helpful for nonpsychiatric trained physician to diagnose delirium quickly and accurately. CAM consists of four components:
  1. Acute onset mental status changes fluctuating course
  2. Inattention
  3. Disorganized thinking
  4. Altered level of consciousness.

  First two components are mandatory and either of two from rest of two are necessary for the diagnosis of delirium.
- Laboratory and radiology test **(Table 3)**.

Computer tomography of head is not indicated in all cases of acute confusional state but more helpful in elderly group of patients. Noncontrast CT is usually sufficient and necessary in paients who are on anticoagulation and history of trauma.

Lumbar puncture and cerebrospinal fluid examination should be considered in patient with fever and confusion. Urine drug screen should be used cautiously due to false positive and negative results.

MANAGEMENT OF AGITATION IN EMERGENCY DEPARTMENT

Physical or chemical restrain of patients are required whenever there is a possibility of "self-harm" and agitated behavior dangerous to hospital staff. Close observation of patient is required to record changes in tone, speech, irritability, clinched jaw, and fist for intervention at the right time. Physician must record the GCS before applying any measures for agitation control. Various drugs used in management of agitation are described in **Table 4**.

Haloperidol (antipsychotic agent) commonly used as first-line medication for delirium.

Haloperidol: Given in 2–5 mg intramuscular; olanzapine: 2.5–5 mg orally once a day; risperidone: 0.5 mg orally twice daily; quetiapine: 12.5–25 mg orally twice daily, and benzodiazepine: lorazepam 2 mg intravenous is also used commonly alone or with haloperidol.

Diazepam is the drug of choice when delirium is suspected due to alcohol withdrawal.

Medical Management

- Withdraw or reduce the drug causing confusion or delirium
- Correct electrolyte abnormalities
- Antibiotic to treat the infection
- *Pain management*: Adequate pain management reduces the agitation.

Table 3 Investigations and causes of acute confusional state

Laboratory and radiology investigations	Clue about causes of acute confusional state/delirium
Complete hemogram	• Acute anemia (hemorrhage) • Leukopenia • Leukocytosis (infection) • Thrombocytosis • Thrombocytopenia
Kidney functions and electrolytes	• Hyponatremia • Hypoglycemia • Hyperglycemia • Acute kidney injury • Uremia
Liver functions test, ammonia levels, and lipase	• Jaundice • Hepatic failure • Hepatic encephalopathy • Pancreatitis
Thyroid function test	• Myxedema or thyroid storm
Arterial blood gases	• Hypoxia • Hypercapnia • Metabolic acidosis
Electrocardiogram	• Myocardial infarction • Arrhythmias • Drug toxicity
Cardiac enzyme	• Myocardial infarction
Chest X-ray	• Pneumonia • Pulmonary edema • Heart failure
Computed tomography (CT) abdomen	• Appendicitis • Pancreatitis • Obstructive uropathy
Noncontrast CT head	• Stroke • Mass lesion
Lumbar puncture and cerebrospinal fluid examination	• Meningitis and encephalitis

Table 4 Specifications of drugs used in treatment of acute confusional state

	Haloperidol	Lorazepam
Qualities	• High potency antipsychotic • Less sedative and less chances of exacerbation of delirium	Short acting
Doses	• Mild/moderate cases 0.5–2 mg orally bd/tds • Severe cases 2–5 mg IM every 8 hours	0.5–2 mg orally/intramuscularly (IM)/intravenously (IV) every 2–4 hour
Precautions	Monitor for extrapyramidal symptoms hypotension rise in temperature central nervous system (CNS) depression	Can cause hypoxic cardiac arrest; use cautiously in elderly severely ill and patient with low pulmonary reserve, and myasthenia gravis
Contraindications	Severe depression, comatose, hypersensitivity, Parkinson's disease	Hypotension, sleep apnea, severe respiratory insufficiency, CNS depression
Interactions	Raises tricyclic antidepressant concentration and hypotensive action of antihypertensive drugs	Raises toxicity when used with alcohol, phenothiazine, and barbiturates

Supportive Management

Team of doctors, nurses, social workers, and managers is required to give supportive care. These measures reduce the need of antipsychotics and benzodiazepines drugs. The following measures should be instituted:
- Avoid long stay of patient in emergency department
- Monitoring device that may irritate the patient should be avoided
- Vitals can be checked intermittently, IV fluid can also be given intermittently as bolus instead of continuous infusion
- False alarm of monitoring devices can also irritate and disorient the patient
- Urinary catheters also increase agitation and risk of infection, and increase length of hospitalization; there is always risk of traumatic self-removal of catheters
- Physical restrain also increases agitation and delirium, use only for brief period if necessary
- Adequate lighting of surroundings
- Presence of family members and close friends
- Placing white board/clock/calendar in room displaying date and time for orientation
- Increase mobilization by avoiding physical restrain
- Minimize sleep disruption and provide calm environment
- Handle gently
- Avoid frequent ward transfers and multispecialty complexity
- Provide glasses and hearing aids if necessary
- Avoid sedation if possible they increase confusion and risk of falls.

EFFECTS OF ACUTE CONFUSIONAL STATE/DELIRIUM

According to various studies acute confusional state or delirium is a marker of severity of illness and multiple comorbidities and also associated with in-hospital and long-term mortality. Acute confusional state adversely affects the patient quality of life. These patients are more to develop hospital acquired infections, pressure sores, malnutrition, fractures, and repeated hospitalization.

Disposition

Most of the patients of acute confusional state need hospitalization once they are identified in emergency department. A very few patient can be discharged if closed supervision and monitoring can be arranged at home but frequent hospitalization are reported in these patients.

CONCLUSION

- Acute confusional state or delirium is common in emergency department especially in elderly with comorbid conditions
- This nonspecific type of presentation actual has serious underlying pathology
- If there is missed diagnosis or delay in management, leads to poor outcome and high in hospital mortality.
- Confusion assessment method is the best tool for emergency department for assessment of delirium.
- Delirium is acute change in mental status fluctuation in attention, awareness and cognition
- Physical examination, trauma evaluation, and stroke scale evaluation
- Diagnostic evaluation to confirm diagnosis
- Treatment of underlying cause
- Apply supportive and nonpharmacological measures
- Haloperidol for hyperactive delirium and control agitation, quetiapine for hypoactive delirium
- In view of high morbidity, mortality, and poor outcome, patient should be admitted and managed aggressively.

BIBLIOGRAPHY

1. Agnoletti V, Ansaloni L, Catena F, et al. Postoperative delirium after elective and emergency surgery: analysis and checking of risk factors. A study protocol. BMC Surg. 2005;28;5:12.
2. Burns A, Gallagley A, Byrne J. Delirium. J Neurol Neurosurg Psychiatry. 2004;75(3):362-7.
3. Brendel RW, Stern TA. Psychotic symptoms in the elderly. Prim Care Companion J Clin Psychiatry. 2005;7(5):238-41.
4. Brown TM, Boyle MF. Delirium. BMJ. 2002;325(7365):644-7.
5. Fong TG, Tulebaev SR, Inouye SK. Delirium in elderly adults: diagnosis, prevention and treatment. Nat Rev Neurol. 2009;5(4):210-20.
6. Gleason OC. Delirium. Am Fam Physician. 2003;67(5):1027-34.
7. Maletta GJ, Agronin ME. Principles and Practice of Geriatric Psychiatry. 2011.
8. Han JH, Wilson A, Ely EW. Delirium in the older emergency department patient: a quiet epidemic. Emerg Med Clin North Am. 2010;28(3):611-31.
9. International Statistical Classification of Diseases and Related Health Problems 10th Revision (ICD-10) - 2015; World Health Organization Version for 2015.
10. Jonathan Potter, Jim George. The prevention, diagnosis and management of delirium in older people: concise guidelines. Clin Med. 2006;6:303-8.
11. Meagher DJ. Delirium: optimising management. BMJ. 2001;322(7279):144-9.
12. NICE. (2010). Delirium: prevention, diagnosis and management. [online] Available from *nice.org.uk/guidance/cg103*. [Accessed February, 2017].
13. Vidal EI, Villas Boas PJ, Valle AP, et al. Delirium in older adults. BMJ. 2013;346:f2031.
14. Violence: The short-term management of disturbed or violent behaviour in in-patient psychiatric settings and emergency departments; NICE Clinical Guideline 2005.
15. Young J, Inouye SK. Delirium in older people. BMJ. 2007;334(7598):842-6.

CHAPTER 49

Acute Stroke

Arun Garg, Devendra Richhariya

INTRODUCTION

Brain attack or stroke occurs when blood supplying blood vessels to specific part of the brain suddenly become blocked by clot or get ruptured, leading to brain infarction or hemorrhage. Most strokes are ischemic 80-85% (not getting blood to part of the brain). Hemorrhage 15-20% within the cranial cavity, whether intraparencyhmal, subarachnoid, subdural, or epidural is also considered a stroke.

Rapid evaluation is critical in these patients. Most common diagnostic modality to differentiate between two is a noncontrast computed tomography (CT) of the head. Noncontrast CT head helpful in differentiating the ischemic stroke from the hemorrhagic stroke (**Fig. 1**).

RISK FACTORS

- Older age
- Males
- Asians Indians more prone to stroke than western populations
- Family history of stroke, and heart disease
- Hypertension, diabetes, obesity, and high cholesterol
- Heart disease, atrial fibrillation, and carotid artery disease
- Smoking, drug abuse, e.g. cocaine, and physical inactivity

ISCHEMIC STROKE

Three possible mechanisms of ischemic stroke:
1. Thrombosis
2. Embolism from carotid artery, aortic arch, or heart
3. Hypoperfusion.
   Etiology of ischemic stroke are described in **Table 1**.

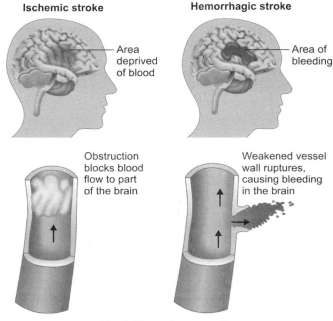

Fig. 1 Types of acute strokes

Causes of Ischemic Stroke

Thrombotic ischemic stroke:
- Atherosclerosis
- Vasculitis
- Small vessel disease.

Embolic ischemic stroke:
- Atrial fibrillation
- Mechanical heart valve

Table 1 Etiologies of most common ischemic stroke

Etiology	Clinical features
Large vessel atherosclerosis	• Plaque rupture results in situ large artery thrombosis or artery-to-artery thromboembolism • Often occurs in early morning hours/on waking • History of transient ischemic attacks (TIAs) in same vascular distribution • Symptoms may fluctuate
Cardioembolism	• History or clinical features of heart disease • Stroke symptoms are maximal at onset as clot is preformed • TIA symptoms are usually different from one another, representing emboli to different vascular distributions • Often occurs during waking hours • Can be associated with Valsalva • Caused by embolism, usually from left atrial appendage (in the setting of atrial fibrillation) or left ventricle (in the case of akinetic segment) • May have strokes of different ages in different vascular territories
Small vessel vasculopathy	• Strong association with hypertension and diabetes • Diameter <1.5 cm • Occurs in subcortical regions such as basal ganglia, thalamus, or brainstem • Never see cortical findings (aphasia, neglect) • Symptoms may fluctuate dramatically • May have TIAs with similar symptoms • Occlusion of small penetrating arteries is not always due to small vessel etiology—alternate etiologies must be evaluated

- Low cardiac ejection fraction
- Endocarditis
- Atrial septal defects
- Cervical artery dissection (i.e. carotid or vertebral arteries).

Injury to carotid and vertebral arteries can cause stroke, suspect in those with neck trauma (including even minor trauma) or cervical spine fractures, young patients (less than 45 years old), and those with neck pain. Horner's syndrome may be seen with carotid injury.

Cardiac conditions associated with stroke include atrial fibrillation or flutter, mechanical valves, septic emboli, and marantic endocarditis. Patent foramen ovale (PFO) remains controversial as a cause of stroke and is not considered a likely cardioembolic source unless left-to-right shunting and a venous clot can be demonstrated. Cases in which no specific cause is identified are called cryptogenic.

Hypercoagulability, arterial dissection, and cardiac abnormalities are the main causes of stroke in young patients.

PRESENTATION OF ACUTE STROKE IN EMERGENCY DEPARTMENT (BOX 1)

Acute onset of focal weakness of face, arm, and leg numbness, facial asymmetry, or speech dificulties are classic presentations. Headache dizziness, confusion, and loss of balance may occur.

Altered level of consciousness, vertigo, and cranial nerve deficits are often seen with posterior circulation (vertebrobasilar or brainstem), and cerebellar strokes. Diminished level of consciousness is unusual for ischemic strokes.

Box 1 Presentation of acute stroke in emergency department

Presenting features of stroke in emergency department
- Headache
- Vomiting
- Hypertension
- Mental changes like confusion disorientation
- Memory impairment
- Aphasia (left CVA)
- Perceptual defect (right CVA)
- Hemiparesis or hemiplegia
- Respiratory problem (decrease neuromuscular control)
- Decrease cough and swallowing reflex
- Agnosia
- Incontinence
- Seizure
- Emotional lability
- Visual changes (homonymous hemianopsia)
- Horner's syndrome (Ptosis of upper eyelid)
- Apraxia (decrease learned movement)

Focal neurological signs and symptoms
- Paralysis
  - Sensory loss
  - Language disorder
  - Reflex changes

TIA (Transient ischemic attack)
- Confusion
- Vertigo dysarthria
- Transient hemiparesis
- Temporary vision changes
- Symptoms last few minutes to 24 hours

Differentiating features of right and left CVA

Right CVA
- Left side paralysis
- Special perceptual deficit
- Short attention span
- Visual field deficit
- Impaired judgment
- Impaired time concept impulsive

Left CVA
- Right side paralysis
- Impaired speech and language
- Visual field defect
- Aware of deficit depression anxiety
- Impaired comprehension

Stroke and transient ischemic attack (TIA) are diagnosed clinically, and no imaging correlation is required for the acute diagnosis. Imaging studies are performed to rule out other causes such as tumor and to determine whether there is brain hemorrhage. Focal neurologic deficits with sudden onset should be considered vascular (e.g. stroke or TIA) until proven otherwise because of the possibility of recurrence or progression of the deficit.

TYPES OF STROKE SYNDROMES AND THEIR SYMPTOMS

- *Anterior cerebral artery*: Contralateral leg > arm numbness and weakness; akinetic mutism or abulia (especially bilateral infarcts)
- *Middle cerebral artery*: Ipsilateral eye deviation; face and arm weakness of opposite side, sensory loss, contralateral hemianopsia; aphasia (left) or neglect (right)
- *Posterior cerebral artery*: Contralateral hemianopsia and memory loss
- *Top of the basilar*: Coma or somnolence or inattention, and cortical blindness
- *Brain stem infarction*: Ataxia, vertigo, diplopia, crossed findings, and contralateral weakness with ipsilateral cranial nerve deficits, cerebellar infarction, ataxia (unilateral appendicular or truncal), vertigo, and nausea or vomiting
- *Lateral medullary (Wallenberg's) syndrome*: Pain and temperature sensation lost from the opposite side of body and same side of face; dysarthria, dysphagia, ataxia, and hiccups
- *Pure motor**: Weakness of opposite side of face arm and leg
- *Pure sensory**: Sensory loss of opposite side of face arm leg
- *Sensorimotor**: Weakness and sensory loss of opposite side of face arm leg
- *Ataxic hemiparesis**: Contralateral ataxia out of proportion to mild weakness
- *Clumsy hand dysarthria**: Weak face and clumsy ipsilateral hand, dysarthria, and dysphagia.

APPROACH TO STROKE PATIENT IN EMERGENCY DEPARTMENT

Team for stroke management:
- Emergency physician and staff nurse trained in stroke management
- Stroke neurologist
- Intervention neuroradiologist
- Diagnostic neuroradiologist
- Neurosurgeon.

Following points are important for attending emergency physician (**Figs 2A and B, Flow chart 1**).
- Early recognition of stroke features by emergency physician by using face arms speech time (FAST) scale
- Time of onset of symptom is critical for thrombolytic therapy and must be documented

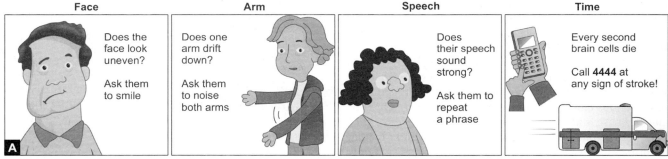

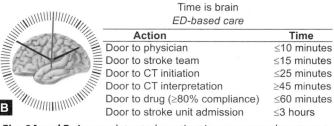

Figs 2A and B Approach to stroke patient in emergency department

---

*The five classic lacunar syndromes result from occlusion of a single penetrating artery, which may be caused by small vessel vasculopathy, cardioembolism, or large artery atherosclerosis.

CHAPTER 49 Acute Stroke

Flow chart 1 Approach to stroke patient in emergency department

① Identify signs and symptoms of possible stroke activate emergency response

② Critical EMS assessments and actions
- Support ABC's; if needed give oxygen
- Perform prehospital stroke assessment
- Notate onset of symptoms
- Alert hospital
- Triage to stroke center
- Check glucose (if possible)

NINDS time goals this color

③ Immediate general assessment and stabilization
- Evaluate ABC's, vital signs
- Provide oxygen if hypoxemic
- Obtain IV access/perform lab assessments
- Check glucose; treat as needed
- Perform neurologic screening assessment
- Activate stroke team
- Order MRI or emergent CT scan
- Obtain 12-lead ECG

ED arrival 10 minutes

④ Neurologic assessment by stroke team
- Go over patient history
- Complete neurologic examination (Canadian neurological scale or NIH stroke scale)
- Note symptom onset (last known normal)

ED arrival 25 minutes

⑤ Does CT scan display hemorrhage?

ED arrival 45 minutes

- **No hemorrhage** →
- **Hemorrhage** →

⑥ Possible acute ischemic stroke; consider fibrinolytic therapy
- Check for fibrinolytic exclusions
- Repeat neurologic exam; are deficits improving to normal?

⑦ Consult neurosurgeon to neurologist; consider transfer if not available

⑧ Is patient still a candidate for fibrinolytic therapy? — Not candidate → **⑨ Give aspirin**

↓ Candidate

⑩ Go over risks/benefits with patient or family
If satisfactory:
- No anticoagulant or antiplatelet treatment for 24 hours
- Administer rtPA

ED arrival 60 minutes

⑪
- Admit to stroke intensive care unit
- Start stroke or hemorrhage pathway

⑫
- Start post-rtPA stroke pathway
- Admit to stroke or intensive care unit
- Frequently monitor;
  – Neurologic deterioration
  – BP per protocol

ED arrival 3 hours

Abbreviations: ABC, airway breathing and circulation; IV, intravenous; CT, computed tomography; ECG, electrocardiogram; ED, emergency department; NIH, National Institutes of Health; NIND, Institute of Neurological Disorders and Stroke; rtPA, recombinant tissue plasminogen activator.

- If no witness is present then time when the patient was last seen to be normal is used. If the patient awakens from sleep with stroke-like symptoms, then the last time when the patient was awake and normal is considered the time of onset
- Manage airway, breathing, and circulation (ABC), intravenous (IV) cannulation, and monitoring
- Early activation of stroke team and preparation for CT or magnetic resonance (MR), management depends on type of stroke (ischemic or hemorrhagic)
- Many hospitals have dedicated stroke protocols and stroke teams. It is important to be familiar with your institution's practice. In cases of suspected stroke in window period—patients come to emergency within 3 hours of symptom onset, speed dial the *code brain rescue* team
- Emergency physician must know the conditions that mimic the stroke like postictal state, hypoglycemia, brain tumor, and conversion reaction.

TRANSIENT ISCHEMIC ATTACK

Transient ischemic attack produce stroke like symptoms which resolves in less than 24 hours although most TIAs resolves within 1 hour. TIAs herald the possibility of a completed stroke—appropriate intervention may prevent strokes and thus permanent disability. There are several scoring systems that can be used to prognosticate the patient's subsequent risk of having an ischemic stroke. One of the most widely studied and used prognostic score is the ABCD score **(Table 2)**.

The results of the score can help predict the likelihood of having an infarct in the next 48 hours. Although many hospitals admit patients with TIA, there are increasing number of hospitals that use emergency department-based observation units to accomplish the workup. Some hospitals even have outpatient-based TIA clinics to rapidly perform the necessary diagnostic studies and initiate care.

Laboratory Tests in Acute Stroke

Whereas no laboratory testing can confirm a cerebrovascular accident (CVA), but a number of tests are important.

Arterial Blood Gas Analysis

A basic metabolic panel can help assess for electrolyte derangements that are known to cause neurologic symptoms, such as hyponatremia, hypoglycemia, and hyperglycemia. Hypoglycemia is a well-known cause of neurologic symptoms and can cause focal neurologic deficits mimicking a stroke. Hypoglycemia and hyperglycemia are contraindications to thrombolytic therapy.

Prothrombin Time (PT)/International Normalized Ratio (INR)

Studies of coagulation can help guide or exclude patients from therapy in both hemorrhagic and ischemic stroke. A complete blood count can be helpful to evaluate the platelet count in patients with hemorrhagic stroke.

Complete Ischemic Stroke Workup (Box 2)

Patients with anterior circulation strokes need urgent carotid imaging. Intracranial as well as extracranial imaging is performed in most cases. Magnetic resonance imaging (MRI) is useful for detecting strokes not apparent on head CT: small strokes in multiple vascular distributions point to a cardioembolic source. In patients with suspected cardio-

Table 2 ABCD scoring in TIA

	Score
A–Age ≥ 60	1 point
B–BP: Initial SBP ≥ 140 or DBP ≥ 90	1 point
C–Clinica features Unilateral weakness, Speech impairment without weakness, Other	2 points, or 1 point, or 0 points
D–Duration of TIA ≥ 60 min 10–59 min <10 min	2 points, or 1 point, or 0 points
D–Diabetes (2-day stroke risk) High: Total 6–7 pts (8.1% risk) Moderate: Total 4–5 pts (4.1% risk) Low: Total 0–3 pts (1.0% risk)	1 point

Abbreviations: TIA, transient ischemic attack; BP, blood pressure; SBP, systolic blood pressure; DBP, diastolic blood pressure; pts, patients.

Box 2 Recommended tests in acute stroke

Acute evaluation (should be focused to allow thrombolytic therapy if indicated):
- **CT scan** of the brain without contrast to evaluate for acute intracerebral hemorrhage
- **Laboratory data:** Glucose, CBC, platelet count, serum electrolytes, coagulation studies, lipid panel, cardiac enzymes, oxygen saturation
- **Electrocardiogram (ECG)** with continued telemetry monitoring

Etiology and risk factor evaluation:
- **Laboratory data in appropriate clinical setting:** Erythrocyte sedimenation rate (ESR), antinuclear antibody (ANA), homocysteine
- **Carotid artery imaging** (Duplex ultrasound or magnetic resonance angiography [MRA]) for anterior circulation symptoms
- **Transthoracic echocardiogram**
- **Echocardiogram** with "bubble study" to assess for intra-atrial shunt, if indicated
- **Evaluation of hypercoagulable state**, if indicated: Protein C, protein S, Factor V Leiden, prothrombin gene mutation

embolism, electrocardiogram (ECG) **(Figs 3A and B)** is indicated. All patients should have telemetry for atrial fibrillation identification—ECGs are inadequate for detection of this important risk factor. Implantable event monitors reveal subclinical atrial fibrillation in a substantial proportion of patients with cryptogenic stroke and are warranted in cases where clinical suspicion is high.

RADIOLOGICAL INVESTIGATIONS IN ACUTE STROKE

Computed Tomography

Urgent CT of brain is obtained under stroke protocol with angiography of head and neck vessels. The most important

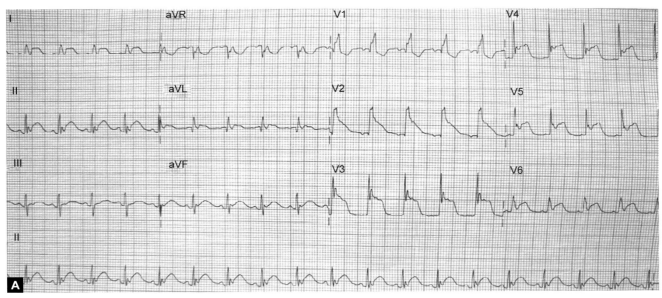

12-lead ECG of a patient with a stroke, showing large deeply invered T-waves

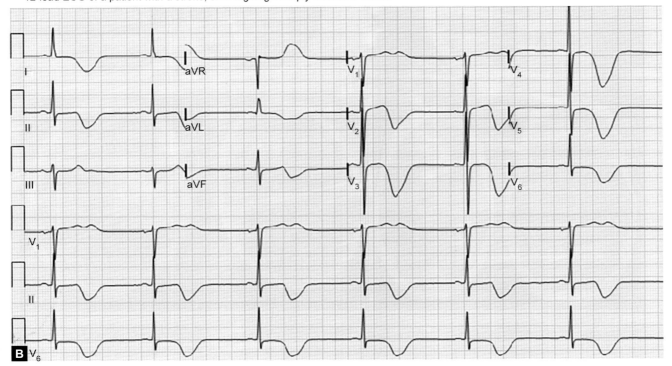

Figs 3A and B (A) Electrocardiogram (ECG) changes, resembling those of an ST segment elevation myocardial infarction in a woman who had an acute central nervous system injury from a subarachnoid hemorrhage; (B) 12-lead ECG of a patient with a stroke, showing large deeply inverted T-waves

early imaging test is noncontrast CT of the brain. This helps with one of the first branch points of therapy, which is distinguishing hemorrhagic stroke from ischemic stroke. Some hospitals use emergent MRI to evaluate patients with possible stroke, but this is much less common. Rapidly obtaining a noncontrast CT of the head should be a priority in working up the patient with suspected CVA. Head CT rules out hemorrhage, subdural hematoma, and tumor. It is the first and most important test when evaluating for thrombolysis. On CT, most ischemic strokes eventually become visible as hypodensities of the brain parenchyma, but CT is largely normal for at least 6 hours. The earliest CT signs are loss of the cortical ribbon and gyral edema **(Figs 4A to E)**.

Magnetic Resonance Imaging

On MRI, strokes will appear hyperintense on T2-weighted sequences. Diffusion-weighted imaging (DWI) detects cytotoxic edema that accompanies ischemic cell death and can appear very shortly after onset of ischemia. True diffusion positivity will appear dark on the apparent diffusion coefficient (ADC) map sequence. Onset of DWI positivity may be delayed up to 48–72 hours, particularly in the brain stem, and typically lasts 10–14 days.

Digital Subtraction Angiography

This is the most accurate in diagnosis of most of the diseases of blood vessels. A small tube (catheter) is guided from the leg blood vessel in to the blood vessel we wish to study followed by dye (contrast) injections to obtain the images. CT/MR angiography is also an option in some cases **(Figs 5A to C)**.

TREATMENT OF ACUTE STROKE IN EMERGENCY DEPARTMENT

Hemorrhagic stroke therapy is centered on reducing hemorrhage. Ischemic stroke therapies are centered on restoring the

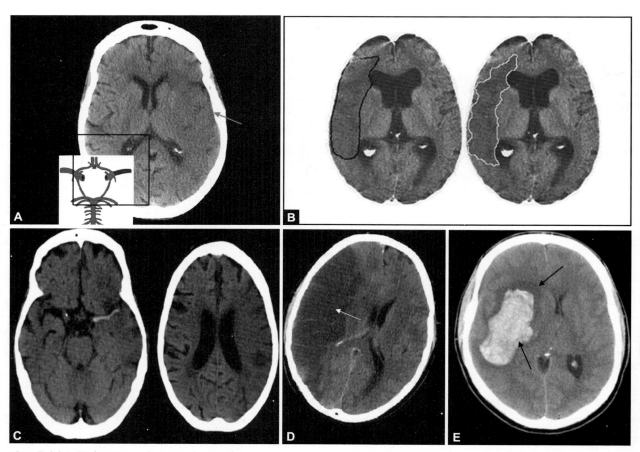

Figs 4A to E (A) A CT showing early signs of a middle cerebral artery stroke with loss of definition of the gyri and gray white boundary; (B) CT scan—darkened area is ischemia in acute stroke; (C) Dense media sign in a patient with middle cerebral artery infarction shown on the left. Right image after 7 hours; (D) CT scan of the brain with an MCA infarct; (E) CT scan of intraparenchymal bleed (bottom arrow) with surrounding edema (top arrow)

Abbreviations: CT, computed tomography; MCA, middle cerebral artery.

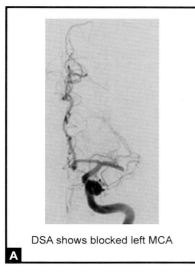
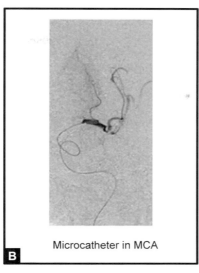
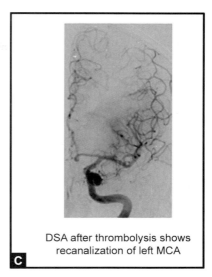

Figs 5A to C (A) Digital subtraction angiography (DSA) shows blocked left middle cerebral artery (MAC); (B) Microcatheter in MCA, and (C) DSA after thrombolysis shows recanalization in MCA

blood flow in blocked vessels. The only medication currently approved by the Food and Drug Administration (FDA) for acute ischemic stroke is intravenous tissue plasminogen activator (IV tPA), administered within 3–4.5 hours of onset of symptom. Only alteplase is approved for acute stroke thrombolysis.

CONCEPT OF THROMBOLYSIS (FIG. 6)

When the blood flow to the brain stops suddenly, brain cells start dying immediately, but few cells in *penumbra* area can survive for few hours with low oxygen or low energy state. If blood flow is restored in this area within window period then these cells can be salvaged and become functional. Favorable outcome are achieved in 30–50% of cases. Major risk of treatment is symptomatic brain hemorrhage.

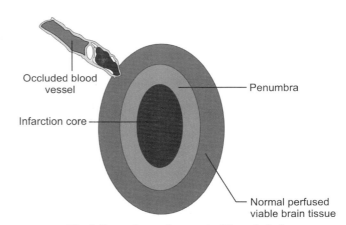

Fig. 6 Penumbra and concept of thrombolysis

Inclusion Criteria for Thrombolysis

- Clinical presentation of stroke
- Presenting within 3–4.5 hours of onset
- No hemorrhage on CT/MRI
- If patient comes after 4.5 hours of onset of symptoms but before 8 hours he can still be candidate for endovascular therapy.

Exclusion Criteria

- Less than 18 years of age
- Arterial puncture at noncompressible site less than 1 week
- Surgery or serious trauma in past 2 weeks
- Significant gastrointestinal and genitourinary (GI/GU) bleed in pat 3 weeks
- Myocardial infarction less than 3 weeks
- Head injury or large stroke in past 3 months
- Subarachnoid hemorrhage (SAH) or intracranial hemorrhage (ICH)
- Active bleeding site
- INR greater than 1.7
- Activated partial thromboplastin time (aPTT) greater than 35 seconds
- Platelet less than 100,000.

Relative Contraindications

- Seizure at onset
- Recent stroke less than 3 months
- Diagnosed brain tumors aneurysm and arteriovenous malformation (AVM)

- "Wake up stroke"
- Blood glucose less than 50 or greater than 400
- Blood pressure systolic greater than 180 mm Hg and diastolic greater than 110 mm Hg
- Known pregnancy.

Blood Pressure Management (Thrombolytic Candidate)

- Labetelol (if no bradycardia, and bronchospasm): 5–10 mg IV every 5 minutes. If not controlled in less than four doses start infusion
- Nicardipine infusion: 5–15 mg/h
- Hydralazine (if bradycardia, and bronchospasm): 5–20 mg IV every 5 minutes. if there is no control in less than four doses then change to nicardipine infusion.

Blood Pressure Management (Not a Candidate for Thrombolysis)

- *Ischemic stroke*: Treat only blood pressure (BP) greater than 230/120 or end organ failure
- *Hemorrhagic stroke*: Goal MAP less than 130
- *SAH*: Goal mean arterial pressure (MAP) less than 100
- MAP = Pulse pressure + 1/3 of diastolic pressure
- Max reduction less than 20%.

Administering tPA

- Tissue plasminogen activator should be prepared in sterile water for IV infusion concentration 1 mg/mL
- *Dose*: 0.9 mg/kg give 10% of total dose over 1 minute and remaining 90% over 60 minutes, total dose not greater than 90 mg.

Monitoring

- *Monitor BP closely in first 24 hours*: Every 15 minutes in first 2 hours, every 30 minutes in next 6 hours and hourly for next 16 hours
- Maintain euglycemia 100–140 mg%
- Monitor for severe headache, vomiting, worsening sensorium, dilated pupil, worsening of motor sensory cerebellar signs.

Suspected Hemorrhage

- *Stop thrombolysis*: Urgent plain CT of head, if hemorrhage confirmed send blood for PT/INR, aPTT, and platelet
- Arrange 6–8 units of cryoprecipitate or fresh frozen plasma, and 6 unit of platelets
- Urgent neurosurgical consultation.

Post-thrombolytic Management

- Transfer to intensive care unit (ICU)
- Do not order aspirin, clopidogrel, and heparin including low molecular weight heparin (LMWH) or warfarin for 24 hours

Box 3 Various ways to perform dysphagia screening

How to perform dysphagia screening
- Patient should be in sitting position
- Patient should be asked to hold the cup independently
- Administer 90 mL of water via cup

Dysphagia screen is failed if:
- Patient coughs after swallow or attempts to clear throat
- Change in voice (hoarse)
- Nasal regurgitation/shortness of breath
- Patient should be watched for at least 3 minutes
If failed: Keep nil per oris (NPO)

- Avoid intramuscular (IM) injection and venipuncture at noncompressible site
- Continuous BP monitoring, avoid automated BP cuffs
- Avoid any discontinuation of arterial or venous access site for 24 hours
- No nasogastric tube placement for 24 hours
- No urinary catheter placement for 30 minutes after tPA
- Nil orally till dysphagia screen (**Box 3**).

General Precautions

- Keep head of bed 15–30° elevated
- Intranasal O_2 in all patients of moderate to severe stroke
- Regularly check for deep vein thrombosis (DVT) signs (leg pain, swelling, and redness)
- DVT pumps in bedridden patients
- Use alpha mattress to prevent bed sores
- *Heel protectors*: Use gloves filled with water
- Provide mouth care regularly
- Patients should be motivated to move paretic or plegic extremity with normal extremity
- Neuro- and chest-physiotherapy, occupational therapy, and speech therapy.

General Management

- Normal saline at 1–2 mL/kg/h
- Heparin 5,000 units subcutaneously every 8 hours or enoxaparin 1 mg/kg subcutaneously once daily
- Pantoprazole oral or IV twice daily
- Goal blood sugar less than 140
- If fever, give paracetamol round the clock
- Lactulose 30 mL/d
- Start antithrombotic (aspirin) or anticoagulants after 24 hours of thrombolysis.

If there is no response in 30 minutes (or patient reports 4.5–8 hours) then:
- Consider shifting the patient to a hospital having facility for endovascular treatment
- CT/MR angiography to confirm major vessel occlusion
- Penumbra imaging to look for salvageable tissue
- Intra-arterial thrombolysis up to 6 hours.
- Mechanical thrombectomy up to 8 hours.

Intra-arterial Thrombolysis

In many tertiary-care medical centers, there is a protocol for catheter-based intra-arterial thrombolysis or clot extraction or both in acute large vessel stroke that involve the middle cerebral artery or its branches and the basilar artery. Interventional procedures for acute stroke remain promising and are undergoing current evaluation through investigational protocols.

When should intra-arterial (IA) therapy be used for acute ischemic stroke?

The role for IA therapy is rapidly evolving. IA therapy with stent retriever devices is reasonable in patients with device-accessible proximal large vessel occlusions without early ischemic changes on brain imaging. Given the dangers of reperfusion injury and device-related complications (11–16%), rapid therapy and careful patient selection are vital **(Figs 7A to F)**.

Advantages

- Higher recanalization rate
- Symptomatic brain hemorrhage:
  - 8.3% in the carotid system
  - 6.5% in vertebrobasilar territory
  - No higher than those in IV thrombolysis.

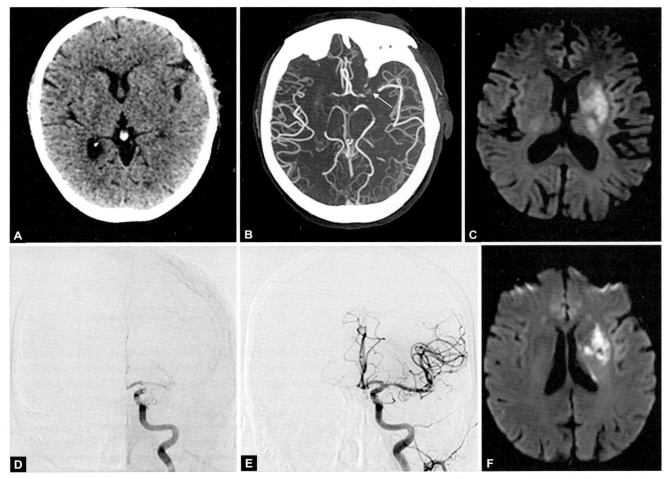

Figs 7A to F Illustrative images from an acute stroke case in which a previously healthy 70-year-old woman presented with a National Institutes of Health Stroke Scale (NIHSS) of 22. Her last known well time was 5 hours previously. (A) Initial noncontrast CT was negative for hemorrhage; (B) CT angiography (axial maximal intensity projections) shows occlusion of the left middle carotid artery (arrow); (C) Diffusion-weighted imaging (DWI), obtained immediately following the CT scan, shows a small established core infarct. Patient was deemed a good candidate for intervention; (D) Initial catheter angiographic image, anteroposterior view, shows opacified internal carotid artery (ICA), a filling defect at the terminus of the carotid artery, and faint opacification of the anterior cerebral artery (ACA) consistent with an ICA-T occlusion; (E) After mechanical thrombectomy, the ICA terminus, middle carotid artery, and ACA filled normally, indicating complete recanalization; (F) Follow-up MRI DWI at 24 hours shows no change in size of the core infarct following recanalization. The patient improved to NIHSS 4 and was NIHSS 2 at time of discharge on day 3 postoperative. She had no deficits at her 3-month follow-up

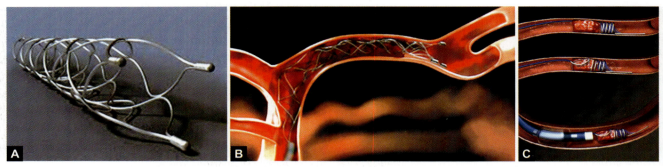

Figs 8A to C MERCI retriever
Abbreviation: MERCI, mechanical embolus removal in cerebral ischemia.

Disadvantages

- Ready availability of neurointerventionalists, a stroke team, and a stroke ICU
- Additional time required to begin treatment compared to IV thrombolysis.

Mechanical Thrombectomy

It is now strongly recommended for patients in whom large arteries within the brain are blocked **(Figs 8A to C)**.

TYPES OF HEMORRHAGIC STROKE

Intracerebral hemorrhage (ICH), which causes approximately 70% of hemorrhagic strokes, or SAH, which is responsible for approximately 30% of hemorrhagic strokes. The most common etiologies of ICH are anticoagulants, hypertension, bleeding disorders, amyloid angiopathy, illicit drug use (usually sympathomimetics), and vascular malformations. Cerebral aneurysms are the most common cause of SAH, accounting for approximately 80%. However, SAH may also be caused by arteriovenous malformations, and vertebral artery dissection.

Hypertensive hemorrhages occur most frequently in patients with a history of poorly controlled hypertension. They are associated with small vessel ischemic changes and microbleeds of the basal ganglia, deep white matter, brain stem, and cerebellum.

Acute Subarachnoid Hemorrhage

The most well-described complaint is that of a thunderclap headache or sudden onset of the worst headache. Up to 15% of patients with sudden onset of the worst headaches of their lives have SAH. However, patients with SAH can have seizure, syncope, depressed mental status, or even focal neurologic deficits **(Figs 9 and 10)**.

It is important if the patient complains of headache to assess whether the headache is new or different for the patient. Additionally, it is helpful to ask for the timing between headache onset and maximal intensity. The literature is evolving with regard to the sensitivity of noncontrast CT as the technology for CT scanning improves. It is also dependent on who is reading the imaging; however, a reasonable estimate is 95% within 24 hours, 80% in 48 hours, 70% in 72 hours, and 50% in 5 days. It is important to note that the literature is consistent in demonstrating a decreasing sensitivity of head CT from headache onset. A more recent study has suggested that if the time from headache to CT scan is 6 hours or less, the sensitivity is as high as 100%; however, this result has not been replicated yet.

Most neurologists still recommend a lumbar puncture when CT scan is negative in SAH. The reasoning is based upon the fact that the noncontrast head CT lacks 100% sensitivity, and the risk for missing one patient with SAH could be catastrophic. CT angiography of the brain can be

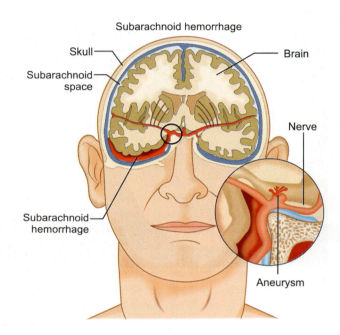

Fig. 9 Subarachnoid hemorrhage

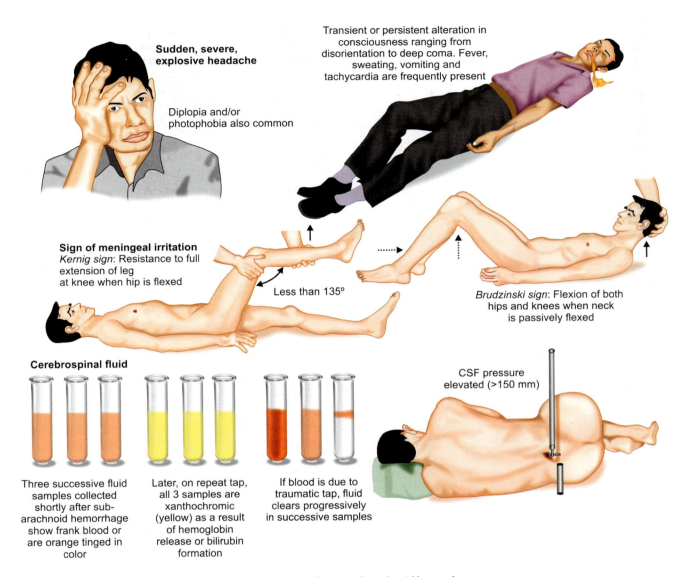

Fig. 10 Evaluation of acute subarachnoid hemorrhage

used to assess for aneurysmal SAH (the most common type of SAH). The absence of aneurysms on CT angiography would reduce the risk of aneurysmal bleeding and effectively rule out SAH **(Fig. 11)**.

If an aneurysm is discovered, urgent intervention to secure the aneurysm via surgical clipping or intravascular coiling is typically indicated and monitoring for vasospasm in an intensive care unit setting for up to 2 weeks **(Figs 12A and B)**.

Complications of Subarachnoid Hemorrhage

Complications of SAH have been shown in **Flow chart 2**.

Parenchymal Hemorrhage (Intracranial Hemorrhage)

Patients with ICH are typically diagnosed by CT scan without contrast. Unless the hemorrhage is in a classic location for hypertensive hemorrhage and the patient has a clear history of uncontrolled hypertension, both immediate and delayed (4–8 weeks) contrasted imaging by CT or MRI are indicated to evaluate for the presence of underlying pathology that may have caused the bleed. Any coagulopathy (iatrogenic or intrinsic) should be reversed promptly and anticoagulant and antiplatelet agents should be held. Trials of procoagulant administration have failed to show improvement in

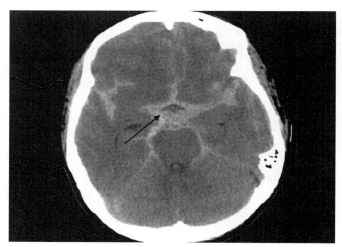

Fig. 11 CT scan of the brain showing subarachnoid hemorrhage as a white area in the center and stretching into the sulci to either side (arrow)

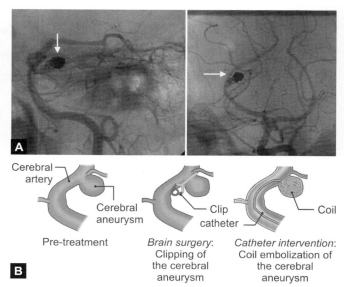

Figs 12A and B Intracranial aneurysm coiling or embolization. Arteriogram showing a partially coiled aneurysm (arrows), of the posterior cerebral artery with a residual aneurysmal sac. Patient was a 34-year-old woman initially treated for a SAH

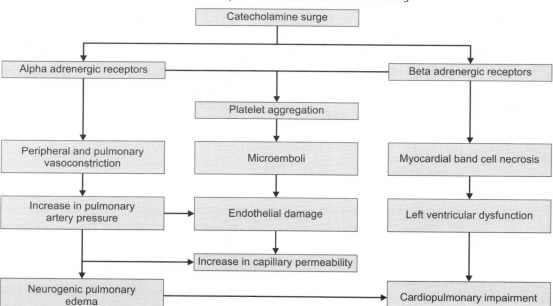

Flow chart 2 Complications of subarachnoid hemorrhage

outcomes. BP should be managed typically to maintain a systolic pressure of 120–140 mm Hg.
- General management principles remain the same (IIv fluids, O_2, DVT pump, physiotherapy, etc.)
- Prophylactic antiepileptic medications are usually not indicated
- Contrast CT scan and CT angiography should be done in all the cases to establish the etiology
- Mannitol or Lasix are indicated in case of significant edema or midline shift
- Surgical intervention or external ventricular drain (EVD)—decision needs to be taken in consultation with neurosurgeon

Identify Risk Factors

- High blood pressure
- Heart disease:
  - Atrial fibrillation (AF), dilated cardiomyopathy (DCM), valvular heart disease, and acute myocardial infarction
- Diabetes
- High-cholesterol or homocysteine levels
- Excess alcohol intake
- Sedentary lifestyle
- Obesity
- Smoking.

Risk Factor Screening

- Lipid profile
- Homocysteine
- 2D echocardiography or transesophageal echocardiography
- Holter monitoring
- Carotid Doppler or computed tomography angiography/ magnetic resonance angiography of head and neck vessels
- Coagulation profile, connective tissue serology, and digital subtraction angiography in selected patients.

Discharge Plan

- Smoking cessation advice
- Antiplatelet or antithrombotic
- *Antihypertensive*: Target BP less than 140/90 mm Hg (less than 130/80 mm Hg for diabetes mellitus)
- *Statins*: Target low-density lipoprotein less than 70 mg/%
- Insulin or oral hypoglycemic agents
- Diet advice by dietician and nutritionist
- Physiotherapy, occupational therapy, and speech therapy
- Elastic stockings in plegic or paretic limb
- Physical activity tailored for patient.

CRYPTOGENIC STROKE

Cryptogenic stroke can be defined as, if no probable cause is identified for ischemic stroke after complete standard diagnostic evaluation. Cryptogenic stroke are about 10–35% of all ischemic stroke but with availability of advanced testing in higher center, this percentage has declined to 10–15%. Cryptogenic stroke are mostly embolic in origin either from heart or right to left shunt. In young adult, patent foramen ovale and in elderly group occult paroxysmal atrial fibrillation is commonly found as a source of cryptogenic stroke **(Flow chart 3)**.

SUMMARY

Management of stroke is improving day-by-day. Emergency physician are now offering treatment option to stroke patient which improving the quality of life. Top priority is immediate recognition of stroke, conditions mimicking the stroke and immediate and effective management of stroke. Following the stroke protocol. Completing the NIHSS score and interpretation on of laboratory and radiological results are crucial. Ischemic stroke is the significant contributor of disability maximum benefit if patient receives the treatment within 4.5 hours. Door to needle time of 60 minute for ischemic stroke should be maintained. Blood pressure and blood glucose management according to guidelines. Evaluation of patient should be done by neurologist as well as neurointerventional consultant. Endovascular therapy for patients who are not the candidates for thrombolysis.

Flow chart 3 Algorithm for evaluation of stroke and cryptogenic stroke

- History and physical examination
- Features of stoke /TIA
- Proceed for standard evaluation for stroke

↓

Standard evaluation for stroke

- *Stroke protocol*: CT/MRI brain
- CT/MR angiography
- Carotid Doppler
- Trans-cranial Doppler
- *Cardiac*: Transthoracic/transesophageal echocardiography 12 lead ECG/ holter

- Hematological testing
- Complete blood count
- Platelet count
- PTT/INR

↓

Advanced evaluation for cryptogenic stroke

- Prolonged cardiac rhythm monitoring (2–4 weeks)
- Cardiac CT/MRI

- Catheter angiography
- Transcranial Doppler
- CSF examination
- Brain biopsy

- Hematologic testing for occult malignancy
- Hypercoagulability tests
- Test for vasculitis
- Genetic testing for mitochondrial disease, Fabry's disease

BIBLIOGRAPHY

1. Adams HP Jr, del Zoppo G, Alberts MJ, et al. Guidelines for the early management of adults with ischemic stroke: a guideline from the American Heart Association/American Stroke Association Stroke Council, Clinical Cardiology Council, Cardiovascular Radiology and Intervention Council, and the Atherosclerotic Peripheral Vascular Disease and Quality of Care Outcomes in Research Interdisciplinary Working Groups: the American Academy of Neurology affirms the value of this guideline as an educational tool for neurologists. Stroke. 2007;38(5):1655-711.
2. Ahmed N, Davalos A, Eriksson N, et al. Association of admission blood glucose and outcome in patients treated with intravenous thrombolysis: results from the Safe Implementation of Treatments in Stroke International Stroke Thrombolysis Register (SITS-ISTR). Arch Neurol. 2010;67(9):1123-30.
3. Broderick JP. Endovascular therapy for acute ischemic stroke. Stroke. 2009;40 (3 Suppl 1):S103-6.
4. Bruno A, Levine SR, Frankel MR, et al. Admission glucose level and clinical outcomes in the NINDS rt-PA stroke trial. Neurology. 2002;59(5):669-74.
5. Capes SE, Hunt D, Malmberg K, et al. Stress hyperglycemia and prognosis of stroke in nondiabetic and diabetic patients. Stroke. 2001;32(10):2426-32.
6. Caplan LR. Intracranial branch atheromatous disease: a neglected, understudied, and underused concept. Neurology. 1989;39(9):1246-50.
7. Carter AM, Catto AJ, Mansfield MW, et al. Predictive variables for mortality after acute ischemic stroke. Stroke. 2007;38(6):1873-80.
8. Castillo J, Leira R, Garcia MM, et al. Blood pressure decrease during the acute phase of ischemic stroke is associated with brain injury and poor stroke outcome. Stroke. 2004;35(2):520-6.
9. Clark WM, Albers GW, Madden KP, et al. The rtPA (alteplase) 0- to 6-hour acute stroke trial, part A (A0276g): results of a double-blind, placebo-controlled, multicenter study. Thrombolytic therapy in acute ischemic stroke study investigators. Stroke. 2000;31(4):811-6.
10. Clark WM, Wissman S, Albers GW, et al. Recombinant tissue-type plasminogen activator (Alteplase) for ischemic stroke 3 to 5 hours after symptom onset. The ATLANTIS Study: a randomized controlled trial. Alteplase Thrombolysis for Acute Noninterventional Therapy in Ischemic Stroke. JAMA. 1999;282(21):2019-26.
11. Cucchiara BL, Jackson B, Weiner M, et al. Usefulness of checking platelet count before thrombolysis in acute ischemic stroke. Stroke. 2007;38(5):1639-40.
12. del Zoppo GJ, Saver JL, Jauch EC, et al. Expansion of the time window for treatment of acute ischemic stroke with intravenous tissue plasminogen activator: a science advisory from the American Heart Association/American Stroke Association. Stroke. 2009;40(8):2945-8.
13. Donnan GA, Davis SM, Chambers BR, et al. Streptokinase for acute ischemic stroke with relationship to time of administration: Australian Streptokinase (ASK) Trial Study Group. JAMA. 1996;276(12):961-6.
14. Edlow JA, Newman-Toker DE, Savitz SI. Diagnosis and initial management of cerebellar infarction. Lancet Neurol. 2008;7(10):951-64.
15. Falluji N, Abou-Chebl A, Rodriguez Castro CE, et al. Reperfusion strategies for acute ischemic stroke. Angiology. 2012;63(4):289-96 [Epub 2011 Jul 6].
16. Ferro JM, Canhao P, Stam J, et al. Delay in the diagnosis of cerebral vein and dural sinus thrombosis: influence on outcome. Stroke. 2009;40(9):3133-8.
17. Ferro JM, Canhao P, Stam J, et al. Prognosis of cerebral vein and dural sinus thrombosis: results of the International Study on Cerebral Vein and Dural Sinus Thrombosis (ISCVT). Stroke. 2004;35(3):664-70.
18. Fiebach JB, Schellinger PD, Jansen O, et al. CT and diffusion-weighted MR imaging in randomized order: diffusion-weighted imaging results in higher accuracy and lower interrater variability in the diagnosis of hyperacute ischemic stroke. Stroke. 2002;33(9):2206-10.
19. Fisher CM. Capsular infarcts: the underlying vascular lesions. Arch Neurol. 1979; 36(2):65-73.
20. Fisher CM. Lacunar strokes and infarcts: a review. Neurology. 1982;32(8):871-6.
21. Fonarow GC, Saver JL, Saver JL, et al. Improving door-to-needle times in acute ischemic stroke: the design and rationale for the American Heart Association/American Stroke Association's target: stroke initiative. Stroke. 2011;42(10):2983-9.
22. Frendl A, Csiba L. Pharmacological and non-pharmacological recanalization strategies in acute ischemic stroke. Front Neurol. 2011;2:32.
23. Frendl DM, Strauss DG, Underhill BK, et al. Lack of impact of paramedic training and use of the Cincinnati Prehospital Stroke Scale on stroke patient identification and on-scene time. Stroke. 2009;40(3):754-6.
24. Furlan A, Higashida R, Wechsler L, et al. Intra-arterial prourokinase for acute ischemic stroke. The PROACT II study: a randomized controlled trial. Prolyse in Acute Cerebral Thromboembolism. JAMA. 1999;282(21):2003-11.
25. Goldstein LB, Samsa GP. Reliability of the National Institutes of Health Stroke Scale. Extension to non-neurologists in the context of a clinical trial. Stroke. 1997;28(2):307-10.
26. Goldstein LB, Simel DL. Is this patient having a stroke? JAMA. 2005;293(19): 2391-402.
27. Groysman LI, Emanuel BA, Kim-Tenser MA, et al. Therapeutic hypothermia in acute ischemic stroke. Neurosurg Focus. 2011;30(6):E17.
28. Hacke W, Donnan G, Fieschi C, et al. Association of outcome with early stroke treatment: pooled analysis of ATLANTIS, ECASS, and NINDS rt-PA stroke trials. Lancet. 2004;363(9411):768-74.
29. Hacke W, Kaste M, Bluhmki E, et al. Thrombolysis with alteplase 3 to 4.5 hours after acute ischemic stroke. N Engl J Med. 2008;359(13):1317-29.
30. Hacke W, Kaste M, Fieschi C, et al. Intravenous thrombolysis with recombinant tissue plasminogen activator for acute hemispheric stroke. The European Cooperative Acute Stroke Study (ECASS). JAMA. 1995;274(13):1017-25.
31. Hacke W, Kaste M, Fieschi C, et al. Randomised double-blind placebo-controlled trial of thrombolytic therapy with intravenous alteplase in acute ischaemic stroke (ECASS II). Second European-Australasian Acute Stroke Study Investigators. Lancet. 1998;352(9136):1245-51.
32. Hommel M, Boissel JP, Cornu C, et al. Termination of trial of streptokinase in severe acute ischaemic stroke. Lancet. 1995;345(8941):57.

33. Jauch EC, Cucchiara B, Adeoye O, et al. Part 11: adult stroke: 2010 American Heart Association Guidelines for Cardiopulmonary Resuscitation and Emergency Cardiovascular Care. Circulation. 2010;122(18 Suppl 3):S818-28.
34. Kallmunzer B, Kollmar R. Temperature management in stroke—an unsolved, but important topic. Cerebrovasc Dis. 2011;31(6):532-43.
35. Kang DW, Chalela JA, Dunn W, et al. MRI screening before standard tissue plasminogen activator therapy is feasible and safe. Stroke. 2005;36(9):1939-43.
36. Keir SL, Wardlaw JM. Systematic review of diffusion and perfusion imaging in acute ischemic stroke. Stroke. 2000;31(11):2723-31.
37. Kidwell CS, Chalela JA, Saver JL, et al. Comparison of MRI and CT for detection of acute intracerebral hemorrhage. JAMA. 2004;292(15):1823-30.
38. Kidwell CS, Starkman S, Eckstein M, et al. Identifying stroke in the field: prospective validation of the Los Angeles Prehospital Stroke Screen (LAPSS). Stroke. 2000;31(1):71-6.
39. Kothari R, Barsan W, Brott T, et al. Frequency and accuracy of prehospital diagnosis of acute stroke. Stroke. 1995;26(6):937-41.
40. Kothari RU, Pancioli A, Liu T, et al. Cincinnati Prehospital Stroke Scale: reproducibility and validity. Ann Emerg Med. 1999;33(4):373-8.
41. Lansberg MG, Bluhmki E, Thijs VN. Efficacy and safety of tissue plasminogen activator 3 to 4.5 hours after acute ischemic stroke: a metaanalysis. Stroke. 2009;40(7):2438-41.
42. Latchaw RE. The roles of diffusion and perfusion MR imaging in acute stroke management. Am J Neuroradiol. 1999;20(6):957-9.
43. Lees KR, Bluhmki E, von Kummer R, et al. Time to treatment with intravenous alteplase and outcome in stroke: an updated pooled analysis of ECASS, ATLANTIS, NINDS, and EPITHET trials. Lancet. 2010;375(9727):1695-703.
44. Leonardi-Bee J, Bath P, Phillips SJ, et al. Blood pressure and clinical outcomes in the international stroke trial. Stroke. 2002;33(5):1315-20.
45. Martin-Schild S, Albright KC, Tanksley J, et al. Zero on the NIHSS does not equal the absence of stroke. Ann Emerg Med. 2011;57(1):42-5.
46. Maulaz AB, Bezerra DC, Bogousslavsky J. Posterior cerebral artery infarction from middle cerebral artery infarction. Arch Neurol. 2005;62(6):938-41.
47. Meyers PM, Schumacher HC, Connolly ES Jr, et al. Current status of endovascular stroke treatment. Circulation. 2011;123(22):2591-601.
48. Mokin M, Kass-Hout T, Kass-Hout O, et al. Blood pressure management and evolution of thrombolysis-associated intracerebral hemorrhage in acute ischemic stroke. J Stroke Cerebrovasc Dis. 2011 Jun 22. [Epub ahead of print].
49. Mullins ME, Schaefer PW, Sorensen AG, et al. CT and conventional and diffusion weighted MR imaging in acute stroke: study in 691 patients at presentation to the emergency department. Radiology. 2002;224(2):353-60.
50. Murray V, Norrving B, Sandercock PA, et al. The molecular basis of thrombolysis and its clinical application in stroke. J Intern Med. 2010;267(2):191-208.
51. Nadeau S, Jordan J, Mishra S. Clinical presentation as a guide to early prognosis in vertebrobasilar stroke. Stroke. 1992;23(2):165-70.
52. Ntaios G, Egli M, Faouzi M, et al. J-shaped association between serum glucose and functional outcome in acute ischemic stroke. Stroke. 2010;41(10):2366-70.
53. Okumura K, Ohya Y, Maehara A, et al. Effects of blood pressure levels on case fatality after acute stroke. J Hypertens. 2005;23(6):1217-23.
54. Ramanujam P, Guluma KZ, Castillo EM, et al. Accuracy of stroke recognition by emergency medical dispatchers and paramedics—San Diego experience. Prehosp Emerg Care. 2008;12(3):307-13.
55. Rha JH, Saver JL. The impact of recanalization on ischemic stroke outcome: a meta-analysis. Stroke. 2007;38(3):967-73.
56. Roger VL, Go AS, Lloyd-Jones DM, et al. Heart disease and stroke statistics—2011 update: a report from the American Heart Association. Circulation. 2011;123(4):e18-209.
57. Ropper AH, Samuels MA, editors. Adams and victor's principles of neurology, 9th edition. The McGraw-Hill Companies, Inc; 2009.
58. Rost NS, Masrur S, Pervez MA, et al. Unsuspected coagulopathy rarely prevents IV thrombolysis in acute ischemic stroke. Neurology. 2009;73(23):1957-62.
59. Runchey S, McGee S. Does this patient have a hemorrhagic stroke? clinical findings distinguishing hemorrhagic stroke from ischemic stroke. JAMA. 2010;303(22):2280-6.
60. Sacco SE, Whisnant JP, Broderick JP, et al. Epidemiological characteristics of lacunar infarcts in a population. Stroke. 1991;22(10):1236-41.
61. Sandset EC, Bath PM, Boysen G, et al. The angiotensin-receptor blocker candesartan for treatment of acute stroke (SCAST): a randomised, placebo-controlled, double-blind trial. Lancet. 2011;377(9767):741-50.
62. Saposnik G, Barinagarrementeria F, Brown RJ, et al. Diagnosis and management of cerebral venous thrombosis: a statement for healthcare professionals from the American Heart Association/American Stroke Association. Stroke. 2011;42(4): 1158-92.
63. Schwamm LH, Pancioli A, Acker JE 3rd, et al. Recommendations for the establishment of stroke systems of care: recommendations from the American Stroke Association's Task Force on the development of stroke systems. Stroke. 2005; 36(3):690-703.
64. Singhal AB. Oxygen therapy in stroke: past, present, and future. Int J Stroke. 2006;1(4):191-200.
65. Sorensen AG, Copen WA, Ostergaard L, et al. Hyperacute stroke: simultaneous measurement of relative cerebral blood volume, relative cerebral blood flow, and mean tissue transit time. Radiology. 1999;210(2):519-27.
66. Stam J. Thrombosis of the cerebral veins and sinuses. N Engl J Med. 2005;352(17):1791-8.
67. Tissue plasminogen activator for acute ischemic stroke. The National Institute of Neurological Disorders and Stroke rt-PA Stroke Study Group. N Engl J Med. 1995;333(24):1581-7.
68. Tomandl BF, Klotz E, Handschu R, et al. Comprehensive imaging of ischemic stroke with multisection CT. Radiographics. 2003;23(3):565-92.
69. Vemmos KN, Tsivgoulis G, Spengos K, et al. U-shaped relationship between mortality and admission blood pressure in patients with acute stroke. J Intern Med. 2004;255(2):257-65.
70. Walter S, Kostopoulos P, Haass A, et al. Point-of-care laboratory halves door-totherapy- decision time in acute stroke. Ann Neurol. 2011;69(3):581-6.
71. Woo D, Broderick JP, Kothari RU, et al. Does the National Institutes of Health Stroke Scale favor left hemisphere strokes? NINDS t-PA Stroke Study Group. Stroke. 1999;30(11):2355-9.

CHAPTER 50

Status Epilepticus and Refractory Status Epilepticus

Atma Ram Bansal, Yeeshu Singh Sudan

INTRODUCTION

Status epilepticus (SE) is the most extreme form of seizure in which aggressive approach can save many lives. Delay in treatment can lead to significant morbidity and mortality. SE is a very common medical emergency in day-to-day critical care and emergency care practice. Annual incidence rates for generalized SE range from 3.6 to 6.6 per 100,000 in European countries. The incidence rate is significantly high if all kinds of SE are included and is about 41 per 100,000 in United States.[1-4] Reported mortality rate is 17–26% and significant morbidly including disabling neurological deficits range from 10% to 23% among the cases who survived SE.[5] It is very important to recognize and treat SE at an early stage as longer the duration of seizures, higher the chances of landing it into refractory SE. In emergency settings, the treating physician is the first contact and should be familiar with various steps of management of SE. He or she should not wait for the specialist to start treatment for SE. An early and aggressive treatment can lead to early control of seizures and a state of refractory status can be avoided. For further management of SE, especially refractory SE, a team of neurologist (epileptologist with expertise in electrophysiology) and critical care expert is required as such patients require continuous monitoring in intensive care unit (ICU) including continuous electroencephalogram (EEG).

DEFINITION OF STATUS EPILEPTICUS

Convulsive Status Epilepticus

Generalized convulsive SE in adults and children older than 5 years is operationally defined as "greater than and equal to 5 minutes of (1) continuous seizure or (2) two or more discrete seizures between which there is incomplete recovery of consciousness". Though traditionally duration of 30 minutes or more continuous seizures was taken as SE, the duration has been reduced considering the fact that majority of generalized seizures terminate spontaneously within 2–3 minutes and seizures that do not cease in 5–10 minutes will need aggressive intervention to get controlled.[6,7]

Nonconvulsive Status Epilepticus

Nonconvulsive status epilepticus (NCSE) is defined as a state when in an obtunded or comatose patient there are no ongoing obvious clinical seizures but the seizure activity is well seen on the EEG. The duration required to label NCSE is still more than 30 minutes. It is important to rule out NCSE in any patient with unexplained altered sensorium especially with reasonably normal radiological and biochemical parameters. Subtle SE may be seen in patients treated for convulsive SE. If convulsions are no longer there but the patient is comatose then a possibility of NCSE should be considered. However, discrete (*subtle*) clinical manifestations like perioral twitching or nystagmus or fixed gaze may be present in such patients.

DIAGNOSIS OF STATUS EPILEPTICUS

Early diagnosis of SE is very important for good outcome. The convulsive SE can be identified by ongoing tonic-clonic seizures. If the seizure is of more than 5 minutes, we should start the treatment on emergency basis. Multiple systemic complications can occur in generalized SE. It includes cardiac arrhythmia, congestive heart failure, metabolic issues like electrolyte imbalance, etc. In prolonged SE renal dysfunction or even multiorgan failure can be seen. Central nervous system (CNS) complications like diffuse cerebral edema, hypoxic brain damage, and cerebrospinal fluid (CSF) pleocytosis may occur.

In a patient with altered or fluctuating sensorium, certain clinical features may help in making a diagnosis of nonconvulsive status. These include perioral or eyelid twitching, sustained head and eye deviation to one side, nystagmoid eye movements and hippus. Subtle tonic posturing or clonic jerks in any limb may also me a manifestation of NCSE. An emergent EEG monitoring is required in such patients for confirmation of diagnosis.

Status Epilepticus in Children

The definition and management of SE are more or less same as in adult population. The main difference is in the etiology. In pediatric population, especially in neonates and early infants, symptomatic causes like metabolic, infections, and structural lesion in the brain are more common. The prognosis depends upon the primary pathology but seems to be better. Every child with SE must undergo workup for metabolic causes like hypocalcemia, hypoglycemia, and hypomagnesemia. Early identification of the etiology can result in aggressive specific management of cause. Other investigations may include complete blood count, renal function test, liver function test, serum calcium, serum magnesium, serum electrolyte, blood urea nitrogen, glucose, and antiepileptic drug levels, as well as a toxicology screening.

Brain imaging is an important part of investigation especially in pediatric age group. Magnetic resonance imaging is the ideal investigation but in emergent condition it may be more convenient to do computed tomography head. CSF should be done in cases of suspicion of brain infection.

MANAGEMENT OF STATUS EPILEPTICUS

Treatment of seizure needs to be initiated possibly at home by care giver. Prehospital management includes both, first aid during seizures and pharmacotherapy. Benzodiazepines like diazepam and midazolam can be used by a care giver. Nowadays intranasal midazolam spray is commercially available which is very convenient to use and is as effective as rectal diazepam and socially more acceptable.

Management of SE in the hospital should start immediately after the clinical diagnosis. After securing airway and breathing, next step is to secure two intravenous (IV) lines and withdrawing blood samples for serological investigations including routine hematology and basic metabolic parameter and electrolytes (including calcium level) and antiepileptic drug levels in a patient who is already under treatment for epilepsy **(Table 1)**.[8]

Early Status Epilepticus (0–10 Minutes)

The first-line antiepileptic drug of choice is benzodiazepine. In view of prolonged action, lorazepam 4 mg (up to 0.1 mg/kg) in adults and 2 mg in children is the drug of choice and can be repeated another half of this dose if patient is still seizing. Midazolam 5– 10 mg (up to 0.2 mg/kg) is another benzodiazepine but it is relatively short-lasting. Diazepam is almost equally effective and can be used as an alternative especially in the peripheral centers where storage of medication is an issue, as it can be easily stored at room temperature.

Established Status Epilepticus (10 Minutes to 30–60 Minutes)

After giving benzodiazepine, a loading dose of long-acting antiepileptic drug is required for sustained action. Parental conventional automated external defibrillators (AEDs) include phenytoin (fosphenytoin), valproic acid, and phenobarbitone while levetiracetam and lacosamide are newer ones. Fosphenytoin may be a better choice than phenytoin as it can be given faster and with fewer side effects. Levetiracetam may be preferred in patients with liver disease or multisystem involvement. Lacosamide is especially effective in ongoing focal seizures. After giving loading dose, another half loading dose can be given of the same AED if seizures are still not controlled. If still there are ongoing seizures, then loading with other parenteral AEDs can be tried **(Table 2)**.

Table 1 Management algorithm of status epilepticus		
	Immediate treatment (first 5–10 minutes)	
1.	Monitoring of vitals	Airway, oxygen, and cardiac monitor
2.	Securing IV lines	Two lines for blood samples and starting treatment
3.	To start IV fluids	Fluid of choice is normal saline To give 100 mg IV thiamine and 50 mL of 50% dextrose in patients with history of alcoholism
4.	First antiepileptic	To give lorazepam or midazolam or diazepam IV *0.1 mg/kg bolus dose of IV lorazepam* in equal volume of diluent by slow IV push at ~2 mg/min
5.	Repeat dose if seizure persist	Repeat another half of the bolus dose if seizures are not controlled

Abbreviation: IV, intravenous.

Table 2 Management algorithm of established status epilepticus

		Early treatment for next 10–60 minutes
1.	Loading antiepileptic second-line IV agent	• *Phenytoin*: IV infusion 15 mg/kg at 50 mg/min • *Fosphenytoin*: IV infusion 15 mg PE/kg at 100 mg PE/min • *Valproate*: IV infusion 25 mg/kg at 3–6 mg/kg/min • *Phenobarbital*: IV infusion 10 mg/kg at a maximum rate of 100 mg/min • *Levetiracetam*: 20 mg/kg bolus of over 15 minutes
2.	If seizure persist then two options	• Repeat half dose of any of the above mentioned AEDs • To load with any of the other antiepileptic drug

Abbreviations: AEDs, automated external defibrillator; IV, intravenous; PE, phenytoin equivalents.

Refractory Status Epilepticus

If despite giving loading doses of AEDs the seizures are going on, then the patient is considered to be in refractory SE. At this stage there are two options to treat. Such patients will need the use of anesthetic agents like midazolam, propofol or thiopentone sodium. Midazolam may be preferred with strict monitoring in cases where intubation is to be avoided. If ICU facility with ventilator support is available then stronger anesthetic drugs like thiopentone sodium or propofol may be a better choice **(Table 3)**.

If a patient with convulsive SE is having altered sensorium with no ongoing convulsions then it may be due to nonconvulsive status and an urgent EEG monitoring is required.

Super-refractory Status Epilepticus

If the seizures are not controlled in 24 hours or recur 24 hours or more after the onset of anesthetic therapy then this is called super-refractory SE. If seizures recur on stopping or reducing anesthetic agents, then also it will be termed super-refractory SE.[9] This condition requires aggressive therapies like ketamine, hypothermia, ketogenic diet, and immunotherapy like immunoglobulin. This will help in controlling seizures, preventing excitotoxicity and providing neuroprotection **(Table 4)**.[9]

HOW TO DO ELECTROENCEPHALOGRAM MONITORING IN A PATIENT WITH STATUS EPILEPTICUS?

Electroencephalogram monitoring is helpful in all the patients with SE. It can be done for short period or as continuous monitoring to rule out electrographic seizures. Continuous EEG monitoring is especially required in conditions where the patient has not recovered even after the control of convulsions to rule out electrographic seizures. In a patient with refractory SE, EEG monitoring may help in optimizing the dose of anesthetic agent with a target to achieve burst suppression pattern (BSP) on EEG. A suppression period of more than 10 seconds of the electrical activities on EEG will indicate adequate doses of anesthetic agents. The tapering of these agents should be considered only after 24 hours of BSP and then also it should be slow withdrawal.

Table 3 Management algorithm of refractory status epilepticus

		Refractory status epilepticus (>60 minutes on going convulsions)
1.	Midazolam infusion (possible to avoid ventilator support)	*Loading*: 0.2 mg/kg by slow IV bolus *Maintenance cIV dose*: 0.1–0.4 mg/kg/h *Maximum cIV dose*: 2.0–3.0 mg/kg/h
2.	Thiopental sodium	*Loading*: 3–5 mg/kg at 0.2–0.4 mg/kg/min *Maintenance cIV dose*: 3.0–5.0 mg/kg/h *Maximum cIV dose*: 5.0 mg/kg/h
3.	Propofol infusion	*Loading dose*: 1–2 mg/kg at 10 mg/min *Maintenance cIV dose*: 2–10 mg/kg/h *Maximum cIV dose*: 15 mg/kg/h

Abbreviation: cIV, continuous intravenous.

Table 4 Management algorithm of super-refractory status epilepticus

		Super-refractory status epilepticus (seizures >24 hours)
1.	Magnesium infusion	*Loading*: 2–6 g/h *Maintenance*: 3.5 mmol/L
2.	Hypothermia	32–35°C for <48 h Endovascular cooling vs external cooling
3.	Immuno-therapy	• IV Methylprednisolone 1 g/day × 5 days • IV Immunoglobulins 0.4 g/kg/day × 5 days • Plasma exchange
4.	Ketogenic diet	• 1:1 or 1:4 ketogenic diet • To avoid glucose containing fluids
5.	Epilepsy surgery	Consider surgery in special circumstances with documented brain lesions responsible for status

Abbreviation: IV, intravenous.

REASONS FOR FAILURE OF TREATMENT IN STATUS EPILEPTICUS[10]

Treatment of SE can fail due to following reasons:
- *Underdosing of antiepileptics*: Treating SE half-heartedly by going half-loading dose may frequently result in failure and should be avoided. A full-loading dose is quite safe to give in a patient with SE.
- *Early stoppage of treatment*: If only emergency therapy or loading dose of AEDs is given, then patient may develop recurrence of seizure as most of the AEDs work for about 12 hours after loading, so maintenance antiepileptic therapy should always be given.
- *Proper diagnosis*: It is very important to keep a high index of suspicion for NCSE in a patient with unexplained altered sensorium as early treatment can result in good outcome and delayed treatment may result in refractory status.

CLINICAL TIPS IN MANAGING STATUS EPILEPTICUS

- Treat fever aggressively as it can precipitate seizure recurrences especially in pediatric population.
- Always look for metabolic factors like hypoglycemia, hyperglycemia, and hypocalcemia and correct it
- In case of difficult IV access phenobarbitone, midazolam and fosphenytoin can be given intramuscularly.
- Automated external defibrillator level monitoring during SE is useful to determine optimal doses.
- Oral AEDs the patient already taking should be continued during the management of SE. Oral route can be changed to IV if drug is available.
- Cerebrospinal fluid pleocytosis can also be seen in SE without any CNS infection.
- Avoid phenytoin in patient with myoclonic epilepsy.
- In patients with chronic liver disease, levetiracetam is a safer option.
- In renal disease, phenytoin or fosphenytoin can be used safely.

REFERENCES

1. Coeytaux A, Jallon P, Galobardes B, et al. Incidence of status epilepticus in french-speaking Switzerland:(EPISTAR). Neurology. 2000;55(5):693-7.
2. Knake S, Rosenow F, Vescovi M, et al. Incidence of status epilepticus in adults in Germany: a prospective, population-based study. Epilepsia. 2001;42(6):714-8.
3. Vignatelli L, Tonon C, D'Alessandro R; Bologna Group for the Study of Status Epilepticus. Incidence and short-term prognosis of status epilepticus in adults in Bologna, Italy. Epilepsia. 2003;44(7): 964-8.
4. DeLorenzo RJ, Hauser WA, Towne AR, et al. A prospective, population-based epidemiologic study of status epilepticus in Richmond, Virginia. Neurology. 1996;46(4):1029-35.
5. Arif H, Hirsch LJ. Treatment of status epilepticus. Semin Neurol. 2008;28(3):342-54.
6. Lowenstein DH, Bleck T, MacDonald RL. It's time to revise the definition of status epilepticus. Epilepsia. 1999;40(1):120-2.
7. Shinnar S, Berg AT, Moshe SL, et al. How long do new-onset seizures in children last? Ann Neurol. 2001;49(5):659-64.
8. Walker M. Status epilepticus: an evidence based guide. Br Med J (Clin Res Ed). 2005;331(7518):673-7.
9. Shorvon S, Ferlisi M. The treatment of super-refractory status epilepticus: a critical review of available therapies and a clinical treatment protocol. Brain. 2011;134(10):2802-18.
10. Shorvon S, Baulac M, Cross H, et al. The drug treatment of status epilepticus in Europe: Consensus document from a workshop at the first London Colloquium on Status Epilepticus. Epilepsia. 2008;49(7):1277-88.

SECTION 6

Gastrointestinal Emergencies

- **Gastrointestinal Bleed in Emergency**
  Neeraj Saraf

- **Hepatic Encephalopathy**
  Rahul Rai, Sanjiv Saigal

- **Acute Pancreatitis**
  Rajesh Puri, Randhir Sud

- **Acute Appendicitis**
  Mukund Khetan, Anand Yadav

- **Perforation and Peritonitis**
  Sharad Manar, Hashim Mozzam, Sudhir BS

- **Intestinal Obstruction**
  Ashok Kumar Puranik, Devendra Richhariya

CHAPTER 51

Gastrointestinal Bleed in Emergency

Neeraj Saraf

INTRODUCTION

Gastrointestinal bleeding (GIB) is one of the most common presentations in emergency department. This can be presented as two extreme conditions, small amount of blood in vomit or in stool or as hemorrhagic shock after massive bleeding in vomitus or in the stools. GI hemorrhage is about 1–2% of all acute admissions. The annual incidence of approximately 170 cases per 100,000 adults increases steadily with advancing age, and is slightly more common in men than women. The bleeding may range from trivial to massive and can originate from almost any region of the GI tract, including the pancreas, liver, and biliary tree.

Managing GIB requires a multidisciplinary approach, involving emergency medicine, gastroenterology, intensive care, surgery, and interventional radiology. In addition to aiding in the resuscitation of the unstable patient, in some settings the surgical endoscopist establishes the diagnosis and initiates therapy. Even when the gastroenterologist assumes this role, early collaboration with the surgeon permits the establishment of goals and limits for initial nonoperative therapy. Ultimately, 5–10% of patients hospitalized for bleeding require an operative intervention. Most patients with an acute GI hemorrhage, bleeding stops spontaneously. Improvements in the management of such patients, primarily by means of early endoscopy and directed therapy, have reduced duration of hospitalization.

Hemorrhage can originate from any region of the GI tract and is typically classified based on its location relative to the ligament of Treitz. Bleeding proximal to the ligament of Treitz is termed as upper GI hemorrhage which is about 80% cases of bleeding. Peptic ulcer disease and variceal hemorrhage are the most frequent causes. Most of lower GI bleed is from the colon diverticula and angiodysplasias. Small bowel is situated between the ligament of Treitz and the ileocecal valve and is responsible for 5% of GI bleed. The small bowel is called "the dark area of the GI tract" because it is unapproachable to endoscopists, due to its intraperitoneal location, excess mobility, and long length. Obscure bleeding is defined as hemorrhage that persists or recurs after negative endoscopy. Patient with occult bleeding usually present with symptoms related to the anemia. Determination of the site of bleeding is important for directing diagnostic interventions with minimal delay. However, attempts to localize the source should never precede appropriate resuscitative measures.

APPROACH TO THE PATIENT

The presentation of GIB depends upon the location of the lesion and rate of bleeding. Presentation of upper GI bleeding (UGIB) is hematemesis, coffee-ground emesis, and melena. Presentation of lower GI bleeding (LGIB) is hematochezia or bleeding per rectum (PR). Although the melanotic appearance typically results from gastric acid degradation which converts hemoglobin to hematin, and from the actions of digestive enzymes and luminal bacteria in the small intestine, blood loss from the distal small bowel or right colon may have this appearance, particularly if transit is slow enough. *Peptic ulcer disease (PUD), esophageal varices, Dieulafoy's lesions* are the most common causes for massive UGIB. Nonsteroidal anti-inflammatory drugs (NSAIDs) develop ulcers in significant number of users especially in older individuals. About 30% of NSAIDs users hospitalized for UGIB. Few NSAID users remain clinically asymptomatic but have peptic ulcers on endoscopic examination. Depletion of prostaglandins is the main cause for ulcer development in NSAIDs users. *Diverticulosis* or *angiodysplasias (common in cecum and right colon)* are the main causes for massive LGIB **(Table 1)**.

Table 1 Clue about gastrointestinal bleed on the basis of history

Bleeding location	Cause	Clues from history
Upper gastrointestinal bleed (UGIB)	Peptic ulcer	Known peptic ulcer disease (PUD), chronic epigastric pain, heavy alcohol use, gastrotoxic medications, e.g. nonsteroidal anti-inflammatory drugs (NSAIDs), aspirin (ASA), or steroids
UGIB	Esophageal varices	Severe liver disease, alcoholism, hemorrhoids on physical examination (external evidence of possible portal hypertension)
UGIB	Aortoenteric fistula	History of aorta repair
UGIB	Mallory-Weiss tear	Vomiting or retching preceding hematemesis
Lower gastrointestinal bleed (LGIB)	Diverticulosis	Known diverticular disease, massive and painless bleed per rectum (PR)

Symptoms such as dizziness, syncope, shortness of breath, or chest pain are suggestive of large amount of blood loss. Clinical parameters, like obtundation, agitation, and hypotension (systolic blood pressure less than 90 mm Hg in the supine position), associated with cool clammy extremities, are consistent with hemorrhagic shock and suggest a loss of more than 40% of the patient's blood volume. A resting tachycardia (100 beats/min), with a decreased pulse pressure, implies a 20%–40% volume loss. In patients without shock, postural changes should be elicited.

The hematocrit is not a useful parameter for assessing the degree of hemorrhage in the acute setting because the proportion of red blood cells and plasma initially remain constant. The hematocrit level does not fall until plasma is redistributed into the intravascular space and resuscitation with crystalloid solution is begun. Similarly, the absence of tachycardia may be misleading; some patients with severe blood loss may actually have bradycardia secondary to vagal slowing of the heart or some elderly patients may be on β-blockers. The rectal examination is important in evaluation of GIB, check stool color (brown vs. black vs. maroon) and the presence of gross or occult blood. Also inspect for any masses, hemorrhoids, or fissures.

Risk Stratification

Not all patients with GIB require hospital admission or emergent evaluation. For example, the patient with a small amount of rectal bleeding that has ceased can generally be evaluated on an outpatient basis. Clearly, in many patients, the decision making is less straightforward. Others required admission and observation but may be further evaluated with endoscopy on a more *selective* basis.

The Rockall scoring system is used to assess risks of recurrent bleeding and death. Clinical factors and two endoscopic findings are used for assessment **(Box 1)**.

Scores ranging from 0 to 11 are divided into three risk categories: low risk ≤2; moderate risk 3–5; high risk ≥6 (Rockall TA, et al).

Box 1 Rockall scoring system for assessing risks of recurrent bleeding and death

Variables	Points
Age (years)	
<60	0
60–79	1
≥80	2
Hemodynamic shock	
Heart rate >100 bpm	1
Systolic blood pressure <100 mm Hg	2
Coexisting illnesses	
Heart failure, ischemic heart disease	2
Renal failure, hepatic failure, metastatic cancer	3
Endoscopic signs (diagnostic)	
No lesion observed, or Mallory—Weiss tear	0
Peptic ulcer, erosive disease, esophagitis	1
Cancer of the upper gastrointestinal tract	2
Endoscopic signs (hemorrhagic)	
Clean-base ulcer or flat, pigmented spot	0
Visible blood, active bleeding, visible vessel, adherent clot	2

Active bleeding, hypotension, raised prothrombin time, altered consciousness, used as red flags in emergency department and triaging should be done appropriately and categorized as high risk patients.

Always look for signs of portal hypertension.

It is important for emergency physician to check for possible undiagnosed liver disease. Look for icterus, jaundice, hepatomegaly, ascites, and spider naevi. All GI bleeding patients should be managed in intensive care unit for and with highest priority, even if they are hemodynamically stable.

DIAGNOSTIC TESTING

Complete hemogram, renal function and liver tests, and coagulation profile and blood grouping typing and cross-matching for blood transfusion are required in patients with acute GIB.

Various studies are unable to demonstrate any benefit from nasogastric tube (NGT) placement in UGIB. Sometimes NGT lavage is used to clarify if a patient has ongoing bleeding and thus early endoscopy may be beneficial; however, a negative NGT lavage does not mean that the patient does not have UGIB.

UPPER GASTROINTESTINAL BLEED

Blood Transfusions

Blood transfusions decision should be taken on the basis of clinical features and severity of the bleeding. Young patients without comorbid illness require blood transfusion when hemoglobin falls below 7 g/dL; in older patients with many and severe comorbid illnesses such as coronary disease, hemoglobin level should be maintained 9 g/dL or above.

Stopping of all anticoagulants and antiplatelet agents, in patients with GI bleeding, reduces risk of bleeding.

Sometime it is unfortunate situation when patient of GI hemorrhage present with acute myocardial infarction (MI). Acute massive bleeding causes hypovolemia, hemodynamic compromise, and hypoperfusion which precipitate acute MI. Drugs given to treat coronary artery disease (anticoagulant, antiplatelet, and thrombolytic agents) also causes GI bleeding.

Acid Suppression

Healing of ulcers are suppressed by the presence of acid. Acidic environment suppress the platelet aggregation and clot formation. Therefore maintaining the gastric pH 6 or more may stabilize clots and helps in stopping the bleeding.

Proton Pump Inhibitors

Proton pump inhibitors (PPIs) act by inhibiting the hydrogen-potassium adenosine triphosphatase, and reduce secretion of acid. PPIs control bleeding from ulcers, reduce duration of stay in hospital, and the requirement for endoscopic therapy also reduced. Start intravenous proton pump inhibitor in upper GI bleeding before endoscopy.

Proton pump inhibitors also reduce the recurrence of peptic ulcer bleeding, blood transfusions need, and surgery, but not the mortality rate. The recommended dose of omeprazole for patients is 80 mg bolus followed by an 8 mg/h infusion for 72 hours. Oral therapy can be started once the patient's condition stabilizes.

Somatostatin Analogs

An analog of the somatostatin hormone like octreotide is helpful in treating UGIB due to varices, by decreasing the splanchnic blood flow, secretion of gastric acid and pepsin.

Octreotide is safe to use and can be useful in patients with bleeding other than varices and who are waiting for endoscopy.

Diagnostic Endoscopy

Endoscopy is important for identification and treatment of the bleeding lesion helpful in reducing the risk of recurrent bleeding. Patients should be hemodynamically stabilized in emergency department before UGI endoscopy. Major complications due to endoscopy are hemorrhage, aspiration, pneumonia, oversedation, hypoventilation, vasovagal episodes, MI, bowel perforation, and cardiopulmonary events. Endoscopy is more informative and helpful in managing the bleed when it is done within 24 hours of UGIB. Endoscopy is the main stay of care, but how early endoscopy is required, is debatable. Erythromycin and metoclopramide (promotility agents) are used as premedication for better visualization. Endoscopy is helpful in diagnosing the bleeding lesion, assessing risk, and safe discharge.

Therapeutic Endoscopy

Endoscopic procedures are performed for the treatment of UGIB. Various methods are used and various agents like epinephrine, normal saline, or sclerosant are used in procedure; other methods like thermal cautery, electrocautery or banding are also used to stop bleeding, and results are more promising when combinations of these therapies are used.

Before doing the endoscopy, start somatostatin analog (for variceal bleeding octreotide 50 μg intravenous bolus, followed by a 50 μg/h infusion for 5 days) which reduces the portal pressure, and antibiotics reduce the risks of infection. Combination of therapeutic endoscopy and medication therapy in patients with variceal bleeding is proven better than single therapy. In refractory cases of recurrent variceal bleeding, transjugular intrahepatic portosystemic shunt (TIPS) is indicated.

LOWER GASTROINTESTINAL BLEED

Lower gastrointestinal bleeding is usually less severe than UGIB but sometimes it can be difficult to locate bleeding lesion and frustrating to both the clinician and the patient. The main objective in emergency department is to hemodynamically stabilize the patients, apply the measures to identify and locate the lesion, and provide specific appropriate treatment. Adequate resuscitation of the patient should be done by using intravenous fluid, and blood product before any intervention like colonoscopy.

SECTION 6: Gastrointestinal Emergencies

Adequate safety measures should be in place like adequate sedation, and appropriate monitoring device during and postprocedure. Once the lesion is identified, management strategies and available treatment options need to be specific for each individual case. A lower GI endoscopy is main diagnostic modality in patient with acute LGIB. In 75–88% of patients with LGIB, lower GI endoscopy is helpful in locating the lesion **(Flow chart 1)**.

Management of Severe Hematochezia

Emergency colonoscopy (within 12 hours of admission) is safe and effective. Early intervention, for massive diverticular hemorrhage, reduces the need for surgery. Early diagnostic intervention like colonoscopy is helpful in early diagnosis, early control of bleeding, reduce the duration, and cost of hospitalization **(Flow chart 2)**.

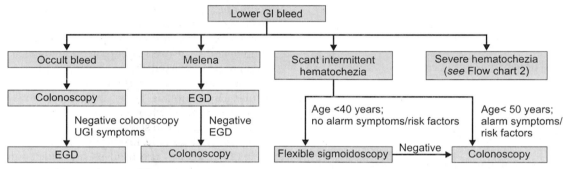

Flow chart 1 Initial approach toward lower gastrointestinal bleed

Abbreviations: GI, gastrointestinal; EGD, esophagogastroduodenoscopy; UGI, upper gastrointestinal.

Flow chart 2 Management of severe hematochezia

Abbreviations: CBC, complete blood count; UGI, upper gastrointestinal; EGD, esophagogastroduodenoscopy; NGT, nasogastric tube; RBC, red blood cells.

Radiography

Multidetector row computed tomography (CT) scan and mesenteric angiography are superior (detect very minute bleeding at a rate of 0.5 mL/min or less) for LGIB evaluation and management of severe bleeding patients who are hemodynamically unstabilized or/and for those with failed endoscopic management. Accurate arterial images are obtained in very less scan time and evaluated for any blood leak into any portion of the GI tract.

Surgery

A small number of patient require surgery indications for surgery are:
- Persistent and refractory bleeding
- Requirement of blood transfusion more than 6 units
- Recurrence of bleeding
- Despite aggressive resuscitation patient remain hemodynamically unstable.

Surgical intervention is required in 15–20% of patients. The overall postoperative mortality rate for emergency surgery in case of LGIB is 10%, despite improved methods. Age is the single most important factor associated with increase comorbidity, and for postoperative mortality.

CONCLUSION

The emergency department evaluation and management of patients with GIB has improved considerably over the past 10 years. Resuscitation and hemodynamic stabilization is the main objective. Applications of the existing diagnostic and therapeutic modalities improve the outcomes. Clinicians are encouraged to use the optimal dose of PPI following endoscopic therapy and latest endoscopic techniques of hemostasis. Surgery may be helpful in refractory cases.

BIBLIOGRAPHY

1. Adam V, Barkun AN. Estimates of costs of hospital stay for variceal and nonvariceal upper gastrointestinal bleeding in the United States. Value Health. 2008;11(1):1-3.
2. Angtuaco TL, Reddy SK, Drapkin S, et al. The utility of urgent colonoscopy in the evaluation of acute lower gastrointestinal tract bleeding: a 2-year experience from a single center. Am J Gastroenterol. 2001;96(6):1782-5.
3. Bardou M, Toubouti Y, Benhaberou-Brun D, et al. Meta-analysis: proton-pump inhibition in high-risk patients with acute peptic ulcer bleeding. Aliment Pharmacol Ther. 2005;21(6):677-86.
4. Barkun AN, Cockeram AW, Plourde V, et al. Review article: acid suppression in non-variceal acute upper gastrointestinal bleeding. Aliment Pharmacol Ther 1999;13(12):1565-84.
5. Barnert J, Messmann H. Lower intestinal bleeding disorders. In: Classen M, Tytgat GN, Lightdale CJ (Eds.) Gastroenterological Endoscopy, 2nd edition. New York: Thieme Medical Publishers; 2010. pp. 641-57.
6. Bjorkman DJ, Zaman A, Fennerty MB, et al. Urgent vs. elective endoscopy for acute non-variceal upper-GI bleeding: an effectiveness study. Gastrointest Endosc. 2004;60(1):1-8.
7. Blatchford O, Murray WR, Blatchford M. A risk score to predict need for treatment for upper-gastrointestinal haemorrhage. Lancet. 2000;356(9238):1318-21.
8. Barkun A, Bardou M, Marshall JK. Consensus recommendations for managing patients with nonvariceal upper gastrointestinal bleeding. Ann Intern Med. 2003;139(10):843-57.
9. Bhatt DL, Scheiman J, Abraham NS, et al. ACCF/ACG/AHA 2008 expert consensus document on reducing the gastrointestinal risks of antiplatelet therapy and NSAID use: a report of the American College of Cardiology Foundation Task Force on Clinical Expert Consensus Documents. Circulation. 2008;118(18):1894-909.
10. Chan FK. NSAID-induced peptic ulcers and *Helicobacter pylori* infection: implications for patient management. Drug Saf. 2005;28(4):287-300.
11. Chung IK, Kim EJ, Lee MS, et al. Endoscopic factors predisposing to rebleeding following endoscopic hemostasis in bleeding peptic ulcers. Endoscopy. 2001;33(11):969-75.
12. Dorward S, Sreedharan A, Leontiadis GI, et al. Proton pump inhibitor treatment initiated prior to endoscopic diagnosis in upper gastrointestinal bleeding. Cochrane Database Syst Rev. 2006;18(4):CD005415.
13. de Franchis R. Evolving consensus in portal hypertension. Report of the Baveno IV consensus workshop on methodology of diagnosis and therapy in portal hypertension. J Hepatol. 2005;43(1):167-76.
14. Dusold R, Burke K, Carpentier W, et al. The accuracy of technetium-99m-labeled red cell scintigraphy in localizing gastrointestinal bleeding. Am J Gastroenterol. 1994;89(3):345-8.
15. Eisenberg MJ, Richard PR, Libersan D, et al. Safety of short-term discontinuation of antiplatelet therapy in patients with drug-eluting stents. Circulation. 2009;119(12):1634-42.
16. Farrell JJ, Friedman LS. Gastrointestinal bleeding in the elderly. Gastroenterol Clin North Am. 2001;30(2):377-407.
17. Fiorito JJ, Brandt LJ, Kozicky O, et al. The diagnostic yield of superior mesenteric angiography: correlation with the pattern of gastrointestinal bleeding. Am J Gastroenterol. 1989;84(8):878-81.
18. Green BT, Rockey DC, Portwood G, et al. Urgent colonoscopy for evaluation and management of acute lower gastrointestinal hemorrhage: a randomized controlled trial. Am J Gastroenterol. 2005;100(11):2395-402.
19. Hochter W, Weingart J, Kuhner W, et al. Angiodysplasia in the colon and rectum. Endoscopic morphology, localisation and frequency. Endoscopy. 1985;17(5):182-5.
20. Hunt RH, Bazzoli F. Review article: should NSAID/low-dose aspirin takers be tested routinely for *H. pylori* infection and treated if positive? Implications for primary risk of ulcer and ulcer relapse after initial healing. Aliment Pharmacol Ther. 2004;19(1):9-16.
21. Jensen DM, Machicado GA. Endoscopic hemostasis of ulcer hemorrhage with injection, thermal, and combination methods. Techniques in Gastrointestinal Endoscopy. 2005;7(3):124-131.
22. Jalan R, Hayes PC. UK guidelines on the management of variceal haemorrhage in cirrhotic patients. British Society of Gastroenterology. Gut. 2000;46(suppl 3-4):III1-III15.

23. Jensen DM, Machicado GA, Jutabha R, et al. Urgent colonoscopy for the diagnosis and treatment of severe diverticular hemorrhage. N Engl J Med. 2000;342(2):78-82.
24. Kaassis M, Oberti E, Burtin P, et al. Argon plasma coagulation for the treatment of hemorrhagic radiation proctitis. Endoscopy. 2000;32(9):673-6.
25. Katz LB. The role of surgery in occult gastrointestinal bleeding. Semin Gastrointest Dis. 1999;10(2):78-81.
26. Kwan V, Bourke MJ, Williams SJ, et al. Argon plasma coagulation in the management of symptomatic gastrointestinal vascular lesions: experience in 100 consecutive patients with long-term follow-up. Am J Gastroenterol. 2006;101(1):58-63.
27. Lau JY, Leung WK, Wu JC, et al. Omeprazole before endoscopy in patients with gastrointestinal bleeding. N Engl J Med. 2007;356(16):1631-40.
28. Lin HJ, Lo WC, Cheng YC, et al. Role of intravenous omeprazole in patients with high-risk peptic ulcer bleeding after successful endoscopic epinephrine injection: a prospective randomized comparative trial. Am J Gastroenterol. 2006;101(3):500-5.
29. Lightdale (Eds.) Gastroenterological endoscopy. 2nd edition. Thieme, New York; 2010. pp. 641-57.
30. Marmo R, Rotondano G, Bianco MA, et al. Outcome of endoscopic treatment for peptic ulcer bleeding: Is a second look necessary? A meta-analysis. Gastrointest Endosc. 2003;57(1):62-7.
31. O'Neill BB, Gosnell JE, Lull RJ, et al. Cinematic nuclear scintigraphy reliably directs surgical intervention for patients with gastrointestinal bleeding. Arch Surg. 2000;135(9):1076-81.
32. Pallin DJ, Saltzman JR. Is nasogastric tube lavage in patients with acute upper GI bleeding indicated or antiquated? Gastrointest Endosc. 2011;74(5):981-4.
33. Parra-Blanco A, Kaminaga N, Kojima T, et al. Hemoclipping for postpolypectomy and postbiopsy colonic bleeding. Gastrointest Endosc. 2000;51(1):37-41.
34. Peura DA, Lanza FL, Gostout CJ, et al. The American College of Gastroenterology Bleeding Registry: preliminary findings. Am J Gastroenterol. 1997;92(6):924-8.
35. Rockall TA, Logan RF, Devlin HB, et al. Risk assessment after acute upper gastrointestinal hemorrhage. Gut. 1996; 38(3):316-21.
36. Rockey DC. Gastrointestinal bleeding. Gastroenterol Clin North Am. 2005;34(4):581-8.
37. Rossini FP, Ferrari A, Spandre M, et al. Emergency colonoscopy. World J Surg. 1989;13(2):190-2.
38. Sobrino-Faya M, Martinez S, Gomez Balado M, et al. Clips for the prevention and treatment of postpolypectomy bleeding (hemoclips in polypectomy). Rev Esp Enferm Dig. 2002;94(8):457-62.
39. Sung JJ, Lau JY, Ching JY, et al. Continuation of low-dose aspirin therapy in peptic ulcer bleeding: a randomized trial. Ann Intern Med. 2010;152(1):1-9.
40. Villavicencio RT, Rex DK, Rahmani E. Efficacy and complications of argon plasma coagulation for haematochezia related to radiation proctopathy. Gastrointest Endosc. 2002;55(1):70-4.
41. Villanueva C, Colomo A, Bosch A, et al. Transfusion strategies for acute upper gastrointestinal bleeding. N Engl J Med. 2013;368(1):11-21.
42. Winstead NS, Wilcox CM. Erythromycin prior to endoscopy for acute upper gastrointestinal hemorrhage: a cost-effectiveness analysis. Aliment Pharmacol Ther. 2007;26(10):1371-7.
43. Wu WC, Rathore SS, Wang Y, et al. Blood transfusion in elderly patients with acute myocardial infarction. N Engl J Med. 2001;345(17):1230-6.

CHAPTER 52

Hepatic Encephalopathy

Rahul Rai, Sanjiv Saigal

INTRODUCTION

Brain function becomes abnormal if liver fails. Acute-onset liver failure without any preexisting liver disease presents with brain edema and coma. Acute-onset (fulminant) liver failure associated with rise in blood ammonia levels and hepatic encephalopathy (HE) is difficult to manage because of acute-onset brain swelling and brainstem injuries. While acute on chronic liver failure presents with behavioral and cognitive abnormalities and usually manageable and can be controlled easily. HE indicates the deterioration of medical condition and advanced liver disease, mortality rates are high in patient with acute-onset HE. HE or overt HE (OHE) usually present with jaundice, variceal bleed, and ascites in a decompensated phase of chronic liver disease and is associated with poor prognosis, the survival rate is 42% at 1 year and 23% at 3 years of follow-up. Various terminology related to hepatic encephalopathy are described in **Table 1**.

PATHOPHYSIOLOGY

Hepatic encephalopathy is a multifactorial disease process. Critical factor in pathogenesis of HE is ammonia. Moreover, a synergistic role with ammonia in modulating HE; oxidative stress, gut flora and inflammation also contribute to pathogenesis of HE along with ammonia.

Ammonia is mainly produced in the gut; thought to be arising predominantly from colonic urease producing gram-negative bacteria. Urease enzymes metabolize urea from the bloodstream to produce ammonia. Research has shown that ammonia is also generated by enterocytes within the small bowel by glutamine metabolism. Ammonia is then carried through the splanchnic venous system into the liver where it is detoxified via urea cycle; urea thus produced is excreted by the kidneys. In chronic liver disease, multiple factors contribute to hyperammonemia, like reduction of the metabolic capacity of the urea cycle and portosystemic shunt (PSS) of blood (either by spontaneous extrahepatic portosystemic collaterals or iatrogenic shunts). The exact mechanism by which ammonia contributes to HE is not very clear. Ammonia changes the phenotype of astrocytes to Alzheimer type II astrocytosis causing neurological dysfunction. Also in astrocytes, ammonia is converted into glutamine by glutamine synthetase which acts as an intracellular osmole, causing an influx of water into the astrocytes causing low-grade cerebral edema.

Table 1	Current terminology for the classification of hepatic encephalopathy (HE)		
Type	Description	Subcategory	Subdivision
A	Encephalopathy associated with acute liver failure	–	–
B	Encephalopathy with portosystemic bypass and no intrinsic hepatocellular disease	–	–
C	Encephalopathy associated with cirrhosis or portal hypertension or portosystemic shunts	Episodic HE	Precipitated Spontaneous Recurrent
		Resistant HE	Mild Severe Treatment dependent
		Minimal	

Ammonia also induces nitroso-oxidative stress in astrocytes which subsequently cause mitochondrial dysfunction. Many other neurotoxic molecules are also implicated in the pathogenesis of HE like gamma-aminobutyric acid (GABA), indoles and oxindoles, short-chain fatty acids, octopamine, manganese, etc.

There is decrease in effective arterial volume and splanchnic arterial vasodilatation in patients with cirrhosis and portal hypertension, leads to activation of the renin-angiotensin system and vasopressin (antidiuretic hormone) leading to dilutional hyponatremia. In astrocytes, intracellular organic osmolytes normally provide a defense against intracellular swelling. In chronic hyponatremia, astrocytic osmolytes are depleted leading to loss of cellular defenses against cerebral edema during hyperammonemia or inflammatory stress.

The fact that infection commonly precipitates HE suggests that inflammation plays an important role in its pathogenesis. Experiments have suggested that inflammation in the background of hyperammonemia precipitates HE. Systemic inflammatory responses produce deleterious brain effects but the mechanisms are unclear.

CLINICAL PRESENTATION

An alteration in consciousness and a generalized motor disturbance are two classic clinical manifestation of HE. A clue to the diagnosis of HE is the finding of one or more factors known to precipitate bouts of OHE **(Box 1)**.

In very initial stages of HE patient is apparently asymptomatic, and routine neurological and psychological assessments are essentially normal. There is subtle alteration of cognitive domains of attention, working memory, psychomotor speed, visuospatial ability, etc. which can only be detected by specialized psychometric and neurophysiological tests. The development of any neuropsychiatric symptoms or signs marks the onset of OHE. Abnormal behavior, irritability, and alteration in sleep cycle are usually noted by the patient's relatives. As HE progresses, obvious alterations in consciousness occur. The patient may progressively develop confusion with disorientation to time and place, stupor, and finally coma. Various stages of hepatic encephalopathy are described in **Table 2**.

Motor system abnormalities like flapping tremors (asterixis) are frequently seen in earlier stages of OHE. Pyramidal signs like hypertonia, hyperreflexia, and a positive Babinski sign are rarely seen; however deep tendon reflexes may be lost in coma. Rarely focal neurological deficits and seizures can also be seen, but the presence of these signs warrant exclusion of organic brain syndromes by appropriate testing like electroencephalography (EEG) and/or computerized tomography (CT) or magnetic resonance imaging (MRI). Extrapyramidal symptoms such as slow speech, bradykinesia, dyskinesia, rigidity, and tremors can be rarely seen. Peripheral neuropathies are frequently seen in patients with chronic alcohol abuse. In patients with severe cerebral edema both decerebrate and decorticate posturing can be seen which a bad prognostic sign.

DIAGNOSIS

As stated earlier, HE is a diagnosis of exclusion. Stroke, mass lesion, infection of brain, and electrolyte abnormalities are common differential diagnosis. In a doubtful case, empiric treatment for HE is warranted; an improvement in neuropsychological dysfunction confirms the diagnosis of HE. On the other hand, no response within 72 hours or clinical deterioration warrants a prompt search for other etiologies, and reconsideration of treatment options.

Box 1 Precipitating factors for hepatic encephalopathy

- Constipation
- *Electrolyte imbalance*: Hyponatremia, hypokalemia, alkalosis
- Gastrointestinal bleeding
- Infection
  - Spontaneous bacterial peritonitis
  - Pneumonia
  - Urinary tract infections
  - Skin and soft tissue infections
- Sedative drugs, psychotropic medicines, benzodiazepines, morphine
- Renal failure
- Surgery
- Dehydration
  - Diuretics
  - Diarrhea
  - Vomiting
  - Excessive paracentesis
  - Fluid restriction
- Alcohol

Table 2 West Haven criteria for staging hepatic encephalopathy

Grade	Features
Grade 0	No abnormality detected
Grade 1	• Trivial lack of awareness • Euphoria or anxiety • Shortened attention span • Impaired performance of addition
Grade 2	• Lethargy or apathy • Minimal disorientation for time or place • Subtle personality change • Inappropriate behavior • Impaired performance of subtraction
Grade 3	• Somnolence to semi-stupor, but responsive to verbal stimuli • Confusion • Gross disorientation
Grade 4	Coma (unresponsive to verbal or noxious stimuli)

MANAGEMENT

The history and clinical examination are the key for diagnosis of OHE. Supportive laboratory and radiological assessment are required to confirm the diagnosis. HE severity can be assessed by various clinical scales. Patients with stupor or coma are difficult of manage; and need highly specialized care or intensive care management including enteral nutrition, prophylactic systemic antibiotics, airway protection, and mechanical ventilation. Assessment of hepatic encephalopathy are described in **Box 2**.

Diagnosing the subtle cognitive dysfunction in HE is difficult. Specific tests like neuropsychological tests, computerized tests and neurophysiological (for example EEG) tests are needed which are performed by a trained examiner and need appropriate tools or equipment.

Investigations in Hepatic Encephalopathy

Neuropsychological Testing

Number connection test-A (NCT-A), number connection test-B (NCT-B), and figure connection test (FCT)-A and FCT-B are used for psychomotor testing.

Electroencephalography

Cortical cerebral activity is recorded by the EEG. Other causes of altered sensorium like seizures can be ruled out. Hyponatremia and various drugs can alter the EEG results. So other tests are required for definitive diagnosis. EEG is nonspecific for HE.

Blood Ammonia Testing

The diagnosis of HE is questionable if ammonia level is normal. Ammonia levels can be measured regularly in intensive care to monitor the efficacy of various interventions. There is no diagnostic, grading or prognostic value of high blood ammonia levels in HE patients with the chronic liver disease.

Brain Imaging

Computerized tomography or MRI is considered to rule out various intracerebral pathology not for diagnosis or grading the severity of HE. Features of brain edema can be appreciated on CT in early hepatic encephalopathy.

TREATMENT

Goals of treatment are reduction of the ammonia absorption and removal of precipitating factors **(Box 3)**.

INTENSIVE CARE MANAGEMENT

Patient should be admitted in intensive care unit and specific measures should be taken in these patients as changes in mental status are rapid and disorientation leads to self-inflicted injuries and fall.

In higher grades of HE, prophylactic tracheal intubations is considered in order to protect the airway and prevent aspiration; prophylactic antibiotics are also justified in such patients. Normal protein intake is advised in these patients. Protein restriction may contribute to poor muscle mass and other nutritional deficiencies which can worsen HE. Zinc deficiency is noticed in most cirrhotic patients; so zinc

---

Box 2 Assessment of patent with hepatic encephalopathy in emergency department

- Assess for nonhepatic causes of altered mental status, such as delirium, intoxication, alcohol withdrawal, and hypoglycemia. Consider non-contrast CT scan head to assess for acute intracranial process if new focal neurologic findings are found
- Assess for clinical and neurological examination findings consistent with HE. Grade the severity of HE by West Haven criteria or Glasgow Coma Scale
- *Triage for patient safety*: Consider hospital admission and monitoring in ICU. Consider intubation if patient is unable to protect airway
- Assess for precipitating causes of HE and treat accordingly: thorough clinical examination, laboratory (e.g. electrolytes, glucose, renal function, cell counts, cultures, urine drug screen, stool for *C. difficile*), and imaging
- Treat HE with lactulose (peroral, nasogastric tube, or rectum) ± rifaximin
- Assess need for long-term therapy for prevention of recurrent HE
- Assess need for liver transplant evaluation

Abbreviations: CT, computed tomography; HE, hepatic encephalopathy; ICU, intensive care unit.
Source: Bajaj JS. Review article: the modern management of hepatic encephalopathy. Aliment Pharmacol Ther. 2010;31(5):537-47.

Box 3 Treatment of hepatic encephalopathy

- Supportive care of unconscious or confused patient
- Identification and treatment of concomitant disease
- Careful search for and correction of precipitating factors
- Reduction of ammonia production and absorption
  - Lactulose, lactitol, and lactose orally or in enema form
  - Restriction of dietary protein
  - Disaccharide inhibitors
  - Probiotics
- Promotion of nitrogen excretion
  - L-ornithine, aspartate IV and PO
  - Sodium benzoate IV and PO
- Correction of neurotransmitter abnormalities in the brain
  - Flumazenil
  - Branched-chain amino acid enriched formulations
  - Zinc replication (many possible modes of action)
- Portosystemic shunt suppression
- Liver support systems
- Liver transplantation

Abbreviations: IV, intravenous; PO, per oral.

supplementation may helpful in improving the condition. Measures should be taken to reduce the ammonia level in HE which is the main factor for cerebral edema. Ammonia level 150–200 micromol/L increases the risk for brain edema and intracranial hypertension. Management of hypovolemia, shock, coagulopathy, thrombocytopenia, and renal failure is equally important. CT scan can be done to document the features of cerebral edema and measures to control the raised intracranial tension can be implemented. Mannitol or hypertonic bolus saline are recommended if evidence of cerebral edema on CT scan.

MANAGEMENT OF PRECIPITATING FACTORS

Infections and gastrointestinal bleeding commonly precipitates HE so both factors should be promptly evaluated and treated medically or endoscopically as per local availability. Dehydration in the setting of aggressive diuresis and overzealous lactulose therapy, and electrolyte disturbances like hypokalemia and hyponatremia are common precipitants of HE; such derangements should be promptly treated by appropriate fluid and electrolyte replenishment. Dilutional hyponatremia (usually associated with increased extracellular fluid compartment manifesting as ascites and peripheral edema) requires fluid restriction (usually less than 1.5 L/day). Vasopressin antagonists (for example Tolvaptan) are newer agents for patients with euvolemic or hypervolemic hyponatremia, but should be used cautiously in refractory cases with monitoring of renal functions. In clinical practice constipation is also a common precipitant of HE. The reason is unclear, and probably decrease in colonic transit causes increase in absorption of ammonia. Routine prescription of osmotic stool softeners and appropriate hydration can prevent constipation. Anxiety, depression, sleep disturbances or body ache or leg cramps are also common in these patients. These patients may self-administer sedating medications like benzodiazepines and opiates which can precipitate HE. In the case of non-improvement of HE, a detailed drug history can be rewarding and patients can be treated with appropriate antidotes.

REDUCTION OF THE NITROGENOUS LOAD FROM THE GUT

Cathartics, nonabsorbable disaccharides, and antibiotics are used to reduce nitrogenous load from the gut. Various laxatives are used, but nonabsorbable disaccharides like lactulose are the treatment of choice. The acidification of the colon by lactulose decreases the absorption of ammonia into the bloodstream. Acidification also helps in reduction of urease producing gut bacteria thus decreasing the formation of ammonia. Lactulose 40–50 mL is given orally every hourly until evacuation occurs then every 8 hourly until 2–3 bowel movements per day. Administration of lactulose enema per rectally can be given in patients unable to tolerate it orally, or in comatose patients.

Rifaximin, a recent drug has broad antibacterial activity against both aerobes and anaerobes. Rifaximin typically lowers the bacterial load in the small bowel. Dose of rifaximin in HE treatment is 550 mg twice daily.

MODULATION OF FECAL FLORA

As described bacterial flora has important role in the pathogenesis of HE, and modulation of this flora either through antibiotics, probiotics, or prebiotics may have a role in the management of HE. Probiotics are defined as live organisms that, when ingested in adequate amounts, exert a health benefit to the host. Prebiotics (like lactulose and fermentable fibers) are important for growth of beneficial bacteria. Thus, prebiotics and probiotics indirectly reduce the influence of potentially more harmful resident flora (i.e. urease-producing species). Probiotics been studied (either alone or with prebiotics) for the treatment of HE and have shown some benefits.

LONG-TERM MANAGEMENT OF HEPATIC ENCEPHALOPATHY

Recurrence of HE are common in cirrhotic patients. Thus, patients with cirrhosis are on secondary prophylaxis indefinitely or until they undergo liver transplantation. Lactulose and rifaximin are mainly used for prophylaxis. Long-term lactulose therapy produces gastrointestinal adverse effects. Rifaximin is recommended as an add-on to lactulose and is well tolerated. Ornithine-L-aspartate (oral dose of 6 g three times daily) is recommended for secondary prophylaxis by some authors.

LIVER TRANSPLANTATION

Indications

- Hepatic encephalopathy with a poor liver function.
- Recurrent HE not responding to standard medical therapy.
- End-stage liver disease is the indications for liver transplantation.
- Molecular adsorbent recirculating system (MARS) can be used in patient with fulminant hepatic failure while preparing the patient for liver transplant.

CONCLUSION

The pathogenesis of HE is multifactorial. Alteration of gut flora and release of products such as ammonia, endotoxin, indoles, oxindoles, etc. may lead to development of HE. Current treatments for HE, such as lactulose, antibiotics, and others, also rely on manipulation of the gut flora. Prebiotics and probiotics are newer and specific therapeutic targets to modulate gut flora, thereby reducing inflammation and paving the way for comprehensive management of HE. Lactulose and rifaximin are helpful in HE with underlying cirrhosis (gradual onset HE). While in fulminant hepatic failure, aggressive management is required for cerebral edema with osmotic diuresis to prevent brainstem damage.

BIBLIOGRAPHY

1. Bajaj JS. Review article: the modern management of hepatic encephalopathy. Aliment Pharmacol Ther. 2010;31(5): 537-47.
2. Blei AT, Córdoba J. Practice Parameters Committee of the American College of Gastroenterology. Hepatic Encephalopathy. Am J Gastroenterol. 2001;96(7):1968-76.
3. Córdoba J. New assessment of hepatic encephalopathy. J Hepatol. 2011;54(5):1030-40.
4. Dhiman RK, Saraswat VA, Sharma BK, et al. Minimal hepatic encephalopathy: consensus statement of a working party of the Indian National Association for Study of the Liver. J Gastroenterol Hepatol. 2010;25(6):1029-41.
5. Dhiman RK. Gut microbiota and hepatic encephalopathy. Metab Brain Dis. 2013;28(2):321-6.
6. Ferenci P, Lockwood A, Mullen K, et al. Hepatic encephalopathy-definition, nomenclature, diagnosis, and quantification: final report of the working party at the 11th World Congresses of Gastroenterology, Vienna, 1998. Hepatology. 2002;35(3): 716-21.
7. Frederick RT. Current concepts in the pathophysiology and management of hepatic encephalopathy. Gastroenterol Hepatol (N Y). 2011;7(4):222-33.
8. Mullen KD. Clinical consequences of liver disease: hepatic encephalopathy. In: Boyer TD, Marves MP, Sanyal AJ (Eds). Zakim and Boyer's Hepatology: A Textbook of Liver Disease. India: Elsevier; 2008. pp. 311-31.
9. Mullen KD. Pathogenesis, clinical manifestation, and diagnosis of hepatic encephalopathy. In: Cores CJ, Bruix J (Eds). Seminars in Liver Disease. India: Thieme Medical Publishers; 2007. pp. 3-9.
10. Vilstrup H, Amodio P, Bajaj J, et al. Hepatic encephalopathy in chronic liver disease: 2014 Practice Guideline by the American Association for the Study of Liver Diseases and the European Association for the Study of the Liver. Hepatology. 2014;60(2):715-35.

CHAPTER 53

Acute Pancreatitis

Rajesh Puri, Randhir Sud

INTRODUCTION

Acute pancreatitis (AP) is a common admitting gastrointestinal emergency. Its clinical spectrum ranges between a mild disease requiring an admission in a ward, to a fulminant course requiring extensive critical care. Its reported incidence is around 13–45 cases per 100,000 persons.[1]

Around 15–25% of cases of AP develop a severe course. With the advent of better intensive care in last few decades, the mortality has been decreasing. Between 1988 and 2003, mortality from AP decreased from 12% to 2%, according to a large epidemiologic study from the United States.[2] However, there still remains certain population group in whom mortality remains high.

In a triage setting, it is very imperative that the diagnosis is ascertained and appropriate treatment instituted to prevent further organ damage.

Revised Atlanta Criteria are used in defining AP and its severity for use in clinical practice as per the latest international consensus which were published after the International Association of Pancreatology or American Pancreatic Association (IAP or APA) symposium which took place in 2012.[3]

In an intensive care setting, management of AP requires an algorithmic approach with identification of parameters which will predict higher mortality. The ability to predict its severity can help to identify patients at increased risk for morbidity and mortality, thereby assisting in appropriate early triage to intensive care units (ICU) and selection of patients for specific interventions.

ETIOLOGY, PATHOPHYSIOLOGY, AND DEFINITION

As per the IAP or APA consensus, the revised Atlanta criteria, diagnosis of AP requires presence of at least two out of three criteria, namely pain abdomen, three times raised enzymes (amylase or lipase) and imaging diagnosis of AP.

Imaging studies [by using transabdominal ultrasonography, computed tomography (CT) or magnetic resonance imaging (MRI)] are not essential for diagnosis and going for them while patients awaits resuscitation can lead to higher mortality. Imaging studies are required in cases where diagnosis is not clear, clinical suspicion of duodenal perforation, or a prolonged period between onset of symptoms and scenarios where cross-sectional imaging may be required in patients where there is clinical suspicion of AP but enzymes have normalized and patients is not in a state of giving clear history.

There are other markers which can be used for diagnosis of AP in a doubtful setting. Tests like urinary trypsinogen levels are sensitive in this setting. In a meta-analysis in 2013, usefulness of urinary trypsinogen-2 (UT-2) for diagnosis of AP was assessed. A total of 18 studies were assessed. The pooled sensitivity and specificity of UT-2 for the diagnosis of AP were 80 and 92%, respectively [area under the curve (AUC) = 0.96, diagnostic odds ratios (DOR) = 65.63, 95% confidence interval (CI) = 31.65–139.09]. The diagnostic value of UT-2 was comparable to serum amylase but was weaker than serum lipase. They concluded that UT-2 as a rapid test could be potentially used for the diagnosis of postendoscopic retrograde cholangiopancreatography (ERCP) pancreatitis and, to an extent, AP.[4]

The clinical use of UT-2 may be in the setting where rapid diagnosis is required, e.g. in a triage setting with the use of urinary dipsticks.

Etiological workup should go on parallel to the resuscitation of the patient. On admission, detailed history to elicit history of gall stones in past, alcoholism, any endoscopic procedure like ERCP, known dyslipidemia in family and hypercalcemia is important. Family history of pancreatic disease should also be asked, especially in young patients where hereditary pancreatitis may be seen. Some treatment decisions depend upon the etiological diagnosis of AP (e.g. cholecystectomy for biliary pancreatitis and de-addiction for alcoholic pancreatitis).

A deranged liver function test (LFT) suggests biliary cause of pancreatitis. An elevated alanine aminotransferase (ALT) level greater than 150 U/L within 48 hours after onset of symptoms discriminates biliary pancreatitis from other causes.[5-7]

In the study by Liu et al.,[6] after multivariate analysis, female sex, age more than 58 years and serum alanine aminotransferase greater than 150 U/L were independent predictive factors for biliary cause of AP. Using these three factors for prediction of biliary cause, the sensitivity was 93% and overall accuracy was 85%.

In the study by Moolla et al.,[5] AP was diagnosed in 464 patients. The disease was related to alcohol in 275 cases, gallstones in 81 cases, human immunodeficiency virus (HIV) in 49 cases, dyslipidemia in 42 cases and it was idiopathic in 17 cases. When compared to patients with nonbiliary causes of pancreatitis, patients with gallstone pancreatitis had greater median (range) serum amylase activity [1,423 U/L (153–7,500 U/L) vs 589 U/L (58–11,144 U/L); $p < 0.001$] and ALT activity [153 U/L (8–13,233 U/L) vs 31 U/L (6–421 U/L); $p < 0.001$].

CLINICAL PRESENTATION

The clinical presentation can vary from mild pain in epigastrium to severe pain with anuria and loss of consciousness depending on severity of the disease.

Usually, patient complaints of abdominal pain—upper or generalized, typically severe, may radiate to back. Other common symptoms to consider include nausea, vomiting and diaphoresis. There will be abdominal tenderness and abdominal distension.

In severe pancreatitis-hypotension, a bluish discoloration around the umbilicus (Cullen's sign) or the flank (Grey-Turner's sign) is sometimes associated with hemorrhagic pancreatitis (a late, serious complication).

RISK FACTORS TO CONSIDER

Common risk factors are:
- Gallstones (50% of cases)
- Ethanol (20–25%)

Other risk factors are:
- Endoscopic procedures (complicates up to 10% of ERCP)
- Trauma
- *Infections*: Viral, bacterial, fungal and parasitic
- Autoimmune diseases
- *Metabolic*: Hypercalcemia, hyperlipidemia, hypothermia
- *Vascular*: Vasculitis, ischemia, embolism
- Genetic
- Pancreatitis may be idiopathic.

ASSESSING SEVERITY OF ACUTE PANCREATITIS

There are many scoring systems that have been developed over the years for assessing the severity of AP. But the most useful in the emergency setting are the Bedside Index for Severity in Acute Pancreatitis (BISAP) index. This can be rapidly applied in the triage itself and patient can be categorized as severe or mild. Another such similar score is the Harmless Acute Pancreatitis Score (HAPS).

The HAPS and BISAP scores are enormously helpful in assessing severity early on, unlike the Ranson criteria and Acute Physiology and Chronic Health Evaluation (APACHE-II) score, which are tedious and complicated, and take up to 48 hours to complete.

The HAPS can be measured within 30 minutes of hospital admission. There are three criteria for a "harmless" HAPS score: (1) a normal hematocrit; (2) normal serum creatinine; and (3) absence of rebound tenderness. The presence of all three criteria has 96% specificity and 99% positive predictive value for a nonsevere disease course.

The BISAP awards one point each for the presence of five possible findings: (1) a urea nitrogen level in excess of 25 mg/dL, indicative of third spacing; (2) impaired mental status defined by a Glasgow Coma Score of even a single point less than the normal 15; (3) age over 60; (4) pleural effusion; and (5) the presence of systemic inflammatory response syndrome (SIRS).

Sixty percent of patients with AP have SIRS on admission. It resolves within 24 hours in half of the cases. Persistent or worsening SIRS is associated with an 11–25% mortality rate. SIRS is defined by two or more of the following: tachycardia, tachypnea, hypocarbia, fever, and either an elevated or depressed white blood cell count.

A patient with a BISAP score of one has less than a 2% risk of mortality. In contrast, a BISAP score of three is associated with a 22% mortality rate.

As per revised Atlanta criteria, AP is divided into the following:
- Mild AP which is characterized by the absence of organ failure and local or systemic complications.
- Moderately severe AP which is characterized by transient organ failure (resolves within 48 hours) and/or local or systemic complications without persistent organ failure (>48 hours).
- Severe AP which is characterized by persistent organ failure that may involve one or multiple organs.

Local complications of AP include acute peripancreatic fluid collection, pancreatic pseudocyst, acute necrotic collection and walled-off necrosis.

Organ failure is defined as a score of two or more for any one of three organ systems (respiratory, cardiovascular, or renal) using the modified Marshall scoring system.[8]

Further on, there were various clinical predictors which suggest higher morbidity and mortality. These include, obesity, older age and shorted time to symptom onset. In a meta-analysis done by Martinez et al.[9] 799 patients were included. Severe AP was significantly more frequent in obese patients [odds ratio (OR) = 2.9; 95% CI = 1.8–4.6). Furthermore, those patients developed significantly more systemic (OR = 2.3; 95% CI = 1.4–3.8] and especially local complications (OR = 3.8; 95% CI = 2.4–6.6). In this analysis, mortality was also higher in obese patients (OR = 2.1; 95% CI = 1.0–4.8). These concluded that obesity was not only a risk factor for severe disease but also an independent risk factor of mortality.

In laboratory variables, high hematocrit values are suggestive of severe disease and predict higher fluid resuscitation.[10]

In the study of Larvin et al. for study of C-reactive protein (CRP) levels as predictors of severe pancreatitis, they found that at 48 hours, CRP above 150 mg/L has a sensitivity, specificity, positive predictive value and negative predictive value of 80%, 76%, 67%, and 86%, respectively, for severe AP.[11]

In other parameters, blood urea nitrogen was an important predictor of severity. In a large hospital-based cohort,[12] it was showed that for every increase in the blood urea nitrogen (BUN) of 5 mg/dL during the first 24 hours, the adjusted OD for mortality was 2.2. In one study of 129 patients, a peak creatinine of greater than 1.8 mg/dL during the first 48 hours had a positive predictive value of 93% for the development of pancreatic necrosis.[13] Other markers that have been studied include procalcitonin, urinary trypsinogen activation peptide (UTAP), polymorphonuclear elastase, pancreatic-associated protein, amylase, lipase, serum glucose, serum calcium, procarboxypeptidase B, carboxypeptidase-B activation peptide, serum trypsinogen-2, phospholipase A-2, serum amyloid protein-A, substance P, antithrombin III, platelet-activating factor, interleukins 1, 6, and 8, and tumor necrosis factor-α or soluble tumor necrosis factor receptor. There is no consensus yet on these markers, especially in their clinical applications especially in critical care setting.

In a practical viewpoint, identification of pancreatic infection early in the course of pancreatitis is the area which requires much more studies. In a study from China, high serum lactate dehydrogenase (LDH) levels, elevated procalcitonin, higher BUN levels and organ failure predicted pancreatic infection as compared to extrapancreatic infection. This may direct the use of antimicrobials in AP.

Imaging modalities in the use of assessment of severity of pancreatitis has been a topic of much debate. A contrast-enhanced CT imaging will help to identify necrosis and extrapancreatic disease in AP, but its superiority in predicting mortality over clinical scores is doubtful. A retrospective analysis of the performance of several CT scoring systems for the severity of AP found that none was statistically superior to the APACHE II or BISAP scoring systems.[14] The more important thing to understand is that pancreatic necrosis takes time to develop and in the first week of management, it does not change the treatment algorithm. As per the revised Atlanta criteria, presence or absence of necrosis is not used in classifying patients with severe disease. Only presence of persistent organ failure as per Marshall Scoring system classifies severe disease.

The CT severity index (CTSI)[15] was developed for correlating presence of necrosis and extrapancreatic collections with mortality. It has been developed based upon the degree of necrosis, inflammation and the presence of fluid collections. In an initial validation study, mortality was 23% with any degree of pancreatic necrosis and 0% with no necrosis. In addition, there was a strong association between necrosis greater than 30% and morbidity and mortality. The original CTSI or the Balthazar was later modified by the same group to be called as modified CT severity index (M-CTSI) which predicted mortality better.

Admission to ICU requires a severe disease especially in terms of the earlier parameters described.

In summary, following recommendations can be made for admission to ICU:
- Patients with severe AP
- Patients with AP and one or more of the following parameters:
  - Pulse less than 40 beats/min or greater than 150 beats/min
  - Systolic arterial pressure less than 80 mm Hg or mean arterial pressure less than 60 mm Hg or diastolic arterial pressure greater than 120 mm Hg
  - Respiratory rate greater than 35 breaths/min
  - Serum sodium less than 110 mmol/L or greater than 170 mmol/L
  - Serum potassium less than 2.0 mmol/L or greater than 7.0 mmol/L
  - Partial pressure of alveolar oxygen (PaO_2) less than 50 mm Hg
  - pH less than 7.1 or greater than 7.7
  - Serum glucose greater than 800 mg/dL
  - Serum calcium greater than 15 mg/dL
  - Anuria
- APACHE II score greater than 8 in the first 24 hours of admission
- Persistent (>48 hours) SIRS
- Elevated hematocrit (>44%), BUN (>20 mg/dL), or creatinine (>1.8 mg/dL)
- Age greater than 60 years
- Underlying cardiac or pulmonary disease, obesity.

MANAGEMENT OF ACUTE PANCREATITIS

Initial Management

Fluid Therapy

Aggressive hydration is one of the mainstays of initial management of patients with AP. The primary aim of fluid therapy is to limit or prevent pancreatic necrosis. Any patient with AP has the potential to progress to severe disease.

Hydration at a rate of 5-10 mL/kg per hour of isotonic crystalloid solution (e.g. normal saline or lactated Ringer's solution) to all patients with AP, unless cardiovascular, renal, or other related comorbid factors preclude aggressive fluid replacement, may be required. Fluid requirements should be assessed at regular intervals, initially at 6 hours, then at 24-48 hours. More careful monitoring with the use of various parameters like inferior vena cava respiratory variability, central venous pressure monitoring may be required especially in patients with comorbid conditions like coronary artery disease with systolic dysfunction and patients with poor kidney reserves. Adequate fluid replacement can be assessed by an improvement in vital signs (goal heart rate <120 beats/min, mean arterial pressure between 65 and 85 mm Hg), urine output (>0.5 to 1 cc/kg/hour) and reduction in hematocrit (goal 35-44%) and BUN over 24 hours, particularly if they were high at the onset.

The evidence of aggressive fluid therapy is not of very high quality. Aggressive fluid resuscitation was defined by the Mayo Clinic group to constitute greater than or equal to 33% of the total volume in 72 hours of infusion performed in the first 24 hours.[16] Chinese researchers have used more objective criteria of 15 mL/kg per hour infusion as aggressive resuscitation, as compared to controlled resuscitation, which they defined as 5-10 mL/kg per hour.[17]

In few of the recent publications, better outcomes have been shown with controlled fluid therapy as compared to liberal fluid replacement. de-Madaria et al.[18] analyzed 247 patients prospectively who were divided into three groups depending on the fluid received in the initial 24 hours. Administration of greater than 4.1 L during the initial 24 hours was found to be associated with persistent organ failure and acute collections, while administration between 3.1 L and 4.1 L was associated with an excellent outcome. A Japanese study analyzed the demographics of fluid resuscitation in 9,489 patients and found that those with higher volume infused in the first 48 hour had higher respiratory complications and higher mortality.[19]

The ideal fluid for resuscitation in AP is yet to be determined. The choice is primarily between a colloid and a crystalloid. Variability in the results of initial studies with fluid resuscitation could be attributed to different types of fluids used. Crystalloids are recommended by the American Gastroenterological Association, and colloids (packed red blood cells) are considered in cases of low hematocrit (<25%) and low serum albumin (<2 g/dL). Among the crystalloids, Ringer's lactate solution is preferred over normal saline. In one small randomized trial of 40 patients, patients who received lactated Ringer's had significantly lower mean CRP levels compared with patients who received normal saline (52 mg/dL vs 104 mg/dL) and a significant reduction in SIRS after 24 hours (84% vs 0%).[20]

Inadequate fluid resuscitation leads to higher necrosis and higher chances of developing acute tubular necrosis. Continued aggressive fluid resuscitation after 48 hours may not be advisable as overly vigorous fluid resuscitation is associated with an increased need for intubation and increased risk of abdominal compartment syndrome.

Pain Control

Pain is the presenting symptom in most of the patients. Adequate pain control is important in overall management of the patients. Again, fluid resuscitation is of importance for pain control as well inadequate fluid replacement leads to higher tissue ischemia and pain from lactic acidosis.

Opioids are safe and required in patients with severe AP. Adequate pain control requires the use of intravenous opiates, usually in the form of a patient-controlled analgesia pump. Fentanyl is now being increasingly used in control of pain in patients of AP, provided patient has adequate respiratory reserves. It can be used both as intravenous or bolus dosing. The typical dose for the bolus regimen ranges from 20 μg to 50 μg with a 10-minute lock-out period.

Monitoring

Patients with acute severe pancreatitis should be closely monitored, especially in first 24-48 hours. Oxygen saturation levels, respiratory rate, electrolytes, glucose levels and acidosis should be routinely monitored. Electrolytes should be monitored frequently in the first 48 -72 hours and especially with aggressive fluid resuscitation. Hypocalcemia should be corrected if ionized calcium is low or if there are signs of neuromuscular irritability (Chvostek's or Trousseau's sign). Low magnesium levels can also cause hypocalcemia and should be corrected. Patients in the ICU should be monitored for potential abdominal compartment syndrome with serial measures of urinary bladder pressures.

Nutrition

Maintaining patient's nutrition is one of the important parameters for management of AP. There have been numerous studies comparing various forms of nutrition in AP. It has been shown in various studies that enteral nutrition is better than parenteral nutrition in these patients. The whole approach is designed in a way to expedite enteral nutrition either oral or through nasogastric (NG) or nasojejunal (NJ) feeds. It has been shown to decrease the rate of infections and early recovery.

Patients with mild AP can be managed with intravenous hydration alone since recovery is expected to occur early without much nutritional depletion of the patient. Oral diet can be instituted early in the course of illness. In the absence of ileus, vomiting and decreasing pain, oral diet can be started in patients with mild pancreatitis. In the beginning, low-residue, low-fat soft diet can be instituted and diet can be increased as the patient tolerates. More recent data suggest that early refeeding when patients are subjectively hungry, regardless of resolution of abdominal pain and normalization of pancreatic enzymes, may be safe.[21]

The difficulty comes in patients of moderate or severe pancreatitis where early initiation of oral therapy may be difficult. In moderately severe to severe pancreatitis, oral feeding is frequently not tolerated due to postprandial pain, nausea or vomiting related to gastroduodenal inflammation and/or extrinsic compression from fluid collections leading to gastric outlet obstruction. Patients usually require enteral or parenteral feeding. However, when the local complications start improving, oral feeds can be initiated and advanced as tolerated.

The next question that arises is that when enteral feeding should be started in patients with severe pancreatitis. There have been various studies and guidelines which advocate early start of feeding in these patients. They state that this decreases the rate of infections although clear evidence is lacking for this assumption.[22,23]

In a randomized trial, 208 patients with severe AP were assigned to early nasoenteric tube feeding (within 24 hours of randomization) or an oral diet at 72 hours with on-demand nasoenteric tube feeding if an oral diet was not tolerated at 96 hours. There was no difference in the primary endpoint (composite of major infection or death at 6 months) between patients who received early or on-demand nasoenteric tube feeding (30% vs 27%, relative risk (RR) = 1.07; 95% CI = 0.8–1.4).[24]

Enteral feeding requires placement of NG or NJ tube. NJ tube would require radiological or endoscopic placement as the tip has to be placed beyond ligament of treitz. There have been studies which have compared NG versus NJ tube placement. Two controlled trials comparing NG with NJ feedings found no significant differences in APACHE II scores, CRP levels, pain, or analgesic requirements. However, another small study comparing NG feeding with total parenteral nutrition noted increased pulmonary and total complications in the nasogastric group.[25-27] More studies are required for conclusive evidence.

Enteral feeding should preferably be high-protein, low-fat, semi-elemental diet. Start at 25 mL per hour and advance as tolerated to at least 30% of the calculated daily requirement (25 kcal/kg ideal body weight), even in the presence of ileus. Signs that the formula is not tolerated include increased abdominal pain, vomiting (with NG feeding), bloating, or diarrhea (>5 watery stools or >500 mL per 24 hours with exclusion of *Clostridium difficile* toxin and medication-induced diarrhea) that resolves if the feeding is held.

Enteral feeding prevents the bacterial translocation from the gut and helps to reduce the overall infection rate. Another advantage is prevention of complications associated with parenteral feeding like sepsis and electrolyte disturbances. Consistent with prior meta-analysis, a 2010 meta-analysis of eight trials demonstrated that enteral nutrition significantly reduced mortality, multiple organ failure, systemic infections, and the need for surgery as compared with those who received parenteral nutrition.[28]

Parenteral nutrition should be started in only those patients who do not tolerate oral feeding.

Antibiotics

Prophylactic antibiotics are not recommended for use in AP especially in the first week of illness. This is regardless of the type or severity of pancreatitis. Only in the cases of proven infected pancreatic necrosis, antibiotics will be required. Empirical treatment of pancreatic necrosis should be done with use of fluoroquinolones or carbapenems, as pancreatic penetration is good with this drugs. Cultures should always be taken in management of AP.

Around 20% of patients develop extrapancreatic infectious complications. Extrapancreatic infectious complications are associated with higher mortality.[29]

Fungal infections occur in approximately 9% of necrotizing pancreatitis. However, it is not clear if they are associated with higher mortality.[30]

CONCLUSION

To summarize, AP is an important diagnosis in emergency setting as early resuscitation can alter the course of the illness. Bedside indices of severity of AP should be applied and patient should be triaged as per the severity. Early resuscitation with intravenous fluids is of utmost importance in managing patients with AP and preventing organ failure.

REFERENCES

1. Yadav D, Lowenfels AB. The epidemiology of pancreatitis and pancreatic cancer. Gastroenterology. 2013;144:1252-61.
2. Fagenholz PJ, Castillo CF, Harris NS, et al. Increasing United States hospital admissions for acute pancreatitis, 1988-2003. Ann Epidemiol. 2007;17:491-7.
3. Banks PA, Bollen TL, Dervenis C, et al. Classification of acute pancreatitis-2012: revision of the Atlanta classification and definitions by international consensus. Gut. 2013;62:102-11.
4. Jin T, Huang W, Jiang K, et al. Urinary trypsinogen-2 for diagnosing acute pancreatitis: a meta-analysis. Hepatobiliary Pancreat Dis Int. 2013;12(4):355-62.

5. Moolla Z, Anderson F, Thomson SR. Use of amylase and alanine transaminase to predict acute gallstone pancreatitis in a population with high HIV prevalence. World J Surg. 2013;37:156-61.
6. Liu CL, Fan ST, Lo CM, et al. Clinico-biochemical prediction of biliary cause of acute pancreatitis in the era of endoscopic ultrasonography. Aliment Pharmacol Ther. 2005;22:423-31.
7. Tenner S, Dubner H, Steinberg W. Predicting gallstone pancreatitis with laboratory parameters: a meta-analysis. Am J Gastroenterol. 1994;89:1863-6.
8. Marshall JC, Cook DJ, Christou NV, et al. Multiple organ dysfunction score: a reliable descriptor of a complex clinical outcome. Crit Care Med. 1995;23:1638-52.
9. Martínez J, Johnson CD, Sánchez-Payá J, et al. Obesity is a definitive risk factor of severity and mortality in acute pancreatitis: an updated meta-analysis. Pancreatology. 2006;6(3):206-9.
10. Brown A, Orav J, Banks PA. Hemoconcentration is an early marker for organ failure and necrotizing pancreatitis. Pancreas. 2000;20:367.
11. Larvin M. Assessment of clinical severity and prognosis. In: Beger HG, Warshaw AL, Buchler MW (Eds). The Pancreas. Oxford: Blackwell Science; 1998.
12. Wu BU, Johannes RS, Sun X, et al. Early changes in blood urea nitrogen predict mortality in acute pancreatitis. Gastroenterology. 2009;137:129-35.
13. Muddana V, Whitcomb DC, Khalid A, et al. Elevated serum creatinine as a marker of pancreatic necrosis in acute pancreatitis. Am J Gastroenterol. 2009;104:164-70.
14. Bollen TL, Singh VK, Maurer R, et al. A comparative evaluation of radiologic and clinical scoring systems in the early prediction of severity in acute pancreatitis. Am J Gastroenterol. 2012;107:612-9.
15. Balthazar EJ, Robinson DL, Megibow AJ, et al. Acute pancreatitis: value of CT in establishing prognosis. Radiology. 1990;174:331-6.
16. Gardner TB, Vege SS, Chari ST, et al. Faster rate of initial fluid resuscitation in severe acute pancreatitis diminishes in-hospital mortality. Pancreatology. 2009;9:770-6.
17. Mao EQ, Tang YQ, Fei J, et al. Fluid therapy for severe acute pancreatitis in acute response stage. Chin Med J (Engl). 2009;122:169-73.
18. de-Madaria E, Soler-Sala G, Sánchez-Payá J, et al. Influence of fluid therapy on the prognosis of acute pancreatitis: a prospective cohort study. Am J Gastroenterol. 2011;106:1843-50.
19. Kuwabara K, Matsuda S, Fushimi K, et al. Early crystalloid fluid volume management in acute pancreatitis: association with mortality and organ failure. Pancreatology. 2011;11:351-61.
20. Wu BU, Hwang JQ, Gardner TH, et al. Lactated Ringer's solution reduces systemic inflammation compared with saline in patients with acute pancreatitis. Clin Gastroenterol Hepatol. 2011;9:710-7.
21. Eckerwall GE, Tingstedt BB, Bergenzaun PE, et al. Immediate oral feeding in patients with mild acute pancreatitis is safe and may accelerate recovery—a randomized clinical study. Clin Nutr. 2007;26:758-63.
22. Mirtallo JM, Forbes A, McClave SA, et al. International consensus guidelines for nutrition therapy in pancreatitis. J Parenter Enteral Nutr. 2012;36:284-91.
23. McClave SA, Martindale RG, Vanek VW, et al. Guidelines for the Provision and Assessment of Nutrition Support Therapy in the Adult Critically Ill Patient: Society of Critical Care Medicine (SCCM) and American Society for Parenteral and Enteral Nutrition (A.S.P.E.N.). J Parenter Enteral Nutr. 2009;33:277-316.
24. Bakker OJ, van Brunschot S, van Santvoort HC, et al. Early versus on-demand nasoenteric tube feeding in acute pancreatitis. N Engl J Med. 2014;371:1983-93.
25. Singh N, Sharma B, Sharma M, et al. Evaluation of early enteral feeding through nasogastric and nasojejunal tube in severe acute pancreatitis: a noninferiority randomized controlled trial. Pancreas. 2012;41:153-9.
26. Kumar A, Singh N, Prakash S, et al. Early enteral nutrition in severe acute pancreatitis: a prospective randomized controlled trial comparing nasojejunal and nasogastric routes. J Clin Gastroenterol. 2006;40:431-4.
27. Eckerwall GE, Axelsson JB, Andersson RG. Early nasogastric feeding in predicted severe acute pancreatitis: A clinical, randomized study. Ann Surg. 2006;244:959-65.
28. Al-Omran M, Albalawi ZH, Tashkandi MF, et al. Enteral versus parenteral nutrition for acute pancreatitis. Cochrane Database Syst Rev. 2010;(20):CD002837.
29. Wu BU, Johannes RS, Kurtz S, et al. The impact of hospital-acquired infection on outcome in acute pancreatitis. Gastroenterology. 2008;135:816-20.
30. Trikudanathan G, Navaneethan U, Vege SS. Intra-abdominal fungal infections complicating acute pancreatitis: a review. Am J Gastroenterol. 2011;106:1188-92.

CHAPTER 54

Acute Appendicitis

Mukund Khetan, Anand Yadav

INTRODUCTION

Acute appendicitis is the most common general surgical emergency, and early surgical intervention improves the final outcome. The diagnosis is at times deceptive, and high index of suspicion is important to prevent serious complications.

ANATOMY

Embryologically, the appendix and cecum develop as outpouchings of the caudal limb of the midgut loop. At birth, the appendix is located at the tip of the cecum, but the adult appendix typically originates from the posteromedial wall of the cecum. The appendix measures 5–9 cm in length, with its outside diameter ranging from 3 mm to 8 mm and lumen ranging from 1 mm to 3 mm. The base of the appendix is consistently found by following the teniae coli of the colon to their confluence at the base of the cecum. The appendicular tip, however, can vary significantly in location **(Figs 1A and B)**.

The arterial supply of the appendix comes from the appendicular branch of the ileocolic artery. Lymphatic drainage flows to the lymph nodes along the ileocolic artery **(Figs 1A and B)**.

HISTORY

The first description of the appendix dates to the 16th century. Appendix was formally described in 1524 by da Capri[1] and in 1543 by Vesalius.[2] The first description of a case of appendicitis was by Fernel[3] in 1554. Amyand[4] is credited with the first

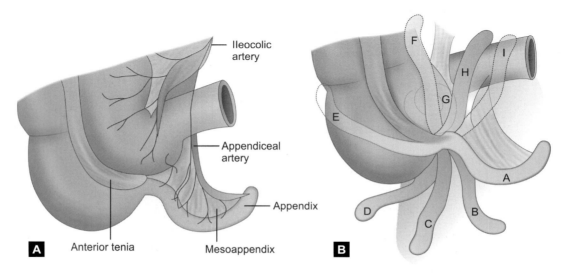

Figs 1A and B Anatomical position of appendix

appendectomy in 1736. Lawson Tait[5] in London presented in 1880 the first successful transabdominal appendectomy for gangrenous appendix. In 1886, Reginald Fitz[6] of Harvard Medical School first described the natural history of the inflamed appendix, coining the term "appendicitis".

In 1889, Chester McBurney described characteristic migratory pain as well as localization of the pain along an oblique line from the anterior superior iliac spine to the umbilicus. Laparoscopic appendectomy was first reported by the gynecologist Kurt Semm in 1982.

ETIOLOGY AND PATHOPHYSIOLOGY

Obstruction of the appendiceal lumen is believed to be the major cause of acute appendicitis.[7] This may be secondary to inspissated stool (fecalith or appendicolith), lymphoid hyperplasia, vegetable matter, parasites, or a neoplasm. A fecalith is typically composed of inspissated fecal material, calcium phosphates, bacteria and epithelial debris.

Obstruction of the appendiceal lumen contributes to bacterial overgrowth, and continued secretion of mucus leads to increased intraluminal pressure and distension. Luminal distension produces typical periumbilical pain. Further impairment of lymphatic and venous drainage leads to mucosal ischemia. This in turn promotes a localized inflammatory process that may progress to gangrene and perforation. Perforation, although there is much variability, occurs after at least 48 hours from the onset of symptoms, and is accompanied by an abscess cavity walled off by the surrounding omentum and small intestine. Various pathophysiologic changes in acute appendicitis are demonstrable in USG finding **(Figs 2A to D)**.

Although appendiceal obstruction is widely accepted as the primary cause of appendicitis, evidence suggests that this may be only one of many possible etiologies. First, some patients with fecalith have a histologically normal appendix, and the majority of patients with appendicitis show no evidence for a fecalith.[8-10]

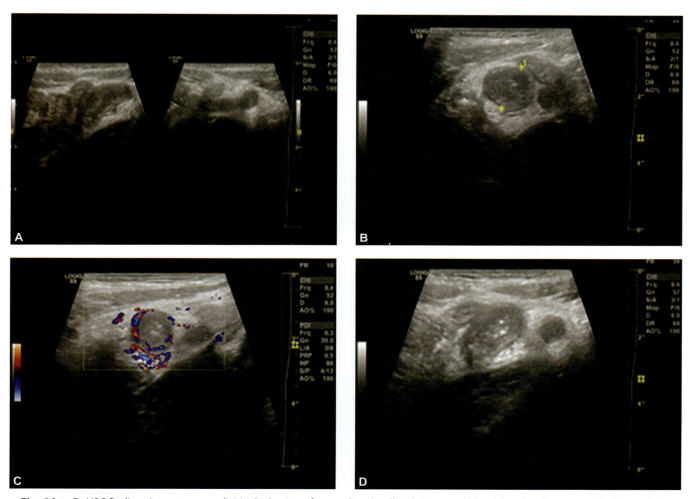

Figs 2A to D USG findings in acute appendicitis-thickening of appendiceal wall with increased blood flow (leading to so called ring-of-fire appearance), loss of wall compressibility, increased echogenicity of the surrounding fat, and loculated pericecal fluid

The flora in the normal appendix is very similar to that in the colon, with a wide variety of facultative aerobic and anaerobic bacteria. *Escherichia coli*, *Streptococcus viridans*, *Bacteroides* and *Pseudomonas* are frequently isolated.

PRESENTATION

Perhaps the most common surgically correctable cause of abdominal pain, still the diagnosis of acute appendicitis remains difficult in many instances.

The classic presentation of acute appendicitis begins with crampy, intermittent abdominal pain which may be either periumbilical or diffuse and difficult to localize. This is typically followed shortly thereafter with nausea. If nausea and vomiting precede the pain, patients are likely to have another cause for their abdominal pain. Classically, the pain migrates to the right lower quadrant (RLQ) due to inflammation of peritoneal lining in RLQ due to transmural migration from appendix. This usually occurs within 12–24 hours from the onset of the symptoms. The character of the pain thus changes from dull and colicky to sharp and constant.

Movement or Valsalva maneuver often worsens the pain, so that the patient typically desires to lie still. Patients may report low grade fever up to 101°F (38.3°C). Patients who have appendicitis commonly report anorexia; appendicitis is unlikely in those with normal appetite.

Typically, two clinical syndromes of acute appendicitis can be apprehended, acute catarrhal (nonobstructive) appendicitis and acute obstructive appendicitis. The latter is characterized by a much more acute course.

The surgeon is constantly reminded that, the classic presentation is not present in all patients. Patients may have none or only few symptoms just described. When the pain becomes constant, it may localize to other quadrants of the abdomen due to an alteration in appendiceal anatomy as in late pregnancy or malrotation. In patients with a retrocecal appendix, the pain may never localize until generalized peritonitis from perforated appendicitis occurs. Urinary or bowel frequency may be present due to appendiceal inflammation irritating the adjacent bladder or rectum.

Perforated Appendicitis

It is a not uncommon that if left untreated, appendiceal inflammation will progress inevitably to necrosis and then to perforation. The time course of this progression varies among patients. Longer duration of prehospital delay is the major contributor to perforation.[11,12] Perforation after presenting to surgical attention appears to be uncommon.

The pain usually localizes to RLQ if perforation has been walled off, but may be diffuse if generalized peritonitis occurs. Patients with perforation often have rigors and high fevers to 102°F (38.9°C) or above. Other rare presentations do occur, most likely in the very young and very old, who cannot express their symptoms and often present late in the course of their disease. Abscesses can also form in the retroperitoneum due to perforation of retrocecal appendix, or in the liver from hematogenous spread of infection through the portal venous system. Pylephlebitis (septic portal vein thrombosis) presents with high fevers and jaundice, and can be confused with cholangitis.

DIAGNOSIS

History and Physical Examination

The patient should be asked about the classic symptoms of appendicitis, but the surgeon should not be deterred by the absence of many of the symptoms. A previous appendectomy does not exclude the diagnosis of appendicitis, as "stump appendicitis" (appendicitis in the remaining appendiceal stump after appendectomy), although rare, has been described.[13]

On examination, patient looks slightly ill and may have mildly elevated temperature and pulse. The clinician should systematically examine the entire abdomen, starting in the left upper quadrant. Maximal tenderness is typically in the RLQ, at or near McBurney's point, located one-third of the way from the anterior superior iliac spine to the umbilicus. This tenderness is often associated with localized muscle rigidity including rebound, shake, or tap tenderness. RLQ tenderness is the most consistent of all signs of acute appendicitis.[14,15]

The patient is asked to point to where the pain began and where it moved (pointing sign). Pain in the RLQ on palpation of the left lower quadrant, results from localized peritoneal inflammation (Rovsing's sign). Pain with the flexion of the leg at the right hip, can be seen with a retrocecal appendix due to inflammation adjacent to psoas muscle (psoas sign). Pain with rotating the flexed right thigh internally, indicates inflammation adjacent to the obturator muscle (the obturator sign) **(Table 1)**.

In case of perforated appendicitis, if sepsis has developed, blood pressure can be depressed. Perforation walled off by surrounding structures can create abscess or phlegmon leading to palpable mass. Free intraperitoneal rupture can lead to signs of generalized peritonitis with diffuse rebound tenderness.

Table 1 Symptoms and signs of appendicitis

Symptoms	Signs	Signs to elicit
Periumbilical colic	Pyrexia	Pointing sign
Pain shifts to right iliac fossa	Localized tenderness in right iliac fossa	Rovsing's sign
Anorexia	Muscle guarding	Psoas sign
Nausea	Rebound tenderness	Obturator sign

Laboratory Studies

The white cell count is typically slightly elevated in nonperforated appendicitis but may be quite elevated in the presence of perforation. A completely normal leukocyte count and differential is found in about 10% of patients with acute appendicitis, particularly in early cases.

A urinary tract infection is not uncommon in patients with appendicitis. Its presence does not exclude the diagnosis of acute appendicitis, but it should be identified and treated.

Measurement of serum liver enzymes and amylase can be helpful in diagnosing liver, gallbladder, or pancreatic disease in patients with mid-abdominal pain. In women of childbearing age, the urine beta-human chorionic gonadotropin (β-hCG) should be checked to alert the clinician to the possibility of ectopic or concurrent pregnancy.

Diagnostic Scores

Diagnostic scoring systems have been developed in an attempt to improve the diagnostic accuracy of acute appendicitis. The most widely used scoring system is the Alvarado score.[9,16] This scoring system gives point for symptoms (migration of pain, anorexia and nausea), physical signs (RLQ tenderness, rebound tenderness and pyrexia) and laboratory values (leukocytosis with a left shift). With the recent improvement in imaging studies, these scores play a smaller role in diagnosis.

Imaging Studies

The potential imaging modalities for diagnosis of acute appendicitis include plain radiographs, ultrasound (US) and computed tomography (CT).

On plain radiographs, fecaliths are non-pathognomonic for appendicitis. Plain radiographs are indicated in elderly patients with severe abdominal pain, in whom a perforated viscus is included in the differential diagnosis.

Abdominal ultrasonography is a popular imaging modality, and findings that suggest appendicitis include thickening of appendiceal wall with increased blood flow (leading to so called ring-of-fire appearance), loss of wall compressibility, increased echogenicity of the surrounding fat, and loculated pericecal fluid. Noncompressible luminal structure seen in cross-section as a target lesion. US is highly operator dependent, and it is frequently unable to visualize the normal appendix.

Computed tomography benefits from a high diagnostic accuracy for appendicitis and visualization and diagnosis of many of the other causes of abdominal pain that can mimic appendicitis.[17] The radiographic findings of appendicitis on CT include a dilated (>6 mm), thick-walled appendix that does not fill with enteric contrast or air, as well as surrounding fat stranding to suggest inflammation.[18] CT demonstrated a sensitivity of 0.94 and a specificity of 0.95.[17] Mural stratification referring to the layers of enhancement and edema within the wall, referred to as target sign **(Figs 3A and B)**.

An algorithm for evaluation of patients with suspected acute appendicitis **(Flow chart 1)**. Patient's history physical examination and laboratory studies suggestive of appendicitis should undergo appendectomy. In those with an evaluation suggestive but not convincing for appendicitis, further imaging is warranted.

In these patients, transabdominal US or abdominopelvic CT should be considered.

SPECIAL CONSIDERATIONS

Children

Appendicitis most commonly affects children aged 10–19 years. Infants aged 0–4 months have the lowest incidence,

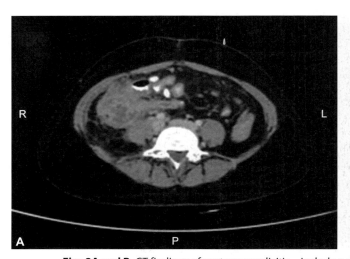
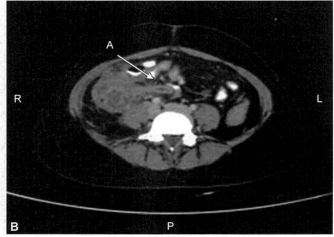

Figs 3A and B CT findings of acute appendicitis—include a dilated (>6 mm), thick walled appendix that does not fill with enteric contrast or air, as well as surrounding fat stranding to suggest inflammation

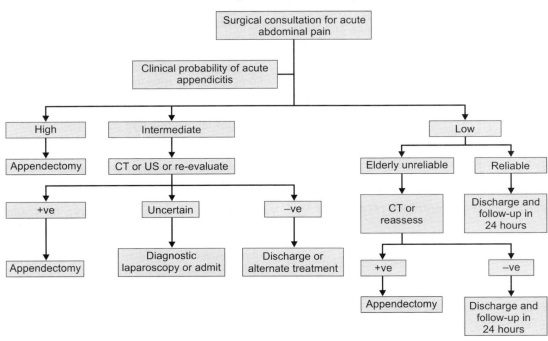

Flow chart 1 Evaluation and management of patients with possible acute appendicitis

Abbreviations: CT, computed tomography; US, ultrasound.

but up to two-thirds will present with perforation.[19] In children with an equivocal history and physical examination, imaging with either a CT scan or US can significantly reduce the negative appendectomy rate. As with adults, both CT and US have been shown to be highly accurate in diagnosing appendicitis in children, although CT scan is believed to have a higher specificity and sensitivity.

Elderly

Because of a diminished inflammatory response, the elderly can present with less impressive symptoms and physical signs, longer duration of symptoms and decreased leukocytosis.[20] Perforation is thus more common, occurring in as many as 50% of patients older than 65.[21] Prompt CT scan is advocated when the diagnosis is in dilemma.

Pregnancy

The diagnosis can be challenging, as nausea, anorexia and abdominal pain may be symptoms of both appendicitis and normal pregnancy. The gravid uterus can displace the abdominal viscera, shifting the location of appendix. It can occur in any trimester, with perhaps a slight increase in frequency in the second trimester.[22,23] Perforation is more common in the third trimester. US is accurate in pregnancy and is a useful first radiological tool. Rectal contrast CT has also been shown to be highly accurate. Although ionizing radiation has risks to the fetus, the radiation from a typical abdominopelvic CT is below the threshold of 5 rad at which teratogenic effects can be seen.[24] Additionally, magnetic resonance imaging (MRI) has been recently used to aid in the diagnosis of appendicitis in the pregnant patient when US results are equivocal. To date, however, no adverse effects of MRI on the developing fetus has been reported.[25]

Immunocompromise

The immunocompromised state alters the response to acute infection and wound healing. Appendicitis affects all types of patients and must be considered in those who have undergone organ transplant, are receiving chemotherapy, or are infected with the human immunodeficiency virus (HIV).

DIFFERENTIAL DIAGNOSIS (BOX 1)

Box 1 Differential diagnosis of acute appendicitis

- *Children*: Gastroenteritis, mesenteric enteritis, Meckel's diverticulitis, intussusception, Henoch-Schönlein purpura, lobar pneumonia
- *Adult*: Regional enteritis, ureteric colic, perforated peptic ulcer, torsion of testis, pancreatitis, rectus sheath hematoma
- *Adult female*: Pelvic inflammatory disease, pyelonephritis, ectopic pregnancy, torsion of ovarian cyst, endometriosis
- *Elderly*: Diverticulitis, intestinal obstruction, colonic carcinoma, torsion appendix epiploicae, mesentric infarction, leaking aortic aneurysm

TREATMENT

Nonoperative or Medical Management

Appendicitis has long been a surgically treated disease, recently few studies of nonsurgical management of the surgical literature. Based on higher rate of failure with antibiotics alone, nonoperative management of acute appendicitis has not been recommended.[26,27] Nevertheless, antibiotic treatment may be a useful temporizing measure in environments with no surgical expertize.

Intravenous antibiotics have been shown to reduce the incidence of postoperative wound infection and intra-abdominal abscess. Antibiotic should be administered 30 minutes prior to skin incision. As the typical flora of appendix resembles that of colon, a second-generation cephalosporin or a combination of antibiotics directed at Gram negatives and anaerobes will suffice. In nonperforated appendicitis, a single preoperative dose, and in cases of perforation, an extended course of at least 5 days of antibiotics is advocated.

Open or Laparoscopic Appendectomy

Once the diagnosis of appendicitis is confirmed, the surgeon must decide whether to perform an open or laparoscopic appendectomy. Meta-analysis and systematic reviews have addressed the controversy **(Table 2)**.[28,29]

Based on the data available, one cannot convincingly recommend either open or laparoscopic appendectomy over the other. One situation in which laparoscopic appendectomy may be advisable is when diagnosis of appendicitis is in doubt.

Open Appendectomy

If open approach is chosen, the surgeon must then decide on the location and type of incision. If a mass representing the inflamed appendix can be palpated, the incision must be centered at that location. If the appendix cannot be visualized, it can be located by following the teniae coli of the cecum to the cecal base. Care should be taken to avoid perforation of appendix, with spillage of pus or enteric contents into the abdomen. In excising the appendix, the surgeon must decide whether or not to invert the appendiceal stump. Recent studies show no advantages to appendiceal stump inversion.[30,31] No matter how the appendix is divided, the residual appendiceal stump should be no longer than 3 mm to minimize the possibility of stump appendicitis in the future. If base of the cecum is also inflamed but there is sufficient uninflamed cecum between the appendix and the ileocecal valve, an appendectomy with partial cecectomy can be performed using a stapling device.[32]

Laparoscopic Appendectomy

Multiple port placements for laparoscopic appendectomy exist. The authors utilize a three-port technique, with one umbilical and one suprapubic port and the third port can be placed in either the left or right lower quadrant. The appendix should be placed in a retrieval bag and removed through the umbilical port site to minimize the risk of wound infection **(Figs 4A to D)**.

POSTOPERATIVE CARE

Patients with nonperforated appendicitis require a shorter (24–48 hours) hospital stay. Postoperative care for both the laparoscopic and open approaches is similar. Patients can be started on a clear liquid diet after 4 hours, and their diet can be advanced as tolerated. Patients can be discharged when they tolerate a regular diet.

SPECIAL CONSIDERATIONS DURING APPENDECTOMY

Perforated Appendicitis

When appendicitis progresses to perforation, management depends on the nature of the perforation. If perforation is contained, it can lead to a mass or phlegmon, or may result into a pus filled abscess cavity. Appendectomy proceeds as described earlier. Peritoneal drains are not necessary, as they do not reduce the incidence of wound infection or abscess, but the final decision is of operating surgeon.[33,34] Patients are often continued on broad-spectrum antibiotics for 5–7 days and should remain in hospital until tolerating a regular diet.

In patients with a solid inflammatory mass in the RLQ, without evidence of abscess cavity, suggesting a phlegmon, appendectomy can be difficult due to dense adhesions and inflammation.

In such circumstances to reduce potential complications, many support an initially nonoperative approach. Conservative treatment failure, as evidenced by bowel obstruction, sepsis, or persistent pain, or leukocytosis, requires immediate appendectomy.

Normal Appendix

Because of the difficulty in diagnosing appendicitis, it is not uncommon for a normal appendix to be found at

Table 2 Laparoscopic versus open appendectomy	
Favors open appendectomy	Favors laparoscopy
• Shorter operating room time • Lower operating room costs • Fewer intra-abdominal abscesses • Lower hospital cost	• Diagnosis of other conditions • Decreased pain and analgesic requirement • Reduced length of stay • Fewer wound infections • Quicker return to activities • Lower societal cost

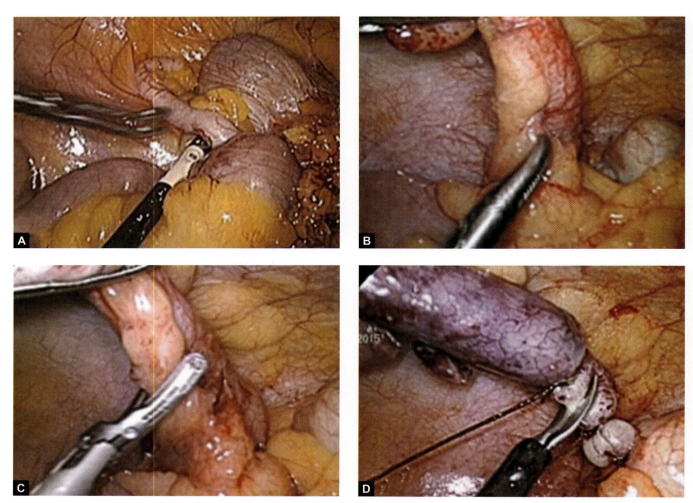

Figs 4A to D Laparoscopic appendectomy: (A) Localization; (B) Dissection of mesoappendix; (C) Harmonizing mesoappendix; (D) Endo-loop ligation and division of appendix

appendectomy. This can occur more than 15% of the time, with considerably higher percentage in infant, the elderly and young women. For many reasons, it is advisable to remove the grossly normal appendix. When a normal appendix is discovered at appendectomy, it is important to search for other possible causes of the patient's symptoms.

Interval Appendectomy

Factors to be considered when advising patients on interval appendectomy include a relatively low incidence of future appendicitis (8–10% and often associated with an appendicolith) and a morbidity associated with an interval appendectomy of approximately 11%.[35]

Chronic or Recurrent Appendicitis

Patients do not present with the typical symptoms of acute appendicitis. Instead, they complain of recurrent and infrequent RLQ pain. When questioned, they may describe an initial episode with more classic symptoms of acute appendicitis, with no treatment delivered.[36] Because the diagnosis is often uncertain preoperatively, laparoscopy is a useful tool to allow exploration of the abdomen.

RECENT ADVANCES

Literature Review

Appendectomy versus antibiotic treatment for acute appendicitis, a Cochrane review, prepared and maintained by the Cochrane Collaboration and published in the Cochrane Library 2011, issue 11. Authors conclude that appendectomy remains the standard treatment for acute appendicitis. Antibiotic treatment might be used as an alternative treatment in a good quality randomized controlled trial or in specific patients or conditions where surgery is contraindicated.

Pure transvaginal appendectomy is emerging as a safe and well-tolerated procedure for women with acute nonperforated appendicitis that reduces the burden of pain and has faster recovery times when compared with laparoscopic approaches.

Guidelines

The American College of Surgeons, the Society for Surgery of the Alimentary Tract, and the World Society of Emergency Surgery all describe appendectomy (either laparoscopic or open) as the treatment of choice for appendicitis.

Regarding an antibiotic-first strategy the American College of Surgeons patient information guide indicates that it "may be effective, but there is higher chance of recurrence"; the Society for Surgery of the Alimentary Tract patient care guidelines suggest that it is "not a widely accepted treatment"; and the World Society of Emergency Surgery states that "this conservative approach features high rates of recurrence and is therefore inferior to the appendectomy … Nonoperative antibiotic treatment may be used as an alternative for specific patients for whom surgery is contraindicated."

CONCLUSION

Appendicitis is one of the common cause of abdominal pain of less than a week duration presenting to emergency department. Appendicitis can occur in any age. In spite of advances in imaging accuracy, appendicitis remains a high-risk disease for delayed or missed diagnosis, because of the its varied presentation, absence pathognomonic sign or symptom, the poor predictive value of associated laboratory testing. Appendicitis continues to be a high-risk for missed and delayed diagnosis specially in extreme of young and elderly. Delayed or missed diagnosis in the emergency department and rupture appendix are the important cause for increase in morbidity and mortality. No specific history, physical finding or laboratory test can make the definitive diagnosis of appendicitis. Ultrasound is helpful when positive but not accurate in excluding appendicitis or identifying the rupture. CT is accurate and also helpful in indentifying the other cause of abdominal pain. Combination of findings can increase the likelihood of disease diagnosis and helpful in further management.

REFERENCES

1. Da Capri JB. Commentaria cum amplissimus additionibus super anatomia mundini una cum texta ejusudem in pristinum et verum nitorem redanto. Bolonial Imp. per H. Benedictus. 1521:528.
2. Vesalius A, Liber V. De Humani Corporis Fabrica. Basel, Switzerland: Johanes Oporinu; 1543. pp. 361-2.
3. Major RH. Classic description of disease. Springfield: Universa Medicina; 1932. pp. 614-5.
4. Amyand C. Of an inguinal rupture, with a pin in the appendix caeci, incrusted with stone, and some observations on wounds in the guts. Phil Trans R Soc Lond. 1736;39:329-42.
5. Tait L. Surgical treatment of typhlitis. Birmingham Med Rev. 1890;27:26-34.
6. Fitz RH. Perforating inflammation of the vermiform appendix; with special reference to its early diagnosis and treatment. Am J Med Sci. 1886;92:321-46.
7. Prystowsky JB, Pugh CM, Nagle AP. Current problems in surgery. Appendicitis. Curr Probl Surg. 2005;42:688-742.
8. Jones BA, Demetriades D, Segal I, et al. The prevalence of appendiceal fecaliths in patients with and without appendicitis. A comparative study from Canada and South Africa. Ann Surg. 1985;202:80-2.
9. Teicher I, Landa B, Cohen M, et al. Scoring system to aid in diagnoses of appendicitis. Ann Surg. 1983;198:753-9.
10. Nitecki S, Karmeli R, Sarr MG. Appendiceal calculi and fecaliths as indications for appendectomy. Surg Gynecol Obstet. 1990;171:185-8.
11. Hale DA, Jaques DP, Molloy M, et al. Appendectomy. Improving care through quality improvement. Arch Surg. 1997;132:153-7.
12. Pittman-Waller VA, Myers JG, Stewart RM, et al. Appendicitis: why so complicated? Analysis of 5755 consecutive appendectomies. Am Surg. 2000;66:548-54.
13. Mangi AA, Berger DL. Stump appendicitis. Am Surg. 2000;66: 739-41.
14. Wagner JM. Likelihood ratios to determine 'Does this patient have appendicitis?': Comment and clarification. JAMA. 1997; 278:819-20.
15. Wagner JM, McKinney WP, Carpenter JL. Does this patient have appendicitis? JAMA. 1996;276:1589-94.
16. Alvarado A. A practical score for the early diagnosis of acute appendicitis. Ann Emerg Med. 1986;15:557-64.
17. Terasawa T, Blackmore CC, Bent S, et al. Systematic review: computed tomography and ultrasonography to detect acute appendicitis in adults and adolescents. Ann Intern Med. 2004;141:537-46.
18. Rao PM, Rhea JT, Rattner DW, et al. Introduction of appendiceal CT: impact on negative appendectomy and appendiceal perforation rates. Ann Surg. 1999;229:344-9.
19. Bratton SL, Haberkern CM, Waldhausen JH. Acute appendicitis risks of complications: age and Medicaid insurance. Pediatrics. 2000;106:75-8.
20. Watters JM, Blakslee JM, March RJ, et al. The influence of age on the severity of peritonitis. Can J Surg. 1996;39:142-6.
21. Addiss DG, Shaer N, Fowler BS, et al. The epidemiology of appendicitis and appendectomy in the United States. Am J Epidemiol. 1990;132:910-25.
22. Tamir IL, Bongard FS, Klein SR. Acute appendicitis in the pregnant patient. Am J Surg. 1990;160:571-5.
23. Mourad J, Elliott JP, Erickson L, et al. Appendicitis in pregnancy: new information that contradicts long-held clinical beliefs. Am J Obstet Gynecol. 2000;182:1027-9.
24. Brent RL. The effect of embryonic and fetal exposure to X-ray, microwaves, and ultrasound: counseling the pregnant and nonpregnant patient about these risks. Semin Oncol. 1989;16:347-68.
25. Basaran A, Basaran M. Diagnosis of acute appendicitis during pregnancy: a systemic review. Obstet Gynecol Surv. 2009;64:481-8.
26. Bauer T, Vennits B, Holm B, et al. Antibiotic prophylaxis in acute nonperforated appendicitis. The Danish Multicenter Study Group III. Ann Surg. 1989;209:307-11.
27. Danish Multicenter Study Group. A Danish multicenter study: cefoxitin versus ampicillin + metronidazole in perforated appendicitis. Br J Surg. 1984;71:144-6.

28. McCall JL, Sharples K, Jadallah F. Systematic review of randomized controlled trials comparing laparoscopic with open appendicectomy. Br J Surg. 1997;84:1045-50.
29. Sauerland S, Lefering R, Neugebauer EA. Laparoscopic versus open surgery for suspected appendicitis. Cochrane Database Syst Rev. 2004;4:CD001546.
30. Watters DA, Walker MA, Abernethy BC. The appendix stump: should it be invaginated? Ann R Coll Surg Eng. 1984;66:92-3.
31. Engstrom L, Fenyo G. Appendicectomy: assessment of stump invagination versus simple ligation: a prospective, randomized trial. Br J Surg. 1985;72:971-2.
32. Poole GV. Management of the difficult appendiceal stump: how I do it. Am Surg. 1993;59:624-5.
33. Greenall MJ, Evans M, Pollock AV. Should you drain a perforated appendix? Br J Surg. 1978;65:880-2.
34. Petrowsky H, Demartines N, Rousson V, et al. Evidence-based value of prophylactic drainage in gastrointestinal surgery: a systematic review and meta-analysis. Ann Surg. 2004;240:1074-85.
35. Andersson RE, Petzold MG. Nonsurgical treatment of appendiceal abscess or phlegmon: a systematic review and meta-analysis. Ann Surg. 2007;246:741-8.
36. Mattei P, Sola JE, Yeo CJ. Chronic and recurrent appendicitis are uncommon entities often misdiagnosed. J Am Coll Surg. 1994;178:385-9.

CHAPTER 55

Perforation Peritonitis

Sharad Manar, Hashim Mozzam, Sudhir BS

INTRODUCTION

Gastrointestinal perforation is a formation of hole or defect in all the way through the stomach, large bowel, or small intestine. Perforation can be due to a number of different diseases, including appendicitis, diverticulitis, gallbladder, and trauma (blunt or penetrating injuries). A hole in your gastrointestinal system or gallbladder can lead to peritonitis. Peritonitis is the inflammation of the peritoneum and peritoneal cavity. Most commonly due to a localized, and generalized infection. Peritoneum is a thin double layer of serous membrane in the abdominal cavity and divides all organs as intraperitoneal, mesoperitoneal, and extraperitoneal. Innervation of parietal peritoneum is by the sensitive somatic nerves as a result of which peritoneum irritation pain is localized. The pelvic peritoneum has no somatic innervation. The visceral peritoneum has vegetative innervations (sympathetic, and parasympathetic) and its irritation does not localizes pain.

Inflammatory destructive diseases of peritoneal cavity organs are the most common causes of different form of peritonitis (gastric and duodenal ulcer 30%, destructive appendicitis 22%, large and small intestine diseases 21% and 13%, respectively). Another group belongs to patient with post-traumatic injury to abdomen. Various risk factors for perforation and peritonitis are described in **Box 1**.

Box 1 Risk factors for perforation and peritonitis

- Abdominal surgery
- Ectopic surgery
- Trauma
- Ulcer
- Appendix rupture
- Diverticulum

CLASSIFICATIONS

The following working classifications of peritonitis are considered as:
- *Primary peritonitis*: Due to direct spread of an infection from blood and lymph nodes to the peritoneum (rarely less than 1%)
- *Secondary peritonitis*: Spread of bacterial infection or enzymes from gastrointestinal tract
  - Perforation peritonitis can arise from biliary tree, uterus, splenic and liver abscess, and intestinal amebiasis
  - *Postoperative peritonitis*: Due to leak of an anastomosis
- *Tertiary peritonitis*: Peritonitis caused by recurrent peritoneal inflammation and is also known as recurrent peritonitis.

Classification as per Character of Exudate

- Serous
- Fibrinous
- Fibrinopurulent
- Purulent
- Hemorrhagic
- Biliary
- Chemical.

STAGES OF PERFORATION PERITONITIS

Stages of perforation peritonitis as per duration are:
- Initial (reactive) stage (up to 24 hours)
- Toxic stage (24–72 hours)
- Terminal stage (after 72 hours).

CLINICAL MANIFESTATION OF PERFORATION PERITONITIS

Clinical manifestations are **Box 2**:
- Acute abdominal pain, abdominal tenderness, and abdominal guarding, which are exacerbated by moving the peritoneum, e.g. coughing (forced cough may be used as a test), flexing one's hips, or eliciting the Blumberg sign (rebound tenderness) meaning that pressing a hand on the abdomen elicits less pain than releasing the hand abruptly, which will aggravate the pain, as the peritoneum snaps back into place
- Anorexia, malaise, nausea, and vomiting are common associated features
- Constipation is usually present, unless a pelvic abscess develops (which can cause diarrhea).

PHYSICAL EXAMINATION

Patient with peritonitis may presents with signs of systemic inflammatory response syndrome (SIRS) or features of sepsis or septic shock **(Fig. 1)**. Physical examination findings in peritonitis patient are described in **Box 3**.

Box 2 Clinical manifestation of perforation and peritonitis

- Fever
- Tachycardia
- Hypotension
- Nausea
- Vomiting
- Anorexia
- Dehydration
- Abdominal distension and rigidity
- Abdominal pain
- Decreased bowel sounds

Box 3 Physical examination findings in peritonitis patients

Physical examination findings in patient of peritonitis
- The patient will lie supine and relativeley motionless with shallow respiratory excursions
- The knees are flexed and drawn up in order to reduce tension in the abdominal wall
- In diffuse peritonitis spasm of the abdominal musculature will result in board like rigidity of abdomen
- Abdominal palation will show tenderness, guarding and rebound tenderness; the site of maximum tenderness is usually related to the site of pathology
- Specific pathognomonic signs of disease may be clinically evident (e.g. Rovsing's sign in acute appendicitis)
- Digital rectal examination will elicit anterior tenderness in pelvic peritonitis
- Auscultation will confirm increasing ileus as bowel sounds diminish and eventually cease

INVESTIGATION AND RADIOLOGICAL IMAGING IN PATIENT WITH PERFORATION PERITONITIS

Investigation and radiological imaging include:
- *Complete blood count*: Leukocytosis
- *Renal function test*: Electrolyte imbalance and acute kidney failure
- *Serum amylase*: A raised serum amylase is diagnostic of acute pancreatitis, but a moderately elevated concentration can be caused by perforated duodenal ulcer.
- *Arterial blood gas*: Low arterial CO_2 and metabolic acidosis
- *Blood grouping and cross-matching*: In view if surgical treatment is initiated, cross-matched blood will be required
- *Chest X-ray*: Pneumoperitoneum as an indicator of gastrointestinal perforation in about 70–80% of visceral perforations **(Fig. 2)**
- *Abdominal X-rays*: It may reveal dilated and edematous intestine **(Fig. 3)**
- *Ultrasound abdomen*: Confirming or excluding specific diagnoses (e.g. abscess) **(Fig. 4)**
- *Computerized tomography (CT)*: More accurate than ultrasound **(Fig. 5)**

DIFFERENTIAL DIAGNOSIS

Differentiate from other causes of severe abdominal pain (e.g. intestinal obstruction, ureteric or biliary colic).

TREATMENT

Management of perforation peritonitis needs to be initiated with intravenous fluids administration (crystalloids or colloids) according to central venous pressure (CVP) monitoring, early use of antibiotic therapy, correction of existing serum electrolyte disturbances or coagulation

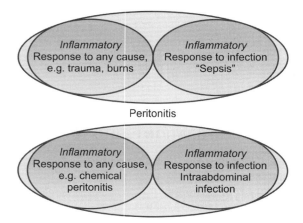

Fig. 1 Systemic inflammatory response syndrome

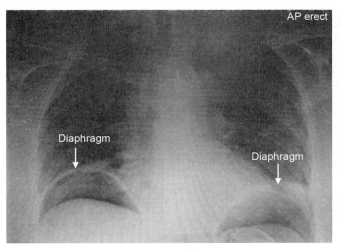

Fig. 2 X-ray of chest

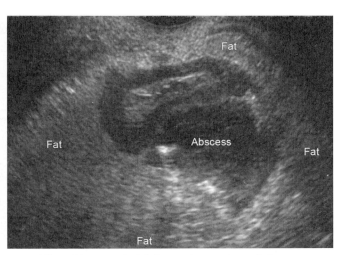

Fig. 4 Ultrasound of abdomen: intraperitoneal abscess

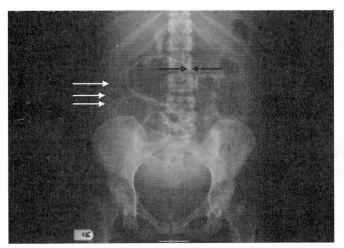

Fig. 3 Abdominal X-ray: dilated and edematous intestine

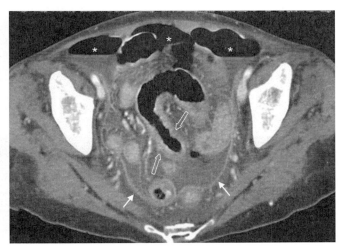

Fig. 5 CT of abdomen showing inflammation with arrow marking, star markings showing free gas

abnormalities. Ideally perforation peritonitis is the most common surgical emergency in India. Therefore early closure of defect or perforation is recommended. The surgical treatment of perforative peritonitis is based on three basic principles, viz.:
1. To eliminate the source of bacterial contamination by treating the underlying pathologic process
2. To decrease the degree of bacterial contamination in the peritoneal cavity
3. To prevent recurrent or residual infection.

Factors associated with more severe sepsis or high mortality in peritonitis are increased age, nonappendicular site, certain pre-existing diseases, and extent of peritonitis.

Most common microorganisms causing peritonitis and used antibiotic therapy are mentioned in **Table 1**.

Impact of timing of antibiotics on survival in patients with severe sepsis or septic shock in whom early goal-directed therapy was initiated in emergency department is described in **Table 2**.

CONCLUSION

Perforation peritonitis is a surgical emergency. Surgical exploration is the cornerstone of the management of peritonitis. Delay in procedure leads onto further complications and increased mortality rate. Early exploration can be a lifesaving procedure in some complicated cases.

Table 1 Type, etiology, and medication of peritonitis

Types	Etiology		Medication
Primary	Gram-positive	• Escherichia coli (40%) • Klebsiella pneumoniae (7%) • Pseudomonas spp. (5%) • Proteus spp. (5%)	Cephalosporin III–IV Aminoglycosides II–III
	Gram-negative	• Streptococcus spp. (15%) • Staphylococcus spp. (3%) • Anaerobes (<5%)	
Secondary	Gram-positive	• E. coli • Enterobacter spp. • Klebsiella spp. • Proteus spp.	Cephalosporin III-II, antianaerobic medications, quinolones, and carbapenems
	Gram-negative	• Streptococcus spp. • Enterococcus spp.	
	Anaerobics	• Bacteroides fragilis • Bacteroides spp. • Eubacterium spp. • Clostridium spp. • Anaerobic Streptococcus	
Tertiary	Gram-positive	• Enterobacter spp. • Pseudomonas spp. • Enterococcus spp.	Cephalosporin IV and carbapenems
	Gram-negative	• Staphylococcus spp.	Vancomycin and Linezolid
	Fungal	• Candida spp.	Fluconazole and amphotericin B

Table 2 Impact of timing of antibiotics on survival

Time	Mortality
Time from triage to appropriate antibiotic therapy <1 hour	19.5%
Time from triage to appropriate antibiotic therapy >1 hour	33.2%
Time from diagnosis to appropriate antibiotic therapy <1 hour	25.0%
Time from diagnosis to appropriate antibiotic therapy >1 hour	38.5%

BIBLIOGRAPHY

1. Anaya DA, Nathens AB. Risk factors for severe sepsis in secondary peritonitis. Surg Infect (Larchmt). 2003;4(4):355-62.
2. Townsend C, Beauchamp RD, Evers BM, Mattox K (Eds). Sabiston Textbook of Surgery, 20th edition. Elsevier; 2016.
3. Gupta SK, Gupta R, Singh G, Gupta S. Perforation peritonitis: A two-year experience. JK Science. 2010;12(3):141-44.
4. Jhobta RJ, Attri AK, Kaushik R, Sharma R, Jhobta A. Spectrum of perforation peritonitis in India review of 504 consecutive cases. World Journal of Emergency Surgery. 2006,1:26.
5. Kapoor S, Kumar A, Singh A, et al. Early And Late Management of Perforation Peritonitis—A Comparative Study of 50 Cases. IOSR Journal of Dental and Medical Sciences. 2016;15(4):50-60.
6. Dani T, Ramachandra L, Nair R, et al. Evaluation of prognosis in patients' with perforation peritonitis using Mannheim's peritonitis index. IJSRP 2015;5(5):1-35.

CHAPTER 56

Intestinal Obstruction

Ashok Kumar Puranik, Devendra Richhariya

INTRODUCTION

Intestinal obstruction is one of the common presentations in emergency department. Intestinal obstruction is about 10–15% of all acute abdominal pain. Nowadays variety of diagnostic tests are available for diagnosis, so morbidity and mortality has decreased but still remains a challenging surgical issue in emergency department. Intra-abdominal adhesion, malignancy, and hernia are common causes for intestinal obstruction. Nausea, vomiting, abdominal pain, and unable to pass flatus are common complaints from the patient. Radiology is (abdominal X-ray erect and supine) often informative about intestinal obstruction. Contrast computed tomography (CT) can be helpful if X-ray is negative. Bowel ischemia perforation and electrolyte abnormalities are common complications. Intravenous fluid, correction of electrolyte abnormalities, rest to bowel, antiemetics, antispasmodics, and antisecretory drugs are used for the management of uncomplicated intestinal obstruction. Bowel ischemia perforation or peritonitis is an indication for surgery.

DEFINITION

Inability of the intestinal contents to pass distally in the lumen of intestine either from a mechanical barrier or absence of peristalsis without any mechanical barrier is known as intestinal obstruction.

CLASSIFICATION

Intestinal obstruction can be classified in many ways:
- Depending upon the nature of obstruction:
  - Dynamic obstruction
  - A dynamic obstruction (paralytic ileus, mesenteric ischemia)
- Depending upon the cause of obstruction:
  - Intraluminal causes
    - Gallstones
    - Ileus
    - Food bolus obstruction
    - Roundworm mass
    - Foreign body
  - In the wall of the gut
    - Strictures
    - Crohn's disease
    - Carcinomas
    - Adhesions
  - Outside the wall of the gut
    - Volvulus
    - Intussusception
    - Obstructed hernia
    - Congenital bands
- Depending upon severity
  - Acute obstruction
  - Subacute obstruction
  - Chronic obstruction
  - Acute on chronic obstruction
- Depending upon blood supply
  - Simple obstruction
  - Strangulated obstruction
- Depending upon the site
  - Small bowel obstruction
  - Large bowel obstruction
- Common causes
  - Adhesions
  - Hernia
  - Paralytic ileus
  - Strictures
  - Malignancy.

PATHOPHYSIOLOGY

Irrespective of the etiology and acuteness of onset, in dynamic obstruction the proximal bowel dilates and develops an altered motility.

Dilation

Obstruction leads to proximal dilation due to accumulation of intestinal secretions and swallowed air. This bowel dilation stimulates cell secretory activity resulting in more fluid accumulation and progressive dilatation.

Altered Motility

Accumulation of secretion in the intestine lumen stimulates increased peristalsis both above and below the obstruction. Below the obstruction increased peristalsis leads to frequent loose stools and flatus early in the course of disease.

Above the obstruction increased peristalsis try to overcome the obstruction, if the obstruction is not relieved the bowel begins to dilate causing a reduction in the peristaltic strength ultimately resulting in flaccidity and paralysis.

The distention proximal to obstruction is caused by two factors:
1. *Gas*: Obstruction leads to significant proliferation of both aerobic and anaerobic organisms resulting in considerable gas production, nitrogen being the predominant (90%) gas along with hydrogen sulfide.
2. *Fluid*: Fluid is made up of various digestive juices, e.g. 1,500 mL of saliva/day, 2 L of gastric juice/day, 3 L of intestinal secretion/day, 1 L of pancreatic juice and bile/day. Following obstruction fluids accumulates in the bowel wall and any excess fluid is secreted in the lumen. Because absorption is retarded, dehydration and electrolytes disturbance is inevitable. Causes include reduced oral intake, defective intestinal absorption, result of vomiting, and sequestration in bowel lumen.

Interference with Blood Supply

As the tension within the bowel loops become more and more, venous congestion takes place resulting in edema of bowel wall. If the obstruction is not relieved, capillary rupture and hemorrhage take place. In case of volvulus, and intussusception, arterial compromise takes place fast that causes gangrene of bowel wall very early.

Transmigration of Organisms

Both aerobic and anaerobic organisms transmigrate through the gangrenous bowel and results in peritonitis. The organisms release powerful endotoxins, which are absorbed from peritoneal surface and cause gram-negative shock or septic shock, which carries high mortality.

Clinical Features

There are four cardinal features of dynamic obstruction:
1. Colicky pain
2. Distention
3. Vomiting
4. Absolute constipation.

The clinical features are also influenced by the "site of obstruction" whether small bowel or large bowel and on the "onset of obstruction" whether acute or chronic.

- *In high small bowel obstruction*: Vomiting occurs early and is profuse with rapid dehydration. Distention is minimal with little evidence of fluid levels on abdominal radiograph.
- *In low small bowel obstruction*: Pain is predominant with central distention. Vomiting is delayed. Multiple central fluid levels are seen in abdominal radiograph. Abdominal pain may be visceral or colicky in nature. In between, patient can be asymptomatic later it becomes more constant and site depends on the level of obstruction. Vomiting in intestinal obstruction is gastric bilious or feculent.
- *In large bowel obstruction*: Distention is early and pronounced. Pain is mild, vomiting, and dehydration is late. The proximal colon and cecum are distended on abdominal radiograph.

Figure 1A showing various site of pain in intestinal obstruction and **Figure 1B** showing distension in intestinal obstruction.

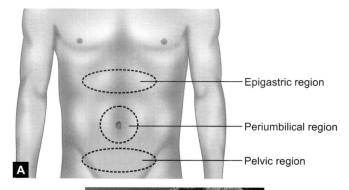

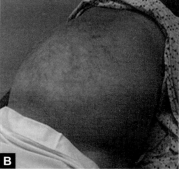

Figs 1A and B (A) Site of pain; (B) Central distension

- *Other features*
  - *Dehydration*: Most common in small bowel obstruction because of repeated vomiting, and fluid sequestration. Signs of dehydration appear early.
  - *Hypokalemia*: It is not a common feature in simple mechanical obstruction. An increase in serum potassium, amylase, and lactate dehydrogenase may be associated with the presence of strangulation along with leukocytosis or leukopenia.
  - *Pyrexia tachycardia hypotension*: In the presence of obstruction, pyrexia tachycardia hypotension indicates—
    - Onset of ischemia
    - Intestinal perforation
    - Inflammation associated with obstructing disease.
  - *Hypothermia*: Indicates septic shock.
  - *Abdominal tenderness*: Localized tenderness indicates pending, and established ischemia.
  - *Signs of peritonitis*: Indicates overt infarction or perforation.
- *Feature of strangulation*: It is important to distinguish strangulating from nonstrangulating obstruction because the former is a surgical emergency. The diagnosis is entirely clinical. Features include:
  - Constant pain
  - Tenderness with rigidity
  - Guarding and absent bowel sound
  - Features of septic shock
  - In case of external hernia the lump is tense, tender, and irreducible with no expansile cough impulse.

Pain is never completely absent in strangulation. Symptoms usually commence suddenly and recur regularly. Any tenderness present is of great significance and need frequent reassessment.

INVESTIGATIONS

Investigations include:
- *Complete blood picture*: Low Hb% indicates underlying malignancy. Increased total white blood cells count indicates infection or sepsis.
- *Electrolytes*: Most of the electrolytes are low in cases of intestinal obstruction.
- *Plain X-ray abdomen*: In erect position, it is an important investigation in cases of intestinal obstruction. Plain X-ray may demonstrate gall stone ileus or foreign body.
- Normal X-ray (**Figs 2A and B**).
- *Multiple gas fluid levels*: These are pathognomonic of intestinal obstruction. Gas level appears earlier than fluid levels.
- *Multiple fluid levels* (**Figs 3A and B**).
- *Small bowel obstruction and large bowel obstruction* (**Figs 4A and B**)
- Combined small and large bowel obstruction paralytic ileus (**Fig. 5**)

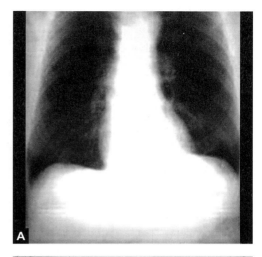
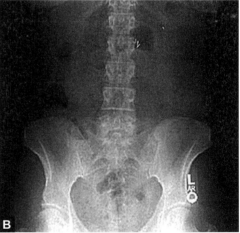

Figs 2A and B Normal X-ray

Sigmoid volvulus appears as a large dilated loop like in large bowel obstruction.

Jejunum is characterized by regularly placed mucosal folds called "valvulae conniventes" placed opposite to each other. They are produced by valves of Kerckring.

Large bowel is characterized by "Haustrations". Incomplete mucosal folds are not placed opposite to each other. They are large. Cecum has no haustrations. However, it appears as a round gas shadow in right iliac fossa (RIF).
- *Haustrations* (**Fig. 6**)
- *CT scan abdomen*: Indicated in patient when physical examination and X-ray of abdomen are negative but high clinical suspicion. Noncontrast CT abdomen especially with oral contrast is helpful in diagnosing as well as in identifying cause and level of obstruction. CT abdomen is highly sensitive and specific but in some cases like partial obstruction, contrast fluoroscopy is helpful. Other variation of contrast fluoroscopy is small bowel followed through study where patient drinks contrast then serial

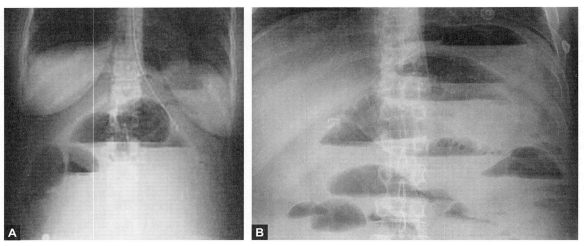

Figs 3A and B Multiple fluid levels

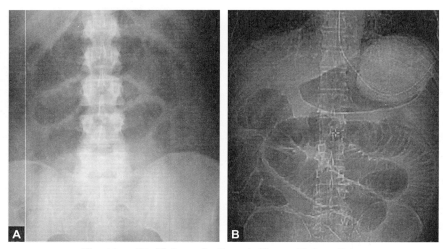

Figs 4A and B (A) Centrally distended loops; (B) Cut-off sign

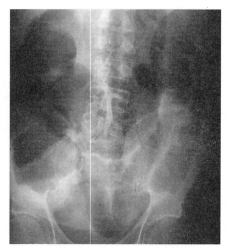

Fig. 5 Paralytic ileus with combined small and large bowel obstruction

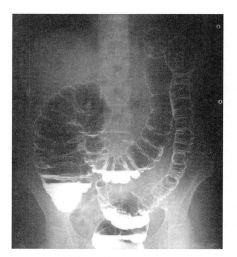

Fig. 6 Haustrations

abdominal X-rays are taken and evaluated. Enteroclysis is more superior to contrast fluoroscopy.

Differential Diagnosis

Differential diagnosis includes:
- Gastroenteritis
- Bowel ischemia
- Perforation
- Acute pancreatitis
- Intussusception in children
- Tuberculosis
- Nongastrointestinal condition
- Myocardial infarction.

TREATMENT OF ACUTE INTESTINAL OBSTRUCTION

Conservative Management

Main measures used to treat acute intestinal obstruction are:
- Gastrointestinal drainage (nasogastric decompression)
  - 4 hourly aspiration and continuous drainage
  - Decompression proximal to obstruction
  - Reduce the risk of aspiration.
- *Fluid and electrolyte replacement*: Common metabolic disorders are dehydration, hypotension, acute kidney injury, hyponatremia, hypokalemia, and acidosis
  - Intravenous fluid
  - Volume depends on clinical criteria
  - Hourly urine output monitoring
  - Vitals monitoring.
- Antibiotics in presence of fever and leukocytosis.

If patient improves with nasogastric decompression then conservative management decision should be taken "not to operate". Conservative management is helpful in relieving the obstruction in 50–70% of cases especially in partial obstruction. If patient is unresponsive to supportive management within 24–48 hours then there is a high possibility of developing the complications, then surgical option should be considered.

Surgical Management

To initiate surgical treatment for intestinal obstruction is difficult, but it should be delayed until resuscitation is complete, provided there are no signs of strangulation or evidence of closed-loop obstruction.

Indications of early surgical intervention:
- Complete obstruction
- Strangulation of hernia
- Acute obstruction
- Persistent abdominal pain despite nasogastric decompression
- Signs of strangulation of bowel
- Peritonitis
- Pneumoperitoneum
- Closed-loop obstruction
- Large bowel obstruction.

Management of Intestinal Obstruction (Flow chart 1)

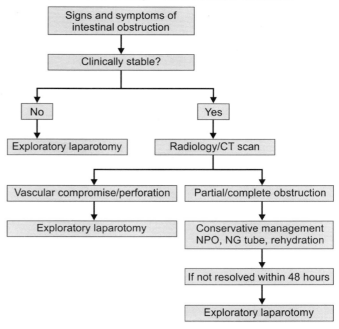

Flow chart 1 Management of intestinal obstruction

CONCLUSION

Interruption of forward flow of intestinal contents leads to intestinal obstruction. Intestinal obstruction ac occur at any level of the GI tract. Intra-abdominal adhesions, malignancy are the most common cause for intestinal obstruction. Nausea vomiting abdominal pain inability to pass flatus are common clinical presentation. Radiologic imaging can confirm the diagnosis. Uncomplicated intestinal obstruction can be managed by conservative management. Evidence of vascular compromise or perforation, or failure to resolve with adequate bowel decompression is an indication for surgical intervention.

BIBLIOGRAPHY

1. Furukawa A, Yamasaki M, Furuichi K, et al. Helical CT in the diagnosis of small bowel obstruction. Radiographics. 2001;21(2):341-55.

2. Irvin TT. Abdominal pain: a surgical audit of 1190 emergency admissions. Br J Surg. 1989;76(11):1121-5.
3. Lappas JC, Reyes BL, Maglinte DD. Abdominal radiography findings in small-bowel obstruction: relevance to triage for additional diagnostic imaging. Am J Roentgenol. 2001;176(1):167-74.
4. Maglinte DD, Heitkamp DE, Howard TJ, et al. Current concepts in imaging of small bowel obstruction. Radiol Clin North Am. 2003;41(2):263-83.
5. Rana SV, Bhardwaj SB. Small intestinal bacterial overgrowth. Scand J Gastroenterol. 2008;43(9):1030-7.
6. Shelton BK. Intestinal obstruction. AACN Clin Issues. 1999;10(4):478-91.
7. Stoker J, van Randen A, Laméris W, et al. Imaging patients with acute abdominal pain. Radiology. 2009;253(1):31-46.
8. Suri S, Gupta S, Sudhakar PJ, et al. Comparative evaluation of plain films, ultrasound and CT in the diagnosis of intestinal obstruction. Acta Radiol. 1999;40(4):422-8.
9. Wangensteen OH. Understanding the bowel obstruction problem. Am J Surg. 1978;135(2):131-49.
10. Wright HK, O'Brien JJ, Tilson MD. Water absorption in experimental closed segment obstruction of the ileum in man. Am J Surg. 1971;121(1):96-9.

SECTION 7

Renal and Genitourinary Emergencies

- **Electrolyte Imbalance**
  Vishal Saxena
- **Acute Kidney Injury in Sepsis**
  Manish Jain, Ashish Nandwani
- **Emergencies in Renal Failure and Dialysis Patients**
  Salil Jain, Sucheta Yadav
- **Urinary Tract Infections**
  Ashish Nandwani, Manish Jain
- **Hematuria**
  Puneet Ahluwalia, Varun Mittal, Rajiv Yadav
- **Acute Urinary Retention**
  Rakesh Khera, Varun Mittal, Puneet Ahluwalia

CHAPTER 57

Electrolyte Imbalance

Vishal Saxena

INTRODUCTION

Electrolytes play an important role in maintaining the homeostatic environment inside the body. They are helpful in maintaining neurological and cardiac function, also helpful in fluid, oxygen, and acid-base balance. Electrolyte imbalance is either increased intake or decreased removal of an electrolyte. The most common cause of electrolyte disturbances is kidney failure.

Most common electrolyte disorders involve sodium, potassium, and calcium. Others like magnesium and phosphorus although important are relatively less common. Electrolytes basically help in maintaining voltages across cell membranes and also help in carrying nerve impulses to heart, nerves, and muscles. It is the function of kidneys to maintain the electrolyte concentration in blood constantly. During illnesses like diarrhea and vomiting, kidneys try to maintain electrolytes and their loss by maintaining the tonicity of urine.

HYPONATREMIA

Hyponatremia is commonly defined as a serum sodium concentration below 135 mEq/L.

$$\text{Plasma tonicity} = \frac{(\text{Extracellular solute} + \text{Intracellular solute})}{\text{TBW (total body water)}}$$

Classification

Classification is given in **Table 1**.

Causes

Causes of hyponatremia are given in **Table 2**.

Table 1 Hyponatremia: Basis and classification

Basis	Classification type
Osmolality	Hyponatremia with low serum osmolality defined as a serum osmolality less than 275 mOsmol/kg
	Hyponatremia with a normal or high osmolality
Hyponatremia with a low serum osmolality (further classified on the basis of either volume or ADH level)	Antidiuretic hormone (ADH) levels (elevated or suppressed)
	According to volume status (hypovolemia, normovolemia, or hypervolemia)

Abbreviation: ADH, antidiuretic hormone.

Table 2 Causes and diseases of hyponatremia

Causes	Diseases
True volume depletion	Vomiting or diarrhea Thiazide diuretics Advanced renal failure
Decreased tissue perfusion	Low cardiac output in heart failure Cirrhosis
ADH disturbances	Increase in ADH release in the syndrome of inappropriate ADH (SIADH) secretion

Abbreviation: ADH, antidiuretic hormone

Treatment

Determine whether the hyponatremia is due to depletion (gastrointestinal losses, renal or adrenal causes) or dilution [excess administration of fluids or syndrome of inappropriate antidiuretic hormone (SIADH) which may be due to infection, cardiovascular, respiratory, central nervous system or drug therapy]. The distinction between depletional hyponatremia and dilutional hyponatremia may be made by reviewing biochemical results; serum potassium, urea, and albumin likely to be low in dilutional hyponatremia. Blood pressure is likely to be normal or high in dilutional hyponatremia and is often low in depletional hyponatremia.

Investigations (Box 1)

Box 1 Investigations of hyponatremia

- Urea and electrolytes
- Plasma and urine osmolality
- Glucose
- Thyroid function tests
- Urinary sodium concentration
- Consider Synacthen test to exclude Addison's disease

Dilutional Hyponatremia

- Restrict fluid, potentially to less than 1 L/day depending on severity
- Stop causative agents, e.g. drugs and hypotonic fluids
- Administration of hypertonic sodium chloride will only be required in exceptional circumstances and the decision should be made by a consultant, see earlier for dose
- Check serum sodium concentration at least every 2–4 hours
- Raising sodium levels too rapidly may cause harm
- Aim to increase sodium levels by 0.5–1.0 mmol/L/hr to a maximum of 12 mmol/L in a 24-hour period. In high-risk patients a slower correction may be necessary.

Syndrome of Inappropriate Antidiuretic Hormone

In SIADH patients may have hyponatremia due to respiratory infection, cardiovascular disease, central nervous system pathology or other causes. Serum osmolality will be low, e.g. less than 275 mOsmol/kg and urine osmolality will be concentrated, e.g. above 300 mOsmol/kg.

Treatment is fluid restriction to less than 1 L/day.

Management of hyponatremia is well-described in **Flow chart 1**.

HYPERNATREMIA

Hypernatremia results from disturbances in the renal concentrating mechanism **(Flow chart 2)**.

Treatment

- Minimizing the large ongoing water loss if present should be the first concern. This can be done by correcting the underlying cause, e.g. in diabetics correction of blood sugars and in central diabetes insipidus **(Box 2)** using vasopressin spray may prove beneficial.
- Water replacement by adding free water or adding intravenous (IV) 5% dextrose can be a way of replenishing water loss **(Table 3)**
- A half-isotonic saline solution is used to correct hypernatremia
- Patients with hypotension 0.9% sodium chloride solution must be infused rapidly
- Use of half-isotonic saline at a rate less than 0.5 mEq/L/hr prevent cerebral edema, intracranial hypertension and herniation of the brain
- Intravenous administration of 5% dextrose (or glucose) in water and free water through nasogastric tube can also be used.

HYPERKALEMIA

Hyperkalemia is common in emergency department. Every emergency physician should know the treatment of hyperkalemia. Increased potassium release from the cells and reduced excretion of potassium through urine is the main cause of hyperkalemia **(Table 4)**.

Hyperkalemia is raised serum potassium level:
- *Mild*: K^+ = 5.5 – 5.9 mmol/L
- *Moderate*: K^+ = 6 – 6.4 mmol/L
- *Severe*: K^+ > = 6.5 mmol/L or if electrocardiogram (ECG) changes or symptoms present.

Measurement of 24-hour urinary potassium excretion is of *limited utility* in patients with persistent *stable* hyperkalemia, and the transtubular potassium gradient (TTKG) is *not* a reliable test for the diagnosis of hyperkalemia.

Clinical Features

Hyperkalemia can cause increased cardiac depolarization, and muscle excitability which leads to arrhythmias ventricular fibrillation or cardiac asystole and death. Rapid ECG changes also occur with rise of K^+ values greater than 6.5 mmol/L. The clinical presentation of hyperkalemia is highly variable ranging from acute illness in some patients while others may be asymptomatic **(Table 5)**. Clinical suspicion of hyperkalemia should be considered with patients with arrhythmias, muscular weakness or paresthesia. The clinical course is unpredictable and sudden death can occur in the absence of typical ECG changes.

Treatment of Hyperkalemia (Flow chart 3)

- Pseudohyperkalemia should be excluded first
- All potassium supplements (IV and oral) should be stopped

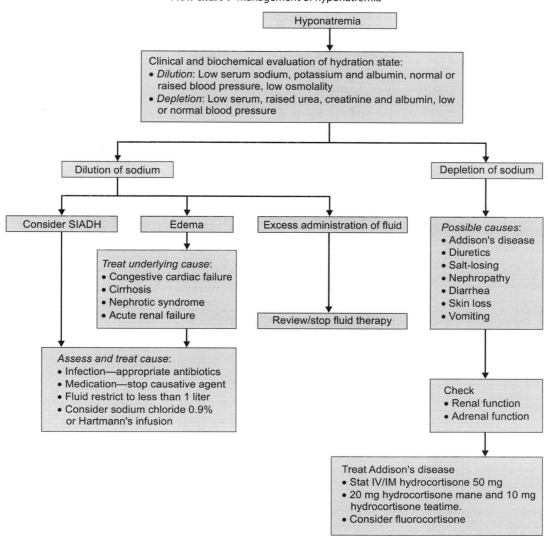

Flow chart 1 Management of hyponatremia

Abbreviations: IM, intramuscular; IV, intravenous; SIADH, syndrome of inappropriate antidiuretic hormone.

- Medication which contribute to hyperkalemia and/or acute renal failure should be evaluated and stopped
- Prescribe low dietary intake of potassium
- Maintain adequate hydration and urine output
- If potassium greater than 6.5 mmol/L or ECG changes monitor patient's cardiac rhythm until it is stable and potassium level is in range. Consider hemodialysis.

HYPOKALEMIA

Severity of hypokalemia is given in **Table 6** and causes and conditions of hypokalemia are given in **Table 7**.

Clinical Features

Clinical features of hypokalemia have been described in **Table 8**.

Treatment (Table 9)

- Try to identify the causes and remove it
- Slow replacement of potassium (via oral route) is preferred, oral potassium should be taken with plenty of fluid, with or after meals
- Replace potassium carefully in patients with renal dysfunction (risk of hyperkalemia secondary to impaired potassium excretion)

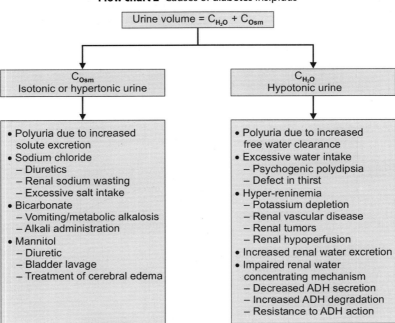

Flow chart 2 Causes of diabetes insipidus

Abbreviation: ADH, antidiuretic hormone.

Box 2 Clinical features of diabetes insipidus

- Abrupt onset
- Equal frequency in both sexes
- Rare in infancy, usual in second decade of life
- Predilection for cold water
- Polydipsia
- Urine output of 3–15 L/day
- Marked nocturia but no diurnal variation
- Sleep deprivation leads to fatigue and irritability
- Severe life-threatening hypernatremia can be associated with illness or water deprivation

- 0.9% sodium chloride is the preferred infusion fluid as 5% glucose may cause transcellular shift of potassium into cells
- Check magnesium levels
- An ECG is strongly recommended in patients with severe or symptomatic hypokalemia, cardiac disease or renal impairment **(Table 9)**.

HYPERCALCEMIA

Usually in normal physiological conditions serum calcium concentration is nicely controlled. Parathyroid function, bone resorption, renal calcium reabsorption or dihydroxylation of vitamin D abnormalities may cause rise in serum. Serum calcium is bound to albumin, and measurements should be adjusted for serum albumin.

Causes

Most of the cases of hypercalcemia are due to primary hyperparathyroidism or malignancy.

Less Common Causes

For less common causes of hypercalcemia, *See* **Table 10**.

Clinical Manifestations of Hypercalcemia

Clinical manifestations with sign and symptoms of various systems have been described in **Table 11**.

Investigation

Investigation of hypercalcemia is given in **Table 12**.

Management

Management of hypercalcemia is given in **Table 13**.

HYPOCALCEMIA

Acute hypocalcemia needs urgent treatment as it can be life-threatening in many cases. In emergency department, IV calcium is the mainstay of initial therapy but important to find out the underlying cause and start specific therapy as early as possible.

Table 3 Water deprivation test for diabetes insipidus*

Diagnosis	Urine osmolality with water deprivation (mOsm/Kg H$_2$O)	Plasma arginine vasopressin (AVP) after dehydration	Increase in urine osmolality with exogenous AVP
Normal	>800	>2 pg/mL	Little or none substantial
Complete central diabetes insipidus	<300	Indetectable	
Partial central Diabetes insipidus	300–800	<1.5 pg/mL	>10% of urine osmolality after water deprivation Little or none
Nephrogenic Diabetes insipidus	<300–500	>5 pg/mL	
Primary polydipsia	>500	<5 pg/mL	Little or none

*Water intake is restricted until the patient loses 3–5% of weight or until three consecutive hourly determines of urinary osmolality are within 10% of each other (Caution must be exercised to ensure that the patient does not become excessively dehydrated). Aqueous (5 U subcutaneous) is given, and urine osmolality is measured after 60 minutes. The expected responses are given above.

Table 4 Causes and conditions of hyperkalemia

Causes	Conditions
Increased potassium release from cells	• Pseudohyperkalemia (mechanical trauma during venipuncture) • Metabolic acidosis • Insulin deficiency, hyperglycemia, and hyperosmolality • Increased tissue catabolism • Beta-blockers • Exercise • Hyperkalemic periodic paralysis • Red cell transfusion • Various drugs including digitalis
Reduced urinary potassium secretion	• Reduced aldosterone secretion • Reduced response to aldosterone (aldosterone resistance) • Reduced distal sodium and water delivery • Acute and chronic kidney disease • Ureterojejunostomy

Table 5 Clinical features of hyperkalemia

Cardiac	• Abnormal ECG • Cardiac arrhythmias • Pacemaker dysfunction
Neuromuscular	• Paresthesias • Weakness • Paralysis
Endocrine	• Decreased renal NH$_4^+$ production • Natriuresis
Others	• Increased aldosterone secretion • Increased insulin secretion

Table 6 Severity of hypokalemia

Severity of hypokalemia	Serum level (mmol/L)
Mild	3.0–3.5
Moderate	2.5–3.0
Severe	<2.5

Causes

In hospital setting, disruption of parathyroid gland function due to total thyroidectomy is common cause of acute symptomatic hypocalcemia. Hypocalcemia may be temporary or permanent.

Other Causes

Other causes of hypocalcemia are listed in **Table 14**.

Clinical Features

Clinical features occur when adjusted serum calcium levels are below approximately 1.9 mmol/L. However, symptoms depend on the rate of fall **(Table 15)**.

Investigations

- Serum calcium (adjusted for albumin)
- Phosphate
- Parathyroid hormone (PTH)
- U+E
- Vitamin D
- Magnesium.

Management (Table 16)

Hypocalcemia can be managed by:
- Calcium ranges
  – Normal adult (total) calcium range = 2.20–2.60 mmol/L (adjusted for albumin)

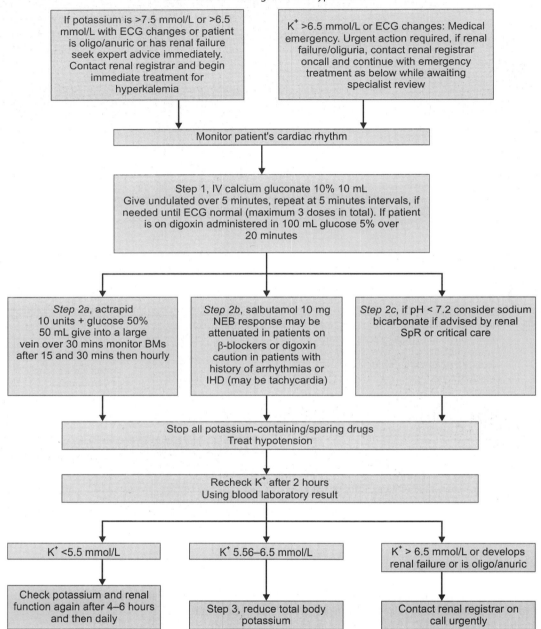

Flow chart 3 Management of hyperkalemia

Mild Hypocalcemia

- Oral calcium supplements should be considered.
- In asymptomatic patients or patients with parathyroidectomy, repeat calcium after 24 hours; patient can be discharged if calcium is greater than 2.1 mmol/L with regular follow-up
- Even after calcium supplement, if patient remain hypocalcemic then start 1-alfa calcidol 0.25 µg/day
- Vitamin D supplementation in case of vitamin D deficiency
- If other cause of hypocalcemia, treat underlying condition.

Severe Hypocalcemia

- Should be treated urgently with IV calcium gluconate
- Start 10–20 mL 10% calcium gluconate in 50–100 mL of 5% dextrose IV over 10 minutes with ECG monitoring
- Repeat the dose till the patient is asymptomatic, followed by calcium gluconate infusion

- Dilute 100 mL of 10% calcium gluconate (ten vials) in 1 liter of normal saline or 5% dextrose and infuse at 50–100 mL/hr (Calcium chloride is an alternative, but it is irritant to veins so infusion only through central lines)
- Frequent blood tests are required during initial phase of treatment
- Treatment of the underlying cause.

Table 7 Causes and conditions of hypokalemia

Cause	Conditions
Increased potassium loss	• *Drugs*: Diuretics (thiazides, loop diuretics), laxatives, glucocorticoids, fludrocortisone, penicillins, amphotericin, aminoglycosides • *GI losses*: Diarrhea, vomiting, ileostomy, intestinal fistula • Renal causes, dialysis • *Endocrine disorders*: Hyperaldosteronism (Conn's syndrome), Cushing's syndrome
Transcellular shift	• Insulin/glucose therapy • Salbutamol and other beta-agonists • Theophylline • Metabolic alkalosis
Decreased potassium intake	
Magnesium depletion (associated with increased renal potassium loss)	

Table 8 Signs and symptoms of hypokalemia

System	Signs and symptoms
Cardiovascular	Bradycardia or tachycardia, hypotension, arrhythmias, cardiac arrest and palpitations ECG changes (U waves, T-wave flattening, ST-segment changes)
Respiratory	Respiratory distress and respiratory failure, hypoventilation
Musculoskeletal	Cramps, tetany, reduced deep tendon reflexes, reduced muscle strength
General	Peripheral edema, lethargy, constipation, nausea, vomiting, abdominal cramping paresthesia

Table 9 Treatment of hypokalemia

Hypokalemia	Treatment	Comments
Mild 3.0–3.4 mmol/L	Oral replacement *Sando-K* 2 tablets TDS (72 mmol/day), or if not tolerated *Kay Cee L* 25 mL TDS (75 mmol/day)	Usually asymptomatic Monitor K+ daily and adjust treatment accordingly Consider IV if patient cannot tolerate PO
Moderate 2.5–2.9 mmol/L		
No or minor symptoms	Oral replacement *Sando-K* 2 tablets QDS (96 mmol/day), or if not tolerated : *Kay Cee L* 25 mL QDS (100 mmol/day)	Monitor K+ daily and adjust treatment accordingly Consider IV if patient cannot tolerate PO
Severe <2.5 mmol/L or symptomatic		
	Intravenous replacement 40 mmol KCl in 1L* 0.9% NaCl BD or TDS (glucose 5% may be used but see notes above) Standard infusion rate 10 mmol/hr Maximum infusion rate 20 mmol/hr Check Mg²⁺ level (reported automatically if K <2.8 mmol/L if patient hypomagnesemic: initially give me 4 mL MgSO₄ 50% (8 mmol) diluted to 10 mL with NaCl 0.9% over 20 min, then start first 40 mmol KCl infusion, followed by magnesium replacement as per hypomagnesemia policy	Monitor K+ level after each 40 mmol and adjust treatment accordingly *In exceptional circumstances (e.g. patient fluid overloaded, severe heart failure, etc.) it may be appropriate to give a higher concentration of potassium (e.g. 40 mmol KCl in 500 mL). Concentrations greater than 40 mmol/L are painful and may cause severe phlebitis: give via the largest suitable peripheral vein using an infusion pump and monitor the infusion site very closely—seek senior guidance first. Alternatively, considered giving via a central line. Monitor patient's fluid status.
Unstable arrhythmias	Resuscitation team call 2222	

Abbreviations: IV, intravenous; PO, per os; QDS, 4 times a day; TDS, 3 times a day.

HYPOPHOSPHATEMIA

Hypophosphatemia can be due to decreased intestinal absorption and increased urinary phosphate excretion.

Treatment

Symptoms of hypophosphatemia occur only when the serum phosphate concentration is less than 2 mg/dL, most of patients will not require therapy.
- *Asymptomatic* patients with a serum phosphate less than 2.0 mg/dL, need oral phosphate therapy.
- *Symptomatic* patients treated with oral phosphate if the serum phosphate is 1.0–1.9 mg/dL.

Intravenous Therapy

If the serum phosphate is less than 1.0 mg/dL, IV phosphate should be given under monitoring as this can produce a variety of adverse effects including hypocalcemia due to binding of calcium; renal failure due to calcium phosphate precipitation in the kidneys, and possibly fatal arrhythmias. The serum phosphate concentration should be monitored every 6 hours when IV phosphate is given, and the patient should be switched to oral replacement when the serum phosphate concentration reaches 1.5 mg/dL.

HYPERPHOSPHATEMIA

Renal failure is a common cause of diminished phosphate excretion. Urinary excretion may not keep pace with

Table 10 Less common causes of hypercalcemia

Drugs	• Thiazide diuretics • Theophylline toxicity • Hypervitaminosis D • Lithium • Hypervitaminosis A
Endocrine	• Tertiary hyperparathyroidism • Thyrotoxicosis • Adrenal insufficiency • Pheochromocytoma
Others	• Rhabdomyolysis • Immobilization • Non-malignant granulomatous disease • Milk-alkali syndrome • Familial hypocalciuric hypercalcemia

Table 11 Signs and symptoms of hypercalcemia

System	Signs/symptoms
Cardiovascular	• Short QT- interval on ECG • Arrhythmias (rare) • Bradycardia • Hypertension • Bundle branch • Cardiac arrest (if severe)
Neuromuscular	• Confusion • Delirium • Psychosis • Stupor • Muscle weakness • Headache • Seizures (rare)
Renal	• Polyuria • Polydipsia • Nocturia • Hypercalciuria • Nephrolithiasis • Nephrocalcinosis • Renal failure
Gastrointestinal	• Nausea/vomiting • Anorexia • Constipation • Abdominal pain • Peptic ulcers • Pancreatitis
Skeletal	• Bone pain/arthralgia • Osteopenia/osteoporosis in cortical bone (often seen in wrist)
Other	• Shock • Death

Table 12 Investigation of hypercalcemia

History	Examination	ECG	Bloods
Symptoms of hypercalcemia and duration • Symptoms of underlying causes, e.g. weight loss, night sweats, cough • Family history • Drugs including supplements and over-the-counter preparations	Assess for cognitive impairment • Fluid balance status • For underlying causes: including neck, respiratory, abdomen, breasts, lymph nodes	Look for shortened QT interval or other conduction abnormalities	• Calcium adjusted for albumin • Phosphate • PTH • Urea and electrolytes

Abbreviation: PTH, parathyroid hormone.

CHAPTER 57 Electrolyte Imbalance

Table 13 Management of hypercalcemia

Intervention	Important points
Normal saline 3–6 liters IV daily for 1–3 days	Closely monitor for fluid overload in patient of renal dysfunction and elderly
Furosemide 10–20 mg IV (for use in severe cases, and only in well hydrated)	Loop diuretics used only if fluid overload develops; not effective for reducing serum calcium
Zoledronic acid 4 mg IV over 15 minutes Pamidronate 60–90 mg IV over 2–4 hr	• Give slowly and low dose in renal dysfunction patient • Monitor serum calcium response—careful in vitamin D deficiency or suppressed PTH can cause hypocalcemia
Calcitonin 4–8 IU/kg IM injection every 6–8 hr	If poor response to bisphosphonates
Glucocorticoids 200–300 mg IV hydrocortisone daily for 3–5 days • Prednisolone 40 mg daily	Usually effective in 2–4 days
Dialysis	If severe renal failure
Parathyroidectomy, if severe hypercalcemia in acute presentation of primary hyperparathyroidism and resistant to other therapy	

Table 14 Other causes of hypocalcemia

Drugs	• Bisphosphonates • Cinacalcet • Citrated blood transfusions • Calcitonin • Foscarnet • Glucocorticoids • Ketoconazole • Phosphates • Phenytoin • Colchicine overdose • Antineoplastic agents
Endocrine and electrolyte disturbances	• Hyperphosphatemia • Hypoparathyroidism • Calcium malabsorption • Pseudohypoparathyroidism • Hypomagnesemia • Vitamin D deficiency • Postparathyroidectomy • Inadequate dietary calcium intake
Others	• Renal tubular disease: Renal failure • Acute pancreatitis: Septic shock • Over hydration • Hypoalbuminemia • Rhabdomyolysis • Malignant disease • Massive blood transfusion: Hyperventilation

Table 15 Signs and symptoms of hypocalcemia

System	Signs/symptoms
Cardiovascular	• Dyspnea • Symptoms of congestive heart failure • Prolonged QT interval • Cardiac arrhythmias • Hypotension
Neuromuscular	• Irritability • Impaired intellectual capacity • Depression • Personality changes • Fatigue • Seizures • Other uncontrolled movements • Numbness and paresthesia in the perioral area or in the fingers and toes • Muscle cramps and muscle weakness • Wheezing • Dysphagia • Laryngospasm • Tremors • Tetany
Other	• Coarse hair • Brittle nails • Dry skin • Psoriasis • Coagulation irregularities • Chvostek and Trousseau signs • Bronchospasm

Table 16 Severity of hypocalcemia

Severity of hypocalcemia	Serum level (mmol/L) (adjusted for albumin)
Mild	2.00–2.20; often asymptomatic
Severe	≤1.9; may be asymptomatic

phosphate intake when the glomerular filtration rate (GFR) falls below 20–25 mL/min.

Treatment

Severe hyperphosphatemia with symptomatic hypocalcemia can be life-threatening. Phosphate excretion can be increased by saline infusion, if renal function is intact.

Hemodialysis is often indicated in patients with symptomatic hypocalcemia, particularly if renal function is impaired.

CONCLUSION

Electrolyte imbalances are common clinical problems. Electrolyte imbalance are associated with significant morbidities and mortalities so appropriate and rapid treatment is mandatory.

BIBLIOGRAPHY

1. Alfonzo A, Soar J, MacTier R, et al. Clinical practice guidelines. Treatment of acute hyperkalaemia in adults. UK Renal Association; 2014. pp. 104.
2. Alfonzo AV, Isles C, Geddes C, et al. Potassium disorders—clinical spectrum and emergency management. Resuscitation. 2006;70:10-25.
3. André Gougoux. Practical approach to patients with electrolyte disorders. The Canadian Journal of CME. 2001;51-60.
4. Gell J. 2013. Guideline for the management of acute hyperkalaemia in adults. [online] NUHS website. Available from *http://www.odpskills.co.uk/pdf/hyperkalaemia*. [Accessed February, 2017].
5. Guideline for the Management of Hypokalaemia in Adults. NHS Foundation Trust. Medicines Information. 2010. Available from *http://www.gloshospitals.nhs.uk/SharePoint110/Antibiotics%20Web%20Documents/TG/Hypokalaemia%20Guidelines.pdf*. [Accessed February, 2017].
6. Hughes D, Bowen-Jones D. Hyponatraemia management. Clinical Guideline. NHS Trust. 2012.
7. HDH/KGH Pharmaceuticals and Therapeutics Committee. (2003). Hypocalcemia: treatment guidelines. [online] Available from *http://im-mmc.synthasite.com/resources/Hypocalcemia%20guideline.pdf*. [Accessed February, 2017].
8. Liamis G, Rodenburg EM, Hofman A, et al. Electrolyte disorders in community subjects: prevalence and risk factors. Am J Med. 2013;126:256-63.
9. Nottingham University Hospitals Trust. Guidelines for the treatment of hypocalcaemia in adults. [online]. Available from *https://www.nuh.nhs.uk/nuh-guidelines-app/guidelines-update/*. [Accessed February, 2017].
10. Schrier RW. Treatment of hyponatremia [review]. N Engl J Med. 1985;312:1121-3.
11. Shane E, Irani D. Hypercalcemia: pathogenesis, clinical manifestations, differential diagnosis, and management. American Society for Bone and Mineral Research. 2006; 176-9.
12. Society for Endocrinology's Clinical Committee. 2013. Acute Hypercalcaemia. Emergency Endocrine Guidance. Bristol, UK. [online] Available from *https://www.rcem.ac.uk/docs/External%20Guidance/10R.%20Acute%20Hypercalcaemia%20-%20Emergency%20Guidance%20(Society%20for%20Endocrinology,%20Jan%202014).pdf*. [Accessed February, 2017]
13. Spasovski G, Vanholder R, Allolio B, et al. Clinical practice guideline on diagnosis and treatment of hyponatraemia. Intensive Care Med. 2014;40:320-31.

CHAPTER 58

Acute Kidney Injury in Sepsis

Manish Jain, Ashish Nandwani

INTRODUCTION

Acute kidney injury is a common and serious complication of sepsis in intensive care unit as well as in emergency department. It is associated with high morbidity and mortality. AKI severity is associated with increased in-hospital mortality and overall higher costs.

Acute renal failure (ARF) had more than 30 definitions in literature before 2004. This caused discrepancies in ARF incidence and prevalence.

In 2004, first consensus definition of ARF was published—RIFLE criteria (risk, injury, failure, loss, end-stage kidney disease) which provided three grades of severity (class R, I, F) and two outcome classes (class L, E). This classification was based on changes in either serum creatinine, estimated glomerular filtration rate (eGFR) or urine output from baseline.[1]

The acute kidney injury network (AKIN) group in 2007 proposed AKI instead of ARF to cover entire spectrum of ARF from asymptomatic changes in laboratory parameters to life-threatening disorders. AKIN group supported the RIFLE criteria but with minor modifications. They decreased the threshold for change in creatinine to 0.3, eliminated the eGFR criteria. Loss and end-stage kidney or renal disease (ESRD) were outcomes, so they were eliminated from definition.

Kidney disease: Improving Global Outcomes (KDIGO) proposed the most recent consensus definition of AKI as rise in serum creatinine concentration of 0.3 mg/dL or more within 48 hours, or greater than 50% increase within 7 days or reduction in urine output less than 0.5 mL/kg/hour for 6 hours.[2]

SEPSIS

Sepsis, till recently, was defined as suspected or proven infection and a systemic inflammatory response syndrome like fever, tachycardia, tachypnea and leukocytosis, while severe sepsis was defined as sepsis with organ dysfunction (hypotension, oliguria, metabolic acidosis, thrombocytopenia or obtundation).

Recently, the definition of sepsis has been revised and a new definition has been recommended. Accordingly, sepsis is defined as life-threatening organ dysfunction caused by dysregulated host response to infection.

Organ dysfunction is identified as an acute change in total sepsis-related organ failure assessment (SOFA) score of more than two points consequent to infection.

Septic shock is defined as a subset of sepsis in which underlying circulatory and cellular metabolism abnormalities are profound enough to substantially increase mortality.[3]

INCIDENCE

The incidence of AKI increases according to sepsis severity. The reported incidence is 4.2%, 22.7% and 52.8% for sepsis, severe sepsis and septic shock, respectively.[4]

Sepsis-associated AKI (SA-AKI) accounts for approximately 50% of cases of AKI in ICU.[5]

Septic AKI is associated with more severe illness, higher aberrations in hemodynamic and laboratory parameters, concomitant other organs dysfunction, need of mechanical ventilation and vasoactive therapy. Septic AKI is associated with higher in-hospital case fatality rate as compared to nonseptic AKI (70.2% vs 51.8%).[6]

RISK FACTORS

The various risk factors associated with SA-AKI are following:
- Elderly patients
- *Sources of sepsis*: Blood stream infections, abdominal and genitourinary sepsis, infective endocarditis has higher incidence of AKI

- Delayed antimicrobial therapy administration
- *Baseline comorbidities*: Chronic kidney disease, diabetes mellitus, heart failure, liver disease increases susceptibility to SA-AKI
- *Concomitant use of contrast agents and drugs*: Nonsteroidal anti-inflammatory drugs, cyclooxygenase 2 inhibitors, calcineurin inhibitors, angiotensin converting enzyme inhibitors, angiotensin receptor blockers, aminoglycosides, etc.

PATHOPHYSIOLOGY

Pathophysiology of AKI in sepsis is complex and multifactorial. This includes:
- Intrarenal hemodynamic changes
- Endothelial dysfunction
- Intraglomerular thrombosis
- Infiltration of inflammatory cells in renal parenchyma
- Obstruction of tubules with necrotic cells and debris.[7]

Sepsis-induced immune response leads to activation of proinflammatory markers followed by anti-inflammatory mechanisms. After initial host microbial interaction, there is activation of innate immune response leading to secretion of various cytokines [interleukin (IL)-1, IL-6, TNF-α], which progresses to state of cytokine storm, hemodynamic instability, organ dysfunction and septic shock. This proinflammatory state is followed by compensatory anti-inflammatory immune response in which there is altered cytokine production, decreased lymphocyte proliferation and increased apoptosis.[8]

DIAGNOSTIC MARKERS

Serum Creatinine

Serum creatinine is a late and insensitive marker because of number of reasons.
- Increments in serum creatinine lag decrements in glomerular filtration rate by hours, so creatinine is not an ideal marker.
- Hemodilution in hypotensive patients receiving fluid resuscitation masks serum creatinine increments—delays AKI diagnosis.
- Patients who are on diuretics may have good urine output, so may not meet AKI diagnosis criteria based on reduced urine output.

Biomarkers

Serum creatinine starts increasing after the window of opportunity for effective therapy has already passed. It is essential to have biomarkers that predict the early detection of AKI and thus timely interventions that would prevent and decrease the morbidity and mortality related to renal failure.

Emerging biomarkers for early detection of AKI are as follows:

Urinary biomarkers: Liver-type fatty acid binding protein (L-FABP), IL-18, kidney injury molecule-1 (KIM-1), netrin-1, neutrophil gelatinase-associated lipocalin (NGAL).

Plasma biomarkers: Cystatin C, NGAL.

TREATMENT

- Treatment is dependent mainly on source control of sepsis, antibiotics and use of organ support, if necessary
- Tissue perfusion and hemodynamic stability are important goals of therapy
- Avoid nephrotoxic medication and contrast agents unless there is absolute indication
- Nutritional support is important but often overlooked aspect of patient care
- Renal replacement therapy
- Septic AKI has higher proinflammatory and anti-inflammatory markers, so extracorporeal techniques which remove inflammatory mediators from the circulation may provide a potential therapy for this condition.

Fluid Resuscitation

Aggressive fluid resuscitation should be done initially and this fluid challenge should be continued as long as there is response and hemodynamic improvement. Fluids should be stopped once there is no response.

There is controversy regarding which fluid should be used for resuscitation. KDIGO guidelines suggest that isotonic crystalloids should be used instead of colloids (starch and albumin).

Godin et al. proposed a strategy for fluid resuscitation:
- *Phase A*: 0–6 hours—aggressive volume resuscitation
- *Phase B*: 6–36 hours—decelerating fluid resuscitation; fluid boluses should be administered to compensate for extravascular sequestration
- *Phase C*: 36–48 hours—equilibrium phase; stop administering intravenous fluids
- *Phase D*: 48–72 hours—mobilization fluids; withhold fluids and allow spontaneous diuresis (or diurese if necessary).[9]

Vasopressors

In patients who are unresponsive to fluid therapy, vasopressors should be started to avoid fluid accumulation. Norepinephrine is the first choice vasopressor for septic patients, dobutamine should be used if there is myocardial dysfunction or if signs of hypoperfusion are present.

In the past, low-dose dopamine was used as it increases renal blood flow and diuresis but dopamine can depress respiratory drive (trigger tachyarrhythmias and myocardial ischemia) and can accelerate intestinal ischemia. Dopamine use is no longer recommended.

Renal Replacement Therapy

The different renal replacement therapy (RRT) modalities used are intermittent hemodialysis, continuous renal replacement therapy (CRRT), sustained low efficiency dialysis (SLED) and acute peritoneal dialysis (PD). Timing of RRT initiation is controversial.

Indications of Renal Replacement Therapy

Absolute indications for renal replacement therapy:
- Metabolic acidosis with pH less than 7.15. Unresponsive to medical therapy
- *Hyperkalemia*: K greater than 6 mmol/L plus electrocardiogram changes
- *Pulmonary edema*: Not responsive to diuresis or to prevent need for ventilator support
- *Uremic complications*: Encephalopathy, pericarditis, neuropathy, bleeding.

Nonemergent indications for renal replacement therapy:
- *Solute control*: No universally accepted levels of urea or creatinine
- *Fluid removal*: Oliguric or anuric patients to prevent fluid overload
- *Nutritional support*: Better parenteral nutritional support with RRT
- Modified ultrafiltration in patients with cardiorenal syndrome and during cardiac surgeries to decrease the preload.

Intermittent Hemodialysis

Intermittent hemodialysis is used in hemodynamic stable patients. It results in faster removal of solutes and fluid usually in 4 hours. This is same therapy as used in regular chronic kidney patients who are on dialysis.

Continuous Renal Replacement Therapy

Continuous renal replacement therapy involves slow, continuous passage of blood over 24 hours, taken from either an arterial or a venous source which is passed through a filter. This prolonged treatment results in better solute control in hemodynamic unstable patients. This includes continuous hemodialysis, hemofiltration and hemodiafiltration.

Continuous hemodialysis includes continuous arterio-venous hemodialysis (CAVHD) and continuous venovenous hemodialysis (CVVHD) depending upon vascular access. The dialysis solution is passed through the dialysate compartment of the filter continuously and at a slow rate (15–35 mL/min). The amount of fluid ultrafiltered across the membrane is low (0–4 L/day). Diffusion is the primary method of solute removal.

Continuous hemofiltration includes continuous arterio-venous hemofiltration (CAVH) and continuous venovenous hemofiltration (CVVH).

No dialysis solution is used in this method. The urea clearance and ultrafiltration is highest with this method. Large volume of replacement fluid is infused into inflow or outflow blood line (predilution or postdilution mode). Convection is the primary method of solute removal along with ultrafiltration.

Continuous hemodiafiltration includes *continuous arterio-venous hemodiafiltration (CAVHDF) and continuous venovenous hemodiafiltration (CVVHDF)*.

This is the combination of both dialysis and filtration method using dialysis solution and replacement fluid. Daily volume of fluid ultrafiltered across the membrane is high, but not as high as with continuous filtration, as the volume of replacement fluid used in much lower in hemodiafiltration.

Sustained Low-efficiency Dialysis

This is a form of hybrid therapy where regular dialysis machine is used with decreased blood and dialysate flows. It is usually performed for 8–12 hours a day in patients who have borderline blood pressures and in whom regular hemodialysis cannot be performed.

Acute Peritoneal Dialysis

Acute PD is usually done for pediatric patients or in adults in developing countries where other modalities are not available.

Extracorporeal Therapies

The timings for commencement of extracorporeal therapies in AKI are yet to be established. There are no guidelines when and where these therapies should be used.
- *Endotoxins and bacterial fragments removal*: Hemoadsorption, plasma exchange
- *Cytokine removal*: Coupled plasma filtration adsorption.

Hemadsorption

Hemadsorption involves the placement of resin-based adsorbent in direct contact with blood via extracorporeal circuit. Sorbent attracts solutes through hydrophobic interactions, ionic attraction and hydrogen bonding and thus are eliminated from the circulation.

Polymyxin B is the most extensively studied sorbent. Polymyxin B-immobilized polystyrene-derived fibers

(*Toraymyxin*) bind and neutralize the endotoxins and then remove these endotoxins from the blood.

Cytosorb

Cytosorb is composed of highly adsorptive biocompatible porous polymer beads which remove inflammatory mediators from blood. This is based on pore capture and surface adsorption. Substances larger than pores (such as blood cells) do not enter pores and go around the beads.

Cytosorb is indicated in "cytokine storm"—pancreatitis, postgastrointestinal surgery, trauma and alcoholic hepatitis.

Coupled Plasma Filtration Adsorption

Coupled plasma filtration adsorption is a hybrid technology which involves plasma separation followed by adsorption over sorbents.

Principle: Coupled plasma filtration adsorption (CPFA) first separates plasma from the blood by plasma filter. This plasma first circulates through sorbent, which leads to adsorption of inflammatory mediators, and finally returns to the blood, where second blood filter is used for renal support. CPFA is beneficial in gram-negative sepsis.

Emerging Therapies

Emerging therapies focus on targeting early proinflammatory and later anti-inflammatory processes on basis of better understanding of pathogenesis of SA-AKI. Various agents like peroxisome proliferator-activated receptor alpha (PPARα) agonists, endocannabinoids, inflammatory antagonists, antioxidants and cell-based therapies are underway.[10]

As sepsis induced acute kidney injury remains one of the leading causes of morbidity and mortality, it is prudent to recognize it at an early stage with newer biomarkers. This can be done by maintaining the hemodynamics, avoiding nephrotoxic agents and treating the underlying cause and source of sepsis.

CONCLUSION

Severe sepsis and shock are the common cause for acute kidney injury. Development of AKI in sepsis is associated with low mean arterial pressure. Restoration of hemodynamic by fluid resuscitation and vasoactive drugs are the basics of the management. Apart from the life threatening indications renal replacement therapy initiation is mainly clinical judgment. The short-term and long-term mortality rate in these patient are still high.

REFERENCES

1. Bellomo R, Ronco C, Kellum JA, et al. Acute Dialysis Quality Initiative workgroup. Acute renal failure—definition, outcome measures, animal models, fluid therapy and information technology needs: the Second International Consensus Conference of the Acute Dialysis Quality Initiative (ADQI) Group. Crit Care. 2004;8(4):R204-12.
2. Kidney Disease: Improving Global Outcomes (KDIGO) Acute Kidney Injury Work Group. KDIGO Clinical practice guideline for acute kidney injury. Kidney Inter. 2012;Suppl 2:1-138.
3. Singer M, Deutschman CS, Seymour CW, et al. The Third International Consensus Definitions for Sepsis and Septic Shock (Sepsis-3). JAMA. 2016;315(8):801-10.
4. Lopes JA, Jorge S, Resina C, et al. Acute kidney injury in patients with sepsis: a contemporary analysis. Int J Infect Dis. 2009;13(2):176-81.
5. Uchino S, Kellum JA, Bellomo R, et al. Acute renal failure in critically ill patients: a multinational, multicenter study. JAMA. 2005;294(7):813-8.
6. Bagshaw SM, Uchino S, Bellomo R, et al. Septic acute kidney injury in critically ill patients: clinical characteristics and outcomes. Clin J Am Soc Nephrol. 2007;2(3):431-9.
7. Wan L, Bagshaw SM, Langenberg C, et al. Pathophysiology of septic acute kidney injury; what we really know? Crit Care Med. 2008;36(4 Suppl):S198-203.
8. Zarjou A, Agarwal A. Sepsis and acute kidney injury. J Am Soc Nephrol. 2011;22(6):999-1006.
9. Godin M, Murray P, Mehta RL. Clinical approach to the patient with AKI and sepsis. Semin Nephrol. 2015;35(1);12-22.
10. Swaminathan S, Rosner M, Okusa M. Emerging therapeutic targets of sepsis-associated acute kidney injury. Semin Nephrol. 2015;35(1):38-54.

CHAPTER 59

Emergencies in Renal Failure and Dialysis Patients

Salil Jain, Sucheta Yadav

INTRODUCTION

It is not uncommon to find a patient with renal dysfunction in emergency. Though stabilization of cardiac and pulmonary status takes precedence, renal dysfunction has significant impact on patient's survival. Kidney disease in itself is a marker of poor prognosis. Acute kidney injury (AKI) if it can be prevented the mortality and morbidity of patients coming to emergency can be significantly reduced. If not detected in time, the renal injury might progress to a stage where patient might require dialysis and such severe injury ultimately results into chronic kidney disease (CKD). CKD has further implication on patient's health with increased risk of morbidity as well as mortality. Thus, timely diagnosis and management of renal emergencies is of paramount importance.

The patients presenting with renal emergency can be broadly classified in three groups:
1. Those with no known renal dysfunction in past
2. Those with known CKD or patients on hemodialysis (HD), peritoneal dialysis (PD)
3. Renal allograft recipients.

NO KNOWN RENAL DYSFUNCTION IN PAST

Acute Kidney Injury

The term acute renal failure (ARF) which was used in past has been replaced by AKI. Kidney disease improving global outcomes (KDIGO) defines AKI as an increase in serum creatinine of 0.3 mg/dL or more within 48 hours of observation or 1.5 times baseline or greater which is known or presumed to have occurred in 7 days, or a reduction in urine volume below 0.5 mL/kg/hr for 6 hours **(Table 1)**.

The causes of AKI can be divided into three broad categories **(Table 2)**:
1. Prerenal (caused by renal hypoperfusion)
2. Renal (involving: glomerulus, tubules, vessels and interstitial)
3. Postrenal (caused by obstruction of urinary tract)

Whenever we see a patient in emergency (ER), we need to integrate the findings of history, physical findings and appropriate laboratory and imaging studies to find the etiology of AKI.

History

- Events preceding AKI
- Renal or extrarenal losses (diarrhea, excessive sweating, vomiting, hemorrhage)
- Sepsis, fever, shock, dysuria or flank pain

Table 1 Kidney disease improving global outcomes (KDIGO) composite staging of acute kidney injury

Stage	Serum creatinine	Urine output
1	1.5–1.9x baseline; or ≥0.3 mg/dL (≥26 µmol/L) increase	<0.5 mL/kg/hour for 6–12 hour
2	2.0–2.9x baseline	<0.5 mL/kg/hour for ≥12 hour
3	3.0x baseline; or Increase in serum creatinine to ≥4.0 mg/dL (≥352 µmol/L); or Initiation of renal replacement therapy; OR, in patients younger than 18 years, decrease in eGFR to <35 mL/min/1.73 m²	<0.3 mL/kg/hour for ≥24 hour; or Anuria for ≥12 hour

Abbreviation: eGFR, estimated glomerular filtration rate

Table 2 Prerenal, renal and postrenal causes of acute kidney injury

PRERENAL CAUSES

Intravascular volume depletion
- Hemorrhage—trauma, surgery, postpartum, gastrointestinal
- Gastrointestinal losses—diarrhea, vomiting, nasogastric tube loss
- Renal losses—diuretic use, osmotic diuresis, diabetes insipidus
- Skin and mucous membrane losses—burns, hyperthermia
- Nephrotic syndrome
- Cirrhosis
- Capillary leak

Reduced cardiac output
- Cardiogenic shock
- Pericardial diseases—restrictive, constrictive, tamponade
- Congestive heart failure
- Valvular diseases
- Pulmonary diseases—pulmonary hypertension, pulmonary embolism
- Sepsis

Systemic vasodilation
- Sepsis
- Cirrhosis
- Anaphylaxis
- Drugs

Renal vasoconstriction
- Early sepsis
- Hepatorenal syndrome
- Actue hypercalcemia
- Drugs—norepinephrine, vasopressin, nonsteroidal anti-inflammatory drugs, angiotension-converting enzyme inhibitors, calcineurin inhibitors
- Iodinated contrast agents

RENAL CAUSES

Tubular injury	
• Ischemia due to hypoperfusion	Hypovolemia, sepsis, hemorrhage, diarrhea congestive heart failure
• Endogenous toxins	Myoglobin, hemoglobin, paraproteinemia, uric acid
• Exogenous toxins	Antibiotics, chemotherapy agents, radiocontrast agents, phosphate preparations

Tubulointerstitial injury	
• Acute allergic interstitial nephritis	Nonsteroidal anti-inflammatory drugs, antibiotics
• Infections	Viral, bacterial, and fungal infections
• Infiltration	Lymphoma, leukemia, sarcoid
• Allograft rejection	

Glomerular injury	
• Inflammation	Antiglomerular basement membrane disease, antineutrophil cytoplasmic autoantibody disease, infection, cryoglobulinemia, membranoproliferative glomerulonephritis, immunoglobin A neophropathy, systemic lupus erythematosus
• Hematologic disorders	Henoch-Schönlein purpura, polyarteritis nodosa, hemolytic uremic syndrome, thrombotic thrombocytopenic purpura, drugs

Renal microvasculature	Malignant hypertension, toxemia of pregnancy, hypercalcemia, radiocontrast agents, scleroderma, drugs

Large vessels	
• Arteries	Thrombosis, vasculitis, dissection, thromboembolism, atheroembolism, trauma
• Veins	Thrombosis, compression, trauma

Contd...

Contd...

POSTRENAL CAUSES
Upper urinary tract extrinsic causes • Retroperitoneal space—lymph nodes, tumors • Pelvic or intra-abdominal tumors—cervix, uterus, ovary, prostate • Fibrosis—radiation, drugs, inflammatory conditions • Ureteral ligation or surgical trauma • Granulomatosis diseases • Hematoma **Lower urinary tract causes** • Prostate—benign prostatic hypertrophy, carcinoma, infection • Bladder—neck obstruction, calculi, carcinoma, infection (schistosomiasis) • Functional—neurogenic bladder secondary to spinal cord injury, diabetes, multiple sclerosis, stroke, pharmacologic side effects of drugs (anticholinergics, antidepressants) • Urethral—posterior urethral valves, stricture, trauma, infections, tuberculosis, tumors
Upper urinary tract intrinsic causes • Nephrolithiasis • Strictures • Edema • Debris, blood clot, sloughed papillae, fungal ball

- Radiocontrast or nephrotoxic medication available over the counter drugs exposure [nonsteroidal anti-inflammatory drugs (NSAIDs), renin-angiotensin-aldosterone antagonists, nephrotoxic antibiotics, alternative and herbal medication]
- Snake bite, excessive exercise, rhabdomyolysis, trauma, intravascular hemolysis
- Urinary hesitancy, poor urinary stream, nocturia, pelvic or flank pain, overflow incontinence, renal colic
- Thrombosis
- Hematuria, decreased urine output, skin rash, oral ulcers, joint pains
- Recent history of aortic catheterization, endovascular procedure, atrial fibrillation
- Diabetes, hypertension, connective tissue disease, malignancy, heart disease, liver disease, pregnancy
- History of recent travel to endemic areas (e.g. malaria, schistosomiasis)
- Detailed review of past medical documents.

Physical Examination

- Assessment of volume status is the most important step. Presence of dehydration, orthostatic hypotension, poor capillary refill, tachycardia, collapsed jugular pulse point towards a prerenal cause of AKI. *But what needs to be remembered is that patient may appear volume overloaded in presence of prerenal AKI due to intravascular depletion, e.g. nephrotic syndrome, congestive heart failure, cirrhosis*
- *Abdominal examination*: Tender distended bladder, abdominal mass, bruit
- Cardiovascular examination for heart failure or possible source of emboli
- Any focus of infection
- Rash, petechiae, livedo reticularis, discolored toes, joint examination
- *Ophthalmologic examination*: Hollenhorst plaques, retinopathy.

Laboratory Investigations

- *Blood urea nitrogen (BUN)* and serum sodium, potassium, bicarbonate, and creatinine levels
- *Complete blood count and peripheral smear*: Presence of anemia can be seen in CKD, hemolysis, hemorrhage. Rouleaux formation is a pointer towards plasma cell dyscrasia. Thrombocytopenia may be seen in systemic lupus erythematosus (SLE), disseminated intravascular coagulation (DIC), thrombotic microangiopathy, and certain infections like dengue virus. Eosinophilia may be seen in atheroembolic renal disease, acute interstitial nephritis or eosinophilic granulomatosis with polyangiitis.
- *Immunological tests*: C3, antinuclear antibody (ANA), antineutrophil cytoplasmic antibodies (ANCA), ds-DNA, antistreptolysin O (ASO), anti-DNAse B, antiglomerular basement membrane (anti-GBM) antibody, cryoglobulins
- *Serum calcium, phosphate, uric acid*: Hypercalcemia can be seen in sarcoidosis, multiple myeloma, vitamin D intoxication and malignancy. Rhabdomyolysis is indicated by hyperphosphatemia, hypocalcemia, and raised serum uric acid.
- *Urine routine microscopy*: Normal urine sediment contains few cells or casts ("bland" sediment). In early prerenal AKI urine examination is normal with occasional hyaline casts. Muddy-Brown granular casts and renal tubular epithelial cells in the urine are suggestive of acute tubular necrosis (ATN)-related AKI. Presence of red blood cell (RBC) casts is diagnostic of glomerulonephritis. White

Table 3 Difference between prerenal and renal acute kidney injury

	Prerenal	Renal
History	GI, urinary, skin volume loss, blood loss, or third spacing	Drugs or toxin exposure, hemodynamic change
Clinical presentation	Hypotension or volume depletion	No specific symptoms or signs
Laboratory studies		
BUN/S_{cr}	>20	<20
Sediment	Normal to few casts	Muddy-Brown casts
U_{osm} (mmol/kg)	>500	<350
Proteinuria	None to trace	Mild to moderate
U_{Na} (mmol/L)	<20	>40
FE_{Na} (%)	<1	>1
FE_{Urea} (%)	<35	>35
Novel biomarkers	None	KIM-1, cystatin C, NGAL, CYR61, others

Abbreviations: BUN, blood urea nitrogen; GI, gastrointestinal; KIM-1, kidney injury molecule-1; NGAL, neutrophil gelatinase-associated lipocalin.

blood cell (WBC) casts indicate pyelonephritis. Broad waxy casts are often seen in CKD. Eosinophiluria may be seen in acute interstitial nephritis, cystitis, prostatitis, pyelonephritis, and atheroembolic disease. Uric acid crystals accompanying high serum phosphorus levels in a patient undergoing chemotherapy may indicate tumor lysis syndrome.

- *Urinary indices*: It includes fractional excretion of (sodium, urea and uric acid), urine sodium concentration, urine specific gravity and urine osmolarity. These are useful in presence of oliguria only and their role lies in differentiating renal from prerenal AKI, which has been summarized in the **Table 3** later.
- *USG, KUB and Doppler*: To look for size, echogenicity, corticomedullary differentiation, to rule out obstruction, renal calculi, flow and patency of renal vessels
- *Plain X-ray abdomen*: To look for radiopaque calculi and nephrocalcinosis
- *Intravenous pyelography*: Best avoided in AKI as contrast causes further worsening of renal function
- *Arteriography and venography*: For diagnosis and confirmation of renal artery and vein thrombosis
- *Renal biopsy*: Biopsy should be considered in cases of undiagnosed renal AKI after ruling out prerenal and postrenal causes by appropriate investigations.

One should be aware of the epidemiology of AKI in different settings such as community acquired, hospital setting or intensive care unit (ICU). Community acquired usually carries a better prognosis than one in critically ill patient in ICU with multiple comorbidities, where it is more likely to be multifactorial.

Differentiating AKI from CKD: Majority of the times, it is difficult to determine, if patient has AKI or AKI superimposed on pre-existing CKD. A prior report of serum creatinine is invaluable to differentiate AKI from CKD but is often unavailable in clinical practice. Other evidences which suggest CKD are small scarred kidneys on ultrasound (USG), normocytic anemia, hyperparathyroidism, hyperphosphatemia, hypocalcemia, presence of proteinuria in past, renal osteodystrophy and broad waxy casts in urine. It needs to be kept in mind that normal-sized kidneys do not exclude CKD absolutely.

Acute Kidney Injury in Specific Settings

Prerenal Azotemia

- *Clinical features*: Weight loss, thirst, tachycardia, postural hypotension, dry mucous membranes, low jugular venous pressure
- *Investigation*: Hyaline casts, FE_{Na} less than 1%, urine Na less than 10 mmol/L, urine specific gravity greater than 1.018
- *Management*: Rapid resolution of AKI with restoration of renal perfusion with intravenous fluid.

Renal Artery Thrombosis

Clinical features: History of recent myocardial infarction, atrial fibrillation, and thrombotic disorder. Such patients usually present with nausea, vomiting, hematuria and flank pain.

Investigation: Urine shows proteinuria, RBC, elevated lactate dehydrogenase (LDH), Doppler of renal vessels, renal arteriogram and magnetic resonance angiography (MRA) are diagnostic. Echocardiography to look for atrial or mural thrombi, valvular lesions should be done in all cases.

Evaluations for underlying hypercoagulable state to be done in consultation with hematologist.

Management: Systemic anticoagulation is indicated if the underlying cause is a hypercoagulable state or embolism from a central source. Patient will require renal angiography with intrarenal thrombolytic therapy or percutaneous endovascular revascularization if thrombosis is of recent onset.

Renal Vein Thrombosis

Clinical features: It may occur in setting of nephrotic syndrome, renal cell carcinoma, pulmonary embolism.

Investigation: Urine shows proteinuria and hematuria. Doppler of renal vessels and MRI venogram are diagnostic.

Management: Indication of thrombolytic is unclear. If present in association with pulmonary embolism, anticoagulation to be continued till nephrotic syndrome is present. Surgical treatment is indicated if bilateral RVT is present or if pulmonary emboli are present and anticoagulation is contraindicated. Inferior vena cava filter may be needed. Surgery will be needed if thrombosis occurs in association with renal cell carcinoma.

Atheroembolism

Clinical features: It usually occurs in elderly patients with history of recent arterial manipulation in vascular procedure. Patient may have signs and symptoms of atherosclerosis, e.g. claudication, angina, myocardial infarction, stroke, and transient ischemic attack. Spontaneous atheroembolism may occur in patients with extensive atherosclerosis with unstable plaques after administration of thrombolytic agents. Examination includes palpable purpura, subcutaneous nodules, livedo reticularis, and retinal plaques.

Investigation: Urine shows occasional casts and eosinophiluria. Other suggestive investigations are echocardiography, Doppler studies, skin biopsy and kidney biopsy. Eosinophilia and hypocomplementemia can be commonly seen in these patients.

Management: There is no specific therapy, prevention is the best strategy. Distal embolic protection device should be used if feasible. Further endovascular interventions should be avoided. Labile hypertension should be controlled with use of angiotensin-converting enzyme (ACE) inhibitors. Corticosteroids have been used with some success. Anticoagulation is to be avoided.

Acute Interstitial Nephritis

Acute interstitial nephritis (AIN) is caused by idiosyncratic allergic response to various agents. The most commonly implicated agents are drugs, with antimicrobials and NSAIDs being the most common. Other less common causes are leukemia, lymphoma, bacterial infections (e.g. *E.coli*), and viral infections [e.g. cytomegalovirus (CMV)]. Antibiotic-associated AIN commonly shows fever, rash, and eosinophiluria.

Investigation: Urine routine examination shows proteinuria usually less than a gram, microscopic hematuria and eosinophiluria.

Management: The mainstay of treatment is withdrawal of causative agent and short course of steroids.

Acute Tubular Necrosis

Clinical features: Ischemic and septic ATN is the most common cause of intrinsic or renal AKI. Diagnosis is suggested by history of recent hypotension, exposure to nephrotoxic agents or sepsis.

Investigation: Urine microscopy shows muddy brown coarse granular casts. FE_{Na} greater than 1%, UNa greater than 20 mEq/L, specific gravity 1.010. Its definitive diagnosis is made by kidney biopsy.

Management: Treatment of underlying cause and optimization of hemodynamic status.

Glomerulonephritis or Vasculitis

Clinical features: History of recent infection, sinusitis, lung hemorrhage, oral ulcers, skin rash, arthralgia, and hypertension.

Investigation: Urine routine—RBC or granular casts, RBCs, WBCs, proteinuria. Low complement levels; positive antineutrophil cytoplasmic antibodies, antiglomerular basement membrane antibodies, ASO antibodies, antideoxyribonuclease, cryoglobulins. Renal biopsy is diagnostic and should be done at the earliest.

Management: Treatment varies depending on the exact etiology and includes steroids and other immunosuppressive agents.

Malignant Hypertension

Clinical features: Presence of severe hypertension, retinopathy, headache, papilledema, and cardiac failure.

Investigation: Urine routine examination may be normal though occasionally RBCs, proteinuria and rarely RBC casts may be seen. ECG shows left ventricular hypertrophy.

Management: Patient should be shifted to ICU. Use of intravenous antihypertensive agents with close monitoring of blood pressure. Blood pressure control resolves AKI in majority of cases. Presence of altered sensorium or localizing features should prompt for a CT head to rule out intracranial bleeding or infarct.

Obstructive Nephropathy

Clinical features: Flank pain, abdominal pain, and palpable bladder

Investigation: Urine examination is usually normal but in presence of renal calculus or prostatic hypertrophy may show RBC or WBC. USG KUB (kidneys, ureters, and urinary bladder) and CT abdomen without contrast will usually reveal the cause and level of obstruction.

Management: Urgent urology opinion should be taken. Patient will require urethral catheterization, DJ stenting, percutaneous nephrostomy (PCN) depending on the level of obstruction.

Rhabdomyolysis

Clinical features: The classical triad of rhabdomyolysis consists of myalgias, generalized weakness and dark-colored urine. Physical findings may reveal muscular tenderness; crush injury, pressure necrosis of skin and soft tissue swelling.

Investigations: Blood investigations reveal high CPK, low calcium and high phosphorus level. Urine is positive for blood but no RBC is seen. Urine myoglobin should be done in suspected cases.

Treatment: Correction of inciting cause and fluid resuscitation should be initiated promptly. Urinary alkalinization, mannitol and loop diuretics are to be used. Correction of electrolyte and acid-base abnormalities may require dialysis.

Contrast Nephropathy

Clinical features: History of contrast administration 24–48 hours prior to presentation is usually present. AKI is usually nonoliguric. Other causes of renal dysfunction, e.g. cholesterol embolization should be ruled out.

Investigations: Serum creatinine starts rising within 24 hours of contrast exposure, peaks between 3 days and 5 days and returns to baseline in 7–10 days.

Treatment: Prevention is best strategy and is achieved by intravenous hydration and use of N-acetylcysteine. Once the injury has occurred, hydration should be optimized. Any further insult to kidneys by nephrotoxic agents or contrast administration should be avoided.

CHRONIC KIDNEY DISEASE/ON HEMO/ PERITONEAL DIALYSIS

Uremic Encephalopathy

Clinical features: Inadequate dialysis, drowsiness, seizure, irritability, and coma.

Investigation: Elevated urea, creatinine, metabolic acidosis, and hyperkalemia.

Management: Resolves with adequate dialysis. If BUN is greater than 100, first session of dialysis should be less than 2 hours to prevent development of dialysis disequilibrium syndrome.

Pulmonary Edema

Clinical features: History of low urine output, noncompliance to fluid restriction, inadequate dialysis, breathlessness, orthopnea, basal crepitations.

Investigation: Chest X-ray suggestive of pulmonary edema.

Management: Diuretics, injection lasix, fluid removal in dialysis and fluid restriction.

Arteriovenous Fistula Bleeding

Hemodialysis fistula is a surgically created communication between the native artery and vein in an extremity. Patients with arteriovenous fistula may rarely present with life-threatening aneurysmal rupture or bleeding.

Management: Compression at site of bleeding will stop bleeding in ER. Vascular surgeon opinion should be taken. Subsequently, patient may require ligation or banding of fistula. If heparin was given during dialysis patient may benefit from protamine.

Pericardial Effusion or Tamponade

Clinical features: Tachycardia, pulsus paradoxus, hypotension, pericardial friction rub, muffled heart sounds, jugular venous distension and positive Ewart's sign in a patient with known renal dysfunction.

Investigation: ECG and echocardiography is the imaging modality of choice.

Treatment: Pericardiocentesis is indicated in pericardial tamponade. Optimization of HD in cases of uremic pericardial effusion.

Hypertensive Encephalopathy

Auto-regulation of cerebral blood flow is maintained within specific limit, e.g. if mean arterial pressure (MAP) is maintained between 60–120 mm Hg. With increase in MAP, cerebral perfusion decreases due to cerebral vasoconstriction. At MAP 180 mm Hg autoregulation overwhelmed and cerebral edema occurs due to cerebral vasodilatation.

Hypertensive encephalopathy is acute organic brain syndrome (acute encephalopathy or delirium) occurring as result of autoregulation breakthrough.

Clinical features: Patient may present as acute or sub acute onset of lethargy, confusion, headache, visual disturbance and focal or generalized seizures.

Investigation: ECG echocardiography CT head.

Treatment: Antihypertensive agent.

Peritoneal Dialysis Peritonitis

Clinical features: Fever, abdominal pain, loose stools, cloudy peritoneal fluid, ultrafiltration failure, and hypotension.

Investigation: Peritoneal fluid microscopy, gram stain and culture, blood culture, USG abdomen to look for any loculation or catheter tunnel infection.

Management: Peritoneal and intravenous antibiotics. Peritonitis which fails to respond to treatment or fungal peritonitis will require removal of PD catheter.

RENAL ALLOGRAFT RECIPIENTS

This group of patients may present with an emergency seen in otherwise healthy person, but few emergencies are specific to this subset of patients.

Acute Rejection

Patients with acute rejection usually present with rapidly rising serum creatinine. Few factors correlated with increased risk of rejection are presence of preformed antibodies, sensitized recipient, history of multiple blood transfusions, and unrelated donor. Any history of noncompliance to medication needs to be sought. History of recent change in medication needs to be noted (e.g. initiation of enzyme inducers like rifampicin).

Investigation: Graft biopsy is the gold standard.

Management: Treatment involves intensification of immunosuppression, intravenous steroids, plasmapheresis, intravenous immunoglobulins (IVIg), bortezomib, etc.

Infection

Infection in renal allograft recipients can be a life-threatening emergency because of their immunosuppressed state. It is important to keep in mind that these patients may not show typical signs and symptoms of infection and so a high index of suspicion is needed. Infection with unusual organisms at unusual sites is not uncommon. All possible efforts should be made to diagnose the focus of infection.

Management: Empirical antibiotics to be started at the earliest after sending appropriate cultures. Antimetabolite agent should be decreased or discontinued in presence of severe life-threatening infection. A high incidence of fungal infections necessitates early initiation of antifungal in event of no response.

CONCLUSION

Renal failure is irreversible loss of renal failure resulting in accumulation of the toxins. Uremia is the clinical syndrome resulting from the renal failure and usually fatal without renal replacement therapy.

BIBLIOGRAPHY

1. Anderson RJ, Barry DW. Clinical and laboratory diagnosis of acute renal failure. Best Pract Res Clin Anaesthesiol. 2004;18(1):1-20.
2. Bellomo R, Ronco C, Kellum JA, et al. Acute renal failure-definition, outcome measures, animal models, fluid therapy and information technology needs: the Second International Consensus Conference of the Acute Dialysis Quality Initiative (ADQI) Group. Crit Care. 2004;8(4):R204-212.
3. Johnson RJ, Feehally J, Floege J. Comprehensive Clinical Nephrology, 5th edition. Canada: Elsevier; 2015. p. 1320.
4. Levin A, Warnock DJ, Mehta RL, et al. Improving outcomes from acute kidney injury: report of an initiative. Am J Kidney Dis. 2007;50(1):1-4.
5. McGee S, Abernethy WB, 3rd, Simel DL. The rational clinical examination. Is this patient hypovolemic? JAMA. 1999;281(11):1022-9.
6. Mehta RL, Kellum JA, Shah SV, et al. Acute kidney injury network: Report of an initiative to improve outcomes in acute kidney injury. Crit Care. 2007;11(2):R31.
7. Turner NN, Lameire N, Goldsmith DJ, Winearls CG, Himmelfarb J, Remuzzi G (Eds). Oxford Textbook of Nephrology, 4th edition. Oxford University Press; 2015.
8. Palevsky PM, Liu KD, Brophy PD, et al. KDOQI US commentary on the 2012 KDIGO clinical practice guideline for acute kidney injury. Am J Kidney Dis. 2013;61(5):649-72.
9. Perazella MA, Coca SG, Kanbay M, et al. Diagnostic value of urine microscopy for differential diagnosis of acute kidney injury in hospitalized patients. Clin J Am Soc Nephrol. 2008;3(6):1615-9.
10. Skorecki K, Chertow GM, Marsden PA, et al. Brenner and Rector's The Kidney, 10th edition; 2016. p. 2748.
11. Szwed JJ. Urinalysis and clinical renal disease. Am J Med Technol. 1980;46(10):720-5.
12. The Kidney Disease Improving Global Outcomes (KDIGO) Working Group. Definition and classification of acute kidney injury. Kidney Int. 2012:(Suppl 2);19-36.

CHAPTER 60

Urinary Tract Infections

Ashish Nandwani, Manish Jain

INTRODUCTION

Urinary tract infections (UTIs) are inflammatory response of the urothelium to the invading infective microorganisms leading to spectrum of clinical diseases ranging from asymptomatic bacteriuria or pyuria to acute pyelonephritis or urosepsis. Normal urine is sterile. UTI can occur in men and women of all ages and lead to significant morbidity and mortality. UTIs can be symptomatic or asymptomatic. Symptomatic UTI can involve kidney, bladder, urethra or may present as urosepsis. Early diagnosis and treatment usually lead to resolution of infection and cure of the disease; however, delay in instituting proper antibiotics may lead to pyelonephritis, pyonephrosis, or urosepsis.

INCIDENCE AND EPIDEMIOLOGY

Urinary tract infections are among the most common bacterial infectious diseases with substantial financial burden on the society. These account for more than 100,000 hospital admissions annually, most frequently for pyelonephritis. Bacteriuria is more common in young women than men; bacteria in women increases with age.[1]

Incidence is highest among young women, followed by infants and the elderly population. UTIs are also the common causes of the nosocomial infections accounting for approximately 38% of the 2 million nosocomial infections. Among these, catheter-associated UTIs are the most common due to indwelling Foley's catheter. Patients with diabetes mellitus, spinal cord disorders, multiple sclerosis, and patients on immunosuppressive drugs have increased incidence of UTIs.[2]

CLASSIFICATION AND DEFINITIONS OF URINARY TRACT INFECTIONS

Practically, UTIs have been divided in uncomplicated and complicated UTIs. UTIs are classified as:
- *Urethra*: Urethritis
- *Urinary bladder*: Cystitis
- *Kidney*: Pyelonephritis
- *Bloodstream*: Urosepsis.

Bacteriuria is the presence of bacteria in the urine, which is normally sterile. It is either due to bacterial colonization of the urothelium or contamination of specimen during collection. Bacteriuria can be symptomatic or asymptomatic.

Pyuria is the presence of white blood cells in the urine. It represents the inflammatory response of urothelium to bacterial invasion, stone or catheter. Bacteriuria without pyuria is usually indicative of bacterial colonization but not UTI. If pyuria is there without bacteriuria then evaluate for tuberculosis, stones, or malignancy.

Cystitis and *urethritis* represent the involvement of lower urinary tract by infection leading to symptoms of frequency, urgency, and dysuria.

Acute pyelonephritis is acute infection of the kidney with flank pain and fever.

Uncomplicated UTIs occur in structurally and neurologically normal urinary tract, whereas *complicated UTIs* occur in the presence of factors that predispose to persistent or relapsing infections such as structural abnormalities of urinary tract, e.g. stones, renal mass, stricture, etc. Also underlying diabetes, immunosuppressed state like organ transplant recipient, neurologic conditions causing retention of urine, pregnant women, men and children are predisposed for complicated UTI.

Some patients may have *recurrent UTI*, which may be due to relapse or reinfection. *Relapse* is recurrence of bacteriuria with the same organism.

Reinfection is recurrence of bacteriuria with different microorganism from the original infecting organism.

Urosepsis is systemic sepsis syndrome caused by UTI leading to bacteremia.

PATHOGENESIS

The human urinary tract is normally sterile and urothelium prevents invading bacteria. The high urine flow rates, various physical barrier such as the mucosal epithelium, normal vesicoureteral junction, length of urethra, local immunoglobulin A (IgA) production, antibacterial action of the prostatic fluid in male, osmolality of urine, absence of glucose, uromucoid antibacterial constituents of urine, acidic pH of urine, and low vaginal pH prevent colonization of bacteria in urinary tract. Infection of the urinary tract occurs when pathogen, often originating from bowel flora, enters urethra and ascends upwards. Although continuous cycles of urine production, storage and evacuation of bladder relentlessly expel invading organism, pathogens are able to migrate to urinary bladder and cause symptomatic cystitis or asymptomatic bacteriuria. Pyelonephritis manifests when pathogen ascends further up to kidney, colonizing tubules of the nephron. Virulence of pathogens is associated with presence of fimbriae or pili on uropathogenic strain of *Escherichia coli*. These fimbriae promote adherence to uroepithelium. Direct invasion by microorganisms from adjacent organs may take place through lymphatics such as from bowel infection or retroperitoneal abscess.[3,4]

MICROBIOLOGY

Escherichia coli is responsible for 80% of community-acquired cases of UTI and 50% of hospital-acquired UTI.[5] Other Gram-negative bacterias are *Klebsiella, Pseudomonas*, and *Proteus*. Gram-positive bacterias include *Staphylococcus saprophyticus* and *Enterococcus faecalis*.

HOST FACTORS PREDISPOSING FOR URINARY TRACT INFECTION

Host factors predisposing for UTI are:
- Urinary tract obstruction
- Vesicoureteral reflux
- Diabetes mellitus
- Immunodeficiency state
- Pregnancy
- Spinal cord injury with high pressure bladder.

CLINICAL MANIFESTATIONS OF URINARY TRACT INFECTION

Frequency, urgency, and dysuria in cystitis. Suprapubic pain and hematuria may be present in few cases.

Flank pain, renal tenderness, fever, and chills in acute pyelonephritis and is associated with bacteremia.

Diagnosis

On the basis of signs and symptoms of the cystitis or pyelonephritis and is supported by laboratory evidence of bacteriuria and/or pyuria and imaging studies.[6]

Urinalysis

Urine analysis provides the rapid method to identify bacteria and pyuria in the urine sample. Mid-stream urine sample is recommended to decrease the risk of contamination. Pyuria in the voided sample has sensitivity of 80–95% and specificity of 50–75%. Sterile pyuria may be associated with tuberculosis, staghorn calculi, and other small-sized stones. Microscopic hematuria is present in 40–60% of cases.[7,8]

Dipsticks can detect leukocyte esterase and nitrites, suggestive of active ongoing infection with sensitivity of 75% and specificity of 82% for detection of UTIs.

Urine Culture

Urine culture is used to detect the causative organism and antimicrobial susceptibility. It is important to get urine culture in cases of complicated UTI, which are recurrent or relapsing as antimicrobial resistance is rising. Colony count is useful in differentiating contamination of sample from true infection. Colony count more than 10^5 is significant and even 10^3 in symptomatic patients is diagnostic of UTI.[9]

Imaging Studies

Previously, imaging was not routinely used for the diagnosis of uncomplicated UTIs in adult patients. Computed tomography (CT) or magnetic resonance imaging (MRI) improves the diagnostic accuracy.
- To detect the structural abnormalities in urinary tract
- To detect the extent of disease and severity
- To detect the complications like renal abscess formation or pyonephrosis or perinephric collection
- To detect the site of obstruction in cases with renal or ureteric stones
- To evaluate the renal damage subsequent to resolution of acute infection.

Ultrasound

It is helpful in diagnosing renal stones, hydronephrosis, pyonephrosis, and perinephric collections. Ultrasonography (USG) is widely available at low cost, no radiation, and no contrast. However, it can miss subtle changes of mild early pyelonephritis and perinephric fat stranding. Microbubble contrast agent is used to increase the sensitivity of ultrasound to detect the early changes in pyelonephritis. Ultrasound can also detect the changes of cystitis and prostatic enlargement. Postvoid residue can also be measured by USG.

Computed Tomography

Computed tomography is the imaging study of choice and superior modality for patients with unusual presentation of pyelonephritis, nonresponders to therapy within 72 hours. It detects the radiolucent stones, renal or perinephric abscess, or emphysematous pyelonephritis. The use of intravenous contrast provides additional functional information of the kidney.

Magnetic Resonance Imaging

Magnetic resonance imaging and magnetic resonance urography (MRU) are useful in patients who are at risk for contrast-induced nephrotoxicity or have history of allergy to iodinated contrast agents. MRU can distinguish among acute pyelonephritis, renal scarring, and renal dysplasia. Diffusion-weighted sequences can differentiate between pyonephrosis and hydronephrosis.

Radionuclide Scan

Technetium-99m dimercaptosuccinic acid (^{99m}Tc DMSA) renal scintigraphy is used to detect renal scars, which are result of fibrosis following acute pyelonephritis.

Other Imaging Studies

Abdominal radiographs [kidneys, ureters, bladder (KUB) X-ray] are of very limited use nowadays and are used to detect renal stones.

MANAGEMENT OF URINARY TRACT INFECTIONS

All symptomatic UTIs need clinical and laboratory evaluation to establish the extent and severity of infection. Asymptomatic bacteriuria usually does not warrant antimicrobial treatment except in pregnant patients. All symptomatic UTIs should be confirmed by urine cultures and appropriate antibiotics should be started at the earliest. Patients with acute pyelonephritis should be evaluated for possible complications and need of parenteral antibiotic therapy.[10]

Supportive Care

In patients with UTIs, hydration of the patient is an important component of overall management. Urinary analgesic, e.g. phenazopyridine hydrochloride has little role in the management of the symptomatic UTIs.[11] Cranberry extracts have been used for symptomatic relief.

Antimicrobial Therapy

In patients with uncomplicated cystitis, the commonly used antimicrobials are:[12]
- *Nitrofurantoin*: 100 mg twice daily for 5–7 days duration
- Trimethoprim-sulfamethoxazole: One double strength tablet twice daily for 3–7 days
- Fosfomycin given as single dose (3 g)
- *Fluoroquinolones*: Ciprofloxacin, ofloxacin, and levofloxacin.

Patients with acute pyelonephritis should be evaluated for hypotension and systemic infection.[13-15] Inpatient treatment is advisable if patient has high grade fever, dysuria, and pain, and for pregnant and elderly patients. The commonly used antibiotics are:[16]
- *Fluoroquinolones*: Ofloxacin, ciprofloxacin, and levofloxacin
- *Aminoglycosides*: Amikacin
- *Extended spectrum cephalosporin*: Cefoperazone and ceftriaxone
- *Carbapenem*: Meropenem and ertapenem.

In conclusion, severity of UTIs varies from asymptomatic bacteriuria to acute pyelonephritis leading to renal dysfunction and urosepsis. Hence timely detection and treatment is necessary to prevent the morbidity and mortality. With the emergence of antibiotic resistance, detection and sensitivity pattern of pathogens are important for instituting proper antibiotic therapy. Imaging studies help in detecting underlying structural abnormalities, which may warrant urological intervention for the eradication of the infections.

REFERENCES

1. Foxman B. Epidemiology of urinary tract infections: incidence, morbidity, and economic costs. Am J Med. 2002;113 Suppl 1A:5S-13S.
2. Lo E, Nicolle L, Classen D, et al. Strategies to prevent catheter-associated urinary tract infections in acute care hospitals. Infect Control Hosp Epidemiol. 2008;29 Suppl 1:S41-50.
3. Hooton TM, Stamm WE. Diagnosis and treatment of uncomplicated urinary tract infection. Infect Dis Clin North Am. 1997;11(3):551-81.
4. Schaeffer A, Jones DM, Dunn JK. Association of in vitro E. coli adherence to vaginal and buccal epithelial cells with susceptibility of women to recurrent urinary tract infections. N Engl J Med. 1981;304(18):1062-6.
5. Johnson JR, Stamm WE. Diagnosis and treatment of acute urinary tract infections. Infect Dis Clin North Am. 1987;1(4):773-91.
6. Johnson JR, Stamm WE. Urinary tract infections in women: diagnosis and treatment. Ann Intern Med. 1989;111(11):906-17.
7. Fihn SD. Clinical practice. Acute uncomplicated urinary tract infection in women. N Engl J Med. 2003;349(3):259-66.

8. Wigton RS, Hoellerich VL, Ornato JP, et al. Use of clinical findings in the diagnosis of urinary tract infection in women. Arch Intern Med. 1985;145(12):2222-7.
9. Jenkins RD, Fenn JP, Matsen JM. Review of urine microscopy for bacteriuria. JAMA. 1986;255(24):3397-403.
10. Gupta K, Hooton TM, Naber KG, et al. International clinical practice guidelines for the treatment of acute uncomplicated cystitis and pyelonephritis in women: a 2010 update by the Infectious Diseases Society of America and the European Society for Microbiology and Infectious Diseases. Clin Infect Dis. 2011;52(5):e103-20.
11. Gupta K, Hooton TM, Stamm WE. Increasing antimicrobial resistance and the management of uncomplicated community-acquired urinary tract infections. Ann Intern Med. 2001;135(1):41-50.
12. Shimizu M, Katayama K, Kato E, et al. Evolution of acute focal bacterial nephritis into a renal abscess. Pediatr Nephrol. 2005;20(1):93-5.
13. Wan YL, Lee TY, Bullard MJ, et al. Acute gas-producing bacterial renal infection: correlation between imaging findings and clinical outcome. Radiology. 1996;198(2):433-8.
14. Shu T, Green JM, Orihuela E. Renal and perirenal abscesses in patients with otherwise anatomically normal urinary tracts. J Urol. 2004;172(1):148-50.
15. Lorentzen M, Nielsen HO. Xanthogranulomatous pyelonephritis. Scand J Urol Nephrol. 1980;14(2):193-200.
16. Esparza AR, McKay DB, Cronan JJ, et al. Renal parenchymal malakoplakia: Histologic spectrum and its relationship to megalocytic interstitial nephritis and xanthogranulomatous pyelonephritis. Am J Surg Pathol. 1989;13(3):225-36.

CHAPTER 61

Hematuria

Puneet Ahluwalia, Varun Mittal, Rajiv Yadav

INTRODUCTION

"Hematuria" in simple term means "blood in urine". In normal urine less than 3 RBCs/hpf (per high-power field) can be present. Isolated hematuria can sometimes be observed without any associated obvious underlying condition (e.g. cystitis, ureteral stone) or may the presenting symptoms of a serious condition like underlying malignancy in urinary tract. The cause for hematuria (and the tests needed for evaluation) vary with the age of presentation. Therefore, it is important to know the basic "workup" of the patient presenting with this symptom.

DEFINITION OF HEMATURIA

Hematuria may be classified as:
- *Gross hematuria* (macroscopic hematuria or which is visible to naked eyes) or
- *Microscopic hematuria* (detected only on urine examination) **(Flow chart 1)**.

Gross Hematuria

Gross hematuria is suspected in patients with history of passing red or brown-colored urine. Patients with gross hematuria are usually frightened by the sudden onset of blood in the urine and frequently present to the emergency department for evaluation, fearing that they may be bleeding excessively. Therefore, a detailed history of consumption of any coloring agent or medications should be taken. Gross hematuria, however, with passage of clots almost always indicates a lower urinary tract source.

Microscopic Hematuria

Microscopic hematuria when blood [either red blood cells (RBCs) or hemoglobin] is found on a laboratory urine examination or dipstick test. Repeated episodes of microscopic hematuria need evaluation. The level of investigation depends upon the risk profile of patient and the level of suspicion regarding the presence of urinary tract abnormality. Although the presence of 3 or more RBCs/hpf in a spun urine sediment is considered abnormal, there is no "safe" lower limit below which significant disease can be excluded.

CONFIRMATION OF HEMATURIA

Urine Examination

First step in any patient presenting with suspected hematuria is to confirm the finding with urine examination. A simple and easily available "dipstick test" is the first step. A positive dipstick for blood in the urine most commonly indicates *either of the three conditions*: (1) hematuria, (2) hemoglobinuria, or (3) myoglobinuria. Peroxidase-like activity of hemoglobin detects the presence of blood in urine and leads to change in color as per the degree and amount of oxidation.

Hemoglobinuria and myoglobinuria can be distinguished from hematuria by the microscopic examination of centrifuged urine. The diagnosis of hematuria is established by the presence of a large number of erythrocytes. Examination of the serum, in the absence of erythrocytes in urine, distinguishes hemoglobinuria from myoglobinuria. In centrifuged specimen, pink supernatant indicates hemoglobinuria. This is due to affinity of free hemoglobin in the serum to bind haptoglobin. The complex has a high-molecular weight, is water insoluble and remains in the serum, causing a pink color. Once all the haptoglobin-binding sites are saturated, free hemoglobin appears in the urine. Myoglobin on the other hand is of low-molecular weight and is water soluble.

Hematuria, defined as more than 3 RBCs/hpf can be identified with urinary dipsticks with sensitivity of more

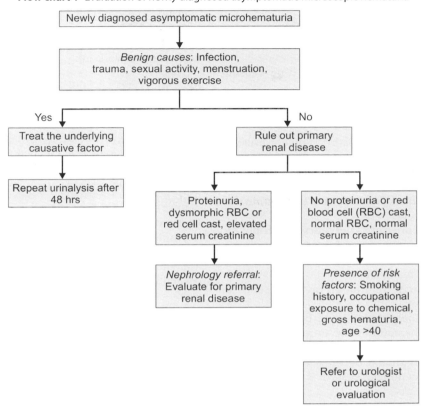

Flow chart 1 Evaluation of newly diagnosed asymptomatic microscopic hematuria

than 90%. Conversely, dipstick method has a high false-positive rate for hematuria leading to lower *specificity as compared with microscopy*. Contamination of the urine specimen with menstrual blood is the most common cause of false-positive dipstick results. Increased concentration of erythrocytes and hemoglobin in dehydration with resultant high specific gravity urine is another cause of false-positive result. First morning voided specimen is also more likely to yield false-positive result due to high specific gravity. Vigorous exercise can sometimes increase the number of erythrocytes in the urine leading to false-positive results. Efficacy of dipstick in hematuria screening to identify significant urologic disease remains somewhat controversial. Confirmation of dipstick result with microscopic examination of the centrifuged urinary sediment is imperative before proceeding to more complicated studies.

HISTORY AND INITIAL EVALUATION

In the initial evaluation of hematuria, several questions should always be asked. The answers to the following questions will enable the urologist to target the subsequent diagnostic evaluation efficiently:

- *Gross or microscopic hematuria*: Patients with gross hematuria generally have definitive pathology while negative evaluation in microscopic hematuria.
- *Hematuria occurs in beginning or end of stream or during entire stream*: Initial hematuria due to urethral inflammation, terminal hematuria due to bladder neck or prostatic urethra inflammation, and total hematuria mainly due to bladder and upper urinary tract inflammation.
- *Pain with hematuria*: It signify inflammation (cystitis) or obstruction (clots, calculi).
- *Any clots with hematuria*: If present, it is significant hematuria.
- *Transient or persistent hematuria*: Transient microscopic hematuria is a common problem in adults. In most patients with transient hematuria, no obvious etiology is identified. Fever, infection, trauma, and exercise are potential causes of transient hematuria. Transient hematuria can also occur with urinary tract infection (UTI) (e.g. cystitis or prostatitis). In this setting, hematuria is typically accompanied by pyuria and bacteriuria and patients often complain of dysuria. Typically benign nature of transient hematuria occurs in older patients (40 years of age) in whom even transient hematuria carries an increased risk of malignancy.

It cannot be overemphasized that hematuria should be considered as symptom of malignancy until proved otherwise, particularly in the adults. Presence of hematuria in adults mandates immediate urologic examination. Bladder

cancer is the most common cause of gross hematuria in a patients older than age 50 years.
- *Glomerular or nonglomerular hematuria*: Dysmorphic RBCs protein more than 500 mg/day and brown and cola-colored urine
- *Medication history*: Anticoagulation and drug causing nephritis cause hematuria.

SOME CLUES

Immunoglobulin A (IgA) nephropathy (Berger disease): Children and young adult (male) having low-grade fever. Hereditary nephritis, polycystic kidney disease, or sickle cell disease—family history.
- Ureteral obstruction, flank pain radiating to the groin due to a calculus or blood clot
- Prostatic obstruction, present as hesitancy and dribbling, may be present in older men
- Urinary tract infection, pyuria, and dysuria but may also be present in bladder malignancy
- Recent vigorous exercise or trauma in the absence of another possible cause.
- Endometriosis of urinary tract should be suspected in women with cyclic hematuria that is most prominent during and shortly after menstruation. Contamination with menstrual blood should be ruled out by a repeat sample when menstruation has ceased.

STEPWISE APPROACH FOR EVALUATION

Hematuria may be due to variety of causes. Urolithiasis, UTI, neoplasms of the urinary tract (including both renal cell carcinoma and urothelial tumors), urinary tract trauma, and medical renal disease are among the more common causes.

Step I: Rule Out Benign Causes

History, physical examination, and laboratory examination to rule out benign causes such as infection, menstruation, vigorous exercise, medical renal disease, viral illness, trauma, or recent urological procedures. If a "benign" cause for microscopic hematuria is suspected, the patient should undergo repeat urinalysis 48 hours after cessation of the activity.

Urine Culture

In patients with bacteriuria or pyuria, a urine culture should be ordered to confirm UTI.

Step II: Baseline Renal Function: Evaluation for Primary Renal Disease

Estimate of renal function including serum creatinine, blood urea nitrogen, and calculated estimated glomerular filtration rate (eGFR) is obtained once benign causes are excluded.

Contrast or gadolinium radiologic studies are contraindicated in patients with renal dysfunction.

The presence of any of the parameters suggestive of renal parenchymal or glomerular disease warrants concurrent nephrological work-up.

Step III: Urological Evaluation (Flow chart 2)

Urine Cytology

Urinary cytology or cystoscopy may be used. Cystoscopy is required, if cytology shows malignant or atypical/suspicious cells.

Imaging

In a patient with otherwise unexplained hematuria, once nephrological or glomerular causes of bleeding are excluded, the diagnostic workup should be directed toward urological evaluation and include a search for lesions in the kidney, collecting system, ureters, bladder or urethra. The diagnostic yield is directly proportional to age and may be higher for gross hematuria than for microscopic hematuria.

Computed Tomography Urography

Computed tomography urography is the investigation of choice for evaluation of hematuria.

Magnetic Resonance Urography

For patients with relative or absolute contraindications that preclude use of multiphasic computed tomography (CT) (such as renal insufficiency, contrast allergy, pregnancy), magnetic resonance urography (MRU) [without or with intravenous (IV) contrast] is an acceptable alternative imaging approach.

Intravenous Pyelography

Intravenous pyelography (IVP) is less sensitive in detecting kidney stones and renal masses (particularly small masses) and has largely been replaced with CT urography. Some clinicians believe that IVP is best able to characterize lesions in the urothelium. However, increasing evidence suggests detection rates for urothelial neoplasm with IVP are between 40% and 65%.

Ultrasonography

Ultrasonography is excellent for detection and characterization of renal cysts but is less sensitive in detecting transitional cell carcinoma, small solid lesions (<3 cm), and calculi.

However, the combination of ultrasonography and CT may improve the characterization of small-sized renal masses.

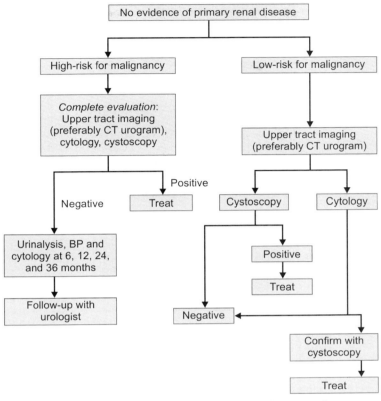

Flow chart 2 Urologic evaluation of hematuria

Abbreviations: BP, blood pressure; CT, computed tomography.

ROLE OF CYSTOSCOPY

Gross Hematuria

Patients who have gross (macroscopic) hematuria without any evidence of either glomerular disease or infection should undergo cystoscopy, since it permits direct visualization of bladder and can detect malignant or other sources of bleeding. Cystoscopy should also be done in patients who have gross hematuria with blood clots even if they have evidence of a glomerular lesion since blood clots are virtually never associated with glomerular bleeding. The presence of blood clots in these patients suggests the concurrent presence of disease in the upper or lower collecting system **(Flow chart 3)**.

Microscopic Hematuria

Cystoscopy should also be done in all patients with microscopic hematuria who have no evidence of glomerular disease or other benign causes such as infection or exercise and who are at increased risk for malignancy.

Cystoscopy allows visualizing entire bladder wall for malignancy or any other abnormality. Cystoscopy may also identify the source of the bleeding among patients with gross hematuria. Moreover, cystoscopy is the only modality that permits visualization of the prostate and urethra **(Flow chart 4)**.

Unexplained Hematuria

In cases of unexplained hematuria, particularly in young and middle-aged patients, glomerular disease or a stone disease is the most likely reason of isolated hematuria. In these patients with persistent isolated hematuria, evaluation with history, cystoscopy and imaging is often not conclusive and may be normal.

FOLLOW-UP AFTER INITIAL NEGATIVE EVALUATION

Patients who have a negative evaluation for hematuria generally require follow-up with cytology, urinalysis, blood pressure monitoring, and in some cases with repeat imaging and cystoscopy. The necessity for repeat imaging and cystoscopy largely depends upon whether hematuria was transient or persistent, and upon the patient's risk for malignancy.

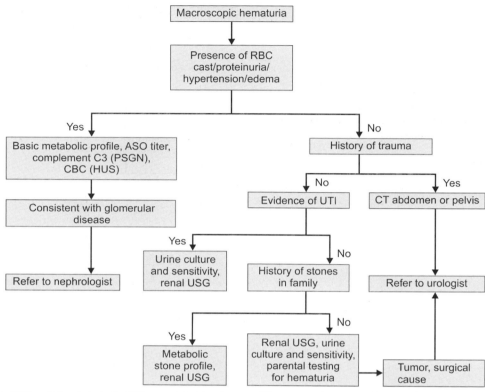

Flow chart 3 Evaluation of macroscopic hematuria in children

Abbreviations: ASO, antistreptolysin O; CBC, complete blood count; CT, computed tomography; HUS, hemolytic-uremic syndrome; PSGN, poststreptococcal glomerulonephritis; RBC, red blood cell; USG, ultrasonography; UTI, urinary tract infection.

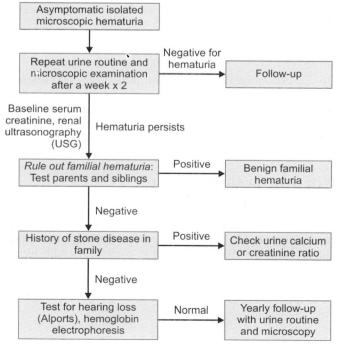

Flow chart 4 Evaluation of asymptomatic isolated microscopic hematuria in a child

Follow-up of Patients with Transient Hematuria

Patients who have even one episode of hematuria and are at high-risk for malignancy require close follow-up following a negative evaluation.

Follow-up of in Cases of Persistent Hematuria

In a patient with unexplained persistent hematuria, it is imperative to rule out the presence of an underlying malignancy. An undiagnosed carcinoma is potentially the most serious disorder in these patients. The combination of negative imaging, cytology, and cystoscopy most likely rules out the presence of a malignant pathology. However, in few patients, careful follow-up is necessary to reveal the cause of persistent hematuria. Recommended follow-up for patients with asymptomatic microhematuria includes monitoring with annual urinalysis.

- If two consecutive annual urinalysis are negative in patients with persistent asymptomatic microhematuria, then the follow-up can be concluded
- Complete initial urological workup is recommended if microhematuria persists for 3–5 years.

CONCLUSION

Hematuria may signify disease anywhere in the genitourinary symptoms or may be sign of nonurologic disease or may be factitious. Many conditions causing hematuria but systematic approach makes the differential diagnosis simple.

Hematuria with proteinuria suggest glomerular diasease while painless hematuria without the proteinuria suggest coagulation disorders, structural abnormalities, and malignancy. If initial evaluation remain inconclusive, imaging studies and cystoscopy are necessary.

BIBLIOGRAPHY

1. Amendola MA, Bree RL, Pollack HM, et al. Small renal cell carcinomas: resolving a diagnostic dilemma. Radiology. 1988;166(3):637-41.
2. Andres A, Praga M, Bello I, et al. Hematuria due to hypercalciuria and hyperuricosuria in adult patients. Kidney Int. 1989;36(1):96-9.
3. Britton JP, Dowell AC, Whelan P. Dipstick haematuria and bladder cancer in men over 60: results of a community study. BMJ. 1989;299(6706):1010-2.
4. Browne RF, Meehan CP, Colville J, et al. Transitional cell carcinoma of the upper urinary tract: spectrum of imaging findings. Radiographics. 2005;25(6):1609-27.
5. Caoili EM, Cohan RH, Korobkin M, et al. Urinary tract abnormalities: initial experience with multi-detector row CT urography. Radiology. 2002;222(2):353-60.
6. Case records of the Massachusetts General Hospital. Weekly clinicopathological exercises. Case 33-1992. A 34-year-old woman with endometriosis and bilateral hydronephrosis. N Engl J Med. 1992;327(7):481-5.
7. Collar JE, Ladva S, Cairns TD, et al. Red cell traverse through thin glomerular basement membranes. Kidney Int. 2001;59(6):2069-72.
8. Cowan NC, Turney BW, Taylor NJ, et al. Multidetector computed tomography urography for diagnosing upper urinary tract urothelial tumour. BJU Int. 2007;99(6):1363-70.
9. Culclasure TF, Bray VJ, Hasbargen JA. The significance of hematuria in the anticoagulated patient. Arch Intern Med. 1994;154(6):649-52.
10. American Urological Association (AUA) (2017). Diagnosis, evaluation, and follow-up of asymptomatic microhematuria (AMH) in adults. [online] Available from www.auanet.org/content/media/asymptomatic_microhematuria_guideline.pdf. [Accessed February, 2017].
11. Ezz el Din K, Koch WF, de Wildt MJ, et al. The predictive value of microscopic haematuria in patients with lower urinary tract symptoms and benign prostatic hyperplasia. Eur Urol. 1996;30(4):409-13.
12. Fowler KA, Locken JA, Duchesne JH, et al. US for detecting renal calculi with nonenhanced CT as a reference standard. Radiology. 2002;222(1):109-13.
13. Froom P, Ribak J, Benbassat J. Significance of microhaematuria in young adults. Br Med J (Clin Res Ed). 1984;288(6410):20-2.
14. Gray Sears CL, Ward JF, Sears ST, et al. Prospective comparison of computerized tomography and excretory urography in the initial evaluation of asymptomatic microhematuria. J Urol. 2002;168(6):2457-60.
15. Grossfeld GD, Wolf JS, Litwan MS, et al. Asymptomatic microscopic hematuria in adults: summary of the AUA best practice policy recommendations. Am Fam Physician. 2001;63(6):1145-54.
16. Hall CL, Bradley R, Kerr A, et al. Clinical value of renal biopsy in patients with asymptomatic microscopic hematuria with and without low-grade proteinuria. Clin Nephrol. 2004;62(4):267-72.
17. Hebert L. Glomerular diseases: The American College of Physicians Nephrology Medical Knowledge Self Assessment Program (MKSAP). Philadelphia: American College of Physicians-American Society of Internal Medicine; 1998.
18. Iseki K, Miyasato F, Uehara H, et al. Outcome study of renal biopsy patients in Okinawa, Japan. Kidney Int. 2004;66(3):914-9.
19. Jamis-Dow CA, Choyke PL, Jennings SB, et al. Small (< or = 3 cm) renal masses: detection with CT versus US and pathologic correlation. Radiology. 1996;198(3):785-8.
20. Kalra MK, Maher MM, Sahani DV, et al. Current status of multidetector computed tomography urography in imaging of the urinary tract. Curr Probl Diagn Radiol. 2002;31(5):210-21.
21. Kawashima A, Glockner JF, King BF. CT urography and MR urography. Radiol Clin North Am. 2003;41(5):945-61.
22. Khadra MH, Pickard RS, Charlton M, et al. A prospective analysis of 1,930 patients with hematuria to evaluate current diagnostic practice. J Urol. 2000;163(2):524-7.
23. Kluner C, Hein PA, Gralla O, et al. Does ultra-low-dose CT with a radiation dose equivalent to that of KUB suffice to detect renal and ureteral calculi? J Comput Assist Tomogr. 2006;30(1):44-50.
24. Leyendecker JR, Gianini JW. Magnetic resonance urography. Abdom Imaging. 2009;34(4):527-40.
25. Lisanti CJ, Toffoli TJ, Stringer MT, et al. CT evaluation of the upper urinary tract in adults younger than 50 years with asymptomatic microscopic hematuria: is IV contrast enhancement needed? Am J Roentgenol. 2014;203(3):615-9.
26. Loo RK, Lieberman SF, Slezak JM, et al. Stratifying risk of urinary tract malignant tumors in patients with asymptomatic microscopic hematuria. Mayo Clin Proc. 2013;88(2):129-38.
27. Maher MM, Kalra MK, Rizzo S, et al. Multidetector CT urography in imaging of the urinary tract in patients with hematuria. Korean J Radiol. 2004;5(1):1-10.
28. Mariani AJ, Mariani MC, Macchioni C, et al. The significance of adult hematuria: 1,000 hematuria evaluations including a risk-benefit and cost-effectiveness analysis. J Urol. 1989;141(2):350-5.
29. McGregor DO, Lynn KL, Bailey RR, et al. Clinical audit of the use of renal biopsy in the management of isolated microscopic hematuria. Clin Nephrol. 1998;49(6):345-8.
30. Messing EM, Young TB, Hunt VB, et al. Home screening for hematuria: results of a multiclinic study. J Urol. 1992;148 (2 Pt 1):289-92.
31. Messing EM, Young TB, Hunt VB, et al. The significance of asymptomatic microhematuria in men 50 or more years old: findings of a home screening study using urinary dipsticks. J Urol. 1987;137(5):919-22.
32. Miller MI, Puchner PJ. Effects of finasteride on hematuria associated with benign prostatic hyperplasia: long-term follow-up. Urology. 1998;51(2):237-40.

33. Mohr DN, Offord KP, Melton LJ. Isolated asymptomatic microhematuria: a cross-sectional analysis of test-positive and test-negative patients. J Gen Intern Med. 1987;2(5):318-24.
34. Mohr DN, Offord KP, Owen RA, et al. Asymptomatic microhematuria and urologic disease. A population-based study. JAMA. 1986;256(2):224-9.
35. Murakami S, Igarashi T, Hara S, et al. Strategies for asymptomatic microscopic hematuria: a prospective study of 1,034 patients. J Urol. 1990;144(1):99-101.
36. Nakamura K, Kasraeian A, Iczkowski KA, et al. Utility of serial urinary cytology in the initial evaluation of the patient with microscopic hematuria. BMC Urol. 2009;9:12.
37. Nieuwhof C, Doorenbos C, Grave W, et al. A prospective study of the natural history of idiopathic non-proteinuric hematuria. Kidney Int. 1996;49(1):222-5.
38. O'Connor OJ, McSweeney SE, Maher MM. Imaging of hematuria. Radiol Clin North Am. 2008;46(1):113-32.
39. Piper JM, Tonascia J, Matanoski GM. Heavy phenacetin use and bladder cancer in women aged 20 to 49 years. N Engl J Med. 1985;313(5):292-5.
40. Praga M, Alegre R, Hernández E, et al. Familial microscopic hematuria caused by hypercalciuria and hyperuricosuria. Am J Kidney Dis. 2000;35(1):141-5.
41. Rodgers M, Nixon J, Hempel S, et al. Diagnostic tests and algorithms used in the investigation of haematuria: systematic reviews and economic evaluation. Health Technol Assess. 2006;10(18):iii-iv.
42. Schröder FH. Microscopic haematuria. BMJ. 1994;309(6947):70-2.
43. Shaw ST, Poon SY, Wong ET. 'Routine urinalysis'. Is the dipstick enough? JAMA. 1985;253(11):1596-600.
44. Sigala JF, Biava CG, Hulter HN. Red blood cell casts in acute interstitial nephritis. Arch Intern Med. 1978;138(9):1419-21.
45. Silverman SG, Leyendecker JR, Amis ES. What is the current role of CT urography and MR urography in the evaluation of the urinary tract? Radiology. 2009;250(2):309-23.
46. Sutton JM. Evaluation of hematuria in adults. JAMA. 1990;263(18):2475-80.
47. Szeto CC, Lai FM, To KF, et al. The natural history of immunoglobulin a nephropathy among patients with hematuria and minimal proteinuria. Am J Med. 2001;110(6):434-7.
48. Tiebosch AT, Frederik PM, van Breda Vriesman PJ, et al. Thin-basement-membrane nephropathy in adults with persistent hematuria. N Engl J Med. 1989;320(1):14-8.
49. Topham PS, Harper SJ, Furness PN, et al. Glomerular disease as a cause of isolated microscopic haematuria. Q J Med. 1994;87(6):329-35.
50. Tsili AC, Efremidis SC, Kalef-Ezra J, et al. Multi-detector row CT urography on a 16-row CT scanner in the evaluation of urothelial tumors. Eur Radiol. 2007;17(4):1046-54.
51. van Paassen P, van Breda Vriesman PJ, van Rie H, et al. Signs and symptoms of thin basement membrane nephropathy: a prospective regional study on primary glomerular disease-The Limburg Renal Registry. Kidney Int. 2004;66(3):909-13.
52. Warshauer DM, McCarthy SM, Street L, et al. Detection of renal masses: sensitivities and specificities of excretory urography/linear tomography, US, and CT. Radiology. 1988;169(2):363-5.

CHAPTER 62

Acute Urinary Retention

Rakesh Khera, Varun Mittal, Puneet Ahluwalia

INTRODUCTION

Acute urinary retention (AUR) is the sudden painful inability to void, with relief of pain following drainage of bladder. It is one of the most common emergencies encountered in urology.[1] A combination of reduced or absent urine output with lower abdominal pain is not enough to make a diagnosis of AUR. Sometimes, a surgical condition with lower abdominal pain and reduced urine output due to fluid depletion can give a false impression of AUR. Therefore, central to the diagnosis of AUR is the presence of large volume of urine. What actually defines this large volume has not been strictly described but volumes of 500–800 mL are typical. In men, the most common cause of AUR is benign prostatic hyperplasia (BPH). AUR is rarely encountered in women.[2] It is imperative to know the etiopathogenesis and management of AUR. The present chapter focuses on both the aspects.

EPIDEMIOLOGY

Acute urinary retention is common in men. The incidence increases with age, occurring most frequently in men over age 60 years.[2-4] The reported incidence is about 0.5–2.5% person years. The risk is cumulative and increases with age. It is estimated that over a 5-year period, approximately 10% of men over the age of 70 years and almost one-third of men in their 80s will develop AUR.[2] In contrast, women rarely present with AUR.[5] It is estimated that there are 3 cases of AUR per 100,000 women per year.[6] The female to male incidence rate ratio is 1:13.[7]

ETIOPATHOGENESIS

Various pathophysiologic mechanisms play a role in the development of AUR. There is no specific etiology and usually it is multifactorial. Etiologic factors responsible for AUR are divided into following broad categories:[8]
- *Obstructive causes*: Outflow obstruction with increased urethral resistance.
- *Neurogenic causes*: Neurologic impairment, interruption of sensory or motor innervations of the bladder.
- *Myogenic causes*: Inefficient detrusor muscle contraction with low bladder pressure.
- Others.

Outflow Obstruction

Obstruction is the most common cause of AUR. A range of mechanical and dynamic factors are responsible for the outflow obstruction. Mechanical obstruction refers to a physical narrowing at any level in urethral channel from bladder neck to external urethral meatus.[9] Dynamic obstruction refers to increased sphincteric activity with increased muscle tone within and around the urethra.[8]

In men, the most common cause of obstruction is bladder outlet obstruction due to BPH.[10] In a study of 310 men over a 2-year period, urinary retention was caused by BPH in 53% of patients. Other obstructive causes accounted for another 23%.[8] Risk factors for developing AUR in patients with BPH include advanced age, severity of lower urinary tract symptoms (LUTS), enlarged prostate gland and decreased urinary flow rate.[4,11]

Age

Several well-controlled studies provided considerable insights into the risk factors for AUR. Perhaps the most significant of these risk factors is age. Studies demonstrate a nearly linear increase in the age-specific incidence of AUR for men ranging in age from 40 years to older than 80 years.[12]

Lower Urinary Tract Symptoms

Increased symptom severity is associated with increased risk of AUR in several large population-based or cohort studies. The Olmsted County study focused on age, symptom severity, maximum flow rate and prostate volume. Incidence rates per 1,000 patient year increased from 2.6 to 9.3 for men in their 40s to their 70s if they had mild symptoms and from 3.0 to 34.7 if they had more than mild symptoms.[13]

Urodynamic Parameters

The relative risk increased for older men, men with moderate to severe symptoms (3.2×), those with a flow rate under 12 mL/sec (3.9 times) and those with a prostate volume greater than 30 mL by real-time transrectal ultrasonography (TRUS) (3.0 times), all compared with a baseline risk of 1.0 time for the corresponding groups.

Prostate Volume and Serum Prostatic Specific Antigen Levels

In the Proscar Long-term Efficacy and Safety Study (PLESS) and Medical Therapy of Prostatic Symptoms (MTOPS) study, a linear relationship between risk of AUR and prostate volume and serum prostatic specific antigen (PSA) has been demonstrated. An analysis revealed a combination of factors such as serum PSA, frequency, symptom severity index, maximum urinary flow rate and hesitancy as being only slightly superior to PSA alone in predicting AUR.[14]

Other causes of outflow obstruction in men include urethral stricture, urolithiasis, cancer prostate, phimosis, or paraphimosis and bladder cancer. Urinary retention from bladder tumors is usually caused by blood clots from intravesicular bleeding and often presents with painless hematuria.[15]

In women, obstruction is generally secondary to anatomic distortion due to various reasons as pelvic organ prolapsed, pelvic masses, or rarely urethral diverticulum.

Fecal impaction and gastrointestinal or retroperitoneal masses large enough to cause extrinsic bladder neck compression can also sometimes present with retention of urine **(Table 1)**.

Neurologic Impairment

Normal functioning of the bladder and lower urinary tract depends on a complex interaction between the brain, autonomic nervous system, and somatic nerves supplying the bladder and urethra.[3] Interruption along these pathways can result in unsustained detrusor muscle contraction or incomplete relaxation of sphincter leading to urinary retention. Neurogenic or neuropathic bladder is defined as any defective functioning of the bladder muscle due to impaired innervation. Urinary retention from neurologic causes occurs equally in both sexes. Although most patients with neurogenic bladder experience incontinence, a significant number might also have urinary retention.[16] Up to 56% of patients who have suffered a stroke experience urinary retention, primarily because of detrusor hyporeflexia. In a prospective study, 23 out of 80 patients with ischemic stroke developed AUR. AUR can occur with spinal cord injuries from trauma, infarct or demyelination, epidural abscess and epidural metastasis, Guillain-Barré syndrome, diabetic neuropathy and stroke.[9] Up to 45% of patients with diabetes mellitus and 75–100% of patients with diabetic peripheral neuropathy experience bladder dysfunction and include urinary retention.[17] Voiding dysfunction tends to correlate with the severity of multiple sclerosis and occurs in up to 80% of patients, with urinary retention being present in approximately 20%.[18] AUR is typically accompanied by back pain and/or other neurologic deficits **(Table 2)**.

Table 1 Obstructive causes of acute urinary retention

Sex	Etiology
Males	- Benign prostatic hyperplasia - Meatal stenosis - Urethral stricture - Phimosis - Paraphimosis
Females	- Pelvic organ prolapse (cystocele, rectocele, uterine prolapse) - Pelvic mass (gynecologic malignancy, uterine fibroid, ovarian cyst) - Retroverted impacted gravid uterus
Both	- Urolithiasis (bladder stone) - Bladder tumor - Constipation with fecal impaction - Retroperitoneal mass - Gastrointestinal malignancy - Foreign body

Inefficient Detrusor Muscle

Inefficient detrusor contraction leading to AUR can be due to multiple factors including neurologic disease as mentioned earlier affecting the detrusor contraction or long-standing untreated obstruction leading to detrusor failure. Sometimes a precipitating event results in an acute distended bladder (e.g. with a fluid challenge, during general or epidural analgesia without an indwelling catheter).[8,9,19] This most often occurs in patients with some unrecognized obstructive urinary symptoms at baseline.

Other Causes

Acute urinary retention is most often secondary to mechanical outflow obstruction.[10] Other etiologies include medication,

Table 2 Neurogenic causes of acute urinary retention	
Neurologic level	Etiology
Autonomic system	• Autonomic neuropathy • Dabetes mellitus • Guillain-Barré syndrome • Herpes zoster virus • Lyme disease • Pernicious anemia • Poliomyelitis • Radical pelvic surgery • Sacral agenesis • Spinal cord trauma • Tabes dorsalis
Brain	• Cerebrovascular episode • Multiple sclerosis • Brain tumor • Hydrocephalus • Parkinson's disease • Shy-Drager syndrome
Spinal cord	• Intervertebral disk disease • Dysraphic lesions • Spina bifida occulta • Meningomyelocele • Multiple sclerosis • Spinal cord hematoma or abscess • Spinal cord trauma • Spinal stenosis • Transverse myelitis • Conus medullaris or cauda equina tumors or masses

Table 3 Infectious causes of acute urinary retention	
Sex	Etiology
Males	• Prostatitis • Prostatic abscess • Periurethral abscess • Balanitis
Females	• Acute vulvovaginitis • Vaginal lichen planus • Vaginal lichen sclerosis • Vaginal pemphigus
Both	• Urethritis • Bacterial cystitis • Tubercular cystitis • Guillain-Barré syndrome • Herpes simplex virus encephalitis • Varicella zoster virus • Lyme disease • Transverse myelitis • Bilharziasis • Echinococcosis

infection, trauma, postoperative and pregnancy-related urine retention.

Medications

Multiple medications are implicated as a cause of urinary retention; most common among these are the anticholinergic and sympathomimetic drugs.[20] These medications lead to AUR through a variety of mechanisms. Patients taking opioids and anticholinergic medications are at higher risk for AUR due to decreased bladder sensation. Anticholinergic medications also reduce detrusor contractility.[21] Nasal decongestants that contain sympathomimetic agents increase smooth muscle tone in the region of the bladder neck. Nonsteroidal anti-inflammatory drugs (NSAIDs) are sometimes responsible for AUR. NSAID-induced urinary retention is thought to occur by inhibition of prostaglandin-mediated detrusor muscle contraction.[22]

Infection

Infections may lead to AUR in the setting of inflammation that causes obstruction. The most common cause of infectious AUR is acute prostatitis. Acute prostatitis is usually caused by gram-negative organisms, such as *Escherichia coli* and *Proteus* species, and results in swelling of the acutely inflamed gland.[23] For example, an acutely inflamed prostate gland from acute prostatitis can cause AUR, particularly in men who already have BPH. Urethritis from urinary tract infection (UTI) or urethritis can cause urethral edema and can result in AUR. Genital herpes may cause AUR both from local inflammation as well as sacral nerve involvement. Other infections that have been associated with AUR include varicella zoster and vulvovaginitis (**Table 3**).[24]

Trauma

Patients with trauma to the pelvis, urethra, or penis may develop AUR from mechanical disruption. AUR may also occur in postoperative period (**Table 4**).[9]

Postoperative Urinary Retention

Multiple factors as pain, traumatic instrumentation, bladder over distension and pharmacological agents (particularly opioid narcotics, prazosin) thought to play a role. After rectal surgery, patients will experience urinary retention up to 70% of the time.[25] As many as 78% of patients who have had total hip arthroplasty and up to 25% of patients who have had outpatient gynecologic surgery will develop urinary retention.[26,27] During hemorrhoidectomy, the use of selective pudendal nerve block rather than spinal anesthesia may decrease urinary retention (**Table 4**).

Pregnancy-associated Urinary Retention

Urinary retention during pregnancy is usually the result of an impacted retroverted uterus obstructing the internal

Table 4	Other causes of acute urinary retention
Sex	Etiology
Males	Penile trauma
Females	Pregnancy associated Postpartum complication External urethral sphincter dysfunction
Both	• Disruption of posterior urethra and or bladder neck in pelvic fracture • Postoperative complication • Psychogenic cause

urethral meatus and is most often encountered at 16 weeks' gestation.[28] In postpartum period, the incidence of AUR is reported to be 1.7–17.9%. Risk factors include nulliparity, prolonged labor, instrumental delivery, epidural anesthesia and cesarean section **(Table 4)**.[24,29,30]

From a clinical and prognostic point of view, AUR has been divided into two broad categories: (1) spontaneous and (2) precipitated. Precipitated AUR refers to the inability to urinate after a triggering event such as nonprostate-related surgery, e.g. hemorrhoidectomy, catheterization, anesthesia, ingestion of drugs as sympathomimetic, anticholinergics or antihistamines, excessive fluid intake, etc. All other episodes of AUR are classified as spontaneous AUR. The clinical significance of differentiating the two types of AUR lies in the final outcomes of these patients. In a study by Roehborn et al. after an episode of spontaneous AUR, 15% of patients had another episode of spontaneous AUR and a total of 75% underwent surgery, whereas after precipitated AUR only 9% had an episode of spontaneous AUR, and 26% underwent surgery.[24,31]

CLINICAL PRESENTATION

Acute urinary retention generally presents as an inability to pass urine. It is typically associated with lower abdominal and/or suprapubic discomfort.[9] Affected patients are often restless and may appear in considerable distress. These manifestations may be less pronounced when AUR is superimposed upon chronic urinary retention. Chronic urinary retention is often painless. Acute-on-chronic urinary retention may present with overflow incontinence. The patients may complain of incontinence rather than the inability to pass urine. Patients with AUR are likely to present initially to an emergency department or the office of a primary care clinician. Most common emergency scenarios encountered by an emergency physician are the bladder outlet obstruction caused by BPH or neurogenic bladder. Hospitalized patients may develop AUR, often related to medications or after surgical procedures.[24]

EVALUATION

Detailed history, physical examination and diagnostic testing can help determine the etiology of urinary retention.

History

The patient history should focus on age of presentation, sex, previous history of retention or LUTS, prostate disease (hyperplasia or cancer), pelvic or prostate surgery, radiation, or pelvic trauma. Patients will generally give history of multiple lower urinary tract voiding or storage symptoms, including frequency, urgency, nocturia, straining to void, poor urinary stream, hesitancy, sensation of incomplete bladder emptying and intermittent urinary stream. The patient should also be asked about the presence of incontinence, hematuria, dysuria, fever, low back pain, neurologic symptoms, or rash. The physician should inquire about precipitating factors, including alcohol consumption, recent surgery, UTI, genitourinary instrumentation, constipation, large fluid intake, cold exposure and prolonged travel. Finally, a complete list of medications, including over the counter medications should be obtained.

Young age group, a history of cancer or intravenous drug abuse, and the presence of back pain or neurologic symptoms suggest the possibility of spinal cord injury or compression. Therefore, a history of neurologic disease, spinal trauma or tumor, and any change in baseline neurologic status is important and should be carefully noted. However, patients with spinal pathology generally do not present primarily with AUR. These patients will most often have other signs and symptoms of spinal cord pathology with AUR being one part of clinical picture. Patients can also present with overflow incontinence and have a history of recurrent UTI. History of long-standing diabetes mellitus is also important, but most patients present with painless retention because of diabetic cystopathy. History of presence of pain in any form as restlessness or suprapubic discomfort is important as it may point towards etiology of retention. Acute urine retention of obstructive etiology is usually painful.

Physical Examination

In patients with AUR of unknown etiology, the physical examination should include the following: general physical examination including vitals, general well-being and systemic examination.

Systemic examination should focus on lower abdominal palpation. The urinary bladder may be palpable or percussible. Usually urinary bladder is percussible or palpable if it contains 150–200 mL of urine. In obese patients, this may not be appreciable but deep suprapubic palpation will provoke discomfort.

A digital rectal examination (DRE) should always be done in both sexes. This is important for detailed evaluation of prostate, masses, fecal impaction, perianal sensation and rectal sphincter tone. In men a normal prostate examination does not exclude BPH as a cause of obstruction, as size of prostate does not correlate the presentation. Prostatic abscess should be looked for in DRE as a hot boggy tender prostate. In women with urinary retention, it is imperative to do per vaginal examination.

In addition to the above, neurological examination should be done in patients with suspected neurogenic bladder to test the integrity of sacral nerve roots that subserve the bladder function. This includes a general neurologic examination, as well as specific examinations related to bladder function. These include the cremasteric reflex, bulbocavernosus reflex (BCR), voluntary contractions of the pelvic floor, anal sphincter tone and perianal sensation in the S2 to S4 dermatomes. BCR is done by squeezing the glans penis while performing a DRE. Presence of contraction of anus on examination indicates that afferent and efferent sacral nerves and sacral cord are intact. In females after catheterization, same reflex can be elicited by gently tugging the catheter onto the bladder neck while doing DRE, when the contraction of anus indicates integrity of afferent and efferent sacral nerves and sacral cord.

Laboratory Studies

A urine sample should be obtained and sent for urinalysis and urine culture. The urine sample is collected with standard sterile precautions after catheter insertion.

The need for other laboratory testing should be determined based upon findings from the patient's history and physical examination. Most patients who present to the emergency room with concern for urinary retention have serum electrolytes and creatinine checked. These should be checked in any patient whose history suggests acute-on-chronic urinary retention, to evaluate for renal failure. Other laboratory tests that may be helpful include a complete blood count for suspected infection. Blood gas analysis sample should be sent in patients presenting with sepsis with or without renal failure to look for metabolic acidosis. Serum prostate-specific antigen (PSA) testing is not recommended in the setting of AUR as it is expected to be elevated during the episode.

Radiological Investigation

This includes an ultrasound kidney, ureter, bladder with prostate and urine retention volume. Upper tracts are to be looked for hydroureteronephrosis. All these basic investigations help tailoring the emergency management of a patient presenting with AUR.

INITIAL MANAGEMENT OF ACUTE URINARY RETENTION

Urethral catheterization is the mainstay of initial management of AUR. This is for immediate decompression with relief of pain due to overdistended bladder. Standard transurethral catheters are readily available and can usually be easily inserted. If urethral catheterization is unsuccessful or contraindicated, the patient should be referred immediately to a physician trained in advanced catheterization techniques, such as placement of a firm, angulated coude catheter or a suprapubic catheter. Record the volume drained which will confirm the diagnosis, determines the subsequent management and provide prognostic information with regard to outcome.

LABEL ACUTE OR ACUTE ON CHRONIC RETENTION

Elderly people are not aware of but they actually have urine retention. This has been particularly defined as chronic retention. This has been further subdivided into low or high pressure chronic retention. In 1984, Mitchell defined high pressure chronic retention (HPCR) of urine as maintenance of voiding, with a bladder volume of greater than 800 mL and intravesical pressure of greater than 30 cm of H_2O, often accompanied by hydronephrosis.[32] This over the time may lead to renal failure. On the contrary, low pressure chronic retention is maintenance of voiding with a bladder volume of greater than 800 mL but with low normal intravesical pressure and without upper tract changes. The patient continues to void spontaneously without sensation of incomplete voiding. Often the first symptom is bed wetting and inspection of the abdomen reveals a grossly distended bladder, confirmed by palpation and/or percussion.

Sometimes a patient with HPCR is suddenly unable to pass urine, called as acute on chronic retention. Patient presents with palpable bladder, raised serum creatinine and bilateral hydroureteronephrosis on ultrasound. On catheterization, a large volume of urine is drained, often amounting to 1–2 L.

As mentioned above recording of volume of urine is important as it holds differentiating two groups of patient, those with acute retention of urine with retention volume of less than 800 mL and those with acute on chronic retention with retention volume of greater than 800 mL. All these patients may develop postobstructive diuresis and it is imperative to keep regular watch on vitals, urine output and electrolytes.[33]

WHAT TO DO NEXT?

Further plan depends on the type of retention whether precipitated or spontaneous and etiology of AUR. Precipitated urine retention often does not recur and should be managed with a trial without catheter after exclusion of the precipitating factor. Spontaneous retention often recurs. In case of BPH, usually it is advisable to give a trial without catheter (TWOC) and not to proceed straight to transurethral resection of the prostate (TURP). American Urological Association (AUA) guidelines recommend at least one attempted trial of voiding after catheter removal before considering surgical intervention.[34] In these patients the optimal amount of time to leave a catheter in place is unknown. Up to three-fourth of men will have recurrent urinary retention within 1 week, if the bladder is simply drained.[35] One-fourth of men will void successfully after a TWOC.[36] Of those with successful TWOC, about 50%, 60% and 70% develop AUR within 1 week, 1 month and after 1 year, respectively. Factors affecting the failure of TWOC are maximal flow rate of less than 5 mL/sec and average voided volume of less than 150 mL.[33] An alpha blocker started 24–72 hours before TWOC increase the likelihood of successful voiding.[37-39] The duration of alpha-blockers after successful TWOC has not been determined yet. Also, it is not known whether continued use prevents further risk of AUR. Usually alpha-blockers are continued after successful TWOC and finasteride or dutasteride is combined with them in case of prostate more than 40 g.[40] A TWOC is clearly not indicated in patients with back pressure changes on the kidneys.[33]

Patients with chronic urinary retention with inefficient detrusor contraction, especially those with neurogenic bladder, can be managed with clean, intermittent self-catheterization. This technique is considered first-line treatment for managing urinary retention caused by neurogenic bladder and can reduce complications, such as renal failure, upper urinary tract deterioration and urosepsis.[36] Further definitive management of urinary retention depends upon the underlying etiology and may involve surgical and medical treatment. A basic algorithm of managing a male patient presenting with AUR is provided in **Flow chart 1**.

CONCLUSION

Acute urinary retention is most common urologic emergency. BPH is most common cause for AUR in men while in AUR women is uncommon. AUR usually painful. History physical examination routine laboratory radiological tests should be used to determine the cause. While uncommon but serious cause of aute urinary retention like cauda equina and cord compression should not be missed.

REFERENCES

1. Marshall JR, Haber J, Josephson EB. An evidence-based approach to emergency department management of acute urinary retention. Emerg Med Pract. 2014;16:1-20.

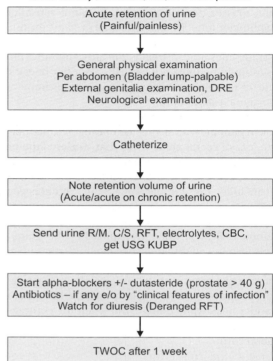

Flow chart 1 Algorithm for emergency management in case of acute urinary retention (AUR) in a male patient

Abbreviations: CBC, complete blood count; C/S, culture and sensitivity; DRE, digital rectal examination; e/o, effect of; R/M, routine microscopy; RFT, renal function tests; TWOC, trial without catheter; USG KUBP, ultrasound kidney, ureter, bladder and prostate

2. Fong YK, Milani S, Djavan B. Natural history and clinical predictors of clinical progression in benign prostatic hyperplasia. Curr Opin Urol. 2005;15:35-8.
3. Murray K, Massey A, Feneley RC. Acute urinary retention--a urodynamic assessment. Br J Urol. 1984;56:468-73.
4. Kaplan SA, Wein AJ, Staskin DR, et al. Urinary retention and post-void residual urine in men: separating truth from tradition. J Urol. 2008;180:47-54.
5. Ramsey S, Palmer M. The management of female urinary retention. Int Urol Nephrol. 2006;38:533-5.
6. Klarskov P, Andersen JT, Asmussen CF, et al. Acute urinary retention in women: a prospective study of 18 consecutive cases. Scand J Urol Nephrol. 1987;21:29-31.
7. Barrisford GW, Steele GS. (2010). Acute urinary retention. [online] UpToDate website. Available from: www.uptodate.com/contents/acute-urinary-retention [Accessed November, 2016].
8. Choong S, Emberton M. Acute urinary retention. BJU Int. 2000;85:186-201.
9. Thomas K, Chow K, Kirby RS. Acute urinary retention: a review of the aetiology and management. Prostate Cancer Prostatic Dis. 2004;7:32-7.
10. Curtis LA, Dolan TS, Cespedes RD. Acute urinary retention and urinary incontinence. Emerg Med Clin North Am. 2001;19:591-619.

11. Roehrborn CG, McConnell JD, Lieber M, et al. Serum prostate-specific antigen concentration is a powerful predictor of acute urinary retention andneed for surgery in men with clinical benign prostatic hyperplasia. PLESS Study Group. Urology. 1999;53:473-80.
12. Cathcart P, van der Meulen J, Armitage J, et al. Incidence of primary and recurrent acute urinary retention between 1998 and 2003 in England. J Urol. 2006;176:200-4.
13. Jacobsen SJ, Jacobson DJ, Girman CJ, et al. Natural history of prostatism: risk factors for acute urinary retention. J Urol. 1997;158:481-7.
14. Roehrborn CG, Malice M, Cook TJ, et al. Clinical predictors of spontaneous acute urinary retention in men with LUTS and clinical BPH: a comprehensive analysis of the pooled placebo groups of several large clinical trials. Urology. 2001;58:210-6.
15. Fuselier HA. Etiology and management of acute urinary retention. Compr Ther. 1993;19:31-6.
16. Fowler CJ, O'Malley KJ. Investigation and management of neurogenic bladder dysfunction. J Neurol Neurosurg Psychiatry. 2003;74(Suppl 4):iv27-iv31.
17. Sasaki K, Yoshimura N, Chancellor MB. Implications of diabetes mellitusin urology. Urol Clin North Am. 2003;30:1-12.
18. Barbalias GA, Nikiforidis G, Liatsikos EN. Vesicourethral dysfunction associated with multiple sclerosis: clinical and urodynamic perspectives. J Urol. 1998;160:106-11.
19. Dolin SJ, Cashman JN. Tolerability of acute postoperative pain management: nausea, vomiting, sedation, pruritus, and urinary retention. Evidence from published data. Br J Anaesth. 2005;95:584-91.
20. Verhamme KM, Sturkenboom MC, Stricker BH, et al. Drug-induced urinary retention: incidence, management and prevention. Drug Saf. 2008;31:373-88.
21. Raz S, Zeigler M, Caine M. Pharmacological receptors in the prostate. Br J Urol. 1973;45:663-7.
22. Verhamme KM, Dieleman JP, Van Wijk MA, et al. Nonsteroidal anti-inflammatory drugs and increased risk of acute urinary retention. Arch Intern Med. 2005;165:1547-51.
23. Meyrier A, Fekete T, Calderwood SB. (2007). Acute and chronic bacterial prostatitis. [online] UpToDate website. Available from: *www.uptodate.com/contents/acute-bacterial-prostatitis* [Accessed November, 2016].
24. Selius BA, Subedi R. Urinary retention in adults: diagnosis and initial management. Am Fam Physician. 2008;77:643-50.
25. Kim J, Lee DS, Jang SM, et al. The effect of pudendal block on voiding after hemorrhoidectomy. Dis Colon Rectum. 2005;48:518-23.
26. Iorio R, Whang W, Healy WL, et al. The utility of bladder catheterization in total hip arthroplasty. Clin Orthop Relat Res. 2005;432:148-52.
27. Hershberger JM, Milad MP. A randomized clinical trial of lorazepam for the reduction of postoperative urinary retention. Obstet Gynecol. 2003;102:311-6.
28. Cardozo L, Cutner A. Lower urinary tract symptoms in pregnancy. Br J Urol. 1997;80:14-23.
29. Glavind K, Bjork J. Incidence and treatment of urinary retention postpartum. Int Urogynecol J Pelvic Floor Dysfunct. 2003;14:119-21.
30. Yip SK, Sahota D, Pang MW, et al. Postpartum urinary retention. Obstet Gynecol. 2005;106:602-6.
31. Roehrborn CG, Bruskewitz R, Nickel GC, et al. Urinary retention in patients with BPH treated with finasteride or placebo over 4 years. Characterization of patients and ultimate outcomes. The PLESS Study Group. Eur Urol. 2000;37:528-36.
32. Mitchell JP. Management of chronic urinary retention. Br Med J (Clin Res Ed). 1984;289:515-6.
33. Reynard J. Lower urinary tract emergencies. In: Urological Emergencies in Clinical Practice. Springer: London; 2013. pp. 11-24.
34. McVary KT, Roehrborn CG, Avins AL, et al. Update on AUA guideline on the management of benign prostatic hyperplasia. J Urol. 2011;185:1793-803.
35. Breum L, Klarskov P, Munck LK, et al. Significance of acute urinary retention due to intravesical obstruction. Scand J Urol Nephrol. 1982;16:21-4.
36. De Ridder DJ, Everaert K, Fernandez LG, et al. Intermittent catheterization with hydrophilic-coated catheters (Speedi Cath) reduces the risk of clinical urinary tract infection in spinal cord injured patients: a prospective randomised parallel comparative trial. Eur Urol. 2005;48:991-5.
37. Hastie KJ, Dickinson AJ, Ahmad R, et al. Acute retention of urine: is trial without catheter justified? J R Coll Surg Edinb.1990;35:225-7.
38. McNeill SA, Hargreave TB, Members of the Alfaur Study Group. Alfuzosin once daily facilitates return to voiding in patients in acute urinary retention. J Urol. 2004;171:2316-20.
39. Lucas MG, Stephenson TP, Nargund V. Tamsulosin in the management of patients in acute urinary retention from benign prostatic hyperplasia. BJU Int. 2005;95:354-7.
40. McConnell JD, Bruskewitz R, Walsh P, et al. The effect of finasteride on the risk of acute urinary retention and the need for surgical treatment among men with benign prostatic hyperplasia. N Engl J Med. 1998;338:557-63.

SECTION 8

Endocrinal Emergencies

- **Hypoglycemia**
  JS Wasir, MS Kuchay, P Aggarwal

- **Diabetic Ketoacidosis in Adults**
  Beena Bansal, Tarannum

- **Thyroid Emergencies**
  Dheeraj Kapoor, Ruchi Kapoor, Mona Dhingra

- **Acute Adrenal Crisis**
  Devendra Richhariya, Sunil Kumar Mishra

CHAPTER 63

Hypoglycemia

JS Wasir, MS Kuchay, P Aggarwal

INTRODUCTION

Hypoglycemia is a clinical syndrome with diverse causes characterized by low levels of plasma glucose eventually leading to neuroglycopenia. It is not an uncommon presenting feature in the emergency care settings and should be considered in all patients presenting with episode(s) of confusion, altered behavior, impaired sensorium, or seizure. It can cause serious morbidity, and if severe or prolonged, can even be fatal.

In patients without diabetes, it is a clinical syndrome in which low plasma glucose can lead to symptoms and signs, with resolution of these symptoms and signs when plasma glucose concentration is raised.[1] A workgroup of American Diabetes Association and Endocrine Society has defined hypoglycemia in diabetic patients as any episode of abnormally low plasma glucose concentration (may be without symptoms) that expose the individual to harm.[2] It is most commonly drug induced (oral hypoglycemic drugs and insulin), or by exposure to other drugs, including alcohol. **Box 1** highlights the various causes of hypoglycemia in adults.

No specific blood glucose concentration absolutely defines hypoglycemia. Physiologically, it is a state of blood glucose concentration sufficiently low to cause the release of counter regulatory hormones and impair central nervous system functioning. The classical *Whipple's triad* is seen in hypoglycemia, which establishes this event most precisely: (1) symptoms consistent with hypoglycemia (discussed later), (2) a low plasma glucose concentration measured with a precise method (not a glucometer), and (3) relief of symptoms after raising the plasma glucose concentration.

It is important to understand that people with diabetes should become concerned about the possibility of developing hypoglycemia when the self-monitored blood glucose level is less than or equal to 70 mg/dL, leaving apart various clinical definitions and cut-off values of different guidelines. As compared to type 2 diabetes, hypoglycemia is more common in type 1 diabetes, especially in patients receiving intensive insulin therapy. Studies report that overall event rate for severe hypoglycemia that required assistance in insulin-treated type 2 diabetes was about one-third of that in type 1 diabetes (35 vs 115 episodes per 100 patients per year).[3] An estimated 6–10% of people with type 1 diabetes mellitus (DM) die as a result of hypoglycemia. Cases of refractory, prolonged hypoglycemia of unknown etiology require admission to an intensive care unit.

PATHOPHYSIOLOGY

Normal plasma concentration of glucose is usually between 60 mg/dL and 100 mg/dL in the fasting state, with slight excursions after a meal. Hepatic glycogen stores are usually sufficient to maintain plasma glucose levels for about 8 hours, however this period is shortened by exercise or during illness or starvation. The human brain is almost entirely dependent on glucose as a fuel (obligate metabolic fuel), and it cannot synthesize or store more than few minutes' supply as glycogen. Thus, if there is a fall in arterial blood glucose concentration below physiological levels, it impairs brain energy metabolism and function almost instantly.

Normally, counter regulatory mechanisms prevent an event of hypoglycemia by rapidly correcting it. **Table 1** highlights the physiological response to lowered blood glucose in our body.[4] There is a physiological hierarchy seen among the defense mechanisms, and in fact the counter regulatory processes begin well before the symptoms of hypoglycemia are felt by the subject.

Thus, based on the protective physiological responses, hypoglycemia is an uncommon clinical event, and would

Box 1 Causes of hypoglycemia

Ill-appearing or Medicated Individual
- *Drugs*: Insulin, insulin secretagogues (sulfonylureas, nonsulfonylureas), alcohol, and others (ACE inhibitors, ARBs, beta-blockers, quinolone antibiotics, indomethacin, quinine, sulfonamides)
- *Critical illness*: Hepatic, renal or cardiac failure, sepsis, and inanition
- *Hormone deficiency*: Cortisol, glucagon, and epinephrine (in insulin-deficient diabetes)
- Nonislet cell tumor

Apparently Well Individual
- Endogenous hyperinsulinism:
  – Insulinoma
  – Functional β-cell disorder (nesidioblastosis), noninsulinoma pancreatogenous hypoglycemia, and postgastric bypass hypoglycemia
  – *Insulin autoimmune hypoglycemia*: Antibody to insulin, antibody to insulin receptor
  – Insulin secretagogues
- Accidental (pharmacy error), surreptitious or malicious hypoglycemia
- Analytical error in measurements (glucometer or laboratory)—rarer

Adult presentation:
- Inborn errors of metabolism (common in infancy)
- *Fasting hypoglycemia*: In glycogen storage disease type 0, I, III and IV
- *Postprandial hypoglycemia*: Glucokinase, SUR1 and Kir 6.2 potassium channel mutations, congenital disorders of glycosylation and inherent fructose intolerance
- Exercise-induced hypoglycemia (increased activity of monocarboxylate transporter 1 in β-cells)

Abbreviations: ACE, angiotensin-converting enzyme; ARB, angiotensin-receptor blocker; SUR1, sulfonylurea receptor 1.

Table 1 Counter regulatory physiological responses to hypoglycemia

S. No.	Response	Glycemic threshold (mg/dL)	Role or mechanism
1.	Decrease in insulin	80–85	First defense against hypoglycemia. Most important regulatory hormone response
2.	Increased glucagon	65–70	Second defense, most important counter-regulatory hormone response. Acts at liver, stimulates glycogenolysis and gluconeogenesis from amino acids and glycerol (thus normal functioning of liver is necessary for an adequate glucagon response)
3.	Increased epinephrine	65–70	Third defense, critical if glucagon is deficient. Acts via β2-receptors, has similar hepatic effects as glucagon. Also increases delivery of gluconeogenic substrates from the periphery, inhibits glucose utilization by tissues and also inhibits insulin secretion (via α receptors)
4.	Increased cortisol and growth hormone	65–70	Defense against prolonged hypoglycemia, not critical. Limit glucose utilization and enhance hepatic glucose production
5.	Symptoms	50–55	Sweating, anxiety, palpitations, hunger and tremor. Behavioral responses of patient trigger food intake
6.	Decreased cognition	<50	Compromises the behavioral response. More severe neurological symptoms, including obtundation, seizures, and coma occur with progressive hypoglycemia. Profound and prolonged hypoglycemia can cause brain death

usually be seen in situations with an underlying pathology, or in patients with a history of use of drugs that lower glucose levels. The latter is more frequently seen in diabetics who are on insulin or insulin secretagogues (sulfonylureas or a glinide).

Insulin, a sulfonylurea (gliclazide, glimepiride, etc.; insulin secretagogues) or a glinide (repaglinide, nateglinide; insulin secretagogues) are known to cause hypoglycemia by virtue of their mechanism. Other antidiabetics (metformin, thiazolidinedione, dipeptidyl peptidase IV inhibitors, glucagon-like peptide-1 analogues, sodium-glucose co-transporter-2 inhibitors, α-glucosidase inhibitors) do not in themselves cause hypoglycemia, however, can accentuate the hypoglycemic effects when prescribed in combination with insulin, sulfonylurea or a glinide. Ethanol inhibits gluconeogenesis but not glycogenolysis.[5] Thus, an alcohol-induced hypoglycemia would usually precede a history of several days of binge drinking and less food intake. It can be both a cause and contributing factor to severe hypoglycemia.

Hormone Deficiency

Hypoglycemia can occur in prolonged fasting states in patients with primary adrenocortical failure (Addison's disease) or hypopituitarism. Anorexia and weight loss would be seen in chronic cortisol deficiency. Growth hormone deficiency can also cause hypoglycemia. In malaria endemic areas (travel history), it should be kept in mind that hypoglycemia can occur from malaria or its treatment.[6]

Risk Factors

A relative or absolute insulin excess forms the basis of hypoglycemia, and can occur in the following situations which must always be carefully examined in any patient with a history of hypoglycemia:[7]
- *Insulin or insulin secretagogue dosing*: Excessive, ill-timed, or wrong dose
- *Reduced oral intake or exogenous glucose*: Overnight fast, missed meals
- *Increased insulin-independent glucose utilization*: Exercise
- *Increased sensitivity to insulin*: Improved glycemic control, postexercise, weight loss
- *Reduced endogenous glucose production*: Alcohol ingestion
- *Reduced insulin clearance*: Renal failure.

CLINICAL PRESENTATION

The glucose deprivation of central nervous system produces neuroglycopenic responses to hypoglycemia. Common signs of hypoglycemia are diaphoresis and pallor. Tachycardia and raised systolic pressure is also seen, but less often in those with history of repeated events of hypoglycemia.

The symptoms can be classified as:
- Adrenergic (mediated by norepinephrine released from sympathetic postganglionic neurons and epinephrine from adrenal medulla): Including palpitations, tremors, and anxiety.
- Cholinergic (mediated by acetylcholine released from sympathetic postganglionic neurons): Which are sweating, hunger, and paresthesias.

Symptoms are clinically nonspecific, thus their concomitant existence with features that complete the classical triad only attribute the event to hypoglycemia in the individual. A blood test to check random sugars should be a routine protocol for any patient presenting with such features, either in emergency or outpatient settings. It is not uncommon to find patients without diabetes being treated for neurological and psychiatry differentials for years, before a final diagnosis of recurrent hypoglycemia was made attributable to an underlying pathology in the pancreas (insulin secreting tumor).

Hypoglycemia Unawareness

Some patients do not develop the early warning symptoms (mediated by adrenergic and cholinergic mechanisms) of hypoglycemia, thus preventing the corrective responses for aborting early an episode of impending neuroglycopenia. This happens due to a defective glucose counter regulatory mechanism by offsetting (lowering) the glycemic threshold for sympathoadrenal response to hypoglycemia (hypoglycemia-associated autonomic failure or HAAF). Such patients are potentially at a higher risk for severe (and recurrent) iatrogenic hypoglycemia if under aggressive glycemic therapy for diabetes (both in type 1 DM, and type 2 DM patients with intensive insulin regimens). The sympathoadrenal responses to a given level of hypoglycemia can also be blunted in patients with autonomic neuropathy, a complication of long-standing uncontrolled diabetes.[8]

MANAGEMENT

Hypoglycemia cases presenting to the emergency or triage can pose unique diagnostic challenges. It is very important for the physician to examine all medical record, talk to the patient and relatives, and attempt a quick clinical examination to elicit the exact underlying cause behind hypoglycemia. The most useful classification of hypoglycemia is the one described in **Box 1**, as it has more clinical and practical significance.

Diagnostic Approach

Hypoglycemia is suspected in patients with typical symptoms, or in clinical settings in which hypoglycemia is known to occur. Blood sample should be drawn (if possible) before administration of glucose, however, in emergency settings this may not be feasible and usually the peripheral capillary blood reading is a trigger to initiate prompt glycemia correction. A normal glucose level would exclude and a low glucose level would confirm hypoglycemia as the cause provided Whipple's triad is fulfilled.

When a distinctly low plasma glucose concentration in a patient is observed with no corresponding symptoms or suggestive history, one should rule out the possibility of an artifact (pseudohypoglycemia). Analytical errors in measuring levels of blood glucose are rare, however, should be kept in mind. Glucometers commonly used are not quantitative methods of estimating blood glucose levels particularly at low glucose levels. Laboratory-based quantitative methods can also produce artifactual hypoglycemia in cases where an antiglycolytic agent (fluoride) is not present in the blood collection tube and processing is delayed, particularly in samples of patients with leukocytosis, severe hemolytic disease or erythrocytosis.

Evaluation

It is pertinent to review patient's history in detail, including nature and the timing of symptoms. Where feasible, ask for any underlying illnesses or conditions, medications taken by the individual or family members, and brief social history. Wherever the cause of hypoglycemia is not clearly evident, laboratory evaluation in detail is needed. Wherever possible, a laboratory sample sent at time of symptoms for blood glucose should be done to establish Whipple's triad. Such a sample should be sent in a collection tube with an inhibitor of glycolysis and processed without delay. In persons without diabetes, other tests that may be sent during the episode of hypoglycemic symptoms, from a sample obtained at time of documented low plasma glucose (<55 mg/dL) are: Insulin polypeptides [serum insulin, serum proinsulin and connecting peptide (C-peptide) levels], β-hydroxybutyrate, sulfonylurea, and glinide drug screen (if available).[9,10]

The findings of symptoms, signs or both with plasma glucose less than 55 mg/dL, plasma insulin concentration of greater than or equal to 3.0 μU/mL (≥18 pmol/L), plasma C-peptide of greater than or equal to 0.6 ng/mL (≥0.2 nmol/L) and plasma proinsulin of greater than or equal to 5.0 pmol/L, document hyperinsulinism. Serum β-hydroxybutyrate levels of less than or equal to 2.7 mmol/L and an increase in plasma glucose of at least 25 mg/dL after intravenous (IV) glucagon indicate mediation of hypoglycemia by insulin or insulin-like growth factor.[8]

Increased plasma C-peptide distinguishes endogenous from exogenous hyperinsulinemia. Plasma β-hydroxybutyrate value is lower in insulinoma patients than in normal subjects due to antiketotic effects of insulin. Drug screen would be positive for a drug-induced hypoglycemia. Presence of insulin or insulin receptor antibody distinguishes insulin autoimmune hypoglycemia from insulinoma. Plasma insulin, C-peptide, and proinsulin values are also elevated in noninsulinoma pancreatogenous hypoglycemia syndrome (NIPHS), which is due to islet hypertrophy and nesidioblastosis. High plasma insulin levels with low C-peptide and low proinsulin values will be seen in cases of exogenous insulin administration. Nonislet cell tumors can also cause hypoglycemia via excess production of insulin-like growth factor-II. Insulinomas are uncommon (yearly incidence ~1 in 250,000). More than 90% are benign, thus are a treatable cause of potentially fatal hypoglycemia. The tumors are usually small (<2 cm in diameter in majority of cases). Localization studies are performed once there is demonstrated evidence of endogenous insulin-mediated hypoglycemia. Insulinomas may be detected by contrast enhanced computed tomography (CT), magnetic resonance imaging (MRI) or transabdominal ultrasonography, however a negative imaging result does not exclude an insulinoma, as it may not be visible with initial imaging. An endoscopic ultrasonography is usually required for localization in such situations before proceeding for a surgical management. In complex cases of endogenous hyperinsulinemic hypoglycemia and negative radiologic localization studies, a selective arterial calcium stimulation test with hepatic venous sampling can be done to distinguish between an insulinoma (usually focal) and islet cell hypertrophy or nesidioblastosis (diffuse process). ^{111}In-pentetreotide imaging and fluorine-18-L-dihydroxy phenylalanine positron emission tomography (18F-DOPA PET) are also other noninvasive procedures available at some centers.

TREATMENT IN EMERGENCY SETTINGS

Glucose

In a conscious patient, who is able to eat, oral treatment with glucose tablets, glucose containing fluids, or candy is seemingly congruous. An initial dose of about 20 g glucose is appropriate. In an unwilling, or unconscious patient, parenteral therapy is necessary. A bolus of 25% dextrose given IV (100 mL) can be followed by a continuous glucose infusion (5% or 10% dextrose) guided by repeated blood glucose measurements. All such measures only raise the blood glucose transiently, and patients should always be encouraged to eat in order to sustain euglycemia. Drug-induced hypoglycemias (particularly sulfonylurea induced) can last for longer duration (up to few days) and this should be kept in mind. Such patients should ideally be admitted to the hospital and given continuous IV glucose infusion. Hypoglycemia in patients taking α-glucosidase inhibitor class of drugs should be treated with IV glucose infusion because the drugs will inhibit or delay the absorption on orally given glucose.

A comatose diabetic patient in triage may be having marked hyperglycemia (with or without ketoacidosis), which should be ideally distinguished from hypoglycemia by a rapid glucose estimation (glucometer). If the same is not available, glucose can be given empirically as it will correct the hypoglycemia (observable clinical improvement), and not be particularly harmful if the blood glucose was high. Blood glucose should be monitored 1–3 hourly and serum glucose concentration maintained at a target level of at least 100 mg/dL.

Glucagon

Induction of glucagon for management of hypoglycemia is less common. It is useful in emergency settings if hypoglycemic coma occurs in a patient without an IV access and is most effective in patients who have sufficient liver glycogen reserves. Since glucagon, in addition to glycogenolysis, stimulates insulin secretion, its use in type 2 diabetes may be considered for those patients with advanced disease who are receiving intensive insulin therapy. A 1 mg dose of glucagon (reconstituted in 1 mL of sterile water) is recommended for adults and children over 25 kg in weight or children aged 6–8 years or above and a half dose (0.5 mL) is recommended for children below 25 kg in weight or younger than 6–8 years of age. Glucagon can be administered by subcutaneous (SC) or intramuscular (IM) injection.

In all situations, one must definitely determine the precipitating factor since none of the measures above treat the cause. A patient should not be discharged from the emergency settings without outlining the underlying process in pathophysiology of hypoglycemic event in that patient. The cause should be clearly identified and an appropriate follow-up plan should be formulated.

PREVENTING FUTURE HYPOGLYCEMIA

Treatment of recurrent hypoglycemia is based on the underlying mechanism, which must be elucidated through a detailed evaluation of each patient. These days continuous glucose monitoring devices (CGMS) are available for eliciting the fluctuations in blood glucose levels in a diabetic patient's daily schedule. These, however, cannot give an early warning for a falling level of blood glucose, as their analysis report is only generated at end of monitoring period, with a purpose to adjust medications accordingly.

In case of a drug-induced hypoglycemia, the drugs can be either discontinued or their doses reduced. Underlying critical illnesses, or hormone deficiencies (cortisol, growth hormone) should be addressed and treated by involving appropriate clinical teams.

In all measures, the most critical therapy is also a detailed patient and relative or caregiver counseling, preferably by a trained diabetic educator so as to keep a preventive approach toward the problem. Needless to say, hypoglycemia being a condition with potential serious morbidity and even mortality, documentation of these steps taken by the physician is as pertinent as the treatment, from the medicolegal point of view.

CONCLUSION

Hypoglycemic disorder is a relatively common presenting feature in emergency care settings. A high index of suspicion is needed to recognize hypoglycemia as a cause of abnormal sensorium, abnormal behavior or an episode of seizure. For every patient presenting to the emergency department with such symptoms, a blood glucose measurement (glucometer and laboratory) must be done. Proper evaluation is mandatory in all patients in whom Whipple's triad is documented. In persons with diabetes, the practice of hypoglycemia risk factor reduction—addressing the issue of hypoglycemia, education regarding management of hypoglycemia at home—should be emphasized. In persons without diabetes, proper evaluation of hypoglycemic disorder including expert evaluation for establishing the cause, localization in cases of endogenous hyperinsulinism, and appropriate medical or surgical management should be done.

REFERENCES

1. Cryer PE, Axelrod L, Grossman AB, et al. Evaluation and management of adult hypoglycemic disorders: and Endocrine Society Clinical Practice Guideline. J Clin Endocrinol Metab. 2009;94:709-28.
2. Seaquist ER, Anderson J, Childs B, et al. Hypoglycemia and Diabetes: a report of a workgroup of the American Diabetes Association and the Endocrine Society. J Clin Endocrinol Metab. 2013;98:1845-59.
3. Donnelly LA, Morris AD, Frier BM, et al. Frequency and predictors of hypoglycemia in type 1 and insulin-treated type 2 diabetes: a population based study. Diabet Med. 2005;22:749-55.
4. Melmed S, Polonsky K, Larsen PR, et al. William's Textbook of Endocrinology, 12th edition. New York: Elsevier; 2012.
5. Marks V, Teale JD. Drug induced hypoglycemia. Endocrinol Metab Clin North Am. 1999;28:555-77.
6. Murad MH, Coto-Yglesias F, Wang AT, et al. Clinical review: Drug induced hypoglycaemia: a systematic review. J Clin Endocrinol Metab. 2009;94:741-5.
7. Cryer PE, Davis SN. Hypoglycemia. In: Kasper DL, Fauci AS, Hauser SL (Eds.) Harrison's Principles of Internal Medicine, 19th edition. Philadelphia: McGraw-Hill; 2015.
8. Bottini P, Boschetti E, Pampanelli S, et al. Contribution of autonomic neuropathy to reduced plasma adrenaline responses to hypoglycemia in IDDM: evidence for a nonselective defect. Diabetes. 1997;46:814-23.
9. Gonzalez R, Zweig S, Rao J, et al. Octreotide therapy for recurrent refractory hypoglycemia due to sulfonylurea in diabetes-related kidney failure. Endocrine Practice. 2007;13:417-23.
10. Krentz AJ, Boyle PJ, Justice KM, et al. Successful treatment of severe refractory sulfonylurea-induced hypoglycemia with octreotide. Diabetes Care. 1993;16:184-6.

CHAPTER 64

Diabetic Ketoacidosis in Adults

Beena Bansal, Tarannum

INTRODUCTION

Diabetic ketoacidosis (DKA) and hyperglycemic hyperosmolar states (HHS) are the two life-threatening complications of diabetes. DKA primarily affects patients with type 1 diabetes mellitus, but can also occur in type 2 diabetes. HHS is exclusively seen in elderly type 2 diabetes patients. This chapter focuses on the management of DKA in adults.

EPIDEMIOLOGY

World Health Organization (WHO) in 2016 reported that globally approximately 422 million adults have diabetes mellitus.[1] Type 2 diabetes constitutes about 85–90% of all cases.[2] Low and middle income countries have the highest increase in prevalence of diabetes mellitus. Data available from the National Diabetes Surveillance Program suggests that hospital discharges for DKA in 2009 in the United States were 140,000 compared to 80,000 in 1988.[3] Recent studies show that number of hospitalizations for DKA are increasing, particularly as recurrent cases.[4] In DKA mortality is less than 1% in young adult subjects whereas in older adults and in patients with comorbidities have higher mortality rates of more than 5%.[5] The reported mortality rates for those between age group of 65 years and 75 years are about 10–20%.[5] Common causes of mortality among adult patients include hypokalemia, infections such as pneumonia, sepsis, and cardiovascular accidents.

PRECIPITATING FACTORS

The most common precipitating factors are infections which occur in about 30–40% of cases and discontinuation of or inadequate insulin therapy. Other factors are summarized in **Table 1**.

Table 1 Various precipitating factors

Precipitating factors	Remarks
Infections	Pneumonia, urinary tract infection, sepsis
Discontinuation of insulin or inadequate insulin therapy	It is commonly seen in patients treated with insulin
New-onset diabetes	20–25% of patients with type 1 DM
Acute illness	Cerebrovascular accidents, myocardial infarction, pulmonary embolism, acute pancreatitis, trauma, alcohol abuse
Drugs	Corticosteroids, thiazides, sympathomimetic agents, terbutaline, pentamidine, clozapine/olanzapine, cocaine, lithium, SGLT2 inhibitors
Psychological problems	Eating disorders, depression, and anxiety. Eating disorders are associated with recurrent DKA
Pump malfunction	Uncommon now, because of improvement in technology and better education of patients

Abbreviations: DM, diabetes mellitus; SGLT2, sodium-glucose co-transporter 2; DKA, diabetic ketoacidosis.

Cocaine abuse has been implicated in recurrent DKA. Unprovoked DKA has been reported in adult subjects with type 2 diabetes more commonly among African, Americans, and Hispanics.[6] Over half of newly diagnosed adult African, American, and Hispanics present with DKA. Pregnant women with diabetes are also at higher risk of developing DKA. Ketosis-prone diabetes comprises a group of diabetes syndromes characterized by severe β-cell dysfunction manifested by presentation with DKA and a variable clinical course. These syndromes are classified in various ways according to presence or absence of beta-cell function and autoantibodies.

PATHOGENESIS

The most important factor leading to DKA is reduced insulin secretion and its action and increased levels of counterregulatory hormones including glucagon, growth hormone, cortisol, epinephrine, and norepinephrine. The insulin deficiency of DKA can be absolute, as in type 1 diabetes or relative as in type 2 diabetes. Altogether these result in increased ketone formation, hyperglycemia, and metabolic acidosis.

Ketogenesis

As a result of insulin deficiency and elevated levels of counterregulatory hormones there is increased lipolysis leading to release of free fatty acids into the circulation which enters into the liver to form fatty acyl coenzyme A (CoA). Acyl CoA enters into the mitochondria with the help of carnitine palmitoyltransferase-1 (CPT 1) where beta-oxidation occurs leading to formation of ketone bodies. Increased concentration of glucagon also reduces the hepatic levels of malonyl CoA which inhibits the activity of CPT 1. Because of increased fatty acyl CoA and CPT 1 activity in DKA there is increased ketone formation in liver **(Flow chart 1)**.

Hyperglycemia

Hyperglycemia in DKA occurs as a result of three processes: increased gluconeogenesis, accelerated glycogenolysis, and impaired glucose utilization by peripheral tissues **(Flow chart 1)**.

CLINICAL PRESENTATION

Syndrome of DKA evolves rapidly over a period of 24 hours. Usually there is few days history of polyuria, polydipsia, and weight loss. Patients often present with gastrointestinal symptoms including nausea, vomiting, and abdominal pain sometimes mimicking acute abdomen. Signs of dehydration include dry mucous membrane, reduced skin turgor, low

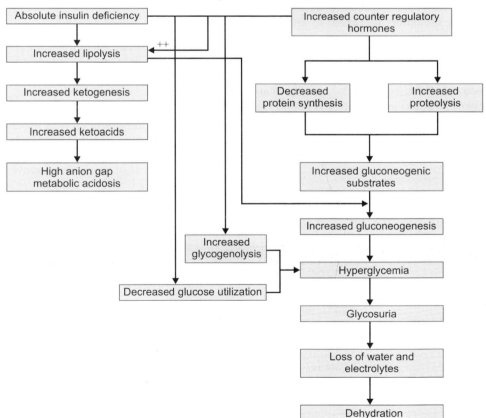

Flow chart 1 Pathogenesis of diabetic ketoacidosis

jugular venous pressure, tachycardia, and hypotension. There is fruity odor due to exhaled acetone in breath. Kussmaul respiration is noted which is characterized by rapid, deep breathing and is seen in adults with severe metabolic acidosis. There is progressive deterioration of neurological condition depending on the severity and duration of hyperglycemia.

Diagnostic Evaluation

Patient should be evaluated in detail particularly focusing on volume and cardiovascular status. History and physical examination should be directed toward search of precipitating factors.

Laboratory evaluation includes measurement of serum glucose, electrolytes, blood count, urinalysis and urine ketones, plasma osmolality, serum ketones, glycated hemoglobin, arterial blood gas, and electrocardiogram. Other investigations depend on the clinical presentation of the patient, e.g. blood or urine cultures, chest X-ray should be obtained if there are findings suggestive of infection. One should be careful in evaluating these patients as infection may exist in the absence of fever.

Laboratory Findings

Diabetic ketoacidosis is a triad of hyperglycemia, ketonemia, and metabolic acidosis. American Diabetes Association has classified DKA as mild, moderate, or severe as shown in **Table 2**.

Hyperglycemia

The serum glucose in DKA patients is usually 300–500 mg/dL. Euglycemic DKA has been described in patients with poor oral intake, prior insulin treatment, pregnant women, alcohol abuse, and liver failure.

Serum Ketones

Ketone bodies produced in DKA are beta-hydroxybutyrate, acetoacetate, and acetone. Although beta-hydroxybutyrate is the major ketone produced in DKA, the most commonly performed test for estimating ketones, i.e. nitroprusside test, measures only acetoacetate and acetone. False positive nitroprusside urine ketone can occur with drugs containing free sulfhydryl groups that react with nitroprusside, e.g. captopril, penicillamine, mesna, etc. Direct assay of beta-hydroxybutyrate is preferred particularly for monitoring response to therapy.

Anion Gap Acidosis

Increased anion gap metabolic acidosis occurs as a result of accumulation of ketoacids. Anion gap is calculated using the formula:

$$Serum\ anion\ gap = serum\ Na^+ - (serum\ Cl^- + HCO_3^-)$$

Normal value of anion gap is 10±2 and an anion gap greater than 12 mEq/L indicates increased anion gap metabolic acidosis. Patients may also present with mixed acid-base disorders. During treatment patients may develop hyperchloremic metabolic acidosis which is transient and resolves slowly.

Plasma Osmolality

Patients with DKA have fluid volume deficit usually in the range 4–10%. Effective osmolality is the best guide to estimate volume deficit. It is calculated as follows:

$$Effective\ osmolality = 2\ (sodium) + glucose\ (mg/dL)/18$$

Levels greater than 320 mmol/L are frequently associated with impaired mental status. This level is typically seen in hyperosmolar state.

Serum Electrolytes

Serum sodium on presentation in these patients is usually low due to transcellular shift created by hyperosmolality due to hyperglycemia. Serum sodium levels decline by 1.6 mEq/L for every 100 mg/dL of glucose level above the normal. Serum sodium should be corrected using following formula:

$$Corrected\ sodium = measured\ sodium + [1.6\ (glucose - 100)/100]$$

Table 2 Classification of diabetic ketoacidosis (DKA)			
Laboratory parameters	Mild DKA	Moderate DKA	Severe DKA
Plasma glucose (mg/dL)	>250	>250	>250
Arterial pH	7.25–7.30	7.00–7.24	<7.00
Serum bicarbonate (mEq/L)	15–18	10–15	<10
Urinary ketone	Positive	Positive	Positive
Serum ketone	Positive	Positive	Positive
Serum osmolality (mOsm/kg)	Variable	Variable	Variable
Anion gap	>10	>12	>12
Sensorium	Alert	Alert/drowsy	Stupor/coma

Serum potassium on admission is normal or elevated in one-third of patients because of shift of potassium out of cells caused by metabolic acidosis, insulin deficiency, and hyperosmolality. The estimated deficit of total body potassium averages 300–600 mEq/L. Serum levels of phosphate may be normal or increased due to metabolic acidosis.

Other Laboratory Findings

Patients usually present with leukocytosis, however, a leukocyte count greater than 25,000 mm³ or the presence of more than 10% neutrophil bands is suggestive of infection. Most patients have elevation of blood urea and creatinine levels as a result of hypovolemia. Nonspecific elevation of serum lipase and amylase levels is reported in DKA.[7] Patients with DKA may present with hyperlipidemia as a result of lipolysis. DKA is a proinflammatory state causing elevated levels of cytokines including tumor necrosis factor alpha and interleukins. These levels return to normal within 24 hours of insulin therapy and resolution of hyperglycemia.

TREATMENT

Intravenous fluid therapy and insulin infusion are the two important aspects in the management of DKA. The other important issue in the management includes correction of electrolyte abnormalities and treatment for precipitating cause.

Vital signs, volume and rate of fluid administration, insulin dosage, urine output, and response to treatment should be frequently monitored. Serum glucose should initially be measured every hour until stable. Serum electrolytes, blood urea nitrogen (BUN), creatinine, and venous pH should be measured every 2–4 hours. A flow sheet of laboratory and clinical parameters should be used to document as it allows better evaluation of the clinical picture throughout the treatment of DKA.

Fluid Management

The fluid therapy restores circulatory volume, corrects electrolyte abnormalities, helps in clearance of ketones and improves insulin sensitivity by reducing circulating counterregulatory hormones. The estimated water deficit in patients with DKA is about 100 mL/kg.[8] Water deficit can be calculated using formula:

(0.6) (Body weight in kg) × [1 − (Corrected sodium/140)].

The goal is to replace the total volume loss within 24–36 hours with half of the estimated deficit within 24 hours. Use of crystalloid fluid is preferred over colloids and isotonic saline (0.9% NaCl) should be the initial fluid of choice. According to recent critical care consensus colloids should be avoided as their use is seen to increase mortality and morbidity.[9] Initial rate of infusion of isotonic saline is 15–20 mL/kg/hour (500–1,000 mL/hour in an average adult) for 1–2 hours subsequently, and rate of infusion and choice of fluid depend on hemodynamic status, urine output, and serum electrolytes. If corrected serum sodium is normal or elevated then half normal saline (0.45% NaCl) is used usually at a rate of 250–500 mL/hour. However, if corrected serum sodium is low isotonic saline should be continued. Rate of fluid replacement should be modified in patients with heart failure, chronic kidney disease, and elderly. Once the plasma glucose is 250 mg/dL, 5–10% dextrose is added to replacement fluids. This is done to avoid hypoglycemia due to continuous insulin infusion which is required for resolution of ketonemia.

The administration of isotonic saline as resuscitation and maintenance fluid can lead to hyperchloremic acidosis. There have been few studies with use of Ringer's lactate which have shown reduced incidence of hyperchloremic acidosis with their use but have not shown any difference in outcome or duration of hospital stay as compared to administration with normal saline.[10]

Insulin Therapy

Insulin therapy is the integral part of management of DKA. Insulin administration leads to peripheral glucose utilization, inhibition of gluconeogenesis, and glycogenolysis as well as suppression of ketogenesis. Treatment with insulin is started only if serum potassium is more than 3.3 mEq/L. In patients with serum potassium levels less than 3.3 mEq/L, potassium should be replaced before initiating insulin as it can worsen hypokalemia by causing shift of potassium from extracellular to intracellular compartment. After an initial intravenous bolus of regular insulin 0.1 unit/kg, continuous infusion of regular insulin is started at a rate of 0.1 unit/kg/hour. However, a recent study has suggested that insulin bolus is not required if initial insulin infusion rate is 0.14 units/kg/hour.[11] Serum glucose should be monitored hourly and insulin infusion rate is adjusted depending on glucose readings. If serum glucose does not decrease by 50–75 mg/dL in 1 hour then infusion site should be examined for any technical fault and once these have been excluded as possible cause then the rate of insulin infusion should be doubled until a steady decline in serum glucose is achieved. When the serum glucose value falls to 200–250 mg/dL, then insulin infusion rate is reduced to 0.05 units/kg/hour and at this time dextrose is added to the replacement fluid.

Patients with mild DKA can be treated with subcutaneous rapid-acting insulin analogs provided there is trained staff in the general medical ward for frequent glucose monitoring.[12] Insulin regimen being followed in these studies is administration of initial subcutaneous (SC) dose of 0.2–0.3 units/kg, followed by 0.1 or 0.2 units/kg every 1 or 2 hours till the resolution of ketoacidosis.

Potassium Replacement

The estimated deficit of potassium in adult DKA patient is 3–5 mmol/kg. The goal of treatment is to maintain serum potassium levels within the range of 4–5 mEq/L.[7] Insulin therapy and correction of acidosis decrease potassium levels by increasing cellular uptake of potassium and by increasing urinary excretion. When initial serum potassium is less than 3.3 mEq/L, intravenous potassium chloride (IV KCl) 20–40 mEq/L should be added to each liter of saline. If the initial serum potassium is between 3.3 mEq/L and 5.3 mEq/L, IV KCl (20–30 mEq) is added to each liter of IV replacement fluid and continued until the serum potassium concentration has increased to the 4.0–5.0 mEq/L range. However, if serum potassium is more than 5.3 mEq/L, then replacement should be delayed until levels are decreased.

Bicarbonate Therapy

Bicarbonate therapy is not indicated unless there is severe metabolic acidosis (pH < 6.9) which can cause decreased cardiac contractility, cerebral vasodilatation, and coma. In such case 50–100 mmol of sodium bicarbonate should be given as an isotonic solution (in 200 mL of water) every 2 hours until the pH increases to 6.9–7.0. Bicarbonate therapy increases risk for hypokalemia and cerebral edema and reduces tissue oxygen uptake, and is not recommended in patients with arterial pH more than 7.

Phosphate and Magnesium Therapy

The serum phosphate concentration may initially be normal or elevated due to transcellular shift of phosphate out of the cells. The routine use of phosphate replacement in the treatment of DKA is not recommended. Phosphate replacement is done in patients with severe hypophosphatemia with levels lower than 1.0–1.5 mg/dL.[7] Patients with DKA have magnesium deficits of 1–2 mEq/L. Magnesium replacement should be considered in patients with symptoms of hypomagnesemia and levels below 1.8 mg/dL.

Criteria for Resolution of Ketoacidosis in Diabetic Ketoacidosis

Criteria include:
- Blood glucose less than 200 mg/dL
- Serum bicarbonate more than equal to 18 mEq/L
- Venous pH more than 7.3.

Transition to Subcutaneous Insulin

When DKA has resolved and patient is able to take orally, transition to SC insulin is initiated. Insulin infusion should be continued at least for 2 hours after SC insulin is started because abrupt discontinuation of IV insulin may result in recurrence of hyperglycemia and/or ketoacidosis. SC insulin should be administered in divided doses of 0.5–0.8 units/kg/day. Patients previously treated with insulin can resume their previous regimen. The basal and bolus insulin is the preferred treatment regimen after the resolution of DKA.

COMPLICATIONS

The most common complications of the treatment of DKA are hypoglycemia and hypokalemia. Other complications are cerebral edema which is seen particularly in children, hypoxemia, noncardiogenic pulmonary edema, and rhabdomyolysis.

REFERENCES

1. World Health Organization. Global Report on Diabetes. [online] WHO website. Available from *apps.who.int/iris/bitstream/10665/204871/1/9789241565257_eng.pdf* [Accessed February, 2017].
2. Australian Indigenous Health Info Net. (2015). Chronic Conditions: Diabetes. [online] Australian Indigenous Health Info Net website. Available from *www.healthinfonet.ecu.edu.au/chronic-conditions/diabetes* [Accessed February, 2017].
3. Centers for Disease Control and Prevention. Diabetes Public Health Resource. [online] CDC website. Available from *www.cdc.gov/diabetes/statistics/hospitalization_national.htm* [Accessed March, 2014].
4. Faich GA, Fishbein HA, Ellis SE. The epidemiology of diabetic acidosis: a population-based study. Am J Epidemiol. 1983;117(5):551-8.
5. Kitabchi AE, Umpierrez GE, Miles JM, et al. Hyperglycemic crises in adult patients with diabetes. Diabetes Care. 2009;32(7):1335-43.
6. Umpierrez GE, Casals MM, Gebhart SP, et al. Diabetic ketoacidosis in obese African-Americans. Diabetes. 1995;44(7):790-5.
7. Umpierrez G, Freire AX. Abdominal pain in patients with hyperglycemic crises. J Crit Care. 2002;17(1):63-7.
8. Kitabchi AE, Umpierrez GE, Murphy MB, et al. Management of hyperglycemic crises in patients with diabetes. Diabetes Care. 2001;24(1):131-53.
9. Reinhart K, Perner A, Sprung CL, et al. Consensus statement of the ESICM task force on colloid volume therapy in critically ill patients. Intensive Care Med. 2013;38(3):368-83.
10. Van Zyl DG, Rheeder P, Delport E. Fluid management in diabetic-acidosis—Ringer's lactate versus normal saline: a randomized controlled trial. QJM. 2012;105(4):337-43.
11. Kitabchi AE, Murphy MB, Spencer J, et al. Is a priming dose of insulin necessary in a low-dose insulin protocol for the treatment of diabetic ketoacidosis? Diabetes Care. 2008;31(11):2081-5.
12. Umpierrez GE, Latif KA, Cuervo R, et al. Subcutaneous aspart insulin: a safe and cost effective treatment of diabetic ketoacidosis. Diabetes Care. 2004;27(8):1873-8.

CHAPTER 65

Thyroid Emergencies

Dheeraj Kapoor, Ruchi Kapoor, Mona Dhingra

INTRODUCTION

Thyroid emergencies though uncommon, are life-threatening conditions which result from either acute or severe deficiency of [thyroxine (T4) or triiodothyronine (T3), referred to as myxedema coma] or, on the other side of the spectrum caused by, decompensated hyperthyroidism wherein there is an increased action of T4 and T3 overshooting the metabolic demands, referred to as thyroid storm (TS). In view of the life-threatening nature, it is only prudent to understand the pathophysiology of these conditions, so that timely recognition of signs and symptoms, may aid in prompt diagnosis and appropriate treatment be instituted.

The present chapter reviews thyroid emergencies: myxedema coma, TS, as regards to etiology, pathogenesis, clinical features, diagnostic dilemmas and finally prognosis.

THYROID STORM

Thyroid storm is a rare condition that generally affects hyperthyroid patients who have been inadequately treated for hyperthyroidism. TS is less commonly seen today possibly because of early and accurate diagnosis and treatment of the underlying thyroid condition, thereby reducing the risk of progression to crisis. Nonetheless, it is still seen in 1–2% of hospital admissions of hyperthyroidism. Hyperthyroidism[1] is more frequent in the females, who are thrice as commonly affected as males.[2]

Pathophysiology

Thyroxine, the major thyroid hormone in circulation accounts for 90% of the total, while T3 contributes the remaining 10%. Of these, T3 is the active hormone while, T4 needs to be converted into T3 before it can act physiologically. TS is a clinical syndrome which results from the overexposure of tissues to supranormal levels of thyroid hormones because of thyroid gland overactivity (**Fig. 1**).

Etiology

Graves' disease, the most common cause of TS, is an autoimmune disorder caused by circulating thyroid-stimulating hormone (TSH)-receptor stimulating antibodies.

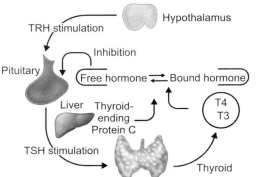

The thyroid hormones, (thyroxine (T4) and tri-iodothyronine (T3) are secreted under the stimulatory influence of pituitary thyrotropin (thyroid-stimulating hormone or TSH). TSH secretion is primary regulated by a dual mechanism:
• Thyrotropin-releasing hormone (TRH);
• Thyroid hormone
Thyroid hormone exits in circulation in both free and bound form. The thyroid gland is the sole source of T4 and only 20% of T3 is secreted in the thyroid. Approximately 80% of T3 in blood is derived from peripheral tissue (mainly hepatic or renal) deiodination of T4 to T3

Fig. 1 Pathophysiology of thyroid gland hormones

SECTION 8 Endocrinal Emergencies

Box 1 Triggering factors for thyroid storm

- Withdrawal of thyrostatic drugs
- Major surgical stress
- Iodide compounds or radioactive iodine ablation (^{131}I or ^{123}I) for Graves' disease or autonomous thyroid nodules
- Trauma
- Systemic infections
- Pregnancy
- Parturition
- Infection
- Diabetic ketoacidosis
- Severe emotional stress
- Cerebrovascular disease
- Pulmonary thromboembolism
- Unaccustomed exercise
- Use of tyrosine-kinase inhibitors

Table 1 Diagnostic criteria for thyroid storm

Criteria	Score
Thermoregulatory dysfunction	
Temperature 99–99.9°F (37.2–37.7°C)	5
Temperature 100–100.9°F (37.8–38.2°C)	10
Temperature 101–101.9°F (38.3–38.8°C)	15
Temperature 102–102.9°F (38.9–39.3°C)	20
Temperature 103–103.9°F (39.4–39.9°C)	25
Temperature 104°F (40°C) or higher	30
Central nervous system effects	
Absent	0
Mild agitation	10
Delirium, psychosis, lethargy	20
Seizure or coma	30
Gastrointestinal dysfunction	
Absent	0
Diarrhea, nausea, vomiting, abdominal pain	10
Unexplained jaundice	20
Cardiovascular dysfunction (beats/min)	
90–109	5
110–119	10
120–129	15
130–139	20
140	25
Congestive heart failure	
Absent	0
Mild (edema)	5
Moderate (bibasilar rales)	10
Severe (pulmonary edema)	15
Atrial fibrillation	
Absent	0
Present	10
History of precipitating event	
Absent	0
Present	10

Calculated on basis of total score, the possibility of the condition being thyroid storm is: unlikely if less than 25, impending 25–44 and highly likely more than 45.

Other causes of hyperthyroidism which can precipitate a TS are, toxic multinodular goiter and toxic adenoma. Amongst rare causes, withdrawal of antithyroid therapy can also lead to the condition.[3,4] Rarely the storm can also be precipitated by thyroiditis or thyrotoxicosis factitia—intentional thyroxine overdose.[5,6]

Irrespective of the underlying thyroid disorder, an additional superimposed insult is generally required to precipitate TS. Infection is the most common precipitating factor, however precipitants like trauma, surgery, myocardial infarction (MI), diabetic ketoacidosis (DKA), pregnancy and parturition have also been described **(Box 1)**.

Diagnosis of TS requires a high-index of suspicion. Clinical findings may be nonspecific and treatment should not be delayed waiting for investigations. Also the hormone profile of TS patients is almost similar to those with uncomplicated thyrotoxicosis. The usual picture is that of elevated T3 and T4 in the face of suppressed TSH. The exception is that of a thyrotroph adenoma where in all the three hormones are elevated.

Clinical Diagnosis

Signs and symptoms are an exaggeration of the classical ones observed in thyrotoxicosis. Multiorgan decompensation may also be observed. Burch and Wartofsky **(Table 1)** suggested a scoring system for evaluating end-organ dysfunction, on the basis of which a thyrotoxic patient may be said to be in TS.

Recently, Akamizu et al.[2] have come up with diagnostic criteria of TS based on Japanese patient survey data. However, this criterion offers no added advantage over Burch HB, and Wartofsky L criteria.

Management

Acute Intervention

If TS is suspected the patient should be admitted in intensive care unit. Prompt assessment of the ABCDEs should be done (i.e. airway, breathing, circulation, disability, i.e. conscious level, and examination) and the patient managed accordingly. Those at a high-risk for severe hypoxemia and tissue ischemia should be put on oxygen inhalation. Most patients will eventually need intubation and mechanical ventilation. Fluid management and electrolyte correction are integral to an uneventful recovery.

Specific Treatment

Treatment for TS should be started early and should focus at decreasing thyroid hormone synthesis and release, and to decrease the peripheral hormone action. Treatment of the suspected precipitating condition should start simultaneously. The treatment is essentially on the lines of thyrotoxicosis, except that higher and more frequent dosing may be required.

The cornerstone of therapy would still be antithyroid drugs, beta-blockers and corticosteroids. Propylthiouracil which blocks the conversion of T4 to T3 is to be preferred. Iodine and amiodarone may be rarely required to block hormone release and control heart rate respectively. Cholestyramine which blocks enterohepatic circulation may also be considered.

Thyrostatics

Methimazole in a dose of 20–30 mg is given every 6 hours or propylthiouracil given as a loading dose of 500–1000 mg and subsequently 250 mg given 4 hourly.[7,8] Propylthiouracil should be preferred in this situation, as it reduces the peripheral conversion of T4 to T3. Both agents can be administered orally by nasogastric tube if the patient is unconscious. Rectal route is also an alternative. One should wait for at least an hour after thionamide administration before giving iodine to block release of preformed hormone.

Saturated solution of potassium iodide (SSKI) may be given 6–8 hourly in a dose of 250 mg iodide 5 drops. Lugol's iodine solution is another alternative in a dose of 5–10 drops every 6 hourly.

In the absence of contraindications, beta-blockers should be started immediately to block the adrenergic surge. Propanol which is short-acting and approved use is the preferred drug. 40–80 mg may be given orally at 4–6 hourly intervals. Esmolol should be used in patients with heart failure. In case of chronic obstructive pulmonary disease (COPD) or bronchial asthma cardioselective beta-blocker should be used like metoprolol. Alternatively, diltiazem 60–90 mg may be given 3–4 times a day. Corticosteroids have been shown to improve survival. They act by inhibiting the peripheral conversion of T4 to T3. Hydrocortisone, in a dose of 100 mg 6-hourly or alternatively, dexamethasone given in a dose of 2 mg given every 6 hours should be administered intravenously or intramuscularly and should be continued till TS resolves. Lithium carbonate, can be used in a dose of 300 mg given every 8 hours, if there is a contraindication to thionamide use or there is a history of previous toxicity to thionamide therapy.

Therapy Directed at Systemic Decompensation

Intravenous fluids with dextrose and electrolytes may needed to control hypotension. In hypotension refractory to adequate hydration, vasopressors or glucocorticoids may be required. In febrile patients, acetaminophen is preferred to salicylates, as it does not inhibit the binding of thyroid hormone to thyroxine-binding globulin (TBG). Hyperthermia responds well to external cooling with sponging, cooling blankets, and ice packs. Congestive heart failure (CHF), if present should be adequately treated with diuretics and angiotensin-converting enzyme (ACE) inhibitors. Lastly therapy directed at the precipitating illness **(Fig. 2)**.

With treatment of the comorbid conditions and fluid replacement, the patient starts to improve within 24–72 hours.

Newer Therapies

Extracorporeal plasmapheresis may occasionally be required in patients who do not respond to conventional therapy.[9] Phenobarbital which increases thyroid hormone metabolism may benefit. L-carnitine, has been shown to have some benefit in clinical trials.[10] Charcol hemoperfusion has also been tried. Antimonoclonal antibodies like rituximab which depletes B lymphocyte which have shown benefits in Graves' ophthalmopathy has not shown benefits in frank thyrotoxicosis.

Prognosis

Even with early diagnosis mortality ranges from 10% to 75% in hospitalized patients.[1,11,12] However with early interventions, mortality has been reduced to 20% in elderly. The most common cause of death in elderly has been cardiopulmonary failure if patient succumbs to death.

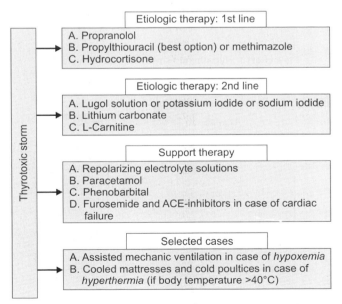

Fig. 2 Treatment for thyrotoxic storm
Abbreviation: ACE, angiotensin-converting enzyme

HYPOTHYROID COMA (MYXEDEMA COMA)

Myxedema coma although rare is a life-threatening form of decompensated hypothyroidism.[13] It usually has an underlying precipitant. Mortality ranges from 25% to 60% even in the best of care.[14-18] It has an annual incidence of 0.22 per million[15] and is most commonly seen in hospitalized elderly females who have long history of hypothyroidism. 80% of cases occur in women, 60 years or older. Myxedema crisis may actually be more appropriate a term as only a few patients are frankly comatose; most patients are obtunded. Myxedema coma is an endocrine emergency that is best managed in an intensive care unit (ICU) setting.

Etiology and Precipitating Factors

The main underlying cause of myxedema coma is a long-standing untreated hypothyroidism. Almost all these patient have been taking L-thyroxine for a long time and have abruptly withdrawn it on their own. Secondary or tertiary hypothyroidism is rare and is seen in about 5–15% of patients.[19]

Infections and septicemia are the most common precipitating factors.[15,16] Cerebral stroke, CHF, gastrointestinal bleed, and sedatives drugs may also precipitate myxedema crisis.

Myxedema coma is common in winter months and infact external cold may be a precipitating factor.[17,20] Hypoglycemia, hypercalcemia, hyponatremia, hypercapnia and hypoxemia may also precipitate myxedema coma. Moreover, the drugs like sedatives, antidepressants and tranquilizers may precipitate or compound hypothyroid patient into myxedematous crisis **(Flow chart 1)**.[21]

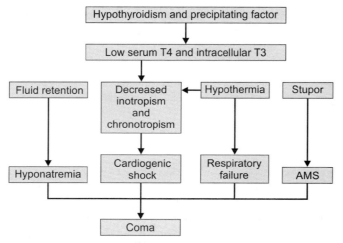

Flow chart 1 Hypothyroidism and precipitating factor

Abbreviations: AMS, altered mental status; T3, tri-iodothyronine; T4, thyroxine

Pathogenesis

The primary pathology of myxedema crisis is the low intracellular T3 activity because of underlying hypothyroidism which in turn leads to hypothermia and a suppressed cardiac activity.[22,23] Low T3 levels render the central nervous system (CNS) less sensitive to hypoxia and hypercapnia which leads to respiratory failure. Frank T3 deficiency leads to respiratory muscle dysfunction and pleural effusion resulting in compromised lung volume which may exacerbate respiratory failure.[24] Finally myxedema of the respiratory tract, particularly the larynx and the pharynx along with macroglossia may worsen the situation. Altered vascular permeability leads to anasarca. T3 deficiency and a concomitant increase in vasopressin level also lead to increase in fluid retention by decreasing the glomerular filtration rate (GFR) and the decreased delivery to the distal tubule respectively.[25-27]

Fulminating sepsis and a coexisting adrenal insufficiency may impair gluconeogenesis and may precipitate hypoglycemia. Seizures, focal or even generalized may result from the coexisting hyponatremia, hypoxia, or hypoglycemia and may worsen the already depressed consciousness levels **(Flow chart 2)**.

Clinical Features

The management of myxedema crisis should focus upon the search for the precipitating cause. Frank hypothyroid features like hypothermia, hung tendon reflexes, nonpitting edema and bradycardia are often present.[18] Skin is usually dry. Voice may be hoarse and macroglossia may be present. Neck should be examined for goiter or for a surgical scar which suggests thyroidectomy.

Hypothermia and impaired consciousness levels are the two cardinal manifestations of myxedema coma. Temperature as low as 80°F (26.7°C) have been observed.

Electrocardiogram (ECG) findings may range from sinus bradycardia, low voltage complexes, QT prolongation, bundle branch blocks or even complete heart blocks. Nonspecific ST-T changes may occasionally be seen.[17,28] Patient may not be frankly comatosed and depression, paranoia, or hallucinations (myxedema madness) are observed more commonly. Cerebellar signs may also be observed. About a fourth of patients may have seizures. Hypoxia, hyponatremia and hypoglycemia have been incriminated. Gastrointestinal manifestation include ascites, gastric atony, impaired peristalsis, or even frank paralytic ileus. Atony of the urinary bladder with retention is not uncommon. Decreased oxygen requirement and erythropoietin may manifest as normocytic normochromic anemia on general blood picture **(Box 2)**.[29]

Laboratory Parameters

Laboratory parameter may reveal hypoxemia and hypercapnia on blood gas analysis. Hemogram may be suggestive of

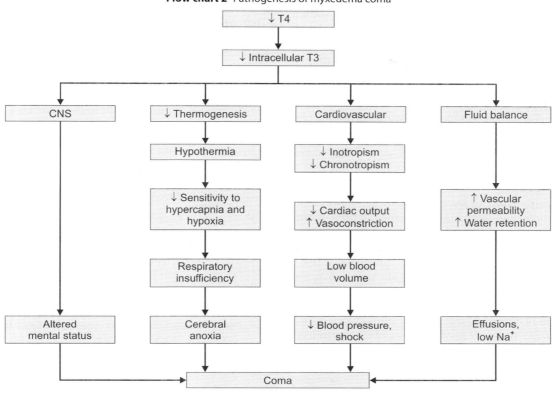

Flow chart 2 Pathogenesis of myxedema coma

Abbreviation: CNS, central nervous system

Box 2 Symptoms and signs peculiar to hypothyroid coma

- Coma status
- Hypothermia (frequently severe, without shivering)
- Dyspnea
- Generalized edema with yellow and dry cutis
- Macroglossia
- Bradycardia
- Weak wrists
- Reduced cardiac sounds
- Constipation
- Reduced reflexes
- Thin and dry hairs
- Focal and general seizures (rare)

anemia; polymorphonucleocytosis may be seen if infection is present. Hyponatremia, hypercholesterolemia, and elevated serum lactate dehydrogenase and creatine kinase levels may been seen in routine biochemical examination. Free T4 (FT4) and free T3 (FT3) levels are usually in the subnormal zone, with serum TSH concentrations being far above the normal range. However in recent onset hypothyroidism and secondary hypothyroidism TSH may not be very high. Precipitating causes should be aggressively looked for and relevant investigations should be done. White blood cell counts, urine examination and culture, blood culture, renal function tests, X-ray chests and ECG should be done.

Treatment

Treatment of myxedema coma should be prompt and a multidisciplinary approach should be employed:
- Patient should be kept under intensive care treatment and may require ventilator support
- Adequate and appropriate fluid replacement should be done for management of hypotension and dyselectrolytemia
- Precipitating factors should be looked for aggressively
- Adequate thyroid hormone replacement should be done
- Steroids supplementation may be required.

General Supportive Treatment

These patients generally require ventilatory support during the initial 36–48 hours. Fluid resuscitation should be done more cautiously because on the one hand more fluids may be required for hypotension whereas hyponatremia may actually mandate fluid restriction. In mild hyponatremia, a rational approach will be to advise fluid restriction commensurate enough with replacement to cover daily losses. However, care should be taken to supplement glucose and electrolytes adequately.[30] In case of severe hyponatremia, 3% sodium chloride should be administered along with furosemide, to avoid fluid overload. Hypotension management requires dextrose saline infusion. Sometimes vasopressors may be needed. Due to relative adrenal deficiency in patients it is advisable to start low dose hydrocortisone at the rate of 10 mg/hr or 50 mg/6 hourly.

Hypothermia can be corrected by external warming with precaution to prevent vasodilatation that may exacerbate hypotension.

Thyroid Hormone Replacement

The major cornerstone of treatment in myxedema coma is thyroid hormone supplementation. Injectable preparations of either T4 or T3 are however not freely available. They are to be given intravenously. Although liothyronine or T4 can be administered by nasogastric tube, it does carry a risk of aspiration in a comatose patient. Drug absorption may also be an issue if the patient has gastric atony.

A bolus of T4 is given in a dose of 300–500 µg initially to replenish the body stores. It is then continued in a dose of 50–100 µg daily. T4 levels may rise acutely to supranormal levels and it then slowly gets converted to its active metabolite T3.[31] Alternatively liothyronine may be given initially (T3) at a dose of 10–20 µg as an intravenous bolus and then followed up by 10 µg every 4 hours for the first 24 hours and subsequently every 6 hours for 2–3 days, and then oral administration may be started. Advantages of T3 over T4 are rapid onset of action with significant clinical improvement within 24 hours and early beneficial effects on neuropsychiatric functions. However poor availability, adverse effect on cardiac function may limit its use. Combination therapy of T3 and T4 has also been used with success. Alternatively, T4 can be started at a dose of 4 µg/kg/day in lean subjects and then followed by 100 µg 24 hours later and subsequently 50 µg daily either intravenously or orally. Liothyronine may also be started concomitantly with an initial dose of 10 µg intravenously and be repeated every 8–12 hours till the patient can accept T4 orally.[14]

HASHIMOTO'S ENCEPHALOPATHY

It would only be appropriate at this point to discuss Hashimoto's encephalopathy which though rare, is a well-documented complication of Hashimoto's thyroiditis.[32] It may have variable presentations ranging from myoclonus and tremors[33] to frank seizures.[34] Stroke-like episodes may also be a presenting feature in some patients. Interestingly, most patients of Hashimoto's encephalopathy are euthyroid and are usually steroid responsive.[35]

CONCLUSION

Thyroid emergencies like thyroid storm and myxedema coma causes significant morbidity and mortality. Thyroid storm is most severe form of thyrotoxicosis usually present with altered mental status. Diagnosis can be difficult because symptoms mimic the other conditions who present with altered sensorium. Emergency physician who can rapidly recognize the features of thyroid storm and myxedema, identify the precipitating factors, appropriatly begin the medical management will definitely save a life.

REFERENCES

1. Dillmann WH. Thyroid storm. Curr Ther Endocrinol Metab. 1997;6:81-5.
2. Akamizu T, Satoh T, Isozaki O, et al. Diagnostic criteria, clinical features, and incidence of thyroid storm based on nationwide surveys. Thyroid. 2012;22(7):661-79.
3. Gavin LA. Thyroid crises. Med Clin North Am. 1991;75(1):179-93.
4. Shaked Y, Samra Y, Zwas ST. Graves' disease presenting as pyrexia of unknown origin. Postgrad Med J. 1988;64(749):209-12.
5. Swinburne JL, Kreisman SH. A rare case of subacute thyroiditis causing thyroid storm. Thyroid. 2007;17(1):73-6.
6. Yoon SJ, Kim DM, Kim JU, et al. A case of thyroid storm due to thyrotoxicosis factitia. Yonsei Med J. 2003;44(2):351-4.
7. Klubo-Gwiezdzinska J, Wartofsky L. Thyroid emergencies. Med Clin North Am. 2012;96(2):385-403.
8. Hampton J. Thyroid gland disorder emergencies: thyroid storm and myxedema coma. AACN Adv Crit Care. 2013;24(3):325-32.
9. Koball S, Hickstein H, Gloger M, et al. Treatment of thyrotoxic crisis with plasmapheresis and single pass albumin dialysis: a case report. Artif Organs. 2010;34(2):E55-8.
10. Benvenga S, Ruggeri RM, Russo A, et al. Usefulness of L-carnitine, a naturally occurring peripheral antagonist of thyroid hormone action, in iatrogenic hyperthyroidism: a randomized, double-blind, placebo-controlled clinical trial. J Clin Endocrinol Metab. 2001;86(8):3579-94.
11. Burch HB, Wartofsky L. Life-threatening thyrotoxicosis. Thyroid storm. Endocrinol Metab Clin North Am. 1993;22(2):263-77.
12. Tietgens ST, Leinung MC. Thyroid storm. Med Clin North Am. 1995;79(1):169-84.
13. Leow MK, Loh KC. Fatal thyroid crisis years after two thyroidectomies for Graves' disease: is thyroid tissue auto transplantation for post-thyroidectomy hypothyroidism worthwhile? J Am Coll Surg. 2002;195:434-5.
14. Wartofsky L. Myxedema coma. Endocrinol Metab Clin North Am. 2006;35(4):687-98.
15. Rodríguez I, Fluiters E, Pérez-Méndez LF, et al. Factors associated with mortality of patients with myxoedema coma: prospective study in 11 cases treated in a single institution. J Endocrinol. 2004;180(2):347-50.
16. Yamamoto T, Fukuyama J, Fujiyoshi A. Factors associated with mortality of myxedema coma: report of eight cases and literature survey. Thyroid. 1999;9(12):1167-74.

17. Dutta P, Bhansali A, Masoodi SR, et al. Predictors of outcome in myxoedema coma: a study from a tertiary care centre. Crit Care. 2008;12(1):R1.
18. Reinhardt W, Mann K. Incidence, clinical picture and treatment of hypothyroid coma. Results of a survey. Med Klin (Munich). 1997;92(9):521-4.
19. Mathew V, Misgar RA, Ghosh S, et al. Myxedema coma: a new look into an old crisis. J Thyroid Res. 2011;2011:493462.
20. Chu M, Seltzer TF. Myxedema coma induced by ingestion of raw bok choy. N Engl J Med. 2010;362(20):1945-6.
21. Gardner DG. Endocrine emergencies. In: Gardner DG, Shoback D (Eds). Greenspan's Basic and Clinical Endocrinology, 8th edition. New York: McGraw-Hill; 2007.
22. Ladenson PW, Goldenheim PD, Ridgway EC. Prediction and reversal of blunted ventilatory responsiveness in patients with hypothyroidism. Am J Med. 1988;84(5):877-83.
23. Wilson WR, Bedell GN. The pulmonary abnormalities in myxedema. J Clin Invest. 1960;39:42-55.
24. Massumi RA, Winnacker JL. Severe depression of the respiratory center in myxedema. Am J Med. 1964;36:876-82.
25. Derubertis FR, Michelis MF, Bloom ME, et al. Impaired water excretion in myxedema. Am J Med. 1971;51(1):41-53.
26. Skowsky WR, Kikuchi TA. The role of vasopressin in the impaired water excretion of myxedema. Am J Med. 1978;64(4):613-21.
27. Chen YC, Cadnapaphornchai MA, Yang J, et al. Nonosmotic release of vasopressin and renal aquaporins in impaired urinary dilution in hypothyroidism. Am J Physiol Renal Physiol. 2005;289(4):F672-8.
28. Polikar R, Burger AG, Scherrer U, et al. The thyroid and the heart. Circulation. 1993;87(5):1435-41.
29. Das KC, Mukherjee M, Sarkar TK, et al. Erythropoiesis and erythropoietin in hypo- and hyperthyroidism. J Clin Endocrinol Metab. 1975;40(2):211-20.
30. Verbalis JG, Goldsmith SR, Greenberg A, et al. Hyponatremia treatment guidelines 2007: expert panel recommendations. Am J Med. 2007;120(11 Suppl 1):S1-21.
31. Ridgway EC, McCammon JA, Benotti J, et al. Acute metabolic responses in myxedema to large doses of intravenous L-thyroxine. Ann Intern Med. 1972;77(4):549-55.
32. Brain L, Jellinek EH, Ball K. Hashimoto's disease and encephalopathy. Lancet. 1966;2(7462):512-4.
33. Pozo-Rosich P, Villoslada P, Canton A, et al. Reversible white matter alterations in encephalopathy associated with autoimmune thyroid disease. J Neurol. 2002;249(8): 1063-5.
34. Cantón A, de Fàbregas O, Tintoré M, et al. Encephalopathy associated to autoimmune thyroid disease: a more appropriate term for an underestimated condition? J Neurol Sci. 2000;176(1):65-9.
35. Peschen-Rosin R, Schabet M, Dichgans J. Manifestation of Hashimoto's encephalopathy years before onset of thyroid disease. Eur Neurol. 1999;41(2):79-84.

CHAPTER 66

Acute Adrenal Crisis

Devendra Richhariya, Sunil Kumar Mishra

INTRODUCTION

Acute adrenal crisis is categorized under important challenging emergencies for emergency physician which is easily missed due to its nonspecific presentation. Acute adrenal crisis should be diagnosed early and managed with appropriate treatment to reduce the mortality. In the recent time, more and more focus is on diagnosing this condition in the setting of severe sepsis HIV (human immunodeficiency virus) infection and patient who are on steroid therapy and with unexplained shock. Acute adrenal crisis mimic to several emergencies due to its nonspecific presentation, so emergency physician should consider this entity as important differential diagnosis.

High index of suspicion on the basis of history, physical examination and laboratory finding is important for emergency physician. Understanding about basic physiology of adrenal gland, pathophysiolgy, etiology and therapy of disease helpful in effective management of acute adrenal crisis.

BASIC ANATOMY AND PHYSIOLOGY OF ADRENAL GLAND

Adrenal gland is capsulated retroperitoneal organ divided into two zones—outer part known as adrenal cortex and outer adrenal medulla. Various part of adrenal gland and their related hormone are described in **Table 1**.

Adrenal cortex is further subdivided into three zones:
1. Zona fasciculata which secretes glucocorticoid (cortisol)
2. Zona reticularis secretes the dehydroepiandrosterone acetate (DHEA) which is the intermediate metabolite for sex steroids androgen and estrogen
3. Zona glomerulosa secretes mineralocorticoids (aldosterone).

Adrenal medulla secretes catecholamines, epinephrine, and norepinephrine.

Various functions of adrenal hormone are described in **Table 2**.

Glucocorticoid (Cortisol)

Cortisol is important for normal functioning of all tissues. Cortisol gives cardiovascular stability by maintaining adequate circulatory volume, cardiac contractility, and vascular tone, thus stimulating cardiac function. Cortisol enhances the action of catecholamines, epinephrine, and norepinephrine. Release of vasodilators from endothelium is also reduced by cortisol. Thus, cortisol-deficient patient presents with circulatory collapse/shock which is the hallmark of acute adrenal crisis.

Table 1 Division of adrenal glands and their hormones

Adrenal gland is divided into two zones			
Adrenal cortex (outer area) subdivided into three zones			Medulla (inner area)
Zona fasciculata	Zona reticularis	Zona glomerulosa	
Secretes glucocorticoids	Secretes DHEA (dehydroepiandrosterone acetate) metabolite for sex steroid	Secrets mineralocorticoids	Catecholamines
Cortisol	Androgen and estrogen	Aldosterone	Epinephrine Norepinephrine

CHAPTER 66 Acute Adrenal Crisis

Table 2 Important functions of adrenal hormone

Cardiovascular	Endocrine	Immune/inflammatory	Metabolic	Renal
Maintain cardiac contractility, cardiac function, and vascular tone thus provide cardiovascular stability	Inhibit insulin secretion, epinephrine synthesis	Maintain inflammatory homeostasis, anti-inflammatory action of cortisol, reduce circulating leukocyte and cytokines response, eosinophils and lymphocytes	Gluconeogenesis lipolysis, muscle protein catabolism Raise plasma glucose during stress	Increase in glomerular filtration rate (GFR)

Box 1 Stress/trauma and response of hypothalamic pituitary adrenal axis and cortisol

- Stress/trauma → in response to tissue injury, pain, hypotension, hypoxia, hypoglycemia → signals are generated and sent to central nervous system (hypothalamus)
- Hypothalamus release the CRH (corticotropin-releasing hormone)
- CRH reaches the pituitary gland and stimulate adrenal corticotropin hormone (ACTH)
- ACTH stimulates release of cortisol from adrenal cortex

Box 2 Role of aldosterone in volume expansion

- Volume depletion → response of aldosterone → volume expansion
- Volume depletion → stimulates the release of renin from juxtaglomerular cells
- Renin converts angiotensin to angiotensin I and angiotensin I converted to angiotensin II by angiotensin-converting enzyme
- Angiotensin II stimulates adrenal cortex to release aldosterone
- Aldosterone causes sodium absorption and potassium excretion by acting on thick ascending limb of loop of Henle → Volume expansion

---

Glucocorticoid is important for glucose, lipid and protein metabolism and regulates energy storage and utilization. Thus, in glucocorticoid-deficient patient, loss of appetite, weight loss, and cachexia are present.

Glucocorticoid also facilitates healing of damaged tissue due to its anti-inflammatory action; its absence or deficiency results in increase in inflammation, and patient presents with fever, arthralgia, myalgia, and lethargy.

Cortisol release is controlled by hypothalamic pituitary adrenal axis (HPA axis) and is released during trauma, infection, and stress **(Box 1)**.

Mineralocorticoid (Aldosterone)

Main function of aldosterone is sodium reabsorption in exchange of potassium at the level of distal convoluted tubule and to maintain sodium, potassium, and water balance. Thus, aldosterone deficiency causes sodium loss and potassium retention, and rapid loss of salt and water during vomiting and diarrhea leads to coma or death. Aldosterone release is regulated by renin-angiotensin-aldosterone system. Hypotension, hemorrhage, low perfusion pressure, volume depletion, and sodium loss are the trigger factors for renin release **(Box 2)**.

After understanding the basics about anatomy, physiology, and function of adrenal gland, one point is clear that adrenocortical hormone deficiency results in reversal of these hormonal effects and produces acute adrenal crisis. Hormone of importance in acute adrenal crisis is coritsol. various causes of adrenal insufficiency are listed in **Table 3**.

Adrenal Hemorrhage and Infarction

Adrenal glands do not have direct arterial blood supply, so they are more prone for infarction and damage during systemic hypotension. Adrenal cortex receives the blood supply from subcapsular arteriolar plexus. Bilateral massive adrenal hemorrhage (BMAH) occurs under severe stressful conditions like myocardial infarction, severe sepsis with shock, trauma, burn, surgery, and complicated pregnancy. Coagulopathy, thrombocytopenia, and anticoagulants are also responsible for adrenal hemorrhage. Adrenal infarction is common in sepsis by meningococcemia, *Pseudomonas, Escherichia coli, Staphylococcus* infections.

Sudden Discontinuation of Long-term Glucocorticoid Therapy

Risk of acute adrenal crisis is more in patient who is on long-term glucocorticoid therapy due to underlying adrenal atrophy and adrenal corticotropin hormone (ACTH) suppression. Adrenal crisis can occur with single use, topical preparation, even with inhaled steroid.

FACTORS CONTRIBUTING TO SHOCK IN ACUTE ADRENAL CRISIS

There are two possibilities in developing the acute adrenal crisis: first adrenal crisis due to minor precipitant with underlying chronic insufficiency and second due to acute adrenal destruction (adrenal infarction and hemorrhage) resulting in catastrophic circulatory shock **(Flow chart 1)**.

Table 3	Causes of adrenal insufficiency	
	Primary	*Secondary*
Vascular	Adrenal infarction and hemorrhage	Pituitary infarction
Infiltrative	Granulomatous disease, sarcoidosis	Sarcoidosis histiocytosis hemochromatosis
Neoplasm	Metastasis	Pituitary adenoma metastasis
Infective	Tuberculosis meningococcal disease, fungal, human immunodeficiency virus	Tuberculosis fungal infection
Autoimmune	Autoimmune adrenalitis Polyglandular autoimmune syndromes I and II	
Traumatic	Blunt trauma abdomen, back trauma	Brain injury
Drugs	Ketoconazole etomidate	Sudden discontinuation of prolonged glucocorticoid therapy

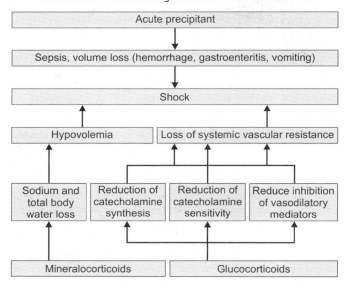

Flow chart 1 Contributing factors in acute adrenal crisis

Box 3 Clinical features of acute adrenal crisis

Circulatory shock is the hallmark of acute adrenal crisis
- Hypotension shock tachycardia
- Fever, fatigue, dehydration, arthralgia, myalgia, nausea, anorexia, vomiting, poor concentration, depression, disorientation
- Abdominal pain (rebound, tenderness, rigidity), flank pain, back pain, lower chest pain

Empiric Treatment for Adrenal Crisis before Confirming Laboratory Results

- Hydrocortisone is the drug of choice; it has both glucocorticoid and mineralocorticoid properties
- Empiric antibiotics can be started depending on underlying conditions
- Fresh frozen plasma to reverse coagulopathy
- Hyperkalemia should be corrected
- Thyroxine supplementation requirement in primary HPA axis failure (clinical hypothyroidism)
- Correction of dehydration and hypoglycemia
- Vasopressors.

DIAGNOSIS

Adrenal crisis is endocrine emergency and should be considered in acutely unwell patient with profound unexplained circulatory shock **(Box 3)**. Severity depends on level of defect, primary or secondary etiology (HPA axis) **(Table 4)**. Initial diagnosis is completely based on clinical evaluation. Detailed history, physical examination, and investigation are helpful in evaluating the patient (subacute, chronic symptoms) in outpatient department but not very helpful in emergency department. High index of suspicion is important for diagnosis of adrenal crisis in emergency department. Emergency physician should start the empiric treatment immediately even before receiving the confirmatory laboratory results. One may not get classic laboratory results in acute adrenal failure like adrenal hemorrhage.

Confirmatory Diagnostic Testing

Patients with all forms of adrenal deficiency have low cortisol level. Low serum cortisol level and inadequate response to stimulation test confirm the diagnosis.
- First step is early morning serum cortisol less than 3 µg/dL which confirms the adrenal deficiency while diagnosis is doubtful when cortisol level is more than 15 µg/dL.
- Second step is to find out if cortisol deficiency is due to ACTH or CRH (corticotropin-releasing hormone); give 250 µg of synthetic ACTH (Cosyntropin) and measure the serum cortisol if serum cortisol is more than 8 µg within 30 minutes; consider normal response, and exclude primary adrenal deficiency, but basal corticotropin level is required to differentiate between primary and secondary

Table 4 Clinical and laboratory features of adrenal insufficiency

	Primary adrenal insufficiency	Secondary adrenal insufficiency
Clinical features	• Hyperpigmentation, vitiligo, weight loss, hypotension, postural dizziness, and syncope shock • Weakness, fatigue, myalgia, arthralgia, anorexia, vomiting, constipation, abdominal pain, diarrhea • Amenorrhea, infertility, salt craving • Depression psychosis	• Weight gain, thin axillary and pubic hair, decrease libido, infertility, amenorrhea • Weakness, fatigue • Headache, visual disturbances • Anorexia, vomiting, constipation, abdominal pain, diarrhea, myalgia, arthralgia • Depression psychosis
Laboratory features	Hyponatremia, hyperkalemia, hypochloremia, and acidosis, mildly elevated blood urea nitrogen (BUN), mild hypoglycemia, anemia, B_{12} deficiency, type 1 diabetes	• Hypernatremia or hyponatremia • Hypokalemia or normal potassium, normal serum chloride, normal BUN, marked hypoglycemia
Risk of acute adrenal crisis	Very high	Low

adrenal deficiency. Corticotropin level is high in primary and low or normal in secondary adrenal deficiency. Insulin tolerance test is the test of choice for suspected secondary adrenal failure.

• But in emergency department and in crisis situation, both above methods of diagnosis, early morning cortisol level and stimulation test are not practical; random serum cortisol level more than 34 µg/dL excludes the adrenal deficiency while random cortisol level below 15 µg/dL in patient with severe sepsis or shock is suggestive of acute adrenal crisis.

Other Investigations

Few more laboratory tests and radiology are required to identify the treatable cause (sepsis) of acute adrenal failure. Computed tomography (CT) abdomen can be done to find out tuberculosis-associated calcification, adrenal hemorrhage, infiltration, while CT head may give clue to destruction of pituitary gland (empty sella syndrome).

TREATMENT

All patients of acute adrenal crisis should be admitted in intensive care unit for restoration of intravascular volume, electrolyte and hemodynamic monitoring, glucocorticoid replacement, and treatment of underlying cause **(Table 5)**.

Long-term hormone replacement therapy should be initiated once patient is recovered from crisis; intravenous steroid should be changed to oral preparation and prednisolone with longer half-life is required only once daily. Fludrocortisone (mineralocorticoid) is usually given in patient with primary adrenal failure. Androgen transdermal DHEA 25–50 mg is also added for primary adrenal failure.

DIFFERENTIAL DIAGNOSIS

Severe sepsis with shock.

Table 5 Treatment guidelines for acute adrenal crisis

Fluid resuscitation	At least 2–3 L of normal saline to restore volume and normal sodium balance
Intravenous steroids	Intravenous hydrocortisone 100 mg bolus followed by 100 mg two or three times per day (300–400 mg daily is initial regimen)
Antibiotics	Broad spectrum antibiotics for febrile patient
Vasopressors	In case of refractory shock
Glucose	50% dextrose may be used if required
In stabilized patient	Oral prednisolone fludrocortisone and androgen replacement Patient education regarding steroid management during acute febrile illness (double the dose of steroid for 3 days) regular follow-up with physician

SUMMARY

Acute adrenal crisis is not common but important endocrine emergency. Severity depends on the underlying etiology; there should be high index of suspicion in severe stressful conditions like trauma, burn sepsis, myocardial infarction and patients who present to emergency with unexplained circulatory shock with history of long-term steroid therapy. Empiric therapy should be started immediately. Prompt diagnosis and treatment is the key for better outcome.

BIBLIOGRAPHY

1. Annane D, Sebille V, Charpentier C, et al. Effect of treatment with low doses of hydrocortisone and fludrocortisone on mortality in patients with septic shock. JAMA. 2002;288(7):862-71.
2. Bouachour G, Tirot P, Varache N, et al. Hemodynamic changes in acute adrenal insufficiency. Intensive Care Med. 1994;20(2):138-41.

3. Hahner S, Allolio B. Therapeutic management of adrenal insufficiency. Best Pract Res Clin Endocrinol Metab. 2009;23(2):167-79.
4. Hahner S, Loeffler M, Bleicken B, et al. Epidemiology of adrenal crisis in chronic adrenal insufficiency: the need for new prevention strategies. Eur J Endocrinol. 2010;162(3):597-602.
5. Lamberts SW, Bruining HA, deJong FH. Corticosteroid therapy in severe illness. N Engl J Med. 1997;337(18):1285-92.
6. Loriaux DL, Fleseriu M. Relative adrenal insufficiency. Curr Opin Endocrinol Diabetes Obes. 2009;16(5):392-400.
7. Smans LC, Van der Valk ES, Hermus AR, et al. Incidence of adrenal crisis in patients with adrenal insufficiency. Clin Endocrinol (Oxf). 2016;84(1):17-22.
8. White K, Arlt W. Adrenal crisis in treated Addison's disease: a predictable but under-managed event. Eur J Endocrinol. 2010;162(1):115-20.
9. Yang S, Zhang L. Glucocorticoids and vascular reactivity. Curr Vasc Pharmacol. 2004;2(1):1-12.
10. Zuckerman-Levin N, Tiosano D, Eisenhofer G, et al. The importance of adrenocortical glucocorticoids for adrenomedullary and physiological response to stress: a study in isolated glucocorticoid deficiency. J Clin Endocrinol Metab. 2001;86(12):5920-4.

SECTION 9

Obstetrics and Gynecology

- **Vaginal Bleeding**
  Sabhyata Gupta, Shradha Chaudhari

- **Ectopic Pregnancy**
  Sabhyata Gupta

- **Emergency Delivery**
  Sangeeta Kaushik Sharma, Keerti Khetan

CHAPTER 67

Vaginal Bleeding

Sabhyata Gupta, Shradha Chaudhari

INTRODUCTION

In the emergency scenario, when a female presents with bleeding per vaginum, approach must be both quick and comprehensive, so as to make the correct diagnosis and initiate treatment without delay. A stepwise action includes a thorough but quick history, complete general and systemic examination and ordering necessary blood investigations and imaging studies. While the results of the same come in, a hemodynamically unstable patient must be resuscitated by the emergency team. Once the gynecologist ascertains the diagnosis, treatment (which may be medical or surgical) must be performed without delay. Close monitoring of vitals and assessment of further blood loss must continue so as to assess success or failure of therapy.

INITIAL ASSESSMENT

Before the detailed assessment is carried out, one must check for the five crucial parameters:
1. Age
2. Pregnancy (established or unknown)
3. Volume of blood loss
4. Hemodynamic stability
5. Associated acute abdomen.

Based on the earlier information, various differentials are kept in mind while taking history, performing examination and ordering investigations.

Age

A large number of females who present with bleeding in emergency are in the reproductive age group.

Pregnancy must always be ruled out for these women.

Menopausal women who have prolonged vaginal (PV) bleeding may have genital tract malignancies, the most common being cancer endometrium. Cancer endometrium is also prevalent in women above age 35 years with history of heavy menstrual bleeding.[1] Endometrial biopsy with or without hysteroscopy must be performed in all these women before initiating therapy. Other differential diagnoses to be kept in mind for menopausal causes of bleeding are atrophic endometritis, urinary infection, or bleeding per rectum.

Prepubertal girls presenting with PV bleeding are less common. Causes in this age group include trauma, endocrine tumors, and rare genital tract tumors.

Pregnancy

Pregnancy could be intrauterine or ectopic.
- Ectopic pregnancy is associated with small volume of bleeding with or without preceding amenorrhea. Pain in abdomen is invariably present and of mild to severe intensity. In initial phase of rupture, patient's vital parameters may be well compensated, thus this differential must always be borne in mind even in stable patients who do not give history of amenorrhea.[2,3] The ectopic pregnancy could be ruptured (requiring immediate surgery) or unruptured (qualifying for expectant/medical/surgical management).
- Threatened or inevitable abortion presents with small volume bleeding with or without pain. Patients are invariably stable. Ultrasound confirms the diagnosis.
- Incomplete or complete abortions are associated with heavy bleeding and pain. Sometimes, patients may be in stage of early compensated hypovolemic shock due to blood loss.
- Second- and third-trimester pregnancy bleeding could be due to placenta previa or abruptio placentae. Bleeding is painless in the former while abruption is associated with painful, slight, brownish or dark or fresh bleeding.

Ultrasound confirms placenta previa but may not be useful to diagnose placental abruption.[4]

Volume of Blood Loss

Following are the common gynecological causes of heavy bleeding:
- Fibroids
- Adenomyosis
- Dysfunctional uterine bleeding
- Polyps
- Trauma
- Bleeding disorders
- Uterine inversion
- Cancers
- Polycystic ovaries.

Following are the common obstetric causes of heavy bleeding:
- Incomplete or complete abortions
- Placenta previa
- Vasa previa
- Placental abruption
- Postpartum hemorrhage.

Following are the common gynecological causes of light or irregular bleeding:
- Polyps
- Polycystic ovaries
- Thyroid dysfunction
- Cancers
- Pelvic inflammatory disease
- Ruptured ovarian hemorrhagic cyst.

Following are the common obstetric causes of light bleeding:
- Ectopic pregnancy
- Threatened abortions
- Placental abruption
- Placenta previa.

Hemodynamic Stability

Patients who present to emergency room with bleeding per vaginum could be in various stages of shock. As in all emergency room protocols, the doctors and nurses must first initiate resuscitation of hemorrhagic shock. Minimum of two wide bore intravenous (IV) access lines must be secured. Blood samples must be drawn for cross-matching packed cells, hematocrit values and prothrombin time-international normalized ratio (PT-INR), activated partial thromboplastin time (APTT). Urine for pregnancy or serum beta-human chorionic gonadotropin (β-hCG) may be ordered if clinically indicated. Bedside ultrasound is the imaging of choice for these patients. While packed red blood cells are being issued by the blood bank, hypovolemia must be corrected with colloids and crystalloids. Foleys catheter may be inserted for intake output monitoring. In case surgical intervention is anticipated, anesthetists and operating room staff are informed in advance.

Once detailed history, examination and necessary investigations confirm the diagnosis, immediate treatment action to eliminate cause of bleeding must be initiated.

In case medical therapy is planned, patient could be transferred to either intensive care unit or wards based on the patient's clinical condition and results of investigations in triage.

Associated Acute Abdomen

Questions must be directed to elicit onset, duration, intensity of pain along with aggravating and relieving factors.

When slight vaginal bleeding is associated with severe pain abdomen, most common causes include ectopic pregnancy, torsion and ruptured hemorrhagic ovarian cyst. Bleeding is invariably an incidental finding and reason for emergency presentation is the pain. Pregnancy-related causes are placental abruption. Nongynecological cause can be ureteric colic with hematuria.

Heavy bleeding with pain abdomen may be encountered in adenomyosis, fibroids and abortions.

Pain may be present in cases of acute pelvic inflammatory disease with incidental PV bleeding.

INITIAL ASSESSMENT

History

Best medical practice always teaches the doctor to always take a complete history of the patient even in emergency setting. Questions must be asked while keeping various causes of the presentation in mind. Vital information to be elicited includes a detailed menstrual history, age, marital status, history suggestive of bleeding disorders, associated amenorrhea, fever, gastrointestinal symptoms, giddiness, and pain.

Menstrual history must include a complete assessment of duration and volume of blood loss, including number of days of heavy and light bleeding. Volume of loss is assessed by the number of sanitary napkins or tampons used. Bleeding lasting more than 7 days and requiring more than 3–4 sanitary napkins a day is abnormal.[5] Passage of large clots indicates heavy bleeding. Clots larger than 1 cm indicate blood loss of more than 80 mL in a cycle.[6,7] Past menstrual cycle pattern including duration and length of cycles must be asked for. In cases of suspected pregnancy-related cause, scanty flow in last menstrual period must be inquired. The gestation may be greater than amenorrhea in cases with implantation bleeding.

When the woman gives prolonged history of menorrhagia, questions must be directed to rule out fibroids (heavy flow on day two of cycle), adenomyosis (dysmenorrhea), polycystic ovaries (irregular cycles, hirsute features, acne, weight gain), thyroid disorders (weight changes, cold or heat intolerance, constipation) and bleeding disorders (easy bruisability).[8]

In cases with history of fever, hemorrhagic cystitis or acute pelvic inflammatory disease may be the etiological factor.

Past medical history must be asked along with details of all medications taken including any hormonal intake or history of being on blood thinners.

General Examination

Upon presentation to triage, patient's vital parameters are obtained with a cardiac monitor. Signs of hemodynamic instability include tachycardia, hypotension, cold clammy extremities, pallor and sweating. Mucosal hemorrhage, purpura or petechial rashes may be present in patients with bleeding disorders. Hirsutism, acne and oily skin are present in polycystic ovarian syndrome. Virilization may indicate an androgen-secreting tumor.

Systemic Examination

Respiratory and cardiovascular systems must be checked. Per abdomen examination must be stepwise including inspection, palpation and auscultation. On inspection, shape and contour of abdomen gives information about pelvic masses or intra-abdominal bleeding which lead to distension. Large fibroids and uterine size in pregnancy can be detected on palpation of the uterus. Presence and location of tenderness on palpation also helps to narrow down the differential diagnosis to suspected causes of painful bleeding. Suprapubic tenderness is present in urinary tract infections and uterine pathology, whereas in tubo-ovarian pathology, the pain is in the iliac fossa. Hepatosplenomegaly may also be present in cases of chronic anemia and malignancies.

Per-speculum Examination

Per-speculum examination must be carried out with all aseptic precautions with a good light source and positioning of the patient. Examination must be gentle. Clots present must be removed gently to assess for cervical lesions like polyps or masses. Care must be taken before dislodging large clots in hemodynamically unstable patients. There can be torrential bleeding once a clot is dislodged, especially in cases of genital trauma and pregnancy. In cases of big vaginal lacerations with heavy bleeding, it is prudent to shift patient to the operating room with adequate blood arranged prior to complete assessment of the laceration. Examination under anesthesia and suturing can be performed simultaneously. In such cases, vaginal packing must be done in triage to reduce blood loss in the duration required to shift the patient to the operating theater.

In cases of incomplete abortions, products of conception are also noticed mixed with the blood clots. Grape-like vesicles are present in cases of complete molar pregnancies. A previous antenatal ultrasound and evaluation in triage can clinch the diagnosis, and the patient is immediately taken for suction curettage without further delay. Molar evacuations are associated with increased complications like bleeding and embolism; hence, such cases must be referred to higher centers with cardiopulmonary backup for curettage.

Bimanual Examination

As with speculum examination, bimanual examination must be very gentle. A careless bimanual examination can result in intra-abdominal bleeding due to dislodgment of clot and worsening of shock in cases of ruptured or impending rupture ectopic.

Uterine size, shape and contour are felt for and adnexal masses are ruled out. Fullness in pouch of Douglas indicates presence of fluid.

Cervical motion tenderness is present in cases of ectopic pregnancy.

Bimanual examination must never be performed in cases of suspected placenta previa.

BLOOD INVESTIGATIONS

After securing good IV access, samples are drawn for the following:
- Blood grouping and Rh typing
- Cross matching of blood products
- Complete blood count with hematocrit
- Prothrombin time-international normalized ratio
- Activated partial thromboplastin time
- Serum β-hCG in indicated cases
- Thyroid profile in indicated cases
- Kidney function test (KFT), liver function test (LFT) in indicated cases
- Viral markers if the patient requires surgery.

IMAGING STUDIES

Ultrasound [transvaginal scan (TVS) where possible] is the diagnostic modality of choice in the emergency setting. Not only is it quick, but also relatively easy and also possible to perform at the bedside if need be. In pregnant women, TVS ultrasound can localize a pregnancy at a minimum β-hCG value of 1,500 IU/mL. Color Doppler studies are useful in cases of ectopic and torsion. Sometimes, magnetic resonance imaging (MRI) may be required if ultrasound is unable to clinch the diagnosis.

TREATMENT

Immediate resuscitation with IV fluids, IV tranexamic acid and IV pain medication is given; antacids and antiemetics too must be given if patient requires anesthesia. Invariably, the patient is not in nil per oral status as required for surgery. Tamponade to the uterus can be given with roller gauze pack, balloon devices as done in postpartum hemorrhage, if need be.

THERAPEUTIC MEASURES

Uterine Curettage

It is the treatment of choice for profuse bleeding in hemodynamically unstable women. Curettage is the best modality of therapy in cases of inevitable abortions and incomplete abortions. Curettage removes all products of conception quickly. Completeness of procedure can be confirmed on ultrasound. In centers where ultrasonography (USG) is not available, the surgeon must look for four signs: (1) grating sensation of all walls; (2) reduction is size of the uterus; (3) bubbles seen at the os; and (4) closing of the os. Misoprostol may be used in conjunction with curettage. Prior usage of misoprostol helps contract the upper cavity and open cervical os. Postprocedure, misoprostol helps to keep the uterus well contracted and also to expel any small piece of conception.

Emergency curettage can be used as treatment modality in nonpregnant women with heavy bleeding and hemodynamic instability who do not respond to initial measures like injectable tranexamic acid. Emergency curettage should be performed if radioimaging shows increased endometrial thickness despite prolonged and profuse bleeding. This immediately relieves the symptoms and also provides histopathological correlation so as to chalk out the further treatment plan to prevent future menorrhagia. Disadvantage of curettage is that if further treatment is not initiated, it cannot prevent future episodes of heavy bleeding.[9,10]

Various studies comparing results of uterine curettage to hormone therapy show that time required for bleeding to subside is more with medical management.[9] Anesthesia is avoided in medical therapy. Medical therapy may be preferred if it yields results without the need of more blood transfusion. It can also be given after curettage to stop bleeding after the procedure.

High-dose Intravenous Estrogen

Mechanism of action of estrogen therapy is promotion of regrowth of endometrium over the bleeding denuded epithelial surface. Estrogen stabilizes lysosomal membranes and stimulates promotion of endometrial ground substance.[9] A randomized control trail of 34 cases was carried out where women with heavy bleeding were treated with IV conjugated equine estrogen (CEE), 25 mg premarin in 5 mL saline was instilled over 2 minutes. The dose was repeated every 3–5 hours if bleeding persisted. In the placebo arm 200 mg of lactulose was given.[11] The difference in the two arms was not statistically significant in the first 3 hours. However, after 72 hours, 72% of patients in the CEE arm showed improvement versus 38% in the placebo arm. Bleeding persisted at 8 hours in two women in the CEE group. There was no correlation between histology on endometrial biopsy and success of therapy. In the CEE arm, 39% women had nausea and vomiting requiring treatment versus 13% in the placebo group.[11]

If bleeding persists beyond 8 hours, estrogen therapy must be stopped and other treatment modalities started.[11]

Maintenance therapy is started once bleeding decreases with IV premarin; 2.5 mg premarin four times a day can be continued for 21 days. A progestin must be given in the next 10 days.

Maintenance therapy can also be started with oral contraceptive (OC) pills containing 35 μg estrogen. Initially, two tablets are given for 5 days, followed by once a day for 20 days.

Potential serious side effects of high-dose estrogen include thrombosis and embolism.[12] Thus, minimum dose to produce desired result must be used. In high-risk category, like women at high-risk for thrombosis, estrogen therapy is contraindicated.

Uterine Artery Embolization

Uterine artery embolization is the first line of management of bleeding due to uterine arteriovenous (AV) malformations. It should not be used as first choice of therapy over emergency hysterectomy due to technical challenges and length of the procedure. However, in higher institutes with good clinical experience of performing the procedure, it can be performed in women who desire future fertility. Current evidence, however, does not establish safety in future pregnancies. Adverse outcomes in pregnancy have been reported after embolization procedure.

Surgical Management of Ectopic Pregnancy

Laparoscopic surgery is invariably feasible in higher centers with good emergency, anesthesia and blood bank facilities. Only in hemodynamically unstable patients where head low position is not possible, laparotomy is considered. Goals of surgery must include correct time management to prevent complications due to the delay. A team approach and good communication with anesthetist is imperative to detect any anticipated complications on time.

Hysterectomy

In obstetric cases, when initial measures like bimanual compression, oxytocics, uterine tamponade, repair of lacerations fail, patient is taken up for emergency laparotomy. A gynecologist must be well versed with anatomy of the iliacs, uterine artery and ureter. A broad ligament hematoma can be treated with uterine artery ligation at its origin. Internal iliac ligation is recommended to control atonic or traumatic postpartum hemorrhage when previous measures fail. When internal iliac ligation fails, obstetric hysterectomy is performed to save the life of the woman.

In gynecological cases of heavy uncontrolled bleeding with hemodynamic instability, when all measures fail, in rare circumstances, emergency hysterectomy may be performed to treat uncontrolled bleeding.

TREATMENT OF BLEEDING PER VAGINUM IN HEMODYNAMICALLY STABLE PATIENTS

Estrogen Therapy

High-dose oral estrogen therapy is most effective in controlling menorrhagia. It carries risk of thrombosis and embolism and should not be used in high-risk patients.[13] Estrogen therapy alone is more effective than combined estrogen-progesterone therapy because progestins inhibit synthesis of estrogen receptors and increase estradiol dehydrogenase, thereby impeding the rapid proliferation of endometrium induced by estrogen.

Estrogen–Progesterone Therapy

This is also used to control heavy and prolonged bleeding. Initial dose is 2 tablets a day for 5 days, followed by once a day for 20 days. Withdrawal bleeding may be slightly heavy but usually stops in 7 days.[14,15]

Progestin Therapy

Medroxyprogesterone 10 mg, two tablets twice a day are started to treat menorrhagia of anovulatory etiology. Progestins inhibit further endometrial growth in women with thickened endometrium. After 5–7 days, the dose is reduced to once or twice a day for a total duration of 25 days.[14] Progesterone causes thinning of endometrium, thus controlling the bleeding. Only progesterone therapy is less effective than estrogen especially in cases where bleeding is due to denudation of the endometrium.[16]

Endometrial Ablation

This is the procedure of choice after endometrial biopsy to confirm benign nature of the disease. Relatively simple and noninvasive, ablation can help to treat the symptom of heavy bleeding without much long-term or short-term complications.

CONCLUSION

Keys to successful outcome in management of emergency vaginal bleeding are thorough knowledge of etiological factors, good time management and emergency team approach to arrive at the correct diagnosis while resuscitating the patient at the same time, followed by administering the appropriate therapy. Speed, close vigilance and time to time reassessment ensure success of therapy.

REFERENCES

1. Clark TJ, Voit D, Gupta JK, et al. Accuracy of hysteroscopy in the diagnosis of endometrial cancer and hyperplasia: a systematic quantitative review. JAMA. 2002;288:1610-21.
2. Kalinski MA, Guss DA. Hemorrhagic shock from a ruptured ectopic pregnancy in a patient with a negative urine pregnancy test result. Ann Emerg Med. 2002;40:102-5.
3. Barnhart K, Mennuti MT, Benjamin I, et al. Prompt diagnosis of ectopic pregnancy in an emergency department setting. Obstet Gynecol. 1994;84:1010-5.
4. Taipale P, Hiilesmaa V, Ylöstalo P. Transvaginal ultrasonography at 18-23 weeks in predicting placenta previa at delivery. Ultrasound Obstet Gynecol. 1998;12:422-5.
5. Mansfield PK, Voda A, Allison G. Validating a pencil-and-paper measure of perimenopausal menstrual blood loss. Womens Health Issues. 2004;14:242-7.
6. Chimbira TH, Anderson AB, Turnbull AC. Relation between measured menstrual blood loss and patient's subjective assessment of loss, duration of bleeding, number of sanitary towels used, uterine weight and endometrial surface area. Br J Obstet Gynaecol. 1980;87:603-9.
7. Warner PE, Critchley HO, Lumsden MA, et al. Menorrhagia I: measured blood loss, clinical features, and outcome in women with heavy periods: a survey with follow-up data. Am J Obstet Gynecol. 2004;190:1216-23.
8. Lane DE. Polycystic ovary syndrome and its differential diagnosis. Obstet Gynecol Surv. 2006;61:125-35.
9. March CM. Bleeding problems and treatment. Clin Obstet Gynecol. 1998;41:928-39.
10. Haynes PJ, Hodgson H, Anderson AB, et al. Measurement of menstrual blood loss in patients complaining of menorrhagia. Br J Obstet Gynaecol. 1977;84:763-8.
11. DeVore GR, Owens O, Kase N. Use of intravenous premarin in the treatment of dysfunctional uterine bleeding—a double-blind randomized control study. Obstet Gynecol. 1982;59:285-91.
12. Zreik TG, Odunsi K, Cass I, et al. A case of fatal pulmonary thromboembolism associated with the use of intravenous estrogen therapy. Fertil Steril. 1999;71:373-5.
13. Speroff L, Fritz M. Postmenopausal hormone therapy. In: Speroff L, Fritz M (Eds). Clinical Gynecologic Endocrinology and Infertility, 7th edition. Baltimore, Maryland: Lippincott Williams & Wilkins; 2005.
14. Munro MG, Mainor N, Basu R, et al. Oral medroxyprogesterone acetate and combination oral contraceptives for acute uterine bleeding: a randomized controlled trial. Obstet Gynecol. 2006;108:924-9.
15. Shwayder JM. Pathophysiology of abnormal uterine bleeding. Obstet Gynecol Clin North Am. 2000;27:219-34.
16. Hickey M, Higham JM, Fraser I. Progestogens with or without oestrogen for irregular uterine bleeding associated with anovulation. Cochrane Database Syst Rev. 2012;(9):CD001895.

CHAPTER 68

Ectopic Pregnancy

Sabhyata Gupta

INTRODUCTION

Ectopic pregnancy is a condition in which a developing blastocyst gets implanted outside the endometrial cavity of uterus. Most common site is ampullary part of fallopian tube (98%). Other possible locations include cervical, interstitial, cornual, ovarian, cesarean scar, abdominal, and heterotopic pregnancies. The incidence of ectopic pregnancy is currently 1–2% and it has been rising in the last decade mainly because of rising incidence of pelvic inflammatory disease (PID) in young teenage girls (due to early commencement of sexual activity), increasing maternal age, and delay in conception leading to more use of assisted reproductive techniques, development of more accurate diagnostic modalities, and increasing awareness. The spectrum of clinical presentation is very wide from completely asymptomatic to a life-threatening condition. There has been a paradigm shift in management of ectopic pregnancy from laparotomy in past to expectant and outpatient management in present day.

ETIOLOGY AND RISK FACTORS

Infection, inflammation, or surgery can cause tubal mucosal and ciliary damage which may impair tubal motility leading to implantation of the blastocyst in fallopian tube.[1]

Factors Contributing to Ectopic Pregnancy

- Previous pelvic surgery
- Previous ectopic pregnancy
- Contraception[2]
- Transperitoneal migration
- Diethylstilbestrol exposure
- Endometriosis
- Infection
- Infertility
- Advanced maternal age
- Hormonal factors
- Previous spontaneous abortion
- Alterations in tubal physiology
- Assisted reproductive technologies
- Uterine curettage.

Pelvic Inflammatory Disease

The risk of an ectopic pregnancy is high after acute salpingitis.[3] The PID and tubal obstruction are closely associated with ectopic pregnancy. *Chlamydia trachomatis* is a common cause of urethritis, cervicitis, and PID.

Previous Ectopic Pregnancy

Many studies reveal that there is high risk of ectopic pregnancy after conservative surgery.

Sterilization

During first year of sterilization, failure rate is 0.1–0.8%, one-third of which are ectopic pregnancies. Sterilization reversal also increases risk for ectopic pregnancy. Exact risk depends on methods of sterilization, site of tubal occlusion, residual tubal length, coexisting disease, and surgical technique.

Intrauterine Devices

Intrauterine device (IUD) works by preventing fertilization as well as implantation, so women using IUD have a lower incidence of ectopic pregnancy.

SIGNS AND SYMPTOMS OF ECTOPIC PREGNANCY

A careful clinical history and strong suspicion of ectopic pregnancy helps in diagnosis. Typically, patients present with classic triad of abdominal pain (most common), irregular bleeding per vaginum, and amenorrhea. Amenorrhea may not be present in a few patients. Patient may also present with vague gastrointestinal symptoms. Early unruptured ectopic pregnancy may be asymptomatic.

Lower abdominal pain and tenderness, shoulder pain, abdominal distension, vomiting, syncope, and shock are common presentations in ruptured ectopic pregnancy. Shoulder pain is secondary to hemorrhagic fluid irritating the diaphragm.

Patient may have tachycardia, hypotension, low hematocrit, and signs of peritoneal inflammation like rebound tenderness secondary to hemoperitoneum.

DIFFERENTIAL DIAGNOSIS OF ECTOPIC PREGNANCY

- Acute appendicitis
- Miscarriage
- Ovarian torsion
- Pelvic inflammatory disease
- Ruptured corpus luteum cyst or follicle
- Tubo-ovarian abscess
- Urinary calculi.

DIAGNOSIS OF ECTOPIC PREGNANCY

Ectopic pregnancy can be diagnosed accurately and at earliest by using serum beta-human chorionic gonadotropin (hCG) and transvaginal ultrasound.[4-6]

Transvaginal Ultrasound

Transvaginal ultrasound (TVS) is most important, safe, acceptable, and extremely cost-effective diagnostic tool for ectopic pregnancy. It has a high level of accuracy.[7,8] Recent studies have reported 94–97% positive predictive value for TVS, low false positive rates, sensitivity rates of around 87–99%, and specificity rates of 94–99%.[9] The accuracy of TVS depends upon skill of the radiologist also.[10]

Serum Beta-human Chorionic Gonadotropin and Serum Progesterone

In the emergency department, serum beta-hCG is important "point of care test" to confirm pregnancy. Pregnancy is diagnosed by determining the urine or serum beta-hCG. This hormone is detectable in urine and blood as early as 1 week before an expected menstrual period. Serum testing detects levels as low as 5 IU/L, whereas urine testing detects levels as low as 20–50 IU/L.[11] Beta-hCG measurement can confirm only pregnancy and for confirmation of location of gestational sac TVS may be needed.

Serum beta-human chorionic gonadotropin is produced by proliferating trophoblast and is expected to double every 48 hours in normal intrauterine pregnancy.[12] Progesterone is secreted by the corpus luteum to maintain the uterine lining for pregnancy and its serum levels remain relatively constant in early pregnancy. In failing pregnancies, beta-hCG will fail to increase normally and progesterone level will be low.

Serial beta-hCG measurements are often used for:
- Women with first-trimester bleeding or pain, or both
- To confirm fetal viability
- Post medical management of ectopic pregnancy.

MANAGEMENT OF ECTOPIC PREGNANCY

It is important to determine best course of treatment in a patient presenting with ectopic pregnancy depending upon symptoms, clinical presentation, and investigations.
- Surgical management
- Medical management.

SURGICAL MANAGEMENT FOR ECTOPIC PREGNANCY

Indications for Surgical Management

- Hemodynamically unstable patient
- Ruptured or suspicion of ruptured ectopic pregnancy
- Presence of hemoperitoneum
- Contraindication to medical management
- Patient cannot come for regular follow-up
- Large size, live ectopic pregnancy
- Patient wants sterilization
- Diagnosis is uncertain
- Associated pelvic pathology like large ovarian cyst, fibroid or adnexal mass.

Management of Acute Abdomen with Ectopic Pregnancy

Whenever a patient of reproductive age group presents in emergency with complaints of abdominal pain, irregular bleeding per vaginum with or without amenorrhea, ectopic pregnancy must be ruled out. In case of ruptured ectopic pregnancy, patient may be hemodynamically unstable and may present in shock.

For patients with known or suspected ruptured ectopic pregnancies, surgical management is the treatment of choice.

Surgical Management

- *Intravenous (IV) access*: Wide bore cannula should be put; IV fluids should be given.
- *Biochemical investigations*: Complete blood counts (CBC), prothrombin time (PT) or international normalized ratio (INR), serum beta-hCG/UPT, and liver or kidney function or viral marker tests.
- Arrange and cross-match blood and other blood products.

Route of Surgery

Laparotomy was the treatment of choice in past, but nowadays, laparoscopy is gold standard for hemodynamically stable patient. Laparotomy may still be needed for a patient in shock and severe anemia.

Tubal ligation in contralateral tube should be offered to those patients who have completed their family.

Laparoscopic Surgery for Ectopic Pregnancy

Salpingectomy versus Salpingostomy

The decision between the two approaches is made intraoperatively after considering the risk factors, patient's desire for future fertility, and hemodynamic condition of the patient.[13,14]

- *Salpingectomy*: It is the segmental or entire removal of the fallopian tube.
  The indications for removing the tube include:
  - Severely damaged and ruptured tube
  - Uncontrolled bleeding (before or after salpingostomy)
  - Recurrent ectopic pregnancy in the same tube
  - Heterotopic pregnancy
  - Lack of desire to bear more children.
- *Salpingostomy*: It is the method of choice in women of reproductive age who wish to preserve their fertility.

Preparation of Patient for Salpingectomy

The patient is placed under general anesthesia and placed in semilithotomy position. After cleaning and draping the patient, a primary trocar is inserted into the umbilical region. In case of patients who had undergone previous surgeries, a primary trocar is inserted at the Palmar's point. Camera port (10 mm) is inserted at umbilicus. Next, two accessory ports (5 mm) are inserted, at lower left iliac region and upper left lumbar area. If required, a third accessory port is made in the right iliac fossa.

Technique of Laparoscopic Salpingectomy

Bipolar coagulation (Robes) forceps and harmonic scalpel/scissors are used and the fallopian tube is excised. The specimen is retrieved by putting an endobag through the 10 mm port, and a 5 mm telescope is inserted through left lumbar port for the retrieval. Hemostasis is ensured.

In the Case of Acute Abdomen and Ruptured Ectopic Pregnancy

If a patient has a hemoperitoneum more than 1 L, 10 mm suction cannula should be used for suction and irrigation thoroughly. The presence of hemoperitoneum may increase the chances of adhesion formation and may decrease future fertility.

Technique of Laparoscopic Salpingostomy

It has been reported to reduce bleeding and operative time in some studies.

Salpingostomy is typically performed by making an incision (linear cut) along the antimesenteric border of the fallopian tube at the point of maximal distension by using monopolar needle cautery followed by suctioning the products of conception. For removing residual products of conception, hydrodissection may be used. It is important to avoid excessive handling of the tube and excessive cautery in order to prevent potential further damage to the fallopian tube. Hemostasis is achieved by continuous irrigation, identifying pinpoint bleeding points and cauterizing them by using microbipolar forceps. Incision is left open to heal by secondary intention.

The rate of subsequent intrauterine pregnancy is improved in patients having linear salpingostomy versus salpingectomy, although the recurrent ectopic pregnancy rate is also higher. Data indicate a beneficial effect of conservative surgery towards subsequent fertility that was not, however, statistically significant in the multivariate analysis.[13]

Patient undergoing salpingostomy should be on close follow-up with serum beta-hCG levels after every 48 weeks for 1 week followed by weekly till value becomes normal. Serum beta-hCG levels may become plateau or may increase due to risk of persistent trophoblastic tissue. Injection methotrexate (MTX) should be given to these patients in postoperative period if serum beta-hCG levels start increasing or become constant.[15]

For cases in which there is risk of persistent trophoblastic tissue and products of conception have not been removed completely, single prophylactic dose of injection MTX should be given in immediate postoperative period.[16] After conservative surgery, patients require longer follow-up and higher risk of recurrent ectopic pregnancy up to 9.8%.

MEDICAL MANAGEMENT FOR ECTOPIC PREGNANCY

Methotrexate therapy is a good option for treatment of hemodynamically stable patients with unruptured ectopic pregnancy.[17] It is equally efficacious and safe with good fertility outcomes. The overall success rate is 91%.[18]

Methotrexate is folic acid antagonist which interferes with deoxyribonucleic acid (DNA) synthesis and cell proliferation. It is effective on highly proliferative tissues such as developing embryo.

Indications for Methotrexate Therapy

- Hemodynamic stability
- Patients with unruptured ectopic pregnancies with size of ectopic mass less than 3.5 cm
- Availability of serial transvaginal ultrasonography (USG) and serum beta-hCG values
- Patients should be willing for regular follow-up for longer time.

Contraindications

- Ruptured ectopic pregnancy or presence of hemoperitoneum
- Immunocompromised patients
- Chronic kidney and liver disease, peptic ulcer disease
- Active pulmonary disease
- Allergic to MTX
- Lack of availability of emergency medical services in case of rupture.

Factors Decreasing Success of Methotrexate Therapy

- Serum beta-hCG levels more than 5,000
- Presence of cardiac activity
- Large ectopic mass size (more than 3.5 cm)
- Presence of peritoneal fluid
- Acute pain in lower abdomen.

Side Effects

Side effects include nausea, vomiting, photosensitivity, bone marrow suppression, acute renal failure, pancytopenia, skin and mucosal damage, oral ulcers, acute respiratory distress syndrome, and impaired liver function.

Methotrexate therapy has comparable efficacy to laparoscopic salpingostomy. It is less invasive, results in similar fertility outcomes and does not decrease ovarian reserve.

Management

Blood investigations like CBC, renal and liver function test, blood group, and coagulation profile should be done.

Patients are counseled in detail about regular follow-up with serum beta-hCG levels and transvaginal USG.

Methotrexate can be given either systemically (intravenously, intramuscularly, orally) or directly by injection into ectopic sac under ultrasound guidance or laparoscopic guidance. The most common approach is intramuscular local injection of MTX for tubal ectopic pregnancy which is rarely used, except in few cases of cervical gestations.

Single-dose Regimen

The most commonly used dose is a single intramuscular injection of MTX 50 mg/m^2 without folic acid. Serum beta-hCG levels are repeated on day 4 and day 7.

Multiple-dose Regimen

In this regimen, MTX is given 1 mg/kg/day intramuscular on days 1, 3, 5, and 7, and oral leucovorin (0.1 mg/kg) on days 2, 4, 6, and 8. hCG levels are drawn on days 1, 3, 5, and 7. Treatment is stopped and surveillance phase begins (serum beta-hCG is measured on weekly basis), if the serum hCG declines more than 15% from the previous measurement. An additional dose of MTX 1 mg/kg intramuscular (IM) is given if hCG declines less than 15% from the previous level.

Both have similar efficacy and success rate. Due to fewer side effects and lower doses required, single-dose regimen is used more often.

Precautions during MTX therapy:[19]

- Avoid vaginal intercourse and new conception until serum beta-hCG levels are undetectable
- Avoid pelvic examinations during surveillance of MTX therapy due to theoretical risk of tubal rupture
- Avoid sun exposure to limit risk of MTX dermatitis
- Avoid foods and vitamins containing folic acid
- Avoid nonsteroidal anti-inflammatory drugs, as the interaction with MTX may cause bone marrow suppression, aplastic anemia, or gastrointestinal toxicity.

Patient receiving medical management should be counseled thoroughly about side effects, reporting signs and symptoms, chances of failure and rupture of ectopic pregnancy. The need for possible surgical intervention in case of rupture or failure of medical management should be explained before starting medical management. Patient should immediately report in case of severe abdominal pain, dizziness, and excessive bleeding per vagina. Patient should be followed up serially with TVS USG for assessment of hemoperitoneum.[20] Patient getting medical management is still at risk of rupture of ectopic pregnancy in spite of decreasing serum beta-hCG levels, so patients should be aware of reporting signs and symptoms.

OVARIAN PREGNANCY

Ovarian pregnancy is a rare and challenging condition to diagnose.

Pathologic criteria developed by Spiegelberg to distinguish primary ovarian pregnancies from other ectopic pregnancies with secondary involvement of the ovary are as follows:[21,22]
- The fallopian tube on the involved side is intact and separate from the ovary
- The gestational sac is in the normal position of the ovary. The ovary with the gestational sac is connected to the uterus by the ovarian ligament
- The specimen has ovarian tissue attached to, and in, the wall of the gestation sac
- The ovary with the gestational sac is connected to the uterus by the ovarian ligament.

During laparoscopy, wedge resection of ovary including gestational products is done, and we try to save maximum amount of healthy ovarian tissues.

CERVICAL PREGNANCY

Cervical ectopic pregnancy is a rare condition with an incidence of less than 0.1% of all ectopic pregnancies.[21,22] It is associated with a high morbidity and mortality potential. Timely intervention is required to preserve fertility and avoid the need for a hysterectomy. Magnetic resonance imaging (MRI) and three-dimensional (3D) ultrasound should be done to make the exact diagnosis.[23]

INTERSTITIAL PREGNANCY

If cornual pregnancy is diagnosed earlier laparoscopic surgery is done. If patient presents with ruptured cornual pregnancy, usually lot of bleeding is present, and laparotomy and cornual resection or hysterectomy may be required if patient presents in shock.

If patient is hemodynamically stable, laparoscopic resection of gestational products by cornuostomy is done.[24] In clinically stable patients, if ultrasound measurements show no cardiac activity and the gestational period is less than 9 weeks, systemic MTX[25] may be tried.

Gestational period more than 9 weeks with the presence of cardiac activity demonstrated on ultrasound in a clinically stable patient may require addition of intra-amniotic potassium chloride in addition to systemic MTX.

Second- or third-trimester diagnosis may warrant hysterectomy.

CONCLUSION

Ectopic pregnancy may have varying clinical presentation and management may change depending upon clinical condition. Availability of TVS USG, serum beta-hCG, and laparoscopy has led to more conservative approach and earlier detection is key to success. Patient's awareness about ectopic pregnancy and earlier reporting to pregnancy units for confirmation and exact localization of pregnancy may save many laparotomies, morbidity, and mortality related to ectopic pregnancy.

REFERENCES

1. Erkkola R, Liukko P. Intrauterine device and ectopic pregnancy. Contraception. 1977;16(6):569-74.
2. Westrom L, Bengtsson LP, Mardh PA. Incidence, trends, and risks of ectopic pregnancy in a population of women. Br Med J. 1981;282(6257):5-17.
3. Paavonen J, Eggert-Kruse W. *Chlamydia trachomatis*: impact on human reproduction. Hum Reprod Update. 1999;5(5):433-47.
4. Sivalingam VN, Duncan WC, Kirk E, et al. Diagnosis and management of ectopic pregnancy. J Fam Plann Reprod Health Care. 2011;37(4):231-40.
5. Yao M, Tulandi T. Current status of surgical and nonsurgical management of ectopic pregnancy. Fertil Steril. 1997;67(3):421-33.
6. Tay JI, Moore J, Walker JJ. Ectopic pregnancy. BMJ. 2000;320(7239):916-9.
7. Kaplan BC, Dart RG, Moskos M, et al. Ectopic pregnancy: prospective study with improved diagnostic accuracy. Ann Emerg Med. 1996;28(1):10-7.
8. Jehle D, Krause R, Braen GR. Ectopic pregnancy. Emerg Med Clin North Am. 1994;12(1):55-71.
9. Kirk E, Papageorghiou AT, Condous G, et al. The diagnostic effectiveness of an initial transvaginal scan in detecting ectopic pregnancy. Hum Reprod. 2007;22(11):2824-8.
10. Winder S, Reid S, Condous G. Ultrasound diagnosis of ectopic pregnancy. Australas J Ultrasound Med. 2011;14(2):29-33.
11. Murray H, Baakdah H, Bardell T, et al. Diagnosis and treatment of ectopic pregnancy. CMAJ. 200511;173(8):905-12.
12. Brennan DF. Ectopic pregnancy—Part I: Clinical and laboratory diagnosis. Acad Emerg Med. 1995;2(12):1081-9.
13. Mol BW, Matthijsse HC, Tinga DJ, et al. Fertility after conservative and radical surgery for tubal pregnancy. Hum Reprod. 1998;13(7):1804-9.
14. Mol F, van Mello NM, Strandell A, et al. Salpingotomy versus salpingectomy in women with tubal pregnancy (ESEP study): an open-label, multicenter, randomized controlled trial. Lancet. 2014;383(9927):1483-9.
15. Gracia CR, Brown HA, Barnhart KT. Prophylactic methotrexate after linear salpingostomy: a decision analysis. Fertil Steril. 2001;76(6):1191-5.
16. Barnhart KT, Gosman G, Ashby R, et al. The medical management of ectopic pregnancy: a meta-analysis comparing "single dose" and "multidose" regimens. Obstet Gynecol. 2003;101(4):778-84.
17. Leeman LM, Wendland CL. Cervical ectopic pregnancy. Diagnosis with endovaginal ultrasound examination and successful treatment with methotrexate. Arch Fam Med. 2000;9(1):72-7.

18. Hajenius PJ, Mol BW, Bossuyt PM, et al. Interventions for tubal ectopic pregnancy. Cochrane Database Syst Rev. 2000;(2):CD000324.
19. Practice Committee of the American Society for Reproductive Medicine. Medical treatment of ectopic pregnancy. Fertil Steril. 2006;86(5 Suppl 1):S96-102.
20. Spiegelberg O. Zur kasuistik der ovarial schwangerschaft. Arch Gyneakol. 1878;13:73.
21. Comstock C, Huston K, Lee W. The ultrasonographic appearance of ovarian ectopic pregnancies. Obstet Gynecol. 2005;105(1):42-5.
22. Kung FT, Chang SY. Efficacy of methotrexate treatment in viable and nonviable cervical pregnancies. Am J Obstet Gynecol. 1999;181(6):1438-44.
23. Singh S. Diagnosis and management of cervical ectopic pregnancy. J Hum Reprod Sci. 2013;6(4):273-6.
24. Tulandi T, Al-Jaroudi D. Interstitial pregnancy: results generated from the Society of Reproductive Surgeons Registry. Obstet Gynecol. 2004;103(1):47-50.
25. Jermy K, Thomas J, Doo A, et al. The conservative management of interstitial pregnancy. BJOG. 2004;111(11):1283-8.

CHAPTER 69

Emergency Delivery

Sangeeta Kaushik Sharma, Keerti Khetan

INTRODUCTION

In pregnancy, labor is defined as the process that begins with the onset of repetitive and forceful uterine contractions sufficient to cause dilation of the cervix and ends with delivery of the infant and placenta.

The management of childbirth is usually the responsibility of gynecologists. Gynecologists are not always available in-house in most of emergency departments (EDs), as they need to be called from OPD or OT in daytime and from their home in nighttime; so emergency physician must know the outlines of management of obstetric emergencies and basic steps of parturition, if situation occurs.

PREHOSPITAL CARE

If such a situation occurs outside the hospital then arrangements must be made to transport the pregnant to the nearby hospital safely and promptly. Under *Janani Suraksha Yojna* for pregnant, Indian Government is providing free transport facility to all pregnant women in labor pains, to nearby hospital for urgent delivery round the clock 24 hours. During prehospital care:
- Provide oxygen
- Obtain intravenous access
- Transfer the patient in left lateral recumbent position, use this position specially if the expectant mother's blood pressure is low (pressure on vena cava reduces the return to the heart)
- Prepare for field delivery, because little can be done to prevent the birth.

EMERGENCY DEPARTMENT CARE

Labor is defined as the initiation of regular and rhythmic contractions that results in serial cervical dilatation and effacement and categorized as four stages of labor **(Box 1)**. The appearance of a slight amount of vaginal blood-tinged mucus is a good indication that labor will begin within the next 24 hours and sequence of labor will start **(Fig. 1)**. Various hormonal factors are contributing in initiation of process of labor **(Flow chart 1)**. The loss of more than a few milliliters of blood at this time, however, must be regarded as being due to a pathological process like placenta previa or abruptio placenta. There are various modes of delivery, e.g. normal, cesarean, vacuum- or forceps-assisted delivery **(Figs 2A to D)**.

Box 1 Stages of labor

First stage (stage of cervical dilatation):
- Begins with onset of regular contraction and ends with complete dilatation
- Latent (0–3 cm) → active (4–7 cm) → transitional (8–10 cm)

Second stage (stage of expulsion):
Begins with complete cervical dilatation and ends with delivery fetus

Third stage (placental stage):
Begins immediately after fetus is born and ends when placenta is delivered

Fourth stage (maternal stabilization stage):
Begins after delivery of the placenta and continues for 1–4 hours after delivery

CHAPTER 69 Emergency Delivery

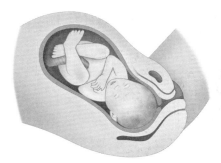
1. Labor begins, membranes intact

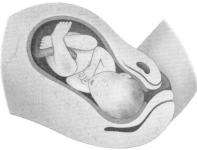
2. Effacement of cervix, which is now partially dilated

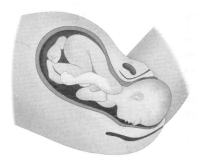
3. Head is rotated, partially extended, and now presents. Membranes are ruptured

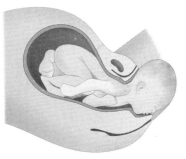
4. Head is almost delivered

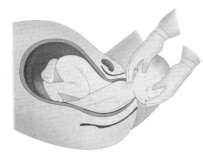
5. Delivery of head

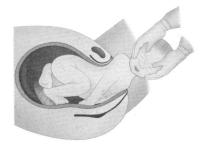
5. Delivery of shoulders

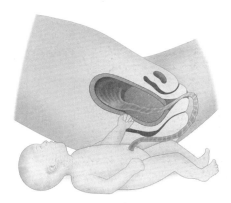
7. Delivery of infant is complete. Uterus begins to contract

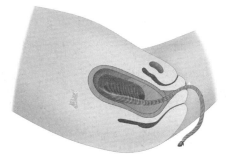
8. Umbilical cord has been lied and cut. Placenta has begun to separate from uterus

Fig. 1 Sequence of labor and childbirth in emergency

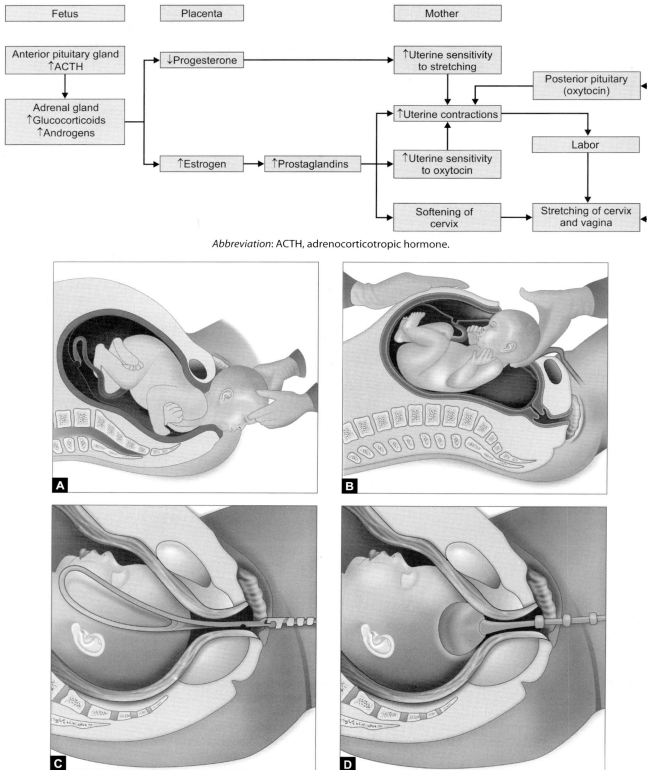

Flow chart 1 Schematic representation of factors believed to have a role in starting labor

Abbreviation: ACTH, adrenocorticotropic hormone.

Figs 2A to D Various modes of delivery. (A) Normal delivery; (B) Cesarean section; (C) Forceps-assisted birth; (D) Vacuum-assisted birth

Following steps are followed for delivery:
A. Swab the perineum with povidone iodine, drap it with towels. Control the baby's head with the nondominant hand. Usually amniotic sac has broken; if not open it now. Note the color and consistency of the amniotic fluid. Once the head emerges, suction the mouth and nose and deep hypopharynx if the amniotic fluid is not clear.
B. Check the neonates neck for the umbilical cord if it is wrapped around the neck; pull it gently over the head. Then deliver the child expeditiously.
C. Gentle traction toward the mothers posterior usually delivers the anterior shoulder.
D. Once the shoulders are out, the rest of the baby slips out quickly; however be careful, because neonates are slippery. Once the baby is out suction the nose and mouth, double clamp the cord 7–10 cm fron the baby and cut the cord between the clamps.
E. If the child starts breathing and moving and appears to be in good health, turn the baby over to nursing personnel. If the birth is complicated by thick meconium, do not stimulate the baby to cry. Instead, use a 3.0 size endotracheal tube, intubate the trachea and suction it then stimulate the baby's breathing.
F. Do not pull the cord; guide the placenta out as it is expelled.
G. If mother and baby are doing well and do not require resuscitation, the ED attending may perform vaginal and perineal repairs under local analgesia. Alternatively, it is generally acceptable to let the obstetrician to finish this portion. Mother and baby can be moved to the obstetrics ward for follow-up care.

Intrapartum and Postpartum Management

- The patient is prepared for the use of cardiac, uterine, and fetal monitors along with intravenous therapy. Maternal vital signs and fetal heart rate (FHR) are monitored. If tocolytic agent (beta-adrenergic drug) is administered intravenously; the infusion rate is increased every 10–30 minutes, depending on uterine response, but never exceeds a rate of 125 mL/hr. Uterine activity is monitored continuously; vital signs and FHR are checked every 15 minutes. Maternal pulse should not exceed 140 beats/min; FHR should not exceed 180 beats/min. When counting respiratory rate, breath sounds are noted, and the lungs are auscultated at least every 8 hours. The patient is assessed for desired response and adverse effects to treatment and is taught about symptoms she may expect and should report. If signs of drug toxicity occur, the medication is stopped. The intravenous line is kept open with a maintenance solution, and the prescribed beta-blocker as an antidote is prepared and administered. The patient is placed in high Fowler's position, and oxygen is administered. Cardiac rate and rhythm, blood pressure, respiratory rate, auscultatory sounds, and FHRs are closely monitored to evaluate the patient's response to the antidote. After birth, check for choking in airway, newborn is dried, covered in sterile cloth and kept in body contact to mother (Kangaroo technique) to prevent hypothermia and to increase mother child bonding.
- If no complications are present, absolute bed rest is maintained throughout the infusion, with the patient in a left-lateral position or supine with a wedge under the right hip to prevent hypotension. Antiembolism stockings are applied, and passive leg exercises are performed. A daily fluid intake of 2–3 L is encouraged to maintain adequate hydration, and fluid intake and output are measured. The patient is weighed daily to assess for overhydration. The patient is instructed in methods to deal with stress. Healthcare providers should respond to parental concern for the fetus with empathy, but never with false reassurance. As prescribed, a glucocorticoid is administered to stimulate fetal pulmonary surfactant production.

Complicated Delivery

Deliveries that occur in the ED are often higher risk than those that occur on the labor floor. The ED sees a higher proportion of women with precipitous deliveries, immigrants and other patients without access to care, and those who are unaware of or in denial of their pregnancies. In addition, the obstetric populations who encounter unexpected complications are more likely to present to the ED rather than an office or labor floor. ED obstetric patients often have little or no prenatal care, and ED births have a higher perinatal mortality. The emergency provider needs to expect the unexpected during a delivery, including precipitous delivery, shoulder dystocia, malpresentation, umbilical cord emergencies, hemorrhage, and multiple gestations.

Call for additional ED staff, along with appropriate external support including obstetrics and pediatrics. Remember that there will soon be two patients, and have the team prepare for neonatal care. This includes obtaining and turning on the infant warmer, opening supplies needed for delivery and neonatal care, and preparing resuscitation equipment including a device to provide positive pressure ventilation for the infant. Obtain intravenous (IV) access in the mother so that oxytocin, fluids, blood, and other medications may be administered as needed during the delivery. Remember to wear personal protective equipment, including a gown, mask, eye protection, shoe covers, and sterile gloves. Although difficult during precipitous deliveries in the ED, try to keep the patient and her family informed about what is happening and what to expect.

If the infant is not crowning [head bulging at the perineum], a brief vaginal examination performed with a sterile-gloved hand reveals if the cervix is dilated (to 10 cm) and/or effaced (thinned to about 1 mm). Additionally, determine the descent of the presenting part relative to the ischial spines (in centimeters) and expressed as + when it is above the ischial spine.

Delivery presentations

Normal delivery

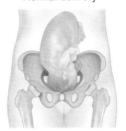

Head-first facing backwards

Abnormal deliveries

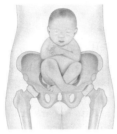 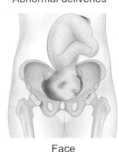 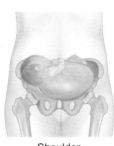

Breech   Face   Shoulder

Identify the presenting part. A smooth surface with a Y configuration of the skull suture lines is the most favorable finding this is lambdoid suture, which indicates presentation of the flexed head

Fig. 3 Various abnormal presentations of deliveries

Various abnormal presentation of deliveries like face, foot, hand, arm or breech presentations are obvious on palpation **(Fig. 3)**. These unexpected presentations can be problematic for the delivery in the ED, because they require special expertise.

General Management of Shoulder Dystocia

- Instruct the mother to stop pushing as soon as shoulder dystocia is recognized.
- Rapidly assign team members to the tasks below as you begin maneuvers to relieve the dystocia.
- Call for additional help, including nurses, obstetrics, pediatrics, and anesthesia.
- Instruct someone to start a timer and call out 60-second intervals.
- Make sure the mother has intravenous access and monitoring, and apply oxygen to maximize oxygenation of the fetus.
- Position the mother with her buttocks flush with the edge of the bed to provide optimal access for executing maneuvers and providing posterior-directed leverage.
- Catheterize the bladder to decompress it and improve any anterior obstruction from distension.
- Ask for a stool for a team member to stand on for the application of suprapubic pressure.
- Assign team members to hold each of the mother's legs for hyperflexion.
- Prepare for neonatal resuscitation—turn on the warmer, open supplies, and designate a team.

The *HELPERR* mnemonic is used by some to assist in remembering the management steps:
- *Help*: Call obstetric, neonatology, anesthesia
- *Empty bladder*: Catheterize to increase AP diameter
- *Legs flexed*: McRobert's maneuver
- *Pressure*: Suprapubic to dislodge anterior shoulder
- *Enter vagina*: Rubin or Woods corkscrew maneuver
- *Remove posterior arm*: Barnum maneuver
- *Roll*: Gaskin maneuver.

Classically, the "E" in HELPERR stood for episiotomy, though in current practice catheterizing and emptying the bladder is a more appropriate step. Episiotomy is no longer routinely recommended. While episiotomy does provide more room for manipulation of the posterior shoulder, it does not relieve the bony obstruction of the anterior shoulder or prevent brachial plexus injury.

Gaskin All-fours Maneuver

- The mother is placed on her hands and knees.
- The fetus may become dislodged during the position change itself.
- The fetus is delivered by gentle downward traction on the posterior shoulder (the shoulder against the maternal sacrum) or upward traction on the anterior shoulder (the shoulder against the maternal symphysis).
- This position increases pelvic diameters plus adds the assistance of gravity.
- Gaskin is a good choice if the patient cannot tolerate internal manipulation.

Breech Presentation

With a normal vertex presentation, the fetus's large head dilates and occludes the cervical opening, clearing space for the body to follow and blocking the umbilical cord from prolapsing. Breech presentations, particularly incomplete breeches, are prone to problems with cervical dilation and umbilical cord prolapse as they lack a good dilating wedge. Asphyxia can result from head entrapment or from umbilical cord prolapse with subsequent compression. Improper attempts at delivery can also cause fetal head and neck trauma from traction, including brachial plexus injuries. Cesarean section is therefore the preferred method of delivery, but likely no longer an option once the delivery is imminent.

Addressing Vaginal Breech Presentation

Prepare for delivery as above, including calling for help. An obstetrician and pediatric provider should be summoned immediately. If the fetus has not yet emerged from the vagina, the mother should be instructed not to push, attempting to delay the delivery until she is transported to the labor floor or an obstetric expert is arrived in the ED. "Panting" by the mother and administration of a beta sympathomimetic drug (like terbutaline) may help limit the pushing and expulsive forces. If any part of the fetus has emerged from the vagina, delivery must proceed as below.

- Place the mother in the dorsal lithotomy position.
- Evaluate for rupture of membranes and prolapsed cord. If the cord is presenting with the breech, pull out a 10–15 cm loop to provide room to work.
- Consider performing a mediolateral episiotomy to provide room for maneuvering, though there is wide practice variation and no data from randomized controlled trials to support this.
- Allow the delivery to happen spontaneously. Support the fetus's body after the umbilicus appears but do not apply traction or squeeze the waist and abdominal organs.
- Wrapping a towel around the fetus provides for better traction after the legs deliver.
- Pull out the 10–15 cm loop of umbilical cord after the umbilicus delivers if not yet already done.
- Keep the fetal sacrum anterior with the fetal face and abdomen away from the symphysis.
- Encourage the mother to bear down strongly until the scapulae are visible.
- Sweep the flexed arms across the chest to deliver each. Rotate the body to deliver the arms, each from an anterior position.
- Perform the Mauriceau-Smellie-Veit maneuver to deliver the head once the fetal chin is at the pelvic inlet. The provider's arm is placed under the fetus with the middle fingers on the fetal maxilla and the fetal legs straddling the forearm. The maxillary fingers plus occipital pressure with the other hand promote head flexion and descent as the body is slightly elevated.
- The fetus should be delivered well within 10 minutes, as the umbilical cord will be compressed during delivery causing acidosis.

Additional vaginal breech delivery maneuvers, if needed:

- The mother can be repositioned in any way that feels most comfortable with the thighs flexed and apart, including crouching or kneeling.
- Use the Pinard maneuver to deliver the legs if they are extended in a frank breech. Apply pressure to the back of the knee and externally rotate the thigh while rotating the fetal pelvis in the opposite direction. This flexes the knee and delivers the foot and leg. Perform it in the opposite direction if needed to extract the other leg.

Precautions during breech delivery and actions to avoid:

- Do not rupture the membranes, as this can cause cord prolapse.
- Do not place traction on or overly squeeze the fetus during delivery, as this can cause injury. Traction causes head extension and squeezing can injure abdominal organs.
- Do not hyperextend the neck, which can cause spinal cord injury or dystocia.
- Do not attempt the Mauriceau maneuver too soon, as it can induce the Moro reflex.
- Do not apply traction to the jaw or mouth during the Mauriceau maneuver, as it can cause temporomandibular joint injury.
- Do not hold the fetal trunk more than 45° above horizontal during delivery, which could apply damaging traction on the cervical spine.
- Compound presentations involve an extremity as the presenting part rather than the head or buttocks. Compound presentations have a 10–20% cord prolapse rate and thus are ideally managed with cesarean rather than vaginal delivery, though this may not be an option in the precipitous delivery. Once a fetal extremity has presented in the vagina, reduction of the presenting part should not be attempted as this increases the risk of cord prolapse.

Umbilical Cord Prolapse (Flow chart 2)

Obstetrician should be called and the mother prepared for emergency cesarean section. However, if labor has progressed far enough that vaginal delivery is imminent, it should be performed as the most rapid method of delivery. If delivery is not imminent, as arrangements are being made for the operating room, care should be focused on reducing pressure on the prolapsed cord. The cord should not be manipulated as this can induce vasospasm and subsequent fetal hypoxia.

Instruct the mother not to push. Position the mother prone in the knee-chest position with the bed in Trendelenburg to enlist the assistance of gravity. Any presenting fetal parts should be manually elevated with a provider's hand to reduce pressure on the cord. The patient should be transported to the operating room and prepared for surgery with the provider's hand still in the vagina. Instillation of 500–700 mL normal saline into the bladder via Foley catheter may also help lift any presenting fetal parts off the cord. If cesarean delivery is not an option at her current location, the mother should be placed knee-chest in Trendelenburg and the bladder filled for transport. The cord should be kept warm and moist, so if it is outside the vagina it should be replaced and held in with moist sterile gauze. Initiate fetal heart monitoring, and administer a tocolytic if fetal bradycardia occurs and persists. If the bradycardia does not resolve with tocolytics, umbilical cord reduction may be the only option, although outcomes have historically been poor. The cord is gently pushed back up towards the uterus above the presenting part. If the head is the presenting part, the head is lifted and the cord is placed over the head into the nuchal area. An assistant providing gentle suprapubic pressure in the cephalad direction may help elevate the fetal head and prevent conversion to a malposition. Nuchal loops and body cords should be anticipated with delivery.

Important Points for Complicated Deliveries

- Complicated deliveries are infrequently performed, high-stress procedures. Call for obstetrics and neonatology early, in addition to extra ED team members. Make sure someone prepares to care for the neonate.
- To relieve shoulder dystocia, avoid excess traction, hyperflex the mothers legs and apply suprapubic pressure, then progress to fetal maneuvering as needed.
- During breech delivery, allow the delivery to happen spontaneously without traction while supporting the fetal body, then prevent excess neck extension while delivering the head.

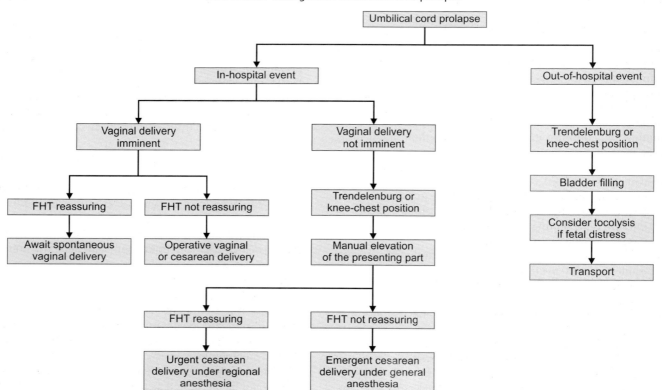

Flow chart 2 Management of umbilical cord prolapse

Abbreviation: FHT, fetal heart tones.

- If cord prolapse occurs, do not manipulate the cord. Minimize pressure on the cord with maternal knee-chest positioning and elevation of presenting parts while preparing for emergency cesarean section.

Postpartum Complications

Postpartum complications have been listed in **Box 2**.

Management of Primary Postpartum Hemorrhage

Preventive: Intramuscular oxytocin at the end of the second stage of labor.

Curative:
- Repeat oxytocin administration
- Check completeness of placenta, if it is not delivered prepare for manual removal
- Bimanual compression
- Intramyometrial prostaglandin E2 or carboprost
- Surgical ligation

Placenta Previa

Placenta previa is a third trimester obstetric complication in which placenta abnormally (partially or completely) covers the internal cervical os.

Symptoms: Bright red, painless, recurrent vaginal bleeding.

Signs: Soft pain free uterus, no fetal distress.

Often fetus is not affected by the first small bleed, but because of high risk after emergency resuscitation shift immediately to obstetric department.

Abruption of Placenta

It means premature separation of placenta.

Box 2 Postpartum complications

Risk factors
- Cesarean delivery
- Prolonged rupture of membrane
- Prolonged labor
- Bladder catheterization

Complications
- Mastitis
- Upper respiratory infection
- Urinary tract infection
- Thrombophlebitis
- Hematoma
- Abscess formation
- Endometritis
- Perineal cellulitis
- Hemorrhage

Symptoms: Abdominal pain, bleeding, and severe shock.

Signs: Shock spasm of uterus fetal part hard to feel, often no fetal heart sound.

All emergency protocol should be considered to shift the patient to obstetric emergency unit.

Maternal Cardiac Arrest and Cardiopulmonary Resuscitation during Childbirth

The first principles of dealing with obstetric emergencies are the same as for any emergency [see to CAB—*C*irculation, *A*irway, *B*reathing, and added *U*terine displacement to left side, so its CABU in managing pregnant with cardiac arrest] **(Flow chart 3)**. CABU in Hindi means controlling the most difficult position. A dying pregnant lady with full-term pregnancy is the most difficult position in emergency, because two lives are involved, and both need to be saved at the same time; the fetus is very vulnerable to maternal hypoxia.

Possible Causes of Maternal Cardiac Arrest

A—Anesthetic complication or accident
B—Bleeding
C—Cardiovascular
D—Drugs
E—Embolic
F—Fever
G—General nonobstetrics causes (5H and 5T)
H—Hypertension.

Any young adult female, who was talking, walking and suddenly collapses on hospital floor or outside in hospital lift lobby, should be suspected pregnant (if no relative of female is available to tell the status), until proven otherwise. To confirm for gravid pregnant uterus, all we have to check is by palpating abdomen at the level of umbilicus, if you can feel any football like bulge at or above umbilicus, this suggest pregnancy above 7 months, capable of causing aortocaval compression, comprising venous return and arterial flow to uterus containing fetus. Now comes to the role of checking response, pulse, breathing in unconscious female. Immediately announce the "Code Blue" team for rescuing both mother and unborn child by calling a team of cardiologist and anesthetist. Since, we have specialists in superspeciality corporate hospitals in metros, so we need to call both pediatric anesthetist with pediatric cardiologist and adult anesthetist with adult cardiologist, along with gynecologist on-spot (inside hospital premises only) to resuscitate both dying victims without wasting anytime in shifting to ED. Because brain is time, it is important to follow the correct sequence of cardiopulmonary resuscitation (CPR) to prevent hypoxic damage to brains of mother and child **(Flow chart 4)**.

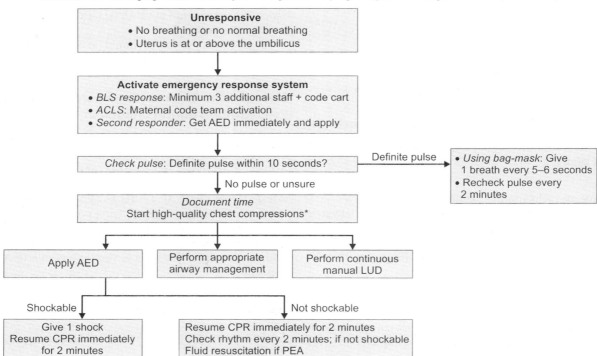

Flow chart 3 Managing cardiac arrest by CABU algorithm in pregnant patient with gravid uterus (>7 months)

*Compress the chest at least 5 cm, chest compression rate 100–120/min and allow complete chest recoil.
Abbreviations: CABU, circulation, airway, breathing, and uterine displacement to left side; BLS, basic life support; ACLS, advanced cardiac life support; AED, automated external defibrillator; LUD, lateral uterine displacement; CPR, cardiopulmonary resuscitation; PEA, pulseless electric activity.

So simply, rescuer has to follow all C's check response by waking up, Code Blue, Call first AID [automated external defibrillator (AED)], Check Pulse and Breathing, Call CAB—Do CAB, Doing CAB stands for Chest Compression, Airway and Breathing artificially by mouth-to-mouth or bag and mask, Calling CAB also stands for calling code blue team, which is lifesaving cab (taxi is the trolley-bed with wheels inside hospitals) for dying pregnant victim.

If the pregnant becomes unconscious, unresponsive, with no pulse and breathing—immediately announce Code Blue to call for help (Anesthetist and Cardiologist) and start the CPR by doing chest compressions in upper-middle part of the chest at flat sternum bone, by compressing one-third part of the chest, allowing full chest recoil. Allow chest compressions at the rate of 100/min. One cycle of CPR include 30 chest compressions followed by two rescue breaths.

Uterine displacement to left side—by applying slight pressure on right side of uterus—to prevent aortocaval compression by gravid uterus. If the fundus height is at or above the level of umbilicus, manual LUD (lateral uterine displacement) is beneficial in relieving the aortocaval compression during chest compression **(Figs 4A and B)**.

Electric Sock in Maternal Cardiac Arrest

Automated external defibrillator is the first aid in cardiac arrest, as soon as available, can be used to identify the rhythm, and if its shockable (VF/VT), 200 Joules shock can be given in pregnant with AED pads attached away from the breast tissue, on the axis of heart, to revert it into sinus rhythm, shock can be repeated every 2 min. Check the pulse or rhythm every 2 minutes.

Perimortem Cesarean Section Delivery

Emergency perimortem cesarean section delivery (PMCS) is performed if the pregnant is not revived after 4 minutes of uninterrupted CPR.

Box 3 shows the list of equipment for PMCS.

Cardiopulmonary resuscitation is given to both mother and child after PMCS to maintain the vitality of brain.

Newborn delivered after PMCS need to be immediately relieved of choking by doing suction from nose and mouth. Give 5 back-blows, 5 chest-thrusts, 5 rescue breaths and start CPR if child is unresponsive. CPR is at the same speed of 100/min as in adults, but more rescue breaths are given

Flow chart 4 Sequence for CPR in pregnant patients

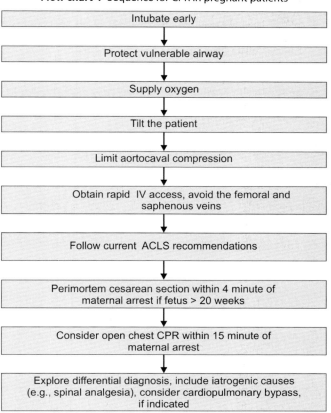

Abbreviations: IV, intravenous; ACLS, advanced cardiac life support; CPR, cardiopulmonary resuscitation.

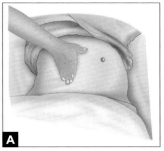 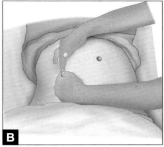

Figs 4A and B Lateral uterine displacement method during chest compression in maternal cardiac arrest
Abbreviation: CPR, cardiopulmonary resuscitation.

as per Neonatal Advanced Life Support guidelines—15:2, i.e. 15 chest compressions and 2 rescue breaths, so the newborn will get four rescue breaths in every cycle of CPR. AED can be used to identify shockable rhythm; electric shock can be given as 2–4 J/kg weight of child.

If the infant is unresponsive with slow pulse less than 60 beats/min, CPR is given to maintain the oxygenation and circulation in brain, as the normal range of heart rate in newborn is 140–160 beats/min.

Box 3 Equipment contents of the emergency cesarean delivery tray

- Scalpel with No. 10 blade
- Lower end of a Balfour retractor
- Pack of sponges
- 2 Kelly clamps
- Needle driver
- Russian forceps
- Sutures and suture scissors

MEDICOLEGAL ISSUES IN EMERGENCY OBSTETRIC CARE

Referral criteria: Shift to hospitals where blood bank, neonatal, and emergency cesarean section facilities are available. Pregnant woman should be shifted in well-equipped ambulance with ventilators, injectable drug kit and a team of qualified doctors, paramedic and nurse, with prior communication to the referral center.

Janani Suraksha Yojana (JSY): Guidelines for Emergency Obstetric Care by MOHFW

1. No pregnant woman in labor or distress should be turned away from the hospital for any reason at any time of the day or night.
2. Every hospital would provide emergency obstetric services free of cost.
3. Every MBBS doctor should be able to deliver in case of emergency delivery.

Clinical Establishment Act (CEA): Standard Treatment Guidelines by MOHFW

It covers medicolegal aspects, preventing negligence in care during emergency deliveries by setting up delivery rooms with all basic facilities and instruments for emergency delivery in every hospital registered under the CEA.

SUMMARY

Every emergency physician should have sound knowledge of the emergency delivery and common obstetrics complications and emergencies.

- First principles of obstetrics emergencies are the same as with any other emergency, maintain circulation, airway, and breathing.
- Left uterine displacement of gravid uterus to prevent aortocaval compression.
- If patient is in second stage of labor, deliver the baby with all due precautions.
- If time permits, shift the patient to obstetric unit after primary resuscitation.

BIBLIOGRAPHY

1. American College of Obstetrics and Gynecology. ACOG Practice Bulletin: Induction of Labor. ACOG Practice Bulletin Number 10. Washington, DC: ACOG; 1999.
2. Kinzie B, Gomez P. Basic Maternal and Newborn Care: A Guide for Skilled Providers. Baltimore: JHPIEGO; 2004.
3. World Health Organization, Department of Reproductive Health and Research. Managing Complications in Pregnancy and Childbirth: A Guide for Midwives and Doctors. Geneva: WHO; 2000.
4. World Health Organization, Department of Reproductive Health and Research. Surgical Care at the District Hospital. Geneva: WHO; 2003.
5. World Health Organization, Fact Sheet 245, Essential Obstetric Care. Geneva: WHO; 2000.
6. World Health Organization, Mother-Baby Package: Implementing Safe Motherhood in Countries. WHO/FHE/MSM/94.11. Geneva: WHO; 1994.

SECTION 10

Pediatric Emergencies

- **Fever in Children**
  Dhiren Gupta, Roop Sharma

- **Vomiting, Diarrhea and Dehydration in Children**
  Prabhat Maheshwari, Devendra Richhariya

- **Febrile Seizure and Status Epilepticus in Children**
  Yeeshu Singh Sudan, Devendra Richhariya

- **Central Nervous System Infections in Children**
  Yeeshu Singh Sudan

- **Diabetes Management in Children**
  Ganesh Jevalikar

- **Pediatric Cardiac Emergencies: Evaluation and Management**
  Aditi Gupta, Munesh Tomar

Chapter 70

Fever in Children

Dhiren Gupta, Roop Sharma

INTRODUCTION

Fever is most often defined as a rectal temperature greater than or equal to 38.0°C (100.4°F). Oral and skin temperatures are lower than rectal temperatures by 0.6°C (1°F) and 1°C (2–2.5°F), respectively. Oral temperatures are not recommended in young children, and skin temperatures obtained from the axilla or forehead are unreliable. Tympanic membrane temperatures are lower than rectal temperatures. Fever most commonly occurs as a response to infection but may be due to immune-mediated or collagen vascular disease and is associated with many malignancies. During infection, moderate fever is probably beneficial, because it enhances host defense reactions. Rapidly rising temperature, however, is associated with febrile convulsions; hyperpyrexia, defined as a core temperature greater than 41.1°C (106°F) can result in complications such as central nervous system damage and rhabdomyolysis. A vast majority of these patients have benign illnesses that are caused by viruses and are therefore self-limited or result from bacterial infections that are amenable to outpatient therapy. A small percentage of patients suffer from life-threatening infections.

The approach to fever in the pediatric patient is age dependent. Neonates and young infants are deficient in the ability to localize and neutralize bacterial infections. The exact age groups are arbitrary and are not based on a scientific understanding of the immune response. Rather, the management of the febrile child is based on cumulative clinical experience and a growing body of research that is challenging traditional treatment.

About 20% of pediatric patients presenting to the emergency room (ER) have fever as a sign or symptom.

There are few questions to be answered when child presents to pediatric emergency:
1. Should I admit the child?
2. Is he/she suffering from viral/bacterial/fungal infection or noninfectious diseases like ambient temperature?
3. Whether disease is going to deteriorate or static?
4. Should I investigate or wait for spontaneous resolution?
Following are few generalizations which can be applicable to children more than 1-year-old:
- During high-grade fever patient response and alertness can be obtunded but if irritability persists during afebrile period then physician should be more alert.
- Child at times becomes irritable in extreme environment, cold and warm, so the importance of comfortable environment during examination is of utmost importance.
- Mere presence of doctor or nurse can trigger the child irritability. To avoid this bias review the patient in presence of caregivers only (view from remote distance).
- There are general red flag signs like—poor oral intake including water, drowsiness, decreased urine output, and fast breathing which are applicable to all febrile and nonfebrile pediatric patients.
- Children more than 8 years maintain good consciousness despite of hypotension, therefore, contrarily to infant adolescent who has come walking to emergency can be preterminal and can deceive ER physician and parents if systemic evaluation is not done.
- Infant less than 6 months may not show any other feature of sepsis except fever and can decompensate. Hypotension is usually late feature.
- Unexplained tachycardia (after ruling out crying, fever) is always bad and deserves thorough detailed evaluation.

THE AGE GROUPS

A febrile infant aged 28–60 days often lack clues on physical examination so general approach to fever in these groups is a high index of suspicion most often due to urinary tract infections (UTIs).

Environmentally acquired encapsulated organisms become the chief pathogens from this period throughout the rest of childhood. The traditional emergency department (ED) approach to febrile infants in this age group has been an aggressive search for bacterial illness, followed by hospitalization and empiric antibiotic therapy until cultures of blood, cerebrospinal fluid (CSF), and urine were negative. Management now includes an effort to define a group of low-risk patients who may be candidates for outpatient management.

Patients between 3 months and 36 months of age constitute the final major category. The immune system has matured to the extent that disseminated infection from a bacterial focus is much less likely. However, up to 5% of patients in this age group with temperatures above 39°C who appear well and have no focus of infection on physical examination will have positive blood culture, termed as occult bacteremia. The management of these patients is a subject of controversy and ongoing investigation. After 36 months of age, the management of the nonimmunocompromised febrile pediatric patient is similar to that of the healthy adolescent and adult.

PRESENTATION

The history of the present illness is obtained from the person most familiar with the patient, usually the mother. Observation of the infant or toddler during the history provides a wealth of information and may be useful in differentiating the "sick" or "not sick" patient. Important information includes the time of onset of the fever and the method of taking the temperature. Temperatures measured by a thermometer may be more accurate than a history that the patient "felt warm". Prior treatment is also important, since antipyretic therapy may result in a normal temperature in the patient with a serious febrile illness. Inappropriate treatment, such as bundling a febrile infant or sponging with alcohol, may also be elicited; the caretaker can then be educated on the proper management of fever. The caretaker is questioned regarding his or her perception of the severity of the patient's illness. Helpful information in neonates and infants includes the patient's level of activity, feeding, and interaction with the environment. In older patients, a history of play activity is helpful. It is important to attempt to elicit a sense of the child's mental status, but it must be remembered that asking about the presence of "irritability" or "lethargy" introduces terminology into the history that may have a different meaning to the caretaker than to the physician. The history of the patient's general behavior is followed by questions regarding associated symptoms.

In infants, difficulty in feeding is the equivalent of dyspnea on exertion and implies significant respiratory distress. Especially in infants, overwhelming infection can cause apnea, which parents may perceive as difficulty in breathing. It is important to realize that apnea can be intermittent and that the patient may appear stable between episodes. Gastrointestinal symptoms are also common in the febrile pediatric patient. Vomiting and diarrhea usually indicate an infectious process involving the gastrointestinal tract. However, they can also occur as nonspecific findings in other infections, including otitis media and pyelonephritis, and may occur in association with life-threatening infections such as meningitis and overwhelming sepsis.

PHYSICAL EXAMINATION

It is impossible to overemphasize the importance of the general assessment in guiding the evaluation and management of the pediatric patient. The general assessment is a combination of observation, experience, and also "clinical judgment". It should be based on objective information. Neonates and very young infants are difficult to assess, even in the most experienced hands. While it is certain that an "ill-appearing" infant has a relatively high probability of having a serious bacterial infection (SBI), a well appearance does not rule out serious illness.

The most important clinical tool is the mental status, evaluated by observing the patient's interaction with the environment and parents. Older infants and children should recognize their parents and demonstrate curiosity about their surroundings. After 5–6 months of age, "stranger anxiety" is appropriate and is not to be construed as irritability. In younger infants, the presence of a social smile is an important finding that implies well-being. In neonates too young to have developed a social smile, the baby's state of alertness and desire to bottle-feed are noted. Virtually all pediatric patients should be consolable. Patients who are inconsolable or appear worse when held or rocked by their parents are truly irritable, which may indicate a central nervous system infection. Anxiousness, listlessness, and lethargy are also signs of serious illness.

The patient's hydration and perfusion are also assessed. In a febrile patient in whom peripheral perfusion is diminished but who has no history compatible with fluid loss, septic shock is likely. In practice, most patients with significantly decreased perfusion will have depressed mental status. Finally, it is important to realize that depressed mental status and signs of impaired perfusion can be intermittent. The cardiovascular system is able to compensate until late in the course of an overwhelming infection. A parent may give a history of an ashen, mottled, or apneic infant at home. Occasionally such patients respond to stimulation alone and may appear relatively well on arrival in the ED. Conversely, a patient who appeared well on arrival in the ED may suddenly appear to decompensate, only to respond in such a way to stimulation or fluid resuscitation that the presence of serious illness is questioned.

MANAGEMENT

Febrile Infants 28 Days to 3 Months Old

Current data support the following approach to the well-appearing febrile patient between 28 days and 3 months of age. The child is evaluated for a focus of infection. Any bacterial infection is considered to be an SBI. Infants with evidence of infection of the soft tissue, joint, or bone are admitted for appropriate antibiotic therapy. If no source of infection is found, laboratory data are obtained to differentiate the low- from high-risk infant. Low-risk criteria include a white blood cell (WBC) count between 5,000/mm^3 and 15,000/mm^3, a band count below 1,500/mm^3, a normal urinalysis, a normal CSF, and, in patients with diarrhea, stool microscopy with less than 5 WBCs per high-power field. WBCs in the stool reflect the potential for *Salmonella enteritidis*. Infants who fulfill the low-risk criteria appear to have a very small probability of having an SBI (<1%). Infants may be discharged from the ER, provided there is close patient follow-up. Empiric therapy with ceftriaxone, 50 mg/kg is begun. Patients receiving ceftriaxone return to the ED in 24 hours for a second dose. Infants with positive cultures of the CSF are admitted for inpatient therapy. Those with positive blood cultures are treated on an individual basis. Low-risk infants may also be discharged without antibiotic treatment. Close follow-up is necessary. Lumbar puncture may not be necessary, because empiric antibiotics are not used. This management option is most often employed by physicians in small practice settings with little laboratory backup and an established family rapport. If reliability is in question, the patient should be admitted.

Infants 3–36 Months of Age

Fever with a Focus of Infection

Certain focal bacterial infections are associated with bacteremia, including epiglottitis, buccal, and periorbital cellulitis, and septic arthritis. The potential for bacteremia always mandates an aggressive workup, including blood cultures and occasionally lumbar puncture. Other infections associated with bacteremia include those caused by *Staphylococcus aureus* and *Salmonella enteritidis*. *S. enteritidis* is especially problematic in younger infants, where it can result in disseminated infection.

Fever without a Focus of Infection

This patient presents a true challenge to the ED physician. The major concern is occult bacteremia, which occurs primarily in patients with a temperature of 39°C or greater. Beyond 39°C, there is a direct correlation between the severity of the fever and the probability of bacteremia, reported to be between 3% and 11%. All socioeconomic groups are equally affected. The most common cause of occult bacteremia is *Streptococcus pneumoniae*, which accounts for about 85% of cases. The second most common is *Haemophilus influenzae* type B (Hib), which is dramatically decreasing since the introduction of conjugate Hib vaccine. *Neisseria meningitidis* accounts for about 3% of cases. The remainder is accounted by a variety of organisms, including *Salmonella*, *S. aureus*, and *S. pyogenes*.

There is no laboratory test that can definitively diagnose bacteremia in the ER. The WBC count has some value as a screening test. The combination of a temperature above 40°C and a WBC more than 15,000/mm^3 increases the probability of bacteremia from about 2.6% to 11%. The erythrocyte sedimentation rate and C-reactive protein have met with limited success and add little to the complete blood count. UTIs account for up to 7% of male patients less than 6 months of age and 8% of female infants less than 1 year of age who have fever without focus. Urine culture must be obtained from catheterization or suprapubic aspiration in order to avoid a contaminated culture. This is especially important, since up to 20% of pediatric patients with UTIs will have an unremarkable urinalysis. A lumbar puncture is indicated in any patient who appears toxic or has clinical findings consistent with meningitis. It is important to remember that in young infants, early meningitis can be extremely subtle, and a liberal approach toward lumbar punctures is indicated. Chest X-rays are helpful in febrile pediatric patients with pulmonary findings, such as cough and tachypnea. Stool cultures are useful only in patients who have bloody diarrhea or more than 5 WBC per high-power field.

The management of the patient between 3 months and 36 months of age who has fever without focus is controversial. Untreated bacteremia with *Pneumococcus* has a 6% risk of the subsequent development of meningitis. *H. influenzae* carries risk of meningitis of up to 26%. Other potential secondary infections include septic arthritis, epiglottitis, and facial cellulitis. Although *Neisseria meningitis* is an infrequent cause of bacteremia, up to half of affected patients develop meningitis or sepsis. With at least some patients with occult bacteremia developing serious sequelae, management algorithms have been devised. Treatment with parenteral antibiotics may be beneficial in preventing the development of meningitis in patients with occult bacteremia as compared with no treatment or treatment with oral antibiotics. Ceftriaxone covers *H. influenzae*, penetrates the CSF and has a long half-life. One option in the well-appearing patient with a temperature above 39°C is to obtain a screening complete blood count. If WBC count is above 15,000/mm^3 blood culture is sent. Male infants less than 6 months of age and females less than 2 years of age have a urinalysis and urine culture. Any patient who appears toxic has a lumbar puncture performed. Empiric therapy with ceftriaxone 50 mg/kg intramuscular is then administered. Another potential strategy is to obtain a blood culture on all patients with a temperature above 39°C and initiate empiric therapy with ceftriaxone. This would result in a large number of patients at low-risk of bacteremia receiving treatment, because of the lack of a screening WBC. Patients who have blood cultures positive for *Neisseria* or *H. influenzae* should be recalled to the ER and hospitalized for treatment. If a lumbar puncture was not performed on the initial visit, it should be done on the patient's arrival. Children with a blood culture positive for *Pneumococcus* who are afebrile can receive a second dose of ceftriaxone and a follow-up course of oral penicillin if not resistant. Patients with pneumococcemia who have persistent fever require a repeat septic workup and admission for parenteral antibiotics. Finally, there are some who feel that neither laboratory evaluation nor empiric antibiotic therapy is indicated in well-appearing febrile children with no focus of infection. All agree that regardless of the ED treatment, close follow-up is the most important factor in assuring a good outcome.

Febrile Child above 36 Months of Age

Beyond 36 months of age, the immune system of the healthy child has developed to the point where disseminated bacterial infection is rare. Even bacteremic patients very uncommonly seed their meninges or develop full-blown sepsis. An exception to this is meningococcemia, which remains a serious disease throughout adulthood. The older febrile child is evaluated for a focus of bacterial infection. Ancillary studies are indicated, depending on the clinical scenario. Examples include throat cultures in patients with pharyngitis and chest X-rays in patients with cough or objective pulmonary findings. UTIs are fairly common in young girls and can at times have somewhat atypical presentations, including vomiting and diarrhea. Thus, a urinalysis is occasionally indicated. Blood counts and blood cultures are rarely indicated except in ill-appearing children. The majority of older febrile patients have viral illness and require no workup.

TREATMENT OF FEVER

Despite the tremendous frequency of the problem, treating fever remains controversial. While there is no doubt that extremely elevated temperatures (>41°C) can be deleterious, the vast majority of patients with fever do well, and lowering the body temperature may obviate some of the potentially beneficial effects off ever. Patients who require aggressive treatment include those with a history of febrile seizures and those who are physiologically unstable. Pharmacologic therapy of fever consists of paracetamol and nonsteroidal anti-inflammatory drugs (NSAIDs). Both normalize the temperature set point, by inhibiting prostaglandin synthesis. Paracetamol is an effective antipyretic and is relatively free of side effects. The dose is 10–15 mg/kg every 4 hours. An advantage of paracetamol is that children are fairly tolerant of overdose. Aspirin is also an effective antipyretic, but, due to a possible link with Reye syndrome, it is generally not recommended. Ibuprofen has been increasingly used as an antipyretic in pediatric patients. It appears to be as effective as acetaminophen, with a slightly longer duration of action. Its use has not been linked to Reye syndrome. The dose is 10 mg/kg every 6 hours. Body temperature can also be reduced by external cooling, which in small children is easily done by bathing. Water temperature should be tepid and not cold enough to induce shivering. Parents should always be informed that sponging with alcohol is dangerous. Bathing or sponging should be combined with pharmacologic therapy.

BIBLIOGRAPHY

1. Al-Eissa YA. Lumbar puncture in the clinical evaluation of children with seizures associated with fever. Pediatr Emerg Care. 1995;11(6):347-50.
2. Alpern ER, Alessandrini EA, Shaw KN, et al. Prevalence, Time to Detection, and Outcome of Occult Bacteremia in an Urban Pediatric Emergency Department (Abstract). New Orleans, LA: Ambulatory Pediatric Association Program and Abstracts; 1998. p. 118.
3. American Academy of Pediatrics. Practice parameter: the neurodiagnostic evaluation of the child with a first simple febrile seizure. Pediatrics. 1996;97(5):769-72.
4. Baker MD, Avner JR, Bell LM. Failure of infant observation scales in detecting serious illness in febrile 4- to 8-week-old infants. Pediatrics. 1990;85(6):1040-3.
5. Baker MD, Bell LM, Avner JR. Outpatient management without antibiotics of fever in selected infants. N Engl J Med. 1993;329(20):1437-41.
6. Baker MD, Fosarelli PD, Carpenter RO. Childhood fever: correlation of diagnosis with temperature response to acetaminophen. Pediatrics. 1987;80(3):315-8.
7. Baker RC, Sequin JH, Leslie N, et al. Fever and petechiae in children. Pediatrics. 1989;84(6):1051-5.
8. Baraff LJ, Bass JW, Fleisher GF, et al. Practice guideline for the management of infants and children 0 to 36 months of age with fever without source. Pediatrics. 1993;92:1-12.
9. Baraff LJ, Osland S, Prather M. Effect of antibiotic therapy and etiologic microorganism on the risk of bacterial meningitis in children with occult bacteremia. Pediatrics. 1993;92(1):140-3.
10. Baskin M, O'Rourke EJ, Fleisher GR. Outpatient treatment of febrile infants 28 to 89 days of age with intramuscular administration of ceftriaxone. J Pediatr. 1992;120(1):22-7.
11. Bass JW, Steele RW, Wittler RR, et al. Antimicrobial treatment of occult bacteremia: a multicenter cooperative study. Pediatr Infect Dis J. 1993;12(6):466-73.
12. Bonadio WA, Hegenbarth M, Zachariason M. Correlating reported fever in young infants with subsequent temperature patterns and rate of serious bacterial infections. Pediatr Infect Dis J. 1990;9(3):158-60.

13. Bonadio WA, Smith DS, Sabnis S. The clinical characteristics and infectious outcomes of febrile infants aged 8 to 12 weeks. Clin Pediatr (Phila). 1994;33(2):95-9.
14. Bramson RT, Meyer TL, Silbiger ML, et al. The futility of the chest radiograph in the febrile infant without respiratory symptoms. Pediatrics. 1993;92(4):524-6.
15. Bulloch B, Craig WR, Klassen TP. The use of antibiotics to prevent serious sequelae in children at risk for occult bacteremia: a meta-analysis. Acad Emerg Med. 1997;4(7):679-83.
16. Curtis N. Non-steroidal anti-inflammatory drugs may predispose to invasive group A streptococcal infections. Arch Dis Child. 1996;75(6):547.
17. Dagan R, Powell KR, Hall CB, et al. Identification of infants unlikely to have serious bacterial infection although hospitalized for suspected sepsis. J Pediatr. 1985;107(6):855-60.
18. Doctor A, Harper MB, Fleisher GR. Group A beta-hemolytic streptococcal bacteremia: historical overview, changing incidence, and recent association with varicella. Pediatrics. 1995;96(3 Pt 1):428-33.
19. Ferrera PC, Bartfield JM, Snyder HS. Neonatal fever: utility of the Rochester Criteria in determining low risk for serious bacterial infections. Am J Emerg Med. 1997;15(3):299-302.
20. Fleisher GR, Rosenberg N, Vinci R, et al. Intramuscular versus oral antibiotic therapy for the prevention of meningitis and other bacterial sequelae in young, febrile children at risk for occult bacteremia. J Pediatr. 1994;124(4):504-12.
21. Green SM, Rothrock SG, Clem KJ, et al. Can seizures be the sole manifestation of meningitis in febrile children? Pediatrics. 1993;92(4):527-34.
22. Hoberman A, Wald ER. Urinary tract infections in young febrile children. Pediatr Infect Dis J. 1997;16(1):11-7.
23. Huebi JE, Barbacci MB, Zimmerman HJ. Therapeutic misadventures with acetaminophen: hepatotoxicity after multiple doses in children. J Pediatr. 1998;132(1):22-7.
24. Huttenlocher A, Newman TB. Evaluation of the erythrocyte sedimentation rate in children presenting with limp, fever, or abdominal pain. Clin Pediatr (Phila). 1997;36(6):339-44.
25. Jacobs RF, Schutze GE. *Bartonella henselae* as a cause of prolonged fever and fever of unknown origin in children. Clin Infect Dis. 1998;26(1):80-4.
26. Jaffe DM, Fleisher GR. Temperature and total white blood cell count as indicators of bacteremia. Pediatrics. 1991;87(5):670-4.
27. Jaffe DM, Tanz RR, Davis AT, et al. Antibiotic administration to treat possible occult bacteremia in febrile children. N Engl J Med. 1987;317(19):1175-80.
28. Jaskiewicz JA, McCarthy CA, Richardson AC, et al. Febrile infants at low risk for serious risk for serious bacterial infection: an appraisal of the Rochester Criteria and implications for management. Pediatrics. 1994;94(3):390-6.
29. Kearns GL, Leeder JS, Wasserman GS. Acetaminophen overdose with therapeutic intent. J Pediatr. 1998;132(1):5-8.
30. Kramer MS, Shapiro ED. Management of the young febrile child: a commentary on recent practice guidelines. Pediatrics. 1997;100(1):128-34.
31. Kuppermann N, Fleisher GR, Jaffe DM. Predictors of occult pneumococcal bacteremia in young febrile children. Ann Emerg Med. 1998;31(6):679-87.
32. Lee GM, Harper MB. Risk of bacteremia for febrile young children in the post-*Haemophilus influenzae* type b era. Arch Pediatr Adolesc Med. 1998;152(7):624-8.
33. Lesko SM, Mitchell AA. An assessment of the safety of pediatric ibuprofen. JAMA. 1995;273(12):929-33.
34. Lieu TA, Baskin MN, Schwartz JS, et al. Clinical and cost-effectiveness of outpatient strategies for management of febrile infants. Pediatrics. 1992;89(8):1135-44.
35. Maller JS, Gorelick MH. Use of monitoring devices. In: Henretig FM, King C (Eds). Textbook of Pediatric Emergency Procedures. Baltimore: Williams & Wilkins; 1997. p. 337.
36. Mandl KD, Stack AM, Fleisher, GR. Incidence of bacteremia in infants and children with fever and petechiae. J Pediatr. 1997;131(3):398-404.
37. Press S. Association of hyperpyrexia with serious disease in children. Clin Pediatr (Phila). 1994;33(1):19-25.
38. Rothrock SG, Harper MB, Green SM, et al. Do oral antibiotics prevent meningitis and serious bacterial infections in children with *Streptococcus pneumoniae* occult bacteremia? A meta-analysis. Pediatrics. 1997;99(3):438-44.
39. Saper CB, Breeder CD. The neurologic basis of fever. N Engl J Med. 1994;330(26):1880-6.
40. Schuchat A, Robinson K, Wenger J, et al. Bacterial meningitis in the United States in 1995. N Engl J Med. 1997;337(14):970-6.
41. Shaw KN, Gorelick M, McGowan KL, et al. Prevalence of urinary tract infection in febrile young children in the emergency department. Pediatrics. 1998;102(2):e16.
42. Shaw KN, McGowan KL, Gorelick MH, et al. Screening for urinary tract infection in infants in the emergency department: which test is best? Pediatrics 1998;101(6):e1.
43. Strait RT, Ruddy RM, Friedland LR, et al. A pilot study of the predictive value of plasma tumor necrosis factor Alpha and interleukin 1 beta for *Streptococcus pneumoniae* bacteremia in febrile children. Acad Emerg Med. 1997;4(1):44-51.
44. Teach SJ, Fleisher GR, Occult Bacteremia Study Group (sup A). Efficacy of an observation scale in detecting bacteremia in febrile children three to thirty-six months of age, treated as outpatients. J Pediatrics. 1995;126(6):177-81.
45. Torrey SB, Henretig F, Fleisher G, et al. Temperature response to antipyretic therapy in children: relationship to occult bacteremia. Am J Emerg Med. 1985;3(3):190-2.

CHAPTER 71

Vomiting, Diarrhea and Dehydration in Children

Prabhat Maheshwari, Devendra Richhariya

INTRODUCTION

Acute diarrhea is important cause of mortality in children less than 5 years of age. About 1.5% of deaths in less than 5 years of age group are due to gastroenteritis. Various viruses bacteria and in some cases parasites are responsible for acute gastroenteritis in children. Rotavirus is most important cause of dehydrating diarrhea in children which require hospitalization. Diarrhea may present in various forms like watery diarrhea, bloody diarrhea, persistent diarrhea, and diarrhea with malabsorption. In majority of cases of uncomplicated diarrhea, oral rehydration solution is sufficient and drug therapy is not required. Children with vomiting and complicated diarrhea should be admitted in hospital, care full assessment for dehydration and management should be given. In young infants breast feeding is best way to prevent dehydration. Rotavirus vaccine is help full in preventing the rotavirus induced severe dehydrating diarrhea. Specialist advice should be taken in cases of persistent diarrhea, food protein allergy, and lactose intolerance diarrhea.

COMMON CAUSES OF VOMITING

Causes include:
- Gastroenteritis
- Gastroesophageal reflux disease
- Overfeeding (in infants)
- Anatomic obstruction (in infants)
- Medication
- Systemic infections.

DIARRHEA

When stool contains more water it become loose and watery. Three or more watery or loose stools in 24 hours considered as diarrhea. Diarrhea causes rapid loss of water and electrolyte through stools. Diarrhea is more common in condition with unfavorable socioeconomic condition, poor sanitation, and hygiene and unsafe drinking water.

Causative Agents and Various Patterns of Diarrhea

Causative agents and pattern of diarrhea are **(Table 1)**:
- *Viral agents*: Rotavirus (common), norovirus, and adenovirus
- *Bacterial agents*: *Escherichia coli*, nontyphoidal *Salmonella*, *Shigella*, *Campylobacter*
- Watery diarrhea is commonly caused by rotavirus and vibrio cholera
- Dysentery (bloody) diarrhea is commonly caused by *Shigella* and toxin producing *E. coli*, *Campylobacter jejuni*, nontyphoidal *Salmonella* and *E. histolytica*.

Table 1 Types of diarrhea

Watery diarrhea	Dysentery diarrhea	Persistent diarrhea	Diarrhea with malnutrition
• Dehydration is main concern last for hours-day • Weight loss can also occur • Death due to dehydration if not treated well	• Blood and mucus present in stool • Dehydration not very prominent • Sepsis and malnutrition common concern	• Diarrhea that last more than 2 weeks or more • Leads to serious infection and malnutrition	• This is serious condition needs special attention to rule out infection, dehydration, heart failure, electrolyte imbalance, mineral and vitamins deficiency

Assessment of Diarrhea and Dehydration in Children (Table 2)

Aims of assessment:
- To identify the types of diarrhea and degree of dehydration (Tables 1 and 3)
- Assess nutritional status and give appropriate treatment
- Identify complications
- Identify causative agents if possible.

History taking is the key when seeking the cause of diarrhea in children:
- Recent medications, especially antibiotics
- History of immunosuppression (e.g. recurrent major infections, history of malnutrition, acquired immunodeficiency syndrome, and recent measles)
- Illnesses in other family members or close contacts
- Travel outside city
- Travel to rural or seacoast areas (i.e. involving the consumption of untreated water, raw milk, or raw shellfish)
- Attendance in day care
- Recent foods
- Presence of family pets
- Food preparation or water source

Children should be seen for the medical evaluation of acute diarrhea:
- Young age (<6 months old or weighing <8 kg)
- History of premature birth, chronic medical conditions, or concurrent illness
- Fever more than or equal to 38°C for infants less than 3 months old or more than or equal to 39°C for children 3–36 months old
- Visible blood in stool
- High output, including frequent and substantial volumes of diarrhea
- Persistent vomiting
- Caregiver's report of signs that are consistent with dehydration
- Change in mental status
- Suboptimal response to oral rehydration therapy or inability of caregiver to administer this therapy.

Severe diarrhea of any cause can lead to dehydration, which can cause significant morbidity and mortality. However, diarrhea can be a sign of a serious associated illness, which in itself can be life-threatening:
- Intussusception
- *Salmonella* gastroenteritis (neonatal or compromised host)
- Hemolytic-uremic syndrome
- Hirschsprung's disease (with toxic megacolon)
- Pseudomembranous colitis
- Inflammatory bowel disease (with toxic megacolon).

Diarrhea in Newborn

In addition to the greater potential for dehydration in a newborn, diarrhea in this age group is more commonly associated with major congenital intestinal defects involving electrolyte transport (e.g. congenital sodium- or chloride-losing diarrhea) or carbohydrate absorption (e.g. congenital lactase deficiency). Although viral enteritis can occur in the nursery, any newborn with true diarrhea warrants thorough evaluation and possible referral to a tertiary center.

Salmonella enteritis so concerning in a child who is less than 12 months old: In older children with *Salmonella* gastroenteritis, secondary bacteremia and dissemination of disease rarely occur. In infants, however, 5–40% may have positive blood cultures for *Salmonella*, and, in 10% of these cases, *Salmonella* can cause meningitis, osteomyelitis, pericarditis, and pyelonephritis. Thus, in infants who are less than 1 year old, outpatient management of diarrhea assumes even greater significance, particularly if *Salmonella* is suspected.

Clinical Features of Dehydration

Clinical features include:
- Sunken fontanelle (infants)
- *Sunken eyes*: Dry mucus membrane and tears

Table 2 Assessment of diarrhea and dehydration in children

History	Following point should be noted: • Onset frequency, quantity of vomiting, and diarrhea • Oral intake, urine output, previous weight, associated symptoms, and medical history
Physical examination	Vitals signs, present body weight, general conditions, sunken eyes, moist or dry mucus-membrane, and respiratory pattern, extremities(capillary filling time), and skin turgor (anterior abdominal wall)
Dehydration	Categorizes severity of dehydration which is helpful for fluid management; commonly used parameters for dehydration are: • Capillary filling time (normal <2 seconds) • Reduced skin turgor • Abnormal respiratory pattern

Table 3 Classification of degree of dehydration (WHO 2005)

Classification	Fluid deficit as % of body weight	Fluid deficit in mL/kg body weight
No signs of dehydration	<3%	<30 mL/kg
Some signs of dehydration	3–9%	30–90 mL/kg
Severe dehydration	>9%	>90 mL/kg

- Excessive thirst but vomiting
- Rapid breathing, increased heart rate
- Irritability, restlessness, lethargy, and weakness
- Poor skin turgor (pinching a fold of abdominal skin and returning slow).
- *Capillary filling time (normal <2 seconds)*: In newborn infants, "capillary refill time" can be measured by pressing on the skin for 5 seconds with a finger or thumb, and noting the *"time"* needed for the color to return once the pressure is released. Common causes of sluggish, delayed, or prolonged capillary refill time are dehydration, shock, and hypothermia.
- Decreased urine output, no wet diapers or little dark urine.

Diagnostic Workup

Laboratory investigations are not helpful if no features of dehydration and in majority of children with uncomplicated diarrhea.

Stool Examination

Stool culture is not routinely indicated. Stool culture is only mandatory in profuse diarrhea (cholera), bloody diarrhea (dysentery), and severe and prolonged diarrhea.

Predictor of bacteria as a cause of diarrhea: Stool polymorphonuclear neutrophils (PMNs) are more reliable indicators of a bacterial etiology than positive stool guaiac tests for blood. Although about 30–50% of patients with blood in the stool will have a bacterial etiology, up to 70% will not. Thus, the presence of blood has a fair specificity but poor sensitivity. Stool PMNs, on the other hand, have a specificity and sensitivity of around 85%, with a positive predictive value of around 60%.

Stool examination for white blood cells: Unlike dipstick testing for urine white blood cells, you must find stool PMNs the old-fashioned way. A thin smear of fresh stool is placed on a slide and air dried. The sample is covered with methylene blue for about 5 seconds, gently rinsed with tap water, and air dried again. The quantity of PMNs seen per high-power microscopic field can be classified as occasional, scattered, or diffuse.

Urine Examination

Specific gravity of urine is helpful in monitoring of response to therapy.

Blood Examination

- *Complete blood count* should be done if sepsis is suspected.
- Eosinophilia as a diagnostic sign of parasitic disease. Normally, the total eosinophil count does not exceed $500/mm^3$. As a screening tool for suspected parasitic disease (e.g. in symptomatic patients returning from travel to villages/slums), it has a very poor positive-predictive value (15–55%). Its negative-predictive value is better (73–96%), particularly if sequential eosinophil counts remain normal.
- *Urea, Na^+, K^+, pH, HCO_3, Ca^{++}, Mg^{++}, and blood sugar monitoring.*

MANAGEMENT OF DIARRHEA AND DEHYDRATION

Aims and objectives of management are:
- Identify the children who may develop severe disease and life threatening complication
- Prevention and correction of severe dehydration and electrolyte imbalance
- Prevention and treatment of metabolic complication and malnutrition
- Diarrhea can be treated as outpatient basis if uncomplicated and not associated with severe dehydration. Children with diarrhea and dehydration should be hospitalized for management if red flags **(Box 1)** are observed.

Rehydration Therapy in Diarrhea and Dehydration

Oral rehydration should be used as first-line therapy in children with diarrhea; oral and enteral rehydration is associated with fewer complications than intravenous hydration **(Table 4)**.

Oral Rehydration Therapy

- Oral rehydration solution should be used for rehydration.
- Oral rehydration should be performed rapidly, ideally 30–90 mL/kg over 2–3 hours.
- For rapid alimentation, an age-appropriate, unrestricted diet is recommended as soon as dehydration is corrected.
- For breastfed infants, nursing should be continued.
- For formula-fed infants, diluted formula is not recommended, and special formula is usually not necessary.
- Additional oral rehydration solution should be administered for ongoing losses through diarrhea.

Box 1 Red flags in diarrhea and dehydration or indications for hospitalization

- Ineffective oral rehydration therapy
- Persistent vomiting
- Severe dehydration shock
- Lethargy seizures
- Features of systemic illness, high fever, and toxic look
- Uncertain diagnosis
- Surgical conditions

Table 4 Therapy in diarrhea and dehydration

No signs of dehydration (<3%)	Some signs of dehydration (3–9%)	Severe dehydration (9%)
• Home management if no vomiting • Continue breastfed in infants • Continue normal food with extra-water in older children	• Still can be managed at home or as outpatient if no vomiting • Oral rehydration solution 30–90 mL/kg over 2–3 hours followed by 10 mL/kg with every diarrhea • Small and frequent feed	• Persistent vomiting and worsening dehydration need hospitalization and intravenous fluid therapy • Immediate hospital admission • Fluid resuscitation with normal saline or Ringer lactate

Table 5 Antibiotic for diarrhea

Shigella	Salmonella	Cholera
Azithromycin day 1: 12 mg/kg Day 2–5: 6 mg/kg Once daily for 5 days	Amoxicillin 30–50 mg/kg thrice daily for 5 days	Doxucycline in >8 kg weight 4.4 mg/kg single dose
Ceftriaxone 50 mg/kg once daily for 2–5 days	Ceftriaxone 50 mg/kg once daily for 2–5 days	Azithromycin day 1: 12 mg/kg Day 2–5: 6 mg/kg once daily for 3 days
Trimethoprim/sulfamethoxazole 10/50 mg/kg twice daily for 5 days	Trimethoprim/sulfamethoxazole 10/50 mg/kg twice daily for 5 days	
	Ciprofloxacin 5–10 mg/kg orally twice daily for 5 days or 5–7 mg/kg iv twice daily for 5 days	

- No unnecessary laboratory tests or medications should be prescribed.
- Many ORS are available in market. Each solution has some advantages and disadvantages. Many home remedies are either very deficient or very excessive in electrolytes or sugar. The main problem with recommended oral rehydration solutions is their low caloric content, but the development of cereal-based and polymer-based solutions, which increase calories without increasing osmolality, is in progress.
- *Mechanism of action of ORS*: Intestinal solute transport mechanisms generate osmotic gradients by the movement of electrolytes and nutrients through the cell, and water passively follows. A coupled transport of sodium and glucose occurs at the intestinal brush border, and this is facilitated by the protein sodium glucose cotransporter. Oral replacement solutions are formulated with sufficient sodium, glucose, and osmolarity to maximize this cotransportation and to avoid problems of excessive sodium intake or additional osmotic diarrhea.

Antibiotics

Most of diarrhea in children are viral origin (rotavirus, adenovirus, norovirus) so antibiotics are not routinely prescribed. Conditions where antibiotics are prescribed in diarrhea are as follows **(Table 5)**:
- Shigella dysentery
- Cholera
- Diarrhea associated with pneumonia and urinary tract infection
- Salmonella gastroenteritis.

Antiemetics and Antidiarrheal Drugs

Drugs have been shown in **Table 6**.

Prevention

Severe dehydrating diarrhea is commonly caused by rotavirus. Rotavirus vaccine is safe and highly efficacious. First dose should be given between 6 and 12 month of age and full schedule should be finished by 6–8 month of the age.

PERSISTENT DIARRHEA

- *Causes*: Lactose intolerance and cow milk protein allergy.
- *Clinical features*: Nausea, abdominal pain, abdominal distension, and persistent watery diarrhea.
- Children with lactose or cow milk protein allergy may present with normal nutritional status or may present with malnourished state.
- *Intervention*: Lactose free diet, consultation with specialist.

SUMMARY

- History is crucial to diagnosis and should include recent medications, ill family contacts, travel, attendance at school or day care, pets, and water sources.

Table 6 Supportive medications for vomiting and diarrhea	
Antiemetics drugs	Not routinely recommended they usually cause sedation and interfere with oral rehydration therapy
Antidiarrheal drugs	
Loperamide activated charcoal	Not effective and not safe for children
Kaolin-pectin, bismuth cholestyramine	Not used in children
Diosmectit, certain probiotics	Generally safe have some effects
Racecadotril	Safe and positive effect
Zinc	Useful in malnourished children

- The three keys to the assessment of dehydration are (1) capillary refill, (2) skin turgor, and (3) respiratory pattern.
- The first line of therapy in infants and toddlers with mild dehydration from diarrhea is oral rehydration with a glucose- or electrolyte-containing solution.
- Salmonella infection is more concerning among infants who are <1 year old because of the increased risk of dissemination (e.g., bacteremia, meningitis).
- Vaccination for rotavirus is helpful in controlling the severe dehydrating diarrhea.

BIBLIOGRAPHY

1. Bonadio WA, Hennes HH, Machi J, et al. Efficacy of measuring BUN in assessing children with dehydration due to gastroenteritis. Ann Emerg Med. 1989;18:755-7.
2. Brown KH, Gastanaduy AS, Saavedra JM, et al. Effect of continued oral feeding on clinical and nutritional outcomes of acute diarrhea in children. J Pediatr. 1988;112:191-200.
3. Brown KH, Peerson JM, Fontaine O. Use of nonhuman milks in the dietary management of young children with acute diarrhea: a meta-analysis of clinical trials. Pediatrics. 1994;93:17-27.
4. DeWitt TG, Humphrey KF, McCarthy P. Clinical predictors of acute bacterial diarrhea in young children. Pediatrics. 1985;76:551-6.
5. Fleisher GR. Diarrhea. In: Fleisher GR, Ludwig S (Eds). Textbook of Pediatric Emergency Medicine, 4th edition. Baltimore: Lippincott Williams & Wilkins; 2000. p. 204.
6. Gryboski J. The child with chronic diarrhea. Contemp Pediatr. 1993;10:71-97.
7. Keating JP. Chronic diarrhea. Pediatr Rev. 2005;26:5-14.
8. King CK, Glass R, Bresee JS, et al. Centers for Disease Control and Prevention. Managing acute gastroenteritis among children: Oral rehydration, maintenance, and nutritional therapy. MMWR Recomm Rep. 2003;52(RR-16):1-16.
9. Ladinsky M, Duggan A, Santosham M, et al. The World Health Organization oral rehydration solution in US pediatric practice: randomized trial to evaluate parent satisfaction. Arch Pediatr Adolesc Med. 2000;154:700-5.
10. Markowitz JE, Bengmark S. Probiotics in health and disease in the pediatric patient. Pediatr Clin North Am. 2002;49:127-42.
11. Mawhorter SD. Eosinophilia caused by parasites. Pediatr Ann. 1994;23:405-13.
12. Mehta DI, Lebenthal E. New developments in acute diarrhea. Curr Probl Pediatr. 1994;24:95-107.
13. Shaw KN. Dehydration. In: Fleisher GR, Ludwig S (Eds). Textbook of Pediatric Emergency Medicine, 4th edition. Philadelphia: Lippincott Williams & Wilkins; 1999. p. 198.
14. Steiner MJ, DeWalt DA, Byerley JS. Is this child dehydrated? JAMA. 2004;291:2746-54.
15. Thielman NM, Guerrant RL. Acute infectious diarrhea. N Engl J Med. 2004;350:38-47.
16. World Health Organization. The Treatment of Diarrhoea—A Manual for Physicians and other Senior Health Workers. World Health Organization, 2005
17. Yassin SF, Young-Fadok TM, Zein NN, et al. *Clostridium difficile*-associated diarrhea and colitis. Mayo Clin Proc. 2001;76:725-30.

CHAPTER 72

Febrile Seizure and Status Epilepticus in Children

Yeeshu Singh Sudan, Devendra Richhariya

INTRODUCTION

A seizure is a single event characterized by the abnormal, excessive, and synchronized firing of cortical neurons that usually results in altered perception or behavior and recurrent unprovoked seizures labeled as epilepsy **(Fig. 1)**.

CLASSIFICATION

Seizure can be classified as: focal, generalized, and unknown. Focal seizure starts from unilateral area of brain while generalized seizures arise from both cerebral hemispheres at once. The manifestations of focal seizures depend on the area of the brain involved. Localized seizures may then spread to adjacent areas or to contralateral or other more distant regions through thalamocortical and interhemispheric pathways, eventually resulting in secondarily generalized seizures **(Flow chart 1)**.

Patients of seizure may present with changes in autonomic systems like changes in pulse rate, sweating, salivation, pupillary dilatation, and incontinence. And patients of generalized tonic-clonic seizures present with an increase in blood pressure and pulse rate, increased autonomic nervous system activation, a metabolic acidosis, a drop in pO_2 and an increase in pCO_2 during the apneic tonic phase, and, rarely, hyperkalemia or rhabdomyolysis. Prolonged generalized tonic-clonic seizures may have serious consequences **(Fig. 2)**.

In seizure, following changes occurs in blood:
- Blood flow to brain and glucose utilization increased
- Increase in lactate, extracellular potassium, serum prolactin, and a decrease in extracellular calcium, helpful in identifying true seizure. Prolactin also may be elevated after syncope and hence cannot differentiate seizures from syncope.

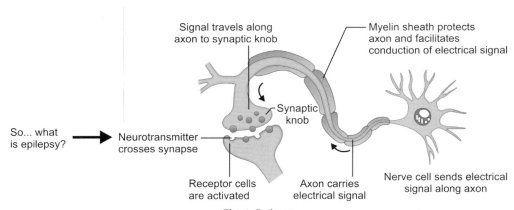

Fig. 1 Epilepsy

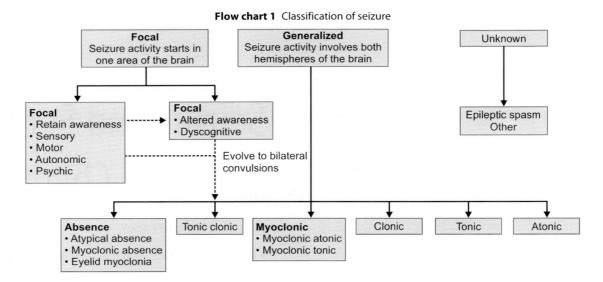

Flow chart 1 Classification of seizure

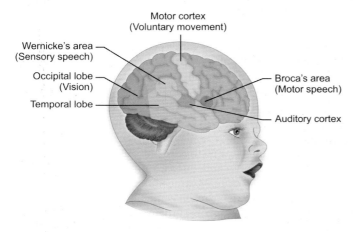

Fig. 2 Brain affected by focal seizures

FEBRILE SEIZURE

- A generalized tonic or tonic-clonic seizure
- 6 months to 5 years of age is involved
- Fever greater than 38°C, but not in the presence of a central nervous system (CNS) infection
- Lasting less than 15 minutes, no focal features, and not recur within 24 hours
- No postictal neurological abnormalities.

Benign febrile seizures (convulsions) are an inherited predisposition to develop a tonic-clonic seizure with a high fever. The description is limited to convulsions associated with high fever in children under the age of 5 years (usually between 6 months and 36 months of age), with no cause for the seizure other than the fever. Benign febrile seizures are common, occurring in 3–5% of children under the age of 5 years. Most of the patients have only one or two seizures. Recent genetic analysis of families with febrile convulsions has defined specific associated gene defects **(Fig. 3)**.

A single, isolated febrile seizure of short duration probably does not greatly influence the later development of epilepsy. In general, if there are no other reasons to suspect recurrent seizures, such children are not treated.

The following features, however, have been identified as risk factors for the development of epilepsy:
- Underlying neurologic or developmental abnormality
- Family history of nonfebrile seizures
- Prolonged febrile convulsions
- Multiple febrile convulsions
- Atypical or focal features (complex febrile seizures).

STATUS EPILEPTICUS

Status epilepticus is a state of continuous seizures without return of normal neurologic functions between them. Any of the classified seizures types may progress to status epilepticus.

Status epilepticus is convulsive or nonconvulsive. Convulsive status epilepticus is a medical emergency that can be produced by either primary generalized or secondary generalized tonic-clonic seizures. Nonconvulsive status epilepticus refers to either absence or complex partial status epilepticus. In either case, the patient does not have major motor seizures but is abnormal cognitively and may appear to be in a fugue state. Absence status appears to have no morbidity (unless injuries occur during the status), but complex partial status may lead to permanent cognitive deficits.

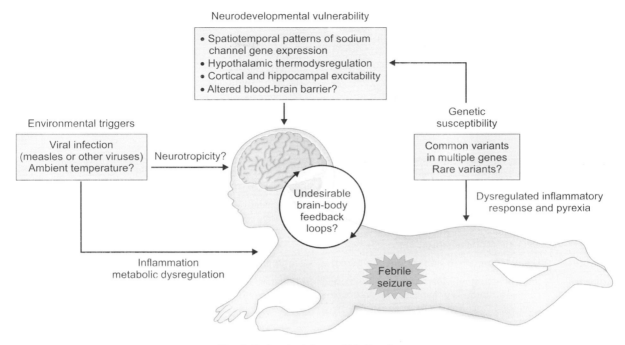

Fig. 3 Pathophysiology of febrile seizure

Causes of Status Epilepticus

- Antiepileptic drugs (AED) withdrawal (most common in emergency department)
- Metabolic abnormalities
- Brain tumors
- Cerebral infarction
- Cerebral hemorrhages
- Meningitis.

Open head trauma produced by bullets or shrapnel is associated with a 50% or greater chance of developing epilepsy. Closed head trauma, such as after automobile accidents or blunt injuries, carries a much lower risk (5% or less). Factors that predispose to the development of epilepsy after head trauma include a seizure within 2 weeks of injury, depressed skull fracture, loss of consciousness for longer than 24 hours, cerebral contusion, subdural hematoma, or subarachnoid blood, and age greater than 65 years.

Metabolic Causes

Metabolic causes include:
- Hypocalcemia
- Hyponatremia
- Hypoglycemia
- Liver failure
- Renal failure
- Anoxia.

Diagnosis

Epilepsy is a clinical diagnosis. Electroencephalogram (EEG) and magnetic resonance imaging (MRI) are helpful in localizing the brain lesions (**Fig. 4**).

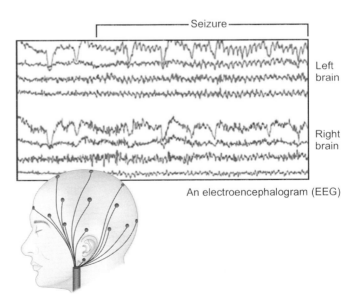

Fig. 4 Electroencephalogram of left and right brain lesion

Treatment

Protocols for the treatment of generalized tonic-clonic status epilepticus are described in **Table 1**.

LOCALIZATION FEATURES AND COMMON CAUSES OF SEIZURES

Features and causes of seizures are described in **Table 2**.

ANTIEPILEPTIC DRUGS

The choice of AED is dictated by the types of seizures that the patient has. If possible, monotherapy should be used.

The above selections are based on side effects as well as effectiveness. Phenobarbital and primidone are as efficacious as phenytoin and carbamazepine but are more likely to produce side effects. Tonic and atonic seizures are often resistant to therapy, and valproate seems to be

Table 1 Protocols for treatment of generalized tonic-clonic status epilepticus	
0–5 minutes	Provide for maintenance of vital signs, maintain airway, give oxygen, observe and examine patient
6–10 minutes	Obtain 50 mL of blood for glucose, calcium, magnesium, electrolytes, blood urea nitrogen, liver functions, anticonvulsant levels, complete blood count, and toxicology screen. Begin normal saline intravenous (IV) and give 50 mL of 50% glucose and 100 mg of thiamine. Monitor electrocardiogram, blood pressure, and if possible, electroencephalogram (EEG)
11–30 minutes	Use IV lorazepam to stop seizures, 0.1 mg/kg at 1–2 mg/min
11–30 minutes	If seizures continue, load with phenytoin using fosphenytoin 20 mg phenytoin equivalents (PE)/kg at 150 mg PE/min. If cardiac arrhythmia or hypotension occurs, slow the infusion rate
31–60 minutes	If seizures persist 10–20 min after administration of phenytoin, give an additional 10 PE/kg. If seizures continue, intubate patient. Consider phenobarbital at a rate of 50–100 mg/min until seizures stop or 20 mg/kg is given. Alternatively move to anesthetic agents
After 60 minutes of status	Review laboratory results and correct abnormalities. Arrange for anesthesia, neuromuscular blockade, and EEG monitoring. Options include midazolam (0.15–0.2 mg/kg load, then 0.06–1.1 mg/kg/h) or propofol (1–2 mg/kg load, then 3–10 mg/kg/h), or barbiturate anesthesia (pentobarbital, 6–15 mg/kg loading dose, then 0.5–5 mg/kg/h) Pentobarbital often causes circulatory collapse, so be prepared to administer a pressor agent such as dopamine

Table 2 Localization features and common causes of seizures			
Region	Typical semiology	Electroencephalogram	Etiology
Frontal	Often nocturnal, occur in clusters, often brief < 30 sec. Other symptoms relate to subregion of frontal lobes (adversive turning). Complex motor automatisms such as bicycling, pelvic thrusting or other sexual gestures. Vocalizations are common, minimal postictal symptoms	Frontal or anterior vertex epileptiform discharges. Occasionally frontal bisynchronous discharges	Trauma, malformations such as cortical dysplasia or cavernous angiomas, strokes, tumors, infections, anoxia. Some genetic syndromes
Mesial temporal	*Common auras include*: Olfactory, gustatory, rising epigastric sensation, déjà vu, experiential phenomena, behavioral arrest, automatisms of the mouth (oroalimentary) and ipsilateral hand (manual). Semipurposeful or repetitive stereotypical movements, contralateral dystonic posturing, and significant postictal confusion	Temporal epileptiform discharges localized to anterior temporal region or sphenoidal electrodes, if used. Rhythmic theta activity	Mesial temporal sclerosis, postinfectious, and trauma
Lateral temporal	Auras more likely to be auditory, vertiginous, visual distortions, and early aphasia symptoms	Lateral temporal epileptiform discharges and rhythmic theta activity	Lateral cortical lesions and dysplasias, cavernous angiomas, genetic
Parietal	Rare. May reflect activity of association, cortex activity and include elementary or unusual formed sensory phenomena, nausea or abdominal, dysphasia or speech arrest	Parietal epileptiform discharges	Usually due to cortical lesions such as infarcts, cortical dysplasia, and malignancies
Occipital	Usually consist of unformed visual phenomena. May be negative visual symptoms	Occipital epileptiform discharges, unilateral, or bisynchronous	Cortical lesions such as infarcts, dysplasia, or malignancies, but also as an idiopathic epilepsy syndrome (benign epilepsy with occipital paroxysms)

Table 3 First-line and second-line drugs for specific type seizures

				Epilepsies	
	Partial seizures and localization-related seizures	Tonic-clonic	Generalized absence	Myoclonic	Atonic or tonic
First-line drugs	• Carbamazepine • Phenytoin • Lamotrigine • Valproate • Oxcarbazepine	• Valproate • Lamotrigine • Phenytoin • Carbamazepine	Ethosuximide valproate	• Valproate • Lamotrigine • Topiramate	• Valproate • Lamotrigine • Topiramate
Second-line drugs	• Primidone • Phenobarbital • Felbamate	• Topiramate • Primidone • Phenobarbital • Felbamate	• Topiramate • Lamotrigine • Clonazepam	• Primidone • Phenobarbital • Clonazepam • Ethosuximide • Felbamate	• Phenytoin • Phenobarbital • Primidone • Clonazepam • Felbamate
Add-on drugs	• Topiramate • Levetiracetam • Zonisamide • Gabapentin • Tiagabine	• Levetiracetam • Zonisamide	• Zonisamide	• Levetiracetam • Zonisamide	• Levetiracetam • Zonisamide

most efficacious. Tonic-clonic seizures may be secondarily generalized, and phenytoin, carbamazepine, lamotrigine, topiramate, and felbamate can be helpful **(Table 3)**.

Decision regarding stopping the antiepileptic should be taken only after consulting the pediatric neurologist.

Recurrence of seizure when following abnormalities are present:
- Neurologic abnormalities
- Mental retardation
- Complex partial seizures
- Consistently abnormal EEGs.

CONCLUSION

Most common problem in pediatric neurology is febrile seizure. Majority of febrile seizure are simple and have excellent prognosis. A very few children who have febrile seizure are at risk of developing epilepsy. Majority of children who have febrile seizure subsequently normal in intellect, neurological function and behavior.

BIBLIOGRAPHY

1. Annegers JF, Hauser WA, Coan SP, et al. A population-based study of seizures after traumatic brain injuries. N Engl J Med. 1998;338(1):20-4.
2. Chang BS, Lowenstein DH. Practice parameter: antiepileptic drug prophylaxis in severe traumatic brain injury: report of the Quality Standards Subcommittee of the American Academy of Neurology. 2003;60(1):10-6.
3. Classification and Terminology of the International League Against Epilepsy: Proposal for revised clinical and electroencephalographic classification of epileptic seizures. Epilepsia. 1981;22:489-501.
4. Devinsky O. Patients with refractory seizures. N Engl J Med. 1999;340(20):1565-70.
5. Engle J, Pedley TA, Aicardi J, Dichter MA, Moshé S, Perruca E, Trimble M. Epilepsy: A Comprehensive Textbook, 2nd edition. Hagerstown, Lippincott-Raven; 1997.
6. Gilbert DL, Sethuraman G, Kotagal U, et al. Meta-analysis of EEG test performance shows wide variation among studies. Neurology. 2003;60(4):564-70.
7. Knudson FU. Febrile seizures: treatment and prognosis. Epilepsia. 2000;41(1):2-9.
8. Kullmann DM, Hanna MG. Neurological disorders caused by inherited ion-channel mutations. Lancet Neurol. 2002; 1(3):157-66.
9. Kwan P, Brodie MJ. Early identification of refractory epilepsy. N Engl J Med. 2000;342(5):314-9.
10. Lowenstein DH, Alldredge BK. Status epilepticus at an urban public hospital in the 1980s. Neurology. 1993;43(3):483-8.
11. Lowenstein DH, Alldredge BK. Status epilepticus. N Engl J Med. 1998;338(14):970-6.
12. Mattson RH, Cramer JA, Collins JF. A comparison of valproate with carbamazepine for the treatment of complex partial seizures and secondarily generalized tonic-clonic seizures in adults. N Engl J Med. 1992;327(11):765-71.
13. Oribe E, Amini R, Nissenbaum E, et al. Serum prolactin concentrations are elevated after syncope. Neurology. 1996;47(1):60-2.
14. Pellock JM, Willmore LJ. A rational guide to routine blood monitoring in patients receiving antiepileptic drugs. Neurology. 1991;41(7):961-4.
15. Pennell PB. Practice Parameter: Management issues for women with epilepsy. Neurology. 1998;51(4):944-8.
16. Pennell PB. The importance of monotherapy in pregnancy. Neurology. 2003;60:S31-8.
17. Temkin NR, Dikmen SS, Wilensky AJ, et al. A randomized, double-blind study of phenytoin for the prevention of post-traumatic seizures. N Engl J Med. 1990;323(8):497-502.
18. Treiman DM, Meyers PD, Walton NY, et al. A comparison of four treatments for generalized convulsive status epilepticus. N Engl J Med. 1998;339(12):792-8.
19. Wilner AN. Epilepsy in Clinical Practice. New York, Demos Medical; 2000.
20. Wyllie E. The Treatment of Epilepsy, 3rd edition. Baltimore, Williams &Wilkins; 2001.

CHAPTER 73

Central Nervous System Infections in Children

Yeeshu Singh Sudan

INTRODUCTION

Childhood neurological emergencies vary from benign disorder like primary headache to serious disorders like status epilepticus, meningoencephalitis, and neurometabolic crisis leading to severe neurological mortality and morbidity with significant sequelae. Infections of the central nervous system (CNS) in childhood are common especially in emergency setting needing prompt diagnosis and management, since delay can be sometimes catastrophic. The most common CNS infections encountered in practice are meningitis and encephalitis or commonly an overlap, i.e. meningoencephalitis.

Any child who presents with neurological signs and symptoms with fever constitutes a medical emergency and should be dealt seriously with immediate assessment and treatment, since children can deteriorate rapidly. Many times, especially in emergency ward, medical management is often empirical based on the clinical features. It is also very important to have knowledge to local epidemics and infections for rapid analysis and medications avoiding unnecessary delay, mortality, and morbidity.

CLINICAL HISTORY, APPROACH, AND INITIAL MANAGEMENT IN EMERGENCY

Fever is present in most of the situations but not in all, therefore, apart from fever other features like irritability, drowsiness, altered sensorium, altered behavior, vomiting, diarrhea, lethargy, neck stiffness, seizures, focal deficit, should raise suspicion of CNS infections. History should include recent travel, contact with infected person, dog bite, etc. It is important to know the temporal semiology of event like duration of illness and appearance of complications which helps in better characterization of syndrome.

Examination of a child with CNS dysfunction most of the times becomes very difficult because of poor cooperation. Occasionally examination may be noncontributory. Important points to note in this scenario may be a search for local infection, checking signs of meningeal irritation, looking for focal deficit, sign of raised intracranial hypertension like papilledema, and finally checking level of consciousness, e.g. Glasgow coma scale (GCS).

DEFINITIONS

- *Meningitis*: Primarily, meningitis is an inflammatory process of the leptomeninges and cerebrospinal fluid (CSF). It is most commonly infective in origin caused by bacteria, viruses, and fungi. As discussed earlier many a times it is associated with involvement of brain parenchyma causing altered sensorium leading to meningoencephalitis.
- *Encephalitis*: Inflammation of brain parenchyma leading to various signs and symptoms like altered level of consciousness, behavior, seizures, and focal deficit. Again there may be considerable overlap with meningitis.
- Acute focal suppurative infection (brain abscess, subdural, and extradural empyema). Usually a complication of bacterial infection.
- *Myelitis*: Inflammation of the spinal cord present as sudden onset of acute paraplegia with bladder bowel symptoms. It may be bacterial, viral, or parainfectious in origin.

ACUTE BACTERIAL MENINGITIS

Majority of the bacterial causes of meningitis is seen during the neonatal, infancy, and early childhood. One important reason could be poor vaccination and immune status

especially in developing countries. All these causative agents may be associated with severe mortality with morbidity. Common pathogens include:
- *Adults*: Streptococcus pneumoniae, Neisseria meningitidis, group B *Streptococcus*
- *Children*: N. meningitidis
- *Infants*: S. pneumoniae, N. meningitidis
- *Neonates*: Group B *Streptococcus*, Escherichia coli.

Emergency department evaluation of bacterial meningitis are shown in **Flow chart 1**.

Complication

Complications occur in 50% acute bacterial meningitis.
- *Infectious*: Cerebritis/abscess, ventriculitis, empyema, and effusion.
- *Vascular*: Ischemia related to arterial spasm or infectious arteritis, and dural venous thrombosis.

SUBACUTE MENINGITIS

Patients with subacute meningitis typically have headache, stiff neck, low-grade fever, and lethargy for days to several weeks before they present for evaluation. Common causative organisms include *Mycobacterium tuberculosis*, *Cryptococcus neoformans*, *Histoplasma capsulatum*, *Coccidioides immitis*, and *Treponema pallidum*.

CHRONIC MENINGITIS

The condition is most commonly diagnosed when a characteristic neurologic syndrome exists for more than 4 weeks and is associated with a persistent inflammatory response in the CSF (white blood cell count >5/L). Common causes include both infectious and noninfectious causes, e.g. meningeal infections, parameningeal infections, malignancy, noninfectious inflammatory disorders, chemical meningitis, and partially treated suppurative meningitis. Most common pathogens include *M. tuberculosis*, Lymes disease, syphilis, Actinomycetes, *Nocardia*, and *Brucella*. Common fungal causes include *C. neoformans*, *C. immitis*, *H. capsulatum*, *Candida*, *Blastomyces*, *Aspergillus*, and *Sporothrix*. Protozoal causes include *Toxoplasma gondii* and trypanosomiasis. Helminth causes include cysticercosis, *gnathostoma spinigerum*, and *Angiostrongylus cantonensis*. Sometimes viruses can cause prolonged illness especially

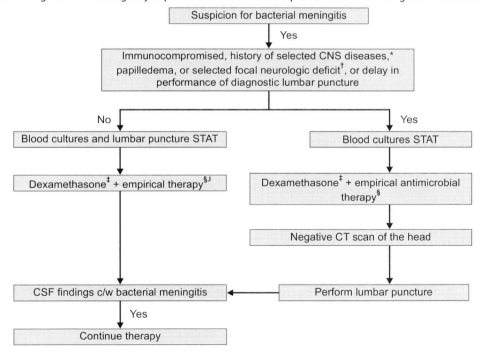

Flow chart 1 Algorithm for emergency department evaluation of suspected bacterial meningitis in infant and children

*Includes those associated with CSF shunts, hydrocephalus or trauma, those occurring after neurosurgery or various space-occupying lesions.
†Palsy of cranial nerve VI or VII is not an indication to delay lumbar puncture.
‡Adjunctive corticosteroid therapy
§See Table 1 for empiric therapy
ӏDexamethasone and antimicrobial therapy should be administered immediately after CSF is obtained.
Abbreviations: CNS, central nervous system; STAT, it indicates that the intervention should be done emergently; CSF, cerebrospinal fluid; CT, computed tomography; c/w, consistent with.

immunocompromised host, common agents include mumps, lymphocytic choriomeningitis, Echo virus, human immunodeficiency virus (HIV), and Herpes simplex virus (HSV).

Clinical Features

Acute onset of fever, headache, photophobia, neck pain, altered sensorium may be seen, although all symptoms may not be present in all. In neonates symptoms may include poor feeding, excessive crying, poor sensorium, and seizures (subtle, tonic, and clonic). On examination neck stiffness is an important sign, focal neurological deficit, cranial nerve palsies seizure and coma are other important presentation. Systemic features include rashes which may be maculopapular, petechial, or purpuric nature. In severe cases shock and organ dysfunction may be present.

Imaging

Conditions Prior to Lumbar Puncture

Conditions in which imaging has to be done prior to lumbar puncture in cases of meningitis are:
- Newly onset seizures
- Evidence of increased intracranial pressure
- An immunocompromised state
- Signs suspicious for space-occupying lesions (such as papilledema and focal neurologic signs)
- Moderate to severe impairment in consciousness.

Both computed tomography (CT) of head and magnetic resonance imaging (MRI) of brain contrast can be done in case of CNS infection, however, MRI brain has much better resolution for better detection. CT head is also beneficial in cases where quick scan is required, in cases of bleed and where affordability is an issue. Always ask for a contrast-enhanced study as plain scan may be normal. In acute cases CT head may reveal exudates in sulci cisterns with mild ventricular enlargement. Imaging studies indirectly aid to differentiate causes of meningitis. CT and MRI of brain may show leptomeningeal enhancement with contrast (differential diagnosis: metastasis, meningioma, infarction, and CSF hypotension), small ventricle due to diffuse cerebral edema, hydrocephalus, cortical infarct, ventriculitis, signs of dural sinus thrombosis, or parameningeal infection (sinusitis, brain abscess, tuberculoma or cryptococcoma). Spinal imaging may show enhancement, encasement of spinal cord (malignancy or infection).

Management

Management includes immediate assessment of cardiovascular and neurological status of the child. Maintaining airway, cardiac output, blood pressure oxygenation should be dealt promptly. Rapid deterioration can happen in neurological, respiratory, and cardiac status, therefore symptomatic care in initial hours must be done on priority basis.
- Fluid management to prevent overload or shock
- Adequate blood pressure to ensure adequate cerebral perfusion
- Metabolic correction including sugar level, calcium, and electrolyte balance.

Administration of antibiotics again must be immediate, more so in cases of suspicion of bacterial meningitis. Empirical broad-spectrum antibiotics with good CNS penetration should be considered (**Table 1**). Duration of the antibiotic should be given according to pathogen isolated in blood culture (**Table 2**). Sometimes antiviral can be added depending upon the clinical condition.

Both clinical and electrographic seizures could be seen which should be managed by loading antiepileptic drugs (benzodiazepines, phenytoin, and phenobarbitone).

Raised intracranial hypertension is again an emergency. Agents like mannitol, 3% saline and steroid should be given to reduce this.

Children with low GCS should be transferred to ICU under critical care experts.

ADJUNCTIVE CORTICOSTEROID THERAPY

The release of bacterial cell-wall components by bactericidal antibiotics leads to the production of the inflammatory cytokines, interleukin 1 (IL-1), and tumor necrosis factor (TNF) in the subarachnoid space. Dexamethasone inhibits the synthesis of IL-1 and TNF decreasing CSF outflow resistance, and stabilizing the blood brain barrier. The rationale for giving dexamethasone 20 minutes before antibiotic therapy is that dexamethasone inhibits the production of TNF by macrophages only if it is administered before these cells are activated by endotoxin. In infants and children dexamethasone should be initiated 10–20 minutes prior to, or at least concomitant with, the first antimicrobial dose, at 0.15 mg/kg every 6 hours for 2–4 days. Adjunctive dexamethasone should not be given to infants and children who have already received antimicrobial therapy, because administration of dexamethasone in this circumstance is unlikely to improve patient outcome.

REPEAT CEREBROSPINAL FLUID ANALYSIS

CSF findings of bacterial viral and fungal meningitis are given in **Table 3**.

Repeated CSF analysis should be performed, however, for any patient who has not responded clinically after 48 hours of appropriate antimicrobial therapy. The neonate with meningitis due to gram-negative bacilli should undergo repeated lumbar punctures to document CSF sterilization, because the duration of antimicrobial therapy is determined, in part, by the result.

Table 1 Empiric antibiotic therapy for bacterial meningitis

	Total daily dose (dosing interval in hours)			
	Neonates age (in days)			
Antimicrobial agent	0–7*	8–28*	Infants and children	Adults
Amikacin[†]	15–20 mg/kg (12)	30 mg/kg (8)	20–30 mg/kg (8)	15 mg/kg (8)
Ampicillin	150 mg/kg (8)	200 mg/Kg (6–8)	300 mg/kg (6)	12 g (4)
Aztreonam	–	–	–	6–8 g (6–8)
Cefepime	–	–	150 mg/kg (8)	6 g (8)
Cefotaxime	100–150 mg/kg (8–12)	150–200 mg/kg (6–8)	225–300 mg/kg (6–8)	8–12 g (4–6)
Ceftazidime	100–150 mg/kg (8–12)	150 mg/kg (8)	150 mg/kg (8)	6 g (8)
Ceftriaxone	–	–	80–100 mg/kg (12–24)	4 g (12–24)
Chloramphenicol	25 mg/kg (24)	50 mg/kg (12–24)	75–100 mg/kg (6)	4–6 g (6)[‡]
Ciprofloxacin	–	–	–	800–1,200 mg (8–12)
Gatifloxacin	–	–	–	400 mg (24)[§]
Gentamicin[†]	5 mg/kg (12)	7.5 mg/kg (8)	7.5 mg/kg (6)	5 mg/kg (8)
Meropenem	–	–	120 mg/kg (8)	6 g (8)
Moxifloxacin	–	–	–	400 mg (24)[§]
Nafcillin	75 mg/kg (8–12)	100–150 mg/kg (6–8)	200 mg/kg (6)	9–12 g (4)
Oxacillin	75 mg/kg (8–12)	150–200 mg/kg (6–8)	200 mg/kg (6)	9–12 g (4)
Penicillin G	0.15 mU/kg (8–12)	0.2 mU/kg (6–8)	0.3 mU/kg (4–6)	24 mU (4)
Rifampin	–	10–20 mg/kg (12)	10–20 mg/kg (12–24)[l]	600 mg (24)
Tobramycin[†]	5 mg/kg (12)	7.5 mg/kg (8)	7.5 mg/kg (8)	5 mg/kg (8)
TMP-SMZ[¶]	–	–	10–20 mg/kg (6–12)	10–20 mg/kg (6–12)
Vancomycin**	20–30 mg/kg (8–12)	30–45 mg/kg (6–8)	60 mg/kg (6)	30–45 mg/kg (8–12)

*Smaller doses and longer intervals of administration may be advisable for very low-birth-weight neonates (<2,000 g).
[†]Need to monitor peak and trough serum concentrations.
[‡]Higher dose recommended for patients with pneumococcal meningitis.
[§]No data on optimal dosage needed in patients with bacterial meningitis.
[l]Maximum daily dose of 600 mg.
[¶]Dosage based on trimethoprim component.
**Maintain serum trough concentrations of 15–20 μg/mL.
Abbreviation: TMP-SMZ, trimethoprim-sulfamethoxazole.

Table 2 Duration of antimicrobial therapy based on the isolated pathogen

Microorganism	Duration of therapy (days)
Neisseria meningitidis	7
Haemophilus influenzae	7
Streptococcus agalactiae	14–21
Aerobic gram-negative bacilli*	21
Listeria monocytogenes	≥21

*Duration in the neonate is 2 weeks beyond the first sterile cerebrospinal fluid culture or 3 weeks, whichever is longer.

Table 3 Cerebrospinal fluid findings of bacterial, viral, and fungal meningitis

Cerebrospinal fluid findings	Bacterial	Viral	Fungal/Tuberculous
White blood cells (per mm³)	>500	<500	<500
Polymorphonuclear neutrophils	>80%	<50%	<50%
Glucose (mg/dL)	<40	>40	<40
Cerebrospinal fluid to blood ratio	<30%	>50%	<30%
Protein (mg/dL)	>100	<100	>100

DIFFERENTIAL DIAGNOSIS

Differential diagnosis for an infant with clinical signs of meningitis and sepsis whose culture results for bacteria are negative.

Two viral infections must be considered. The first is *disseminated HSV with CNS involvement*. One helpful diagnostic clue is the development of skin vesicles, which can also be used as a source from which to isolate virus for diagnosis.

However, about 20% of babies with this form of HSV never develop skin vesicles. Other sources of virus for culture include respiratory secretions, blood, and CSF. The CSF should be cultured for virus, although it is rare to isolate HSV from this source. If infection with HSV is strongly suspected, therapy with acyclovir can begin while viral cultures and other tests remain pending.

The other viral infection associated with such a severe neonatal syndrome is *enteroviral infection*, usually due to coxsackievirus or enteric cytopathic human orphan virus. Pleconaril, a new antiviral agent, has been used to treat life-threatening enteroviral infections.

RECOMMENDED DIAGNOSTIC STUDIES FOR VIRAL MENINGITIS

Recommended diagnostic studies include:
- *Cerebrospinal fluid:*
  - Cell count and glucose concentration
  - Viral culture
  - PCR (RT-PCR) for enteroviruses
  - PCR for HSV-2 DNA, Varicella-zoster virus (VZV) and Epstein-Barr virus (EBV)
  - PCR for HIV-1 RNA
  - Immunoglobulin M (IgM) antibody-capture enzyme-linked immunosorbent assay (ELISA) for arboviruses
  - Anti-VZV IgG
- *Paired acute and convalescent sera:*
  - Heterophil antibody
  - Anti-viral capsid antigen (VCA) IgM antibodies
  - Anti-VCA IgG antibodies
  - Anti-Epstein-Barr nuclear antigen (EBNA) IgG antibodies

- Throat and stool culture
- Pelvic examination.

RECOMMENDATIONS FOR INITIAL EMPIRIC THERAPY OF MENINGITIS IN THE NEONATE

- A regimen of ampicillin and cefotaxime or a combination of a penicillin (e.g., ampicillin) and an aminoglycoside is recommended for initial empiric therapy.
- Ceftazidime is probably as efficacious as cefotaxime but should be reserved for *Pseudomonas aeruginosa* infections.

KEY POINTS: DIAGNOSIS OF NEONATAL INFECTION

- The sensitivity of blood cultures increases with increasing volume
- Meningitis may occur in the absence of a positive blood culture result
- Urine culture specimens should be obtained if infection is evaluated after the first week of life
- No single laboratory test or combination of tests is 100% sensitive or specific for diagnosing infection.

BIBLIOGRAPHY

1. Ashwal S, Perkin RM, Thompson JR, et al. Bacterial meningitis in children: Current concepts of neurologic management. Curr Prob Pediatr. 1994;24:267-84.
2. Feigin RD. Use of corticosteroids in bacterial meningitis. Pediatr Infect Dis J. 2004;23:355-7.
3. Haslam RH. Role of CT in the early management of bacterial meningitis. J Pediatr. 1991;119:157-9.
4. McCracken GH. Current management of bacterial meningitis in infants and children. Pediatr Infect Dis J. 1992;11:169-74.
5. Powell KR. Meningitis. In: Hoekelman RA, Friedman SB, Nelson NM, et al. (Eds). Primary Pediatric Care, 3rd edition. St. Louis: Mosby; 1997. p. 1423.
6. Tunkel AR. Bacterial Meningitis. Philadelphia: Lippincott Williams & Wilkins; 2001.
7. Tunkel AR. Practice Guidelines for the Management of Bacterial Meningitis. CID. 2004;39.
8. Wubbel L, McCracken GH. Management of bacterial meningitis. Pediatr Rev. 1998;19:78-84.

CHAPTER 74

Diabetes Management in Children

Ganesh Jevalikar

INTRODUCTION

Childhood diabetes is one of the most common long-term metabolic diseases in children and is rapidly increasing. According to the atlas of International Diabetes Federation (IDF), children globally are affected with diabetes. Worldwide type 1 diabetes (T1DM) is the most common type of diabetes. But, recent few decades have witnessed significant increase in childhood onset type 2 diabetes (T2DM). This chapter deals with important clinical aspects of diagnosis and management of diabetes in children. A detailed discussion on etiopathogenesis and finer aspects of management is beyond the scope of this book.

DIAGNOSIS AND CLASSIFICATION

The biochemical cut-offs for diagnosis of diabetes in children **(Table 1)** are not different from adults. The categories of impaired fasting glucose (IFG) and impaired glucose tolerance (IGT) represent prediabetic state with potential of progression to overt diabetes. Especially in case of T1DM, diagnosis of diabetes is easy when suspected. Often the delays are due to attribution of typical symptoms to other conditions such as winter season or urinary tract infection. In emergency department, children presenting with altered sensorium, respiratory distress, abdominal pain, vomiting and apparently dehydrated child with "good" urine output

Table 1 Diagnosis of diabetes in children	
Category	Criteria
Diabetes	• Classic symptoms of diabetes[1] or hyperglycemic crisis • With plasma glucose concentration ≥200 mg/dL or • Fasting[2] plasma glucose ≥126 mg/dL or • 2 hours postload[3] glucose ≥11.1 mmol/L (≥200 mg/dL) during an OGTT or • HbA_{1c}[4*] >6.5%
Impaired fasting glucose (IFG)	Fasting plasma glucose 100–125 mg/dL
Impaired glucose tolerance	2 hours postload glucose[3] 140–200 mg/dL

1. Classic symptoms include polyuria, polydipsia, polyphagia and weight loss
2. Fasting is defined as no caloric intake for at least 8 hours
3. The test should be performed using a glucose load containing the equivalent of 75 g anhydrous glucose dissolved in water or 1.75 g/kg of body weight to a maximum of 75 g
4. The test should be performed in a laboratory using a method that is National Glycohemoglobin Standardization Program (NGSP) certified and standardized to the Diabetes Control and Complications Trial (DCCT) assay
* Should not be used as a stand-alone criteria, especially in case of borderline high values
Abbreviations: OGTT, oral glucose tolerance test; DCCT, Diabetes Control and Complications Trial; NGSP, National Glycohemoglobin Standardization Program.

should raise suspicion of diabetes mellitus (DM) as one of the differential diagnosis. If diagnosis is clear by random/fasting/postprandial glucose, oral glucose tolerance test (OGTT) is not necessary and can even be potentially harmful.

Various causes of diabetes in children are listed in **Box 1**. Gestational diabetes is extremely rare and is not discussed in this chapter. Although majority of children have T1DM, a differential of T2DM needs to be considered in an obese adolescent. In selected situations **(Box 2)** other rare types of DM should be suspected. Correct typing of diabetes has significant implications on management as conditions like neonatal diabetes due to KCNJ mutations and maturity-onset diabetes of the young (MODY) can be managed with sulfonylureas.

In an obese adolescent differentiation between T1DM and T2DM is difficult. T2DM is typically seen in children during or after puberty with background of obesity, family history of T2DM, and clinical signs of insulin resistance like acanthosis nigricans, skin tags, and polycystic ovary syndrome (PCOS).

However, none of these features exclude diagnosis of T1DM. In such cases, fasting C-peptide after stabilization of initial hyperglycemia and testing for diabetes autoantibodies [anti-GAD-65, *islet cell antibodies* (ICA), islet antigen-2 (IA2), and zinc transporter-8 (ZnT8) antibodies] can be helpful. Absolute long-term insulin dependency is a reliable sign of T1DM. **Table 2** summarizes common differentiating features between three most common types of pediatric diabetes.

MANAGEMENT OF TYPE 1 DIABETES

Type 1 diabetes is thought to result from autoimmune destruction of insulin producing B-cells of pancreas in genetically susceptible individuals. Increase in incidence has been noted in the past few years worldwide especially in children less than 5 years of age. Therefore, it is increasingly necessary for all physicians to be well versed with basics of T1DM management.

Structure of Care

Successful management of T1DM requires a multidisciplinary team with the patient and family being central to the team. In Indian scenario, a pediatric endocrinologist or physician trained in T1DM along with a diabetes nurse educator and a nutritionist can manage most aspects of diabetes. The presence of a trained psychologist is desirable but often not available, hence well-adjusted senior patients and families can provide important support to newly diagnosed. Every center should have structured formats for assessment and education of patients. A protocol for evaluation and management of ketoacidosis based on evidence-based guidelines should be available. After initial assessment, follow-up visits need to be more frequent in initial months and 3 monthly subsequently.

Insulin Therapy in Type 1 Diabetes

Till date subcutaneous injection of insulin is the only effective way to treat T1DM. A formulation of inhaled insulin has been approved recently for prandial insulin replacement but has not become very popular as of now.

Modern management of T1DM is based on results of the Diabetes Control and Complications Trial (DCCT), a landmark study which established the importance of intensive diabetes treatment [multiple insulin doses, blood glucose (BG) testing, dose adjustments and frequent contact with diabetes team] in reduction of risk of retinopathy, neuropathy, and overt nephropathy by 76%, 60%, and 54%, respectively. In the post-DCCT era, physiologic insulin regimen like basal-bolus insulin therapy or continuous subcutaneous insulin infusion (CSII) has become a standard of care.

Box 1 Etiological classification of diabetes

- Type 1 diabetes
  - Autoimmune
  - Idiopathic
- Type 2 diabetes
- Other specified types of diabetes
  - *Genetic defects of B-cell function*: MODY, neonatal diabetes (transient and permanent), mitochondrial diabetes
  - *Genetic defects of insulin action*: Type A insulin resistance, Rabson-Mendenhall syndrome, lipodystrophy, leprechaunism
  - *Diseases of exocrine pancreas*: Pancreatitis, post-pancreatectomy, fibrocalcific pancreatopathy, cystic fibrosis
  - *Endocrinopathies*: Cushing syndrome, pheochromocytoma, acromegaly, hyperthyroidism
  - *Drug induced*: Glucocorticoids, L-asparaginase, tacrolimus, thiazides, phenytoin, diazoxide
  - *Infections*: Congenital rubella syndrome
  - *Syndromes*: Down syndrome, Klinefelter syndrome, Turner syndrome, Bardet-Biedl syndrome, Prader-Willi syndrome
- Gestational diabetes mellitus

Abbreviation: MODY, maturity-onset diabetes of young.

Box 2 Situations where other types of diabetes (non-type 1 and type 2) should be suspected

- Family history of youth-onset diabetes in parents and first or second degree relatives
- Diabetes in first 6 months of life
- Associated features like deafness, optic atrophy, and mental retardation
- Dysmorphic features
- Repeated abdominal pain, steatorrhea
- Exposure of drugs known to be associated with diabetes

Table 2 Clinical characteristics of common types of pediatric diabetes

Characteristics	T1DM	T2DM	MODY
Age of onset	6 months, adults	During or after puberty	Often postpubertal (except neonatal DM and GCK)
Clinical presentation	Usually acute or subacute	Variable, incidental to severe	Often incidental, severe presentations less common
Autoimmunity	Yes (antibodies may be negative in 20–30%)	No (antibodies may be positive in 5–25%)	No
Ketosis	Common	Uncommon	Rare (except neonatal)
Obesity	Population frequency	Common	Population frequency
Family history	Less common	Common	Common
Genetics	Polygenic	Polygenic	Monogenic

Abbreviations: DM, diabetes mellitus; GCK, glucokinase; MODY, maturity-onset diabetes of young; T1DM, type 1 diabetes mellitus; T2DM, type 2 diabetes mellitus.

Insulin Types, Delivery Devices, Dose and Regimen

Similar to physiological insulin secretion (**Fig. 1**), insulin treatment needs to provide basal insulin coverage to limit hepatic glucose production and prevent ketoacidosis by preventing breakdown of proteins and fat, whereas prandial (bolus) insulin is required to control rise in BG after a meal. A patient of T1DM needs choice of one-basal and one-bolus insulin. Bolus insulin is additionally needed for correction of high sugars, particularly during intercurrent illnesses.

Currently available insulin formulations and their pharmacokinetic properties are enlisted in **Table 3**. In comparison to neutral protamine Hagedorn (NPH), newer basal analogs have a relatively peakless pharmacokinetic profile, thereby reducing the risk of hypoglycemia. Unlike NPH, they are clear solutions hence do not require preinjection mixing thereby reducing day-to-day variability. However, increased cost is their limitation. In such cases, NPH insulin used twice daily can give reasonably good basal insulin coverage.

Several new rapid-acting insulin analogs are available and have a rapid onset of action permitting intake 5–15 minutes before meals, and a faster and higher peak action closer to physiologic insulin. This is especially beneficial in infants and toddlers, and those on insulin pump. However, since the duration of action is shorter, additional boluses are necessary for mid-meal snacks. Both regular and rapid-acting analogs can be given intravenously in ketoacidosis, however the latter does not have any additional advantage by this route.

Premixed insulins (fixed-dose combinations of regular insulin with NPH or rapid-acting analogs with their protaminated forms) are not ideal for most patients with T1DM as separate adjustments of basal and prandial insulin cannot be done. This causes more fluctuations and relatively poor glycemic control. However, they might be required in rare circumstances of poor adherence to multiple doses. Starting insulin at diagnosis is most important, and premixed insulin is commonly used by many physicians. Although this is not recommended as a standard treatment, it is better than not starting insulin at all.

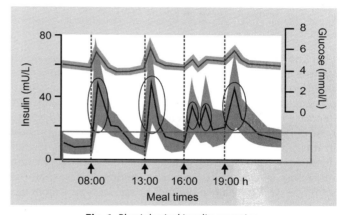

Fig. 1 Physiological insulin secretion
Note: Diagram showing glucose excursions and insulin secretion in a day. Portion highlighted in a square represents basal insulin secretion that limits hepatic glucose output and prevents ketogenesis whereas the ellipsoid areas represent prandial boluses secreted in response to mealtime rise of glucose.

Insulin Dose

- *Prepubertal children at the time of diagnosis*: 0.7–1 units/kg/day
- *Honeymoon phase (partial remission phase)*: Less than 0.5 units/kg/day, in some case insulin might have to be stopped temporarily
- *Puberty*: 1.2–2 units/kg/day.

Table 3 Currently available insulin formulations and their pharmacokinetic properties

Insulin type	Onset	Peak	Duration	Remarks
Rapid acting				
Lispro, Aspart, Glulisine	5–15 min	1 hrs	3–5 hrs	Given 5–15 min before meals. Ideal for use in pumps
Short acting				
Regular (plain/crystalline)	30 min	2–3 hrs	6–8 hrs	Given 30–45 min before meals
Intermediate				
NPH (isophane)	2–4 hrs	5–8 hrs	10–16 hrs	Peak effect necessitates mid-meal snacks
Long acting				
Glargine, detemir	2–4 hrs	Peakless*	24 hrs†	Less risk of hypoglycemia, less day-to-day variability
Degludec	0.5–1.5 hrs	Peakless	>24 hrs	

* Some peak action can be seen especially with detemir
† Duration of action in some patients can be less than 24 hrs
Abbreviations: NPH, neutral protamine Hagedorn.

Soon after the diagnosis dose requirement is usually very high due to excess appetite and glucotoxicity, and may reach up to 1.5–2 units/kg/day, but with settling of appetite dose requirement comes down. A partial remission (honeymoon) phase usually sets in few days to weeks and is characterized by decrease in insulin requirement below 0.5 units/kg/day with near normal glycemic control. BG testing is very important in this phase to pick up end of honeymoon phase. Higher doses are required during puberty due to increase in insulin resistance secondary to growth hormone and sex steroid secretion. It is typically a difficult phase for type 1 diabetics due to factors like erratic meals, behavioral changes, eating disorders, and peer pressures in addition to the insulin resistance.

Of the total daily dose, 40–50% is given as basal insulin and remaining divided as 3–5 bolus doses to cover major meals and snacks. Carbohydrate counting or food exchange lists can be used to vary insulin intake for variations in food thereby giving more flexibility in diet.

Insulin Regimen

Split-mix regimen: This involves NPH and regular insulin mixed in a syringe and administered twice a day. Two-thirds of total dose is given before breakfast and one-third before dinner. Nearly two-third of morning dose and half of evening dose is given as NPH and rest as regular. Matching of insulin syringe to strength of insulin used (40 units or 100 units/mL) and correct mixing (drawing regular insulin first in syringe) is necessary.

Basal-bolus regimen (multiple subcutaneous injections): This involves using single daily dose of long-acting analog or NPH twice daily as a basal insulin and three or more injections of short or rapid-acting insulin taken as meal time boluses. Glargine/detemir/degludec can be given at any time of the day but on the same time every day. A common practice is to give the dose at bedtime in older children and adolescents and in the morning in infants and toddlers.

This regimen is more physiological and provides more flexibility with respect to meal timings and lifestyle.

More frequent self-monitoring (at least 3–4 tests daily) and dose adjustment is required for good glycemic control. This increases the overall cost of the treatment. However, the DCCT study and several other studies have clearly demonstrated the long-term benefits of this approach for better control and reduction in the complications of diabetes.

Continuous subcutaneous insulin infusion: This consists of continuous infusion of rapid-acting insulin with insulin pump. This is infused at a manually programmed basal rate and additional bolus doses taken by pressing a button. The advantages include availability of different basal rates for different time periods of the day and ability to take more boluses without additional pricks. Features like temporary basal rates for exercise/illness or ability to automatically suspend pump in case of low sugars are available in newer pumps. Since back up long-acting insulin is not used, risk of ketoacidosis is higher with interruption of insulin delivery even for short time. Insulin pump therapy is costly at present and needs motivated parents and patients who are willing to do regular BG tests, learn the dose adjustments and count dietary carbohydrates. Improper use can lead to deterioration in glycemic control.

Closed-loop insulin therapy which combines continuous glucose monitoring with automated infusion of insulin with the help of algorithms is being successfully tried and is likely to be an option for T1DM in the near future.

Insulin Delivery Devices

Insulin can be administered by insulin syringe, insulin pen or insulin pump. Since insulin vials are available in two strengths in India (40 units/mL, 100 units/mL), it is important to match insulin syringe with vial. Both disposable and permanent insulin pen are available. For long-term management it is more cost-effective to use permanent pens with refills. Disposable pen can be used at the time of diagnosis to allow more time for family to select insulin for long-term. Insulin pump is costly at present and is not reimbursed under insurance schemes in India, thereby limiting its use. However, when used correctly, it is the most physiologic way of giving insulin.

Equally good glycemic control can be obtained using any of the devices, hence the choice should be individualized. Correct technique of using each device should be taught to families to avoid insulin administration errors.

Insulin Storage

Insulin vial or cartridge in use is stable up to a month when used at room temperature (except in peak summer). However, it should be protected from direct heat exposure. Patients should be instructed not to keep insulin in a parked car or vehicle. Extra insulin vials or cartridges should be stored at 2–8°C (preferably in the middle or lower compartment of fridge). Insulin should never be frozen. If refrigerator is not available, insulin can be kept in earthenware pitcher (matka) in a cool and dry place in the house. During travel in summer, insulin can be carried in cool gel packs or a thermos with few cubes of ice.

Insulin Injection Sites

Insulin can be injected at sites shown in **Figure 2**. Correct rotation of insulin sites should be taught to patient and caregiver during initial education and use of all sites need to be encouraged. Generally, faster absorption is noted from abdomen or an exercising limb.

Monitoring of Glycemic Control

Monitoring of BG is as important as taking insulin. It is most commonly done by testing capillary glucose using a glucometer. Testing frequency needs to be individualized based on variations in lifestyle and affordability of the family. While selecting glucometer cost of the strips should receive consideration rather that initial cost of meter.

Blood glucose testing helps in:
- Identification of abnormal patterns of BG and insulin dose adjustment
- Detection of low BG
- Identification of responses to different foods, exercise, sick days, menses, etc.

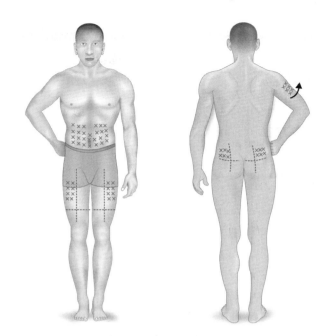

Fig. 2 Insulin injection sites

Generally testing is done before meals, 2 hours after meals and during overnight. Best outcomes in terms of glycosylated hemoglobin (HbA_{1C}) have been documented, if patients are testing BG 4–6 times per day. Post-meal testing is especially important if rapid-acting analogs are being used.

Targets for BG control are mentioned in **Table 4**. These need to be individualized to obtain best glycemic control without causing frequent hypoglycemia. Glycosylated Hb (HbA_{1C}) is assessed every 3 months and is a measure of overall control and a predictor for long-term complications.

All patients and families should have facility for testing urine or blood ketones at home during sick days. Glucometer with ability to test both glucose and ketones are now available and are more sensitive and specific than urine ketone testing.

Continuous glucose monitoring of interstitial fluid is now available. High cost is significant limitation to its continuous use but even intermittent use either retrospectively or real-time can give valuable information of glucose variability and occurrence of hypoglycemia (**Fig. 3**).

Self-adjustment of Insulin Doses

Learning to self-manage insulin doses based on the BG monitoring is the key to successful diabetes management. Fasting morning reading or reading during times when no meal/bolus or correction doses are not taken guide the dose of basal insulin whereas post-meal readings inform adequacy of bolus dose. Basal and bolus insulin doses should be changed on pattern of readings over a period of 3–7 days to prevent high or low BG patterns. More rapid changes may need to be done in case of sick days or ketonuria. In addition,

546　SECTION 10　Pediatric Emergencies

Table 4 Suggested targets for glycemic control*

Level of control		Optimal	Suboptimal (action suggested)	High-risk (action required)
SMBG (mg/dL)	Fasting/pre-meal	70–145	146–162	>162
	Postprandial	90–180	180–250	>250
	Bedtime	120–180	<80 or >180	<75 or >200
	Nocturnal	80–162	<75 or >162	<70 or >200
HbA$_{1C}$ (%)		<7.5	7.5–9	>9

Source: Modified from ISPAD 2014 guidelines.
*These population-based target indicators must be adjusted according to individual circumstances. Different targets will be appropriate for various individuals such as those who have experienced severe hypoglycemia or those with hypoglycemic unawareness
Abbreviations: HbA$_{1C}$, Hemoglobin A$_{1C}$; ISPAD, International Society for Pediatric and Adolescent Diabetes; SMBG, self-monitoring of blood glucose.

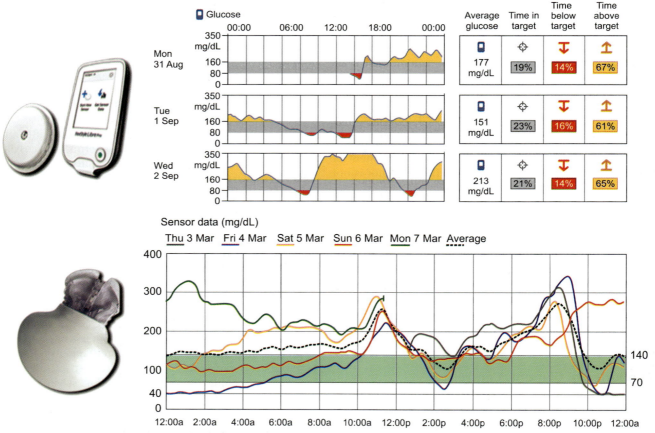

Fig. 3 Continuous glucose monitoring devices and graphs. Continuous glucose monitoring system provides a continuous record of glucose and gives idea of glucose variability, can pick up hypoglycemia and be used as an educational tool

the bolus dose also needs to be adjusted for variations in food, correction for high premeal BG or exercise. Hypoglycemia, if present needs to be corrected first before interpreting high readings.

The distribution of the dose change depends on the time point when the readings are abnormal. Following are some examples for the correlation between the BG reading and the dose to be adjusted **(Table 5)**.

Dietary Management

Diet of a child with T1DM is based on principles of healthy eating suitable for all children and family members. The

Table 5 Examples of insulin adjustments depending on timings of abnormal reading

Readings	Insulin to be adjusted
Before breakfast	Predinner NPH or bedtime long-acting analogue (nocturnal hypoglycemia should be ruled out)
After meals	Premeal short/rapid acting
Before lunch*	Short/rapid-acting insulin at the time of breakfast
Before dinner*	Short/rapid acting at the time of lunch (thrice daily or MSI or CSII) Morning NPH (conventional regimen)

*If the high reading is attributed to a snack not covered with insulin dose, additional bolus dose for the snack might be required for the patients on basal-bolus therapy.
Abbreviations: NPH, neutral protamine Hagedorn; MSI, multiple subcutaneous injections; CSII, continuous subcutaneous insulin infusion.

general goals of dietary management are to promote linear growth, avoid obesity, and cut down intake of simple carbohydrates. The use of terms like "diabetic diet" needs to be avoided and healthy eating should be practiced by the whole family. Consultation with a nutritionist trained in T1DM should be done and at all stages children should be encouraged to be part of the discussion. Unlike commonly advised, 2 hourly eating is not necessary and meal plan should be individualized. Generally, it includes major meals (breakfast, lunch, dinner) and a couple of healthy snacks between meals. It is a common practice to give milk at bedtime for young children and those on NPH insulin to prevent nocturnal hypoglycemia but strong evidence of benefit of this practice is lacking. Small amount of sucrose (up to 10% of total caloric intake) is not harmful. Occasional treats for birthdays and major festivals go a long way to ensure long-term cooperation of the child.

Exercise

Age-appropriate exercise and participation in sports should be actively encouraged for 30–60 minutes daily. Similar to healthy eating, exercise should also be part of family activities. Physical activity should be incorporated in daily routine, like climbing stairs, walking to nearby places, doing household chores, etc. BG testing before and after exercise helps to make an exercise plan to prevent low or high sugars. Exercise can potentially trigger hypoglycemia. To prevent this, insulin dose before exercise can be reduced by 10–20%. Those using insulin pumps can use temporary basal rates (20–50% less) from 1½–2 hours before exercise to few hours after exercise. Additional carbohydrate intake before or immediately after exercise is recommended to prevent hypoglycemia, particularly if preexercise BG is tending to be low or vigorous exercise is anticipated. A fast-acting carbohydrate source (like juice, glucose biscuits or tablets) should be available to treat low glucose. Exercise should be discouraged during sickness and if sugars are very high, as this can trigger ketoacidosis.

Hypoglycemia

Hypoglycemia (capillary BG <70 mg/dL) is an important complication of insulin therapy and a major barrier to successful diabetes management. Presence of hypoglycemia should be actively sought by history, BG record and continuous glucose monitoring system (CGMS) and education on prevention and management of the same should be done. Symptoms of hypoglycemia are a result of autonomic responses (shakiness, sweating, fast heartbeat, excess hunger) and neuroglucopenia (headache, drowsiness, poor concentration, behavioral changes, tantrums). Serious complications include seizures, unconsciousness, and rarely death. Repeated hypoglycemia may induce a state of hypoglycemia unawareness where autonomic symptoms are absent, increasing the risk of serious neurological sequelae. Most commonly hypoglycemia results from insulin, food and exercise-related factors like wrong type or dose of insulin, delayed or missed meals or excess physical activity. Frequent hypoglycemia merits evaluation of comorbid conditions like celiac disease, adrenal insufficiency, hypothyroidism or underlying behavioral or psychiatric problems leading to manipulation of insulin doses. Mild hypoglycemia can be treated with 10–15 grams of fast-acting carbohydrate like glucose, sugar, carbonated drinks (not diet) or sweet candies or juice. Foods containing fat like milk chocolates or ice cream are not ideal for hypoglycemia treatment. Families should be discouraged to use hypoglycemic episode as occasions of "celebrations" as it may promote insulin or food manipulation by the child. In case of unconsciousness or seizures, child should be kept in lateral position, nothing should be forcefully given orally and a dose of glucagon (0.02–0.03 mg/kg or 0.5 mg for children <12 years, 1 mg for children >12 yrs) is given subcutaneously. If glucagon in not available child should be taken to nearby hospital and intravenous 10% glucose should be given in the dose of 2–5 mL/kg.

If BG is still low after 15–20 minutes of initial intervention, treatment should be repeated. In a conscious child initial treatment is followed by a snack if a meal is not due.

All patients with diabetes should carry a medic alert (bracelet, pendent, wrist band or identity card) declaring their acute condition and emergency contacts.

Management of Sick Days

During sick days BG invariably becomes high and risk of diabetic ketoacidosis (DKA) is increased. In some illnesses like gastroenteritis, there is a risk of hypoglycemia. All patients with T1DM should receive written instructions on management of sick days. These rules include the following:
- Do not stop or skip insulin doses
- Frequent monitoring of BG and serum or urine ketones
- Adequate water and salt intake to prevent dehydration

Table 6 Screening of comorbidities and complications of type 1 diabetes

Condition	Screening test	Testing frequency	Potential interventions
Hypothyroidism	TSH	Baseline and annually	Thyroxine
Celiac disease	Anti-TTG IgA*	Baseline and biannually	Gluten-free diet
Dyslipidemia†	Fasting-lipid profile	Annually	Diet, lifestyle Statin therapy
Hypertension	BP measurement	All clinic visits	Diet, lifestyle ACEI/ARB
Retinopathy†	Fundoscopy on dilated pupil	Annually	Glycemic control, Laser
Nephropathy	Urine albumin to creatinine ratio**	Annually	Glycemic control, ACEI/ARB
Neuropathy	Clinical-foot examination‡	Annually	Glycemic control, B12s

*TTG, tissue transglutaminase: Testing at baseline needs to be with total immunoglobulin IgA.
†Start from 10 years of age (or onset of puberty) and >2 years of type 1 diabetes, recommended frequency is minimum and can be more if clinically indicated.
‡Includes palpation of pulses, ankle jerk, monofilament testing, and vibration testing.
**Spot sample, if high on spot samples—need to be done on three consecutive samples or a 24 hrs urine collection.
Abbreviations: ACEI, ACE inhibitor; ARB, angiotensin-receptor blockers; BP, blood pressure; TSH, thyroid-stimulating hormone; TTG, tissue transglutaminase.

- Avoiding exercise
- Treatment of precipitating illness
- Taking supplemental bolus insulin (10–20%) of total daily dose, added to routine doses or taken as extra correction boluses
- Visit hospital if moderate or large ketones, persistent vomiting or abdominal pain, increasing lethargy or respiratory distress.

Psychological Aspects

Patients and families with diabetes have significant psychological issues including depression and eating disorders. Assessment by trained psychologist at baseline and at least annually thereafter should be advised. Where this is not available patient support groups can be helpful.

Screening of Comorbid Conditions and Complications

About 7–10% of patients with T1DM may have comorbid conditions like hypothyroidism or celiac disease. Other conditions like vitiligo, Addison' disease or Graves' disease can also be infrequently seen but are not screened routinely. Regular screening for micro- and macrovascular complications is recommended after onset of puberty (or 10 yrs of age whichever is earlier) and above 2 years of diabetes duration. Details are given in **Table 6**. In addition to these, annual dietary, psychological and dental evaluations are recommended.

Diabetes Education

Diabetes education is the key to successful diabetes management and needs to be done by a trained nurse educator. Initial education focuses on survival skills like giving insulin correctly, testing glucose and managing low BG. Ongoing education equips patients to self-adjust insulin doses, adjust for food, exercise, and sick days. Advanced education includes carbohydrate counting, insulin pump adjustments, and finer aspects of diabetes management. Annual review and repeated reinforcement is necessary. Education should be individualized considering level of education, motivation, background knowledge, culture, and beliefs.

MANAGEMENT OF TYPE 2 DIABETES

Childhood T2DM is increasingly being seen with a background of increased prevalence of obesity. It has variable clinical spectrum from asymptomatic to severe manifestations like DKA. From the available literature, childhood onset T2DM is thought to be an aggressive disease and associated with multiple comorbidities of metabolic syndrome and poor cardiovascular outcomes. Management focuses on dietary and lifestyle management aimed at achieving healthy weight. All children need to be started on pharmacologic management right at the time of diagnosis. Currently metformin and insulin are the only approved medications in children and adolescents; however, in some cases other medications may have to be used in close supervision of an endocrinologist dealing with adult T2DM. Decompensated patients and those where distinction from T1DM is not possible are treated with insulin and metformin is attempted at a later stage, whereas stable patient with mild hyperglycemia (HbA_{1C} <9%) are started on metformin. BG monitoring for patients on metformin alone is done with fasting and 2 hours post-meals at least 2–4 times in a week. Patients are seen and HbA$_{1C}$ is estimated in every 3 months and treatment titrated to obtain HbA$_{1C}$ less than 6.5–7%. Noncompliance with diet and medications is the most important barrier in T2DM treatment and is associated with poor outcomes.

CONCLUSION

Diabetes has the major impact on the life of a child and also on their family and careers diabetes management should include insulin therapy, education and psychological support. Adequate preparation should be done for smooth transition of pediatric diabetes to adult diabetes.

BIBLIOGRAPHY

1. Agus MS, Wolfsdorf JI. Diabetic ketoacidosis in children. Pediatr Clin North Am. 2005;52:1147-63.
2. Akerblom HK, Vaarala O, Hyoty H, Ilonen J, Knip M. Environmental factors in the etiology of type 1 diabetes. Am J Med Genet. 2002;115:18-29.
3. Association AD. Diagnosis and classification of diabetes mellitus. Diabetes Care. 2006;29(Suppl 1):S43-8.
4. Babenko AP, Polak M, Cave H, Busiah K, Czernichow P, Scharfmann R, et al. Activating mutations in the ABCC8 gene in neonatal diabetes mellitus. N Engl J Med. 2006;355:456-66.
5. Balamurugan AN, Bottino R, Giannoukakis N, Smetanka C. Prospective and challenges of islet transplantation for the therapy of autoimmune diabetes. Pancreas. 2006;32:231-43.
6. Barrett TG. Nonautoimmune forms of diabetes: Neonatal diabetes, DIDMOAAD-Wolfram, and related syndromes. In: Sperling MA (Ed). Type 1 diabetes. Totowa: Humana Press; 2003. pp. 163-82.
7. Bode BW, Sabbah HT, Gross TM, Fredrickson LP, Davidson PC. Diabetes management in the new millennium using insulin pump therapy. Diabetes Metab Res Rev. 2002;18(Suppl 1):S14-20.
8. Bottini N, Musumeci L, Alonso A, Rahmouni S, Nika K, Rostamkhani M, et al. A functional variant of lymphoid tyrosine phosphatase is associated with type I diabetes. Nat Genet. 2004;36:337-8.
9. Chang TJ, Lei HH, Yeh JI, Chiu KC, Lee KC, Chen MC, et al. Vitamin D receptor gene polymorphisms influence susceptibility to type 1 diabetes mellitus in the Taiwanese population. Clin Endocrinol (Oxf). 2000;52:575-80.
10. Chowdhury TA, Mijovic CH, Barnett AH. The aetiology of type I diabetes. Baillieres Best Pract Res Clin Endocrinol Metab. 1999;13:181-95.
11. Concannon P, Erlich HA, Julier C, Morahan G, Nerup J, Pociot F, et al. Type 1 diabetes: evidence for susceptibility loci from four genome-wide linkage scans in 1,435 multiplex families. Diabetes. 2005;54:2995-3001.
12. Curtis JR, Bohn D, Daneman D. Use of hypertonic saline in the treatment of cerebral edema in diabetic ketoacidosis (DKA). Pediatr Diabetes. 2001;2:191-4.
13. Dabelea D, D'Agostino RB, Jr., Mayer-Davis EJ, Pettitt DJ, Imperatore G, Dolan LM, et al. Testing the accelerator hypothesis: body size, beta-cell function, and age at onset of type 1 (autoimmune) diabetes. Diabetes Care. 2006;29:290-4.
14. Devendra D, Eisenbarth GS. Interferon alpha—a potential link in the pathogenesis of viral-induced type 1 diabetes and autoimmunity. Clin Immunol. 2004;111:225-33.
15. Devendra D, Liu E, Eisenbarth GS. Type 1 diabetes: recent developments. BMJ. 2004;328:750-4.
16. Dunger DB, Sperling MA, Acerini CL, Bohn DJ, Daneman D, Danne TP, et al. European Society for Paediatric Endocrinology/Lawson Wilkins Pediatric Endocrine Society consensus statement on diabetic ketoacidosis in children and adolescents. Pediatrics. 2004;113:e133-40.
17. Dunger DB, Sperling MA, Acerini CL, Bohn DJ, Daneman D, Danne TP, et al. ESPE/LWPES consensus statement on diabetic ketoacidosis in children and adolescents. Arch Dis Child. 2004; 89:188-94.
18. Fajans SS, Bell GI, Polonsky KS. Molecular mechanisms and clinical pathophysiology of maturity-onset diabetes of the young. N Engl J Med. 2001;345:971-80.
19. Figueroa RE, Hoffman WH, Momin Z, Pancholy A, Passmore GG, Allison J. Study of subclinical cerebral edema in diabetic ketoacidosis by magnetic resonance imaging T2 relaxometry and apparent diffusion coefficient maps. Endocr Res. 2005;31: 345-55.
20. Genuth S, Alberti KG, Bennett P, Buse J, Defronzo R, Kahn R, et al. Follow-up report on the diagnosis of diabetes mellitus. Diabetes Care. 2003;26:3160-7.
21. Giuffrida FM, Reis AF. Genetic and clinical characteristics of maturity-onset diabetes of the young. Diabetes Obes Metab. 2005;7:318-26.
22. Glaser N, Barnett P, McCaslin I, Nelson D, Trainor J, Louie J, et al. Risk factors for cerebral edema in children with diabetic ketoacidosis. The Pediatric Emergency Medicine Collaborative Research Committee of the American Academy of Pediatrics. N Engl J Med. 2001;344:264-9.
23. Glaser NS, Wootton-Gorges SL, Buonocore MH, Marcin JP, Rewers A, Strain J, et al. Frequency of sub-clinical cerebral edema in children with diabetic ketoacidosis. Pediatr Diabetes. 2006;7:75-80.
24. Glaser NS, Wootton-Gorges SL, Marcin JP, Buonocore MH, Dicarlo J, Neely EK, et al. Mechanism of cerebral edema in children with diabetic ketoacidosis. J Pediatr. 2004;145:164-71.
25. Gloyn AL, Odili S, Zelent D, Buettger C, Castleden HA, Steele AM, et al. Insights into the structure and regulation of glucokinase from a novel mutation (V62M), which causes maturity-onset diabetes of the young. J Biol Chem. 2005;280: 14105-13.
26. Gloyn AL, Weedon MN, Owen KR, Turner MJ, Knight BA, Hitman G, et al. Large-scale association studies of variants in genes encoding the pancreatic beta-cell KATP channel subunits Kir6.2 (KCNJ11) and SUR1 (ABCC8) confirm that the KCNJ11 E23K variant is associated with type 2 diabetes. Diabetes. 2003;52:568-72.
27. Goldman-Levine JD, Lee KW. Insulin detemir—a new basal insulin analog. Ann Pharmacother. 2005;39:502-7.
28. Gomez-Perez FJ, Rull JA. Insulin therapy: current alternatives. Arch Med Res. 2005;36:258-72.
29. Gragnoli C, Stanojevic V, Gorini A, Von Preussenthal GM, Thomas MK, Habener JF. IPF-1/MODY4 gene missense mutation in an Italian family with type 2 and gestational diabetes. Metabolism. 2005;54:983-8.

30. Haider S, Antcliff JF, Proks P, Sansom MS, Ashcroft FM. Focus on Kir6.2: a key component of the ATP-sensitive potassium channel. J Mol Cell Cardiol. 2005;38:927-36.
31. Haller MJ, Atkinson MA, Schatz D. Type 1 diabetes mellitus: etiology, presentation, and management. Pediatr Clin North Am. 2005;52:1553-78.
32. Hamilton J, Cummings E, Zdravkovic V, Finegood D, Daneman D. Metformin as an adjunct therapy in adolescents with type 1 diabetes and insulin resistance: a randomized controlled trial. Diabetes Care. 2003;26:138-43.
33. Hirsch IB. Insulin analogues. N Engl J Med. 2005;352:174-83.
34. Hovorka R. Continuous glucose monitoring and closedloop systems. Diabet Med. 2006;23:1-12.
35. Hyoty H. Environmental causes: viral causes. Endocrinol Metab Clin North Am. 2004;33:27-44.
36. Ize-Ludlow D, Sperling MA. The classification of diabetes mellitus: a conceptual framework. Pediatr Clin North Am. 2005;52:1533-52.
37. Katagiri H, Asano T, Ishihara H, Inukai K, Anai M, Miyazaki J, et al. Nonsense mutation of glucokinase gene in late-onset non-insulin-dependent diabetes mellitus. Lancet. 1992;340:1316-7.
38. Kaufman DL, Erlander MG, Clare-Salzler M, Atkinson MA, Maclaren NK, Tobin AJ. Autoimmunity to two forms of glutamate decarboxylase in insulin-dependent diabetes mellitus. J Clin Invest. 1992;89:283-92.
39. Kelly MA, Mijovic CH, Barnett AH. Genetics of type 1 diabetes. Best Pract Res Clin Endocrinol Metab. 2001;15:279-91.
40. Kim MS, Polychronakos C. Immunogenetics of type 1 diabetes. Horm Res. 2005;64:180-8.
41. Klonoff DC. A review of continuous glucose monitoring technology. Diabetes Technol Ther. 2005;7:770-5.
42. Knerr I, Wolf J, Reinehr T, Stachow R, Grabert M, Schober E, et al. The 'accelerator hypothesis': relationship between weight, height, body mass index and age at diagnosis in a large cohort of 9,248 German and Austrian children with type 1 diabetes mellitus. Diabetologia. 2005;48:2501-4.
43. Kordonouri O, Hartmann R. Higher body weight is associated with earlier onset of Type 1 diabetes in children: confirming the 'Accelerator Hypothesis'. Diabet Med. 2005;22:1783-4.
44. Kukreja A, Maclaren NK. Autoimmunity and diabetes. J Clin Endocrinol Metab. 1999;84:4371-8.
45. Lammi N, Karvonen M, Tuomilehto J. Do microbes have a causal role in type 1 diabetes? Med Sci Monit. 2005;11:RA63-9.
46. Lawrence SE, Cummings EA, Gaboury I, Daneman D. Population-based study of incidence and risk factors for cerebral edema in pediatric diabetic ketoacidosis. J Pediatr. 2005;146:688-92.
47. Lonnrot M, Hyoty H, Knip M, Roivainen M, Kulmala P, Leinikki P, et al. Antibody cross-reactivity induced by the homologous regions in glutamic acid decarboxylase (GAD65) and 2C protein of coxsackievirus B4. Childhood Diabetes in Finland Study Group. Clin Exp Immunol. 1996;104:398-405.
48. Mahoney CP, Vlcek BW, DelAguila M. Risk factors for developing brain herniation during diabetic ketoacidosis. Pediatr Neurol. 1999;21:721-7.
49. Menon RK, Sperling MA. Diabetic ketoacidosis. In: Menon RK, Sperling MA (Eds). Pediatric diabetes. Norwell: Kluwer Acedemic Publishers; 2003. pp. 227-42.
50. Menon RK, Sperling MA. Diabetic Ketoacidosis. In: Sperling MA (Ed). Type 1 diabetes. Totowa: Humana Press; 2003. pp. 183-98.
51. Metz C, Cave H, Bertrand AM, Deffert C, Gueguen-Giroux B, Czernichow P, et al. Neonatal diabetes mellitus: chromosomal analysis in transient and permanent cases. J Pediatr. 2002;141:483-9.
52. Motohashi Y, Yamada S, Yanagawa T, Maruyama T, Suzuki R, Niino M, et al. Vitamin D receptor gene polymorphism affects onset pattern of type 1 diabetes. J Clin Endocrinol Metab. 2003;88:3137-40.
53. Mrena S, Virtanen SM, Laippala P, Kulmala P, Hannila ML, Akerblom HK, et al. Models for predicting type 1 diabetes in siblings of affected children. Diabetes Care. 2006;29:662-7.
54. Muir AB, Quisling RG, Yang MC, Rosenbloom AL. Cerebral edema in childhood diabetic ketoacidosis: natural history, radiographic findings, and early identification. Diabetes Care. 2004;27:1541-6.
55. Njolstad PR, Sagen JV, Bjorkhaug L, Odili S, Shehadeh N, Bakry D, et al. Permanent neonatal diabetes caused by glucokinase deficiency: inborn error of the glucose-insulin signaling pathway. Diabetes. 2003;52:2854-60.
56. Njolstad PR, Sovik O, Cuesta-Munoz A, Bjorkhaug L, Massa O, Barbetti F, et al. Neonatal diabetes mellitus due to complete glucokinase deficiency. N Engl J Med. 2001;344:1588-92.
57. Odegard PS, Capoccia KL. Inhaled insulin: Exubera. Ann Pharmacother. 2005;39:843-53.
58. Owen K, Hattersley AT. Maturity-onset diabetes of the young: from clinical description to molecular genetic characterization. Best Pract Res Clin Endocrinol Metab. 2001;15:309-23.
59. Owens DR, Zinman B, Bolli G. Alternative routes of insulin delivery. Diabet Med. 2003;20:886-98.
60. Owerbach D, Pina L, Gabbay KH. A 212-kb region on chromosome 6q25 containing the TAB2 gene is associated with susceptibility to type 1 diabetes. Diabetes. 2004;53:1890-3.
61. Pearson ER, Flechtner I, Njolstad PR, Malecki MT, Flanagan SE, Larkin B, et al. Switching from insulin to oral sulfonylureas in patients with diabetes due to Kir6.2 mutations. N Engl J Med. 2006;355:467-77.
62. Pickup J, Keen H. Continuous subcutaneous insulin infusion at 25 years: evidence base for the expanding use of insulin pump therapy in type 1 diabetes. Diabetes Care. 2002;25:593-8.
63. Pietropaolo M, Trucco M. Genetics of type 1 diabetes. In: Sperling MA (Ed). Type 1 diabetes. Totowa: Humana Press; 2003. pp. 55-70.
64. Porter JR, Barrett TG. Acquired non-type 1 diabetes in childhood: subtypes, diagnosis, and management. Archives of Disease in Childhood. 2004;89:1138-44.
65. Proks P, Arnold AL, Bruining J, Girard C, Flanagan SE, Larkin B, et al. A heterozygous activating mutation in the sulphonylurea receptor SUR1 (ABCC8) causes neonatal diabetes. Hum Mol Genet. 2006;15:1793-800.
66. Pugliese A. Genetics of type 1 diabetes. Endocrinol Metab Clin North Am. 2004;33:1-16.
67. Puliyel JM. Osmotonicity of acetoacetate: possible implications for cerebral edema in diabetic ketoacidosis. Med Sci Monit. 2003;9:BR130-3.
68. Rachmiel M, Perlman K, Daneman D. Insulin analogues in children and teens with type 1 diabetes: advantages and caveats. Pediatr Clin North Am. 2005;52:1651-75.

69. Renard E. Intensive insulin therapy today: 'basal-bolus' using multiple daily injections or CSII? Diabetes Metab. 2005;31: 4S40-44.
70. Report of the Expert Committee on the Diagnosis and Classification of diabetes mellitus. Diabetes Care. 1997;20: 1183-97.
71. Riccardi G, Giacco R, Parillo M, Turco S, Rivellese AA, Ventura MR, et al. Efficacy and safety of acarbose in the treatment of type 1 diabetes mellitus: a placebo-controlled, double-blind, multicentre study. Diabet Med. 1999;16:228-32.
72. Rissanen J, Markkanen A, Karkkainen P, Pihlajamaki J, Kekalainen P, Mykkanen L, et al. Sulfonylurea receptor 1 gene variants are associated with gestational diabetes and type 2 diabetes but not with altered secretion of insulin. Diabetes Care. 2000;23:70-3.
73. Roivainen M. Enteroviruses: new findings on the role of enteroviruses in type 1 diabetes. Int J Biochem Cell Biol. 2006; 38:721-5.
74. Romagnani S. The increased prevalence of allergy and the hygiene hypothesis: missing immune deviation, reduced immune suppression, or both? Immunology. 2004;112:352-63.
75. Rungby J, Brock B, Schmitz O. New strategies in insulin treatment: analogues and noninvasive routes of administration. Fundam Clin Pharmacol. 2005;19:127-32.
76. Ryan C, Gurtunca N, Becker D. Hypoglycemia: a complication of diabetes therapy in children. Pediatr Clin North Am. 2005; 52:1705-33.
77. Schmitz O, Brock B, Rungby J. Amylin agonists: a novel approach in the treatment of diabetes. Diabetes. 2004;53 (Suppl 3):S233-8.
78. Sieg A, Guy RH, Delgado-Charro MB. Noninvasive and minimally invasive methods for transdermal glucose monitoring. Diabetes Technol Ther. 2005;7:174-97.
79. Silverstein J, Klingensmith G, Copeland K, Plotnick L, Kaufman F, Laffel L, et al. Care of children and adolescents with type 1 diabetes: a statement of the American Diabetes Association. Diabetes Care. 2005;28:186-212.
80. Sperling MA. ATP-sensitive potassium channels–neonatal diabetes mellitus and beyond. N Engl J Med. 2006;355:507-10.
81. Sperling MA. Cerebral edema in diabetic ketoacidosis: an underestimated complication? Pediatr Diabetes. 2006;7: 73-4.
82. Sperling MA. Diabetes Mellitus. In: Sperling MA (Ed). Pediatric endocrinology, 2nd edn. Philadelphia: Saunders; 2002. pp. 323-66.
83. Sperling MA. Neonatal diabetes mellitus: from understudy to center stage. Curr Opin Pediatr. 2005;17:512-8.
84. Sperling MA. Neonatal diabetes. In: Menon RK, Sperling MA (Eds). Pediatric diabetes. Norwell: Kluwer acedemic publishers; 2003. pp. 215-25.
85. Stoffers DA, Zinkin NT, Stanojevic V, Clarke WL, Habener JF. Pancreatic agenesis attributable to a single nucleotide deletion in the human *IPF1* gene coding sequence. Nat Genet. 1997;15: 106-10.
86. Tamborlane WV, Fredrickson LP, Ahern JH. Insulin pump therapy in childhood diabetes mellitus: guidelines for use. Treat Endocrinol. 2003;2:11-21.
87. The effect of intensive treatment of diabetes on the development and progression of long-term complications in insulin-dependent diabetes mellitus. The Diabetes Control and Complications Trial Research Group. N Engl J Med. 1993; 329:977-86.
88. The writing team for the Diabetes Control and Complications Trial/Epidemiology of Diabetes Interventions and Complications Research Group. Sustained effect of intensive treatment of type 1 diabetes melllitus on development and progression of diabetic nephropathy. The epidemiology of diabetes intervention and comlications (EDIC) study. JAMA. 2003;290:2159-67.
89. Trajkovski M, Mziaut H, Schwarz PE, Solimena M. Genes of type 2 diabetes in beta cells. Endocrinol Metab Clin North Am. 2006;35:357-69.
90. Ueda H, Howson JM, Esposito L, Heward J, Snook H, Chamberlain G, et al. Association of the T-cell regulatory gene *CTLA4* with susceptibility to autoimmune disease. Nature 2003;423:506-11.
91. Urakami T, Morimoto S, Owada M, Harada K. Usefulness of the addition of metformin to insulin in pediatric patients with type 1 diabetes mellitus. Pediatr Int. 2005;47:430-3.
92. Velho G, Robert JJ. Maturity-onset diabetes of the young (MODY): genetic and clinical characteristics. Horm Res. 2002; 57(Suppl 1):29-33.
93. von Muhlendahl KE, Herkenhoff H. Long-term course of neonatal diabetes. N Engl J Med. 1995;333:704-8.
94. Weintrob N, Benzaquen H, Galatzer A, Shalitin S, Lazar L, Fayman G, et al. Comparison of continuous subcutaneous insulin infusion and multiple daily injection regimens in children with type 1 diabetes: a randomized open crossover trial. Pediatrics. 2003;112:559-64.
95. White NH. The DCCT and its implications for management of diabetes in children and adolescents. In: Menon RK (Ed). Pediatric diabetes. Norwell: Kluwer Acedemic Publisher; 2003. pp. 337-69.
96. Wilkin TJ. The accelerator hypothesis: weight gain as the missing link between type I and type II diabetes. Diabetologia. 2001;44:914-22.
97. Williams RM, Dunger DB. Insulin treatment in children and adolescents. Acta Paediatr. 2004;93:440-6.
98. Wolfsdorf J, Glaser N, Sperling MA. Diabetic ketoacidosis in infants, children, and adolescents: A consensus statement from the American Diabetes Association. Diabetes Care. 2006; 29:1150-9.
99. Wraight PR, Fourlanos S, Morahan G, Harrison LC. Genetics of type 1 diabetes mellitus. In: Menon RK, Sperling MA (Eds). Pediatrics diabetes. Norwell: Kluwer Academic Publishers; 2003. pp. 1-28.
100. Xiao XH, Liu ZL, Wang H, Sun Q, Li WH, Yang GH, et al. Effects of vitamin D receptor gene polymorphisms on susceptibility to type 1 diabetes mellitus. Chin Med Sci J. 2006;21:95-8.

CHAPTER 75

Pediatric Cardiac Emergencies: Evaluation and Management

Aditi Gupta, Munesh Tomar

INTRODUCTION

Cardiac emergencies in children can be either congenital or acquired. Congenital heart disease (CHD) is the major causes of morbidity and mortality. The prevalence of congenital cardiac diseases has been reported to be 8–10/1,000.[1] There are the two major acquired cardiac emergencies, rheumatic heart disease and acute myocarditis.[2,3] All pediatric cardiac emergencies require knowledge and good index of suspicion by the attending pediatrician for diagnosis and to institute an appropriate plan of therapy. Timely identification, management, and stabilization of these patients are important goals.

CARDIAC DISEASES PRESENTING AS EMERGENCY

Cardiac emergencies can be classified into two groups according to the age of presentation:
1. Those presenting in neonatal period
2. In later age group.

Both are further grouped into congenital and acquired causes.

Common causes are given in **Table 1**.

Most neonates with heart disease presenting in emergency have duct-dependent circulation either:[4]
- To ensure adequate mixing as in conditions with parallel nonmixing circulations like complete dextro-transposition of the great arteries (d-TGA)
- To maintain adequate pulmonary blood flow in lesions causing right ventricular outflow tract obstruction (RVOTO) or
- To maintain adequate systemic perfusion as in left ventricular outflow tract obstruction (left-sided LVOTO) or hypoplastic lesions.

These neonates require intervention (surgical or catheter) within the first weeks of life in order to sustain life or prevent major morbidity.

NEONATAL CARDIAC EMERGENCIES: AN OVERVIEW

Heart disease in newborn can have varied presentations. The diagnosis is usually not straightforward because of the nonspecific clinical picture of various congenital heart defects and difficult interpretation of electrocardiogram (ECG) and chest X-ray (CXR). Neonates with pulmonary symptoms unresponsive to standard therapies, indicates strong suspicion for CHD.

They are mainly classified into those who need an immediate intervention (catheter or surgical) and those who have a nonurgent disease and require medical management or close follow-up. In neonates, many patients show acute worsening on day 3–4 of life after discharge due to restriction or closure of ductus arteriosus which compromises the cardiac defects with duct-dependent circulation. Prostaglandin E1 (PGE1) infusions or emergency interventional cardiac catheterization are used as life-saving initial measures.

Presentation

Almost half of CHDs present in the neonatal period with an incidence reported to be around 3–3.5/1,000 live births.[5] The various presentations in the neonatal period include cyanosis, shock, congestive cardiac failure and rarely with arrhythmias.[6,7] As the diagnosis and pick up rate of CHD in antenatal period by level II antenatal fetal scan followed by detailed fetal echocardiography continues to be low because of lack of expertise and resources, majority of the neonates with critical CHD are detected for the first time after birth.

Table 1 Causes of cardiac emergency

	Congenital	Acquired

Neonatal	• Duct-dependent pulmonary blood flow
	   – Critical pulmonary stenosis or pulmonary atresia with ventricular septal defect (VSD) or with intact ventricular septum
	• Duct-dependent systemic blood flow
	   – Critical aortic stenosis
	   – Critical coarctation of aorta or arch interruption
	   – Hypoplastic left heart syndrome
	• Admixture lesion with restrictive interatrial communication
	   – Transposition of great vessels
	   – Total anomalous pulmonary venous connection (TAPVC)
	• Obstructed TAPVC
	• Anomalous origin of the left coronary artery from the pulmonary artery (ALCAPA)
	• Ventricular dysfunction due to inborn error of metabolism, e.g. glycogen storage defects, fatty acid oxidation defects, and mitochondriopathies
		Ventricular dysfunction due to:
		• Sepsis
		• Metabolic and electrolyte imbalance (metabolic acidosis, and hypocalcemia)
		• Hypothermia

Older children	• Severe obstructive lesions (left side or right-sided) with ventricular dysfunction, e.g. severe aortic stenosis, severe pulmonary stenosis, and severe coarctation • Shunt lesions decompensated by infection or arrhythmia • Anomalous origin of the left coronary artery from the pulmonary artery	• Rheumatic heart disease leading to severe valve regurgitation (mitral, aortic and/or tricuspid) or severe stenosis, e.g. mitral stenosis • Bacterial endocarditis • Kawasaki disease
All age groups	• Arrhythmias	• Arrhythmias • Dilated cardiomyopathy • Pericardial tamponade

Neonates with congenital heart defects usually present to the emergency with:
- Cyanosis
- Shock
- Acute congestive heart failure (CHF)
- Tachyarrhythmias or bradyarrhythmias.

Cyanosis

Case scenario: A 2-day-old neonate, born at full-term gestation via normal vaginal delivery was detected to have respiratory distress in the postnatal ward. The baby was referred to tertiary center for further management where at presentation, the baby was found to be lethargic, in distress and had central cyanosis. On auscultation no significant murmur could be appreciated. His arterial blood gas showed severe hypoxemia with metabolic acidosis.

Chest X-ray had mild cardiomegaly with increased pulmonary vascular markings **(Fig. 1)**. Respiratory and cardiac pathologies are the main differential diagnosis with such presentations and it is very important to distinguish between respiratory and cardiac causes of cyanosis so that the management can be done accordingly **(Table 2)**.

Hyperoxia test[5] differentiate cardiac from pulmonary causes of cyanosis. Arterial oxygen tension is measured in the right radial artery (preductal) while the patient on 100%

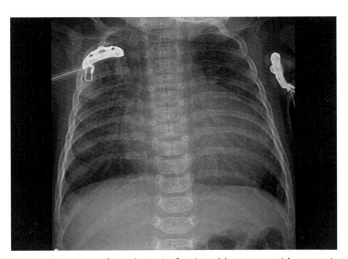

Fig. 1 Chest X-ray (frontal view) of 3-day-old neonate with cyanosis showing cardiomegaly, increased pulmonary blood flow with narrow mediastinum (egg on side appearance)

oxygen for 10 minutes. Oxygen is administered via hood[8] or endotracheal tube if the patient is already intubated.

The preductal oxygen tension while breathing 100% oxygen concentration rarely exceeds 150 mm Hg in cyanotic heart disease and usually exceeds this value in pulmonary

Table 2 Differentiation between cardiac and respiratory causes of cyanosis

	Respiratory	Cardiac
History	History of meconium aspiration, prematurity, and risk factors for sepsis	Diabetic mother, history of previous child affected with CHD
Examination	Respiratory distress, grunting cyanosis, and tachypnea	Cyanosis disproportionate to respiratory distress
Onset	Usually at birth or within hours of birth	Hours or days after birth
Auscultation	Altered air entry, lung crepts or wheeze	Clear lungs, normal air entry, murmur may or may not be present
Blood gas	High pCO_2, and low pO_2	Normal or low pCO_2, and low pO_2
Hyperoxia test	Passed	Failed
Chest X-ray	Lung infiltrates, and normal heart size	Clear lung fields, heart ± enlarged, oligemic or plethoric lung fields
ECG	Normal	May be abnormal

Abbreviations: CHD, congenital heart disease; ECG, electrocardiogram; pCO_2, partial pressure of carbon dioxide; pO_2, partial pressure of oxygen.

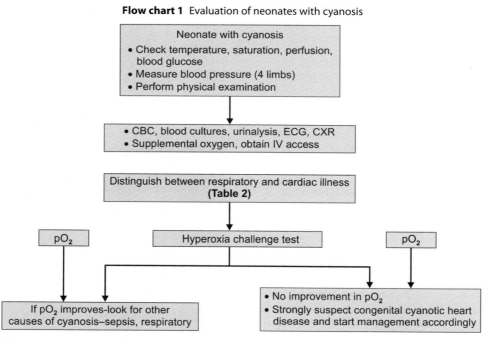

Flow chart 1 Evaluation of neonates with cyanosis

Abbreviations: CBC, complete blood count; CXR, chest X-ray; ECG, electrocardiogram; IV, intravenous; pO_2, partial pressure of oxygen.

disease. In case of failed hyperoxia test, an echocardiogram is needed to establish the underlying diagnosis.

A pulse oximeter should *not* be used for the hyperoxia test because it may not detect an inadequate increase in oxygen tension. Because of the characteristics of the oxygen dissociation curve, normal hemoglobin is fully saturated with oxygen when the arterial partial pressure of oxygen (pO_2) exceeds 70 mm Hg. Therefore, a patient receiving 100% inspired oxygen concentration may have an oxygen saturation of nearly 100% associated with an arterial pO_2 of 75 mm Hg, a value that is abnormal. Thus, discrimination between cardiac lesion and pulmonary disease may be limited **(Flow chart 1)**.

It is useful to remember the most common CHDs that present with neonatal cyanosis include:
- Complete transposition of great arteries
- Tetralogy of Fallot (TOF) [with critical pulmonary stenosis (PS) or pulmonary atresia]

- Obstructive total anomalous pulmonary venous connection
- Single ventricle with critical PS or pulmonary atresia
- Tricuspid atresia with critical PS or pulmonary atresia
- Critical PS or pulmonary atresia with intact interventricular septum.

Management: The definitive diagnosis is readily established by detailed echocardiography.
- Prostaglandin E1 (PGE1) (alprostadil) intravenous (IV) infusion to keep the patent ductus arteriosus (PDA) open (dose 10–60 ng/kg/min, if poor response saturations and acidosis not improving) the dose can be increased to maximum 300–400 ng/kg/min.[9] Apnea is a common side effect of PGE1 so infusion should be started in intensive care unit (ICU) settings with ventilator support available. Flushing, diarrhea, and hypotension are other common side effects
- Intravenous fluid for blood volume expansion 10 mL/kg 0.9% saline bolus, improve preload repeat until liver edge is palpable—enhance further opening of the PDA and pulmonary blood flow through the duct
- Correction of metabolic abnormalities, e.g. hypoglycemia, hypocalcemia, acidosis, and sepsis
- Oxygen to maintain the saturations 75–85% (do not give 100% oxygen by mask in patients with duct-dependent lesions as high level of oxygen triggers closure of ductus arteriosus)
- Inotropes or vasopressors required to maintain adequate systemic perfusion
- If earlier measures are not helpful, intubation and ventilation with adequate sedation required to improve oxygenation and minimize the metabolic demands.

Definitive management includes:
- *Transposition of great vessels*: Arterial switch operation
- *Total anomalous pulmonary venous connection*: Surgical rerouting of pulmonary veins
- *Severe valvular pulmonary stenosis*: Balloon valvotomy.[10]
- Ductal stenting or Blalock-Taussig (BT) shunt for duct-dependent pulmonary circulation.

Shock or Cardiovascular Collapse

Case scenario: A 6-day-old term neonate presented in medical emergency with complaints of lethargy, increased respiratory rates and refusal to feed. The baby was mottled in color with poor peripheral perfusion. While the central pulses were palpable, the lower limb pulses were feeble.

Chest X-ray revealed cardiomegaly with prominent pulmonary vascular markings **(Fig. 2)**.

On echocardiography, the baby was diagnosed to have interrupted aortic arch and restrictive PDA which was supplying descending aorta. Baby also had severe left ventricular (LV) dysfunction with ejection fraction (EF) 15–20% **(Fig. 3)**. Further restriction and impending closure

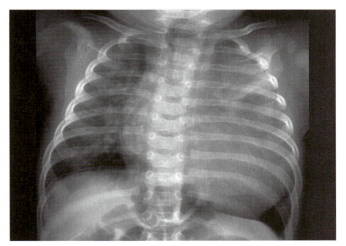

Fig. 2 Chest X-ray (frontal view) of a neonate presenting in emergency with shock. X-ray reveals cardiomegaly, prominent vascular markings with retrocardiac lung collapse

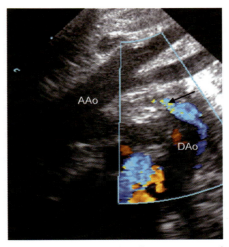

Fig. 3 Echocardiography with color flow mapping of a neonate with aortic arch interruption, restrictive PDA and LV dysfunction. Suprasternal long axis view showing arch interruption, small PDA (arrow) filling descending aorta
Abbreviations: LV, left ventricular; PDA, patent ductus arteriosus; AAo, ascending aorta; DAo, descending aorta

of the ductus on day 5–6 of life had led to acute loss of lower body perfusion causing shock and severe metabolic acidosis.

Patients with this presentation are grouped under lesions with duct-dependent systemic circulation. These babies can present directly with cardiovascular collapse after ductal closure and are therefore often critically ill at presentation.

It is very important to have a high index of suspicion for CHD in neonates presenting with shock as most commonly it is mistakenly diagnosed and managed as neonatal sepsis. While babies with sepsis are medically managed those with duct-

dependent systemic circulation need aggressive resuscitation and prompt intervention usually.

Lesions presenting with duct-dependent systemic circulation include the critical left-sided outflow tract obstructions:
- Critical aortic stenosis (AS)
- Hypoplastic left heart syndrome (HLHS)
- Severe coarctation of aorta and
- Interrupted aortic arch.

Management:
- Prostaglandin therapy
- Blood volume expansion
- Stabilization with inotropes and oxygen and mechanical ventilation in unresponsive cases
- Confirmation of diagnosis by echocardiography followed by relief of obstruction by surgical correction.

Acute Congestive Heart Failure

Case scenario: A 3-week-old neonate presented with tachypnea, tachycardia, and refusal to feed for 3 days. There was hepatomegaly and cardiomegaly on examination. Auscultation revealed gallop rhythm, no significant murmur. CXR frontal view showed cardiomegaly, no parenchymal lesion. 12-lead ECG showed sinus tachycardia, deep Q-wave in I, aVL, V5, V6 with ST-T wave changes **(Fig. 4)**.

Echocardiography revealed severe LV dysfunction with EF 15–20%. On echocardiography left coronary was seen arising anomalously from pulmonary artery and baby was diagnosed to have anomalous origin of the left coronary artery from the pulmonary artery (ALCAPA). The baby underwent successful surgical correction of ALCAPA with slow but complete recovery of ventricular function in postoperative period.

In ALCAPA, the babies usually present with features of CHF due to myocardial ischemia leading to LV dilation and dysfunction. The presentation can be delayed up to 3–4 weeks of age till the pulmonary vascular pressures falls substantially.

Babies with CHF usually present with feeding difficulties and excessive sweating. They are tachypneic and tachycardiac at rest and can have wheeze due to LV failure. Gallop rhythm, hepatomegaly, and cardiomegaly are other important signs.[4]

Cold extremity and low blood pressure are signs of low pulse volume and indicate CHF. However bounding pulses may be present in CHF due to lesions causing aortic runoff like PDA and arteriovenous malformations.

Thoracic roentgenogram is especially useful in evaluation of neonates. Cardiac enlargement is always present if CHF exists, in addition, pulmonary pathologies can also be detected.[10]

It is important to differentiate neonatal CHF from respiratory distress due to lung disease and neonatal sepsis clinically. This differentiation is difficult due to overlapping signs such as rales and rhonchi. The most important signs for diagnosing heart failure are cardiomegaly and hepatomegaly.

Structural causes of CHF in neonatal period include:
- Large left to right shunts:
  - Large ventricular septal defect (VSD) or multiple VSDs
  - Complete atrioventricular (AV) canal defect with AV regurgitation
  - Large PDA (especially in preterm baby)
  - Aortopulmonary window
  - *Arteriovenous malformations*: Vein of Galen malformation
- Heart failure with mild cyanosis (admixture lesions):
  - Total anomalous pulmonary venous connection
  - Truncus arteriosus
  - Single ventricle physiology without PS
- *Ventricular dysfunction*: Coronary anomaly–ALCAPA.

Management:
- Oxygen therapy is very useful in babies with CHF with pulmonary edema as the cause of hypoxia. Oxygen raises the alveolar pO_2 and helps to alleviate hypoxia
- General neonatal care which includes maintenance of temperature and glucose levels
- Nasogastric feeding is preferred over oral feed to avoid aspiration in the distressed infant and also to increase the amount of caloric intake.[4]
- Diuretics, usually furosemide 1–4 mg/kg 8–12-hourly IV (bolus or continuous infusion) or orally with spironolactone 1 mg/kg 12-hourly to decrease pulmonary congestion
- Correction of coexistent metabolic derangements like anemia, hypoglycemia, electrolyte imbalance, and acidosis
- Inotropes or vasodilators such as low-dose dobutamine, dopamine, milrinone to decrease systemic vascular resistance and improve cardiac contractility
- Mechanical ventilation is usually required in heart failure with impending cardiogenic shock.

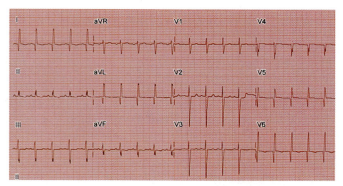

Fig. 4 12-lead ECG of an infant with ALCAPA. Deep Q-waves in leads I, aVL, V5, and V6 and T wave inversion seen in lead I
Abbreviations: ALCAPA, anomalous origin of the left coronary artery from the pulmonary artery; ECG, electrocardiogram

PEDIATRIC CARDIAC EMERGENCIES

The various presentations of pediatric cardiac emergencies include:
- Congestive heart failure
- Cyanotic spell
- Pericardial tamponade
- Arrhythmia or palpitations
- Sudden death.

Among the various presentations CHF and cyanotic spell attributes to 70–80% of pediatric cardiac emergencies. In neonates while structural diseases of the heart are the most common causes of CHF, in older children acquired causes are also attributed. Fluid restriction and inotropic support followed by definitive correction of the established cause is the mainstay of treatment.

Cyanotic CHD like tetralogy of Fallot and pulmonary atresia present with cyanotic spells. They usually occur in the morning and can be provoked by stress, crying, or periods of dehydration. Their presentation can vary from minor spells to seizure to severe life-threatening episodes.

Isolated arrhythmias though relatively less common can present with palpitations or hemodynamic instability in infants and children. Supraventricular tachycardia is the most common presentation in the pediatric population.

Early recognition and appropriate therapy in pediatric cardiac emergencies are essential for better outcomes.

Congestive Heart Failure

Case Scenario

An 8-year-old boy presented to the medical emergency department with complaints of respiratory distress. Patient had history of breathlessness on exertion and orthopnea since months. Patient had past history of swelling in left knee followed by swelling of left ankle 2 months ago.

He had tachycardia, cardiomegaly, and a loud apical pansystolic murmur with radiation to axilla. He also had hepatomegaly with liver 5 cm below costal margin. CXR showed cardiomegaly with straightening of left heart border (left atrial enlargement), LV type of apex and signs of pulmonary venous hypertension **(Fig. 5)**.

Echocardiography revealed rheumatic involvement of mitral valve with thickened leaflets and ruptured chordae leading to severe mitral regurgitation (MR).

Congestive heart failure is common presentation for congenital and acquired heart diseases. Volume or pressure overload on normal myocardium, arrhythmias, pericardial diseases, and combination of metabolic factors can result in CHF.

Congenital cardiac defects most commonly associated with CHF in pediatric age group are:
- Large VSDs
- Complete AV canal defects

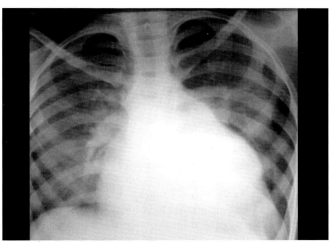

Fig. 5 Chest X-ray frontal view of a 8-year-old child with rheumatic heart disease, severe mitral regurgitation. There is cardiomegaly with pulmonary venous hypertension. Features of left atrial (LA) dilatation, i.e. straightening of left heart border and widening of carinal angle are seen

- Persistent PDA
- Aortopulmonary window
- Truncus arteriosus
- Unobstructed total anomalous pulmonary venous return
- Critical left or right ventricular outflow obstruction with ventricular dysfunction.

Acquired causes of pediatric CHF include:
- Rheumatic heart disease
- *Cardiomyopathy*: Dilated, restrictive or obstructive
- Arrhythmias
- Pericardial tamponade.

Heart failure secondary to CHD is a gradual process while heart failure due to secondary acquired causes is acute process.

Clinical Features

Common manifestations of CHF in the infant in the approximate order of frequency include tachypnea, tachycardia, liver enlargement, cardiomegaly, pulmonary rales and rhonchi, and feeding difficulties. Less common signs and symptoms include peripheral edema, measurable elevated systemic venous pressure, inappropriate diaphoresis at normal room temperature, gallop rhythm, pulsus alternans, and ascites.

Management

- Treatment of the precipitating factors like infective endocarditis, intercurrent infections, anemia, electrolyte imbalances, arrhythmia, pulmonary embolism, and drug toxicity

- Treatment of the congested state includes:
  - Nonpharmacological measures, e.g. modest fluid restriction, propped up posture, supplemental humidified oxygen if desaturated, and optimization of nutrition
  - If the patient is restless or dyspneic, sedatives are used. Morphine sulphate in doses of 0.05 mg/kg subcutaneous (SC) provides effective sedation
  - Diuretics, usually furosemide 1–4 mg/kg 6–12-hourly IV or orally, provide quick relief in systemic and pulmonary venous congestion.[11,12] If child is having grossly edematous or in pulmonary edema, IV infusion of furosemide (0.1–0.4 mg/kg/hour) should be given. After stabilization, shift to bolus doses of furosemide
  - Secondary hyperaldosteronism does occur in infants with CHF and addition of spironolactone 1 mg/kg single dose to other diuretics conserves potassium
  - *Inotropes*: Dopamine, dobutamine, milrinone, and levosimendan.
  - Vasodilators, e.g. angiotensin-converting enzyme (ACE) inhibitors, are useful in the presence of hypertension, mitral or aortic regurgitation. ACE inhibitors are useful in patients with large shunts or in those with an elevated systemic vascular resistance. These drugs contraindicated in patients with obstructive lesions as aortic or mitral stenosis. Enalapril is most commonly used ACE inhibitor in pediatric age group. It is important to ensure normal renal function and potassium (K^+) during therapy
  - Augmenting myocardial contractility by inotropic drugs like digitalis improves cardiac output. Digitalis decreases heart rate and increases myocardial contractility.[13] Oral digoxin is available in 0.25 mg tablets and as digoxin elixir (1 mL contains 0.05 mg)

    The role of digoxin in shunt lesions is controversial. Our policy is to start digoxin in maintenance dose only in large shunt lesions with undue tachycardia. As safety margin of digoxin is very low, the patient should be observed for signs of digitalis toxicity **(Fig. 6)**.
  - *Beta-blocker therapy*: Patients with dilated cardiomyopathy may respond to beta-blockers. Carvedilol is well tolerated in infants with dilated cardiomyopathy and there is significant improvement in their functional status
  - *Electrolyte correction*: In dilated cardiomyopathy, always rule out hypocalcemia and vitamin D deficiency as a cause of dilated cardiomyopathy
  - Treat underlying pathology:
    - *Corrective surgery for structural defect*: The curative therapy is directed toward the cause of CHF, wherever possible, e.g. surgical correction of congenital or acquired heart defects

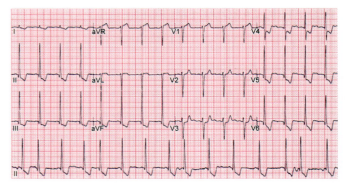

Fig. 6 12-lead electrocardiogram (ECG) of an infant taking high dose of digoxin by mistake. ECG shows digitalis effect, i.e. prolongation of PR interval with sagging of ST segment

  - *Precipitating factors:*
    - Hypertension as cause of dilated cardiomyopathy should always be rule out as it needs aggressive treatment of hypertension and also of cause of hypertension (kidney, endocrinal, drug induced, and Takayasu arteritis)
    - Hypocalcemia secondary to vitamin D deficiency, and hypoparathyroidism
    - Anemia
    - Hyper- or hypothyroidism
    - Beriberi.

Cyanotic Spell

Cyanotic spell is a clinical state of acutely reduced pulmonary blood flow which leads to severe hypoxemia and metabolic acidosis. During the spell the infant becomes hyperpneic and restless. As cyanosis increases, syncope, convulsions or cerebrovascular accidents can develop.[1] Hypoxic spells are a particular problem during the 2nd to 6th month of life. The spells can occur after episodes of stress like vigorous crying and dehydration. They can even occur without a precipitating cause.

Structural anomalies presenting with cyanotic spell are:
- Most common anomaly is TOF
- Double outlet right ventricle with PS
- Tricuspid atresia with PS
- Transposition of great vessels with VSD and PS
- Single ventricle physiology with PS or pulmonary atresia.

Management

Cyanotic spell can be managed by:
- Keep the child calm and quite and to avoid any painful procedures
- Sedation in the form of morphine [0.1–0.2 mg/kg intramuscular (IM)/IV/SC] or ketamine (1–2 mg/kg IV) can be given and repeated as necessary

Table 3 Differentiation between pneumothorax, hemothorax and cardiac tamponade

	Tension pneumothorax	Cardiac tamponade	Hemothorax
Breath sounds	Ipsilaterally decreased	Normal	Ipsilaterally decreased
Percussion note	Hyperresonant	Normal	Dull
Tracheal position	Shifted contralaterally	Midline	Midline or shifted
Neck veins	Distended	Distended	Flat
Heart sounds	Normal	Muffled	Normal

- The infant should be placed in the knee-chest position
- Blood volume expansion with crystalloids like initial IV saline bolus at the rate of 10 mL/kg which can be repeated as per the hydration status until the liver is palpable
- Sodium bicarbonate 1–2 mmol/kg IV which can be repeated according to blood gas

    Metabolic acidosis usually develops when arterial pO_2 falls below 40 mm Hg, rapid correction with IV sodium bicarbonate is especially necessary if the spell is unusually severe and the child shows a lack of response to the ongoing therapy. Once the pH has returned to normal recovery from the spell is usually rapid.
- *Phenylephrine hydrochloride IM (increases systemic vascular resistance)*: 0.01 mg/kg IV slowly or 0.1 mg/kg SC, the dose has to be titrated according to the blood pressure (BP) response
- *Beta-blocker*: Injection metoprolol, 0.1 mg/kg over 5 min, can be repeated every 5 minutes to maximum of three doses, infusion can be given at dose of 1–5 µg/kg/min. Patient can be shifted to oral beta-blocker preferably propranolol once the patient stabilizes
- In refractory cases when there is no response to any of these measures intubation with ventilation and urgent transfer to a tertiary facility where facilities of emergent surgical systemic-to-pulmonary shunt (BT shunt) or definitive corrective procedure are available should be done.

Response of treatment can be assessed in the form of increasing intensity of the ejection systolic murmur and rising oxygen saturations both the signs being reassuring.

Pericardial Tamponade

Cardiac tamponade is one of the life-threatening emergencies which is caused due to slow or rapid accumulation of pericardial fluid, pus, blood which causes compression of the heart and increases the intrapericardial pressure.

Presentation

Chest pain, impalpable apex beat, muffled heart sounds on auscultation, pericardial friction rub or occasionally a "pericardial knock" are the common clinical features, rapid fluid accumulation leads to cardiac tamponade and present as cardiogenic shock. Hypotension, diminished heart sounds, and venous hypertension are three classic findings in cardiac tamponade (Beck's triad).

It is important to distinguish cardiac tamponade from pneumothorax and hemothorax which are also common emergencies and can have similar presentations **(Table 3)**.

Straightening of the left heart border on chest radiograph is a useful finding. A progressively enlarging globular heart also is a reliable indicator of pericardial effusion, but this is characteristically a late finding **(Fig. 7)**. Echocardiography is diagnostic modality of choice for diagnosing and evaluating a pericardial effusion **(Figs 8 and 9)**.

Diastolic collapse of atria and ventricles are considered pathognomonic for cardiac tamponade on echocardiography.

Management

Management includes:
- Urgent decompression of the pericardial space is mandatory and lifesaving if signs of cardiac tamponade are present
- Blood volume expansion with 20 mL/kg crystalloid IV bolus, repeated as necessary.

Arrhythmias

Arrhythmias though relatively rare, are not very uncommon in neonatal and pediatric age-group. They are broadly classified as tachyarrhythmias and bradyarrhythmias. Rhythm disturbances cause hemodynamic compromise in children due to rate abnormalities or loss of synchrony. The most common conditions predisposing to arrhythmias in children are CHD and postoperative cardiac surgery. An appreciation of normal variation and disturbances in pediatric ECG with age and maturation is essential for interpretation of pediatric rhythm disturbances **(Table 4)**.[14]

Tachyarrhythmias

An electrocardiography is essential for critical evaluation of tachycardia.

They are suspected when:
- The heart rate greater than 180/min in children and greater than 220/min in infants and is usually fixed

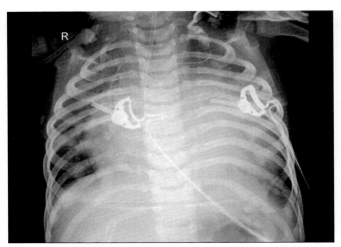

Fig. 7 Chest X-ray (frontal view) showing cardiomegaly with globular heart shadow in a child with large pericardial effusion

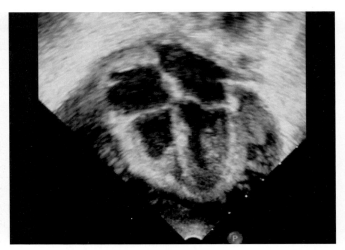

Fig. 9 Echocardiography of a 1 year old child presenting with fever for 1 month and respiratory distress. Apical four-chamber view showing large pericardial effusion all around with multiple strands. On pericardial tap, purulent fluid was drained

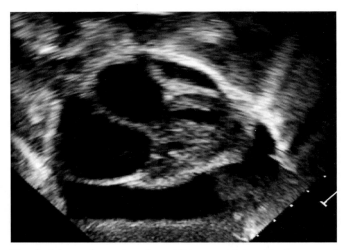

Fig. 8 Echocardiography of a child presenting with features of cardiac failure in emergency. Subcostal coronal view showing large pericardial effusion. On pericardial tap, serous fluid was drained and was of tubercular etiology

between 250–280/min and shows no variability
- Atrioventricular dissociation
- Abnormal P wave axis.

Classification: Tachyarrhythmia is classified into:
- Narrow QRS complex (<90 msec) tachycardias
- Wide QRS complex (>90 msec) tachycardias.

Narrow complex tachycardias: Are due to:
- Atrioventricular re-entrant tachycardia via an accessory pathway [supraventricular tachycardia (SVT)] **(Fig. 10)**
- Nodal or junctional ectopic tachycardia
- Ectopic and multifocal atrial tachycardias
- Atrial flutter **(Fig. 11)**.

Wide complex tachycardia: Wide complex tachycardia in children is ventricular tachycardia (VT) until proven otherwise. So, all monomorphic wide complex tachycardias should be treated as VT without delay, especially if hemodynamically unstable **(Fig. 12)**.

Clinical presentation: Wide range of clinical presentation, asymptomatic to cardiogenic shock and even sudden cardiac death (SCD).

Palpitations are the usual presenting symptom in older children with paroxysmal tachycardia, but other nonspecific symptoms such as light-headedness, syncope, chest pain, pallor or nausea may occur. Tachycardia may go unrecognized for many hours and significant hemodynamic compromise may result. If the duration of the tachycardia exceeds 6–12 hours, symptoms and signs of heart failure (HF) may become apparent.[15]

Management:
- 12-lead ECG recording with a rhythm strip
- Reversible causes of arrhythmias should be identified and treated, e.g. 5 H's and 5 T's [that includes hypoxemia, hypovolemia, hypo- or hyperthermia, hyper- or hypokalemia, acidosis and tamponade (cardiac), tension pneumothorax, toxins, e.g. digoxin, beta-blockers, calcium channel blockers and thrombosis (coronary and pulmonary)].

Narrow complex tachycardia:
- *Atrial flutter*: Adenosine is usually not effective. The treatment of choice is synchronized DC cardioversion, as little as 0.5 J/kg is often enough to cardiovert to sinus rhythm. Pediatric paddles should be used with electrode

Table 4 Heart rates and PR and QRS intervals according to age[14]

Age	Heart rate/minute	PR interval	QRS intervals
0–1 days	94–155 (122)	0.08–0.16 (0.107)	0.02–0.07 (0.05)
1–3 days	91–158 (122)	0.08–0.14 (0.108)	0.02–0.07 (0.05)
3–7 days	90–166 (128)	0.07–0.15 (0.102)	0.02–0.07 (0.05)
7–30 days	96–182 (149)	0.07–0.14 (0.100)	0.02–0.08 (0.05)
1–3 months	120–179 (149)	0.07–0.13 (0.098)	0.02–0.08 (0.05)
3–6 months	105–185 (141)	0.07–0.15 (0.105)	0.02–0.08 (0.05)
6–12 months	108–169 (131)	0.07–0.16 (0.106)	0.03–0.08 (0.05)
1–3 years	89–152 (119)	0.08–0.15 (0.113)	0.03–0.08 (0.06)
3–5 years	73–137 (109)	0.08–0.16 (0.119)	0.03–0.07 (0.06)
5–8 years	65–133 (100)	0.09–0.16 (0.123)	0.03–0.08 (0.06)
8–12 years	62–130 (91)	0.09–0.17 (0.128)	0.04–0.09 (0.06)
12–16 years	60–120 (80)	0.09–0.18 (0.135)	0.04–0.09 (0.07)

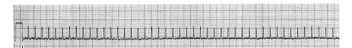

Fig. 10 Supraventricular tachycardia. Heart rate (HR) 270/min with narrow QRS complexes and P waves not seen

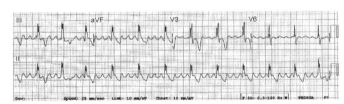

Fig. 11 Atrial flutter: Ventricular rate 75/min with 3:1 atrioventricular (AV) conduction. Saw tooth pattern P waves seen

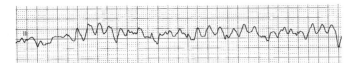

Fig. 12 Torsades de pointes with prolonged QT interval and changing ventricular rate in a child with long QT syndrome (Jervell and Lange-Nielsen syndrome)

jelly and should be correctly applied. Children should be sedated for the comfort

- *Atrioventricular reentry tachycardia*: In hemodynamically stable children, vagal maneuvers should be attempted and if there is no response, adenosine 100 µg/kg should be given as rapid IV bolus increasing by 100 µg/kg every 2 minutes up to a maximum of 500 µg/kg (300 µg/kg for neonates) or 12 mg total dose. In hemodynamically unstable children **(Fig. 13)** synchronized DC cardioversion is the first-line therapy

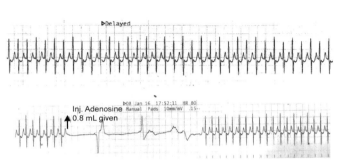

Fig. 13 Supraventricular tachycardia being treated with injected adenosine with only transient response

- Wide complex tachycardia (probable VT) should be treated with immediate synchronized DC cardioversion 1 J/kg increasing to 2 J/kg if no response in hemodynamically unstable patients
- In stable patients consider amiodarone 5 mg/kg IV over 20–30 min, if medical therapy is unsuccessful synchronized cardioversion should be attempted.

Bradyarrhythmias

The three main causes of bradyarrhythmias include (1) sinoatrial (SA) node dysfunction, (2) second-degree AV block, and (3) complete AV block.

Sinus bradycardia: The most common cause of bradycardia is hypoxemia, which is an ominous sign and should be managed aggressively. Other causes include hypothermia, hypothyroidism, raised intracranial pressure and drug intoxication.

The diagnosis of sinus bradycardia is easily made by establishing the 1:1 relationship between P waves and QRS complexes on the surface ECG. An upright P wave in leads

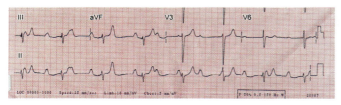

Fig. 14 Complete heart block with no relation between P waves and QRS waves with slow ventricular rate of 50/min

I, II and aVL, and a negative P wave in lead aVR, indicates a sinus origin of the bradycardia. It is vital to exclude other causes of bradyarrhythmias such as AV block.

The main cause of bradycardia in children presenting as cardiac emergency is complete heart block (CHB) **(Fig. 14)**, which is either congenital or acquired.

Clinical presentation: Dizziness or syncope are distressing symptoms occur at a heart rate below 40–45/min may present as cardiogenic shock or SCD.

It may present as HF in congenital heart block.

Management:
- In symptomatic bradycardias drugs used include atropine given at a dose of 20 µg/kg as bolus (minimum dose 100 µg, maximum 600 µg), adrenalin (10 µg/kg bolus) followed by infusions or isoprenaline infusion
- Crystalloid bolus of 10–20 mL/kg IV is given if the patient is hypotensive or in shock
- Patient should be referred to a tertiary care center where expertise for pacing is available and temporary pacing should be promptly instituted
- In refractory cases the definitive treatment is insertion of permanent pacemaker which can be endocardial or epicardial in position.

Common indications of permanent pacemaker include:
- Symptomatic bradycardia with second- or third-degree AV block
- Sinoatrial node dysfunction
- Postoperative advanced second- or third-degree AV block
- Congenital third-degree AV block in an infant with a heart rate lower than 50–55 beats/min
- Congenital third-degree AV block with a wide QRS escape rhythm, complex ventricular ectopy, or ventricular dysfunction.

In the postoperative patients, it is reasonable to observe for a period of 7–10 days to allow sufficient time for AV node recovery before considering permanent pacemaker implantation.

COMMONLY USED DRUGS IN CARDIAC EMERGENCIES

- *Prostaglandin E1 (Alprostadil)*: 60 µg/kg in 50 mL 0.9% saline 0.5–3 mL/hr (starting dose 10–60 ng/kg/min), if poor response (saturations and acidosis not improving) the dose can be increased to maximum 100–200 ng/kg/min
- *Diuretics*:
  - *Furosemide*: 0.5–1 mg/kg (adult 20–40 mg) 6–24 hr oral, IM or IV over 20 minutes. IV infusion 0.1–0.4 mg/kg/hr
  - *Spironolactone*: 1–3 mg/kg 6–12 hourly orally
- *Angiotensin-converting enzyme inhibitor*: *Enalapril*: Test dose 0.05 mg/kg (adult 2.5 mg) oral with BP monitoring, increase over 2 weeks if required to maximum 0.5 mg/kg (adult 5–20 mg) twice daily orally
- *Beta-blockers*:
  - *Propranolol*: 0.2–0.5 mg/kg (adult 10–25 mg) 6–12 hr oral, increase to maximum 1.5 mg/kg (maximum 80 mg) 6–12 hr if required. IV 0.02 mg/kg (adult 1mg) test dose then 0.1 mg/kg (adult 5 mg) over 10 mins
  - *Metoprolol*: Intravenous 0.1 mg/kg (adult 5 mg) over 5 mins, repeat every 5 mins to maximum 3 doses, then 1–5 µg/kg/min. Oral 1–2 mg/kg (adult 50–100 mg) 6–12 hr
  - *Esmolol*: 0.5 mg/kg (500 µg/kg) IV over 1 min, repeated if required. Infusion 25–300 µg/kg/min (undiluted 10 mg/mL solution) rarely given for greater than 48 hrs
  - *Carvedilol*: 0.1 mg/kg (adult 3.125 mg) 12 hr oral, if tolerated increase by 0.1 mg/kg (adult 3.125 mg) every 1–2 weeks to maximum 0.5–0.8 mg/kg (adult 25 mg) 12 hr
- *Inotropes*:
  - *Dopamine*: 5–20 µg/kg/minute IV infusion. Central line preferred
  - *Dobutamine*: 5–20 µg/kg/minute IV infusion. Central line preferred
  - *Milrinone*: 50 µg/kg IV bolus over 10 minutes, 0.3–0.8 µg/kg/minute IV infusion
  - *Levosimendan*: Start with a bolus dose of 12–24 µg/kg IV over 10 min followed by 0.1 µg/kg/min IV infusion. Increase the dose slowly to 0.2 µg/kg/min and usually the total duration of the infusion was 24–48 hrs. The bolus dose may be omitted in unstable hypotensive patients.
- *Digoxin*: For digoxin, see **Table 5**.

CONCLUSION

- There are a number of congenital and acquired heart diseases in neonates, infants and children that may present as life-threatening emergencies
- These may be undiagnosed and present for the first time as emergencies, or they may present with complications in a child with a known diagnosis
- Entertaining the possibility of a cardiac problem in neonates with pulmonary symptoms unresponsive to standard therapies is crucial for successful management of patients with CHD. In addition to ventilatory support, PGE1 infusions or emergency interventional cardiac

Table 5 Digoxin: Digitalizing dose and maintenance dose

Digoxin	Digitalizing dose (mg/kg)	Maintenance dose (fraction digitalizing dose)
Premature, neonates	0.04	1/4th
1 month–1 year	0.08	1/3rd–1/4th
1–3 years	0.06	1/3rd–1/4th
Above 3 years	0.04	1/3rd

catheterization is often a lifesaving initial measure in patients with acutely decompensated congenital cardiac lesions that require a PDA for survival
- Every health practitioner caring for children should be aware of the common diagnoses, expected complications and their immediate management
- The most commonly encountered emergencies are cyanosis or hypercyanotic spells, acute CHF, cardiogenic shock, tachyarrhythmias or bradyarrhythmias and pericardial effusion or cardiac tamponade
- The emphasis should be on early recognition of hemodynamic derangements and immediate appropriate intervention in order to prevent death and significant morbidity
- Early consultation with a pediatric cardiologist is desirable especially if there is doubt as to the diagnosis or poor response to initial treatment
- Once a child is stabilized, prompt referral to a tertiary pediatric cardiac center is usually required for definitive diagnosis and management.

REFERENCES

1. Van Roekens CN, Zuckerberg AL. Emergency management of hypercyanotic crises in tetralogy of Fallot. Ann Emerg Med. 1995;25(2):256-8.
2. Iyer PU. Management Issues in Intensive Care Units for Infants and Children with Heart Disease. Indian J Pediatr. 2015;82(12):1164-71.
3. Manole MD, Saladino RA. Emergency department management of the pediatric patient with supraventricular tachycardia. Pediatr Emerg Care. 2007;23(3):176-85.
4. Zahka KG, Gruenstein DH. Approach to the neonate with cardiovascular disease. In: Martin RJ, Fanaroff AA, Walsh MC (Eds). Fanaroff and Martin's Neonatal-Perinatal Medicine Diseases of the Fetus and Infant, 8th edition. Philadelphia: Elsevier Mosby; 2006. pp. 1215-21.
5. Vetter VL. Pediatric Cardiology: The Requisites in Pediatrics. Philadelphia: Elsevier Mosby; 2006. p. 366.
6. Savitsky E, Alejos J, Votey S. Emergency department presentations of pediatric congenital heart disease. J Emerg Med. 2003;24(3):239-45.
7. Yee L. Cardiac emergencies in the first year of life. Emerg Med Clin North Am. 2007;25(4):981-1008.
8. Frey B, Shann F. Oxygen administration in infants. Arch Dis Child Fetal Neonatal. 2003;88(2):F84-8.
9. Marino BS, Wernovsky G. Preoperative care. In: Chang AC, Hanley FL, Wernovsky G, Wessel DL (Eds). Pediatric Cardiac Intensive Care. Baltimore: Williams and Wilkins; 1998. pp. 151-62.
10. Siwik ES, Erenberg FG, Zahka KG. Tetralogy of Fallot. In: Allen HD, Driscoll DJ, Shaddy RE, Feltes TF (Eds). Moss and Adams' Heart Disease in Infants, Children and Adolescents: Including the Fetus and Young Adult, 7th edition. Philadelphia: Lippincott Williams and Wilkins; 2008. pp. 888-910.
11. Shrivastava S. Congestive heart failure in the neonatal period. Indian J Pediatr. 1980;47(386):245-52.
12. Saxena A, Juneja R, Ramakrishnan S. Drug therapy of cardiac diseases in children. Indian Pediatr. 2009;46(4):310-38.
13. Krishna Kumar R, Tandon R. Disorders of cardiovascular system. In: Ghai OP, Paul VK, Bagga A (Eds). Ghai Essential Pediatrics, 7th edition. New Delhi: CBS Publishers & Distributors (P) Ltd; 2010. pp. 372-439.
14. Davignon A, Rautaharju P, Boisselle E, et al. Normal ECG standards for infants and children. Pediatr Cardiol. 1980;1(2):123-131.
15. Bagri NK, Yadav DK, Agarwal S, et al. Pericardial effusion in children: experience from tertiary care center in northern India. Indian Pediatr. 2014;51(3):211-3.

SECTION 11

Dermatological Emergencies

- **Dermatological Emergencies**
  Ramanjit Singh, Devendra Richhariya

CHAPTER 76

Dermatologic Emergencies

Ramanjit Singh, Devendra Richhariya

INTRODUCTION

Emergencies related to dermatology are not so common but well-recognized entity and are associated with long-term morbidity and mortality. Emergency physician may be the first to see the patient with life-threatening dermatologic conditions. Early recognition and treatment of the conditions help in reducing the morbidity and mortality. Dermatologic emergencies if not treated well and timely, lead to acute skin failure, loss of normal temperature control, and inability to maintain core body temperature, barrier mechanism against foreign material is also compromised, fluid electrolyte and protein loss and other serious complications like sepsis, multiorgan failure pulmonary embolism, can also happen. Understanding the pathogenesis and systemic complication of acute skin failure and aggressive management in intensive care unit significantly reduces the fatality rate due to dermatologic emergencies are classified in **Table 1**.

ACUTE SKIN FAILURE

Acute skin failure is a state of total failure of skin functions due to various dermatological conditions, requires a multidisciplinary, intensive care approach for management.

The major consequences of acute skin failure are:

- *Fluid and electrolyte imbalance*: In normal circumstances water loss through the skin is 0.1 mL/cm²/hour. In patients with acute skin failure, the daily water loss through skin increases to 40 times more than the normal range. This is due to the destruction of skin layer stratum corneum responsible for the barrier function of the skin. If about 50% body surface area (BSA) affected, estimated daily fluid loss of up to 4–5 L, loss of protein (40 g/L), Na (120–150 mmol/L), Cl (10–90 mmol/L), and K (5–10 mmol/L). The manifestations are dehydration and decreased urinary output, electrolyte imbalance (low Na⁺ and high K⁺), and raised serum levels of urea and creatinine.
- *Infection*: Damaged barrier function of the skin supports growth and systemic entry of microorganisms and increases the incidence of septic complications.
- *Hemodynamic alteration*: Persistent inflammation of the skin leads to marked peripheral vasodilatation and increased cutaneous blood flow nearly doubles the cardiac output resulting in high-output cardiac failure in compromised cardiovascular system (elderly, hypertensive, ischemic, or valvular heart disease).
- *Thermoregulatory dysfunction*: Common occurrence that these patients may present as hyperthermia or

Table 1 Possible etiologic classification of dermatologic emergencies

Noninfectious	Infectious	Autoimmune causes
• Stevens-Johnson syndrome (SJS) • Toxic epidermal necrolysis (TEN) • Pyoderma gangrenosum	• Staphylococcal skin syndrome • Necrotizing fasciitis • Fournier's gangrene • Herpes zoster • Meningococcemia • Rocky Mountain spotted fever	Type I (immunoglobulin E dependent) • Anaphylaxis, urticaria angioedema Type II (cytotoxic) • Pemphigus Type III (immune complex) • Vasculitis Type IV (delayed) • Lepra reaction

hypothermia; patients with extensive skin lesion may present with fever even in the absence of infection. This is mediated by interleukin-1 (shivering due to increased interleukin-1). Sudden onset of hypothermia in a relatively stabilized patient may be a premonitory sign of septic shock.
- *Increased energy expenditure*: Hypercatabolic state increases energy expenditure.

Management

The management of patients with acute skin failure requires well-coordinated teamwork. Care should focus on double barrier nursing care; monitoring hemodynamic changes; fluid, electrolyte balance, and nutrition; prevention of complication (e.g. sepsis); prompt identification of risk factors; and topical therapy.

Monitoring Hemodynamic Changes

Due to disruption of barrier mechanism of the skin, continuous loss of water through the body surface, it is important to monitor and maintain an hourly hemodynamic status pulse rate, heart rate, urine output (50–100 mL/hour). Temperature, blood glucose, and gastric content to be monitored every 3 hourly.

Fluid, Electrolyte and Nutrition

Fluid and electrolyte administration to correct and maintain hemodynamic and electrolyte equilibrium. In the initial 24 hours the intravenous (IV) fluid administered contain human albumin 1 mL/kg/%BSA and isotonic saline 0.7 mL/kg/BSA. 1,500–2,000 mL of nasogastric feed should be added. Start with total 1,500–2,000 kcal/day then daily increment of 500 kcal up to 3,500–4,000 kcal/day and 2–3 g/kg/day protein intake in adults (3–4 g/kg/day in children).

Nursing Care and General Measures

The environmental temperature should be maintained at 30–32°C. Regular cleaning and removal of crusts from the oral and nasal cavities, and care of the eyes, genitalia, and perianal region is essential to prevent infections.

Topical Management

Various topical agents like silver sulfadiazine, nonphysiologic lipids (petroleum jelly, lanolin), and physiologic lipids (component mixture of cholesterol, ceramide, and free fatty acids in an optimized ratio of 3:1:1) should be used as barrier repair agents and to accelerate the barrier repair after cleaning.

Antibiotics

Antibiotics should be used judiciously. Few factors to be considered to start antibiotics are direct and indirect signs of sepsis, sudden rise or fall in temperature, increased pulse, oliguria, deterioration of alertness, increased gastric residual volume, accelerated respiration, and bacterial culture. Identification of the causative agents of acute skin failure is very important.

STEVENS-JOHNSON SYNDROME AND TOXIC EPIDERMAL NECROLYSIS

Stevens-Johnson syndrome (SJS) and toxic epidermal necrolysis (TEN) are the blistering diseases of the skin. In 1922 Steven and Johnson described a condition which was characterized by disseminated cutaneous eruption with central necrosis febrile erosive stomatitis and severe purulent conjunctivitis. Adverse reaction of the drugs is the common cause of these complex conditions (SJS and TEN) **(Table 2)**. Adverse drug reaction is the cause in about more than 80% of the cases in TEN and 50% cases in SJS. Condition is associated with widespread erythema necrosis bullous detachment of extensive areas of epidermis. SJS is considered as erythema multiform major. Epidermal detachment in SJS is less than 10% while epidermal detachment in TEN is more than 30%. 10–30% cases overlap between SJS and TEN. Diagnosis is mostly clinical.

Clinical Presentation

Clinical presentation includes fever, malaise, muscle joint pain, acute skin failure, hemorrhagic crust on lips, ocular manifestation like conjunctivitis, clouding symblepharon, corneal erosion, and photophobia. Erosion can spread to

Table 2 Most common drugs associated with Stevens-Johnson syndrome and toxic epidermal necrolysis

Sulfonamides	Anticonvulsants	Antibiotics	Nonsteroidal anti-inflammatory drugs
• Sulfadoxine • Salazine • Cotrimoxazole	• Carbamazepine • Barbiturates • Phenytoin • Lamotrigine	• Fluoroquinolones • Cephalosporin • Vancomycin • Erythromycin • Ethambutol	• Phenylbutazone • Piroxicam diclofenac • Naproxen

gastrointestinal (GI) tract and respiratory tract giving rise to symptoms like dysphagia, diarrhea, pulmonary edema, and bronchopneumonia. Glomerulonephritis represents renal involvement.

Complications

Complications include:
- Electrolyte imbalance
- Bacterial infection progressing to sepsis
- Anemia
- Gastrointestinal hemorrhage
- Hypercatabolic state
- Multisystem involvement in TEN
- Ocular sequelae dryness of eye, keratitis, inturned eyelashes, photophobia, visual impairment, and even blindness.

Prognosis

Stevens-Johnson syndrome (5% mortality) has better prognosis than TEN (30–40% mortality) **(Figs 1 and 2)**.

Management

Stevens-Johnson syndrome and TEN are life-threatening conditions so early recognition and treatment are required.
- Patient should be managed in intensive care unit
- Discontinue all drugs
- *Aggressive fluid management:* IV fluid therapy
- Pain management
- Barrier nursing aseptic handling
- Protection of exposed skin
- Silver sulfadiazine (sulfonamide derivative) should be avoided
- Correcting and maintaining electrolyte balance
- Nutritional support
- Antibiotics
- Use of systemic steroid and intravenous immunoglobulin (IVIG) controversial
- Ophthalmologist, plastic surgeon, respiratory physician, and gastroenterologist should be involved in the management.

PYODERMA GANGRENOSUM

Pyoderma gangrenosum is rare noninfectious dermatosis associated with systemic disease in more than 50% cases. Commonly associated diseases are inflammatory bowel disease, rheumatoid arthritis, and systemic lupus erythematosus.

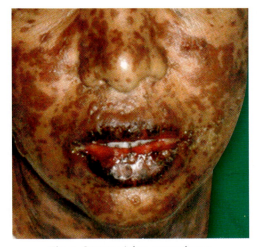

Fig. 1 Stevens-Johnson syndrome

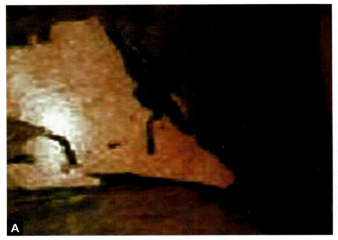
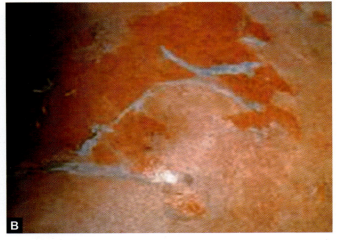

Figs 2A and B Toxic epidermal necrolysis

Pyoderma gangrenosum is characterized by rapid progression of painful necrotic ulceration with irregular margins with papule pustule or bulla associated with severe pain and no evidence of infection.

Diagnosis of pyoderma gangrenosum is based on clinical characteristics. Histopathology is nonspecific, skin biopsy not diagnostic but can rule out other conditions.

Topical steroid or tacrolimus 0.1% is an ointment used for mild cases and severe cases respond to oral corticosteroid (1–2 mg/kg). Cyclosporine acts rapidly in corticosteroid resistant cases.

STAPHYLOCOCCAL SCALDED SKIN SYNDROME

It is commonly seen in infants and children due to toxin released by *Staphylococcus aureus* phage 71. Diffuse erythema, fever, skin tenderness, and large bullae with clear fluid. Extensive loss of skin surface due to epidermal damage by endotoxin. Patient should be admitted and managed in intensive care unit.

NECROTIZING FASCIITIS

Necrotizing fasciitis is necrosis of subcutaneous tissue and rapidly progressive infection of deep fascia **(Fig. 3)**. Diabetes, peripheral vascular disease, trauma, alcohol, and nonsteroidal anti-inflammatory drugs (NSAIDs) are the common risk factors for necrotizing fasciitis. Lower extremities and abdomen perineum are the common sites. Necrotizing fasciitis of perineum and genital is known as Fournier gangrene. Patient of necrotizing fasciitis usually has history of surgery, wound, and trauma. Type 1 necrotizing fasciitis is due to polymicrobial involvement and associated pathogens are streptococci, bacteroides, and Enterobacteriaceae. Type 2 necrotizing fasciitis is caused by single pathogen beta-hemolytic streptococci and *Staphylococcus aureus*.

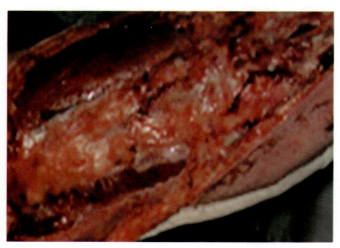

Fig. 3 Necrotizing fasciitis

Fever, chills, erythema, edema, and pain over involved skin are common features, erythematous skin turn into blue discoloration and vesicular and bullous lesion developed over erythematous skin with serosanguineous discharge. After that gangrene develop in next 4–5 days and black eschar by 10 days.

No specific diagnostic test for necrotizing fasciitis, routine blood test should be done. Radiology is used to detect gas within soft tissue and muscle.

Hospitalization, surgical debridement, fluid resuscitation, and broad-spectrum antibiotic therapy are the main steps in the management.

URTICARIA (HIVES), ANGIOEDEMA, AND ANAPHYLAXIS (TABLE 3)

Urticaria is common skin reaction that may be transient for 12–24 hours or lasts long for 6–8 weeks. Urticaria and angioedema have similar mechanism of action histamine and other mediators (anaphylatoxins C3a C5a) are released from mast cell and basophils. Mostly these are type I hypersensitivity reaction mediated by immunoglobulin E (IgE) antibodies. In urticaria mast cells are present in superficial dermis while in angioedema mast cells are present in dermis and subcutaneous tissues. Conditions are self-limiting but when respiratory mucus membranes are involved and produce laryngeal edema indicating the medical emergency. Common trigger factors are allergens, insect envenomation, and physical stimuli like heat, cold, vibration, and pressure. Patient on angiotensin-converting-enzyme (ACE) inhibitors may develop angioedema. Slightly elevated pruritic erythematous papules or plaques are the common presenting clinical features. Relevant history taking and physical examination should be performed to determine cause. Laboratory workup is not helpful unless history and examination suggest some specific cause. Basic laboratory investigations like complete blood count (CBC), erythrocyte sedimentation rate (ESR), thyroid-stimulating hormone (TSH), and antinuclear antibody (ANA) should be done in chronic and recurrent urticaria.

Management strategies include avoidance of triggers, nonsedating H1 antihistamines like loratadine, desloratadine, fexofenadine, and cetirizine are indicated in mild to moderate urticaria. If urticaria is severe and persists for more than 24–48 hours H2 receptor blockers like ranitidine should be added. Corticosteroid can be added for 5–7 days. If angioedema persists with urticaria parenteral corticosteroid and epinephrine 0.3–0.5 mg should be given.

PEMPHIGUS VULGARIS

Pemphigus vulgaris (PV) is an autoimmune disorder (antibodies to pemphigus vulgaris antigen) present with blistering of skin. Blisters are either epidermal or subepidermal. IgG class of antibodies forms cleft in epidermis and widespread

Table 3 Symptoms of urticaria, angioedema, and anaphylaxis		
Urticaria	*Angioedema*	*Anaphylaxis*
• Itching • Edema in dermis • Well-defined • Only skin involved	• Nonitching • Edema in subcutaneous fat • Ill defined • Skin mucous membrane, lips larynx, gastrointestinal (GI) mucosa • Causing upper airway obstruction • Angioedema is emergency	• Type I hypersensitivity urticaria and/or angioedema plus hypotension and tachycardia • *Treatment:* Epinephrine, corticosteroids

skin loss leads to acute skin failure. Young adults and geriatric population are more susceptible for bullous pemphigoid.

Common clinical features are fever, chills, and rigors. Flaccid vesicles are all over the skin. Oral pharyngeal and genital mucous membrane involvements lead to sore throat, dysphagia, dysuria, and vaginal pain. Ruptured blisters causing marked fluid and electrolyte and protein loss, hypoalbuminemia, and life-threatening infections.

Pemphigus vulgaris is a rapidly fatal condition, which requires large doses of corticosteroid methyl prednisolone for first 3–5 days.

Azathioprine cyclophosphamide can also be used with plasmapheresis to prevent autoantibodies rebound. Patient should be managed as per acute skin failure management.

VASCULITIS (FIG. 4)

- Immune complex (type 3 reaction)
- *Three types*: Small-vessel, medium-vessel, and large-vessel vasculitides
- *Most common type*: Leukocytoclastic vasculitis
- *History is important*: Medications (Penicillin, NSAIDs, sulfas, cephalosporins)
- Workup for systemic involvement
- *Treatment*: Eliminate cause, treat infection, steroids, colchicine, and immunosuppressant.

LEPRA REACTION

Lepra reaction occurs during the treatment course of leprosy. Lepra reaction is treated as emergency because this may lead to permanent damage to nerves, limbs, or may cause blindness. There are two types of lepra reaction:
- *Type I reactions:* Type IV hypersensitivity reactions, local existing lesions become more painful, erythematous and prominent paresthesia. Type I reaction is not present in lepromatous type of leprosy. Systemic steroid and NSAIDs are helpful in treating type I reaction.
- *Type II reaction* also known as erythema nodosum leprosum (ENL) is humoral hypersensitivity reaction usually occurs at later stage of treatment and is seen in lepromatous and borderline lepromatous leprosy. Type II reaction presents as tender erythematous nodule associated with fever, joint pain, and malaise. Oral steroid, clofazimine, and thalidomide are useful in treatment of type II lepra reaction.

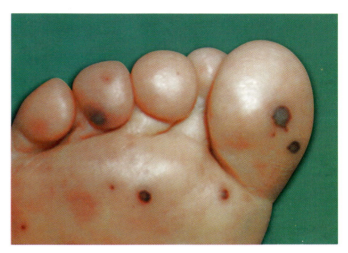

Fig. 4 Vasculitis

CONCLUSION

Emergencies related to skin are important clinical conditions, various pathophysiologic mechanisms lead to acute skin failure and various complications, thus, early identification and prompt management is required to prevent long-term morbidity and mortality.

BIBLIOGRAPHY

1. Ahmed AR. Pemphigus Vulgaris: Clinical features. Clin Dermatol. 1983;1(2):171-7.
2. Ayangco L, Rogers RS. Oral manifestations of erythema multiforme. Dermatol Clin. 2003;21(1):195-205.

3. Chave TA, Mortemer NJ, Sladden MJ, et al. Toxic epidermal necrolysis. Current evidence, practical management and future directions. Br J Dermatol. 2005;153(2):241-53.
4. Criton S, Devi K, Sridevi PK, et al. Toxic epidermal necrolysis—a retrospective study. Int J Dermatol. 1997;36(12):923-5.
5. Irvin C. "Skin failure"—a real entity: discussion paper. J R Soc Med. 1991;84(7):412-3.
6. Lyell A. Toxic epidermal necrolysis (the scalded skin syndrome): a reappraisal. Br J Dermatol. 1979;100(1):69-86.
7. Lyell A. Toxic epidermal necrolysis: an eruption resembling scalding of the skin. Br J Dermatol. 1956;68(11):355-61.
8. Prendville J. Stevens-Johnsons syndrome and toxic epidermal necrolysis. Adv Dermatol. 2002;18:151-73.
9. Rojeau JC, Guillaume JC, Fabre JP, et al. Toxic epidermal necrolysis (Lyell syndrome). Incidence and drug history in France 1981–1985. Arch Dermatol. 1990;126(1):37-42.
10. Ryan TJ. Disability in dermatology. Br J Hosp Med. 1991;46(1):33-6.

SECTION 12

Rheumatological Emergencies

- **Rheumatological Emergencies**
  Shruti Bajad, Naval Mendiratta, Rajiva Gupta

CHAPTER 77

Rheumatological Emergencies

Shruti Bajad, Naval Mendiratta, Rajiva Gupta

INTRODUCTION

Rheumatological disorders are generally considered as chronic diseases in view of their slow onset and gradual evolution. Rarely we encounter a rheumatological disease presenting as an acute emergency situation demanding prompt action. But, since these disorders are known to involve multiple organs and can have catastrophic effects leading to serious events even death, every emergency physician should be aware of such situations and strategies to tackle it in timely manner **(Fig. 1)**.

There can be two situations; one in which patients suffering from rheumatological disorders can present with medical emergencies. First is either due to the medical problem complicating the current disease or due to the drug side effects (steroid-induced psychosis, hyperglycemia, like bone marrow suppression, methotrexate pneumonitis, etc.). Second, rheumatological disorders themselves present as emergency like a patient with systemic lupus erythematosus (SLE) with antiphospholipid syndrome (APS) can present with catastrophic antiphospholipid syndrome (CAPS). The index of suspicion should be high for suspecting an underlying rheumatological disorder especially when we encounter multiple symptom involvement **(Fig. 2)**.

PATHOGENESIS

Two main processes that dominate in the multiple organ involvement and widespread damage are vasculitis and thrombosis of vessels. Vasculitis is leukocytes infiltration into the vessels due to inflammatory response. Pathologically, it is characterized by fibrinoid necrosis of the vessel wall. Thrombosis occurs commonly in APS, thus resulting in ischemia and end organ damage. Direct organ damage can also occur but remains a rarely encountered situation **(Fig. 3)**.[1]

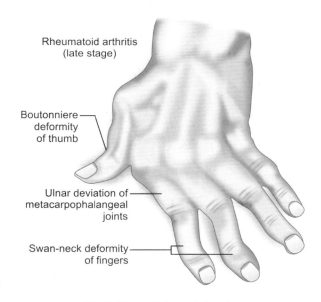

Fig. 1 Rheumatological disorders

WHEN TO SUSPECT?

Index of suspicion should be high when we encounter a patient in emergency presenting with these complaints **(Box 1)**.
- Polyarthritis
- Skin rashes
- Fever
- Multiorgan involvement
- History of acute thrombosis episode
- Young stroke
- Past history of suffering from rheumatological disease

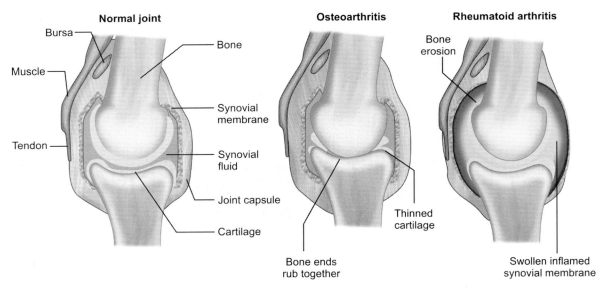

Fig. 2 Differentiating features between osteoarthritis and rheumatoid arthritis

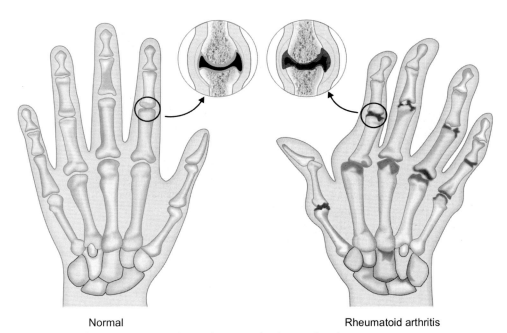

Fig. 3 Rheumatoid arthritis in hand

- History of rheumatological disease in immediate family members
- Not responding to conventional therapy
- Lack of definite diagnosis.

HOW TO EVALUATE AND MANAGE?

In critically sick patients, the fact remains important that the diagnosis needs to be established before starting the therapy keeping in consideration the drugs used in its treatment and degree of immunosuppression. Diagnostic evaluation of rheumatological disease will require a detailed history pertaining to the suspected underlying disease, physical examination, routine blood investigations, urine examination to look for casts, proteinuria, hematuria, inflammatory markers, autoimmune serological tests like antinuclear antibody (ANA), extractable nuclear antigens (ENA) profile, antineutrophil cytoplasmic antibody (ANCA) and tissue biopsy which is the conclusive investigation.

Box 1 Rheumatological emergencies according to disease

Rheumatoid arthritis:
- Acute infections
- Scleritis
- Scleromalacia perforans
- Atlantoaxial dislocation

Systemic lupus erythematosus:
- Pulmonary embolism
- Lupus pneumonia
- Pulmonary hemorrhage
- Pulmonary hypertension
- Shrinking lung syndrome
- Valvular affection
- Premature coronary artery disease with myocardial infarction
- Vasculitis
- Myocarditis
- Pericarditis
- Guillain-Barré syndrome
- Extrapyramidal syndrome
- Organic brain syndrome
- Psychosis
- Transverse myelitis
- Seizures
- Lupus cerebritis
- Cerebrovascular accidents
- Aseptic meningitis
- Rupture of hepatic artery aneurysm
- Bowel ischemia
- Bowel perforation
- Pancreatitis
- Thrombotic thrombocytopenic purpura
- Autoimmune hemolytic anemia
- Thrombocytopenia
- Antiphospholipid (APS) syndrome
- Acute glomerulonephritis
- Rapidly progressive glomerulonephritis (RPGN)
- Hypertensive crisis

Antiphospholipid antibody syndrome:
- Stroke
- Miscarriages
- Intrauterine growth restriction
- Pre-eclampsia

Spondyloarthritis:
- Uveitis
- Amyloidosis

Vasculitis:
- Sudden vision loss
- Stroke
- Mesenteric ischemia
- Renal ischemia
- Diffuse alveolar hemorrhage

Others:
- Acute gout
- Reactive arthritis
- Septic arthritis

A multispecialty approach involving anesthetists, nephrologists, neurologists and other team specialists will be required for successful management.

TREATMENT GUIDELINES

Treatment guidelines will vary according to the underlying disease and condition of the patient. Firstly, rheumatological mimics-like infection, malignancy and other vasculitis mimics need to be ruled out, then only we can institute the immunosuppressive therapy. Here we will discuss the management guidelines for few common conditions that we encounter.

Systemic Lupus Erythematosus

Common clinical features of SLE are shown in **Box 2**.

In the complications arising out of this disease, the mainstay remains the use of high-dose glucocorticoids. It is recommended that initial therapy should be considered in form of either high-dose daily glucocorticoids (1–1.5 mg/kg) in divided doses or intravenous (IV) methylprednisolone pulses (500–1000 mg/d for 3 days) which is followed by oral prednisolone according to body weight. Cyclophosphamide and azathioprine with glucocorticoid have better results than glucocorticoid alone in acute severe SLE.[2] Other newer therapies include use of newer drugs like belimumab, mycophenolate mofetil, intravenous immunoglobulins, and autologous stem cell transplantation. Rituximab is emerging as a new therapy for conventional treatment resistant SLE, but has not been approved for the same.

Antiphospholipid Syndrome

Antiphospholipid syndrome is characterized by vascular thrombosis, complications of pregnancy, presence of lupus anticoagulant and anticardiolipin antibodies.[3] APS may present as deep vein thrombosis (DVT), pulmonary embolism, stroke or transient ischemic attack (TIA), thrombotic microangiopathy, thrombocytopenis, and hemolytic anemia.

Women with APS may present as frequent pregnancy loss and premature deliveries.

Box 2 Clinical features of SLE

Respiratory: Tachypnea, cough pleural effusion
Cardiac: Raynaud's phenomenon pericarditis
Kidney: Lupus nephritis protinuria hematuria
Skin: Photosensitivity erythematous rashes over skin exposed to sunlight, butterfly rash over cheeks
Generalized: Fatigue weight loss, fever arthritis emotional lability hematological and neurological disorders

Catastrophic Antiphospholipid Syndrome

Catastrophic APS is a life-threatening situation which includes involvement of three organ system and multiple occlusions of small and large vessels.[4,5] Venous or arterial thrombosis of large vessels is common in patient with catastrophic APS. Patients with definite APS should be treated with long-term anticoagulation. For venous events, the suggested target for international normalized ratio (INR) is 2.0–3.0, while it is suggested that arterial events should be managed with high-intensity oral anticoagulation (INR 3.0–4.0). In this life-threatening condition, the combination of anticoagulation, steroids, and plasmapheresis or intravenous immunoglobulins (IVIg) is currently recommended.

Vasculitis

The treatment of patient is to be tailor-made for each patient considering the level of involvement of various organs in vasculitis. One of the criteria which can serve as a guide is the Five-Factors Score (FFS): raised creatinine levels (>140 µmol/L), proteinuria (>1 g/day), specific cardiomyopathy, gastrointestinal tract involvement, and central nervous system involvement. High-dose glucocorticoids are the mainstay of treatment for vasculitis and regimen involves daily intravenous pulses of 500–1,000 mg of methylprednisolone for 3–5 days and then the patient is maintained on oral steroids according to the body weight of patient. Intravenous cyclophosphamide (0.5–1 g/m^2 body surface area) is generally started along with the methylprednisolone and then needs to be repeated at intervals of between 4 weeks generally for 6 months. There is some evidence on efficacy of plasma exchange in fulminant disease causing pulmonary–renal failure and for diffuse alveolar hemorrhage. Biological immunomodulatory therapies, namely rituximab and infliximab, have emerged as potential new therapeutic options. Intravenous immunoglobulin is also under consideration for the same and may be the future hope.[6,7]

REFERENCES

1. Wallace DJ, Hahn BH (Ed). Dubois' Lupus Erythematosus, 6th edition. Philadelphia: Lippincott Williams & Wilkins; 2002. pp. 645-62; 693-738; 793-820; 843-62; 917-26; 985-1076.
2. Ortmann RA, Klippel JM. Update on cyclophosphamide for systemic lupus erythematosus. Rheum Dis Clin North Am. 2000;26(2):363-75.
3. Miyakis S, Lockshin MD, Atsumi T, et al. International consensus statement on an update of the classification criteria for definite antiphospholipid syndrome (APS). J Thromb Haemost. 2006;4:295-306.
4. Berman H, Rodríguez-Pintó I, Cervera R, et al. Rituximab use in the catastrophic antiphospholipid syndrome: descriptive analysis of the CAPS registry patients receiving rituximab. Autoimmun Rev. 2013;12(11):1085-90.
5. de Jesus GR, Agmon-Levin N, Andrade CA, et al. 14th International Congress on Antiphospholipid Antibodies Task Force report on obstetric antiphospholipid syndrome. Autoimmun Rev. 2014;13(8):795-813.
6. Specks U, Fervenza FC, McDonald TJ, et al. Response of Wegener's granulomatosis to anti-CD20 chimeric monoclonal antibody therapy. Arthritis Rheum. 2001;44:2836-40.
7. Keogh KA, Wylam ME, Stone JH, et al. Induction of remission by B lymphocyte depletion in eleven patients with refractory antineutrophil cytoplasmic antibody-associated vasculitis. Arthritis Rheum. 2005;52:262-8.

SECTION 13

Hematologic and Oncological Emergencies

◯ **Evaluation and Management of Oncological Emergencies**
Devender Sharma, Pratibha Dhiman, Nintin Sood, Neelam Sharma, Jyoti Wadhwa, Ashok Vaid

◯ **Care of Patients with Hematological Malignancies and Bone Marrow Transplantation**
Mukul Aggarwal, Anjan Shrestha, Narendra Agrawal, Rayaz Ahmed, Dinesh Bhurani

CHAPTER 78

Evaluation and Management of Oncological Emergencies

Devender Sharma, Pratibha Dhiman, Nintin Sood, Neelam Sharma, Jyoti Wadhwa, Ashok Vaid

INTRODUCTION

With advances in therapeutics and enhanced survival of cancer patients, complications of malignancies are an increasingly common reason for admission in emergency. Every healthcare provider should be aware and able to recognize oncologic emergencies. Emergencies in oncology can be life-threatening, event can arise in a known malignancy or individual not previously diagnosed with cancer, or these events can happen during treatment. These life-threatening oncologic emergencies do not have characteristic signs and symptoms, so high degree of suspicion is crucial while dealing with malignancy related complications. Oncologic emergencies should be treated promptly in emergency department.

Oncological emergencies broadly classified into mechanical, metabolic, and hematologic **(Table 1)**.

SUPERIOR VENA CAVA SYNDROME

Superior vena cava (SVC) is the main vessel for drainage of venous blood from upper part of body up to upper thorax. Any obstructions like compression, invasion, thrombosis, or fibrosis of this vessel leads to obstruction of blood flow through the SVC to the right atrium. Despite the collateral pathways, like azygos venous system, internal mammary veins, lateral thoracic veins, and paraspinal veins, the venous pressure is almost always elevated in the upper compartment, if there is obstruction of the SVC **(Figs 1A and B)**.

Incidence and Etiology

Malignancies have accounted for the large majority (nearly 78–86%) of superior vena cava syndrome (SVCS) cases. Out of this, lung cancer comprises nearly 65% cases. Other malignant causes, like lymphoma metastatic cancers, including mesothelioma, thymoma, breast, germ cell, and thyroid cancers, are also responsible for SVCS. Central venous catheters placement including pacemaker catheters are nonmalignant causes of SVCS.

Signs and Symptoms

Onset of SVCS is usually gradual. Common symptoms are:
- Headache
- Feeling of fullness of head and neck region
- Dilated neck and chest veins
- Swelling of arm breast upper chest
- Periorbital edema
- Breathlessness

Table 1 Classification of oncologic emergencies

Mechanical	Metabolic	Hematologic
• Superior vena cava syndrome • Spinal cord compression • Hyperviscosity syndrome • Cardiac tamponade • Malignant pleural effusion • Brain metastasis	• Tumor lysis syndrome • Hypercalcemia of malignancy	Febrile neutropenia

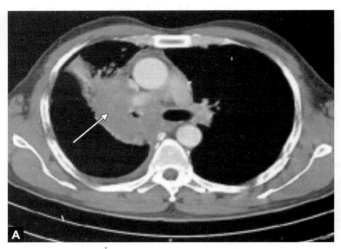 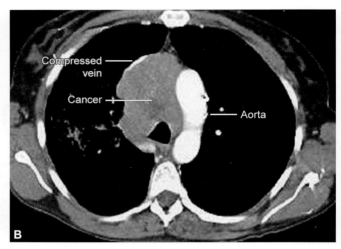

Figs 1A and B Tumor mass compressing superior vena cava

- Cough
- Hoarseness of voice
- Swallowing difficulties
- Respiratory distress, syncope, visual changes, and altered sensorium are late changes.

Diagnosis

A plain chest X-ray shows abnormal enlargement of the mediastinum or may reveal a tumor in the lung. Computed tomography (CT) is helpful in evaluating the SVC, its tributaries, and other critical structures, such as the bronchi and the cord. CT-guided fine-needle biopsy is as an effective and safe alternative to open biopsy. Lymph node biopsy can be done in case of suspected lymphoma.

Treatment

Cure of primary malignant disease and relief of symptoms are the main objectives of the treatment. Lung carcinoma (small cell lung carcinoma) and lymphoma are the main malignant causes of SVCS. Combination of chemotherapy and radiation therapy is the standard treatment for SCLC. Combination therapy is effective in rapidly improving the symptoms of SVCS.

In case there is a thrombus then removal of the central lines and initiation of anticoagulation therapy or thrombolytic therapy would be needed. Thrombolytic therapy should not be used unless brain metastasis has been ruled out. Superior vena caval stenting may be used in those who have failed chemotherapy or radiation therapy. The stent would relieve the symptoms immediately but would have to remain for the rest of the patient's life. In addition, steroids are used to decrease the inflammation and edema surrounding the tumor. Diuretics are also used to reduce the venous return to heart and relieve the pressure symptoms.

SPINAL CORD COMPRESSION

Any cancer can spread to the bone; spinal cord compression (SCC) occurs in about 5% of patients with cancer **(Figs 2 and 3)**. Cancer of lung, breast, prostate, multiple myeloma, and lymphoma (Hodgkin and non-Hodgkin) are associated with SCC. The majority of patients who present with SCC have a known diagnosis of cancer. However in 8–34% cases, it can represent as the initial manifestation of cancer. SCC develops within 3 months of the initial diagnosis of cancer in the majority of cases.

Epidemiology

Patients with lung, prostate, and breast cancer produce the metastatic SCC, and the overall frequency is approximately 5%. SCC is the second most frequent neurological complication of metastatic cancer. Intramedullary lesions make up only 0.8–3.8% of all cases of metastatic SCC.

The most frequent tumor types producing pediatric cord compression are neuroblastoma (7.9–50%), Ewing's sarcoma (15–28.5%), rhabdomyosarcoma (15–28%), osteosarcoma (6–9%), lymphoma (6–7.5%), and leukemia (6%).

Pathophysiology

Hematogenous spread of cancerous cells into vertebral column with epidural extension leads to extrinsic compression. SCC also occurs due to pathologic fracture of vertebra which rapidly progresses to loss of neurological function due to vascular compromise and vasogenic edema. Spinal cord damage and loss of neurological function results from venous stasis, spinal cord edema, reduced capillary blood flow, ischemia, and mechanical compression culminating in infarction.

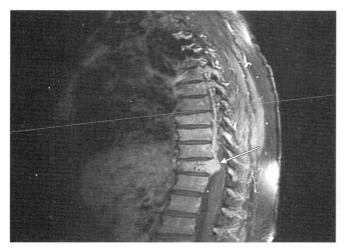

Fig. 2 Spinal cord compression

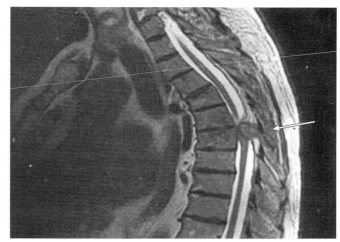

Fig. 3 Intramedullary metastasis

Clinical Presentation

The most common initial symptom of SCC is back pain; sensory and motor deficit are common findings on neurological examination. Cauda equina syndrome develops in half of the patient in which bowel and bladder incontinence is prominent findings. Complete paralysis develops if cauda equina syndrome is not treated well.

Diagnostic Evaluation

A careful history, physical and neurological examination, and radiological evaluation including a magnetic resonance imaging (MRI) survey of the spine are important in evaluation. MRI has become the gold standard for imaging in case of metastatic SCC because it is more sensitive and has specificity and an overall diagnostic accuracy in detecting cord compression. In summary, the investigations of an individual patient shall have to be tailored as per the clinical situation, and one patient may require a combination of diagnostic tests to prove the diagnosis and for effective treatment planning.

Positron emission tomography (PET) is used in identifying metabolic changes in the cervical spinal cord and intramedullary spinal cord metastases.

Treatment

Therapy for the individual patient can be optimized, based on tumor histology and extent, severity and mechanism of spinal compression. The response to nonsurgical therapy and the duration of survival, following treatment can be varied among the different histological tumor types:
- *High dose corticosteroid*: To reduce the vasogenic edema
- *Emergent radiation therapy for radiosensitive tumors*: Prevents the further loss of neurological functions and spinal stability can be preserved. Radiotherapy is the mainstay of treatment in radiosensitive tumors. Radiation therapy is also helpful in reducing the pain. Stereotactic beam radiation therapy is more in use because external beam radiation therapy is associated with high radiation toxicity.

Surgery is indicated if spinal instability and rapid neurological deterioration are present. Rest of the patients should receive primary radiotherapy alone.

Cytotoxic chemotherapy and hormonal therapy have been used to successfully alleviate SCC from prostate cancer, Hodgkin's disease, myeloma, germ cells, tumors, lymphoma, and breast cancer.

HYPERVISCOSITY SYNDROME

High white blood cells (WBCs) count or severe hyperproteinemia can cause high serum viscosity and microcirculatory problems, commonly associated with patients with multiple myeloma or acute leukemia. Increase in circulatory proteins interfere with platelet aggregation.

Classic triad is mucosal bleeding (epistaxis, vaginal or rectal bleeding, and hematuria), visual disturbances, and altered level of consciousness. Increase in serum protein, viscosity, and sausage shaped veins on fundoscopy confirm the diagnosis.

Fluid resuscitation and plasmapheresis are the treatment of choice.

CARDIAC TAMPONADE

Pericardial involvement is seen in about 20–30% cases of cancer patients. Primary malignancies in which pericardium involvement is common are lung, breast, and esophageal cancer and manifest as pericardial effusion. A condition is called cardiac tamponade when cardiac output is compromised due to high intrapericardial pressure. Normal amount of fluid in pericardial space is about 50 mL. Malignant cells can reach the pericardial space either through direct invasion or by hematogenous and lymphatic spread. Acute rise of even more than 200 mL of pericardial effusion can result in hemodynamic compromise and require emergent intervention.

Exertional dyspnea, tachycardia, and chest pain are nonspecific complaints.

Muffled heart sound, hypotension, raised jugular venous pressure (JVP), and pulsus paradoxus are findings on examination.

Right atrial collapse in late diastole is more sensitive and right ventricular collapse in early diastole is most specific findings for cardiac tamponade on echocardiography. On cardiac catheterization, equalization of pressure in both atria is diagnostic gold standard. Electrocardiogram (ECG), X-ray of chest, and CT imaging are also important diagnostic tools.

Ultrasound-guided emergent pericardiocentesis is definitive treatment for acute pericardial tamponade.

MALIGNANT PLEURAL EFFUSION

It is commonly seen with metastatic cancers. 50–65% of malignant pleural effusions are due to lung and breast cancers. Other causes include mesothelioma and lymphoma. Pain and acute or chronic dyspnea are common presenting features. Chest X-ray and/or a chest CT scan, along with an ultrasound are helpful in diagnosis. Send pleural fluid for cytology. Management of malignant pleural effusion includes oxygen therapy pain management and chest tube placement if indicated.

BRAIN METASTASIS

Brain metastasis is common neurological complication of cancer and occurs in about 35–40% of cancers. Melanoma, breast, and lung cancer commonly produce brain metastasis and quickly raise the intracranial pressure. Neurological deterioration can be prevented by early recognition and prompt treatment of intracranial pressure.

Clinical features are nausea, vomiting, seizure, altered sensorium, and coma.

Contrast CT is the initial investigation of choice in emergency department. Contrast MRI has better sensitivity and specificity than CT.

Three main steps in management are steroid therapy, radiation therapy, and measures to reduce the raised intracranial pressure.

TUMOR LYSIS SYNDROME

Tumor lysis syndrome (TLS) is a metabolic disturbances encounter during management of a variety of cancers such as lymphoma and leukemia. TLS is defined as the abrupt release of cellular component in the blood flow as a result of rapid lysis of malignant cells after initiation of chemotherapy. It will lead to a hazardous modification in the usual equilibrium of fluids and electrolytes—the amounts of potassium, phosphate, and uric acid are increased, whereas calcium levels are reduced. This syndrome is a combination of hyperuricemia, hyperkalemia, hyperphosphatemia, hypocalcemia, and metabolic acidosis which is confirmed by the laboratory findings (**Box 1**).

Management

The management of tumor lysis syndrome is shown in **Table 2**.

HYPERCALCEMIA OF MALIGNANCY

Hypercalcemia of malignancy is most common metabolic oncologic emergency associated with almost all malignancies but most frequently seen in multiple myeloma, breast, lungs, and kidney malignancies.

Hypercalcemia is defined as serum calcium greater than 10 mg/dL or ionized calcium greater than 5 mg/dL. Hypercalcemia can be:
- *Mild*: 10–12 mg/dL
- *Moderate*: 12–14 mg/dL
- *Severe*: Greater than 14 mg/dL.

Hypercalcemia in malignancies is seen as a result of bone resorption and calcium release from the bone. Parathyroid hormone-related polypeptide (PTHrP) is responsible in about 80% cases of humoral hypercalcemia of malignancy. Cytokines, chemokines, and PTHrP are responsible for local osteoclastic hypercalcemia.

Clinical feature of hypercalcemia are related to neurological, cardiovascular, gastrointestinal, and renal systems (**Table 3**).

Treatment of hypercalcemia has been shown in **Table 4**.

Box 1 Cairo-Bishop classification system for diagnosing tumor lysis syndrome

Laboratory TLS
Two or more laboratory changes within 3–7 days of chemotherapy
Uric acid >8 mg/dL
Potassium >6 mEq/L
Phosphorus >6.5 mg/dL
Calcium <7 mg/dL
Clinical TLS
Renal involvement: Creatinine >1.5 times the upper limit of normal
Cardiac involvement: Cardiac arrhythmia or sudden death
Neurological involvement: Seizure

Table 2 Treatment of metabolic derangements in tumor lysis syndrome

Problem	Treatment
Hyperphosphatemia	Minimize intake with restriction of milk products
	Phosphate binders (aluminum hydroxide or aluminum carbonate) 30 mL every 6 hours in adults
	Dialysis if no response to oral therapy
Hyperkalemia	Insulin 10U intravenous (IV) with dextrose 50 mL of 50% IV push then infuse 50–75 mL of 5% dextrose over an hour
	Albuterol nebulization
	Diuretics like furosemide
	Dialysis if no response
Hypocalcemia	If patient is symptomatic then IV calcium gluconate
Hyperuricemia	Allopurinol 100 mg/m^2 per dose orally every 8 hours (maximum daily dose: 800 mg)
	Rasburicase 0.15–0.2 mg/kg/d IV. 2nd dose may be based on response seen
Renal insufficiency and hypovolemia	Intravenous fluids normal saline, 3 L/m^2 daily. Use with caution if decreased systolic function
	Dialysis for fluid-unresponsive oliguric renal failure or patients with congestive heart failure

Table 3 Clinical features of hypercalcemia of malignancy

Neurological	Cardiovascular	Gastrointestinal	Renal	Dermatological
• Muscle weakness • Fatigue • Lethargy • Altered mental status and coma	• Short QRS and QT interval • Bradyarrhythmias • Complete heart block • Cardiac arrest	• Nausea • Vomiting • Constipation • Paralytic ileus • Pancreatitis	• Polyurea • Polydipsia • Renal insufficiency due to volume depletion	• Pruritus

Table 4 Treatment of hypercalcemia

Measures	Doses
Normal saline	300–500 mL/h rapid infusion. Use caution in patients with compromised heart function
Furosemide	After adequate hydration 20–40 mg intravenous (IV) furosemide every 12–24 hours
Pamidronate	60–90 mg IV
Zoledronic acid	4 mg IV. Special precaution in renal failure patients
Steroids: Hydrocortisone or prednisolone	*Hydrocortisone:* 100 mg IV every 6 hours *Prednisone:* 60 mg orally daily
Calcitonin	4–8 IU/kg subcutaneously or IV every 12 hours

SIADH

The syndrome of inappropriate antidiuretic hormone secretion (SIADH) is caused either by the sustained release of antidiuretic hormone (ADH) in the absence of stimuli, or by the enhanced action of ADH on the kidneys.

Causes: Small cell carcinoma of lungs and brain tumors. Some chemotherapy drugs (e.g. cyclophosphamide, cisplatin, vincristine, vinblastine, docetaxel, and etoposide) can also produce SIADH.

Patients are present to emergency department with hyponatremia and associated symptoms, such as nausea, vomiting, headache, confusion, cerebral edema, hypertension, urine osmolality, and fluid overload.

Treatment is hypertonic saline and vasopressin receptor antagonists.

Febrile Neutropenia

Fever is one of the most common presentations in emergency department in both adult and pediatric age group. Fever in healthy individuals not always indicate serious illness but fever in patient with neutropenia indicate life-threatening situation for which rapid evaluation and initiation of empiric broad-spectrum antibiotics are indicated to prevent progression of sepsis to severe sepsis, septic shock, and death **(Table 5)**. Febrile neutropenia is a medical emergency and should be treated promptly. Patients who are on repeated cycles of chemotherapy are on higher risk of developing the neutropenia. Cytotoxic therapy causes myelosuppression.

Table 5 Neutropenia [absolute neutrophil count (ANC): cell/μL]

Mild	Moderate	Severe
1,000–1,500	500–1,000	<500

Table 6 Empiric antibiotics options

First-line	Allergic to penicillin	Gram-negative coverage, catheter related infection, and hemodynamically unstable patients
• Cephalosporins • Carbapenem (meropenem imipenem cilastatin) • Piperacillin • Tazobactam	• Aminoglycosides • Fluoroquinolones	• Vancomycin • Linezolid

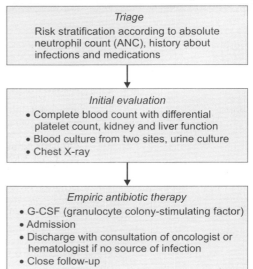

Flow chart 1 Evaluation of febrile neutropenic patients

Oral temperature greater than 38.5°C and an absolute neutrophil count less than $0.5 \times 10^9/l$ is considered as febrile neutropenia.

The severity of neutropenia depends on the absolute neutrophil count (ANC) and is described in **Table 6**.

Typical signs and symptoms of infection may not present in patients who are on chemotherapy. Detail history about various conditions and medication affecting the immune system should be obtained. Laboratory investigations like complete blood count with differential diagnosis and platelet count, kidney function test, and liver function test are suggested. Blood culture should be collected from two different sites and one from the venous catheter. Sputum and urine culture should be obtained. Urine and chest X-ray should also be considered in every patient as typical clinical features are not present in febrile neutropenic patient. Febrile neutopenic patient should be evaluated according to **Flow chart 1** and emperic antibiotic should be started according to **Table 6**.

CONCLUSION

Evaluation and diagnosis of oncologic emergencies in emergency department need high index of suspicion. Patient with history of malignancy, on chemotherapy or with clinical features of malignancies should be attended promptly. Various conditions related to malignancies progress rapidly, so accurate diagnosis and treatment is required in emergency department to reduce the mortality.

BIBLIOGRAPHY

1. Bates T. A review of local radiotherapy in the treatment of bone metastases and cord compression. Int J Radiat Oncol Biol Phys. 1992;23(1):217-21.
2. Cairo MS, Bishop M. Tumour lysis syndrome: new therapeutic strategies and classification. Br J Haematol. 2004;127(1):3-11.
3. Chisholm MA, Mulloy AL, Taylor AT. Acute management of cancer-related hypercalcemia. Ann Pharmacother. 1996;30(5):507-13.
4. Gilbert RW, Kim JH, Posner JB. Epidural spinal cord compression from metastatic tumor: diagnosis and treatment. Ann Neurol. 1978;3(1):40.
5. Ihde DC, Cohen MH, Bernath AM, et al. Serial fiberoptic bronchoscopy during chemotherapy of small cell carcinoma of the lung: early detection of patients at high risk of relapse. Chest. 1978;74(5):531-6.
6. Lewis MA, Hendrickson AW, Moynihan TJ. Oncologic emergencies: Pathophysiology, presentation, diagnosis, and treatment. CA Cancer J Clin. 2011;61(5):287-314.
7. Lewis DW, Packer RJ, Raney B, et al. Incidence, presentation and outcome of spinal cord disease in children with systemic cancer. Pediatrics. 1986;78(3):438-43.
8. Loblaw DA, Laperriere NJ. Emergency treatment of malignant extradural spinal cord compression: an evidence-based guideline. J Clin Oncol. 1998;16(4):1613-24.
9. Maranzano E, Latini P, Beneventi S, et al. Radiotherapy without steroids in selected metastatic spinal cord compression patients. A phase II trial. Am J Clin Oncol. 1996;19(2):179-83.
10. Mundy GR, Guise TA. Hypercalcemia of malignancy. Am J Med. 1997;103(2):134-45.
11. Spinazze S, Caraceni A, Schrijvers D. Epidural spinal cord compression. Crit Rev Oncol Hematol. 2005;56(3):397-406.
12. Stewart AF. Clinical practice. Hypercalcemia associated with cancer. N Engl J Med. 2005;352(4):3739.
13. Viscoli C. The evolution of the empirical management of fever and neutropenia in cancer patients. J Antimicrob Chemother. 1998;41:6580.
14. Wallington M, Mendis S, Premawardhana U, et al. Local control and survival in spinal cord compression from lymphoma and myeloma. Radiother Oncol. 1997;42(1):43-7.

CHAPTER 79
Care of Patients with Hematological Malignancies and Bone Marrow Transplantation

Mukul Aggarwal, Anjan Shrestha, Narendra Agrawal, Rayaz Ahmed, Dinesh Bhurani

INTRODUCTION

Hematological malignancies are disorders of bone marrow, characterized by deficiencies of normal blood cells (erythrocytes, leukocytes and platelets). Most of them share a state of profound immunosuppression due to dysfunctional and abnormal leukocytes, severe neutropenia and side effects of various chemotherapeutic and immunotherapeutic agents. Any sign of infection needs immediate evaluation and management. In addition, severe anemia causing circulatory compromise and severe thrombocytopenia leading to bleeding warrant prompt attention and immediate institution of therapy.

Patients of hematological malignancies present with signs of bone marrow failure (anemia, pallor, bleeding or infections), lymphadenopathy, hepatosplenomegaly or systemic complaints of fever, weight loss, night sweats, malaise, etc. Recognition of these signs and symptoms should make one suspicious of possible hematological disorder and prompt evaluation by complete blood count and peripheral smear. If these are suggestive, patient should be referred to the center experienced in managing such patients at the earliest after stabilization. Patient needs to undergo evaluation for diagnosis and staging. This usually involves bone marrow aspiration and biopsy, flow cytometry immunophenotyping, cytogenetics or fluorescence in situ hybridization (FISH) from bone marrow aspirate or lymph node biopsy, and immunohistochemistry evaluation. In addition, computed tomography-positron emission tomography (CT/PET) scans are needed for staging in many cases.

Central venous access is preferred for administration of many chemotherapeutic agents and vesicant drugs, intensive care unit (ICU) management of sicker patients, administration of large volumes of fluids and frequent sampling. This may be done in the form of peripherally inserted central catheters (PICC), central lines, ports or tunneled catheters. Proper septic precautions are to be adhered with in handling these central venous access devices (CVADs).

Personnel handling these patients should be experienced to take care of various emergencies that may arise including neutropenic fever, tumor lysis syndrome (TLS) and dyselectrolytemia, leukostasis, bleeding, cord compression and in case of bone marrow transplant recipients graft versus host disease, graft failure and infections.

NEUTROPENIC CARE (FLOW CHART 1)

Moderate to severe neutropenia (absolute neutrophil count <1000/μL and <500/μL) is a common event post-chemotherapy for acute leukemia, bone marrow transplant and some lymphomas. Any infection in such patients can have catastrophic consequences.

Neutropenic fever patients should be immediately assessed for vital parameters, state of consciousness and localization of infection. Any sign of hemodynamic instability, confused state or seizure qualifies for ICU admission. These patients should have blood culture and biochemistry sampled immediately on arrival to the emergency. In addition, cultures from any localizing site [like sputum for pneumonia, urine culture (mid stream sample), stool culture including *Clostridium difficile* toxin for diarrhea, pus culture for skin infection, cerebrospinal fluid (CSF) samples for meningitis] should be sent. These patients should be started on broad-spectrum antibiotics (piperacillin–tazobactam or cefoperazone-sulbactam ± aminoglycoside) after taking cultures. Consider adding vancomycin or teicoplanin for patients having skin infections, perineal infections, associated mucositis or suspected CVAD infection. If fever persists, carbapenems need to be substituted and finally antibiotics given as per culture sensitivity report for adequate duration. Neutropenic colitis, a life-threatening complication of severe neutropenia, presents with abdominal pain, diarrhea or distention. Due

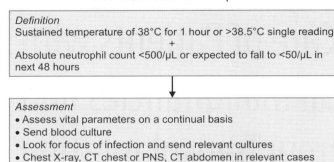

Flow chart 1 Febrile neutropenia

Abbreviations: CT, computed tomography; PNS, paranasal sinus.

to transmigration across gut because of mucositis, infection with gram-negative bacteria, anaerobes, alpha streptococci and candida are common. CT or ultrasound abdomen should be done early to look for bowel wall thickening (usually >4 mm), distention, megacolon or ascites. Antibiotics covering potential organisms should be started at the earliest.

Fungal infections are also common in neutropenic patients especially in whom neutropenia is prolonged (>10 days) or those with dysfunctional neutrophils. Threshold for CT chest for patients with persistent fever or signs of pneumonia should be low. CT of paranasal sinuses for patients with signs of sinusitis or CT abdomen for typhlitis should be done whenever there is suspicion. Infections with *Aspergillus* and *Mucor* species occur more commonly in these settings. One should try biopsy to diagnose suspected lesions for definite diagnosis (not possible in many cases due to hemodynamic instability or deranged hematological parameters). Bronchoalveolar lavage and serial serum galactomannan have shown specificity for *Aspergillus* species. Start treatment with amphotericin B (conventional or liposomal) or voriconazole (in case of suspected *Aspergillus* infection).

TUMOR LYSIS SYNDROME AND DYSELECTROLYTEMIA (FLOW CHART 2)

Tumor lysis syndrome is a metabolic syndrome caused due to accumulation of metabolites produced by excessive breakdown of tumor cells. As tumor cells lysed after chemotherapy or radiotherapy or sometimes spontaneously also, potassium, uric acid, and phosphate are increased in serum and calcium is decreased. These may cause renal failure, arrhythmias, seizure or altered sensorium which if not corrected on time may result in mortality. The risk is enhanced in patients with high tumor load burden or aggressive malignancies (Burkitt's lymphoma, acute leukemia with high blast counts, large tumor masses, etc.), at extremes of age or those with preexisting renal or cardiac dysfunction.

Diagnosis is based on biochemical and clinical criteria as described below. All patients should be started on hydration at the rate of 3 L/m^2 and agents lowering uric acid synthesis including allopurinol or febuxostat as prophylaxis. Those in established biochemical or clinical TLS should ideally receive rasburicase (recombinant uricase) in addition to hydration and diuretics. Patients should have their electrolytes and renal parameters monitored at least twice a day and fluid balance monitored four times a day till TLS is resolved. Patients should be managed by a multidisciplinary team consisting of nephrologist, cardiologist, and intensive care physician in addition to primary oncologist or hematologist. Patients with refractory dyselectrolytemia should undergo hemodialysis on an urgent basis. Peritoneal dialysis is less preferred due to more risks of infection or possible underlying abdominal masses and less efficiency. Mortality with proper care has come down to less than 10% in most series.

LEUKOSTASIS

Leukostasis is a clinical syndrome caused due to very high blood cell counts. Patients with counts more than 1 lac/µL in acute leukemia or greater than 3 L in chronic leukemia are predisposed. Also, it is more commonly seen with myeloid malignancies due to larger size of myeloid blasts and increased adhesion to capillary walls. The blasts cells stick to capillaries and lead to stasis in peripheral circulation and those with end arteries. This leads to precapillary dilatation and rupture of small vessels causing bleeding. This stasis and hemorrhage occurs in cerebral circulation causing altered sensorium or focal deficits; in pulmonary circulation causing cough, dyspnea or hemoptysis; in retinal circulation causing decreased vision, photophobia, etc.; or in renal and penile circulation. Clinically, leukostasis is appreciated best by fundal examination showing dilatation of retinal vessels and focal hemorrhages. Blood viscosity does not always correlate with symptoms.

Management includes hydration and management of fluid and electrolyte balance. Therapeutic leukapheresis may be helpful in lowering leukocyte count in a short span of time, but not resulted in improved overall survival. Therapy for the underlying disease should be started at the earliest, keeping in mind the higher risk of TLS.

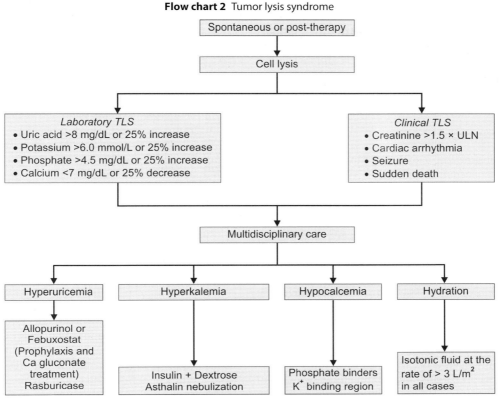

Flow chart 2 Tumor lysis syndrome

Abbreviations: TLS, tumor lysis syndrome; ULN, upper limit of normal.

BLEEDING (THROMBOCYTOPENIC AND COAGULOPATHY)

Moderate to severe thrombocytopenia is a frequent complication of hematological malignancies and their treatment. Many patients have platelet count less than 10,000/µL at diagnosis of acute leukemia and these increases only after treatment, and subsequent bone marrow recovery. During this period, patients are predisposed to bleeding manifestation, which can be life-threatening if it occurs intracranially or into the gastrointestinal tract or respiratory tract. So, these patients should be supported with platelet concentrates or single donor apheresis platelets to keep levels greater than 10,000/µL. In a patient with active bleed, platelet transfusion even at higher platelet counts is indicated.

Active bleeding in hematological patients can be due to disseminated intravascular coagulation (DIC) as well. DIC can occur due to sepsis in sick hematological patients or due to acute promyelocytic leukemia (APML). It leads to consumption coagulopathy of various coagulation factors, increased fibrinolysis, and frequent bleeding manifestations. Treatment of DIC due to sepsis includes supplementation with platelet concentrates and fresh-frozen plasma (FFP) two to three times in a day in addition to broad-spectrum antibiotics. There is no role of tranexamic acid.

Acute promyelocytic leukemia is true hematological emergency, which can be rapidly fatal if not properly managed and at the same time, it is associated with best long-term survival in trained hands. APML is most commonly caused by t(15;17) leading to formation of fusion protein (promyelocytic leukemia gene-retinoic acid receptor alpha) PML-RARα. This protein disturbs the retinoic acid signal transduction in myeloid precursor cells leading to a differentiation block and proliferation of abnormal promyelocytes. These leukemic cells express tissue factor and cancer procoagulant that can initiate coagulation. They also express increased amounts of annexin II that mediates augmented conversion of plasminogen to plasmin. The result is a state of DIC. Management includes supplementation with platelet concentrates and FFP or cryoprecipitates to maintain platelet count at least 30,000/µL and fibrinogen concentration of greater than 180 m%. Commonly, these patients present with short history of bleeding and pancytopenia on blood counts. Checking a peripheral smear for abnormal promyelocytes is very helpful and should lead to start of all-trans-retinoic acid (ATRA) or arsenic trioxide. Bone marrow studies are to be done and cytogenetic studies and PCR for PML-RARα are considered diagnostic. ATRA provides increased retinoic acid and arsenic causes breakdown of PML-RARα fusion protein and apoptosis of promyelocytes, thus removing the differentiation block and allowing normal maturation to proceed. In addition, anthracycline-based therapy should be considered early in treatment. Blood product support should be continued even after coagulation parameters have normalized and at least till complete differentiation and disappearance of promyelocytes from peripheral blood. APML, if properly treated, is associated with best long-term survival and low relapse rates among all acute leukemia.

CORD COMPRESSION

Spinal cord compression causing variable neurological compromise can occur in a host of hematological malignancies, most commonly in multiple myeloma due to vertebral collapse. It can also occur with lymphoma, plasmacytoma or granulocytic sarcoma located near vertebral canal, and compressing upon the spinal cord itself or the exiting nerves. Delay beyond 48 hours after paraparesis has set in, can lead to delayed neurological recovery and even residual paresis. Hence, diagnostic tissue should be obtained at the earliest. Necessary investigations including bone marrow or imaging should be carried out and therapy should be started.

Early consultation with radiation therapist and neurosurgeon is helpful and external-beam radiotherapy should be instituted to involved area. Many patients may require spinal decompression surgery and laminectomy, which can be done while obtaining diagnostic tissue. Steroids, usually dexamethasone are started simultaneously with radiation. In addition, definitive management with chemotherapy should be started soon to obtain systemic control of disease. Lymphoma and acute leukemia patients with paraspinal masses are at risk of central nervous system (CNS) involvement as well, and require CNS prophylaxis to prevent subsequent disease relapse in CNS. Those with positive CNS involvement require systemic chemotherapy regimens usually consisting of high-dose methotrexate with or without cytarabine.

GRAFT VERSUS HOST DISEASE (FLOW CHART 3)

Graft versus host disease (GvHD) is an immune-mediated complication of bone marrow transplant in which immunocompetent donor cells act against normal tissues in an immunocompromised host. The damage is most pronounced in skin, gut and liver in acute GvHD and can occur in any organ in chronic GvHD. Patients present with maculopapular rash in acute skin GvHD; diarrhea, abdominal pain, vomiting or persistent nausea in gut GvHD; jaundice with transaminitis in hepatic GvHD. Early treatment with steroids (usually 2 mg/kg/d of methylprednisolone, acts by direct lymphocyte toxicity and cytokine suppression) is required. Delay in starting treatment may be associated with refractoriness to initial treatment. Immunosuppression needs to be enhanced during the acute episode and continue calcineurin inhibitors (cyclosporine or tacrolimus). In steroid refractory cases, basiliximab (IL-2 receptor antagonist), methotrexate, etanercept (TNF-α inhibitor), and mycophenolate mofetil (inhibitor of inosine monophosphate dehydrogenase) are amongst the treatment options. Chronic GvHD requires long-term immunosuppression in addition to local therapy depending on organ involved. Patients should be continued on antiviral, anti-*Pneumocystis jiroveci*, and antifungal prophylaxis while on immunosuppression.

GRAFT FAILURE AND RELAPSE

Graft failure, i.e. loss of transfused donor cells that establish hematopoiesis in the host, is a dreadful complication of stem cell transplant. It can be primary (donor engraftment

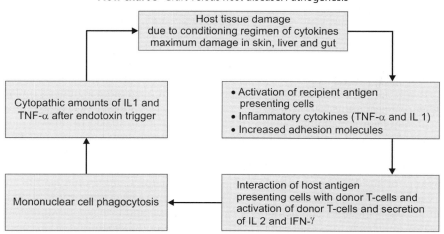

Flow chart 3 Graft versus host disease: Pathogenesis

Abbreviations: IL, interleukin; IFN, interferon; TNF, tumor necrosis factor.

never achieved) or secondary (loss of graft after initial engraftment). The host is severely pancytopenic in both circumstances with very low leukocyte counts and platelet counts less than 10,000/µL. Graft failure, although a rare event, is more frequently associated with cord transplant, haploidentical transplant, inadequate cell dose, inadequate immunosuppression or in multiple transfused host.

Management usually involves urgent second transplant with same donor or preferably another donor, if available. Without second transplant, high-mortality rates usually associated with severe infection or bleeding ensues.

Relapse of the primary disease after transplant also presents in a similar way. Such relapses are usually very aggressive and treatment refractory in nature and present with features of bone marrow infiltration and subsequent cytopenia. Treatment options are limited in most such circumstances. Repeat induction therapy followed by a second transplant or upcoming immunotherapy (chimeric antigen receptor T-cells) may be helpful in selected patients if started early, but most patients succumb to underlying disease.

CONCLUSION

Hematological malignancies are associated with serious complications. These patient are managed in intensive care unit. Post hematopoietic stem cell transplant patient are associated with higher complication rate. Few complication are specific to particular malignancies while many complications occurs all groups of patients.

BIBLIOGRAPHY

1. Ades L, Itzykson R, Fenaux P. Myelodysplastic syndromes. Lancet. 2014;383:2239-52.
2. Azoulay E, Lemiale V. Non-invasive mechanical ventilation in hematology patients with hypoxemic acute respiratory failure: a false belief? Bone Marrow Transplant. 2012;47:469-72.
3. Azoulay E, Mokart D, Lambert J, et al. Diagnostic strategy for hematology and oncology patients with acute respiratory failure: randomized controlled trial. Am J Respir Crit Care Med. 2010;182:1038-46.
4. Azoulay E, Mokart D, Pene F, et al. Outcomes of critically ill patients with hematologic malignancies: prospective multicenter data from France and Belgium—a groupe de recherche respiratoire en reanimation onco-hematologique study. J Clin Oncol. 2013;31:2810-8.
5. Azoulay E. A new standard of care for critically ill patients with cancer. Chest. 2014;146:241-4.
6. Benoit DD, Soares M, Azoulay E. Has survival increased in cancer patients admitted to the ICU? We are not sure. Intensive Care Med. 2014;40:1576-9.
7. Canet E, Lengline E, Zafrani L, Peraldi MN, Socie G, Azoulay E. Acute kidney injury in critically ill allo-HSCT recipients. Bone Marrow Transplant. 2014;49:1121-2.
8. Darmon M, Thiery G, Ciroldi M, Porcher R, Schlemmer B, Azoulay E. Should dialysis be offered to cancer patients with acute kidney injury? Intensive Care Med. 2007;33:765-72.
9. Hanahan D. Rethinking the war on cancer. Lancet. 2014;383:558-63.
10. Hilbert G, Gruson D, Vargas F, et al. Noninvasive ventilation in immunosuppressed patients with pulmonary infiltrates, fever, and acute respiratory failure. N Engl J Med. 2001;344:481-7.
11. Khassawneh BY, White Jr P, Anaissie EJ, Barlogie B, Hiller FC. Outcome from mechanical ventilation after autologous peripheral blood stem cell transplantation. Chest. 2002;121:185-8.
12. Lecuyer L, Chevret S, Guidet B, et al. Case volume and mortality in haematological patients with acute respiratory failure. Eur Respir J. 2008;32:748-54.
13. McDermott U, Downing JR, Stratton MR. Genomics and the continuum of cancer care. N Engl J Med. 2011;364:340-50.
14. Mokart D, Lambert J, Schnell D, et al. Delayed intensive care unit admission is associated with increased mortality in patients with cancer with acute respiratory failure. Leuk Lymphoma. 2013;54:1724-9.
15. Patel JD, Krilov L, Adams S, et al. Clinical cancer advances 2013: annual report on progress against cancer from the American Society of Clinical Oncology. J Clin Oncol. 2013;32:129-60.
16. Peigne V, Rusinova K, Karlin L, et al. Continued survival gains in recent years among critically ill myeloma patients. Intensive Care Med. 2009;35:512-8.
17. Pene F, Percheron S, Lemiale V, et al. Temporal changes in management and outcome of septic shock in patients with malignancies in the intensive care unit. Crit Care Med. 2008;36:690-6.
18. Pene F, Salluh JI, Staudinger T. Has survival increased in cancer patients admitted to the ICU? No. Intensive Care Med. 2014;40:1573-5.
19. Saillard C, Mokart D, Lemiale V, Azoulay E. Mechanical ventilation in cancer patients. Minerva Anestesiol. 2014;80:712-25.
20. Sant M, Minicozzi P, Mounier M, et al. Survival for haematological malignancies in Europe between 1997 and 2008 by region and age: results of EUROCARE-5, a population-based study. Lancet Oncol. 2014;15:931-42.
21. Schmatz AI, Streubel B, Kretschmer-Chott E, et al. Primary follicular lymphoma of the duodenum is a distinct mucosal/submucosal variant of follicular lymphoma: a retrospective study of 63 cases. J Clin Oncol. 2011;29:1445-51.
22. Thepot S, Itzykson R, Seegers V, et al. Azacitidine in untreated acute myeloid leukemia: a report on 149 patients. Am J Hematol. 2014;89:410-6.
23. Thiery G, Azoulay E, Darmon M, et al. Outcome of cancer patients considered for intensive care unit admission: a hospital-wide prospective study. J Clin Oncol. 2005;23:4406-13.
24. van Vliet M, Verburg IW, van den Boogaard M, et al. Trends in admission prevalence, illness severity and survival of haematological patients treated in Dutch intensive care units. Intensive Care Med. 2014;40:1275-84.
25. Winston DJ. Infections in bone marrow transplant recipients. In: Mandell GL, Besett JE, Nolin R (Eds). Principles and Practice of Infectious Disease, 4th edition. Churchill Livingstone, Inc, New York; 1995. pp. 2717-22.

SECTION 14

Trauma

- **Basics of Trauma System**
  Sandeep Jain

- **Code Trauma**
  M Sai Surendar

- **Trauma: Initial Assessment and Management**
  Khusrav Bhajan, Archana Shrivastav

- **Facial Trauma**
  Syed Ahmed Adil

- **Head Trauma**
  Devendra Richhariya, Manish Vaish

- **Spinal Trauma**
  Sudhir Dubey, Ratandeep Bose, Devendra Richhariya

- **Thoracic Trauma**
  Shaiwal Khandelwal, Ali Zamir Khan

- **Abdominal Trauma**
  Ashok Kumar Puranik, Devendra Richhariya

- **Extremity Trauma and Management of Fractures in Emergency**
  Ritabh Kumar

- **Emergency Wound Management and Closure**
  Aditya Aggarwal, Vimalendu Brajesh, Sukhdeep Singh, Umang B Kothari, Rakesh K Khazanchi

- **Radiology in Emergency and Trauma**
  Sonal Krishan

- **Disaster and Mass Casualty Management in Emergency**
  Devendra Richhariya, TS Srinath Kumar, Tamorish Kole

CHAPTER 80

Basics of Trauma System

Sandeep Jain

DEFINITION

Trauma can be defined as any harm imparted to the body of a living organism, by an external physical force having a potential to threaten life or limb. When the trauma involves multiple body parts or organ systems, it is called as polytrauma or multisystem trauma.

Magnitude of Problem

Trauma is one of the leading causes of death and disability worldwide. Accidental deaths are on a rise. In 2014, more than 4.5 lacs deaths were reported due to accidents, both natural and unnatural. An increase of 12.8% in accidental deaths was reported in 2014 as compared to 2013. Every hour 52 deaths are occurring due to trauma. According to World Health Organization report on global burden of disease, by 2020 road traffic accidents will be the third leading cause of death. Trauma usually is the disease of young population between the age group of 15 years and 45 years, thereby depriving the whole family of its breadwinner. This not only causes a loss of life of an individual but many a times leaves the family in huge financial debts incurred for medical treatment of the deceased.

Trimodal Distribution of Death

Trimodal distribution of deaths due to trauma was first described by Donald Trunkey in 1983. The deaths have classically been defined to occur in three distinct phases: (1) immediate, (2) early, and (3) late.

Immediate deaths occur due to the impact at the time of accident, within seconds to minutes after trauma. It is usually caused by severe traumatic brain injury, rupture of great vessels or cardiac chambers and high cervical spine injury. These deaths can only be prevented by injury prevention measures.

Early deaths are those which occur within minutes to hours after the accident. It is usually due to hemorrhage, pneumothorax, airway obstruction, etc. These deaths can be prevented by providing immediate, appropriate, and adequate care, so-called "golden hour" treatment. This needs availability of trained manpower. The focus of prehospital care is in reduction of deaths in this phase only.

Late deaths are those which occur within hours to days after trauma. These occur due to sepsis and multiorgan failure. A good primary resuscitation and critical care is the key to good outcomes.

Epidemiology

Trauma can be caused by natural or unnatural factors.

Natural factors are caused by forces of nature. In 2014, more than 20,000 deaths were caused by natural factors such as lightning, landslides, heat stroke, and exposure to cold. These are mostly seen in poor socioeconomic status people. Factors such as poverty, lack of sanitation, malnutrition, and inadequate access to healthcare are contributory.

Unnatural deaths are due to road traffic accidents, railway accidents, fire, drowning, electrocution, falls, suicides, and homicides. In 2014, more than 3 lacs deaths and more than 5 lacs injuries were reported due to unnatural accidents. Road traffic accidents constitutes the largest group with 1.5 lac deaths. Majority of patients are in the productive age group of 18–45 years with males outnumbering females. In the current scenario, terrorist attacks are also becoming a major cause of trauma deaths.

SYSTEM

Trauma care is a national health issue and the government-controlled system. A trauma system is a coordinated system of healthcare delivery which aims to provide rapid access to optimal trauma care to an injured. Major components are: prehospital care, acute hospital care, and posthospital rehabilitation.

Prehospital Care

Early detection of the injury and activation of emergency medical services (EMS) is paramount in prehospital care. Injuries can occur anywhere and a good prehospital care can ensure better survivals. Most of the injuries are attended first by a relative, friend, passerby or local police. Awareness about early detection and activation of EMS by the members of the society will ensure access to the appropriate medical care within the "golden hour". This needs good ambulance services and methods to access them. Currently, India does not have a robust EMS. There is severe shortage of adequately equipped ambulances and trained personnel. Although 108 ambulance services are available in many states, still the need is much more. There are EMS services in private hospitals but they are usually for interfacility transfers. A centrally coordinated ambulance service with mapping through general packet radio service (GPRS) can help in proper distribution and optimization of the resources.

There is a need to train first responders in basic life support and first aid measures to minimize damage. There is a further need to have trained paramedics in the ambulances and the networking of hospitals, based on the resources available, so that patient can be treated at an appropriately equipped hospital. Structured courses like International Trauma Life support and prehospital trauma life support provide good training in prehospital care.

Acute Hospital Care

After the patient reaches the hospital, it becomes incumbent on the medical team to rapidly triage, resuscitate, and provide definitive treatment to the patient. Round the clock availability of the surgeons with skills to manage injuries, operation theaters, and critical care facility is the main limiting factors in providing optimum trauma care. Majority of the hospitals in India lack these facilities. In USA, all hospitals providing trauma care are designated from level I–IV based on the available resources. Level I is the highest care center with capabilities to provide comprehensive trauma care including training and research. They are equivalent to University Hospitals in India. Level III centers also provide comprehensive trauma care but do not provide training and research. They are equivalent to district hospitals where specialists are available but superspecialists are lacking. Level II centers have basic facilities but lack specialized personnel and equipment. They are equivalent to community health center. A level IV trauma center provides only basic trauma resuscitation and is equivalent to primary health center.

Posthospital Rehabilitation

Majority of severely injured patients needs long convalescence period before a fruitful return to activity. This involves care of hygiene and nutrition along with physical exercises for which patients cannot be hospitalized. Comprehensive trauma care is incomplete, if patients do not get proper post-discharge care. Each hospital has its own support service departments like physiotherapy, occupational therapy, social support and rehabilitation. Polytrauma patients also suffer from post-traumatic psychiatric stress disorder which many a times needs help from psychologists and psychiatrists. To ensure smooth transition from acute care to rehabilitation and follow-up after discharge, dedicated personnel are required at these centers.

MECHANISM OF INJURY

Injury is produced as a result of transfer of energy to the body of patient. Energy can neither be produced nor destroyed and can only change its form. Moreover, the energy produced is the product of mass and the velocity.

$$KE \text{ (kinetic energy)} = \frac{1}{2} m \text{ (mass)} \times v^2 \text{ (velocity)}$$

Therefore, severity and distribution of injuries are dependent on the site of impact, direction of the force vector, mass and velocity of the striking objects. Knowledge of the mechanism of injury helps trauma care professionals in reconstructing the method of energy transfer and look out proactively for the occult injuries, thereby preventing missed injuries and improving survivals.

Injuries are produced due to two main mechanisms: (1) blunt trauma and (2) penetrating trauma.

Blunt Trauma

Blunt trauma is caused due to motor vehicle accidents, automobile-pedestrian injury, assaults, and falls.

Motor Vehicle Accidents

Risk of injury to the occupants of the motor vehicle is dependent on the size and mass of the vehicle, location of the person within the vehicle, use and type of restraint, and the direction of the impact. The injuries are due to sudden loss of inertia of motion as the vehicle along with the body comes to a sudden halt. These are also called as deceleration injuries.

- Higher the mass and size of the vehicle, lesser is the chance of the injury as the vehicle absorbs the majority of energy during the crash.
- Restraints such as seat belts are effective in preventing a serious injury only if they are worn correctly. Unrestrained occupants have a higher chance of injury. Three-point restraints are the best in protecting against significant injuries. Lap belts alone produce a higher incidence

of abdominal injury and chance fractures of lumbar spine. Airbags prevent major injuries during primary frontal-impact collisions but are ineffective in secondary collisions as they are deflated during this time. Helmets worn properly have shown a 50% reduction in the incidence of severe head injuries and have substantially reduced mortality.

- Injuries are produced in a predictable patterns based on the direction of the impact. Crashes have been defined in four categories:
  1. *Frontal impact*: These occur when the vehicle crashes head on. This is the most common type of crash and usually occurs during high-speed driving. Seat belts and airbags are maximally effective in preventing serious injuries in this type of crash. Unrestrained drivers are likely to get injuries to head, face, cervical spine, thorax (steering wheel injury), abdomen, and central fracture dislocation of the hip.
  2. *Lateral impact*: These are side on collisions and can happen either from the driver side or the passenger side. In India, with a right-hand drive system an impact from driver side causes flexion injuries to the cervical spine, chest injuries, and abdominal injuries especially to liver and right kidney along with lateral compression injuries to pelvis and long bones. Passenger side impacts cause injury to the left-sided organs.
  3. *Rear-end impact*: Injuries are less severe when vehicle is hit from behind as the luggage compartment absorbs most of the injuries but this is not true for those vehicles with very small luggage compartment. Passengers get injuries as they are frequently unrestrained and due to the impact are tossed against the front seats. Injuries produced are those to face and cervical spine (whiplash injuries), thorax and lower extremities.
  4. *Rollover collisions*: These produce unpredictable injury patterns as force vectors change directions. In restrained passengers, the injuries are minimized. Unrestrained passengers can be ejected out of the vehicle and cause severe injuries.

Pedestrian Accidents

Pedestrians hit by a moving vehicle produce three types of injuries:
1. *Primary injuries*: These are caused when the vehicle hits the pedestrian, usually causing injuries to lower extremities.
2. *Secondary injuries*: These occur when the pedestrian after the first impact is thrown and hits against the hood or windscreen of the vehicle causing injuries to the head, face, thorax or abdomen.
3. *Tertiary injuries*: These are caused when the victim impacts the ground after being hit and can be run over causing injuries to head, thorax, abdomen, pelvis or extremities.

Falls

Injury patterns depend upon the mass of the victim, height of the fall, body part that impacts the ground and the surface of the ground. Higher the mass and the height of the fall, more severe are the injuries. In falls with landing on feet, the force transmits vertically causing fractures of the calcaneum, tibia, femur, hip, and spine. Head-first impacts cause severe head and cervical spine injuries and have a higher mortality rates. Tumbling on stairs causes multisystem injuries. Comorbidities especially in older people adversely affect the morbidity and mortality.

Assaults

These injuries depend upon the object used, area of the body hit, position of the patient, and the intensity of the attack.

Penetrating Trauma

Penetrating trauma is caused by an object, which penetrates the tissue. The injury severity and pattern depends upon the type of weapon, velocity of the projectiles, and the distance from which it is fired. Based on the velocity, weapons are classified into three categories: (1) high energy, (2) medium energy, and (3) low energy.

1. *High energy*: These weapons transfer energy at a rate higher than 2,000 ft/sec (600 m/sec). Weapons that cause these types of injuries are machine guns, rifles, carbines, and automatic guns. Due to the high speed, the tissue gets damaged not only along the path of the missile but at right angles to the path as well. This is called as cavitation effect. The amount of cavitation is determined by the surface area of the point of impact, the density of the tissue and the speed of the projectile. Higher the surface area and the speed of the projectile, higher is the cavitation and the resultant collateral damage.
2. *Medium energy*: These are weapons with a muzzle velocity of about 1,200 ft/sec (360 m/sec). Shotguns, pistol, and revolver fall predominantly in this category. They use multiple pellets, which gets distributed in a conical fashion after the fire and thus causes injury due to higher surface area of impact. The cavitation effect is lesser and these inflict lethal injuries if fired from close range. They can carry wads and the clothing along the tract.
3. *Low energy*: These weapons have a velocity lower than 600 ft/sec (180 m/sec). Common weapons are knives, needles, daggers or any hand-driven metal weapon. The injury is produced along the path of the blade of the weapon. The depth of the wound is usually more than the width of the wound. If a long object is driven into the body and is still present at the time of presentation to the hospital, it is called as "impalement injury". This object should not be removed outside the operation theater.

Prehospital Care

Prehospital care, ambulance services or EMS is an important component of healthcare delivery. It is the first critical link in "golden hour" treatment of trauma victim. It provides out-of-hospital medical care to the patient during a medical or surgical emergency. The initial treatment received in the field often determines the outcome of the patient. The aim of prehospital trauma care is to provide the basic life support measures to a victim at the site and transport him to the nearest appropriate hospital. Thus, it acts as a bridge between the time of injury and access to definitive care.

Key Elements

There are six key elements of a prehospital care system: (1) detection, (2) activation, (3) response, (4) on-site care, (5) en route care, and (6) transport to a definitive care facility:
1. *Detection*: It is of paramount importance that a person near the victim is able to recognize the need for an EMS. If the passerby ignores the condition and fails to call for help, it leads to delay in getting the care and poor outcome. In India, at present, the situation is grim with most of the public failing to help the trauma victim for fear of trouble by police or the court. This can only be improved with increasing awareness. The upcoming "Good Samaritan Law" which has provisions of avoiding the trouble to the person helping the victim is expected to motivate people.
2. *Activation*: All EMS services can be activated by a simple telephonic call; however, multiplicity of the services and their activation numbers in India is a limiting factor in recall. A single national helpline number for activation is likely to improve the activation rate and time.
3. *Response*: The EMS is expected to respond to the call promptly. With improved communication systems and mapping of the ambulances through global positioning system, the response time can be reduced and care provided early. Also physician presence in the call center helps by providing medical direction till the arrival of care at scene.
4. *On-site care*: The ambulance team is trained to provide basic life support measures such as airway and breathing maintenance, control of hemorrhage, splinting of fractures and then shift the patient to the nearest appropriate facility.
5. *En route care*: As trauma care is a dynamic process, continuous monitoring and treatment during transit provides the continuity of optimum care till arrival in the trauma center. This may include measures such as oxygen supplementation, intravenous fluid, and drug administration, etc.
6. *Transport to definitive care facility*: Best patient outcomes are recorded when the patient is transported to an appropriate facility based on the triage category. Shifting a seriously ill-trauma patient to a hospital which is not equipped to handle such cases results in treatment delays and adversely affects the patient survival.

Levels of Prehospital Care

Out-of the hospital trauma care can be provided at three levels:
1. *First responder care*: Police, fire brigade, community volunteers, and laypersons who are trained in providing immediate first aid provide this care. They are involved in detection and activation of EMS, rescue and assessment of the victim and initiation of basic life support measures.
2. *Basic trauma care*: This care is provided by the volunteers, paramedics or emergency medical technicians who have undergone the formal training in prehospital trauma care, extrication, resuscitation and stabilization, and transportation techniques.
3. *Advanced trauma care*: This care is provided by the formally trained paramedics or nurses with or without a trauma physician who have received advanced training in airway and ventilation management such as intubation, cricothyroidotomy and needle decompression of the chest, hemorrhage control and use of intravenous fluids and drugs.

Principles of Prehospital Care

Most of the EMS systems follow either of the two principles. However, there is no proven benefit of one over the other. Each system has to make a balance based on their own experiences and area of operations.
1. *Scoop and run*: This principle envisages the basic trauma care at scene by trained paramedics and early transport to the trauma center in an equipped ambulance. Further care such as advanced airway techniques, intravenous fluid administration, etc. is provided en route. This is followed all over in US, UK, Australia, and Asian countries. This is intended to prevent delay to definitive care facility.
2. *Stay and play*: In France and Germany, a trained physician accompanies the advanced life support ambulance and patient receives full resuscitation and stabilization at scene before transport to the trauma center.

Modes of Transport

All EMS providers transport the victim by either a road ambulance or the air ambulance. Whatever the mode used, the goal remains early trauma care and rapid transport. Majority of EMS providers across the world are experienced in ground transport by fully equipped ambulances with all lifesaving equipment and drugs along with advanced monitoring devices. This provides good space to provide en route treatment; this is easy to operate and is less expensive. Air transport is provided through either helicopter or fixed-wing aircrafts. This is more resource intensive and needs highly-skilled personnel and thus is more expensive. It has a proven benefit when the site of accident is difficult to reach and the distance to the appropriate trauma center is more.

Prehospital Trauma Care in India

Various prehospital care agencies are working at present in India, both by government and private organizations. However, a uniform emergency medical system is still lacking in the country. Centralized Accident and Trauma Services (CATS) in Delhi was the first such service in country. Emergency Management Research Institute (EMRI) started the first comprehensive EMS system through a public private partnership model in Andhra Pradesh. Through 108 ambulance services this system is being provided in majority of states in south, north and eastern India. Ambulance Motorbike and Rescue Services (AMARS) was started in Punjab and Himachal Pradesh to provide faster care in areas where the ground ambulances cannot reach due to either narrow lanes or difficult terrain. With coming of corporate hospitals in urban areas, majority of the hospitals are providing ambulance services but still the demand is high and distribution uneven. Moreover, there is a scarcity of trained paramedics for these ambulances.

TRAUMA SCORING SYSTEM

All trauma patients need to be transported to a trauma center in a quick time. Appropriate triage is mandatory to optimize resource utilization which is scarce. Undertriage prevents early access to a hospital capable to treat severely injured patient leading to increased mortality and morbidity. Overtriage leads to inundation of hospitals by less severely injured patient, which can be easily managed at a less resource-intensive hospital.

Various trauma scoring systems have been defined to aid paramedics in appropriate triage. These also help in objectively defining the severity of injury, prediction of outcome, statistical analysis of diagnostic and therapeutic interventions and thereby ensuring quality improvement.

The scoring systems are based on measurement of physiological, anatomical or a combination of these parameters.

Physiological Parameters

Glasgow Coma Scale

This scale measures the state of consciousness by measuring eye opening (E), best motor (M), and verbal response (V). Score in each of the component is summed to calculate final score. Minimum score is 3 and maximum score is 15. A score of 8 or less implies deep coma **(Table 1)**.

Although it is a good score but is limited in patients who have been paralyzed, intubated or cannot open eyes due to periorbital injuries. Thus, motor response is the most reliable component.

AVPU Scale

This is a very simple tool for prehospital personnel for evaluating the consciousness level of the patient.
A: Alert
V: Response to verbal commands
P: Response to painful stimulus
U: Unresponsive.

Revised Trauma Score

This score measures Glasgow Coma Scale, systolic blood pressure, and respiratory rate. Each parameter is coded from 0–4 **(Table 2)**. Minimum is 0 and maximum is 12. Any coded value of three or less need a transport to a trauma center.

Pediatric Trauma Score

This score is used to simplify triaging in this population by measurement of critical components needed for initial assessment of severely injured patients. A pediatric trauma score of 8 and more is indicative of good prognosis. It measures weight, status of airway, systolic blood pressure, level of consciousness, presence of fractures, and the state of skin.

Anatomical Parameters

These scores are good for comparative and statistical analysis of injury severity and prediction outcomes, as full extent

Table 1 Glasgow coma scale

Eye opening	Motor response	Verbal response	Score
Spontaneous	Obeys commands	Oriented	1
To verbal commands	Localizes pain	Confused	2
To painful stimuli	Withdraws to pain	Inappropriate words	3
None	Abnormal flexion	Incomprehensible sounds	4
	Extension to pain	None	5
	None		6

Table 2 Revised trauma score

Glasgow coma scale	Systolic blood pressure	Respiratory rate	Coded value
13–15	>89	10–29	4
9–12	76–89	>29	3
6–8	50–75	6–9	2
4–5	1–49	1–5	1
3	0	0	0

can only be known after a thorough diagnostic process. Therefore, they are less useful in the field for triaging. They define injuries based on anatomical regions affected.

Abbreviated Injury Scale

This scale quantifies injury to each of the organs. Each organ injury is graded from 1 (minor injury) to 6 (lethal injury). There are hundreds of injuries thus defined. This score defines the severity of injury in each of the organ system but lacks the grading of injury severity in a patient as a whole.

Injury Severity Score

This score is calculated by summing the squares of three highest injury scales of abbreviated injury scale (AIS) in different anatomic regions: head, neck and face, thorax and abdomen, pelvis and extremities, and external structures. The minimum score is 1 and maximum score is 75. Any AIS score of 6 automatically makes injury severity score (ISS) equivalent to 75 (lethal injury). An ISS score of greater than 16 is considered as severe injury.

CONCLUSION

The ideal trauma system should deliver the wide range of care to all injured patient and is important aspect of public healthcare system. Success of the trauma system is largely determined by the seamless services in each phase of care and improved patient outcome. Trauma system must emphasize the prevention of injuries

BIBLIOGRAPHY

1. American College of Surgeons. Advanced Trauma Life support for Doctors Student Course Manual, 9th edition; 2012. p. 366.
2. Anand LK, Singh M, Kapoor D. Prehospital trauma care services in developing countries. Anaesth Pain & Intensive Care. 2013;17(1):65-70.
3. Champion HR, Sacco WJ, Copes WS, et al. A revision of the trauma score. J Trauma. 1989;29(5):623-9.
4. Gold CR. Prehospital advanced life support vs "scoop and run" in trauma management. Ann Emerg Med. 1987;16(7):797-801.
5. John Campbell. International Trauma Life Support for Emergency Care Providers, 7th edition. Pearson education; 2013.
6. National Crime Records Bureau. (2014). Accidental Deaths and Suicides in India. [online]. Available from *ncrb.nic.in/StatPublications/ADSI/ADSI2014/adsi-2014%20full%20report.pdf.* [Accessed January, 2017].
7. National Highway Traffic Safety Administration. "Star of Life": Emergency Medical Care Symbol-Background: Specifications, and Criteria. US, Washington: Department of Transportation, National Highway Traffic Safety Administration; 1995.
8. Peitzman AB, Rhodes M, Schwab CW, et al. The Trauma Manual, 2nd edition. Philadelphia: Lippincott Williams & Wilkins; 2002.
9. Sasser S, Varghese M, Kellermann A, et al. Prehospital trauma care systems. Geneva: World Health Organization; 2005.

Chapter 81

Code Trauma

M Sai Surendar

INTRODUCTION

Code trauma is the basic need for any emergency department (ED) to handle trauma cases as best as possible in a nation with the highest trauma burden in the world. Indian Emergency physicians play a significant role in reducing the trauma mortality in the country. This chapter will outline the concept of code trauma and how to inculcate code trauma in the hospital to manage trauma patients more effectively.

OVERVIEW

Death due to trauma is the third leading cause of death all over the world. Leading cause of death in age group 20–40 years has a great impact on family, as major population involves students and office goers. Inappropriate use of traffic signs, nonusage of seat belts, and drunken diving are the main reasons in the back drop.

It contributes to the highest medical costs and maximum numbers of life long disabilities. Code trauma is an effort to coordinate and improvise the efforts involved in trauma management in the Indian scenario.

STATISTICS

Statistically, India has the highest number of road accidents in the world. India is the accident capital of the world. With 130,000 deaths annually, the country has overtaken China. World Health Organization (WHO) in its first ever Global Status Report on Road Safety states that speeding, drunk driving, and low use of helmets, seat belts and child restraints in vehicles are the main contributing factors. Every hour, 40 people under the age of 25 die in road accidents around the globe. According to the WHO, this is the second most important cause of death for 5–29-year olds.

WHAT IS GOLDEN HOUR?

The golden hour starts at the time of injury. It is the first hour following a trauma during which aggressive resuscitation can improve the chances of survival, minimize secondary injury, and restore the normal functions. Early prehospital care, early transport, aggressive resuscitation and interventions in ED, and continued care in intensive care unit (ICU) have definite and significant roles in preventing deaths due to trauma in the golden hour, platinum minutes, and the diamond seconds **(Figs 1A and B)**.

Big Threat

- Every 1.9 minutes someone dies of trauma
- 80% accident victims do not access medical care within the golden hour
- 30% of emergency patients die before they reach a hospital
- 69% of road accident victims suffer from traumatic brain injury (TBI)
- 70% of death and injuries occur among men 15–44 years of age.

Trimodal Pattern of Mortality

Three modes of presentation of trauma are:
1. *Prehospital*: Devastating head and major vascular injuries
2. *Emergency department*: Major head, chest, and abdominal injuries
3. *Intensive care unit*: Organ hypoperfusion, systemic inflammatory response syndrome (SIRS), and multiple organ dysfunction (MOD) syndromes.

Deaths commonly occur due to:
- Inadequate prehospital care (delay in scene treatment and safety)

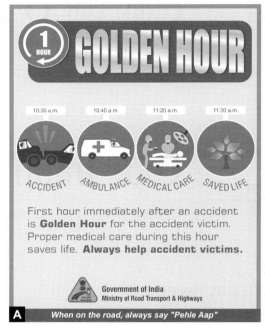
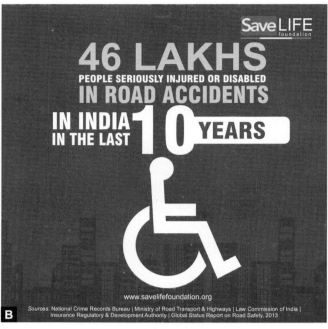

Figs 1A and B (A) Golden hour after trauma; (B) Road accidents in India

- In-hospital delays or delay in coordination between expertise in the golden hour due to multifactorial reasons. Deaths occur more in the golden hour due to the delayed action on scene leading to increase in mortality.

CODE TRAUMA

Definition

The code trauma team consists of a group of doctors, emergency physician and orthopedic, general surgeon and neurosurgeon, nurses, operating theater (OT) assistants, radiographers, and other support personnel who have no other commitment that day but only to receive and treat trauma patients in a coordinated and synchronized fashion. The new lifeline for trauma management for emergency physicians is to provide early evaluation and identification of all the injuries and definitive treatment.

Code Trauma Team

Trauma team can be team of more than 10 people working for a single patient. Ideally trauma team consists of emergency team, surgeons, critical care specialist and other supportive staff as shown in **Table 1**. Members of code trauma team positioned around the trauma victims as shown in **Fig. 2**. Every member of the team should know his/her work. Vital signs should be recorded and informed every 5 minutes.

When do you call a trauma code? For every trauma patient, the answer is a big no. Only when the scope or the magnitude of the trauma satisfies the following criteria:

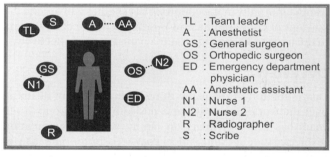

Fig. 2 Positioning of members of code trauma team

- *Criteria for code trauma activation* (**Table 2**):
  - Mechanical factors
  - Anatomical factors
  - Physiological factors
- *Modified trauma team activation criteria*:
  - Injury to extremities with pulse deficit
  - Altered mental status (i.e. head injury or intoxication) that require diagnostic evaluation of the abdomen
  - Burns associated with trauma
  - Two or more proximal long bone fractures
  - Amputation proximal to ankle or wrist
  - Unstable pelvis with possible fracture
  - Multiple (three or more) rib fractures, flail chest, hemothorax or pneumothorax
  - Pregnancy more than 20 weeks
  - Severe mechanism of injury:
    - Collision with ejection
    - Death of occupant in vehicle

Table 1 Code trauma team members

Emergency team	Surgeons	Who need early notification?
• Emergency consultant • Emergency physician • Head nurse • Emergency nurse • Paramedics • Manager • General duty assistant	• General surgeon • Neurosurgeon • Orthopedic surgeon • Thoracic surgeon • Vascular surgeon • Plastic surgeon • Critical care specialist	• Radiologist • Radiographer • Hematologist and biochemist (to receive and process samples) • Blood bank • Radiologist • Computed tomography scanner • Operation theaters

Table 2 Criteria for activation of code trauma team

Mechanical factors	Anatomical factors	Physiological factors
• High speed impact and collision • Fatal accident • Fall from height more than 15 feet	• Airway obstruction • Polytrauma • Penetrating injuries • Head injury • Spinal injury • Vascular injury amputation	• Low GCS • Hypotension • Heart rate >150 beats/min • Respiratory rate <10 or >30 breaths/minute

- Intrusion more than 12 inches into patient compartment or more than 18 inches (any compartment)
- Adult falls more than 20 feet
- Child (<15 years) fall more than 10 feet or 2–3 times height
- Auto versus pedestrian or bicycle with significant impact, speed more than 20 mph or separation of rider from motorcycle.

Roles and Responsibilities

- *Team leader*: Team leader should be most experienced and he/she should be present before arrival of patient and all the members should take the directions from the team leader. Roles of team leader include:
  - Obtain accurate history from paramedics about mechanism of injuries and prehospital care. Talk to relatives who brought the patient
  - Give instruction to all team members
  - Establish priorities and give order for investigation procedures and management
  - Interpret all results of investigations
  - Coordination with other specialties
  - Management of fluid, blood, and blood products
  - Briefing and debriefing the trauma team
  - Closely and regularly monitor the status of the patient.
- *Emergency attending consultant/physician*:
  - Airway management
  - Stabilization of cervical spine
  - Ventilation
  - Intravenous access central line insertion
  - Vital stabilization and monitoring
  - Fluid and drug administration monitoring
  - Pain management
  - Chest tube insertion
  - Urinary catheterization
  - Reassess...Reassess....Reassess.

The mantra of code trauma is to always reassess frequently to avoid and minimize errors.

- *General surgeon*:
  - Primary survey
  - Examination of the thorax, abdomen, and head
  - Identification of head and facial injuries
  - Chest tube insertion
  - Tracheostomy, if needed.
- *Orthopedic surgeon*:
  - Examination of spine and pelvis
  - External fixator application
  - Examination of limb injury
  - Dressing of wounds and stabilization of fractures.
- *Nurse incharge*:
  - One nurse should be entirely dedicated to the orders of the ED physician
  - Help each hands-on surgeon or ED physician and assist in their tasks
  - The nurses should not leave the resuscitation room to fetch equipment other supporting staff should provide this.
- *Radiology assistant*:
  - Start taking all X-rays as per trauma series cervical spine, chest, and pelvis, unless directed otherwise
  - Provide all X-ray films
  - Coordination with computed tomography (CT) scan room.

- *Manager*:
  - To keep the record of the trauma call
  - Arrival time of each member of team
  - Record medicolegal case
  - Coordination with family members and give them support
  - Handing over the belongings
  - *Vital signs*: Urine output, Glasgow coma scale
  - Coordinate with X-rays, CT scan room, and laboratory for early results
  - Coordinate with the OT incharge
  - Disposal of patient.

ADVANTAGES OF CODE TRAUMA

Advantages of code trauma are:
- Team effort reflects as the outcome
- Door to scalpel time reduced
- Hospital stay, morbidity, and mortality reduction
- More team work and team spirit.

GOALS TO KEEP IN MIND IN CODE TRAUMA

Goals to be kept in mind in code trauma are:
- Priorities in management and resuscitation
- Assumption of most serious injuries
- Treatment before diagnosis
- Thorough examination
- Frequent reassessment
- Monitoring
- Every minutes counts
- Right intervention at right time can be lifesaving....!!

CONCLUSION

- As a healthcare personnel, we have to realize the importance of the golden hour
- Code trauma is the need for any ED to handle life-threatening trauma patients
- If delayed, we may lose life because... *time is life*
- Code trauma is needed for every ED in India
- Inculcate code trauma in ED
- Manage trauma in a better way
- Save lives as many as possible in the golden hour.

BIBLIOGRAPHY

1. American College of Surgeons Committee on Trauma. Resources for Optimal Care of the Injured Patient. Chicago, IL: American College of Surgeons Committee on Trauma; 2006.
2. Ehrlich PF, Rockwell, S, Kincaid S, et al. American College of Surgeons, and Committee on Trauma verification review: does it really make a difference? J Trauma. 2002;53(5):811-6.
3. MacKenzie EJ, Rivara FP, Jurkovich GJ, et al. A national evaluation of the effect of trauma-center care on mortality. N Engl J Med. 2006;354(4):366-78.
4. Norwood S, Fernandez L, England J. The early effects of implementing American College of Surgeons level II criteria on transfer and survival rates at a rurally based community hospital. J Trauma. 1995;39(2):240-5.
5. Piontek FA, Coscia R, Marselle CS, et al. Impact of American College of Surgeons verification on trauma outcomes. J Trauma. 2003;54(6):1041-7.

Chapter 82

Trauma: Initial Assessment and Management

Khusrav Bajan, Archana Shrivastav

INTRODUCTION

India, the world's largest democracy and second most populous country, is in the midst of an economic boon and, hence, is in the phase of domestic product growth and hike in standard of living. There is an overall increase in incidence of polytrauma as a consequence of increased urbanization and industrialization. The World Health Organization (WHO) has predicted that trauma-related deaths in India will move up from the ninth position up to the third position by the year 2020.

But unfortunately, despite this overall economic growth, we are still lacking in effective system of delivering trauma care and emergency services to majority of our citizens.

The National Crime Records Bureau in India reported that in 2010, at least 10.1% deaths were due to road traffic accidents and injuries. There were a total of 678,326 cases of accidents, which caused 359,583 deaths and 503,932 people were rendered injured and the affected population belonged to productive age group of 15–44 years.

In this chapter, we will discuss the initial assessment and management of polytrauma patient.

TRAUMA MORTALITY: A TRIMODAL DISTRIBUTION

Immediate Deaths

Immediate deaths usually occur within the first hour and include death on spots. Major vascular, brain, and cardiac injuries are main causes. Approximately 50% of trauma-related deaths are immediate deaths.

Early Deaths

Deaths occurring within hours are included in early deaths. The main causes are hemorrhage and breathing issues.

Late Deaths

Late deaths occur after 3 days and peak at 3–4 weeks. The main causes are sepsis and multiorgan failure **(Figs 1 and 2)**.

Objectives

- To identify the *correct sequence of priorities* for assessment of polytrauma patient and *triage*.
- To know and apply the principles outlined in *primary and secondary surveys*.
- To apply guidelines and techniques to *initial management* and *definitive care*.

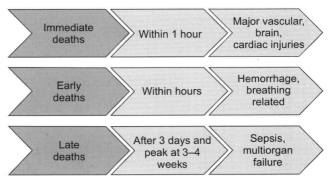

Fig. 1 Trimodal distribution deaths in polytrauma

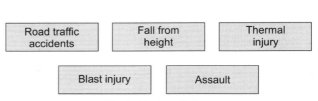

Fig. 2 Modes of injury

- To explain how patient's *medical history* and *mechanism of injury* contribute to the identification of injuries.
- To *re-evaluate*, when patient is not responding appropriately to resuscitation and management.
- To understand importance of *teamwork*.
- To recognize patients who will require *safe transfer* for definitive management.

SYSTEMATIC APPROACH FOR MANAGEMENT OF TRAUMA PATIENT

Systematic approach includes:
- Be prepared
- Triage
- Primary survey
- Resuscitation
- Secondary survey
- Monitoring, definitive treatment and transfer.

Preparation

Preparation for a trauma patient occurs in two different clinical settings:

Prehospital phase: Prehospital phase refers to field management. It includes the following principles:
- To notify the receiving hospital before transport of patient from scene, so as to allow time for mobilization of personnel and resources beforehand only
- Airway maintenance
- Control of external bleeding and shock
- Immobilization of patient
- Immediate transfer to closest healthcare facility, preferably a verified trauma center.

Hospital phase: It includes:
- A resuscitation area should be made available
- Airway equipment should be organized, checked, and placed in accessible location
- Warmed intravenous crystalloid solutions should be made available
- Appropriate monitoring devices should be made available
- To call for additional medical assistance
- To notify laboratory and radiology personnel
- Standard precaution gears are mandatory due to concerns of communicable diseases.

Triage

Triage involves the sorting of patients based on their needs for treatment and the resources available to provide that treatment. It also involves the sorting of patients in the field so that a decision can be made regarding the appropriate receiving medical facility.

Box 1 ABCDE sequences of primary survey

- Airway maintenance with cervical spine protection
- Breathing and ventilation
- Circulation with hemorrhage control
- *Disability*: Neurologic status
- *Exposure or environmental*: Completely undress the patient, but prevent hypothermia

Primary Survey

In primary survey, patient is quickly assessed and treatment priorities are established based on injuries, mechanism of injuries and hemodynamic status of patient. ABCDE sequence needs to be followed in **Box 1**.

Assessment in 10 Seconds

A quick assessment of trauma patient can be made by asking for his or her name, and asking what happened. An appropriate response suggests:

Airway: No major airway compromise—ability to speak clearly.

Breathing: Adequate breathing—ability to generate air movement to permit speech.

Circulation and disability: No major decrease in level of consciousness and adequate perfusion—alert enough to describe.

Airway Maintenance with Cervical Spine Protection

The airway patency should be assessed first in initial assessment of any trauma patient. The following points are of consideration:
- Look for signs of airway obstruction
- Inspect for foreign bodies, facial or tracheal/laryngeal fractures
- For airway patency, chin-lift or jaw-thrust maneuver is recommended with C-spine immobilization **(Figs 3 and 4)**. Chin-lift maneuver should not hyperextend the neck
- As a rule, assume cervical spine instability
- Patients with Glasgow coma score of 8 or less warrant placement of definitive airway
- Loss of cervical spine stability should be assumed till evaluation and diagnosis of specific spine injury in all trauma patients, especially those with blunt multisystem trauma, altered level of consciousness, and blunt injury above clavicle
- Cervical spine should be immobilized by appropriate devices

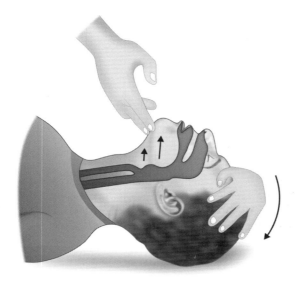

Fig. 3 Chin-lift maneuver

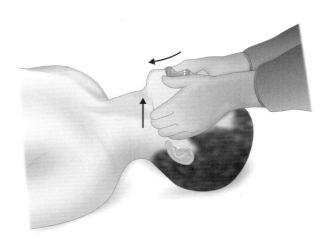

Fig. 4 Jaw-thrust maneuver

- When immobilization device needs to be removed temporarily then C-spine should be manually stabilized **(Figs 5A to D)**
- Frequent re-evaluation for airway patency is necessary.

Breathing and Ventilation

- Patient's neck and chest should be adequately exposed
- Inspect for jugular venous distension, position of trachea, chest wall excursion, and obvious injuries
- Auscultate for air entry bilaterally
- Percussion of thorax
- Tension pneumothorax, flail chest with pulmonary contusion, massive hemothorax, and open pneumothorax should be identified during primary survey, as these can severely impair ventilation in short time.

Circulation with Hemorrhage Control

Once tension pneumothorax has been ruled out as cause of shock, hypovolemia should be considered as the cause of hypotension following trauma, until proven otherwise.
- Level of consciousness, skin color, and pulse are important tools **(Flow chart 1)**.
- The source of bleeding should be identified as either external or internal **(Flow chart 2)**.

Disability

- Assess for patient's level of consciousness, pupillary size and reaction, lateralizing signs, spinal cord injury level.
- Glasgow coma scale is quick and simple method for assessment **(Table 1)**.

- *Altered level of consciousness indicates*: Impaired cerebral oxygenation and perfusion or direct brain injury.

Exposure and Environment Control

- Remove patient's clothing and perform thorough examination and assessment
- Prevent hypothermia by covering the patient with warm blankets or external warming devices
- Infuse warm intravenous fluids
- Provide warm environment by maintaining room temperature.

Resuscitation

- Airway should be addressed first
- Ensure adequate ventilation and oxygenation
- Pulse oximetry should be used for monitoring
- Aim for definitive control of bleeding along with appropriate replacement of intravascular volume
- Establish two wide bore peripheral intravenous accesses
- Consider cutdowns and central line as need be
- At the time of IV insertion, blood should be collected for baseline hematological studies, blood group and cross match, and pregnancy test for all females of childbearing age
- Always infuse warm intravenous fluids. Fluid warmers or microwave oven can be used
- Consider blood transfusion, if patient is unresponsive to initial crystalloid therapy. Blood products should not be warmed in microwave oven
- Prevent hypothermia
- Resuscitation is ineffective, if there is no definitive management of bleeding

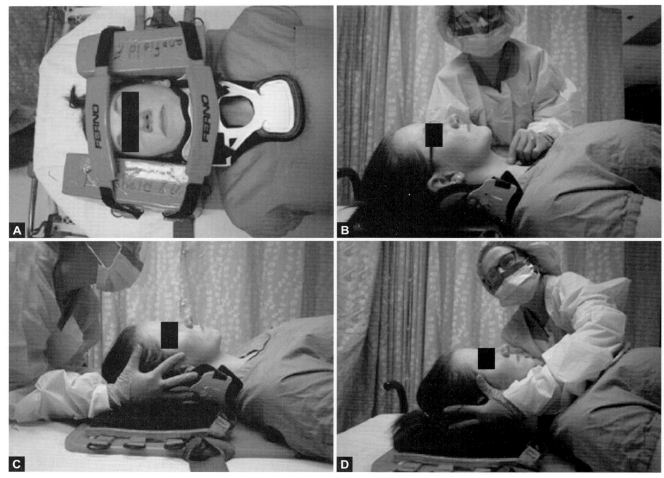

Figs 5A to D Cervical spine protection by immobilization

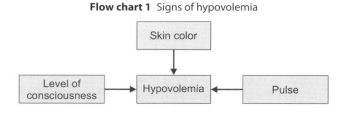

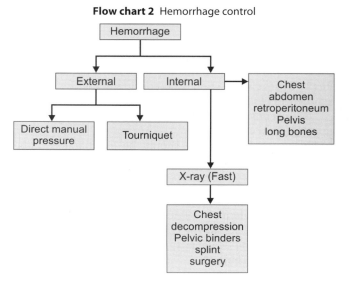

- Definitive control includes surgery, angioembolization, and pelvic stabilization
- *Permissive hypotension*: It aims to defer or restrict fluid resuscitation until hemorrhage is controlled. Balancing the goal of organ perfusion with the risk of rebleeding by accepting lower than normal blood pressure is termed "balanced resuscitation" or "hypotensive resuscitation" or "permissive hypotension".

CHAPTER 82 Trauma: Initial Assessment and Management

Table 1 Glasgow coma scale

		Score
Eye opening	• Spontaneously • To speech • To pain • None	4 3 2 1
Verbal response	• Orientated • Confused • Inappropriate • Incomprehensible • None	5 4 3 2 1
Motor response	• Obeys commands • Localizes to pain • Withdraws from pain • Flexion to pain • Extension to pain • None	6 5 4 3 2 1
Maximum score		15

Adjuncts to Primary Survey

- *Electrocardiogram monitoring*
  - Tachycardia, atrial fibrillation, ST changes—blunt cardiac injury
  - Pulseless electrical activity (PEA)—cardiac tamponade, tension pneumothorax, profound hypovolemia
  - Bradycardia—hypoxia.
- *Urinary catheters*
  - Sensitive indicator of renal perfusion and volume status
  - But transurethral bladder catheterization is contraindicated in suspected urethral injury **(Flow chart 3)**.
- *Gastric catheters*
  - A gastric tube is indicated to decompress stomach, decrease the risk of aspiration, and assess upper gastrointestinal hemorrhage.
  - *Do not put nasogastric tube, if cribriform plate fracture is suspected, put orogastric tube instead*
- *Other monitoring*
  - Arterial blood gas (ABG) levels
  - Pulse oximetry
  - Capnography to confirm endotracheal placement of tube
  - Noninvasive or invasive blood pressure monitoring
  - *Imaging*:
    - Emergency diagnostic X-rays should be done even in pregnant patients
    - Pelvic X-ray **(Figs 6 and 7)** and chest X-ray **(Figs 8 and 9)** are mandatory
    - Focused assessment sonography in trauma (FAST) is essential for identification of intra-abdominal source of bleeding
    - Diagnostic peritoneal lavage can be a useful tool
- *Consider need for patient's transfer.*

Flow chart 3 Suspected urethral injury

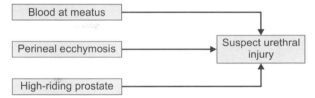

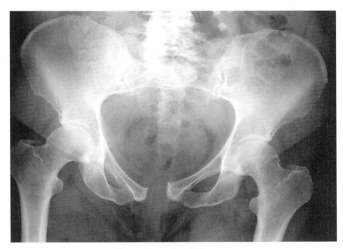

Fig. 6 Open book fracture

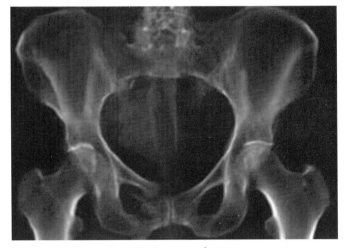

Fig. 7 Pubic ramus fracture

Secondary Survey

The criteria for initiating secondary survey are as follows:
- Primary survey (ABCDE) is completed
- Ongoing resuscitation
- Normalization of vital signs

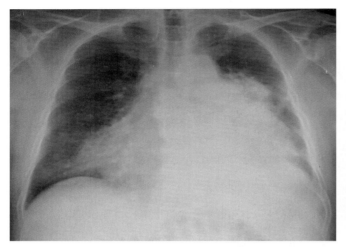

Fig. 8 Cardiac tamponade

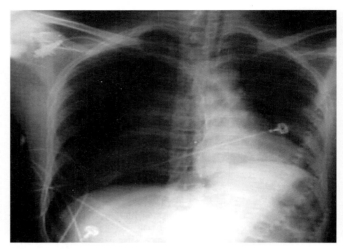

Fig. 9 Tension pneumothorax

- When additional personnel are available, then secondary survey can be conducted simultaneously, when other personnel are attending to primary survey.

Secondary survey includes the following:

History

- The AMPLE history is a useful mnemonic (**Box 2**).
- A history of mechanism of injury should be obtained.
- To know whether *blunt, penetrating* or *thermal injury* is there singly or in combination.
- A history of exposure to chemicals, toxins, and radiation is important as along with deleterious effects on victim, there is a risk of exposure to healthcare providers.

Physical Examination

A complete head to toe physical examination is performed.
- *Head*
  - Examine entire scalp and head for lacerations, contusions, fractures
  - Ophthalmic examination.
- *Maxillofacial structures*
  - Palpation of bony structures to look for fractures
  - Airway obstruction and major bleeding
  - Assessment of soft tissue.
- *Cervical spine and neck*
  - Neck immobilization should be considered until an injury is excluded by diagnostic studies
  - Look for cervical spine tenderness, subcutaneous emphysema, tracheal deviation, laryngeal fractures
  - Auscultate carotid arteries for bruits

Box 2 AMPLE history

- **A**llergies
- **M**edications
- **P**ast illness or pregnancy
- **L**ast meal
- **E**vents or environment

  - If evidence of any arterial bleeding, airway compromise or expanding hematoma, then urgent surgical intervention is indicated.
- *Chest*
  - Look for open pneumothorax, flail segments
  - Palpate clavicles, ribs, and sternum.
  - Percuss and auscultate.
- *Abdomen*
  - Close observation and frequent re-evaluation by same observer
  - Early involvement of surgeon
  - Unexplained hypotension warrants search for intra-abdominal source of bleeding
    - Perform perineal, rectal, and vaginal examination.
    - Inspect extremities for contusions, lacerations, and fractures.
    - Neurological examination.

Adjuncts to Secondary Survey

- We can avoid missed injuries by maintaining a high index of suspicion
- Additional X-ray examinations of spine and extremities

- Computerized tomography scans of head, chest, abdomen, and spine
- Contrast urography and angiography
- Bronchoscopy and esophagoscopy.

Definitive Care

Transfer should be considered whenever the patient's treatment needs exceed the capability of receiving institution.

CONCLUSION

Polytrauma is a major cause of mortality and morbidity, affecting mainly younger population. The heaviest toll of traumatic deaths occurs within the first hour, defined as the golden hour of trauma. Hence, the principle "time is essence" should be religiously followed during the first hour of trauma.

The correct sequence of *preparation, triage, primary survey, adjuncts to primary survey, consider need for patient transfer, secondary survey, adjuncts to secondary survey, re-evaluation* and *definitive care* should be followed. Patient's medical history and mechanism of injury are crucial in identifying injuries. Frequent re-evaluation is a key to success. Understanding one's limitations and identifying patients requiring transfer to higher centers on time, improves outcomes. A good teamwork is absolutely essential to practice the guidelines of trauma management.

BIBLIOGRAPHY

1. Advanced trauma life support. (2008). ATLS, ACS Committee on Trauma. [online] Available from *https://www.facs.org/quality%20programs/trauma/atls* [Accessed December, 2016].
2. Battistella FD. Emergency department evaluation of the patient with multiple injuries. In: Wilmore DW, Cheung LY, Harken AH. Scientific American Surgery. New York, NY: Scientific American; 2000.
3. Kam CW, Lai CH, Lam SK, et al. What are the ten new commandments in severe polytrauma management? Review Article. World J Emerg Med. 2010;1(2):85-92.
4. McIntosh BT, Sheppy B, Rane S. An Indian tragedy: an Indian solution: perspective of managing service quality in EMS in India. J Global Heathcare Syst. 2012;2(1):1-8.
5. Puri P, Goel S, Gupta AK, et al. Management of polytrauma patients in emergency department: an experience of tertiary healthcare institution of northern India. World J Emerg Med. 2013;4(1):15-9.

Facial Trauma

Syed Ahmed Adil

INTRODUCTION

Trauma to the facial region causes injuries to skeletal components, dentition as well as soft tissues from frontal bone superiorly to the mandible inferiorly. Several studies suggest that facial fracture dissipates a lot of force during trauma, in effect protecting the brain.[1]

The mandible was the most frequent site involved. Among maxillary fractures, zygomatic bone and arch fractures were most common.[2] Most common causes are motor vehicle crashes, falls, violent assaults, and crashes during bicycling.

Cervical spine injury should be considered in a maxillofacial trauma patient until proved otherwise.[3] Up to 44% of patients with severe maxillofacial trauma require endotracheal intubation due to mechanical disruption or massive hemorrhage into the airway.[4]

HISTORY

The history indicates the site and direction of force, the possible presence of other injuries, especially to the neck, and other relevant features such as loss of consciousness and head injury. Important issues should be asked or elicited like vision, facial numbness, bite, pain with eye movements, pain with moving the jaw and breathing difficulties.

APPROACH AND MANAGEMENT

Primary Survey

Every trauma patient should be evaluated as per Advanced Trauma Life Support (ATLS) protocol. Primary survey and its management is taken as the topmost priority **(Flow chart 1)**. Do not get distracted with other injuries as long as you have airway, breathing and circulation under control. Next comes life-threatening injuries and then manage facial injuries.

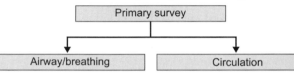

Flow chart 1 Primary survey and its management

- Open airway-jay thrust
- Mandible fracture-tongue pull
- Adequate airway clearing–double suctioning
- Prevent tongue fall–oropharyngeal airway
- Cervical spine stabilization
- Assess airway before intubation
- Adequate seal during bag mask ventilation
- Avoid naso-tracheal intubation
- Sedate but do not paralyse before intubation until alternative in place
- Backup–IMA, combitube, needle or surgical crico set, video laryngoscopy

- Apply direct pressure to external wounds
- Nasal tampon/anterior gauze packing for epistaxis
- Avoid blind clamping
- Cautious use of Foleys catheter for posterior nasal bleed
- Oral cavity packing for oral bleed
- Use hemostatic agents like Ferracylum, fibrin sealants, cellulose, gelatin to arrest bleed

Secondary Survey

- Inspect the face for asymmetry
- Inspect open wounds for foreign bodies
- Palpate the entire face
- Supraorbital and infraorbital rim
- Zygomatic and frontal sutures
- Zygomatic arch
- Oral mucosa.

Sinuses

Frontal bone and sinus injuries usually are result from a direct blow to the frontal bone with a blunt object. This fracture is frequently associated with intracranial injury, secondary to disruption of the posterior table of the sinus. Dural tears are frequent and patients may have associated injuries to the orbital roof.

Look for disruption or crepitance near orbital rim. Palpate for subcutaneous emphysema. Look for lacerations or bulging of forehead.

Those with depressed skull fractures and posterior wall involvement should be admitted. Neurosurgical or oromaxillofacial surgery opinion must be obtained. Foreign bodies and bony injuries must be looked for. Patient with frontal sinus injuries may require head, neck, neurological, ENT (ear, nose and throat) and eye examination. Intravenous antibiotics and tetanus prophylaxis must be considered. Nondisplaced fractures may be treated as outpatients after neurosurgical consultation.

Nose

Nasal fractures account for greater than 50% of all facial fractures in adults.[5] The bones and cartilage of the nose provide both esthetic and structural support for the midface and airway. Therefore, proper evaluation and management are necessary to prevent nasal deformity and nasal airway compromise.[6]

Nasal trauma classification:
Type I: Injury restricted to soft tissue
*Type IIa**: Simple, unilateral, nondisplaced fracture
Type IIb: Simple, bilateral, nondisplaced fracture
Type III: Simple displaced fracture
Type IV: Closed comminuted fracture
*Type V**: Open comminuted fracture

Look for asymmetry, tenderness, crepitus, and mobility of the nasal complex if present, suspect trauma to the nose or medial orbit. Perform bimanual nasal palpation test and check for tenderness over the medial canthus **(Fig. 1)**. Inspect nasal septum for septal hematoma, CSF rhinorrhea or epistaxis may be present. Flattened nasal bridge, widening of the nasal bridge (telecanthus) or a saddle-shaped deformity of the nose suggest nasal bridge fracture with orbital involvement. A septal hematoma appears as a blue or red, boggy, and tender area of swelling along the nasal septum **(Fig. 2)**.

Control epistaxis by either pinching the nose or performing anterior or posterior packing. Topical vasoconstrictors can be used. Make the patient sit straight so that he does not swallow the blood.

Incision and evacuation of the septal hematoma is required to prevent destruction of the cartilage resulting in saddle nose deformity. To drain septal hematoma, first anesthetize the area. Using number 11 blade, incise the inferior portion

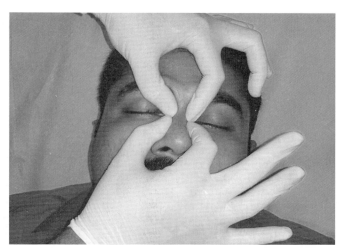

Fig. 1 Bimanual digital palpation of the nose
Source: Dr SA Adil.

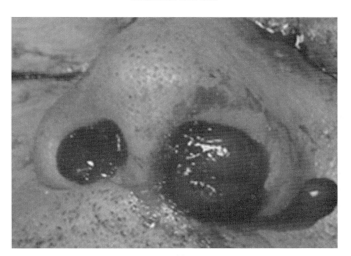

Fig. 2 Septal hematoma

of the hematoma and allow it to drain. Then pack the nose with Vaseline gauze to prevent re-accumulation of blood.

In the absence of epistaxis or deformity, ice and analgesics may be given. Refer to ENT in 2–5 days for reduction. Rhinorrhea, if present must be inspected for CSF leak by testing for β-transferrin, glucose or Halo sign.[7] If suspected a neurosurgical consultation is warranted. Head must be kept elevated and supine positioning should be avoided to allow healing.

Closed reduction is usually reserved for simple, noncomminuted nasal fractures, although exceptions can be made. The key principle is to apply a force opposite to the vector of trauma to achieve fracture reduction. Attention should be paid to the bony nasal pyramid. The Goldman

---

Types II to V: Fracture with cerebrospinal fluid (CSF) rhinorrhea, airway obstruction, septal hematoma, crush injury, numbness, severe displacement or midface involvement.

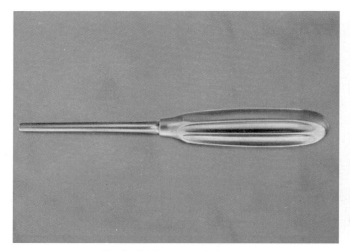

Fig. 3 Goldman septal elevator

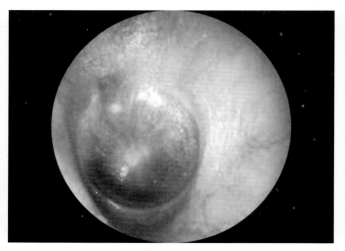

Fig. 4 Hemotympanum

elevator (**Fig. 3**) is applied with upward or outward force with bimanual manipulation of the external nasal bones. Care should be used with this technique over the cribriform plate if injury is suspected.

Ear

- Inspect the external auditory canal for any lacerations, CSF leaks, and hemotympanum (**Fig. 4**)
- Battle sign over mastoid region or auricular hematoma
- Mandibular condylar fracture.

Check for mandibular condylar fracture by inserting a finger into the external auditory canal and asking the patient to gently open and close the mouth (**Fig. 5**).

A number of published studies have shown that the risk of meningitis is significantly reduced when prophylactic antibiotics are used in post-traumatic CSF leakage. Place the patient at bed rest with the head elevated. The basic concept is to decrease intracranial pressure, which in turn should decrease the rate of leakage. Most traumatic leaks will close spontaneously within 7–10 days. If it does not, a neurosurgeon or ENT surgeon should be consulted to consider surgical closure.

Major Bones

Zygomatic arch can fracture in two to three places along the arch. These patients present with depressed cheek with tenderness on palpation. The zygomaticomaxillary fracture (tripod fracture) is rare but complicated fracture (**Figs 6 and 7**). Patients usually present with pain on opening their mouth.

Fractures of the maxilla are high energy injuries. An impact 100 times the force of gravity is required to break the midface.[8] These patients often have significant multisystem

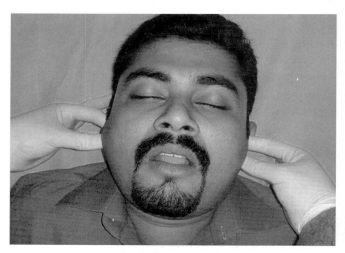

Fig. 5 Finger in ear test
Source: Dr SA Adil.

trauma. The fractures of the maxilla are classified as Le Fort fractures (**Fig. 8**).

Inspect the face from all sides to detect asymmetry in facial structures from zygomatic, orbital, and Le Fort injuries. Palpate the zygoma along its arch and its articulations with the maxilla, frontal and temporal bone. Open patient's mouth and grasp the maxilla arch, place the other hand on the forehead. Push back and forth, up and down and check for movement (**Fig. 9**).

Emergency care for all these fractures involves airway maintenance with intubation or cricothyrotomy if necessary. Airway compromise is probably more common with Le Fort II and III fractures. CSF rhinorrhea is uncommon in Le Fort I fracture but is often seen in Le Fort II and III fractures. If CSF rhinorrhea is present or intracranial air is seen on X-ray

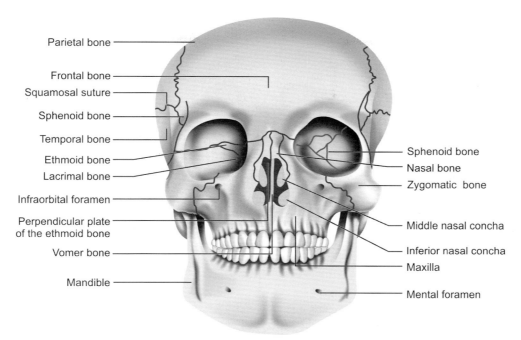

Fig. 6 Facial bones

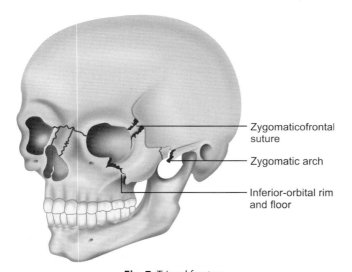

Fig. 7 Tripod fracture

or an open skull fracture is present, the patient should be admitted and placed in a head elevated position (40-60° angle) if possible. Prophylactic antibiotics are often given to these patients. Patients with maxillary fractures also have significant epistaxis requiring nasal packing. Operative intervention may be needed if bleeding does not resolve with packing alone.

Look for associated injuries, especially intracranial, spinal, thoracic, and abdominal. Incidence of blindness is high for Le Fort II and III fractures, so it is important to get ophthalmology consultation. Patients with complex maxillary fractures require admission for open reduction and internal fixation.

Mandible

Mandibular fractures are the third most common type of facial fracture. Because of its ring shape, fractures are often multiple in up to 50% of the cases.[9] The most common areas fractured are the condyle (36%), body (21%), and parasymphyseal region (17%).[10]

A dental line step off or ecchymosis of the floor of the mouth are common findings. There is inability to open the mouth. Periauricular pain while biting is common with condylar fracture. Bilateral body fractures of the mandible may cause airway compromise.

Inspect for malocclusion of teeth and bleeding. Ensure there is no aspiration. Loose and mobile teeth must be counted. Use the tongue blade test to identify fracture of the mandible **(Fig. 10)**.

Bite down on the tongue blade, twist the blade to try to break it. Patients with broken jaw will reflexively open their mouth (*See* **Fig. 9**).

Nondisplaced fractures should be treated with adequate analgesia. Orosurgical consult must be sought.

Displaced fractures, open fractures, and fractures associated with dental trauma need urgent orosurgical consultation. These patients require admission and need either closed reduction or open reduction with internal

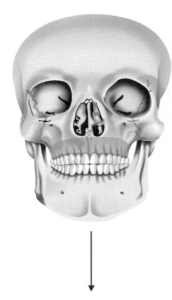
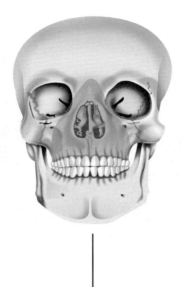

Le Fort 1
- Horizontal fracture of maxilla at level of nasal fossa
- Maxilla moves while nasal bridge is stable
- No hyperthesia
- Facial edema and malocclusion of teeth is present

Le Fort 2
- Pyramidal fracture involving maxilla, nasal bones, medial aspect of the orbits
- Movement of upper jaw with nose
- Marked facial edema is present with nasal flattening, traumatic telecanthus, epistaxis or CSF rhinorrhea

Le Fort 3
- Craniofacial dissociation involving maxilla, zygoma, nasal bones, ethmoid bones and bones of base of skull
- Movement of entire face with distraction
- High-risk of airway obstruction
- DISH face deformity
  – Facial flattening and elongation
  – Swollen eyes
  – Protrusion of mandible

Fig. 8 Types of Le Fort fractures

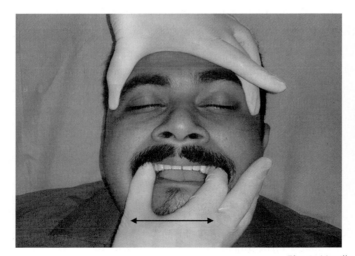
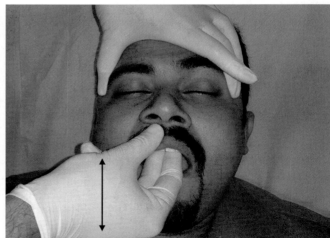

Fig. 9 Maxilla examination
Source: Dr SA Adil.

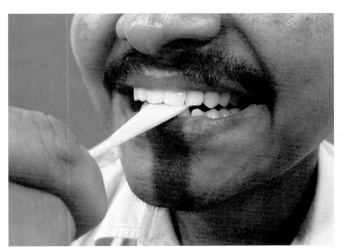

Fig. 10 Tongue blade test
Source: Dr SA Adil.

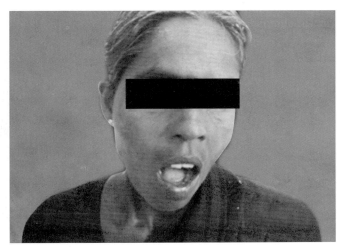

Fig. 11 Temporomandibular joint (TMJ) dislocation
Source: Dr SA Adil.

fixation. All patients with mandibular fractures must be administered antibiotics and tetanus prophylaxis.

Temporomandibular Joint Dislocation

Temporomandibular joint (TMJ) dislocation generally results from a direct blow to chin while the mouth is open, or more commonly during vigorous yawning. The mandible can be dislocated in the anterior, posterior, lateral, and superior plane. Anterior dislocation is the most common and occurs when the condyle is forced in front of the articular eminence.

Once the jaw is dislocated, muscular spasm of the temporalis and lateral pterygoid muscles tend to prevent reduction.[11,12] Dislocations are most frequently bilateral, but they also can be unilateral. Unilateral dislocations result in deviation of the mandible to the unaffected side. Bilateral dislocations cause the mandible to be displaced anteriorly **(Fig. 11)**. Posterior dislocations are rare.

Lateral dislocations are associated with a jaw fracture. Superior dislocations are associated with cerebral contusions, facial nerve palsy, and deafness.

These patients present with the inability to close an open mouth and/or pain, discomfort and facial swelling.

Look for deviation of the mandible or anterior dislocation of the jaw with tenderness and swelling at the angle of the jaw. Paraesthesia or anesthesia of the face signifies nerve injury.

Temporomandibular joint dislocation should be reduced with short acting muscle relaxant and adequate analgesia. Regional block using 2 mL of 2% lidocaine may be given in preauricular depression anterior to tragus.

The patient should be seated. Facing the patient, the examiner places his or hers thumbs in the patient's mouth, over the mandibular molars as far back as possible. The fingers should curve beneath the angle and the body of the mandible. The examiner applies downward and backward pressure with his or her thumbs until the condyle slides back into the articular eminence. A successful reduction must enable the patient to open his or her mouth immediately **(Fig. 12)**.

Newer external methods have been shown in **Figures 13A and B**.

Eyes/Orbit

The orbital rim (frontal, maxillary, and zygomatic bones) protects the globe from direct trauma. The weakest part of the orbit is the medial wall and orbital floor. This fractures first and the orbital soft tissues can pass through the hole created, causing the globe level to drop (hypoglobus) and sink back (enophthalmos). This is called a pure orbital blow-out fracture. Subconjunctival hemorrhage and chemosis occur with orbital fractures.

Visual acuity, light perception, and pupils must be examined. Look for raccoon eyes (bilateral orbital ecchymosis).

Examine the lids for lacerations. Injuries to the medial 3rd of the eyelids can damage the lacrimal apparatus. Test extraocular muscles. Restriction of upward gaze can be seen with zygomatic or infraorbital wall fractures. Examine the cornea for abrasions and lacerations.[13] Examine the anterior chamber for hyphema. Fundoscopy must be performed for posterior chamber and retinal examination.

Palpate entire orbital rim for tenderness or deformity **(Fig. 14)**. Look for hypesthesia of the infraorbital nerve. Look for periorbital tenderness, swelling, subcutaneous air,

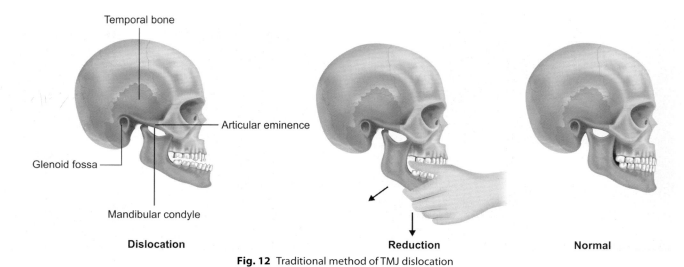

Fig. 12 Traditional method of TMJ dislocation

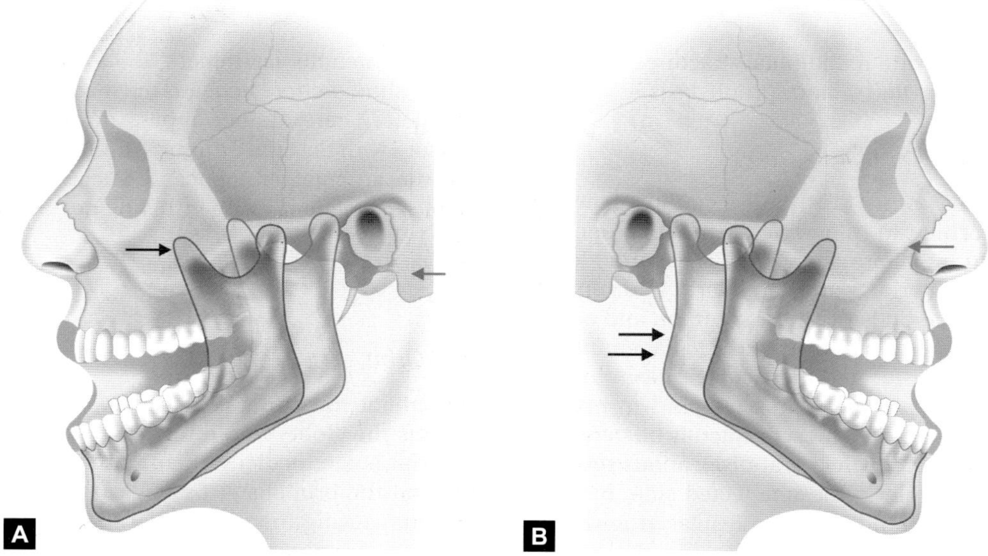

Figs 13A and B (A) To reduce left side, the thumb is placed just above the anteriorly displaced coronoid process (black arrow), and the fingers are placed behind the mastoid process (gray arrow). (B) Simultaneously on the right side, the fingers hold and rotate anteriorly the mandible angle (black arrows) and the thumb is placed over the malar eminence as a fulcrum (gray arrow)

ecchymosis, enophthalmos, and impaired ocular motility. Look for infraorbital anesthesia. Check facial stability. Palpate the medial orbit area to rule out nasoethmoidal orbital (NEO) fracture. Place a cotton bud inside the nose to the medial canthus, place your finger outside the medial canthus, if the bone moves it is known as NEO fractures.

Lacerations

Entrapment injury, pinna laceration or avulsion and intraoral lacerations must be ruled out. Although suturing is preferred for repair, tissue adhesives are similar in patient satisfaction, infection rates, and scarring risk in low skin tension areas.[14]

Surgical consultation for laceration may be warranted in the following:
- Full thickness laceration of the eyelid **(Fig. 15)**, vermilion cutaneous border of the lip or helical rim of the ear, free margin of alar rim
- Lacerations involving nerves, arteries, bones or joints
- Penetrating wounds of unknown depth
- Severely contaminated wounds requiring drainage
- Wounds leading to a strong concern about cosmetic outcome.

Reconstruction of laceration or avulsion tongue injuries is not usually required. Primary wound healing often occurs rapidly because of the rich vascular supply. Lacerations

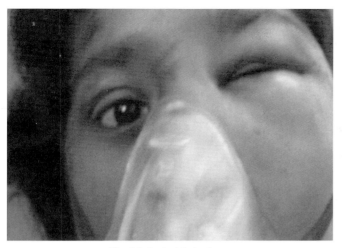
Fig. 14 Periorbital edema

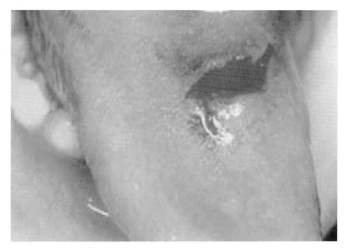
Fig. 16 Laceration of the tongue

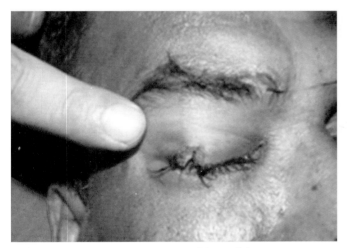
Fig. 15 Laceration of the eyelid

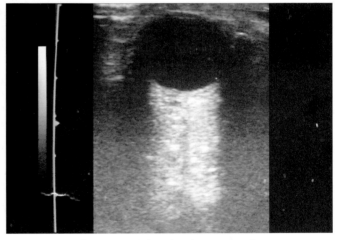
Fig. 17 Normal ocular ultrasonography

larger than 2 cm may require intervention **(Fig. 16)**. Deep lacerations should be sutured in layers.

INVESTIGATION

Imaging Studies

Head computed tomography (CT) with bone window is a good tool in patients with significant findings of frontal fractures, sinuses, and midface fractures. Plain radiographs remain helpful when CT is not available or to exclude injury in the low-risk patient. The Water's view X-ray safely replaces the multiple views in traditional facial series for mid facial fractures. Lateral view for the nose could be helpful. Low suspicion mandible fractures can be found with panorex view but in case of significant findings, mandible CT or facial CT is warranted facial CT with coronal and axial sections is the imaging study of choice for patients with abnormal Water's view or as the initial study with significant clinical findings.[15]

Other diagnostic tool which is very reliable to detect fracture is ultrasonography (USG) **(Fig. 17)**. It has been widely used in detecting superficial facial fractures for example nasal bone fracture **(Figs 18 and 19)**.[16] orbital fracture and zygoma fractures in children.[17] It is also used in finding pupillary reaction through periorbital edema. It can also detect ocular injuries like retrobulbar hemorrhage

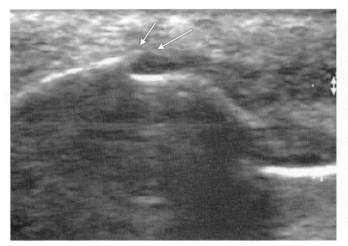

Fig. 18 Longitudinal scan of left nasal bone shows depressed fracture

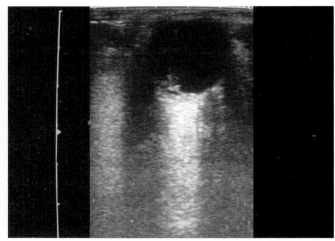

Fig. 21 Ocular scan showing retinal detachment

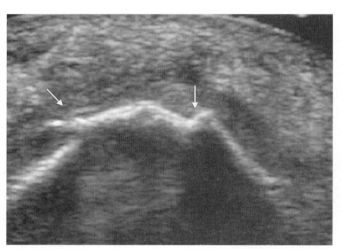

Fig. 19 Marked soft tissue edema and hyperechoic hematoma near depressed fracture lines

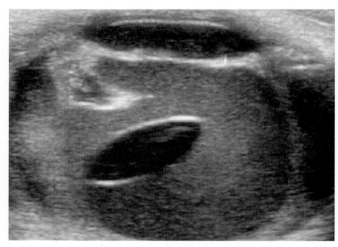

Fig. 22 Scan showing dislocated lens

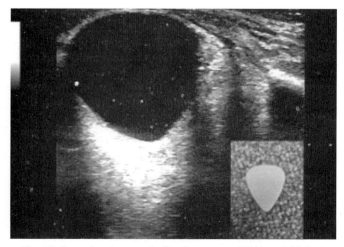

Fig. 20 Scan showing retrobulbar hematoma ("Guitar pick" sign)

which is also known as "Guitar Pick" sign (**Fig. 20**), retinal detachment (**Fig. 21**), and lens dislocation (**Fig. 22**).[18]

Classic tests for CSF rhinorrhea are not accurate in distinguishing CSF from serous nasal discharge in the presence of nasal bleeding. The double ring or halo sign occurs when clear CSF diffuses around blood when dropped on a paper towel. The glucose test is likewise not reliable. Nasal discharge does not contain glucose, whereas CSF does. Blood from the injury may create a false positive test. Beta-2 transferrin assay marker is very specific to CSF. However, the test is expensive and results may take several days to a few weeks.

In the absence of CT scan, X-ray along with USG can detect most of the injuries.

SUMMARY

Approach to facial injuries are summarized in **Flow chart 2**.

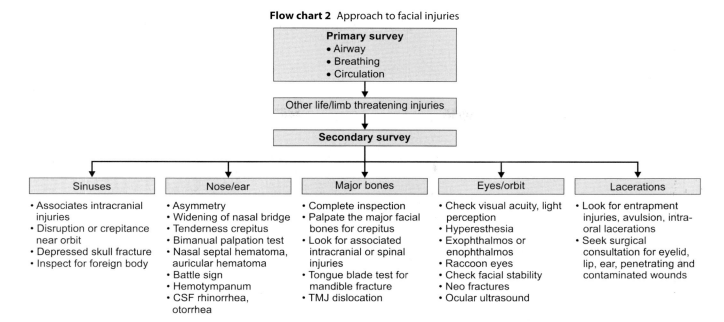

Flow chart 2 Approach to facial injuries

REFERENCES

1. Lee KF, Wagner LK, Lee YE, et al. The impact-absorbing effects of facial fractures in closed-head injuries. An analysis of 210 patients. J Neurosurg. 1987;66(4):542-7.
2. Rajanikanth K, RM Borle, Bhola N, et al. The pattern of maxillofacial fractures in central India A Unicentric retrospective study. IOSR Journal of Dental and Medical Sciences (IOSR-JDMS). 2014;13(1):28-31.
3. Elahi MM, Brar MS, Ahmed N, et al. Cervical spine injury in association with craniomaxillofacial fractures. Plast Reconstr Surg. 2008;121(1):201-8.
4. Alvi A, Doherty T, Lewen G. Facial fractures and concomitant injuries in trauma patients. Laryngoscope. 2003;3(1):102-6.
5. Renner GJ. Management of nasal fractures. Otolaryngol Clin North Am. 1991;24(1):195-213.
6. Kelley BP, Downey CR, Stal S. Evaluation and Reduction of Nasal Trauma. Semin Plast Surg. 2010;24(4):339-47.
7. Higuera S, Lee EI, Cole P, et al. Nasal trauma and the deviated nose. Plast Reconstr Surg. 2007;120(7):64S-75S.
8. Wilson WC, Grande CM, Hoyt DB (Eds). Trauma: Emergency Resuscitation, Perioperative Anesthesia, Surgical Management, Volume I. Radiologic Technology. 2007.
9. Hobbs DL, Mickelsen W. Trauma radiography of the Mandible. Radiologic Technology. 2007;78(4).
10. Atilgan S, Erol B, Yaman F, et al. Mandibular fractures: a comparative analysis between young and adult patients in the southeast region of Turkey. J Appl Oral Sci. 2010;18(1):17-22.
11. Tintinalli JE, Stapczynski JS, O John Ma, Yealy DM, Meckler GD, Cline DM (Eds). Tintnalli Emergency Medicine: A Comprehensive study guide, 8th edition.
12. Ardehali MM, Kouhi A, Meighani A, et al. Temporomandibular Joint Dislocation Reduction Technique A New External Method vs the Traditional. Ann Plast Surg. 2009;63.
13. Semer N (Ed). Facial Lacerations. Practical Plastic Surgery for Nonsurgeons. iUniverse: 2007.
14. Imran S, Amin S, Imran M, Hameed Daula. Imaging in ocular trauma optimizing the use of ultrasound and computerized tomography. Pak J Ophthalmol. 2011;27(3):146-51.
15. Forsch RT. Essentials of Skin Laceration Repair. Am Fam Physician. 2008;78(8):945-51.
16. Hogg K, Maloba M. Best evidence topic report: which facial views for facial trauma? Emerg Med J. 2004;21:79.
17. Hong HS, Cha JG, Paik SH. High-resolution sonography for nasal fracture in children. Am J Roentgenol. 2007;188(1):W86-92.
18. Sallam M, Kahlifa G, Ibrahim F, et al. Ultrasonography vs computed tomography in imaging of complex zygomatic fractures. J Am Science. 2010;6(9).

CHAPTER 84

Head Trauma

Devendra Richhariya, Manish Vaish

INTRODUCTION

Trauma to the central nervous system (the brain and spinal cord) can be classified on the basis of mechanisms of injury, clinical severity, radiological appearance, or anatomic distribution. Education regarding preventive measures of head trauma is important for public, such as the use of helmets and seatbelts.

Main objective in the management of patients with head trauma is the prevention of secondary injury such as ischemia and hypoxia. This chapter includes common neurologic injuries related to trauma; prehospital, in-hospital, and critical care management of these patients.

EPIDEMIOLOGY

Head trauma is critical situation and leading cause of death worldwide. Head trauma leads to brain parenchymal injury which is termed as traumatic brain injury (TBI). In emergency department TBI is due to falls, road traffic accident, blunt head injury, assault, blast injury, and sometimes child abuse. TBI can be classified on the basis of Glasgow coma scale (GCS) as mild GCS 14–15, moderate GCS 9–13, and severe GCS less than 8.

PATHOPHYSIOLOGY OF TRAUMATIC BRAIN INJURY

Normal functioning of brain depends upon the cerebral perfusion pressure (CPP) which is the difference between the mean arterial pressure (MAP) and intracranial pressure (ICP). CPP roughly denotes the cerebral blood flow (CBF). CBF is maintained well when MAP is maintained between 60 mm and 150 mm. Normal CBF is maintained by cerebral blood vessels by its constriction and dilation ability under various physiological conditions this is called autoregulation.

This ability of autoregulation and maintenance of CBF get disrupted when any TBI occurs. Cerebral vasoconstriction occurs due to hypertension, alkalosis, and hypocarbia and cerebral vasodilation occurs due to hypotension, acidosis, and hypercarbia.

After TBI increase in intracranial blood volume (due to vasodilatation) causes brain swelling, this is the compensatory mechanism of brain to maintain optimal CBF in view of damaging brain tissue.

Secondary to TBI various devastating intracranial and extracranial events occur like severe intracranial hypertension, seizures and cerebral edema, hypotension, hypoxia, anemia, and hypercapnia and hypocapnia. These devastating events determine the final outcome in the patient after TBI. Hypotension and hypoxia clearly worsen the patient outcome **(Flow chart 1)**.

Flow chart 1 Series of events in traumatic brain injury

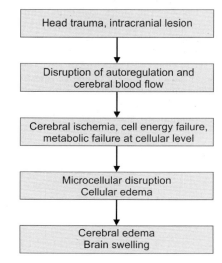

MODES OF TRAUMA AND PATTERN OF BRAIN INJURIES

Blunt Injuries

Acceleration and deceleration of brain after direct blunt impact to head is known as blunt injuries. Blunt impact-induced mechanical forces cause tissue compression, distortion, and shearing, resulting in parenchymal contusions, extra-axial hematomas, and diffuse axonal injury **(Table 1)**.

Penetrating Injuries

Penetrating brain injuries are less common than blunt injuries and are having high mortality rates. Most frequent penetrating brain injury in emergency department is gunshot injury or fire arm injury. High velocity projectile penetrates into the brain and damage the parenchyma.

HEAD TRAUMA ACCORDING TO SEVERITY (TABLE 2)

Mild Traumatic Brain Injury

Concussion

Transient brief disruption of neurologic function after minor blunt trauma to head, with or without a loss of consciousness, usually as a result of acceleration-deceleration forces to the head. Usually patient presents with symptoms of headache, confusion, and amnesia. Headaches, sensory sensitivity, memory or concentration difficulties, irritability, sleep disturbances, or depression, may persist for long periods after a concussion termed as post-concussion syndrome.

Moderate and Severe Traumatic Brain Injury

Moderate TBI patients have a GCS score of 9–13. They present with variety of clinical features like worsening headache and nausea, confusion, seizure initially loss of consciousness but can follow command on arrival to the emergency department. Patient may present with isolated facial trauma or polytrauma associated with focal neurologic deficits. Emergency physician should be more cautious while managing this type of patient. Initially patients are able to talk but gradually their GCS scores deteriorate significantly and consistently with severe TBI (talk-and-deteriorate patient). Most of patients have extra-axial hematomas, epidural or subdural. These patients have better clinical outcomes if detected early and treated rapidly. Successful management depends upon frequent assessment of GCS score, close observation for minor mental status changes or focal neurologic findings, frequent use of computed tomography (CT) scanning, and early neurosurgical intervention.

In emergency department if patient presents with moderate TBI with herniation, immediate intervention like hyperventilation and osmotic therapy should be initiated and consideration should be given for surgical evacuation of hematoma before transferring to definitive care unit. All moderate TBI patients should undergo for CT scan and admitted for observation unit for frequent neurological examination and monitoring and repeat CT scan should be done if required.

Severe TBI is when patient presents acutely with a GCS score of 8 or less. Any intracranial contusion, hematoma, or brain laceration is considered as severe TBI. Patient with severe TBI and with increase in ICP presents with symptoms of progressive hypertension, bradycardia, and shallow or irregular respiration (Cushing's reflex/phenomenon). These features represent the life-threatening raised ICP and require urgent ICP management like hyperventilation, osmotic therapy, and surgical decompression.

Common Extra-axial Hematomas

Epidural hematoma: Epidural hematoma (EDH) develops after direct mechanical force over the skull and skull fracture. The most common site for EDH is temporoparietal region, mostly unilateral and in young individuals. Classic presentation of lucid interval is seen in about 30% of patients. Biconvex lenticular lesion in noncontrast CT scan is shown in **Figure 1**.

Table 1	Blunt trauma and pattern of brain injuries		
	Pathophysiology	Anatomical location	Special features
Parenchymal contusion	Coup/countercoup injury	Frontal or temporal	Can expand within 24 hours
Epidural hematoma	Disruption of middle meningeal vessels diploic vein and venous sinuses	Near skull fracture	Lens shaped (convex)
Subdural hematoma	Bridging vein injury	Cerebrum tentorium and falx	Crescent shaped (concave)
Subarachnoid hemorrhage	Pial vessels injury	Cerebrum basal cistern ventricles	Can be limited to few sulcus fissure or diffuse
Diffuse axonal injury	Shear injury of axonal	At cortex and white matter junction	Axonal swelling and axotomy

Table 2 Risk assessment in head trauma patient in emergency department

High-risk head trauma	Medium-risk head trauma	Low-risk head trauma
• Focal neurologic deficit • Unequal pupils • Skull fracture • Polytrauma • GCS < 8 • Unconsciousness • Post-traumatic confusion • Worsening headache • Vomiting • Post-traumatic seizure • Associated intoxication • Unreliable history of injury • Age older than 60 years or younger than 2 years	• Initial GCS score of 13–15 • Brief period of LOC • Post-traumatic amnesia • Vomiting • Headache • Intoxication	• Asymptomatic • Conscious • Well orientation/memory • Accurate history • No other injuries • Normal neurological examination • Normal pupils • GCS score 15 • Injury >24 hours duration • No/mild headache • No vomiting

Abbreviations: GCS, Glasgow coma scale; LOC, loss of consciousness.

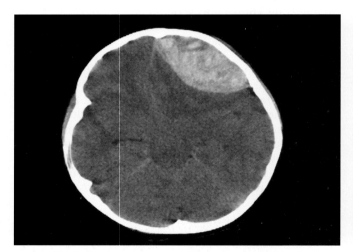

Fig. 1 Noncontrast computed tomography image of epidural hematoma

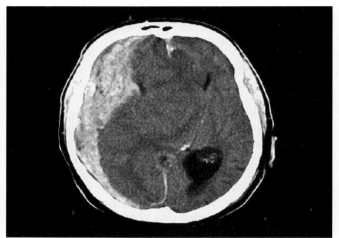

Fig. 2 Noncontrast computed tomography image of subdural hematoma

Subdural hematoma: Subdural hematoma (SDH), developed between dura mater and brain, is mostly due to fall from height and acceleration-deceleration injury due to road traffic accident. SDH is more common than EDH; common in elderly. The clinical features of an SDH depend upon the patient's age, the presence of polytrauma, or the presence of altered mental status from a nontraumatic cause (e.g. alcohol or drug intoxication) **(Fig. 2)**.

RESUSCITATION AND MANAGEMENT OF HEAD TRAUMA IN EMERGENCY DEPARTMENT

Airway Breathing Circulation

Head trauma management started with assessment and stabilization of the airway, breathing, and circulation, like any other critically ill patient. Rapid sequence endotracheal intubation with in-line stabilization of the cervical spine should be considered for airway protection for patients with a GCS less than 8. Maintain PaO_2 (partial pressure of arterial oxygen) more than 60 mm Hg and saturation more than 90%. Hypoxia hypotension is associated with increased mortality. Maintain normocarbia [$PaCO_2$ (partial pressure of arterial carbon dioxide) around 35 mm Hg] and avoid hyperventilation in patients with TBI; hyperventilation produces vasoconstriction and further ischemia which decreases cerebral perfusion. Similarly hypercarbia produces vasodilation and raised intracranial tension and clinical deterioration. Use of hyperventilation should be restricted only to acutely herniating and deteriorating patients while arranging for emergency craniotomy.

Fluid Resuscitation

Choosing the right fluid is important aspect for head trauma management. Maintain normovolemia by intravenous fluid, blood, and blood products. Ringer's lactate and normal saline are ideal solutions for resuscitation of TBI. Hypotonic and glucose-containing fluid should not be used. Normal serum sodium level should be maintained. Hyponatremia causes brain edema. Vasopressor can be used in neurogenic shock due to spinal cord injury.

Measures to Maintain Intracranial Pressure

It is important to maintain equal volume of each compartment [brain, blood, cerebrospinal fluid (CSF)] of skull. If volume of one component is increased [due to space-occupying lesions (SOL), intracranial hemorrhage, edema] then volume of other component should decrease as a compensatory mechanism. Mismatch in compensatory mechanism leads to rise in ICP; decrease in CPP ultimately causes cerebral ischemia.

Intracranial pressure monitoring is preferred in severe traumatic injury by placing external ventricular drain which is helpful in measuring the global ICP and controlling it by CSF drainage **(Box 1)**.

Mannitol is helpful in reducing the raised ICP. Mannitol should not be used in hypotensive patients. Mannitol is highly recommended as bolus (1 g/kg) in acutely deteriorating and herniating patient provided patient is normovolemic normotensive.

Hypertonic saline is also helpful in reducing the raised ICP. 3% concentration is frequently used and hypertonic saline can be used in hypotensive patient.

Barbiturates are also helpful in reducing the raised ICP but should not be used in hypotensive and hypovolemic patient; so not helpful in acute resuscitative phase.

Hypothermia is also helpful in reducing the raised ICP. Prophylactic hypothermia is neuroprotective and beneficial effects are seen in severe TBI.

Anticonvulsant: Possibility of seizure in head trauma increases with increase of severity of head injury. Patients with severe TBI are more prone for seizures. Seizures can be controlled by anticonvulsant like phenytoin. Fosphenytoin, diazepam, and lorazepam are also used in addition. Seizures should be controlled as soon as possible to prevent secondary brain injury. In adult loading dose of phenytoin is 1 g then maintenance dose is 100 mg every 8 hours.

Antibiotics: There is high possibility of infection rate in patient with severe TBI. Prophylactic antibiotics can be used in patient with basal skull fracture and CSF leak in view of risk of meningitis. Risk of infection also exists in patient with external ventricular drain.

Scalp wound: Scalp wound should be inspected carefully and adequately cleaned. Stop hemorrhage by applying direct pressure or bleeding vessels ligation. Sutures or staples can be applied. CT scan head should be performed to exclude or confirm the skull fracture. Neurosurgeon advice should be taken for all cases of open/depressed skull fracture.

Surgical management and surgical decompression in TBI have been discussed in **Table 3**.

Penetrating Brain Injuries

Computed tomography scan is appropriate in locating the bullet foreign bodies and intracranial air. Angiography is helpful in identifying the traumatic aneurysm and arteriovenous fistula. In these cases endovascular management is helpful. Start prophylactic antibiotics and early ICP monitoring.

Do not remove any penetrating objects like knife or arrow before vascular injury assessment or definitive surgical management otherwise fatal hemorrhage may occur.

Box 1 Stepwise approach to maintain intracranial pressure

- Raise head end of bed >30°
- Normalize vitals parameters
- Maintain normothermia
- Adequate sedation and analgesics
- Cerebrospinal fluid drainage
- Mannitol
- Hypertonic saline
- Propofol
- Decompressive craniotomy
- Barbiturate
- Hypothermia

Table 3 Surgical management and surgical decompression in traumatic brain injury

Conditions	Indications for surgery
Epidural hematoma	EDH > 30 cm^3, GCS < 9, and unequal pupil
Subdural hematoma	SDH clot thickness > 10 mm or midline shift > 5 mm, irrespective of GCS. Unequal or fixed and dilated pupils
Parenchymal lesions	Progressive neurologic deterioration, signs of mass effect on CT scan, GCS 6–8 with frontal or temporal contusions >20 cm^3, midline shift >5 mm
Posterior fossa lesions	Mass effect on CT, neurologic dysfunction, and deterioration
Depressed skull fractures	Fracture thickness more than that of cranium intracranial hematoma, depression >1 cm, frontal sinus involvement, gross cosmetic deformity, wound contamination and infection, and pneumocephalus

Abbreviations: EDH, epidural hematoma; SDH, subdural hematoma; GCS, Glasgow coma scale; CT, computed tomography.

GUIDELINES FOR MANAGEMENT OF HEAD INJURIES

Guidelines are for effective clinical assessment and management of patient with head injury. These promote best and appropriate treatment to the persons with head injury and are also useful for their families and their attendants so that they have the knowledge about what should be done for the betterment of the injured person. Also include referral guidelines in cases where specialist care is needed.

Initial Assessment

Initial assessment should start with "GCS" and the score should be recorded or communicated properly on every note.
- *Children with head injury should be assessed and managed according to*
  - Advanced Pediatric Life Support
- *Adults with head injury should be assessed and managed according to*
  - Advanced Trauma Life Support (ATLS) course.

Immediate Care at the Scene

Cervical collar should be applied in case of suspected head injury:
- Glasgow coma scale less than 15 on initial assessment
- Neck pain or tenderness
- Focal neurological deficit
- Paresthesia in the extremities
- Any other clinical suspicion of cervical spine injury
- Manage pain effectively
- Assurance to patient and family
- Support to limb fractures
- Foley's catheterization.

Patient Assessment and Management in the Emergency Department

Assessment of all head injuries of the patients should be done within 15 minutes of arrival:
- Airway, breathing, and circulation (ABC) assessment and management
- Assessment of risk factors
- CT imaging of head and cervical spine and other body areas
- Consciousness of patient should be assessed immediately
- An anesthetist or critical care physician should provide appropriate airway management and assist with resuscitation in patient with GCS 8 or less
- A standard head injury proforma should be used for documentation.

Neurosurgical Consult

Neurosurgeon should be consulted in each and every case of head injury and for follow-up further. Most important indications for urgent neurologic consult are:
- Coma
- Confusion
- Focal neurological deficit
- Seizure
- Penetrating injury
- Skull base fracture with CSF leak.

Investigations for Clinically Important Brain Injuries

Acute clinically important brain injuries should be investigated by CT imaging of the head using minimum radiation dose. Magnetic resonance imaging (MRI) should be performed depending on the need but should not be the primary investigation. No role of X-ray of skull.

Criteria for Performing a CT Head Scan

- GCS less than 13 on initial assessment in the emergency department
- GCS less than 15 at 2 hours after the injury on assessment in the emergency department
- Open or depressed skull fracture
- Features basal skull fracture
- Post-traumatic seizure
- Focal neurological deficit
- Vomiting
- Elderly group
- Any history of bleeding or clotting disorders
- Retrograde amnesia of events immediately before the head injury.

In all of the above mentioned cases, a provisional written radiology report should be made available within 1 hour of the scan being performed.

Communication with Families and Attendants

Medical and paramedical staff should brief the families about overall condition and explain what they are doing. Team of doctors managing the patient should share information about possible complex changes in the patient with family members.

Transfer of Child or Adult from Hospital to a Neuroscience Unit

- Patient should be transferred to a neuroscience unit
- Only after completing the initial resuscitation and stabilization

- Establishing comprehensive monitoring
- Use intubation and ventilation before transfer
- Patient should be accompanied by a trained and experienced doctor and assistant in emergency cases and with clinical staff in nonemergency condition.

During transfer family members must be given full access to the patient as is practical.

Admission and Observation

Head injury should be admitted under the care of a trained neurosurgery team.
- Patients with clinically significant abnormalities on neuroimaging
- Patients with low GCS regardless of the neuroimaging results
- CT scanning could not be done due to patient irritability
- Persistent vomiting, severe headaches
- Drug or alcohol intoxication, suspected nonaccidental injury, meningism, and CSF.

Observation of Admitted Patients

Patient admitted with head injury should be observed only by trained clinicians for neurological observation like GCS; pupil size and reactivity; limb movements; respiratory rate; heart rate; blood pressure; temperature, and blood oxygen saturation. These should be performed and recorded on a half-hourly basis until GCS equal to 15 has been achieved. After that it should be done half-hourly for 2 hours, then 1-hourly for 4 hours and then 2-hourly thereafter. And any deterioration should be informed to supervising team:
- New development of agitation
- Decrease of even 1 point in GCS score
- Severe or increasing headache or persisting vomiting
- New development such as pupil inequality or asymmetry of limb or facial movement

In all of the above cases immediate CT scan should be considered.

Discharge and Follow-up

Patients can be discharged:
- If no indication for CT scan head
- No other factors (like drug or alcohol intoxication, other injuries, shock)
- Patients with normal imaging of the head or cervical spine
- GCS equal to 15 with clinical examination is normal.

Patients admitted after a head injury may be discharged after resolution of all significant symptoms and signs.

Advice on Discharge

Provide printed discharge summary of all the patients with any kind of head injury to their families. Printed summary should focus on:

- Details about head injury and recovery process
- List of dangerous symptoms when they need to contact emergency department
- Contact details of hospital services treating team
- Medication chart.

Follow-up

Any patient who has residual problems should be managed as outpatient by team of neurologist, neurosurgeon, clinical psychologist, and rehabilitation medicine.

BIBLIOGRAPHY

1. Aarabi B, Tofighi B, Kufera JA, et al. Predictors of outcome in civilian gunshot wounds to the head. J Neurosurg. 2014;120(5):1138-46.
2. Bochicchio GV, Lumpkins K, O'Connor J, et al. Blast injury in a civilian trauma setting is associated with a delay in diagnosis of traumatic brain injury. Am Surg. 2008;74(3):267-70.
3. Bullock MR, Chesnut RM, Clifton GL, et al. The Brain Foundation and American Association of Neurological Surgeons. Guidelines for the management of severe traumatic brain injury. J Neurotrauma. 2000;17:471-8.
4. Center NSCIS. Spinal cord injury facts and figures at a glance. [online] NSCIS website. Available from *www.nscisc.uab.edu/PublicDocuments/fact_figures_docs/Facts2013.pdf* [Accessed February, 2017].
5. Centers for Disease Control and Prevention NC for IP and C. Traumatic brain injury: statistics. 2013. [online] CDC website. Available from *www.cdc.gov/traumaticbraininjury/statistics.html* [Accessed February, 2017].
6. Cernak I. Recent advances in neuroprotection for treating traumatic brain injury. Expert Opin Investig Drugs. 2006;15(11):1371-81.
7. Chesnut RM, Marshall LF, Klauber MR, et al. The role of secondary brain injury in determining outcome from severe head injury. J Trauma. 1993;34(2):216-22.
8. Coronado VG, Xu L, Basavaraju SV, et al. Surveillance for traumatic brain injury related deaths—United States, 1997-2007. MMWR Surveill Summ. 2011;60(5):1-32.
9. Cruz J. Severe acute brain trauma. In: Cruz J (Ed). Neurologic and Neurosurgical Emergencies. Philadelphia: Saunders; 1998. pp. 405-36.
10. Davis DP, Meade W, Sise MJ, et al. Both hypoxemia and extreme hyperoxemia may be detrimental in patients with severe traumatic brain injury. J Neurotrauma. 2009;26(12):2217-23.
11. Davis DP, Ochs M, Hoyt DB, et al. Paramedic-administered neuromuscular blockade improves prehospital intubation success in severely head-injured patients. J Trauma. 2003;55(4):713-9.
12. Devivo MJ. Epidemiology of traumatic spinal cord injury: trends and future implications. Spinal Cord. 2012;50(5):365-72.
13. Faden AI, Simon RP. A potential role for excitotoxins in the pathophysiology of spinal cord injury. Ann Neurol. 1988;23(6):623-6.
14. Faul M, Xu L, Wald MM, et al. Traumatic brain injury in the United States: emergency department visits, hospitalizations and deaths 2002–2006. Atlanta (GA): Centers for Disease

15. Ingebrigtsen T, Romner B. Routine early CT-scan is cost saving after minor head injury. Acta Neurol Scand. 1996;93(2-3):207-10.
16. Kim JT, Shim JK, Kim SH, et al. Remifentanil vs. lignocaine for attenuating the haemodynamic response during rapid sequence induction using propofol: double-blind randomised clinical trial. Anaesth Intensive Care. 2007;35(1):20-3.
17. Magnuson J, Leonessa F, Ling GS. Neuropathology of explosive blast traumatic brain injury. Curr Neurol Neurosci Rep. 2012;12(5):570-9.
18. Marmarou A, Signoretti S, Fatouros PP, et al. Predominance of cellular edema in traumatic brain swelling in patients with severe head injuries. J Neurosurg. 2006;104(5):720-30.
19. McHugh GS, Engel DC, Butcher I, et al. Prognostic value of secondary insults in traumatic brain injury: results from the IMPACT study. J Neurotrauma. 2007;24(2):287-93.
20. Narayan R. Closed head injury. In: Rengachary SS, Ellenbogen RG (Eds). Principles of Neurosurgery. London: Wolfe; 1994. pp. 235-92.
21. Robinson N, Clancy M. In patients with head injury undergoing rapid sequence intubation, does pretreatment with intravenous lignocaine/lidocaine lead to an improved neurological outcome? A review of the literature. Emerg Med J. 2001;18(6):453-7.
22. Servadei F, Teasdale G, Merry G. Defining acute mild head injury in adults: a proposal based on prognostic factors, diagnosis, and management. J Neurotrauma. 2001;18(7):657-64.
23. Stein DM, Boswell S, Sliker CW, et al. Blunt cerebrovascular injuries: does treatment always matter? J Trauma. 2009;66(1):143-4.
24. Stein SC, Smith DH. Coagulopathy in traumatic brain injury. Neurocrit Care. 2004;1(4):479-88.
25. Wilberger J. Emergency care and initial evaluation. In: Cooper R, Golfino J (Eds). Head Injury. New York: McGraw-Hill Publishers; 2000. pp. 63-132.

CHAPTER 85

Spinal Trauma

Sudhir Dubey, Ratandeep Bose, Devendra Richhariya

INTRODUCTION

Ten to fifteen percent of head injury cases have coexisting cervical spinal injury, so radiological evaluation of cervical spine is necessary along with head injury. During the evaluation of head injury, there should be high suspicion of spinal injury, adequate immobilization and handling should be done. Proper evaluation and management of spinal injurers are important because if missed or not treated can lead to permanent neurological deficit.

Most common causes of spinal cord injury (SCI) are:
- Vehicular crashes (36.5%)
- Falls (28.5%)
- Violence, primarily gunshot wounds (14.3%)
- Sports (9.2%)
- Other (11.4%).

Spinal cord injury can occur at any level; it can be complete or incomplete. The most common level of SCI injury in adults is C5, followed by C4, C6, C7, T12, and L1. In children, fractures of C1 and C2 are more common. SCI primarily affects young healthy adult, mostly young adult males (80.7% male predominance) and thus is a devastating and life-altering injury. SCI can present from minor symptoms like pain numbness to severe symptoms like paralysis and incontinence. Injury to any one of the seven cervical vertebra can cause quadriplegia (injury at the level of neck). Spinal cord injuries not only damage the sensory and motor system but also cause muscle atrophy, pressure sore, kidney, bladder and bowel problems, cardiac and respiratory dysfunctions.

MODES OF SPINAL INJURIES

Modes of spinal injuries can be seen through **Figures 1 and 2**.

Clues of Spinal Trauma from Mechanism of Injury

- Stabbing/impalement near spine
- Shooting/blast injury to the neck or torso (**Fig. 3**)
- Trauma above the clavicles
- Diving accidents or falls
- Motor vehicle collision or bicycle accidents.

Signs and Symptoms of Spinal Trauma

- Neck or back pain
- Local muscle spasm
- Paralysis
- Loss of movement or weakness
- Sensory dysfunction
- Numbness or tingling.

Physical Examination Findings of Spinal Trauma

- Pain on movement/palpation
- Obvious deformity
- Guarding
- Loss of sensation
- Weak/flaccid muscles
- Incontinence
- Priapism
- Spinal shock.

VARIOUS SYNDROMES IN SPINAL CORD INJURY

Anterior Cord Syndrome

Findings include loss of voluntary motor function and pain and temperature sensation below the level of the injury with preservation of the posterior column functions of position and function.

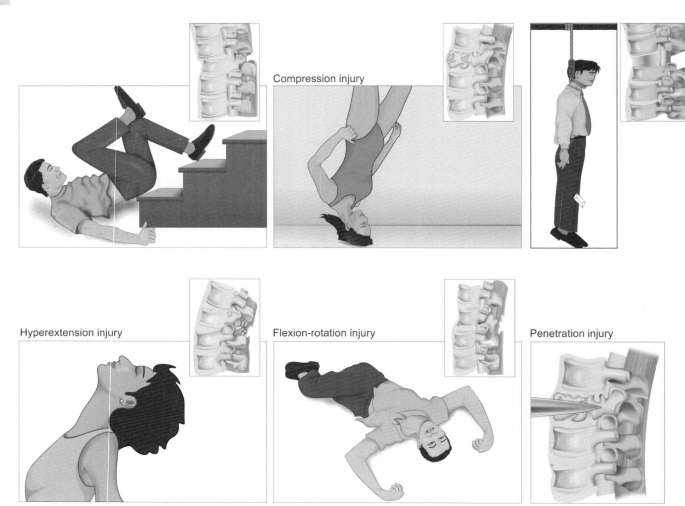

Fig. 1 Types of spinal injury

Central Cord Syndrome

Central part of the cervical cord is usually affected; upper part of body is involved. Bowel or bladder control is usually preserved. The mechanism of injury is due to hyperextension of a cervical spine. Most cases of central cord syndrome will slowly improve if the patient is given time to recover. Therefore, many doctors will treat this injury nonsurgically and instead offer supportive care and physical therapy to speed up functional recovery.

Brown-Séquard Syndrome

Due to penetrating trauma, hemisection of the spinal cord causes loss of pain and temperature on the opposite side, and motor and posterior column functions are lost on the side of the injury.

Cauda Equina Syndrome

Due to injury to lumbar, sacral, and coccygeal nerve roots, there can be motor and sensory loss in the lower extremities, bowel and bladder dysfunction, and loss of pain sensation at the perineum (*saddle anesthesia*).

TYPES OF FRACTURES (TABLE 1)

The types of fractures are:
1. Compression fractures **(Figs 4A and B)**
2. Burst fractures **(Figs 5A and B)**
3. Seat belt fractures **(Figs 6A and B)**.

CHAPTER 85 Spinal Trauma

Table 1 Types of fractures		
Types	Column affected	Stable vs unstable
Wedge fractures	Anterior only	Stable
Burst fractures	Anterior and middle	Unstable
Fracture/dislocation injuries	Anterior, middle, posterior	Unstable
Seat belt fractures	Anterior, middle, posterior	Unstable

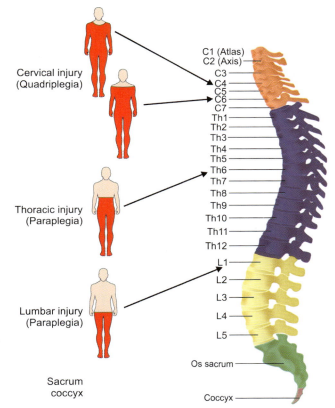

Fig. 2 Sites of spinal injury

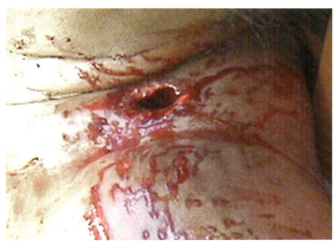

Fig. 3 Shooting injury to the neck

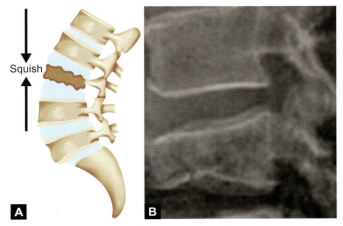

Figs 4A and B Compression fracture

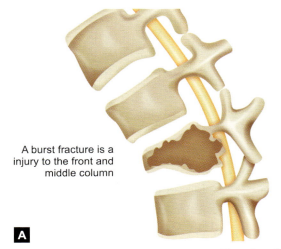

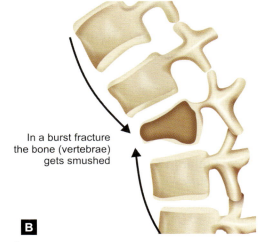

Figs 5A and B Burst fracture

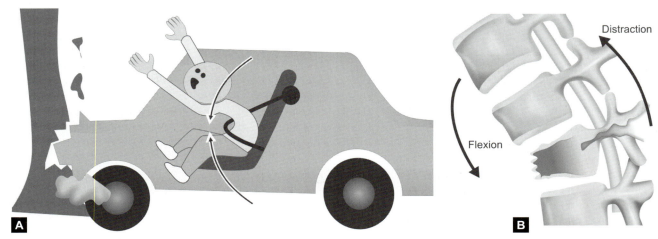

Figs 6A and B (A) Road traffic accident head on collision; (B) Seat belt fracture

PREHOSPITAL CARE AND SPINE IMMOBILIZATION

Patients who need spine immobilization:
- Car rollover
- Fall from height
- Spine pain or tenderness
- Focal neurologic deficit
- Head injury with facial trauma low Glasgow coma scale (GCS).

Technique of Removal of Helmet

Helmet Removal Technique

Two rescuer are involved in this process first rescuer maintain the inline stabilization placing the both side of mandible and apply pressure on the jaw. Second rescuer slide the helmet backward if the helmet is covering the full face, glasses should be removed first and helmet should be expand laterally to clear the ears and moved backward and raised over the nose for soft removal **(Fig. 7)**.

Airway Management in Spinal Trauma

- Stabilize in *neutral position*
- Open and secure airway
- Jaw thrust technique of opening airway during intubation (head tilt chin lift technique is not permitted in suspected cervical spine victim)
- Apply cervical collar.

Apply Cervical Collar in Suspected Cervical Spine Injury

Cervical collar provides excellent support to head when appropriate size is used **(Fig. 8)**.

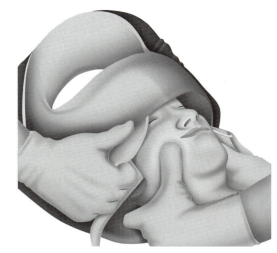

Fig. 7 Helmet removal in suspected spine trauma by supporting neck

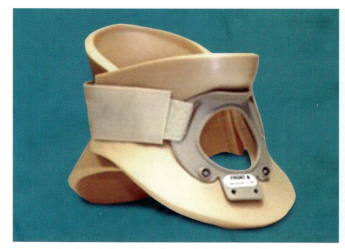

Fig. 8 Cervical collars—Philadelphia collar

CHAPTER 85 Spinal Trauma

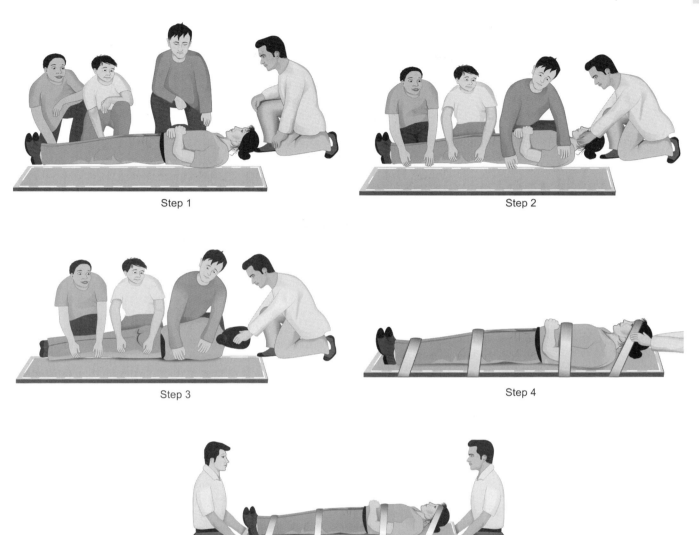

Fig. 9 Technique of logroll in shifting suspected spinal trauma

Technique of Logroll in Shifting Suspected Spinal Trauma

Logroll is the procedure used to put the injured on a stretcher. Four persons are required. Maximum care must be taken to avoid worsening an unstable trauma. The head-neck-chest axis must be kept straight to protect the spine and the first responders must keep the patient's body stable (no movement of the feet) during the lift **(Fig. 9)**.

Spine Boards

Traditionally, when any spinal injury has been suspected, the entire spine has been immobilized onto a long board, along with placement of a rigid collar to immobilize the cervical spine.

Spine boards can cause significant discomfort to the patient, skin breakdown and decubitus ulcers in a relatively short amount of time. It can compromise ventilatory status

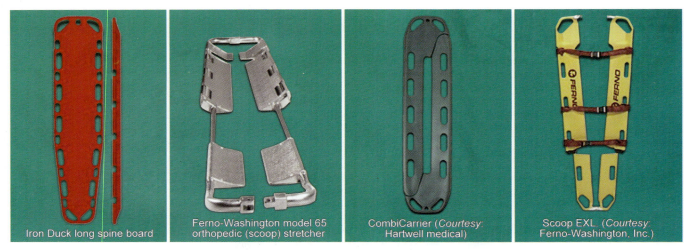

Fig. 10 Spine boards, scoops, CombiCarrier and orthopedic stretcher

in some patients. Thus for all of these reasons, patients who are placed on a backboard initially should be removed from them as soon as possible. The backboard should continue to be used for specific purposes. It is an excellent device to help extricate patients or when patients need to be carried over large distances **(Fig. 10)**.

Ambulatory Care in the Patient with Spinal Cord Trauma

- Airway with high-flow oxygen
- Spinal motion restriction on spine board
- Load-and-go
- Intravenous (IV) access en route
- Monitor cardiac status.

MANAGEMENT IN EMERGENCY DEPARTMENT

- Airway and hemorrhage control
- Early endotracheal intubation is always recommended whenever signs of existing or potential airway compromise, including altered mental status, expanding hematoma, hypoventilation or hypoxia, or direct trauma to the trachea or larynx.
- Tracheostomy by an appropriately trained physician is preferred, if there is an anterior hematoma or visible damage to the larynx and cricoid cartilage.
- Early gastric and bladder decompression are also indicated. Overhydration should be avoided so as to not cause pulmonary edema.
- Emergency department should use full sterile precautions for any procedure, such as urinary catheters or central venous access, when possible.

Emergency Evaluation of Spinal Trauma

A—Altered mental state: Check for drugs or alcohol.
M—Mechanism of injury
U—Underlying conditions: Are high-risk factors for fractures present?
S—Symptoms: Is pain, paresthesias, or neurologic compromise there?
T—Timing: When did the symptoms begin in relation to the event?

Conscious patients:
- *Sensory*—touch fingers and toes
- *Motor*—have patient move fingers and toes.

Unconscious patients:
- May withdraw when you pinch fingers or toes. Document and repeat every 5 minutes
  Spine examination for any pain tenderness deformities
  Neurological examination to assess sensory and motor functions.

Radiological Evaluation of Spine Trauma

X-rays are often the first step in evaluating a spine injury **(Figs 11A to C)**; check for:
- Alignment (smooth line at anterior and posterior vertebral line)
- Bone (vertebral bodies spine process)
- Cartilage (intervertebral disk space)
- Soft tissues.

However, these days emergency rooms that treat high-energy trauma will take patients directly to the computerized axial tomography (CAT) scanner before getting X-rays. CAT

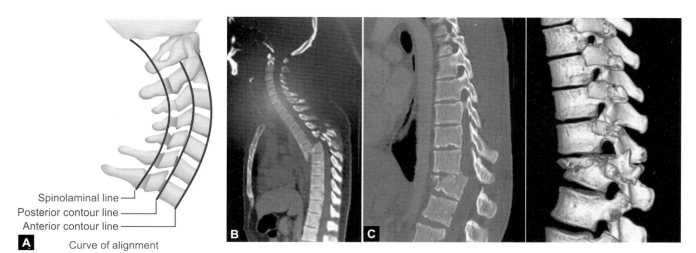

Figs 11A to C X-rays of spine trauma

scans are best thought of as a collection of many X-ray slices, which are taken from multiple angles, which provide a 3D picture of the spine. They are very helpful in showing spine fractures (broken vertebrae) or vertebrae displacement. However, a magnetic resonance imaging (MRI) is often ordered as well to look for injury to the spinal ligaments and the spinal cord itself (a CT scan is great at showing bones, but not very helpful in showing soft tissue injury like tendons, ligaments, and nerves).

In addition to getting all of these images of the spine, a very detailed neurologic examination is necessary to determine the degree of spinal cord damage, and also to localize the site of injury. By assessing where a patient is feeling muscle weakness or numbness, doctors are able to pin point which vertebrae in the spine are likely to be damaged. All of this information is critical when doctors decide on a plan of treatment.

TREATMENT

The primary goal is to protect the spinal cord from further injury (this occurs if the spine is unstable and the vertebral bones slip even further out of position). If spine is not significantly deformed, and there is no significant damage to the posterior spinal ligaments, then patients can be treated safely with a brace that goes around the chest and back to provide stability while the injury heals.

If a patient presents with signs of SCI, and the CT scan or MRI shows a high likelihood of injury to the spinal cord, then surgery is recommended. The surgery is performed to take pressure off the spinal cord, and to stabilize an otherwise unstable spine using metal rods and screws (this prevents the vertebrae from moving further out of position, thus further pressing against the spinal cord).

The fractures will typically heal well when given time. The key is to ensure they heal with good alignment, so there is no pressure on the spinal cord. Often ligaments are very slow to heal, if at all, and that is why rods and screws are used to stabilize the spine. Our natural ligaments are replaced by metal support. Sometimes, there is an injury to the posterior ligaments that is not fully appreciated and the injury is treated without surgery, and then a follow up X-ray taken months or years later can show a progressive spinal deformity called kyphosis (or better known as a hunched back).

Unfortunately, recovery from neurologic injury is less understood. Some people are able to recover, while others see only a partial or sometimes very little recovery. It depends on the force of the initial injury as well as the age of the patient and other variables that doctors do not fully understand.

Prevention of Spinal Cord Injury

- Using safety equipment
- Safety regulations in sports and traffic.

SUMMARY

Effective and efficient management of spinal injury is important in emergency department. Cervical spine protection during initial evaluation and stabilization and prevention of further neurological injury remains the major management principle. Understanding of the spine anatomy; types of spine injury; and associated neurologic, vascular, and soft tissue injuries to manage this potentially devastating injury is paramount importance. Importance should be given to prehospital care of suspected spinal injury. Prehospital providers should be supervised and trained in out of hospital management of spine injury.

BIBLIOGRAPHY

1. Ahn H, Singh J, Nathens A, et al. Pre-hospital care management of a potential spinal cord injured patient: A systematic review of the literature and evidence-based guidelines. J Neurotrauma. 2011;28(8):1341-61.
2. Augustine JJ. Spinal trauma. In: Campbell JR. International Trauma Life Support for Emergency Care Providers. New York, USA: Pearson Education; 2012.
3. Bigelow S, Medzon R. Injuries of the spine: Nerve. In: Legome E, Shockley LW (Eds). Trauma: A Comprehensive Emergency Medicine Approach. Cambridge University Press; 2011.
4. Bracken MB. Steroids for acute spinal cord injury. Cochrane Database Syst Rev. 2012;1:CD001046.
5. Bracken MB. Steroids for acute spinal cord injury. Cochrane Database Syst Rev. 2002;(2):CD001046.
6. Cameron P, Jelinek G, Kelly AM, et al. Textbook of Adult Emergency Medicine, 4th edition. Canada: Elsevier Health Sciences; 2014.
7. DeKoning EP. Cervical spine injuries. In: Sherman S, Weber J, Schindlbeck M, Patwari R. Clinical Emergency Medicine. New York, USA: McGraw-Hill Education; 2014.
8. Fehlings MG, Cadotte DW, Fehlings LN. A series of systematic reviews on the treatment of acute spinal cord injury: A foundation for best medical practice. J Neurotrauma. 2011;28(8):1329-33.
9. Hadley MN, Walters BC, Grabb PA, et al. Pharmacological therapy after acute cervical spinal cord injury. Neurosurgery. 2002;50(Suppl 3):S63-72.
10. Kwan I, Bunn F, Roberts IG. Spinal immobilization for trauma patients. Cochrane Database Syst Rev. 2001;(2):CD002803.
11. Manoach S, Paladino L. Manual in-line stabilization for acute airway management of suspected cervical spine injury: historical review and current questions. Ann Emerg Med. 2007;50:236-45.
12. Marx J, Walls R, Hockberger R. Rosen's Emergency Medicine: Concepts and Clinical Practice, 8th edition. Philadelphia: Elsevier Health Sciences; 2013.
13. Michaleff ZA, Maher CG, Verhagen AP, et al. Accuracy of the Canadian C-spine rule and NEXUS to screen for clinically important cervical spine injury in patients following blunt trauma: a systematic review. CMAJ. 2012;184(16):E867-76.
14. Oteir AO, Smith K, Jennings PA, et al. The prehospital management of suspected spinal cord injury: an update. Prehosp Disaster Med. 2014;29(4):399-402.
15. Pearson AM, Martin BI, Lindsey M, et al. C2 vertebral fractures in the medicare population: incidence, outcomes, and costs. J Bone Joint Surg Am. 2016;98(6):449-56.
16. Shah KH, Egan D, Quaas J. Essential Emergency Trauma. Lippincott Williams & Wilkins; 2012.
17. Song J, Shao J, Qi HH, et al. Risk factors for respiratory failure with tetraplegia after acute traumatic cervical spinal cord injury. Eur Rev Med Pharmacol. 2015;19:9-14.
18. Spine and Spinal Cord Trauma. ATLS (Advanced Trauma Life Support): Student Course Manual, 9th edition. American College of Surgeons; 2012. pp. 174-205.
19. Standard Neurological Classification of Spinal Cord Injury. American Spinal Injury Association and ISCOS. Archived from the original on June 18, 2011. Retrieved 5 November 2015.
20. Stuke LE, Pons PT, Guy JS, et al. Prehospital spine immobilization for penetrating trauma—review and recommendations from the Prehospital Trauma Life Support Executive Committee. J Trauma. 2011;71(3):763-9.
21. Sundstrøm T, Asbjørnsen H, Habiba S, et al. Prehospital use of cervical collars in trauma patients: a critical review. J Neurotrauma. 2014;31(6):531-40.
22. Wyatt JP, Illingworth RN, Graham CA, et al. Oxford Handbook of Emergency Medicine. UK: Oxford University Press; 2012.
23. Yu WY, He DW. Current trends in spinal cord injury repair. Eur Rev Med Pharmacol Sci. 2015;19(18):3340-4.

CHAPTER 86

Thoracic Trauma

Shaiwal Khandelwal, Ali Zamir Khan

INTRODUCTION

Approximately, 20% of all trauma patients sustain injury to their thorax. Penetrating chest injuries often caused by gunshot or stab wounds are obvious at the time of presentation. Sequelae of injury may cause subcutaneous emphysema or sucking chest wounds, which can be easily identified. Alternatively, in blunt chest trauma the signs of injury may be more subtle, presenting solely with tachypnea or tachycardia. A detailed history, if available, is important to understand the mechanism of injury so that the potential injuries can be diagnosed.

Physical examination is a part of initial assessment and is essential in determining injuries. A primary survey is immediately performed as soon as the patient arrives in the emergency department (ED). The goal of the primary survey is to identify immediate, life-threatening injuries that could cause ventilation or hemodynamic instabilities that, if left uncorrected, could lead to the death of the patient.[1] The Advanced Trauma Life Support (ATLS) guidelines as described by American College of Surgeons provides the standard protocols of resuscitation of trauma patients.

The ABC (airway, breathing, and circulation) algorithm is followed so that potentially life-threatening injuries can be recognized before they become lethal: the airway is controlled, then breathing is assessed and assisted with mechanical ventilation if necessary, and third, circulation is supported by establishing reliable, large-bore venous access and initiating fluid resuscitation. Finally, the patient's neurologic disabilities are assessed, and the entire body is exposed to identify any significant deformities or penetrating injuries that might otherwise have been overlooked.

Several diagnostic tests are used for the work up of patients with thoracic trauma.

CHEST X-RAY

Chest X-ray should be done and evaluated urgently in the ED in all patients with suspected thoracic trauma. A systematic review of the film should reveal suspected and unsuspected injures, and the presence of any foreign bodies.

Fractures of the bony thorax, including the ribs, clavicles, spine, and scapulas, should be excluded. Fractures of the thoracic cage indicate significant energy transfer to the patient. Fractures of the upper ribs and scapula may be associated with trauma to the great vessels and fractures of the clavicle may be associated with pulmonary or cardiac contusions. The lung fields should be examined for pneumothorax, hemothorax, or pulmonary contusion. In patients with chest X-ray showing mediastinal widening, pneumomediastinum, or shifting there should be high suspicion for aortic transection, tracheobronchial or esophageal injuries, or tension pneumothorax or hemothorax. The soft tissues may reveal subtle subcutaneous air or foreign bodies. Finally, the width of the cardiac silhouette may raise the suspicion of tamponade.

COMPUTERIZED TOMOGRAPHY SCAN

Computerized tomography (CT) scan should be done when the patient is hemodynamically stable. It can be rapidly done, and may reveal injuries not seen clearly on chest X-ray: aortic disruption, pneumothorax, pneumomediastinum, hemothorax, or pulmonary contusions. It may be useful to screen all patients with blunt trauma and has been shown to be more sensitive than chest X-ray in detecting thoracic injuries such as pulmonary contusions, hemothorax, and pneumothorax. Up to 75% of trauma patients with a normal physical examination and chest X-ray will have an occult injury diagnosed on chest CT, and 5% of these patients will need intervention for their injuries.[2,3] CT chest done in patients with evidence of thoracic trauma in physical examination and chest X-ray, may lead to altered management and therapeutic decisions in up to a third of patients. Three-dimensional (3D) reconstruction of the bony cage increases the sensitivity of detecting the fractures.

FOCUSED ASSESSMENT WITH SONOGRAPHY FOR TRAUMA

Focused assessment with sonography for trauma (FAST) is a rapid bedside ultrasound examination performed by surgeons, emergency physicians, and certain paramedics as a screening test for blood around the heart (pericardial effusion) or abdominal organs (hemoperitoneum) after trauma. The extended FAST (eFAST) allows for the examination of both lungs by adding bilateral anterior thoracic sonography to the FAST examination.[4,5] This allows for the detection of pneumothorax with the absence of normal "lung-sliding" and "comet-tail" artefact (seen on the ultrasound screen). Compared with supine chest X-ray, with CT or clinical course as the gold standard, bedside sonography has superior sensitivity (49–99% versus 27–75%), similar specificity (95–100%), and can be performed in less than a minute. The subxiphoid view is the most accurate in the hands of surgeons for detecting abnormalities in the trauma setting. It is safe, expeditious, repeatable, and effective even in the hands of surgeons from different specialties and can be useful to identify injuries to the heart, and fluid in the pericardium.

ANGIOGRAPHY

Conventional angiography was once the gold standard in the diagnosis of aortic transection or injuries to the great vessels. The present role of conventional arteriography is unclear, as many centers now use highly detailed CT angiography scan with 3D aortic reconstructions alone for diagnosis and operative planning.[6] Others obtain a conventional aortogram if the results of the CT angiogram are equivocal or if the study was technically inadequate. Still others routinely obtain conventional arteriograms to confirm the presence of an aortic injury prior to surgical intervention. When performed, a retrograde femoral arteriogram is the preferred study. The indications for conventional or CT angiography are listed in **Box 1**.

CHEST WALL INJURIES

Blunt trauma to the chest wall can disrupt respiratory mechanics provided by the chest wall and lead to poor pulmonary toilet and significant morbidity. Chest wall trauma alone occurs in only 16% of cases and is more often a marker of more ominous injury to the visceral organs in the chest or in the abdomen.[7]

Box 1 Indications for angiographic studies for potential thoracic injuries

- High-speed deceleration injuries
- Chest radiographic findings:
  - Widened mediastinum
  - Loss of aortic knob shadow
  - Tracheal or esophageal deviation to the right
  - Widening of paraspinal stripe and/or apical capping
  - Downward displacement of left main-stem bronchus
  - Obliteration of the aortopulmonary window
  - Fractured first rib, sternum, or scapula
  - Multiple rib fractures or flail chest
  - Massive hemothorax
- Upper extremity hypertension
- Unexplained hypotension
- Pulse deficits or asymmetry
- Systolic murmur

Rib Fractures

Fracture of the ribs is the most common blunt thoracic injury. Rib fractures are an important indicator of trauma severity. The greater the number of ribs fractured, the higher is the patient's morbidity and mortality, especially if six or more ribs are broken. The number of ribs fractured has been significantly correlated with the presence of hemothorax or pneumothorax if two or more ribs were fractured.[8,9] Fractures of the fourth through the ninth rib are associated with injuries to the lung, bronchus, pleura, and heart, whereas fractures below the ninth rib are indicative of spleen, hepatic, or renal injuries. The main symptoms include pain, tenderness, and sometimes bony crepitus. Chest radiograph alone fails to diagnose rib fractures in over half of trauma patients with fractures, and the addition of CT to the trauma evaluation improves the sensitivity of the diagnosis of rib fractures.[10] Elderly patients (≥65 years old) with simple rib fractures are five times more likely to die than those younger than 65 years.[11] The first rib fracture has particular significance because of the great force required for it to occur and the likelihood that intrathoracic visceral injury has also taken place. CT angiography is indicated to access intrathoracic vasculature. The modern approach to treatment is to provide relief of pain, so that patient can perform chest physiotherapy so as to optimize pulmonary toilet and prevent atelectasis. Interventions used for short-term pain relief include epidural analgesia, intercostal rib blocks, intrapleural instillation of local anesthetic agent, and intravenous opiates as well as oral nonsteroidal anti-inflammatory drugs (NSAIDs).[12-14]

Flail Chest

This injury usually occurs with the fracture of four or more ribs at two sites, either unilateral or bilateral. This leads to instability of the thoracic cage causing paradoxical motion locally.

This impairs respiratory mechanics and results in hypoventilation, poor pulmonary drainage, and atelectasis. Endotracheal intubation is required in more than two-thirds of patients with flail chest and is indicated for a respiratory rate of more than 40 breaths per minute, or a pO_2 of less than 60 mm Hg despite 60% face mask oxygen.[15] Relative indications for intubation include shallow respirations, depressed consciousness, preexisting chronic lung disease, or the presence of associated injuries. It is highly associated with pulmonary contusion, which occurs in about 45% of these patients.[16] Conservative therapy with emphasis on pain relief with thoracic epidural analgesia is the mainstay of treatment. Few intubated patients with no possibility of being weaned from the ventilator because of a large unstable flail segment of chest wall require chest wall stabilization.[17,18]

Sternal Fractures

Isolated fractures of the sternum are seen with increasing frequency in motor vehicle accidents, particularly because of the rapid deceleration, especially in vehicles with absent or malfunctioning airbags.[19] Physical examination may reveal point tenderness, edema, and obvious deformity. A lateral chest radiograph is diagnostic in the majority of patients.

Morbidity and mortality from isolated sternal fractures is low, and surgical repair is uncommon (<2%). Selective repair is indicated in patients with severe deformities or associated chest wall fractures.[20]

Clavicular Fractures

The clavicles are thin and exposed, are often fractures in thoracic trauma. The mid-clavicular shaft, in particular, is often fractured, and this occurs in three of four patients with clavicular fractures.[21] Clinical examination reveals tenderness, deformity, crepitus, and occasionally upper extremity neurovascular injury. Routine chest radiographs often demonstrate the diagnosis. Conservative treatment for pain control using closed reduction and figure of eight slings heals 95% of patients.

Scapular Fracture

Scapular fractures are relatively rare and usually occur only after high kinetic-energy impacts, because the scapula is thick and well protected. They are usually associated with injuries to other sites because of the severe amount of energy needed to produce this injury.[22] Diagnosis is often difficult on physical examination, occasionally identified by localized tenderness, swelling, and hematoma formation over the fracture site. Scapular fractures are often overlooked on supine chest radiographs, and the three-view trauma series of the shoulder is often necessary to reveal the fracture. Conservative treatment with immobilization in a sling with pain relief and early range-of-motion exercises is advocated.

Thoracic Spine

Common causes of thoracic spinal fractures include fall from a height, motor vehicle accidents, and penetrating trauma. The entire spinal column is inspected and palpated on secondary survey. Crepitus or tenderness found on examination, suspicion due to mechanism of injury, or the inability to obtain an adequate examination due to other distracting injuries should prompt additional radiographic study to determine injury to spine. CT scans with 3D reconstructions are helpful in determining if a fracture of the thoracic spine is stable or unstable.[23] Fractures of the vertebral body or transverse process are common whereas unstable fractures are not. There have been several classification systems to describe unstable fractures. The most commonly used classification system was described by Denis et al.[24] This classification system divides the spine into three columns (anterior, posterior, and middle). Disruption of two of the three columns is definitive for an unstable fracture. Unstable fractures require spinal precautions and eventually fixation of spine. Assessment of the spinal canal and injury of the cord often requires magnetic resonance imaging (MRI). In penetrating trauma, there is no role for the administration of steroids for spinal cord injuries. However, in blunt trauma, the administration of steroids for patients with neurologic deficits is controversial. The management of spinal trauma is described in Chapter 85 (Spinal Trauma).

LUNG INJURIES

Pulmonary Contusion

Pulmonary contusion is common due to injuries that impart substantial kinetic energy to the thorax.

In blunt trauma, pulmonary contusion results from the transmission of force across the bony thorax. Children may present with a large pulmonary contusion with little evidence of bony thoracic injury due to the elastic nature of immature bone. In penetrating injury due to gunshot, contusion occurs both due to the direct tissue lacerations and the dissipation of the kinetic energy of the bullet. Pulmonary contusion occur due to hemorrhage into adjacent alveolar spaces rather than injury to the alveolar capillary wall itself, and typically manifest themselves within hours of injury and usually resolve within approximately 7 days. Clinical symptoms, including respiratory distress with hypoxemia and hypercarbia, worsen for the first 24–48 hour.[25] The diagnosis of pulmonary contusion is made by the combination of pulmonary dysfunction and radiographic findings. CT is the study of choice and has been found to be more sensitive than chest X-ray in detecting a pulmonary contusion. All patients with a pulmonary contusion should be observed on supplementary oxygen in a hospital setting. The mortality rate from an isolated pulmonary contusion is low, but when combined with other severe injuries, it rises to as high as 50%.

The main goals of management are pain control, judicious fluid administration, careful hemodynamic monitoring, and aggressive pulmonary toilet. Older patients are particularly susceptible to complications following pulmonary contusion.[26]

Penetrating Lung Injury

The majority of patients with penetrating lung injury can be managed with tube thoracostomy alone.[27] However, 20% of patients who require thoracotomy will need some form of lung resection.[28] The extent of the lung resection has been shown to be an independent predictor of hospital mortality.

The worst outcomes are seen with pneumonectomy.[29] The use of staplers has facilitated rapid and minimal resection thereby reducing mortality. Stapled pulmonary tractotomy has been shown in several series to provide rapid and effective exposure to bleeding pulmonary parenchymal vessels and transected bronchi.[30]

Tracheobronchial Injuries

Tracheobronchial injuries are uncommon, but they occur usually after high-energy impact and are associated with trauma to other vital organs.[31] High-speed motor vehicle accident is the most common cause for tracheobronchial injuries. More than 80% of tracheobronchial injuries are due to blunt trauma and are located within 2.5 cm of the carina.[32] Three potential mechanisms of blunt tracheobronchial disruption have been identified. The first and most common is a forceful anteroposterior compression of the thoracic cage, the so-called dashboard injury, where an unrestrained automobile occupant hyperextends the neck, striking it on the dashboard or steering wheel and producing a crushing injury of the cervical trachea. The second mechanism is a consequence of high airway pressures, and the third is a rapid deceleration. The typical clinical features include respiratory distress, dyspnea, and air leak. Hoarseness or dysphonia is also common. Persistence of an undiagnosed air leak is life-threatening and may lead to hypoventilation and, ultimately, respiratory insufficiency. On physical examination, the most common diagnostic signs are subcutaneous emphysema (35–85%), pneumothorax (20–50%), and hemoptysis (14–25%). The investigation of choice is a flexible bronchoscopy. Effective airway management consists of bypassing the lesion with endobronchial intubation to the healthy bronchus using a single- or double-lumen endotracheal tube. Primary surgical repair of the injured airway is often necessary. More severe injury may even require lobectomy or pneumonectomy. Prompt diagnosis and treatment generally lead to good functional recovery, but if tracheobronchial injuries remain undetected and untreated, late complications such as bronchial stenosis, recurrent pneumonia, and bronchiectasis can develop.

CARDIAC INJURIES

Blunt Cardiac Injury

Blunt cardiac injury is blunt chest trauma that causes contusion of myocardial muscle, rupture of a cardiac chamber, or disruption of a heart valve. Sometimes a blow to the anterior chest wall causes cardiac arrest without any structural lesion (commotio cordis).

Manifestations vary with the injury. Diagnosis is established by electrocardiogram (ECG), echocardiography, and cardiac enzymes. Cardiac markers [e.g. troponin, creatine phosphokinase MB] are most useful to screening and thus help to exclude blunt cardiac injury. If cardiac markers and ECG are normal and there are no arrhythmias, blunt cardiac injury can be safely excluded.

Patients with myocardial contusion causing conduction abnormalities require cardiac monitoring for 24 hour because they are at risk for sudden dysrhythmias during this time. Treatment is mainly supportive (e.g. treatment of symptomatic dysrhythmias or heart failure) and is seldom needed. Surgical repair is indicated for rare cases of myocardial or valvular rupture.

Patients with commotio cordis are treated for their dysrhythmia [e.g. resuscitation with cardiopulmonary resuscitation and defibrillation followed by in hospital observation].

Penetrating Cardiac Injury

Penetrating cardiac trauma is a highly lethal but potentially salvageable injury.[33] Approximately 90% of victims with penetrating cardiac wounds die before reaching the hospital.[34] Factors predicting improved survival include patients who receive prompt diagnosis and surgical intervention, stab wounds versus gunshot wounds, single-chamber versus multiple-chamber injury, and the location of thoracotomy (operating room vs. ED).[35,36] Death occurs as a result of cardiac tamponade or exsanguination. A suspicion of cardiac injury should be made in any patients with a precordial penetrating wound. The diagnosis of tamponade by physical examination can be challenging, since the classic triad of tamponade (hypotension, muffled heart tones, and jugular venous distention) is only present in one-third of patients. The chest radiograph may demonstrate a widening of the cardiac silhouette. Ultrasonography shows presence of blood in the pericardial space. Echocardiography is a rapid, noninvasive, and accurate test for pericardial fluid and is now incorporated into the FAST evaluation. Pericardiocentesis can be both diagnostic and therapeutic, and is reserved for patients with significant hemodynamic compromise without another likely etiology. Cardiac lesions may be initially inapparent. Wounds of the ventricle may be self-sealing, and small lacerations may be contained by clot within the pericardium. Prompt definitive therapy is imperative and based on the patient's hemodynamic status. This includes emergency thoracotomy and suture of the cardiac wound. Emergency department thoracotomy is seldom indicated, being reserved for moribund patients or those whose condition is rapidly deteriorating without time for transfer to the operating room. Left anterolateral thoracotomy is the preferred initial approach because rapid access to the heart can be gained.

Aortic Injury

More than 90% of thoracic great vessel injuries are due to penetrating trauma, gunshots and stab wound are the most common cause of injury.[37] Most of these injuries are lethal because of exsanguinating hemorrhage, massive hemothorax, and pericardial tamponade, which usually occur, resulting in death even in the most efficient trauma center, there is little hope for salvage. Blunt aortic injury (BAI) is the most common of the cardiovascular trauma and is associated with significant morbidity and mortality.[38] BAI is second to head injury as the leading cause of death after road traffic accidents. The vast majority of these injuries are produced from the rapid deceleration mechanism which is encountered in motor vehicle accidents with high-risk collision.[39] However, they may also occur from falls, pedestrian accidents, and crushing chest wounds. BAI should be considered in all patients sustaining injuries due to motor vehicle accidents. Characteristics of high-risk occupant include age more than 60, front-seat occupancy, or unrestrained. A chest X-ray should be the initial screening tool. The most common finding prompting further diagnostic work up includes a widened mediastinum, obscure aortic knob, left pleural effusion, first and/or second rib fracture, tracheal deviation, or depressed left bronchus.[40]

The predominant mechanism of BAI is described as the force of deceleration concentrated at the junction of the fixed and nonfixed segments of the thoracic aorta. The isthmus is the most frequent site of rupture (50–70%) followed by ascending aorta or arch (18%), and the distal thoracic aorta (14%).[41] CT angiography with 3D reconstruction is now preferred over conventional angiography. In the last decade, there have been several significant changes in the diagnosis and management of BAI. Prompt repair of BAI is preferred when there are no other substantial injuries that would otherwise complicate the repair. Medical control of blood pressure with beta-blockers and nitroprusside is recommended until surgery. Endovascular stenting is now shown to be a safe and effective procedure with excellent technical success while maintaining low rates of complication.[42]

Injuries to Other Great Vessels

Most of the injuries to the great vessels are the result of penetrating trauma and require immediate intervention. Diagnostic investigation to determine the precise anatomic localization of injury is appropriate only for hemodynamically stable patients. Proximal vessel injuries (pulmonary hilar, innominate, and superior vena caval injuries) are often diagnosed at exploration done for massive bleeding. More distal vessels (neck, subclavian, and axillary) may be visualized with duplex ultrasonography, CT angiography, and traditional arteriography. Unequal pulses, asymmetrical artery-artery indices, and expanding hematomas should all raise suspicion for arterial injury. Massive bleeding may be seen with both arterial and venous injury. As with other cases of massive hemorrhage, minimizing time between injury and definitive operative management is the key to reducing mortality. All subclavian and axillary injuries should undergo surgical repair except in the most severely unstable patients. Temporary shunting may be necessary in these patients. Due to the difficulty and increased morbidity of achieving exposure to repair injuries to the thoracic outlet, recently there has been interest in using endovascular techniques. In unstable patients, the options are limited to immediate exploration.

ESOPHAGEAL INJURIES

The incidence of esophageal injury after blunt or penetrating trauma is rare. The low incidence is related to several factors. The esophagus lies in the deep location of posterior mediastinum protected by the bony shell of the thoracic cavity. In addition, esophageal injuries are often associated with other injuries, specifically vascular injuries, which require urgent attention and can lead to death prior to arrival at the hospital or missed diagnosis of small perforations. The treatment of blunt or sharp traumatic injuries to the esophagus is determined by several factors. The timing of the injury, the degree of the injury (contained vs noncontained perforation), and the location of the injury collectively guide subsequent intervention.[43] Cervical esophagus is commonly injured in penetrating trauma. Inpatients who are clinically stable with no hemodynamic instability, the esophagus is best evaluated by esophagography.[44] Clinical findings may include subcutaneous emphysema, pneumomediastinum, pleural effusion, or unexplained persistent fever for more than 24 hours following injury. Esophageal injuries identified early are repaired primarily (in layers, if possible) and is often reinforced with tissue-flap coverage (pleural tissue, intercostal muscle, or fundoplication). Those repaired in a delayed manner (>12 hr) require wide drainage with multiple tube thoracostomies. Esophageal diversion is considered especially if there is evidence of mediastinitis.

DIAPHRAGMATIC INJURIES

Traumatic diaphragmatic injury can occur due to penetrating or blunt thoracoabdominal trauma. The incidence of diaphragmatic injuries is difficult to estimate because diaphragmatic hernias are often missed by diagnostic imaging and found as incidental findings later in life.[45] For blunt injury, usually seen on the left side, identification of the nasogastric tube in the left hemithorax on chest X-ray suggests herniation of the stomach and is diagnostic of diaphragmatic disruption. In the case of penetrating trauma, the diaphragmatic defect is often too small for herniation in the acute setting. However, the unrecognized defect exacerbated by the gradient between the negative intrathoracic pressure and positive intra-abdominal pressure, enlarges over time, resulting in subsequent herniation of intra-abdominal contents into the chest.[46] It is not uncommon for patients to present in the nonacute setting with a diaphragmatic hernia and a previous history of penetrating thoracoabdominal trauma.

Due to the potential of developing incarceration of bowel contained in diaphragmatic hernia, surgical exploration is recommended to evaluate diaphragm in case of left-sided thoracoabdominal trauma. Right-sided penetrating diaphragmatic injuries are thought to be of little consequence because right-sided injury is rarely associated with herniation, as the herniation of abdominal contents is prevented by liver.

PNEUMOTHORAX

Pneumothorax frequently occurs following both blunt and penetrating chest trauma. The entry of air in the pleural space results in partial or total collapse of the lungs. Physical findings may include subcutaneous emphysema identified by crepitus over the injured side and diminished or absent breath sounds. Chest X-ray demonstrates collapsed lung and absences of lung markings. The accumulation of air under pressure in the pleural space can lead to a tension pneumothorax. This condition can develop when injured tissue forms a one-way valve, allowing air to enter the pleural space and preventing it from escaping naturally. This is commonly called a "sucking" chest wound or open pneumothorax. To prevent the development of a tension pneumothorax, sterile occlusive gauze should be applied to the chest wall and taped on three sides. This creates a flutter valve that allows air to escape but not to enter the pleural cavity. A tension pneumothorax can also result from positive-pressure ventilation to an injured lung with an initially small air leak. The result of a tension pneumothorax is massive overinflation of the affected side, causing a shift of the mediastinal structures toward the opposite side of the chest as well as the flattening of the diaphragm. The increase in thoracic pressure results in a decrease in venous return to the heart and a subsequent decrease in blood pressure. On physical examination, the trachea may deviate toward the opposite side. The clinical picture associated with a tension pneumothorax should prompt immediate decompression without chest X-ray in most cases. If a chest tube is not immediately available, a large-bore intravenous catheter can be used to access the chest cavity. The needle should be inserted in the second intercostal space in the mid-clavicular line. This temporizing maneuver should be followed by the urgent placement of a thoracostomy tube placed in the fifth intercostal space at the anterior axillary line. Simple pneumothorax is treated by tube thoracostomy alone. For uncomplicated pneumothorax, moderate-sized (28F) tubes are appropriate. The presentation of an uncomplicated pneumothorax is rare because of associated intrapleural hemorrhage due to trauma. This necessitates the use of a larger tube (36F) to allow for better drainage.

HEMOTHORAX

Bleeding into the pleural space can occur with injury to the tissues of the chest wall and pleura, or the intrathoracic structures. Even minor injury to the chest wall can lead to a significant hemothorax. In addition, intra-abdominal bleeding in patients with diaphragmatic injury can manifest as a hemothorax. The initial treatment of hemothorax is tube thoracostomy. A 32-F chest tube or larger should be placed to ensure effective drainage of intrapleural blood and reexpansion of the lung. The reexpansion of the lung often tamponades the bleeding and further treatment is not required. However, if the hemothorax is massive or if the bleeding is ongoing, then the patient should be taken to the operating room for prompt thoracotomy and hemostasis.

Following the insertion of a chest tube, a chest X-ray, upright if possible, should be obtained to evaluate placement of the tube and confirm evacuation of the hemothorax. Occasionally the clotted blood can clog the tube, leading to a false impression that the ongoing bleeding is minimal. The presence of a retained hemothorax and persistent hypotension should raise suspicion that ongoing bleeding is present. Sometimes the chest tube is kinked resulting in occlusion. The simple maneuver of spinning the chest tube before fixing it in place can prevent this from occurring. Both of these clinical scenarios can be detected on X-ray, thereby emphasizing the importance of obtaining a postprocedure X-ray.

Chest Tube Management

Only 10–15% of all chest wounds require thoracotomy, whereas the remaining 85% can be managed with a closed tube thoracostomy. Thoracotomy should be performed for hemodynamically unstable patients with chest trauma that are not responsive to adequate resuscitation. Other indications for thoracotomy are greater than 1,500 mL of blood evacuated initially on chest tube insertion, ongoing blood loss (>200–300 mL/hr for 4 hr), and persistent hemothorax despite adequate drainage with two chest tubes **(Box 2)**. For patients with hemopneumothorax, the chest tube can be removed when the output decreases to less than

Box 2 Indications for thoracotomy

- Penetrating injury with cardiac arrest
- Immediate output of >1,500 mL of blood from the chest tube insertion
- Ongoing blood loss (>200–300 mL of blood per hour over 4 hours)
- Persistent hemothorax despite adequate chest tube placement
- Ongoing massive air leak
- Evidence of esophageal injury
- Evidence of diaphragmatic injury
- Large chest wall defect requiring reconstruction

Box 3 Indications and contraindications for emergency room thoracotomy

Accepted indications
- Unresponsive hypotension [systolic blood pressure (SBP) < 60 mm Hg]
- Rapid exsanguination from indwelling chest tube (>1,500 mL)
- Traumatic arrest with previously witnessed cardiac activity (before or after hospital admission), after penetrating thoracic injuries
- Persistent hypotension (SBP <60 mm Hg) with diagnosed cardiac tamponade, air embolism

Relative indications
- Traumatic arrest with previously witnessed cardiac activity (before or after hospital admission), after blunt trauma
- Traumatic arrest without previously witnessed cardiac activity (before or after hospital admission), after penetrating chest injuries
- Prehospital cardiopulmonary resuscitation: <10 minutes in intubated patient, <5 minutes in nonintubated patient

Contraindications
- Blunt thoracic injuries with no previously witnessed cardiac activity
- Multiple blunt trauma
- Severe head injury

200 mL/24 hr and there is no recurrence of pneumothorax on water seal. Thoracoscopy should be considered for residual hemothorax. A significant complication associated with tube thoracostomy, although rare, is empyema. When a bullet or knife penetrates the chest cavity and enters the pleural space, bacterial contamination occurs. Antibiotics should be used to prevent development of empyema.

EMERGENCY DEPARTMENT THORACOTOMY

Emergency department thoracotomy clearly plays a role in patients having penetrating chest injury particularly in patients who develop cardiac tamponade following penetrating trauma. For patients with blunt chest injuries, the only accepted indication is the patient who arrives with vital signs and suffers a traumatic arrest in the ED. Thoracotomy allows relief of cardiac tamponade, the ability to perform open cardiac massage, and control of ongoing intrathoracic hemorrhage. In addition, by applying a cross-clamp to the thoracic aorta, one can limit intra-abdominal bleeding and improve cerebral and coronary perfusion in the setting of exsanguinating hemorrhage. Patients with penetrating cardiac stab wounds and other penetrating cardiac injuries are the most likely to survive resuscitation with ED thoracotomy. The likelihood of patient survival depends on the duration of time elapsed since trauma to reaching medical facility, the patient's age and comorbidities, and signs of life on arrival to the ED. General guidelines have been recommended for ED thoracotomies by the American College of Surgeons' Committee on Trauma in the setting of thoracic trauma **(Box 3)**.

The surgical approach for thoracotomy is left fouth intercostal space. It provides rapid access to most of the important anatomical structures during resuscitation including the aorta. The incision can also be extended to right side if required. An incision is made along the fourth or fifth intercostal space (between the ribs), intercostal muscles and the parietal pleura are divided, and then the ribs are retracted to provide visualization. When the incision covers both the right and left hemithoraces it is referred to as a "clamshell" thoracotomy. The clamshell thoracotomy is used when there is a right side pulmonary or vascular injury.

Video-assisted Thoracic Surgery for Trauma

The majority of traumatic hemothoraces are adequately treated with tube thoracostomy. However, residual post-traumatic hemothorax may occur in 3–8% of patients. The retained blood products are thought to be a major contributing factor in the development of an empyema and subsequent trapped lung. Video-assisted thoracic surgery (VATS) has a therapeutic role in the evacuation of retained hemothorax. The evacuation of the retained blood products reduces the risk of contamination of the residual blood, development of an empyema, and the chronic changes of a fibrothorax. VATS decortication can be performed at the same time to allow complete lung expansion. VATS evacuation has been shown to be best accomplished within 5 days after injury when the semi-solid clot can be easily suctioned. VATS is an excellent technique to perform stapling of the injured lung for penetrating injuries, assessment of intrathoracic injuries, and removal of foreign bodies from the thoracic cavity. The advantages of VATS are quite obvious in terms of less morbidity, quicker recovery of pulmonary functions, and better cosmesis.

CONCLUSION

Thoracic trauma is common presentation in polytrauma patients associated with high mortality. Systematic approach and management by emergency physician has resulted in improved outcome.

REFERENCES

1. DeArmond D, Carpenter AJ, Calhoun JH. Critical primary survey injuries. Semin Thorac Cardiovasc Surg. 2008;20(1):6-7.
2. Deunk J, Dekker HM, Brink M, et al. The value of indicated computed tomography scan of the chest and abdomen in addition to the conventional radiologic work-up for blunt trauma patients. J Trauma. 2007;63(4):757-63.
3. Omert L, Yeaney WW, Protetch J. Efficacy of thoracic computerized tomography in blunt chest trauma. Am Surg. 2001;67(7):660-4.
4. Körner M, Krötz MM, Degenhart C, et al. Current role of emergency US in patients with major trauma. Radiographics. 2008;28(1):225-42.
5. Kirkpatrick AW, Sirois M, Laupland KB, et al. Handheld thoracic sonography for detecting post-traumatic pneumothoraces: the Extended Focused Assessment with Sonography for Trauma (EFAST). J Trauma. 2004;57(2):288-95.
6. Carpenter AJ. Diagnostic techniques in thoracic trauma. Semin Thorac Cardiovasc Surg. 2008;20:2-5.
7. Shorr RM, Crittenden M, Indeck M, et al. Blunt thoracic trauma. Analysis of 515 patients. Ann Surg. 1987;206(2):200-5.
8. Sharma OP, Oswanski MF, Jolly S, et al. The Perils of rib fractures. Am Surg. 2008;74(4):310-4.
9. Flagel BT, Luchette FA, Reed RL, et al. Half a dozen ribs: the breakpoint for mortality. Surgery. 2005;138(4):723-5.
10. Livingston DH, Shogan B, John P, et al. CT diagnosis of rib fractures and the prediction of acute respiratory failure. J Trauma. 2008;64(4):905-11.
11. Bergeron E, Lavoie A, Clas D, et al. Elderly trauma patients with rib fractures are at greater risk of death and pneumonia. J Trauma. 2003;54(3):478-85.
12. Gabram SG, Schwartz RJ, Jacobs LM, et al. Clinical management of blunt trauma patients with unilateral rib fractures: a randomized trial. World J Surg. 1995;19(3):388-93.
13. Wu CL, Jani ND, Perkins FM, et al. Thoracic epidural analgesia versus intravenous patient-controlled analgesia for the treatment of rib fracture pain after motor vehicle crash. J Trauma. 1999;47(3):564-7.
14. Haenel JB, Moore FA, Moore EE, et al. Extrapleural bupivacaine for amelioration of multiple rib fracture pain. J Trauma. 1995;38(1):22-7.
15. Velmahos GC, Vassiliu P, Chan LS, et al. Influence of flail chest on outcome among patients with severe thoracic cage trauma. Int Surg. 2002;87:240-4.
16. Ciraulo DL, Elliott D, Mitchell KA, et al. Flail chest as a marker for significant injuries. J Am Coll Surg. 1994;178:466-70.
17. Oyarzun JR, Bush AP, McCormick JR, et al. Use of 3.5 mm acetabular reconstruction plates for internal fixation of flail chest injuries. Ann Thorac Surg. 1998;65(5):1471-4.
18. Carbognani P, Cattelani L, Bellini G, et al. A technical proposal for the complex flail chest. Ann Thorac Surg. 2000;70(1):342-3.
19. Knobloch K, Wagner S, Haasper C, et al. Sternal fractures are frequent following high deceleration velocities in a severe vehicle crash. Injury. 2008;39:36-43.
20. Richardson JD, Franklin GA, Heffey S, et al. Operative fixation of chest wall fractures: an underused procedure? Am Surg. 2007;73(6):591-6.
21. Nowak J, Mallmin H, Larsson S. The aetiology and epidemiology of clavicular fractures. A prospective study during a two-year period in Uppsala, Sweden. Injury. 2000;31(5):353-8.
22. Baldwin KD, Ohman-Strickland P, Mehta S, et al. Scapula fractures: a marker for concomitant injury? J Trauma. 2008;65(2):430-5.
23. Gross EA. Computed tomographic screening for thoracic and lumbar fractures: Is spine reformatting necessary? Am J Emerg Med. 2010;28(1):73-5.
24. Denis F. The three column spine and its significance in the classification of acute thoracolumbar spinal injuries. Spine (Phila Pa 1976). 1983;8(8):817-31.
25. Cohn SM, Dubose JJ. Pulmonary contusion: an update on recent advances in clinical management. World J Surg. 2010;34(8):1959-70.
26. Kollmorgen DR, Murray KA, Sulllvan JJ, et al. Predictors of mortality in pulmonary contusion. Am J Surg. 1994;168(6):659-63.
27. Onat S, Ulku R, Avci A, et al. Urgent thoracotomy for penetrating chest trauma: analysis of 158 patients of a single center. Injury. 2011;42(9):900-4.
28. Karmy-jones R, Jurkovich GJ, Shatz DV, et al. Management of traumatic lung injury: a Western Trauma Association Multicenter review. J Trauma. 2001;51(6):1049-53.
29. Martin MJ, McDonald JM, Mullenix PS, et al. Operative management and outcomes of traumatic lung resection. J Am Coll Surg. 2006;203(3):336-44.
30. Velmahos GC, Baker C, Demetriades D, et al. Lung-sparing surgery after penetrating trauma using tractotomy, partial lobectomy, and pneumonorrhaphy. Arch Surg. 1999;134(2):186-9.
31. Johnson SB. Tracheobronchial injury. Semin Thorac Cardiovasc Surg. 2008;20(1):52-7.
32. Lynn RB, Iyengar K. Traumatic rupture of the bronchus. Chest. 1972;61(1):81-3.
33. Kang N, Hsee L, Rizoli S, et al. Penetrating cardiac injury: overcoming the limits set by nature. Injury. 2009;40(9):919-27.
34. Campbell NC, Thomson SR, Muckart DJ, et al. Review of 1198 cases of penetrating cardiac trauma. Br J Surg. 1997;84(12):1737-40.
35. Asensio A, Berne D, Demetriades D, et al. One hundred five penetrating cardiac injuries: a 2-year prospective evaluation. J Trauma. 1998;44(6):1073-82.
36. Tyburski G, Astra L, Wilson RF, et al. Factors affecting prognosis with penetrating wounds of the heart. J Trauma. 2000;48(4):587-90.
37. Mattox KL, Feliciano DV, Burch J, et al. Five thousand seven hundred sixty cardiovascular injuries in 4459 patients. Epidemiologic evolution 1958 to 1987. Ann Surg. 1989;209(6):698-705.

38. Cook CC, Gleason TG. Great vessel and cardiac trauma. Surg Clin North Am. 2009;89(4):797-820, viii.
39. McGwin G Jr, Metzger J, Moran SG, et al. Occupant- and collision-related risk factors for blunt thoracic aorta injury. J Trauma. 2003;54(4):655-60.
40. Fabian TC, Richardson JD, Croce MA, et al. Prospective study of blunt aortic injury: multicenter trial of the American Association for the Surgery of Trauma. Trauma. 1997;42(3):374-380.
41. Jamieson WR, Janusz MT, Gudas VM, et al. Traumatic rupture of the thoracic aorta: third decade of experience. Am J Surg. 2002;183(5):571-5.
42. Hoffer EK. Endovascular intervention in thoracic arterial trauma. Injury. 2008;39(11):1257-74.
43. Bryant AS, Cerfolio RJ. Esophageal trauma. Thorac Surg Clin. 2007;17(1):63-72.
44. Weigelt JA, Thal ER, Snyder WH 3rd, et al. Diagnosis of penetrating cervical esophageal injuries. Am J Surg. 1987;154(6):619-22.
45. Hsee L, Wigg L, Civil I. Diagnosis of blunt traumatic ruptured diaphragm: is it still a difficult problem? ANZ J Surg. 2010;80(3):166-8.
46. Hanna WC, Ferri LE. Acute traumatic diaphragmatic injury. Thorac Surg Clin. 2009;19(4):485-9.

CHAPTER 87

Abdominal Trauma

Ashok Kumar Puranik, Devendra Richhariya

INTRODUCTION

General and trauma surgeons frequently encounter abdominal trauma (AT), mostly penetrating and occasionally blunt. These injuries may be confounded by altered mental status secondary to head trauma, distracting injuries, delayed presentation, inaccessibility of the pelvic organs to palpation and lack of historical information, and hence may present challenges in management.

However, in the last few years, focused assessment by sonography for trauma (FAST), computed tomography (CT) scans, laparoscopy, ability for selected nonoperative management, understanding "damage control", and increased experience have offered new options in treatment. Rapid evacuation and early intervention has also resulted in improved survival.

PENETRATING ABDOMINAL TRAUMA

Background

Improvised explosive devices (IEDs) and mine blasts are causing an increasingly dangerous and different type of penetrating abdominal trauma (PAT) not usually seen with gunshot wounds (GSW). Small bowel, large bowel, and hepatic injuries are often found.

Pathophysiology

The specific characteristics of wounds due to GSW and IEDs are as follows:
- They produce high-energy transfer
- Ricochet injuries due to bullet and bone fragments should be kept in mind
- Thermal and shearing damage lateral to the missile tract can cause significant damage
- Penetration of the abdominal wall by a sharp object causes stab wound.

Initial Assessment

Apply universal precautions against body fluid exposure. Assessment of the patient and basic life support measures are applied at the scene of the incident and en route. Exposed bowel loops should be covered with a sterile towel and not reposted inside the abdomen.

Physical Examination

In evaluating PAT, the abdomen must be taken to extend from the nipples to the knees. Patients with abdominal wound may have secondary wound in axilla, perineum, and chest.

Noting trajectory of GSWs helps to determine the presence of intraperitoneal injury. IED blasts cause multiple irregular shrapnel of varying sizes to wobble and cause severe destruction. In unstable patients consider tension pneumothorax, hemothorax, and pericardial tamponade.

Emergency Management

- At the surgical center, maximal available history is elicited quickly and Advanced Trauma Life Support (ATLS) protocols are initiated
- Manage airway and ventilator support fluid resuscitation [balanced intravenous (IV) fluid]
- Arrange blood product in class III shock (30–40% blood volume loss)
- Efforts should be made to limit hypothermia
- Antibiotics should be administered
- A nasogastric tube and Foley catheter are inserted
- May require chest tube placement.

At this stage the treating surgeon should be able to decide as to whether the patient requires "urgent mandatory laparotomy", "early laparotomy" or "observation".

Urgent Mandatory Laparotomy

Indications include hemodynamic instability, the presence of gross peritoneal signs on physical examination, and evisceration. The patient is rushed to the OT without any investigations.

Early Laparotomy

All these patients should undergo basic laboratory testing. As compared to blunt abdominal trauma (BAT), a significantly larger number of patients with PAT will go for urgent or early laparotomy.

Observation

When the clinical picture is confusing and patient is relatively stable, further evaluation ensues with diagnostic and imaging studies. Here, a major deciding factor for laparotomy is establishing peritoneal penetration. Tangential GSW and stab wounds may not produce peritoneal violation or visceral injury requiring operative intervention. Judicious use of local wound exploration, CT, diagnostic peritoneal lavage (DPL), laparoscopy, and ultrasound (US), coupled with physical examination, can help to select patients appropriate for nonoperative management.

Imaging

Plain radiograph: Chest and abdominal radiographs can reveal air under the diaphragm which indicates peritoneal penetration.

Focused assessment with sonography for trauma: Four standard sonographic windows (right and left hypochondrium, epigastric, and pelvic) are used. Look for free fluid in the abdomen, sign of hemorrhage secondary to liver or splenic laceration **(Figs 1A to D)**.

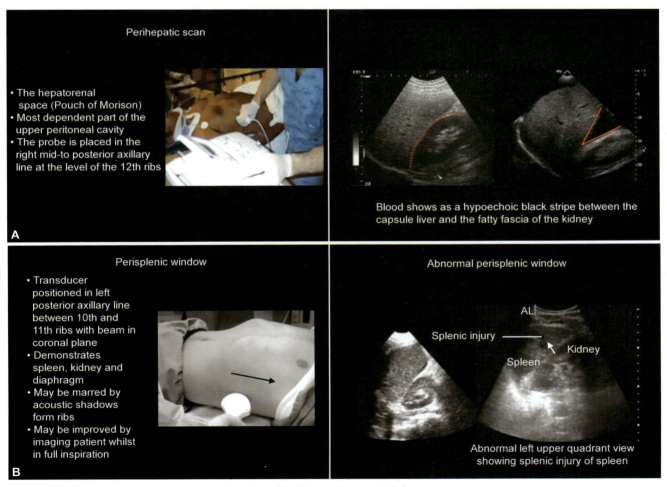

Figs 1A and B (A) Hepatic scan; (B) Splenic scan

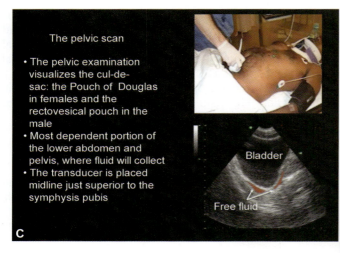

Figs 1C and D (C) Pelvic scan for any bladder injury or free fluid; (D) Cardiac scan for pericardial effusion or any cardiac injury after trauma

Computed tomography scan: Computed tomography in abdominal trauma requires:
- Initial evaluation of:
  - Blunt trauma
  - Penetrating trauma
- Follow-up of nonoperative management
- Rule out injury.

Triple contrast (i.e. oral, intravenous, and rectal) is used to maximize the sensitivity. Specific signs of peritoneal penetration include wound tract outlined by hemorrhage or air, bullet, or bone fragments that clearly extend into the peritoneal cavity, presence of intraperitoneal free air, free fluid, or bullet fragments and obvious intraperitoneal organ injury.

Penetrating injury to kidney is depicted through CT scan in **Figures 2A and B**. **Figures 3A and B** show the renal injury scale and renal injury.

BLUNT ABDOMINAL TRAUMA

Introduction and Incidence

Blunt abdominal trauma (BAT) is occasionally seen in vehicular accidents most commonly injured organ is spleen (Fig. 4). Various mechanisms of injury are as follows (Fig. 5):
- Direct impact or movement of organs
- Compressive, stretching or shearing forces
- Solid organs more than the blood loss
- Hollow organs more than blood loss and peritoneal contamination
- Retroperitoneal more than often asymptomatic initially.

In trauma the liver is the second most commonly involved solid organ in the abdomen after the spleen. However, liver injury is the most common cause of death. This is due to the fact that there are many major vessels in the liver, like the inferior vena cava (IVC), hepatic veins, hepatic artery, and portal vein. It is important to remember, especially if you are doing ultrasound, that the posterior segment of the right liver lobe is the most frequently injured part. This part also involves the bare area and this can lead to retroperitoneal bleeding rather than bleeding into the peritoneal cavity (Fig. 6).

Pathophysiology

Three possible mechanisms: first when rapid deceleration causes differential movement among adjacent structures;

CHAPTER 87 Abdominal Trauma

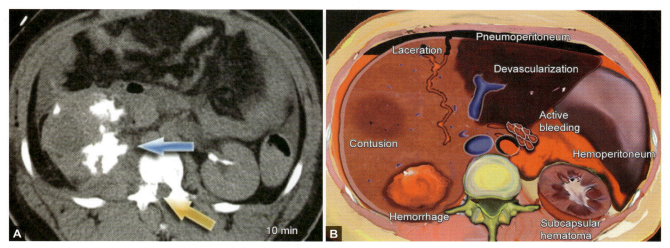

Figs 2A and B (A) Penetrating injury to the kidney on CT scan; (B) Various possible abdominal injury after trauma

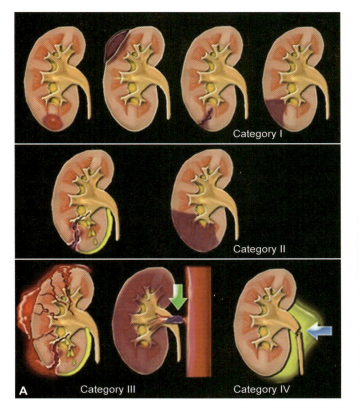

	Renal injury scale
Grade I	Confusion/Subcapsular hematoma No parenchymal laceration
Grade II	Laceration <1 cm depth of renal cortex No urinary extravasation
Grade III	Laceration >1 cm depth of renal cortex No urinary extravasation
Grade IV	Laceration extending through renal cortex, medulla and into collecting system Minor renal artery or vein injury with contained hematoma
Grade V	Shattered kidney Devascularized kidney, hilar avulsion

Figs 3A and B (A) Renal injury; (B) Renal injury scale

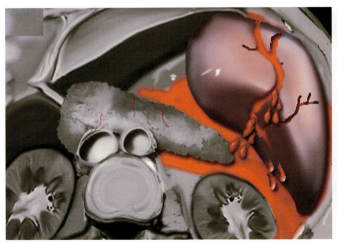

Fig. 4 Patient presenting with abdominal pain and tachycardia after blunt trauma abdomen diagram showing splenic injury

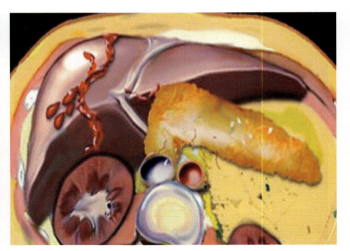

Fig. 6 Liver injury

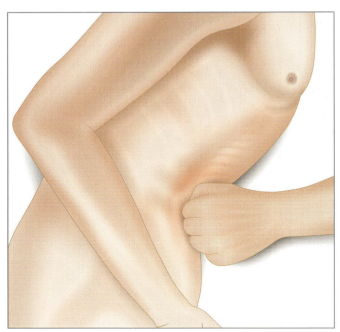

Fig. 5 Mechanism of injury

second when intra-abdominal contents are compressed between the anterior abdominal wall and the vertebral column; and third when external compression causes sudden rise in intra-abdominal pressure.

Physical Examination

Injuries involving the head, respiratory, or cardiovascular system may take priority over an abdominal injury; physical examination is still priority. Ecchymosis across the lower abdomen, the "seat belt sign", indicates intra-abdominal injuries. Palpation to look for local or generalized tenderness, guarding or rigidity which suggests peritoneal injury. A rectal examination should be performed. The objective is to rapidly identify patients who need a laparotomy.

Emergency Management

Severely hypotensive patients with gross abdominal signs should be rushed to the OT without any investigations. Unstable patients with doubtful abdominal signs are rapidly investigated for hemoperitoneum.

Plain Radiograph

The chest and pelvic radiograph may help in the diagnosis of ruptured hemidiaphragm, pneumoperitoneum, and fractures of the thoracolumbar spine **(Fig. 7)**.

Focused Assessment with Sonography for Trauma

It is performed to detect hemoperitoneum.

Computed Tomography Scan

This remains the valuable diagnostic modality for the detection and grading of solid organ injuries. It also detects vertebral and pelvic fractures, retroperitoneal injuries and determines the source of hemorrhage. Solid organ injury grading on CT can help to observe hemodynamically stable patients by nonoperative management with close observation, serial examinations, and hematocrit **(Figs 8 to 14)**.

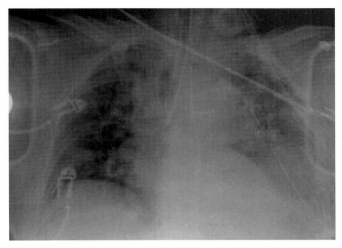

Fig. 7 X-ray of diaphragmatic injury

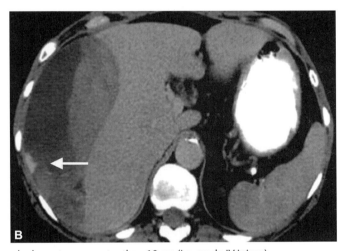

Hepatic CT injury grading scale	
Grade I	Laceration (s) <1 cm deep
	Subcapsular hematoma <1 cm diameter
Grade II	Laceration (s) 1–3 cm deep
	Subcapsular or central hematoma 1–3 cm diameter
Grade III	Laceration (s) 3–10 cm deep
	Subcapsular or central hematoma 3–10 cm diameter
Grade IV	Laceration (s) >10 cm deep
	Subcapsular or central hematoma >10 cm diameter
	Lobar maceration or devascularization
Grade V	Bilobar tissue maceration or devascularization

Figs 8A and B (A) Hepatic injury grading scale; (B) Subcapsular hematoma greater than 10 cm (i.e. grade IV injury). Contrast blush. No associated hemoperitoneum (arrow)

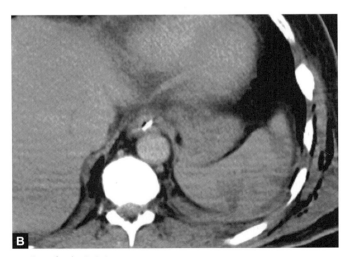

Splenic CT injury grading scale	
Grade I	Laceration (s) <1 cm deep
	Subcapsular hematoma <1 cm diameter
Grade II	Laceration (s) 1–3 cm deep
	Subcapsular or central hematoma 1–3 cm diameter
Grade III	Laceration (s) 3–10 cm deep
	Subcapsular or central hematoma 3–10 cm diameter
Grade IV	Laceration (s) >10 cm deep
	Subcapsular or central hematoma >10 cm diameter
Grade V	Splenic tissue maceration or devascularization

Figs 9A and B CT scan suggestive of splenic injury

Renal injury—blunt mechanism

- 90% due to blunt trauma—10% penetrating
- Kidney is 3rd most common involved organ in adults—10% of solid visceral injury
- Most common injury organ in children
- Evaluation for
  - Parenchymal injuries
  - Vascular injuries
  - Collecting system injuries

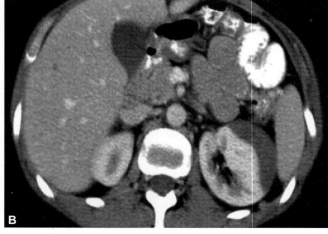

Figs 10A and B (A) Renal injury: blunt mechanism; (B) Subcapsular hematoma, which is also Grade I renal injury

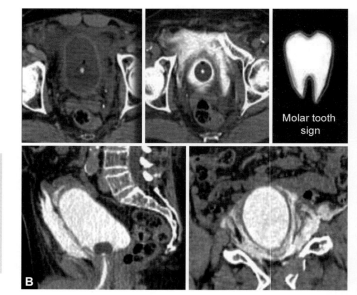

CT cystography

- Drain bladder via indwelling Foley
- Make contrast solution (50 cc IVCM in NS)
- Instill contrast material via Foley catheter until:
  - Flow stops with bag at 40 cm above patient
  - 350–400 cc contrast instilled
  - Patient no longer tolerates
- Image the pelvis

Figs 11A and B (A) *Computed tomography*: cystography; (B) *Bladder injury*: pre-cystogram and post-cystogram images. There is contrast in the bladder surrounding the Foley catheter and there is extravasation of contrast in the prevesical space. This has been referred to as the "molar tooth sign" indicating extraperitoneal bladder rupture

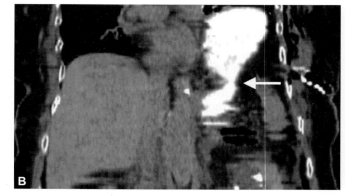

Diaphragmatic injury

Specific signs
- Herniation of abdominal viscera into thorax
- CT "collar" sign

Non-specific signs
- Discontinuity of the crus
- Thickening of the diaphragm
- "Dependent viscera" sign

Figs 12A and B (A) Various signs of diaphragmatic injury; (B) Computed tomography "collar" sign (arrow)

Pneumoperitoneum

Uncommon finding, not diagnostic
Known causes of false positive (FP)
- Peritoneal lavage
- Foley insertion with intraperitoneal bladder rupture
- Translocation from thorax (PTX)

Oral CM and re-scan
- If surgery is not immediately necessary

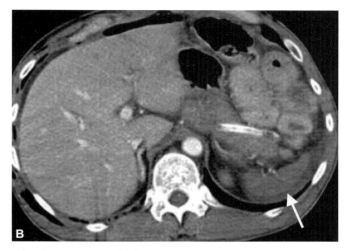

Figs 13A and B CT scan abdomen showing pneumoperitonium

Small bowel injury

Diffuse circumferential thickening
- Hypoperfused "shock" bowel
- Not direct injury

Focal thickening
- Usually nontransmural injury

Specific findings, rare
- OCM or bowel content extravasation
- Focal bowel wall discontinuity

Most common finding
- Unexplained nonphysiologic free fluid (84%)

Other findings
- Mesenteric stranding
- Focal bowel thickening
- Interloop fluid

If in combination, strongly suggestive

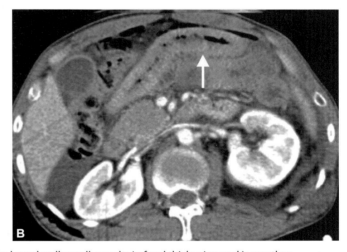

Figs 14A and B (A) Small bowel injury; (B) Direct injury to the bowel wall usually results in focal thickening and is mostly a nontransmural injury. Multiple segments of bowel with diffuse wall thickening (arrow)

MANAGEMENT OF ABDOMINAL TRAUMA

Apply nonoperative management strategies for stable abdominal trauma patient as per common practice in recent years. CT scan should be done in all hemodynamically stable patients to assess the extent of the injury before applying the nonoperative strategies. Patient who are hemodynamically unstable or have peritonitis, immediate surgery referral should be given for operative management.

If nonoperative management is selected, patient should be admitted in area where continuous monitoring, serial clinical assessment and facility for emergent operative intervention is available. If operative intervention ability is not available patient must be transferrd.

Figure 15 shows the summary of the management in case of hemodynamic stability.

LAPAROSCOPY IN PENETRATING AND BLUNT ABDOMINAL TRAUMAS

In spite of significant advances in imaging, 10–15% cases of PAT and BAT undergo unnecessary laparotomy. CT scan can miss hollow viscus injuries, bile leaks in hepatic lacerations, diaphragmatic injuries, and ongoing bleed. In tangential thoracoabdominal stab wounds, diaphragmatic injuries may be missed. GSW with questionable tangential trajectory may not penetrate into the peritoneum as may stab wounds. Laparoscopy may be beneficial in all these cases. However,

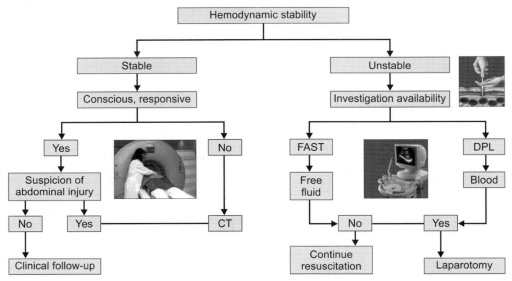

Fig. 15 Management of abdominal trauma

laparoscopy can be carried out if the patient is evacuated to a tertiary center.

Damage Control Surgery

In these cases, the surgeon would control the bleeding and contamination, exteriorize bowel, and opt for a temporary abdominal wall closure. Then patient is shifted to the ICU on ventilator for continued resuscitation and warming. Reconstruction then takes place upon return to the operating room in 24–48 hours.

Complications after Surgery

- *Early postoperative complications*: Bleeding, coagulopathy, and abdominal compartment syndrome. The latter is treated with opening of the abdomen and temporary closure.
- *Late complications*: Acute respiratory distress syndrome, pneumonia, sepsis, intra-abdominal fluid collections, wound infections, and enterocutaneous fistulae. Small bowel obstruction and incisional hernias.

CONCLUSION

Abdominal trauma remain the leading cause of mortality. Abdominal trauma is either blunt or penetrating blunt trauma is common cause of death after head injury. Most common organ injured is spleen followed by liver and bowel. Abdominal injury occurs due to compression or deceleration force. Assessment of abdominal injury is very challenging and often intra-abdominal injuries are missed. While assessing the trauma patient apply systematic approach (primary and secondary survey) with consideration of possible abdominal trauma. Pelvic X-ray, focused assessment of sonography for trauma (FAST) CT abdomen are important aid to diagnosis. Over the last decade use of CT abdomen has become the reliable diagnostic tool for diagnosis of abdominal injuries.

In recent years nonoperative management of stable abdominal injury has become the common practice. Lower hospitalization cost, shorter duration of stay, and fewer complication (infection pleurisy, pneumothorax, intestinal obstruction) are the benefits of nonoperative management in stable abdominal trauma.

BIBLIOGRAPHY

1. Ahmed N, Whelan J, Brownlee J, et al. The contribution of laparoscopy in evaluation of penetrating abdominal wounds. J Am Coll Surg. 2005;201(2):213-6.
2. American College of Surgeons Committee on Trauma. Abdominal Trauma. ATLS Student Course Manual, 8th edition. American College of Surgeons; 2008.
3. Arikan S, Kocakusak A, Yucel AF, et al. A prospective comparison of the selective observation and routine exploration methods for penetrating abdominal stab wounds with organ or omentum evisceration. J Trauma. 2005;58(3):526-32.
4. Brasel KJ, Nirula R. What mechanism justifies abdominal evaluation in motor vehicle crashes? J Trauma. 2005;59(5): 1057-61.
5. Brown CK, Dunn KA, Wilson K, et al. Diagnostic evaluation of patients with blunt abdominal trauma: a decision analysis. Acad Emerg Med. 2000;7(4):385-96.
6. Demetriades D, Murray JA, Brown C, et al. High-level falls: type and severity of injuries and survival outcome according to age. J Trauma. 2005;58(2):342-5.

7. Demetriades D, Rabinowitz B. Indications for operation in abdominal stab wounds. A prospective study of 651 patients. Ann Surg. 1987;205(2):129-32.
8. Deunk J, Brink M, Dekker HM, et al. Predictors for the selection of patients for abdominal CT after blunt trauma. A proposal for diagnostic algorithm. Ann Surg. 2010;251(3):512-20.
9. Ertekin C, Yanar H, Taviloglu K, et al. Unnecessary laparotomy by using physical examination and different diagnostic modalities for penetrating abdominal stab wounds. Emerg Med J. 2005;22(11):790-4.
10. Fakhry SM, Watts DD, Luchette FA, et al. Current diagnostic approaches lack sensitivity in the diagnosis of perforated blunt small bowel injury: analysis from 275,557 trauma admissions from the EAST multi-institutional HVI trial. J Trauma. 2003;54(2):295-306.
11. Ferrera PC, Verdile VP, Bartfield JM, et al. Injuries distracting from intra-abdominal injuries after blunt trauma. Am J Emerg Med. 1998;16(2):145-9.
12. Gonzalez RP, Han M, Turk B, et al. Screening for abdominal injury prior to emergent extra-abdominal trauma surgery: a prospective study. J Trauma. 2004;57(4):739-41.
13. Hackam DJ, Ali J, Jastaniah SS. Effects of other intra-abdominal injuries on the diagnosis, management, and outcome of small bowel trauma. J Trauma. 2000;49(4):606-10.
14. Hankin AD, Baren JM. Should the digital rectal examination be a part of the trauma secondary survey? Ann Emerg Med. 2009;53(2):208-12.
15. Kozar RA, Moore JB, Niles SE, et al. Complications of nonoperative management of high-grade blunt hepatic injuries. J Trauma. 2005;59(5):1066-71.
16. Mitsuhide K, Junichi S, Atsushi N, et al. Computed tomographic scanning and selective laparoscopy in the diagnosis of blunt bowel injury: a prospective study. J Trauma. 2005;58(4):696-703.
17. Moore EE. Staged laparotomy for the hypothermia, acidosis and coagulopathy syndrome. Am J Surg. 1996;172(5):405-10.
18. Murphy JT, Hall J, Provost D. Fascial ultrasound for evaluation of anterior abdominal stab wound injury. J Trauma. 2005;59(4):843-6.
19. Nagy KK, Krosner SM, Joseph KT, et al. A method of determining peritoneal penetration in gunshot wounds to the abdomen. J Trauma. 1997;43(2):242-6.
20. Newgard CD, Lewis RJ, Kraus JF. Steering wheel deformity and serious thoracic or abdominal injury among drivers and passengers involved in motor vehicle crashes. Ann Emerg Med. 2005;45(1):43-50.
21. Ollerton JE, Sugrue M, Balogh Z, et al. Prospective study to evaluate the influence of FAST on trauma patient management. J Trauma. 2006;60(4):785-91.
22. Salim A, Sangthong B, Martin M, et al. Whole body imaging in blunt multisystem trauma patients without obvious signs of injury: results of a prospective study. Arch Surg. 2006;141(5):468-73.
23. Varin DS, Ringburg AN, van Lieshout EM, et al. Accuracy of conventional imaging of penetrating torso injuries in the trauma resuscitation room. Eur J Emerg Med. 2009;16(6):305-11.
24. Velmahos GC, Constantinou C, Tillou A, et al. Abdominal computed tomographic scan for patients with gunshot wounds to the abdomen selected for nonoperative management. J Trauma. 2005;59(5):1155-61.
25. Velmahos GC, Demetriades D, Toutouzas KG, et al. Selective nonoperative management in 1,856 patients with abdominal gunshot wounds: Should routine laparotomy still be the standard of care. Ann Surg. 2001;234(3):395-402.
26. Velmahos GC, Tatevossian R, Demetriades D, et al. The "seat belt mark" sign: a call for increased vigilance among physicians treating victims of motor vehicle accidents. Am Surg. 1999;65:181-5.
27. Woodruff SI, Dougherty AL, Dye JL, et al. Use of recombinant factor VIIA for control of combat-related haemorrhage. Emerg Med J. 2010;27(2):121-4.

Chapter 88

Extremity Trauma and Management of Fractures in Emergency

Ritabh Kumar

INTRODUCTION

Trauma is a time-sensitive but unfortunately neglected disease of modern times. It is the leading cause of avoidable death in the most productive age group, the young adult.[1] Extremity injury is common and often the most visible element of blunt musculoskeletal trauma **(Figs 1A and B)**. This should, however, not distract the physician. Proper management requires attention to the "whole patient" and the injured extremity. The initial assessment following trauma should focus on identification of immediate life threats, with concurrent resuscitation as per the Advanced Trauma Life Support (ATLS) protocol. At this stage, attention to limb injury is limited to control of external active bleeding by direct pressure via compression dressing and splinting. Once the patient is hemodynamically stable, attention is shifted to extremity trauma for a detailed assessment.

FRACTURE CARE

Orthopedic injuries are important because of pain; physical and psychological, limitation of function—often prolonged, dependency for activities of daily living and substantial direct and indirect costs of treatment and follow-up.

The first and perhaps the most crucial element in acute trauma care is the cervical spine status. Cervical spine injury is always assumed to be present following trauma and should be protected in a semi-rigid collar till clearance is given by the orthopedic or spine consultant **(Fig. 2)**. The algorithm for clearing the cervical spine is given below.
- *Conscious alert patient without neck pain*:
  - No head injury
  - No abnormal limb neurology
  - No severe "distracting" injury that may confuse the patient

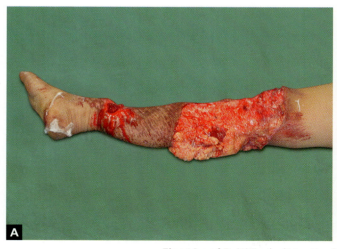
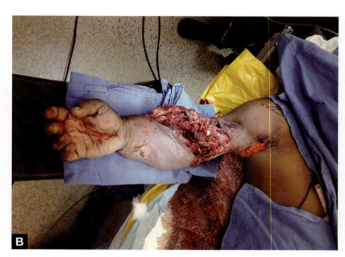

Figs 1A and B (A) Easily distracting limb trauma; (B) Upper limb crush injury

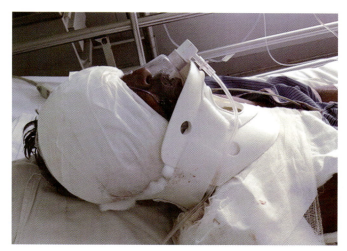

Fig. 2 Cervical spine immobilization

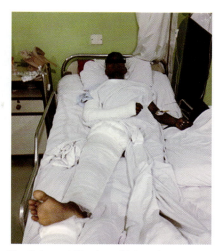

Fig. 3 Immobilization of injured extremities

- Clearance can be given without the need for any imaging.
- *Conscious alert patient with neck pain*:
  - *Radiograph of the cervical spine*: Lateral view with C7-T1 junction visible
  - Computed tomography (CT) scan with 2 mm slices from cervico-occipital junction to T1 vertebral body.
- Unconscious intubated patient:
  - *Radiograph of the cervical spine*: Lateral view with C7-T1 junction visible
  - CT scan with 2 mm slices from cervico-occipital junction to T1 vertebral body.

Protecting the cervical spine in emergency is mandatory. The clearance can be obtained later when the patient is hemodynamically stable.

The general principles of acute fracture care aim to ease pain, reduce bleeding, immobilize the injured extremity and prevent complications. The specific diagnosis can be arrived at later by appropriate radiography.

Pain: The best method to alleviate pain is to splint the extremity. Medication is a useful adjunct and must be administered via the intravenous (IV) route. Paracetamol and diclofenac are safe. Opioids may be administered once head injury is cleared.

Immobilization or splinting: Immobilization of the injured limb avoids further soft-tissue damage by moving bone fragments and also tamponades the ongoing invisible internal bleeding. Where possible, the joint above and below the broken bone must be included in the splint **(Fig. 3)**. The neurovascular (NV) status of the limb must be documented before and after the procedure.

Avoiding complications: Trauma and pain trigger stress reactions—physiological and psychological. H_2-receptor antagonists must be administered early along with tetanus prophylaxis. When the immunization status is known, one shot of tetanus toxoid 0.5 mL intramuscular suffices. Where there is a doubt and wound contamination extensive, it is advisable to give the toxoid in one buttock and the immunoglobulin in the other buttock. Often overlooked, assumed or sometimes neglected, communication with the patient and their attendants is a crucial factor. It may not be possible to predict with accuracy the future course of events but a reasonable road map to recovery (guarded prognosis) must be explained.

In emergency, the musculoskeletal injuries that merit high priority can be divided into two categories: (1) limb threats and (2) serious skeletal injuries **(Table 1)**.

Table 1 High priority extremity trauma

Limb threats	Serious skeletal injury
Vascular injury	*Long-bone fractures*: Lower limb
Compartment syndrome	Dislocations
Open fractures; degloving injury	Pelvic fractures
Mangled extremity (complex trauma)	*Multiple fractures*: Polytrauma

Vascular Injury

The first diagnostic priority in extremity trauma evaluation is the distal NV status. Nerves and vessels travel together and injury to one structure is very likely to be associated with damage to its travelling partner. Vascular injury must be assumed in all patients with extremity injury. The two most common injuries associated with vascular injury are the supracondylar fracture humerus in children and knee dislocation in adults. Vascular injury is very uncommon but if missed unforgiving **(Fig. 4)**. It is seen in less than 1% of all

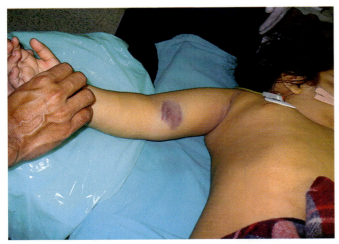

Fig. 4 Supracondylar fracture humerus in child with bruising in cubital fossa region suggesting possible brachial artery injury

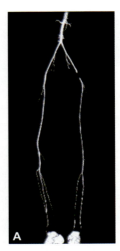

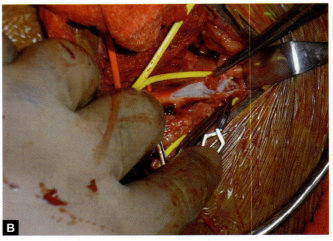

Figs 5A and B (A) Computed tomographic arteriogram showing femoral artery injury; (B) Intraoperative image showing femoral artery injury

extremity traumas, but one of the major determinants of limb salvage. All peripheral pulses must be palpated diligently to rule out vascular injury and the same documented. When obvious signs are missing a high index of suspicion and systematic evaluation of the injured limb can help avoid this potential pitfall. A high index of suspicion must be maintained in penetrating trauma.

Diagnosis

Hard signs of vascular injury are:
- Active external hemorrhage
- Expanding hematoma or pulsatile swelling
- Absent distal pulses with asymmetry (pulse present in opposite limb)
- Cold extremity with asymmetry (opposite limb is warmer)
- Reduced ankle or brachial index.

These signs warrant an urgent vascular surgical referral. Most of the cases are due to soft tissue or bone bleeding, malaligned extremities, tense compartments or traction of the NV bundle. Use of radiological adjuncts, CT arteriogram, and Doppler is strongly recommended and may help clear the cause **(Fig. 5A)**. Where imaging is not possible, it is safe and prudent to go ahead with surgical exploration of the involved NV bundle **(Fig. 5B)**. Extremity trauma is fundamentally a surgical disease and the threshold for surgical intervention must be very low in vascular injury.

Compartment Syndrome

The human locomotor system is an almost perfect machine combining architecture and efficiency. The structures are arranged in closed compartments that may be anatomically distinct but are functionally interdependent. Compartment syndrome (CS) is a condition wherein the muscles and nerves enclosed in a closed compartment become ischemic without an overt vascular injury. The normal compartment pressure is 0 mm Hg. This pressure always increases following injury but rarely exceeds the critical values that threaten the integrity of muscle and nerve. History of prolonged crush or entrapment of the limb amplifies the risk of CS significantly. The incidence of CS is higher in open fractures.[2] Failure to recognize or inadequate treatment within the "window of opportunity" has almost fatal consequences for limb viability and function with medicolegal implications.[3]

Pathophysiology

There are two fundamental mechanisms: (1) a reduction in the size of the compartment (tight dressing, external pressure; **Figs 6A and B**) or (2) increase in the content volume (bleeding) **(Flow chart 1)**.

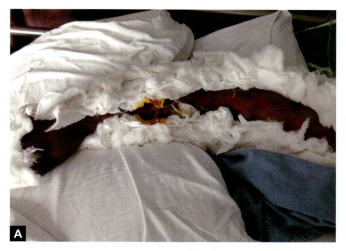
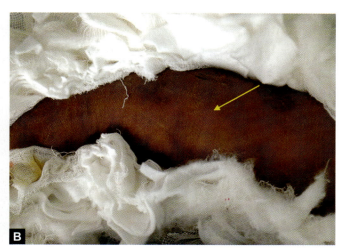

Figs 6A and B (A) Tight dressing that is split open; (B) Constriction

Flow chart 1 Pathophysiology of compartment syndrome

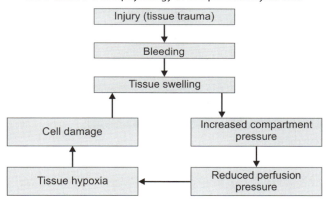

Diagnosis: Clinical features are most important. The classical 6P's are as follows:
1. Pain
2. Pallor
3. *Paresthesias*: Funny feelings
4. *Poikilothermia*: Cooler extremity compared to the other
5. Paralysis
6. Pulselessness.

Pain out of proportion to the injury, increasing with time mandating escalation in analgesic requirements is the most important diagnostic tool. In addition, pain on passive stretch of the involved compartment muscles with tense compartments on palpation suffice justification for going ahead with emergency decompression (fasciotomy; **Figs 7A to D**). Measurement of compartment pressure offers objective evidence but is controversial. The most commonly affected sites are forearm and leg. Mechanism of injury and clinical judgment matters. The fundamental prerequisite is repeated examination. CS is one condition where it is safe to overdiagnose and manage. The time interval from injury to decompression is the main factor that determines the outcome. Delay spells disaster with grave complications for the patient and doctor. An incomplete fasciotomy is the next common cause of failure. Muscle can survive up to 4 hours of ischemia and is definitely dead beyond 8 hours. Opening the compartments then exposes dead tissue to infection and increases the risk of repeat debridement surgery, and finally amputation **(Figs 8A and B)**.[3] Treatment in cases of delay is best expectant with emphasis on maintaining a high urine output to minimize risk of myoglobinuria.

Open Fractures

Wounds that expose bone tissue or the fracture hematoma to environment are classified as open fractures **(Figs 9A and B)**. The concern is infection, delayed bone healing, and prolonged morbidity. Integrity of soft tissues dictates bone healing. The classification given by Gustilo-Anderson is mostly cited to classify open fractures **(Table 2)**.[4]

Fracture is essentially a soft-tissue injury in which bone is incidentally broken. Soft tissue can heal without bone; bone will never heal without soft tissue.

The principles in managing an open fracture are:
- Early administration of broad-spectrum antibiotics, tetanus prophylaxis, and adequate pain relief
- Photograph of the wound
- When the wound is located near the joint or over the joint it must be assumed to communicate with the joint
- Documentation of distal NV status
- Irrigate the wound with saline to reduce contamination and cover with sterile dressing
- Splintage of the limb
- X-rays of the injured bone including the joint above and below

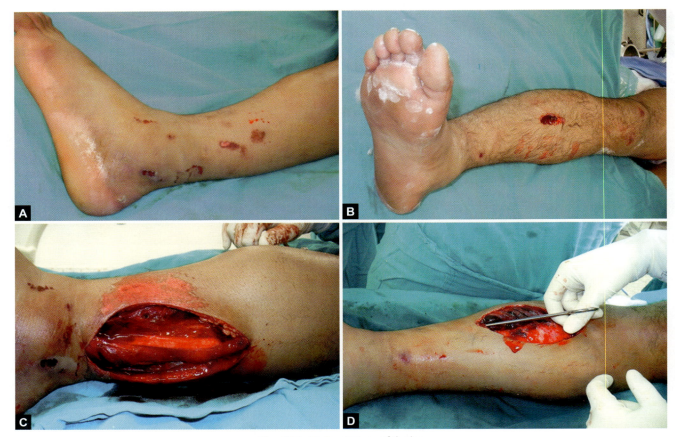

Figs 7A to D Fasciotomy of the leg

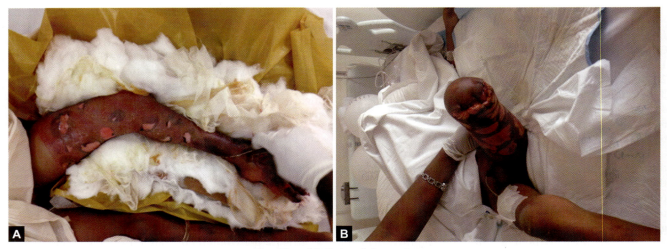

Figs 8A and B Delayed diagnosis

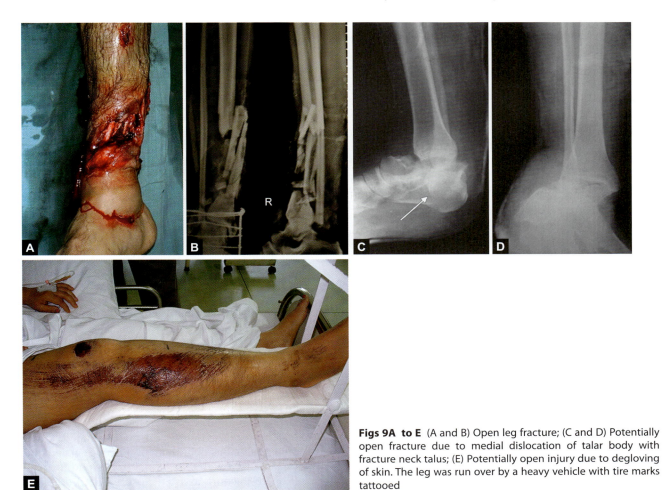

Figs 9A to E (A and B) Open leg fracture; (C and D) Potentially open fracture due to medial dislocation of talar body with fracture neck talus; (E) Potentially open injury due to degloving of skin. The leg was run over by a heavy vehicle with tire marks tattooed

Table 2 The Gustilo-Anderson open fracture classification

Grade	Wound size	Soft tissue	Bone	Contamination
I	<1 cm	–	–	Clean
II	>1 cm	–	–	–
III	Not a consideration	Extensive damage	Segmental fracture	–
A	–	Bone can be adequately covered	–	–
B	–	Periosteal stripping with exposed bone	–	Massive
C	–	Arterial injury that requires repair	–	–

- Urgent orthopedic referral
- Be aware of compartment syndrome.

Management of these injuries should be done on an urgent basis. The patient is prepared for shifting to the operation room for debridement of the wounds, surgical stabilization of the broken bone, and wound cover.

Impending Open Fractures

- Certain fractures by virtue of displacement or the instability, place the overlying soft-tissue envelope at risk of pressure necrosis. The skin is usually intact at presentation but may necroze and exposes the underlying

bone to the environment. These fractures are surgical emergencies. Fractures in the foot and ankle region have limited soft-tissue cover, and the specific injuries to be aware of are as follows:
- Lateral and posterolateral displacement of the ankle joint, this stretches the anteromedial skin overlying the distal leg
- Displaced calcaneal tuberosity fractures that may break open the posterior heel skin
- Talar neck fractures displaced posteromedially **(Figs 9C and D)**
- Displaced tarsal or metatarsal dislocations or fracture dislocations.

Degloving

A history of run over by vehicle or tire tattoo marks on skin should immediately raise suspicion. The skin appears intact but looks obviously damaged **(Fig. 9E)**. The skin and subcutaneous tissue avulses off from the fascia and this may jeopardize the blood supply to the skin. This too is a potentially open injury and must be approached with caution and repeated evaluation.

Mangled Extremity

These are complex and very high energy open injuries with varying degrees of damage to every tissue of the musculoskeletal system: skin, muscle and tendon, nerve, vessels, and bone **(Fig. 10)**. Associated life-threatening injuries add to the complexity. They require a team approach, a prompt objective evaluation of the injured limb and early appropriate management to minimize the morbidity. The fundamental issue is salvage or amputation.

Diagnosis

The mechanism of injury and appearance of the limb suffices. Scoring systems help to quantify a complex condition and attach a numerical value to assist in decision-making **(Table 3)**. Serial evaluations, the overall hemodynamic status, and injury status must be considered in the socioeconomic context to arrive at a decision.

Although scoring systems have been validated, absolute reliability on these criteria is inappropriate. It is difficult to quantify a complex injury objectively with absolute certainty but a very reasonable estimate can be arrived at by the following:
- History
- Clinical evaluation of the limb
- Distal NV status
- Fracture personality
- Physiology of the patient.

It is important to emphasize that repeated clinical evaluation is vital. Bone injury is static. The fragments will remain same in size, shape, and number. It is the soft-tissue

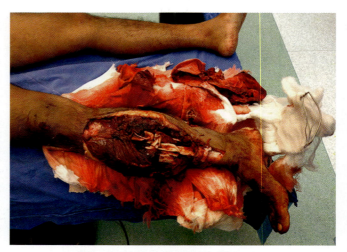

Fig. 10 Mangled leg run over by train

changes that are dynamic and evolve over time. It is prudent to stage the reconstructive procedures.

Some of the risk factors for amputation are:
- Gustilo grade IIIC open distal-limb fractures
- Extensive crush or destructive soft-tissue wounds with severely comminuted fractures or those with segmental bone loss.

If early amputation is decided the wound should not be closed, as most of the injuries are contaminated. If there is any doubt a judicious debridement must be carried out, the skeleton stabilized with an external fixator and the wounds are left open. Vacuum-assisted closure (VAC) dressing is a useful option **(Figs 11A and B)**. Not only are the wounds left open, the negative suction continues to debride the wound. Skin and soft tissues are allowed breathing time to recover from the insult of injury and edema is greatly reduced. It also saves the patient the discomfort of daily dressing. The patient returns to the operating room at an elective date for definitive management.

Long Bone Fractures in the Lower Limb

Fractures of the femur and tibia are common injuries. The violence required to break these bones in the young adult is significant and often associated with injuries to other body regions. Fat embolism (FE) is extremely common after long-bone injury. In fact the reported incidence is greater than 90% after long-bone fractures. However, fat embolism syndrome (FES) is rather uncommon after an isolated long-bone injury with a reported incidence of 0.5–2%. In multiply injured victims, the incidence of FES is reportedly high (5–10%).[5]

Clinical Presentation

The history is usually diagnostic with the patient complaining of severe pain and complete loss of function of the broken

Table 3 Mangled extremity severe score[6]

Group	Characteristics	Injury	Points
Age			
1	<30 years		0
2	>30 and <50 years		1
3	>50 years		2
Skeletal or soft-tissue injury			
1	Low energy	Simple closed fractures, stab injuries	0
2	Moderate energy	Open fractures or dislocations, moderate crush injuries	1
3	High injury	Gustilo IIIB open fractures, extensive crushing injuries, close range gun shots	2
4	Extensive crush	Circumferential degloving, run over by heavy vehicles	3
Ischemia			4
1	None	Pulsatile limb with no sign of ischemia	0*
2	Mild	Diminished pulses without signs of ischemia	1*
3	Moderate	No pulse by Doppler, sluggish capillary refill	2*
4	Severe	Pulseless, cool, paralyzed and numb limb with no capillary refill	3*
Shock			
1	Normal hemodynamics	BP stable in field and OR	0
2	Transient hypotension	BP unstable but responder to fluid resuscitation	1
3	Prolonged hypotension	BP <90 mm Hg systolic but responder to fluids	2

Abbreviations: BP, blood pressure; OR, operating room.
*Note: Multiply by two if ischemia time exceeds 6 hours; score greater than 7 increases the probability of salvage failure.

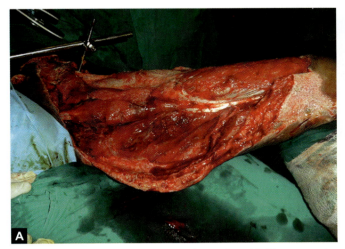 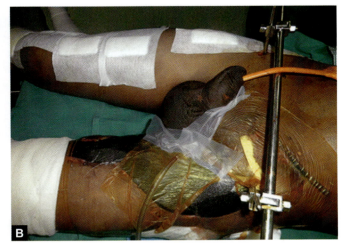

Figs 11A and B Vacuum-assisted closure of degloved thigh wound

extremity **(Figs 12A to C)**. The mechanism of injury gives an idea of the severity of the external forces. The usual modes of injury are road traffic accidents, fall from bikes, fall from height or assault.

Management

The principles of acute fracture management, recognition, and resuscitation followed by splinting, pain relief, and medical adjuvants must be followed. High quality initial care

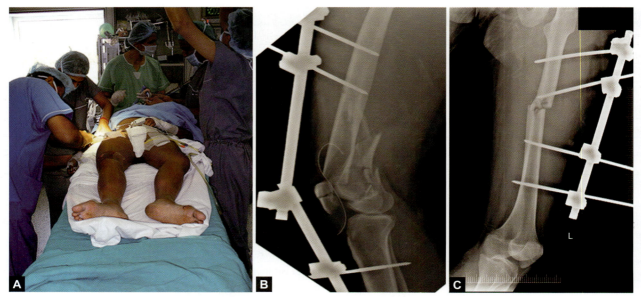

Figs 12A to C Deformity of lower limb following bilateral femur fractures

has a significant bearing on the eventual functional outcome. The incidence of FES reduces dramatically with appropriate early splinting and resuscitation.

Dislocations

The injury leads to complete separation of the congruent articular surfaces of the articulating bone ends. They are true orthopedic emergencies that warrant immediate reduction. These are high-risk injuries with potential for serious complication. Due to proximity of the nerve supplying the joint, neurologic injury is a real threat. Delay in reduction threatens the viability of the articular cartilage with potential for serious long-term disability.

Diagnosis

The obviously deformed and painful limb is usually diagnostic. The classical appearances of the commonly dislocated joints are shown in **Figures 13 to 19**.

Shoulder: Anterior dislocation is the most frequently encountered dislocation in the emergency **(Figs 13A and B)**. Posterior dislocation is very uncommon and frequently missed. Loss of external rotation on clinical examination is highly suggestive and the axial view delineates the dislocation well **(Figs 14A to D)**.

Elbow dislocation is uncommon but the clinical presentation is evident. The joint dislocates posteriorly and the triceps tendon stands out taut **(Fig. 15)**.

Hip dislocation generally occurs posteriorly. The appearance of the injured lower limb is typical, shortened, internally rotated, and adducted **(Figs 16 A to C)**.

Knee dislocation is amongst the most serious of all dislocations with very high incidence of vascular injury (almost 20%).[7] The appearance may be subtle as the dislocated knee springs back. A very index of suspicion must be maintained in the management of this injury **(Figs 17A and B)**. Bruising in the popliteal region indicates potential vascular disruption and threat to limb survival.

When associated with a fracture, the injury is labeled as a fracture-dislocation. The appearance is not classical but the urgency of management remains the same **(Figs 18A and B)**.

Management

Evaluation and documentation of the distal NV status is paramount. The injured limb must be splinted in the position of deformity, adequate analgesia administered, and appropriate radiographs obtained. Orthopedic referral must be sought very early on for prompt reduction of the dislocation.

Pelvis Fracture

This injury is associated with significant internal hemorrhage and a serious threat to life **(Fig. 19)**. Mortality in all types of pelvic fractures is about one in six and in patients of pelvic fractures with hypotension one in four.[8] Foremost in the management is its awareness and recognition. High-energy injury mechanisms must increase the suspicion of the primary care physician toward this injury. Hemorrhage is controllable and an avoidable cause of death following a broken pelvis.

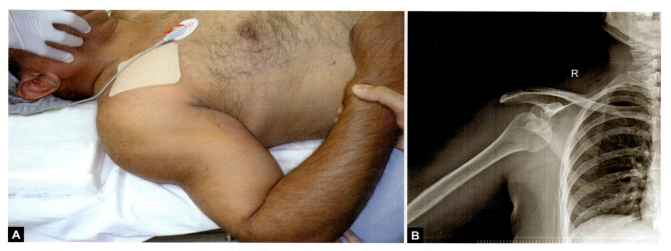

Figs 13A and B Anterior shoulder dislocation

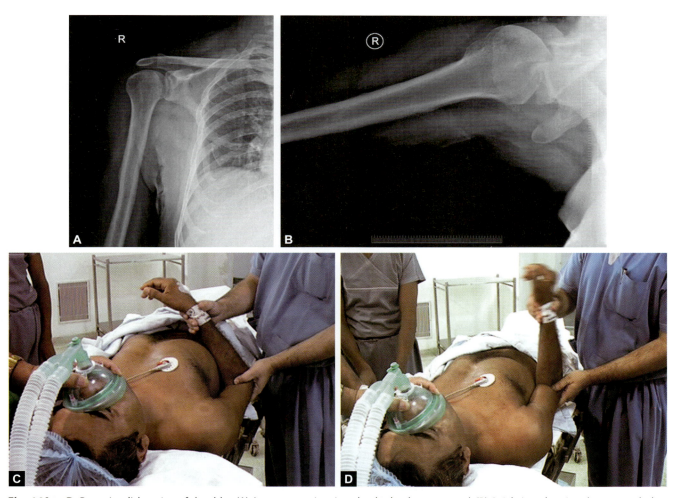

Figs 14A to D Posterior dislocation of shoulder. (A) Anteroposterior view that looks almost normal; (B) Axial view showing the true pathology (C and D) Posterior dislocation: Loss of external rotation of shoulder

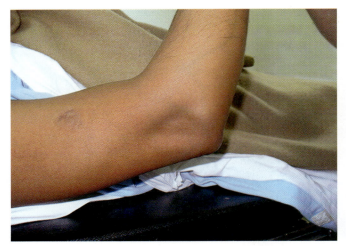

Fig. 15 Posterior elbow dislocation showing prominent taut triceps tendon

Pathophysiology

Disruption of the strong deeply seated cancellous bone ring of the pelvis leads to torrential bleeding from the torn venous plexuses around the bone and from within the bone. Hemorrhage from the internal iliac artery though infrequent may also occur. The pelvic cavity may be likened to a sphere with its contents. The volume of a sphere is $4/3\ \pi r^3$; if the normal width of the average human pelvis is 8 cm, an increase by 4 cm after fracture will increase the volume of contents by a factor of eight **(Figs 20A and B)**.

Management

This requires replacing the lost volume and control of bleeding. Volume supplementation is done in the initial resuscitation phase with warm isotonic saline or Ringer lactate solution via wide bore IV lines. Control of bleeding requires reducing the volume of the pelvis. This can be

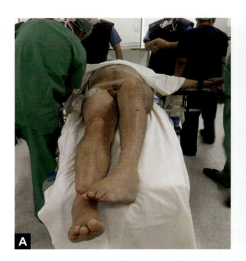
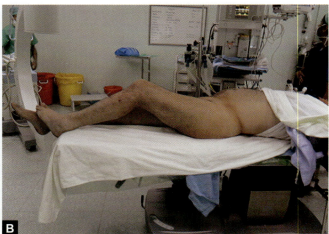
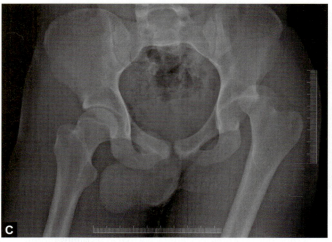

Figs 16A to C (A and B) Posterior hip dislocation: Classical clinical appearance: flexion, adduction and internal rotation; (C) X-ray showing posterior dislocation of left hip

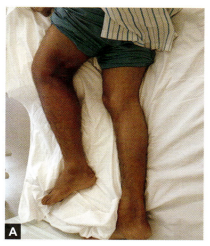
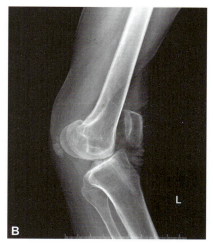

Figs 17A and B Knee dislocation with vascular injury

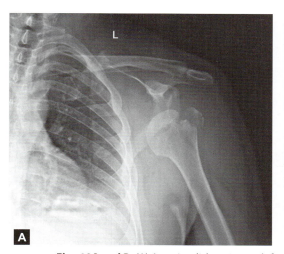
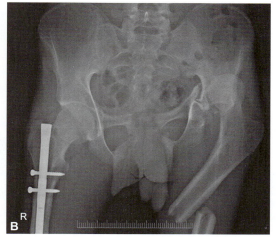

Figs 18A and B (A) Anterior dislocation with fracture shoulder; (B) Posterior hip dislocation with fracture of acetabulum and femur shaft fracture

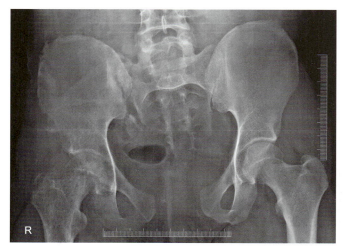

Fig. 19 Open book pelvis fracture with diastasis of symphysis pubis and opening up of right sacroiliac joint

achieved by internal rotation of the lower limbs and tying them together, and the application of pelvic binders. A bed sheet, lumbosacral corset or any other such device can be used as a binder to provide sufficient stability of the fractured pelvis **(Fig. 21)**. These simple maneuvers though temporary are very effective and can be used to save lives even at the primary healthcare level. Definitive management requires a multidisciplinary approach at an elective setting to surgically stabilize the pelvic ring.

Multiple Fractures (Polytrauma)

Injuries to two or more body regions increase the immediate threat to life. Multiple fractures amplify the damage. Multiple direct injuries initiate a cascade of localized inflammatory responses in the damaged extremities that collectively spill into the systemic circulation and threaten remote indirect organ injury, i.e. bilateral fracture femur has a high

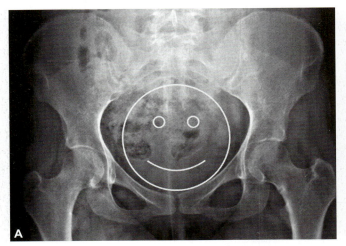
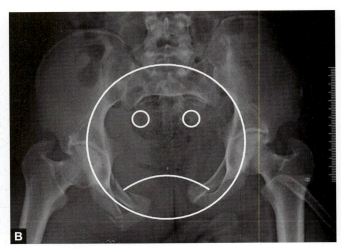

Figs 20A and B Increase in pelvic volume

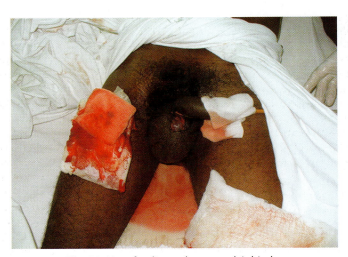

Fig. 21 Use of ordinary sheet as pelvis binder

probability of causing FES and adult respiratory distress syndrome (ARDS).

The six body regions are as follows:
1. Cranium and face
2. Chest and neck
3. Abdomen
4. Pelvis
5. Extremity
6. Spine.

Pathophysiology

Airway obstruction can cause death within seconds. Problems with breathing (ventilation) can lead to death within minutes due to hypoxia. Fortunately, these are uncommon. The main cause of death in polytrauma is bleeding and delay in control of bleeding which is associated with poor prognosis. The fundamental question is from where is the patient bleeding? There are five potential sites: (1) "blood on the floor and four more", external hemorrhage, (2) in the chest cavity (hemothorax), (3) in the abdominal cavity, (4) the pelvis (retroperitoneum), and (5) long bones.

Management

The primary aim is to stop bleeding. Resuscitation is carried out in accordance with well-established principles laid out by ATLS. Repeated evaluation and monitoring of the response to resuscitation is the key **(Table 4)**.

Polytrauma victims are most likely transient or nonresponders. Continued administration of fluid and blood is unlikely to be of meaningful benefit until bleeding is arrested. This is possible only by surgery. The aim is primarily to stop bleeding and not to perform heroic definitive fixation of all fractures. Damage control orthopedics (DCO) is a tactic of aborted surgery and an integral part of resuscitation to

Table 4 Response to fluid resuscitation

Response	Rapid responder	Transient responder	Nonresponder
Approximate blood loss	10–20%	20–40%	>40%
Ongoing bleeding	Nil	Likely	Heavy/?Nonhemorrhagic shock
Blood requirement	Nil	High	Very high
Need for immediate surgery	Nil	Likely	Absolute

help optimize the deranged physiology.[9] Resuscitation in the emergency is continued into the operation room, and thereafter in the intensive care unit till the patient is hemodynamically stable.

CONCLUSION

Evaluation of polytrauma patient is challenging task. Every minute is precious in evaluation and management of polytrauma patient. Main objective of evaluation of trauma patient are rapid identification of life threatening injuries, early initiation of adequate supportive therapy and early transfer to facility that provide definitive therapy.

REFERENCES

1. World Health Organization. (2013). Global status report on road safety: supporting a decade of action. [online] Available from www.who.int. [Accessed December, 2016].
2. Blick SS, Brumback RJ, Poka A, et al. Compartment syndrome in open tibial fractures. J Bone Joint Surg Am. 1986;68(9):1348-53.
3. Reis ND, Michaelson M. Crush injury to the lower limbs. Treatment of the local injury. J Bone Joint Surg Am. 1986;68(3):414-8.
4. Gustilo RB, Anderson JT. Prevention of infection in the treatment of one thousand and twenty-five open fractures of long bones: retrospective and prospective analysis. J Bone Joint Surg Am. 1976;58(4):453-58.
5. Pape HC, Hildebrand F, Pertschy S, et al. Changes in management of femoral shaft fractures in polytrauma patients: from early total care to damage control orthopaedics. J Trauma. 2002;53:452-62.
6. Johansan K, Daines M, Howey T, et al. Objective criteria accurately predict amputation following lower extremity trauma. J Trauma. 1990;30(5):568-72.
7. Medina O, Arom GA, Yeranosian MG, et al. Vascular and nerve injury after knee dislocation; a systematic review. Clin Orthop Related Res. 2014;472(9):2621-9.
8. American College of Surgeons. Abdominal and pelvic trauma. ATLS Student Course Manual: Advanced Trauma Life Support (ATLS), 9th edition. Chicago, IL: American College of Surgeons; 2008. p. 136.
9. Scalea TM, Boswell SA, Scot JD, et al. External fixation as a bridge to intramedullary nailing for patients with multiple injuries and with femoral fracture: damage control orthopaedics. J Trauma. 2000;48(4):613-23.

CHAPTER 89

Emergency Wound Management and Closure

Aditya Aggarwal, Vimalendu Brajesh, Sukhdeep Singh, Umang B Kothari, Rakesh K Khazanchi

WHAT IS A WOUND?

A wound is a discontinuity and breakage of normal structure and function of the skin and its structure.[1] An acute wound has normal wound physiology and the healing follows the normal stages of wound healing, whereas a chronic wound does not heal in the orderly manner and is physiologically impaired.[2,3]

In emergency the following types of wounds may be seen.

Clean Lacerated Wound or Simple Laceration

These are clean cut wounds with clean margins, no dirt or contamination is present in these wounds. These could be superficial (involving the superficial layers of the skin) or deep (involving all layers of the skin). Simple lacerations may be cleaned and closed primarily with tapes, staples or sutures (**Fig. 1**).

Complicated Laceration

Complicated laceration: These lacerations involve deeper layers of tissue such as muscle, tendon, joints, nerves or blood vessel. Complicated lacerations may need cleansing and debridement of the wound. It is not uncommon for the irregular skin edges or skin at sites where such lacerations meet to break down and therefore plastic surgical techniques may be needed to provide an acceptable cosmetic and functional result (**Fig. 2**).

Contaminated laceration: These may be simple or complicated lacerations that are contaminated with dirt or

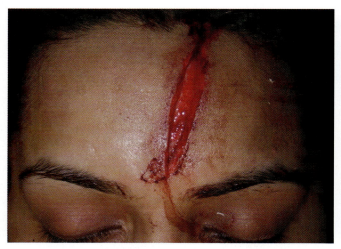

Fig. 1 Clean lacerated wound on the forehead

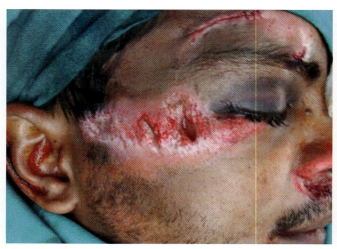

Fig. 2 Complicated laceration of the face

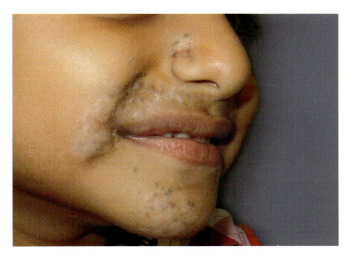

Fig. 3 Post-traumatic tattooing due to inadequate removal of foreign bodies

Table 1 Clinical evaluation of a patient with a laceration		
History	*Clinical examination*	*Local examination*
Time of injury	Vitals	Depth of laceration, and extent of wound
Mechanism of injury	Obesity	Neurovascular or tendon injury
Immunization status for rabies and tetanus	Peripheral arterial disease	Visualization of base of the laceration
Allergies to antibiotics, anesthetics, latex, other drugs	Malnutrition	Presence or absence of foreign body
Ongoing medical therapy and concomitant illnesses	Hypertension, chronic renal failure	Special considerations (injury near/to eye, animal bites)
Any implants (for imaging purposes)	Tendency to form keloids	Cosmetic significance of the wound

saliva (bites), foreign bodies, and other contaminants. These wounds have a potential to become infected or result in post-traumatic tattooing **(Fig. 3)**.

Large-tissue Defect

Large-tissue defects can result from traumatic wounds or the need to remove devitalized tissue due to infection (e.g. Fournier's gangrene). Once the debridement is completed, the wound needs special care until the wound bed allows for skin graft or flap closure.

Burns

Burn wound care depends on many factors including the depth of the burn and anatomic locations.

INITIAL ASSESSMENT OF THE PATIENT

After the initial evaluation of vitals, the assessment of lacerations include determination of time and mechanism of injury, a history of allergies, status of immunization (tetanus, hepatitis, and others), extent of the wound, and the presence of a foreign body and the type of injury (simple or complicated) **(Table 1)**.

The parameters given below may impact the plan for wound repair and its final outcomes and must be evaluated carefully prior to initiating the management of the laceration:

Location of the Injury

In the case of head and facial injuries the healing is relatively independent from the time of injury to time of repair. They can be closed up to 24 hours later if the injury is reasonably clean.[4]

Time of Injury

There is no ideal time between injury and time of laceration but a repair must be attempted at the earliest.

Mechanism of Injury

Understanding the mechanism of injury helps to define the type of laceration (simple or complicated) the presence of a foreign body (contaminated) and thus the prognosis for development of infection or scarring.[5] Injuries such as caused by compressive trauma may have a component of crush injury have the highest risk of infection.[5] Other considerations include the following:
- Bite wounds must be evaluated for associated injuries and risk of infection
- Crush injuries may involve devitalized tissue that must be debrided to decrease the risk of infection
- Stab wounds should be evaluated for depth; surgical consultation may be necessary if underlying structures (e.g. fascia) have been penetrated or damaged.

The Presence of Foreign Body

Identifying and removing foreign bodies is important because retained foreign bodies increase the risk of delayed wound healing and infection.[6,7] Any foreign body that can be easily seen should be removed. If the object can be reliably palpated, the wound should be explored to make an attempt to remove it, provided there is no risk to underlying critical structures. A nonirritant foreign body, such as glass or metal that is not in a critical area (e.g. a joint space) or adjacent to a vital structure (e.g. major blood vessel) and will not

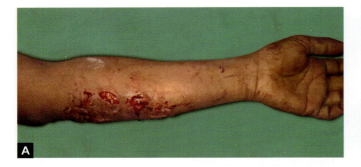
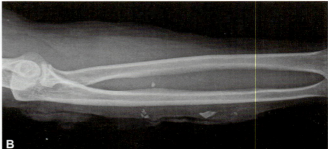
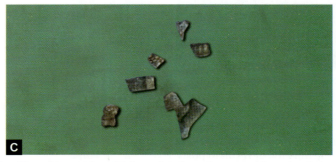

Figs 4A to C (A) Patient with road traffic accident with multiple cut injuries to forearm with retained glass pieces; (B) X-ray showing multiple radiopaque shadows suggestive of retained glass particles; (C) Multiple glass pieces removed from the wound

cause ongoing irritation may be left in place if unable to be removed, and the wound sutured. Irritant material, such as wooden splinters that can be a source of later infection should be removed even if requiring exploration of the base of the wound. Direct wound inspection may fail to detect all foreign bodies, particularly if the base of the wound cannot be seen. Deep wounds, wounds on the head or foot, and wounds due to trauma in a motor vehicle accident or due to glass cut injuries are more likely to contain retained glass.[8,9] Radiologic evaluation by a plain X-ray is helpful, if the foreign body is radiopaque and should be considered as an adjunct to visual inspection, if history indicates a possibility of a foreign body or debris **(Figs 4A to C)**.[10,11]

Extent of Wound

The base of the wound must be identified whenever possible. Injury to underlying structures, such as a fracture beneath a laceration or penetration of a joint space in a finger laceration, has significant implications for management and must therefore be identified.

Neurovascular or Tendon Injury

Careful assessment of circulation and sensation, including two-point discrimination in hand injuries, will identify neurovascular injury. Any wound overlying a tendon should be assessed for tendon function and the base of the wound should be carefully explored, with tourniquet and loupes if necessary, to identify an injured tendon. Tendons must be explored in movement or as the position of body during the injury, as an example, an injury might be missed if a laceration occurred with the finger in flexion and the wound is inspected only with the digit in extension. Similarly, the ends of a tendon that has been completely severed may retract from view. Wounds that involve joints, nerves, tendons, and major blood vessels require operative exploration.[12,13]

INVESTIGATIONS

Investigations are needed if there is an underlying deeper tissue injury or nonvisualization of the base of the wound which may need operative exploration. These investigations may include complete blood counts, coagulation profile, viral markers, a plain X-ray, CT scan or MRI (magnetic resonance imaging) scan of the local region to evaluate and exclude fractures, neurovascular injuries, and any foreign body.

PAIN RELIEF

Local anesthetics: The author suggests use of local anesthetic agents such as xylocaine, sensorcaine, etc. to improve patient cooperation and minimize patient discomfort with the surgical procedure. Procedural or conscious sedation should be considered for repair of wounds in areas that require the patient to be still (e.g. wounds that are near the eye or mouth) or in patients whose inability to cooperate jeopardizes the adequacy of repair.

WOUND MANAGEMENT PLAN

The management of lacerated wounds has two primary aims given as follows:
1. A good approximation to give a functional and cosmetically acceptable resultant scar
2. Minimizing infection.

Once the patient has been examined and necessary investigations are conducted the next steps include the points described next.

Wound Preparation: Irrigation and Hair Removal

Irrigation

Irrigation is an important means of minimizing wound infection as it washes out any soil or small foreign bodies that may remain and reduces the bacterial load.[14,15] However, irrigation is not mandatory and may be avoided in low-risk wounds, especially those in well-vascularized locations.[12] Irrigation should be performed after adequate local anesthesia has been administered or peripheral nerve block has been performed. Consideration must be given to the irrigation solution, pressure, and volume. Isotonic (normal) saline is frequently used for uncomplicated wounds, when easily available, warmed saline may offer a comfort advantage to room-temperature irrigation.[16] Other antiseptic solutions such as chlorhexidine and hydrogen peroxide are no longer used as they may be toxic to wound tissue, impede wound healing, or have other adverse effects.[12,17,18]

Hair Removal

Hair does not need to be shaved in most cases and is best trimmed to avoid interference with wound closure or knot formation.[19,20] Lubrication to comb the hair away from wound margins or simple clipping with scissors is all that is necessary in most cases. Shaving flush to the skin level increases the risk of infection.[21] In case of lacerations around the eyebrow great care must be taken to maintain the hairline of the eyebrow to ensure cosmesis and this hair must not be shaved.

Preoperative Antibiotics and Immunization

For clean lacerated wounds stitched within the first 6 hours of injury no oral or injectable antibiotics are needed. In case of contaminated wounds broad-spectrum coverage for both gram-positive and gram-negative bacteria should be given.

Tetanus Toxoid

Tetanus immunization must be done especially for patients who have either never been vaccinated (250 U of intramuscular human tetanus immune globulin) or did not have tetanus shots in the last 10 years [intramuscular or subcutaneous tetanus toxoid (0.5 mL)].

Rabies

If the laceration is due to the bite of a wild animal, rabies prophylaxis must be given.

If a domestic animal is the culprit, check the rabies immunization status and quarantine the animal for 10 days.

Closure

Clean Lacerated Wounds

Primary closure: Clean lacerated wounds may undergo primary closure at the earliest any time up to 12–18 hours after injury; location on the trunk or proximal extremity and the patient's lack of other risk factors favor success in closure. The wounds of the head and neck have a rich vascularity and may be primarily closed up to 24 hours post-injury **(Figs 5A to C)**.

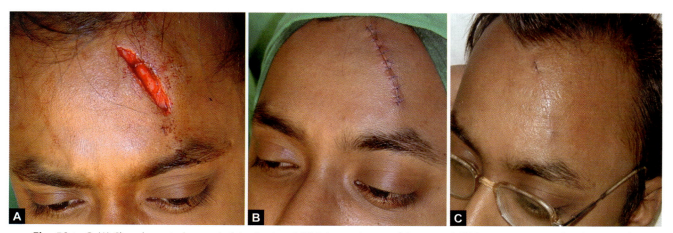

Figs 5A to C (A) Clean lacerated wound of the forehead; (B) Primary closure of the wound; (C) Postoperative results after 4 weeks

Contaminated or Complicated Lacerations

Primary closure: Only in the case of a noncontaminated injury which is recent in origin (<12–18 hrs). Absolute contraindications to a primary wound closure are signs of inflammation (redness, warmth, swelling, and pain). In the absence of these findings, the decision to suture is based upon clinical judgment.

Closure by Secondary Intention

Indications for secondary closure (i.e. by granulation and wound contraction) include:[22]
- Deep stab or puncture wounds that cannot be adequately irrigated
- Contaminated wounds
- Small noncosmetic animal bites
- Abscess cavities
- Presentation after a significant delay (i.e. >24 hrs).

Delayed Primary Closure

Delayed primary closure is considered for uncomplicated wounds that present after the safe period for primary closure. It involves initial cleaning and debridement followed by at least a 4–5 day waiting period. Consideration of the relationship of the laceration to the relaxed or resting skin tension lines (RSTL) is essential. Lacerations that are oblique or perpendicular to these lines are at increased risk of scarring. Therefore, any excision should be parallel to the RSTL. A jagged laceration in which some of the components are parallel to the RSTL may result in a better cosmetic repair than a wound that has been excised.

SPECIFIC WOUND SITES

In addition to routine triage of lacerations **(Table 1)** some special considerations are needed while handling lacerations including ones that are periorbital, ear, nose, lips, tongue, and scalp.

Periorbital

Eyelid lacerations should be carefully evaluated for involvement of the lid margin, and any tissue loss. They tend to follow RSTLs.

Management includes:
- Careful evaluation of injury to the globe
- Protection of the cornea
- Excluding the presence of any foreign body
- Minimizing the risk of infection
- Optimizing cosmesis.

History of the Injury

In addition to standard information carefully ascertain the presence of any foreign body and tissue loss. Animal or human bite wounds may result in infection and should be appropriately managed for rabies, HIV, and hepatitis. In cases of small penetrating lid lacerations, maintain a high index of suspicion for underlying globe trauma. Document carefully the prior visual acuity.

Patients who are inebriated or children may not be good historians, be essentially careful while evaluating them.

Examination of the Eye

Look for any gross injury. Evert the lids only in the absence of globe rupture and flush the fornices. Palpate and examine the lids for foreign bodies, including contact lenses. Examine the cornea for any lacerations, tears or foreign bodies. Carefully observe all ocular movements including intrinsic and extrinsic muscles of the eye.

Damage to the tarsal plate, ptosis, injuries to the lacrimal duct system, canthi or lid margins should be referred to an oculoplastic surgeon for repair.

Investigative Workup

Investigations in addition to the routine must include HIV, hepatitis serology and when needed a CT scan to exclude foreign bodies, retrobulbar hemorrhage, globe rupture, or an orbital fracture.

Treatment

Antibiotics and tetanus prophylaxis may be given as previously discussed.

Anesthesia and Pain Relief

Most adults can be operated for lid repair under local anesthesia (topical anesthetic drops and topical lidocaine gel, anesthetic with epinephrine) in the emergency itself, yet uncooperative patients or children may require general anesthesia. A loupe magnification is useful in wound exploration and repair.

Surgical Management

Assessment and management of eyebrow lacerations: A careful inspection of the orbital rim with a palpation of the circumference can help identify underlying fractures and displacement of the rim. The eyebrow should never be shaved, because the hairline cannot be visualized and that is critical for the correct alignment and additionally regrowth of the hair is unpredictable **(Figs 6 and 7)**.

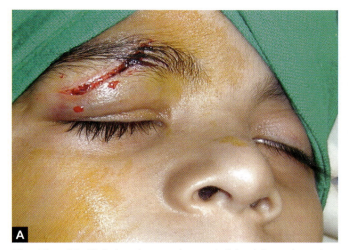
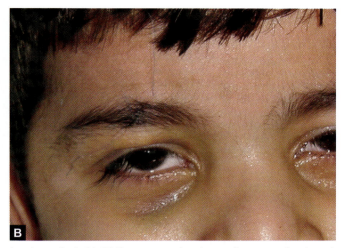

Figs 6A and B (A) A clean lacerated wound of the right eyebrow (no need to shave the hair); (B) Shows a good eyebrow alignment after 1 week

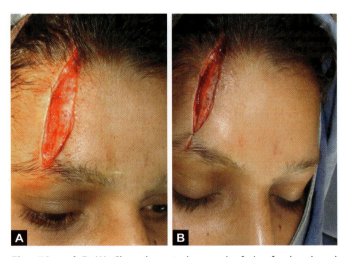

Figs 7A and B (A) Clean lacerated wound of the forehead and eyebrow; (B) A single stitch taken to align the eyebrow prior to a primary repair of the remaining wound

Combined Injuries

If a patient has a ruptured globe and a lid laceration, the globe rupture must be repaired first. If the lid repair must be delayed in favor of more life-threatening injuries ensure adequate corneal lubrication and consider systemic antibiotic coverage.

It is beneficial to try and save all lid tissue as the ocular adnexa has good blood supply, and even ischemic-appearing tissue will often heal (**Figs 8A and B**).

Nasolacrimal Duct Injuries

Suspect these in cases of lacerations near the medial canthus of the eye. Once identified these need to repair under magnification, best done by an oculoplastic surgeon (**Figs 9A and B**).

Cheek Lacerations (Zygoma)

Deep lacerations to the cheek, just anterior to the ear, have the potential to injure the parotid gland or the facial nerve. If the parotid gland is injured, bloody fluid can be seen leaking from the parotid duct via the buccal mucosa at the level of the maxillary second molar (**Fig. 10**).

Ear Lacerations

Wound closure on the ear can proceed in standard fashion when the cartilage is not involved. The cartilage should not be sutured if at all possible because of the risk of infection. If suturing is necessary, the perichondrium must be included in the stitch in order for it to hold. The goal in repairing a wound with exposed cartilage is to cover it with skin as completely as possible. Blunt trauma may cause perforation of the tympanic membrane and a high degree of suspicion must be kept to exclude the same (**Figs 11A and B**).

Nose Lacerations

An injury to the nose is fairly obvious due to deformity of the nose or epistaxis. Performing an adequate and thorough nasal examination is difficult without epistaxis control. The origin of most nosebleeds is the vascular area on the anterior septum. Once the bleeding is controlled, by pinching the same or nasal packing, an intranasal inspection using a nasal speculum should be performed. The nasal septum (for hematomas), turbinates and inferior meatus should be visualized bilaterally. Mucosal lacerations may be the sign of underlying fracture and should be carefully noted. Cerebrospinal fluid (CSF) rhinorrhea should be suspected in case of significant trauma.

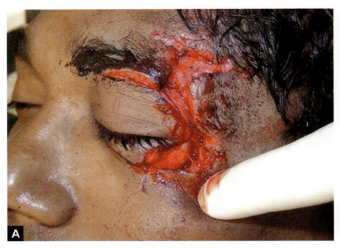
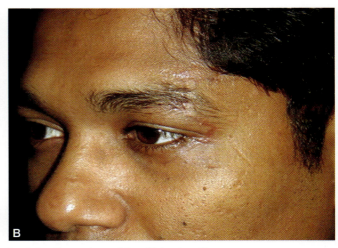

Figs 8A and B (A) Complex periorbital laceration involving the eyebrow, lid and lateral canthus; (B) Results after 6 months: careful anatomical alignment maintained during repair

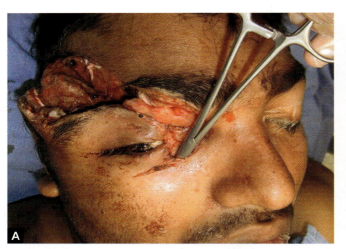
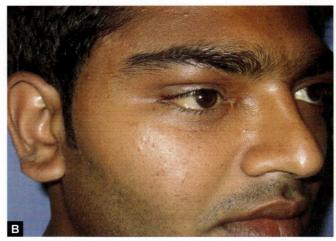

Figs 9A and B (A) Complex periorbital injury showing disruption of the medial canthus with nasolacrimal duct injury and facial skin avulsion following a road traffic accident; (B) Late postoperative (6 months) results of a primary repair and fixation of underlying fractures

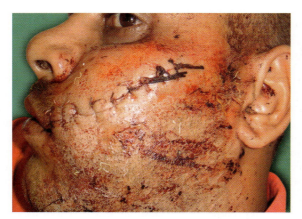

Fig. 10 Poorly stitched oblique cheek laceration with parotid duct injury. The wound was reexplored and parotid duct repaired

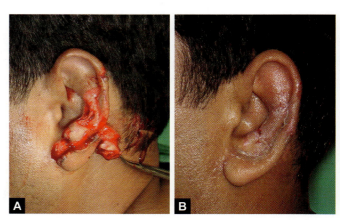

Figs 11A and B (A) Complex ear laceration with exposed cartilage; (B) Well-aligned repair with good healing on postoperative day 7

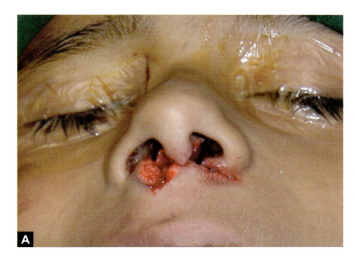
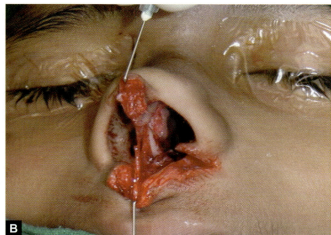
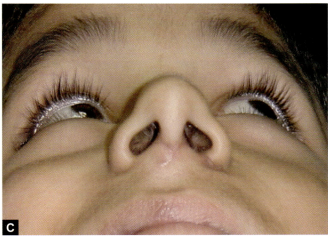

Figs 12A to C (A) Complicated nasal injury following a fall on a sharp object; (B) Identifying the injured structures: septal cartilage, columella, upper lip and the nasal floor; (C) Postoperative (day 30) picture showing good anatomical alignment

Septal hematoma if not identified in time can result in a continuous pressure on the septal cartilage resulting in necrosis and deformity. Septal hematoma is best managed by decompression (by large gauge needle or by incision and drainage) followed by bilateral nasal packing **(Figs 12A to C)**.

Scalp

As it is a highly vascular structure the bleeding may be disproportionate to the size of the injury. After cleaning the wound, hemostasis with direct pressure application must be done to stop the bleeding before further evaluation should be attempted with direct pressure **(Figs 13 to 15)**.

Lip

It is especially critical that lip lacerations are repaired correctly to preserve the cosmetic appearance and functionality of the lip. Disruption of the vermilion border should be noted as a failure to do so can lead to do a significant cosmetic deformity. A step-off of the vermilion border as small as 1 mm is apparent at a close distance.

Inspect inside the mouth and lips in case of every facial injury for any through-and-through wounds, carefully evaluating the parotid duct area and inspecting for any disrupted teeth and hematomas **(Figs 16A and B)**.

Complex Lip Laceration

Unlike the cosmetically important facial lacerations that are almost always closed primarily, certain small intraoral lacerations may be left open and will heal well without repair.[23] Intraoral closure is needed when the mucosal laceration creates a flap or is large enough to trap food particles or is longer than 2 cm **(Figs 17A and B)**.

Vermilion Border

If the vermilion border is involved, approximate it with the first suture placed on facial skin. Use 6-0 Ethilon or Prolene

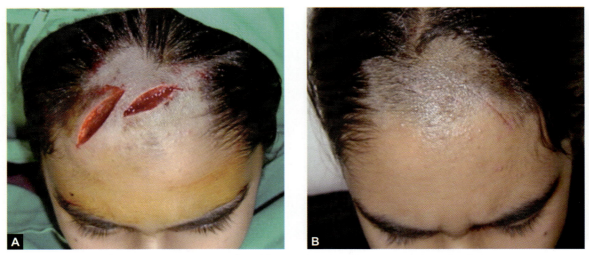

Figs 13A and B (A) Patient referred from primary health center with shaved scalp hair (avoid shaving unless grossly contaminated); (B) Wound on postoperative day 10

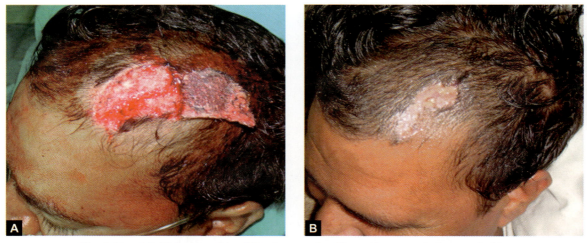

Figs 14A and B (A) Scalp avulsion following a road traffic accident—needed removal of the avulsed skin flap and split skin graft; (B) Postoperative results on day 15

suture. In young children, consider using absorbable sutures for repair of these lacerations.

Intraoral Skin

Intraoral skin may be closed either before or after the facial skin. Approximate the buccal wet mucosa with simple interrupted absorbable sutures (4-0 or 5-0); absorbable sutures fall out or absorb and do not require removal. However, do not use fast-absorbing sutures on mucosal surfaces. Secure each stitch with four or more knots to ensure that the stitches are not untied by the tongue. These sutures can be continued onto the wet and dry vermilion surface of the lip. Silk is best avoided in the mouth, as it can irritate mucosal tissues. Any small intraoral flaps may be excised. If a patient with a lip or oral laceration also has a newly chipped tooth, search diligently for tooth fragments in the oral mucosa as if these are not removed, they may cause wound infections.

Facial Skin

Using 6-0 sutures, approximate the skin with simple interrupted sutures. This suture material can be continued onto the lip. Many prefer absorbable sutures on the dry vermilion surface.

CHAPTER 89 Emergency Wound Management and Closure

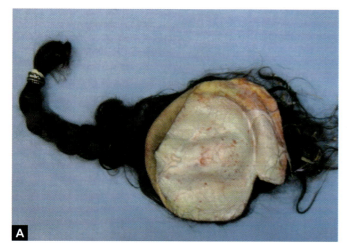
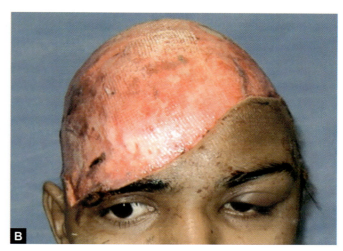
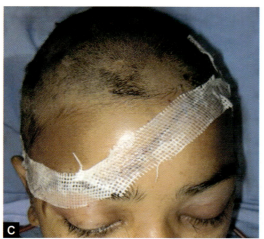

Figs 15A to C (A) Scalp avulsion after hair entanglement in a threshing machine; (B) Scalp defect following the injury; (C) Microvascular reimplantation of the avulsed scalp (postoperative day 4)

Tongue

All tongue lacerations will not need a repair but must be carefully evaluated for depth of the injury and any foreign bodies. An exception is the complete anterior laceration, which should be repaired properly else it can result in a bifid tongue **(Figs 18A and B)**.

Face

In the case of any traumatic accidental injury the face should be inspected and palpated for any asymmetry. The facial expressions and the related nerves should be evaluated by raising eyebrows, closing eyes, smiling, and frowning **(Figs 19A to C)**.

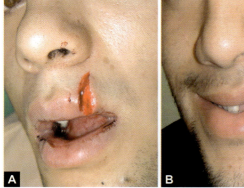

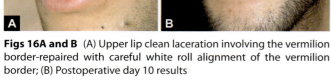

Figs 16A and B (A) Upper lip clean laceration involving the vermilion border-repaired with careful white roll alignment of the vermilion border; (B) Postoperative day 10 results

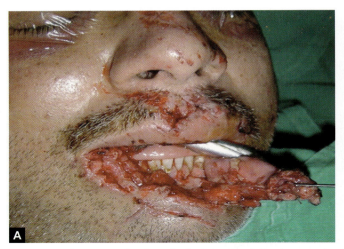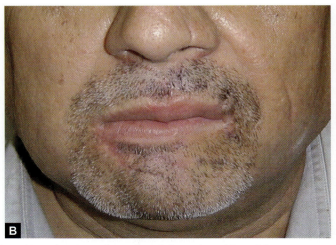

Figs 17A and B Complex lip laceration following a road traffic accident showing a through-and-through avulsion of the lower lip with other facial injuries. A three-layer repair (mucosa, muscle and skin done); (B) Results on postoperative day 30

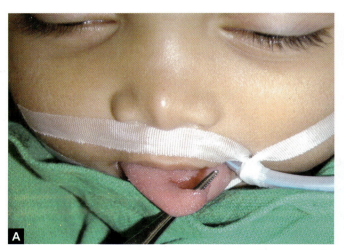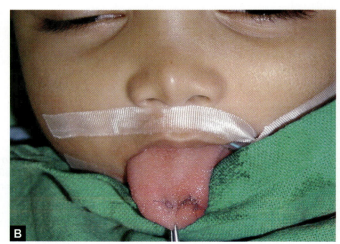

Figs 18A and B (A) Deep through-and-through laceration of the tongue that was repaired by a layered closure with a 5-0 vicryl; (B) Intraoperative results

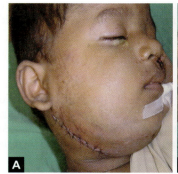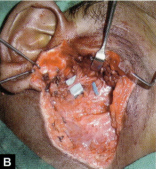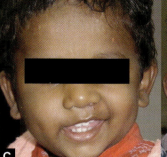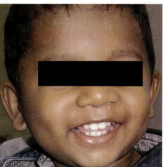

Figs 19A to C (A) Patient reported with a facial nerve palsy following facial laceration repair at a primary care unit; (B) Operative picture showing exploration of the wound and identification of the facial nerve injury; (C) Showing gradual recovery of the repaired facial nerve

Repair

Superficial wounds may be repaired in a single layer but deeper wounds should be repaired in layers. If muscle layers are not repaired they may result in puckering and scarring.[24] When performing a two-layer closure, the deeper layers should be closed with absorbable sutures and the skin with a nonabsorbable monofilament suture.

Dermal adhesives have shown equivalent efficacy for simple clean wounds as sutures.[25] The advantages of dermal adhesive use include a shorter repair time, less pain and no need of follow-up stitch removal. The disadvantages are that they cannot be used on the lips or mucous membranes.

Staples may be conveniently used in scalp lesions, need a shorter repair time and have similar rates of infection. Disadvantages include the lack of precision in alignment of the wound edges thus limiting the use to the scalp.

BITES

Human Bites

Human bites have a preponderance to become infected due to the bacterial inoculum in the saliva and the fact that most injuries involve the hands and hand wounds have a higher rate of infection regardless of etiology.

Recognition of the risk of infectious complications and early aggressive treatment are the thumb rules to prevent serious wound infection.[24]

Human bite wounds occur as two separate entities: (1) clenched-fist injuries and, (2) occlusive bites.

Clenched-fist Injury

These occur when a closed fist strikes the teeth of another individual with force enough to create an injury. The injury usually occurs over the dorsal surface of the third and fourth metacarpophalangeal (MCP) or proximal interphalangeal joints of the dominant hand. As the skin in these areas is thin there may be the penetration of joints and injuries to extensor tendons.

Occlusive Bites

Occlusive bites occur when there is sufficient bite force to break the skin. Such injuries to the hand or finger when a finger is bitten must be carefully evaluated to rule out deeper tendon injuries. Bites to the head and neck can result in avulsion, laceration, and crushing of the tissues.

Such injuries in small children must be reviewed carefully for depth of injury, in addition to legal considerations of suspected abuse.

Wound Characteristics

Assess all bites as: location, shape, size, depth, associated laceration, avulsion, or crush, any retained foreign or particulate matter. Additionally, note for any neurovascular or tendon injury.

Puncture Wounds

Puncture wounds are most common around the head and are difficult to clean due to the depth of the wound. Explore the depth by extension of the neck, irrigation, and investigations such as X-ray or CT scans to identify the presence of any debris.

They are best left open and secondarily closed. As they are prone to infections appropriate antibiotics are necessities.

Bites to the Ear or Nose or Lips

These are best closed in consultation with a plastic surgeon **(Fig. 20)**.

Ear Bites

Ear wounds are also common due to their prominent location. Small bites may be closed primarily and bigger ones may need a wedge excision. It is important to cover any exposed cartilage and restore original shape.

Nose Bites

Nose wounds and resultant nose reconstruction can be challenging and may need a plastic surgeons opinion for the same **(Fig. 21)**.

Wound Closure

In general we do not primarily close deep puncture wounds, hand wounds or those older than 12 hours. They may be closed secondarily or revised at a later date.

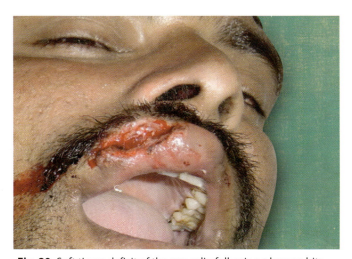

Fig. 20 Soft tissue deficit of the upper lip following a human bite—will require an expert plastic surgical repair

Clean and uncontaminated head and neck wounds younger than 12 hours of age may be closed primarily and heal well due to excellent blood supply. Antibiotic prophylaxis is mandatory in patients with bite wounds.[26,27]

Ensure closure in a simple interrupted fashion with good edge approximation and yet allowing drainage.

Tetanus prevention is recommended as previously discussed.

Special Considerations for Animal Bites (Dog and Cat)

As with human bites primary closure is suggested only in facial wounds younger than 8 hours.

Puncture wounds or contaminated wounds or those older than 12 hours may be better left open for healing with a delayed closure.

Treatment with prophylactic antibiotics for 3–7 days is recommended.

Treatment

- Tetanus immunization as previously discussed
- Rabies immunization
- If the laceration is due to the bite of a wild animal, complete rabies prophylaxis must be given.
- If a domestic pet was the culprit, check the pet's rabies immunization status and quarantine the animal for 10 days. In case it is not possible to quarantine the animal, the bite victim should receive rabies immunization.
- Rabies immunization should begin within 48 hours after the bite and consist of active immune cover with a vaccine and passive immune cover with rabies immunoglobulin **(Figs 22A to C)**.

Limb Injuries

Injuries to limbs may be simple or complex with neurovascular or deeper tissue. They may be caused due to blunt or penetrating trauma or a combination of blunt and penetrating trauma (such as bull goring injuries) **(Figs 23A to C and Table 2)**.

History

Note carefully the time of injury (to evaluate the warm ischemia time), the type of injury (crush or bites are more prone to infections) and any coexisting medical conditions (such as diabetes, immunocompromise, vascular insufficiency that can impair wound healing).

Open avulsion injuries of limbs are severe because skin is the last structure to tear much later than vessels and nerves. Vascular injury should also be suspected in patients with massive soft tissue avulsion or crush injury, displaced long-

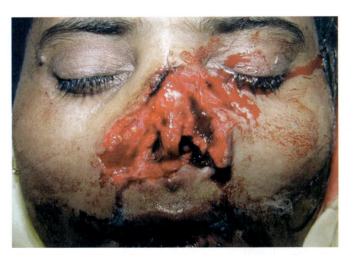

Fig. 21 Human bite on the nose with subtotal nasal loss will require a complex plastic surgical repair

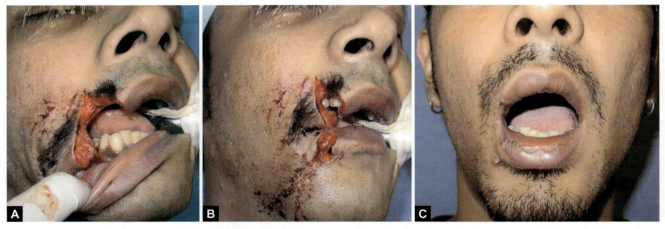

Figs 22A to C (A) Pet dog bite with a through-and-through disruption of the upper and lower lip (front on view); (B) Pet dog bite with a through-and-through disruption of the upper and lower lip (lateral view); (C) Results on postoperative day 30

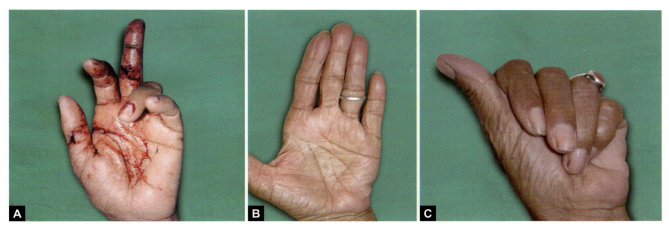

Figs 23A to C (A) Glass cut injury of the left middle finger with tendon and digital neurovascular damage (unable to flex the finger)—carefully explore for any shards of glass in the wound—all injured structures repaired; (B) Postoperative results at 6 months; (C) Good functional recovery with restored sensation after 6 months

Table 2 Clinical evaluation of a limb injury			
Upper limb		*Lower limb*	
Palpate peripheral pulses	Compare strength and quality on both sides	Palpate peripheral pulses	Compare strength and quality on both sides
Movement	Across all joints Flexion and extension	Movement	Across all joints Flexion and extension
Sensation	Compare sensory deficit on both sides	Sensation	Compare sensory deficit on both sides
Suspect missed injuries	Blunt arterial injury, intra-abdominal, diaphragmatic, pulmonary and intracranial injuries	Suspect missed injuries	Blunt arterial injury, intra-abdominal, diaphragmatic, pulmonary and intracranial injuries

bone fractures, electrical or lightning injuries, and severe burns, as well as in those with compartment syndrome from trauma or prolonged immobilization as a result of stroke, coma, drug overdose, or other causes.[28] Large animal bites are particularly prone to arterial injury and wound complications **(Figs 24A to C)**.

Physical Examination

Careful physical examination including palpation of the peripheral pulses and recording blood pressures in both affected and unaffected limbs is important in the diagnosis of nonobvious vascular injury.[28]

Diagnostic Workup

Investigations needed will include complete blood count, renal function tests, coagulation parameters, serum lactate level (as a marker of end-organ perfusion) that can serve as a guide for ongoing resuscitation.

Other investigations may be needed include the following described next.

Plain Radiography

Plain radiographs of the affected extremity to detect fractures, joint penetration, and foreign bodies.

Handheld Doppler and Ultrasound

In case pulses are not palpable in an injured extremity.

Ankle-Brachial Index and Arterial Pressure Index

In an effort to improve on the accuracy of physical examination without relying on expensive and invasive tests such as arteriography, the use of blood pressure in the injured versus the uninjured extremity [arterial pressure index (API)] or the blood pressure in an injured leg at the ankle compared with brachial artery pressure [ankle-brachial index (ABI)]

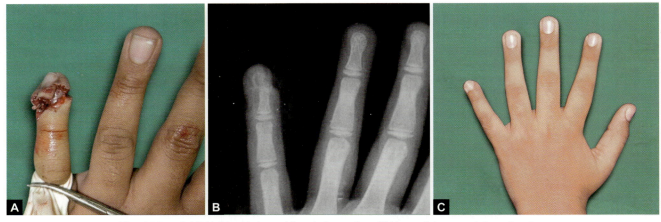

Figs 24A to C (A) Nail bed injury with pulp laceration; (B) X-ray of the same injury showing tuft fracture of the distal phalanx; (C) Postoperative (nail bed and pulp repair) at 8 weeks

was developed and validated in numerous studies as an accurate means of detecting vascular injury.

Computed Tomography and Magnetic Resonance Imaging

Computed tomography (CT) with contrast enhancement (CTA) has become the standard of care for the detection of peripheral vascular injury in most trauma centers. MRI is contraindicated in the presence of iron-containing metallic foreign bodies.

Arteriography

Arteriography and digital subtraction angiography (DSA) may be used for assessing vessels before any surgical exploration.

WOUND CARE

Injured patients present with a myriad of different wounds depending upon the injury mechanism. Upon admission, the location and size of each wound should be documented. Deep and more extensive wounds, particularly those in proximity to major vessels, should be explored in the operating room where lighting is optimal, debridement can be undertaken, and any disrupted vessels can be managed in a controlled fashion. Individual wounds are managed with moist dressings, and closure or coverage, as indicated **(Figs 25 to 27)**.

Detection and management of vascular injuries is done in accordance with established principles of trauma care with the resuscitation of the patient **(Figs 28A and B)**. Once identified the source of bleeding it is compressed with digital pressure.

The classic findings of vascular injury include pulsatile bleeding, loss of distal pulses, audible bruit or palpable

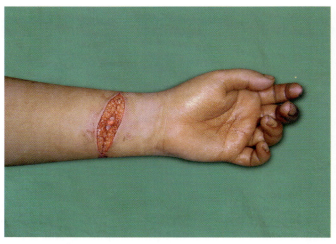

Fig. 25 Glass cut injury forearm needs exploration for possible tendon, nerve and vascular injuries

thrill.[28,29] Findings such as pallor, cyanosis and cold extremities, distension of superficial veins may indicate an arteriovenous (AV) fistula.

Wounds that are close in proximity to neurovascular bundles must be carefully evaluated to rule out vascular injuries **(Figs 29 to 32)**.

Treatment

Initial treatment includes resuscitation of both airways and circulation. Any active vascular hemorrhage can initially be controlled direct digital pressure, clamps may then be applied if the vessel can be clearly visualized. Blind clamping of a bleeding vessel is not recommended due to the risk of damaging adjacent tissue especially nerves. Tourniquets are best avoided in routine due to risk of compression injury

CHAPTER 89 Emergency Wound Management and Closure

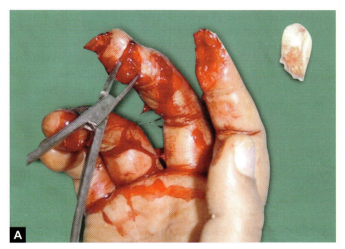
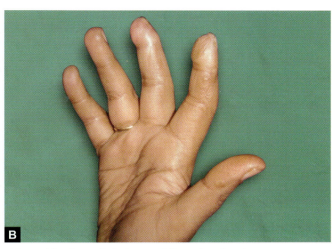

Figs 26A and B (A) Multiple fingertip injury (kitchen accident with mixer-grinder)—carefully explored and repaired with a cross-finger flap for the index finger; (B) Postoperative results at 3 months

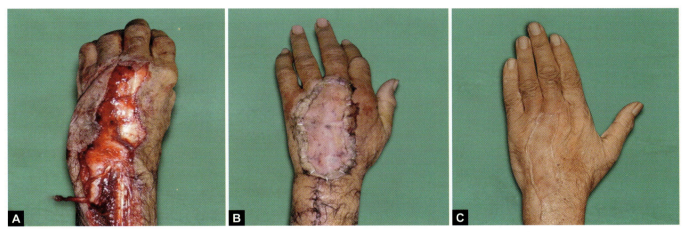

Figs 27A to C (A) Dorsal hand skin avulsion with extensor tendon injury following a road traffic accident; (B) Tendon repair with dorsal split-skin graft (graft secured with staples); (C) Postoperative results at 3 months

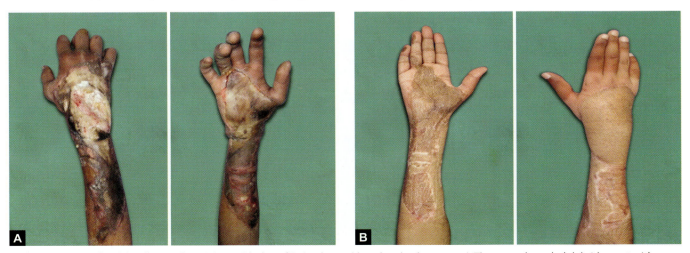

Figs 28A and B (A) Roller machine injury with deep friction burns (dorsal and volar aspects). The wound needed debridement with volar skin graft and dorsal free flap with an extensor tendon repair; (B) Postoperative results at 6 months

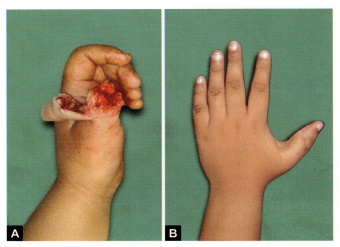

Figs 29A and B (A) Table fan injury with devascularized left thumb—requiring neurovascular and tendon repair; (B) Postoperative results at 3 months

to nerves, occlusion of veins resulting in the compartment syndrome and increased chances of venous thrombosis; yet may be lifesaving in some cases.[30-33]

After identification of the vascular injury, a management strategy should be developed consistent with the clinical condition of the patient, severity of the injuries and the resource availability. In case the patient has to be moved to another center, cooling the ischemic limb will minimize warm ischemia time. For this to be accomplished, the limb is wrapped in towels, and ice in plastic bags is applied around the limb, avoiding direct contact of the ice to the limb, which can result in cold ischemic injury (frostbite) **(Figs 33A to C)**.

Materials that may be Used for Closure of Lacerations

Staples: They can be used best in clean lacerated wounds of the scalp, trunk, arms and legs, especially in mass casualty situation.[34,35] They are best avoided on the face or the neck due to poor approximation of the edges and thus poorer

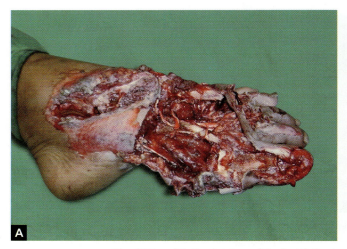
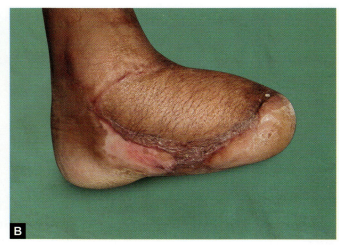

Figs 30A and B Crush injury of the foot following a road traffic accident—forefoot amputation with microvascular free tissue transfer done; (B) Postoperative results at 3 months

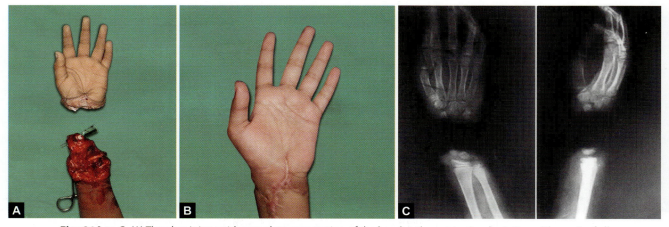

Figs 31A to C (A) Thresher injury with complete amputation of the hand at the wrist-reimplantation with repair of all injured structures; (B) X-ray of the same injury; (C) Postoperative results at 3 months with good hand function

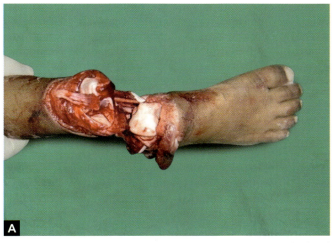
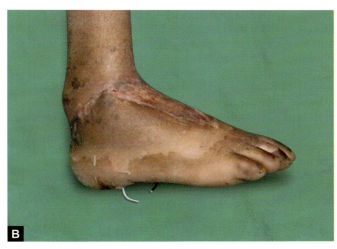

Figs 32A and B (A) Devascularized right foot following a road traffic accident-K wire fixation with neurovascular and tendon repair; (B) Postoperative results at 6 weeks

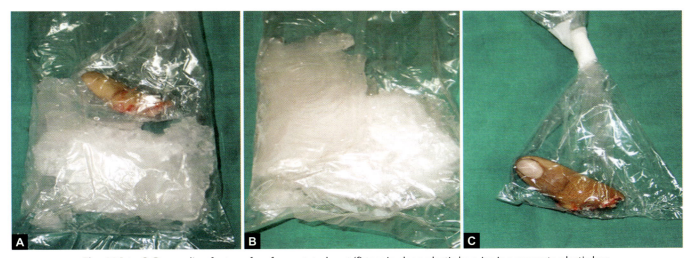

Figs 33A to C Dry cooling for transfer of amputated part (finger in clean plastic bag, ice in a separate plastic bag, bag with finger placed such that the finger does not have a direct contact with the ice)

cosmetic results.[36-38] In patients who may need CT or MRI as part of their care staples are best avoided for scan artifacts and possible avulsion by the powerful magnetic field.[39,40]

Many stapling devices are commercially available. Units which hold between 5 staples and 25 staples can be purchased. The 10-staple unit suffices for most lacerations. The stapling is done after approximation of the adjacent skin margins with eversion of the skin edges using toothed forceps (forceps with teeth) or the thumb and forefinger. Stapler is placed firmly on the skin without indenting it, aligned with the center of the wound and gently squeezed to eject the staple on to the skin, ensuing proper apposition of the wound margins. Staples can be removed within 5-7 days by positioning the staple remover under the staple and depressing its handle to ease the staple out of the skin.

Tissue adhesives (cyanoacrylates) and tapes: Cyanoacrylate tissue adhesives are liquid monomers that upon exposure to moisture (e.g. on the skin surface), change to polymers that form a strong tissue bond.[41] When applied to a laceration, the polymer binds the wound edges together and permits normal healing of the underlying tissue.

Once applied, maximum bonding strength is achieved within 2 minutes of application. The tissue adhesives form a barrier to moisture and microbes over the wound with longer side chain adhesives taking longer to set.[42,43] The bonded adhesives spontaneously slough off within 5-10 days. Compared with wounds closed with either absorbable or nonabsorbable sutures, the tensile strength of wounds closed by tissue adhesives is less at the time of initial application but equalizes by 1 week after repair.[42-45]

We suggest that patients with short (<5 cm) traumatic skin lacerations that are clean have good wound approximation, and are under low wound tension, undergo repair with tissue adhesives rather than sutures. Clinical experience indicates that scalp wounds can also be closed with tissue adhesive, but the hair around the wound needs to be trimmed prior to closure. Adhesives are also helpful for closure of skin tears and flaps in patients with fragile skin that cannot be easily sutured (e.g. elderly patients).[42-45] When wounds are under tension, placement of subcutaneous sutures can often reduce the tension sufficiently to permit the use of tissue adhesives for skin closure.

Tissue adhesives have the following advantages for repair of short, clean, straight, traumatic lacerations[46] with low wound tension when compared with sutures:

- Less painful procedure
- More rapid repair time
- Creation of a waterproof and antimicrobial barrier
- Better acceptance by patients
- No need for suture removal or follow-up
- Cosmetically similar results at 12 months post-repair.

Evidence suggests that wound dehiscence occurs more frequently with tissue adhesives but that the frequency of dehiscence in properly selected wounds is low (baseline frequency 4%).[47] Tissue adhesives are not thought to prevent the formation of keloids but may promote less tissue reaction than sutures when performing closure of small lacerations in susceptible patients.

Tissue adhesives should *not* be used in the following:[42-45]

- Wounds under tension, unless subcutaneous sutures can be placed to lessen tension and permit good wound approximation
- Complex stellate lesions, crush wounds, or other lacerations with poor wound approximation
- Wounds on the hands, feet, or over joints unless the affected areas are immobilized, because repetitive movements could cause the adhesive bond to break before sufficient tensile strength is achieved
- Oral mucosa or other mucosal surfaces (e.g. vagina) or areas of high moisture, such as the axillae and perineum
- Wounds in hairy areas unless the hair is trimmed
- Wounds requiring a high level of precision (e.g. hairline or vermilion border)
- Bite wounds and other wounds at increased risk of infection (e.g. puncture wounds, wounds with devitalized or contaminated tissue).
- Allergy to adhesives (or formaldehyde).

Caution should be used when applying them to wounds in conditions that may delay wound healing such as diabetes mellitus, chronic vascular disease, peripheral vascular disease, decubitus ulcers, prolonged steroid use, etc.[48-51]

Ocular exposure to cyanoacrylates: The eyes should be well protected during repair of adjacent lacerations. If adhesive gets into the eye, under the eyelid, or glues the eyelashes together; generous amounts of ophthalmic antibiotic ointment should be placed within the eye and on the eyelid to break down the adhesive.[52-54] Gentle manual traction typically permits reopening of eyelids that have been glued shut. If manual traction is unsuccessful, an ophthalmologist should be consulted. Once the eyelids are reopened, the patient should be assessed for a corneal abrasion.

Tapes may be used directly in the case of small clean superficial lacerations.

Sutures and Suturing Methods*

Sutures may be monofilamentous (Prolene or Ethilon) or multifilamentous (silk). The designation for suture strength is the number of zeros. The higher the number of zeros (1-0 to 10-0), the smaller the size and the lower the strength. They can also be defined as absorbable (dissolve within 14–180 days) or nonabsorbable **(Table 3)**.

Table 3 Sutures and suturing methods			
Laceration parameters	Type of needle	Type of suture	Special suturing techniques
Superficial facial lacerations	Reverse cutting	Prolene or ethilon (6-0)	Simple interrupted skin sutures
Deep facial lacerations (layered closure)	Reverse cutting	5-0 PDS or monocryl Prolene or ethilon (6-0)	• Subdermal interrupted sutures • Simple interrupted skin sutures
Tongue	Taper cut	4-0 or 5-0 vicryl	Vertical mattress sutures
Oral mucosa	Taper cut	4-0 or 5-0 vicryl	Vertical mattress sutures
Eyelid	Taper cut	6-0 silk or prolene	Simple interrupted skin sutures
Nailbed	Reverse cutting/ Taper cut	6-0 or 7-0 plain catgut	Simple interrupted sutures
Limbs and torso	Reverse cutting	4-0 or 5-0 ethilon or prolene	Simple interrupted sutures or vertical mattress sutures

Abbreviation: PDS, polydioxanone.

*Pediatric injuries are managed similarly but may require general anesthesia.

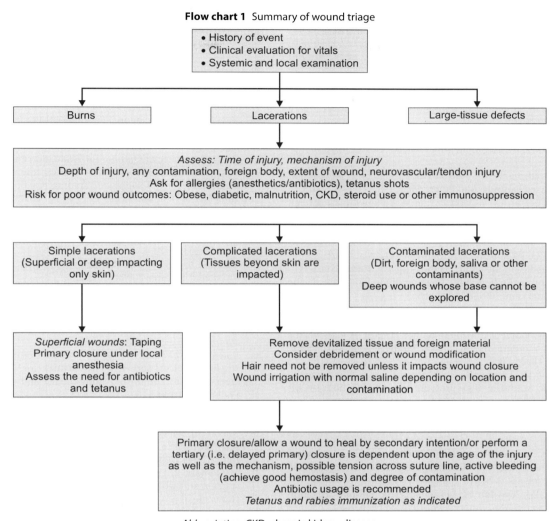

Flow chart 1 Summary of wound triage

Abbreviation: CKD, chronic kidney disease.

Suture removal: The timing of suture removal varies with the anatomic site:[55,56]
- *Eyelids*: 2–3 days
- *Neck*: 3–4 days
- *Face*: 5 days
- *Scalp*: 7–14 days
- *Trunk and upper extremities*: 8–10 days
- *Lower extremities*: 8–10 days

ACKNOWLEDGMENT

To my colleagues in the Department of Plastic, Aesthetic and Reconstructive Surgery at Medanta—The Medicity.

Special thanks to Dr Pooja Sharma, MD (Obstetrics and Gynecology), Senior Scientist in the Medanta Clinical Research, for her invaluable help in researching and preparing the manuscript.

SUMMARY WOUND TRIAGE

The summary of wound triage is described well in **Flow chart 1**.

REFERENCES

1. Atiyeh BS, Ioannovich J, Al-Amm CA, et al. Management of acute and chronic open wounds: the importance of moist environment in optimal wound healing. Curr Pharm Biotechnol. 2002;3:179.
2. Schultz GS, Sibbald RG, Falanga V, et al. Wound bed preparation: a systematic approach to wound management. Wound Repair Regen. 2003;11 (Suppl 1):S1-28.
3. Golinko MS, Clark S, Rennert R, et al. Wound emergencies: the importance of assessment, documentation, and early treatment using a wound electronic medical record. Ostomy Wound Manage. 2009;55(5):54-61.

4. Berk WA, Osbourne DD, Taylor DD. Evaluation of the 'golden period' for wound repair: 204 cases from a Third World emergency department. Ann Emerg Med. 1988;17(5):496-600.
5. Stamou SC, Maltezou HC, Psaltopoulou T, et al. Wound infections after minor limb lacerations: risk factors and the role of antimicrobial agents. J Trauma. 1999;46(6):1078-81.
6. Hollander JE, Singer AJ, Valentine SM, et al. Risk factors for infection in patients with traumatic lacerations. Acad Emerg Med. 2001;8:716.
7. Wheeler CB, Rodeheaver GT, Thacker JG, et al. Side-effects of high pressure irrigation. Surg Gynecol Obstet. 1976;143(5):775-8.
8. Montano JB, Steele MT, Watson WA. Foreign body retention in glass-caused wounds. Ann Emerg Med. 1992;21(11):1360-3.
9. Steele MT, Tran LV, Watson WA, et al. Retained glass foreign bodies in wounds: predictive value of wound characteristics, patient perception, and wound exploration. Am J Emerg Med. 1998;16(7):627-30.
10. Russell RC, Williamson DA, Sullivan JW, et al. Detection of foreign bodies in the hand. J Hand Surg Am. 1991;16(1):2-11.
11. Donaldson JS. Radiographic imaging of foreign bodies in the hand. Hand Clin. 1991;7(1):125-34.
12. Hollander JE, Singer AJ. Laceration management. Ann Emerg Med. 1999;34(3):356-67.
13. Arbona N, Jedrzynski M, Frankfather R, et al. Is glass visible on plain radiographs? A cadaver study. J Foot Ankle Surg. 1999;38(4):264-70.
14. Stevenson TR, Thacker JG, Rodeheaver GT, et al. Cleansing the traumatic wound by high pressure syringe irrigation. JACEP. 1976;5(1):17-21.
15. Rodeheaver G, Pettry D, Turnbull V, et al. Identification of the wound infection-potentiating factors in soil. Am J Surg. 1974;128(1):8-14.
16. Ernst AA, Gershoff L, Miller P, et al. Warmed versus room temperature saline for laceration irrigation: a randomized clinical trial. South Med J. 2003;96(5):436-9.
17. Moscati RM, Reardon RF, Lerner EB, et al. Wound irrigation with tap water. Acad Emerg Med. 1998;5(11):1076-80.
18. Loeb T, Loubert G, Templier F, et al. Iatrogenic gas embolism following surgical lavage of a wound with hydrogen peroxide. Ann Fr Anesth Reanim. 2000;19(2):108-10.
19. Howell JM, Morgan JA. Scalp laceration repair without prior hair removal. Am J Emerg Med. 1988;6(1):7-10.
20. Tang K, Yeh JS, Sgouros S. The influence of hair shave on the infection rate in neurosurgery. A prospective study. Pediatr Neurosurg. 2001;35(1):13-7.
21. Horgan MA, Piatt JH Jr. Shaving of the scalp may increase the rate of infection in CSF shunt surgery. Pediatr Neurosurg. 1997;26(4):180-4.
22. Brancato JC, Babl FE, Vinci RJ. Minor Wound Care. In: Pediastat (CD-ROM), Orenstein JB, Klein BL, Mayer TA (Eds). CMC ReSearch: Portland, OR; 1998.
23. Forsch RT. Essentials of skin laceration repair. Am Fam Physician. 2008;78(8):945-51.
24. Capellan O, Hollander JE. Management of lacerations in the emergency department. Emerg Med Clin North Am. 2003;21:205-31.
25. Singer AJ, Quinn JV, Hollander JE. The cyanoacrylate topical skin adhesives. Am J Emerg Med. 2008;26(4):490-6.
26. Dire DJ, Coppola M, Dwyer DA, et al. Prospective evaluation of topical antibiotics for preventing infections in uncomplicated soft-tissue wounds repaired in the ED. Acad Emerg Med. 1995;2(1):4-10.
27. Hinman CD, Maibach H. Effect of air exposure and occlusion on experimental human skin wounds. Nature. 1963;200:377-8.
28. Frykberg ER, Dennis JW, Bishop K, et al. The reliability of physical examination in the evaluation of penetrating extremity trauma for vascular injury: results at one year. J Trauma. 1991;31(4):502-11.
29. Nance ML. (2012). National Trauma Data Bank Annual Report. [online] NTDB website. *http://www.facs.org/trauma/ntdb/pdf/ntdb-annual-report-2012.pdf* [Accessed October, 2013].
30. Fox N, Rajani RR, Bokhari F, et al. Evaluation and management of penetrating lower extremity arterial trauma: an Eastern Association for the Surgery of Trauma practice management guideline. J Trauma Acute Care Surg. 2012;73(5 Suppl 4):S315-20.
31. Dorlac WC, DeBakey ME, Holcomb JB, et al. Mortality from isolated civilian penetrating extremity injury. J Trauma. 2005;59(1):217-22.
32. Swan KG Jr, Wright DS, Barbagiovanni SS, et al. Tourniquets revisited. J Trauma. 2009;66(3):672-5.
33. Arrillaga A, Bynoe R, Frykberg ER, et al. (2002). EAST Practice Management Guidelines for Penetrating Trauma to the Lower Extremity. [online] *http://www.east.org/content/documents/lower_extremity_isolated_arterial_injuries_from_penetrating_trauma.pdf* [Accessed October 22, 2013].
34. Kanegaye JT, Vance CW, Chan L, et al. Comparison of skin stapling devices and standard sutures for pediatric scalp lacerations: a randomized study of cost and time benefits. J Pediatr. 1997;130(5):808-13.
35. MacGregor FB, McCombe AW, King PM, et al. Skin stapling of wounds in the accident department. Injury. 1989;20(6):347-8.
36. Ritchie AJ, Rocke LG. Staples versus sutures in the closure of scalp wounds: a prospective, double-blind, randomized trial. Injury. 1989;20(4):217-8.
37. McNamara R, DeAngelis M. Laceration repair with sutures, staples, and wound closure tapes. In: King C, Henretig FM. (Eds). Textbook of Pediatric Emergency Procedures, 2nd edition. Philadelphia: Lippincott Williams & Wilkins; 2008. pp.1034.
38. Stockley I, Elson RA. Skin closure using staples and nylon sutures: a comparison of results. Ann R Coll Surg Engl. 1987;69(2):76-8.
39. Kanegaye JT, McCaslin RI. Pediatric scalp laceration repair complicated by skin staple migration. Am J Emerg Med. 1999;17(2):157-9.
40. Brickman KR, Lambert RW. Evaluation of skin stapling for wound closure in the emergency department. Ann Emerg Med. 1989;18:1122.
41. Bruns TB, Worthington JM. Using tissue adhesive for wound repair: a practical guide to dermabond. Am Fam Physician. 2000;61(5):1383-8.
42. Toriumi DM, Bagal AA. Cyanoacrylate tissue adhesives for skin closure in the outpatient setting. Otolaryngol Clin North Am. 2002;35(1):103-18.
43. Yamamoto LG. Preventing adverse events and outcomes encountered using dermabond. Am J Emerg Med. 2000;18(4):511-5.
44. Hollander JE. Use of tissue adhesives in laceration repair. In: King C, Henretig FM. (Eds). Textbook of Pediatric Emergency Procedures, 2nd edition. Philadelphia: Lippincott, Williams, & Wilkins; 2008. p. 1045.

45. Perron AD, Garcia JA, Parker Hays E, et al. The efficacy of cyanoacrylate-derived surgical adhesive for use in the repair of lacerations during competitive athletics. Am J Emerg Med. 2000;18(3):261-3.
46. Farion K, Osmond MH, Hartling L, et al. Tissue adhesives for traumatic lacerations in children and adults. Cochrane Database Syst Rev. 2002;(3):CD003326.
47. Osmond MH, Quinn JV, Sutcliffe T, et al. A randomized, clinical trial comparing butylcyanoacrylate with octylcyanoacrylate in the management of selected pediatric facial lacerations. Acad Emerg Med. 1999;6(3):171-7.
48. Singer AJ, Giordano P, Fitch JL, et al. Evaluation of a new high-viscosity octylcyanoacrylate tissue adhesive for laceration repair: a randomized, clinical trial. Acad Emerg Med. 2003;10(10):1134-7.
49. Man SY, Wong EM, Ng YC, et al. Cost-consequence analysis comparing 2-octyl cyanoacrylate tissue adhesive and suture for closure of simple lacerations: a randomized controlled trial. Ann Emerg Med. 2009;53(2):189-97.
50. Handschel JG, Depprich RA, Dirksen D, et al. A prospective comparison of octyl-2-cyanoacrylate and suture in standardized facial wounds. Int J Oral Maxillofac Surg. 2006;35(4):318-23.
51. Quinn J, Wells G, Sutcliffe T, et al. A randomized trial comparing octylcyanoacrylate tissue adhesive and sutures in the management of lacerations. JAMA. 1997;277(19):1527-30.
52. Resch KL, Hick JL. Preliminary experience with 2-octylcyanoacrylate in a pediatric emergency department. Pediatr Emerg Care. 2000;16(5):328-31.
53. Coutts SJ, Sandhu R, Geh VS. Tissue glue and iatrogenic eyelid gluing in children. Pediatr Emerg Care. 2012;28(8):810-1.
54. Yeilding RH, O'Day DM, Li C, et al. Periorbital infections after dermabond closure of traumatic lacerations in three children. J AAPOS. 2012;16(2):168-72.
55. Ethicon wound closure manual. Dunn DL (Ed). Ethicon, Inc. 1998-2000.
56. Phillips LG, Heggers JP. Layered closure of lacerations. Postgrad Med. 1988;83(8):142-8.

CHAPTER 90

Radiology in Emergency and Trauma

Sonal Krishan

INTRODUCTION

Radiology in emergency and trauma is a broad topic. I have tried to cover here what the clinicians need to know about various imaging modalities available to us. Thorough clinical examination and history is a must for every emergency department (ED) doctor before they decide to order imaging. Imaging must be ordered with a clinical question in mind. For some clinical scenarios, ultrasound sonography (USG) is definitive while for others computed tomography (CT)/ magnetic resonance imaging (MRI) is categorical. The clinician must refrain from ordering all available radiological investigations just because they are available, clinician is not sure or because the clinician wants to be defensive. Abdominal, chest, head and neck, and pediatric major emergencies are covered. Trauma is addressed both as a part of the site-specific emergencies as well as a brief description of role of CT in trauma. The last part of the chapter is dedicated to common fractures and findings on X-ray must for every emergency clinician.

Do not wait for serum creatinine reports in life-threatening situations. However, it is recommended to discuss with the radiologist the best imaging and type of contrast. Hydrating the patients with normal saline or ringer lactate is helpful in certain situations best referred to institutional guidelines and discussed with radiologist.

In brief, radiology is indispensable part of emergency management of patients and there must be active engagement of the radiologist right from the beginning rather than just reporting findings.

ABDOMINAL EMERGENCIES

Right Upper Quadrant Pain

- Ultrasound remains the initial test of choice for imaging patients with suspected acute cholecystitis (AC)—allowing for assessment of intrahepatic and extrahepatic bile ducts, evaluation of the presence or absence of gallstones and any alternative diagnoses.
- However, CT is better for complications such as gangrene, gas formation, and intraluminal hemorrhage.
- In addition, CT is useful in preoperative planning, absent gallbladder wall enhancement, and prior knowledge of these imaging findings often help to guide appropriate surgical approach.
- Other differential diagnoses include peptic ulcer, pancreatitis, gastroenteritis and bowel obstruction, and cholecystitis.
- If USG is negative for AC, CT is useful for establishing alternative diagnosis. In pregnant patients, MRI is the preferred test for right upper quadrant pain when USG is inconclusive.

Right Lower Quadrant Pain

- The most common cause of pain in the right lower quadrant is acute appendicitis (AA).
- Computed tomography has been shown to decrease negative appendicectomy rate; CT is better than USG for identifying complications and in evaluating patients with periappendiceal abscess, especially when the abscesses become large.
- Computed tomography can also triage patients who will benefit from nonsurgical options including antibiotic treatment with small abscesses and percutaneous drainage of larger abscesses.
- Computed tomography is also helpful in establishing alternative diagnosis which includes infectious bowel disease, inflammatory bowel disease, small-bowel obstruction, genitourinary conditions, epiploic appendages, omental and mesenteric inflammation, and gynecological conditions.

- In children, USG is nearly as good in experienced hands and due to lack of ionizing radiation equivocal results can be followed up by CT.
- In pregnant patients also USG is the first imaging test of choice, followed preferably by MRI if the results are equivocal.

Left Lower Quadrant Pain

Diverticulitis of the descending or sigmoid colon is the most common cause. Complications requiring surgery or percutaneous drainage include abscesses, fistulas, obstruction, or perforation. CT is now accepted for evaluating extent of disease and complications. CT can also show other urologic or gynecologic abnormalities which can provide alternative diagnosis. In young women with fever transvaginal sonography should be considered. Suspect ectopic pregnancy in young women as differential diagnosis. Sonography should therefore be the initial imaging in young women. CT may be used when nongynecologic etiology is suspected or USG findings are equivocal.

Acute Abdominal Pain with Fever

The differential diagnoses to consider in acute abdominal pain with fever are:
- Gut obstruction or infarction
- Pancreatitis
- Bowel perforation or inflammation
- Abscesses anywhere in the abdomen **(Fig. 1)**
- Tumor
- Pneumonia
- Hepatobiliary disease.

Care must be taken in neutropenic patients where the diagnosis of the acute abdomen may be delayed because of lack of classical signs and symptoms. Abdominal complications in neutropenia include neutropenic enterocolitis, gut infarction and perforation, *Clostridium difficile* colitis, cytomegalovirus (CMV) colitis, and graft-versus-host disease.

Other conditions to consider are tumors with adenopathy and bowel involvement such as Kaposi's sarcoma and lymphoma of bowel; these can lead to bowel obstruction, intussusception, pneumatosis intestinalis, and perforation. Contrast-enhanced computed tomography (CECT) is the imaging procedure of choice to diagnose gastrointestinal (GI) complications in immunocompromised patients.

Blunt Abdominal Trauma

Multidetector computed tomography (MDCT) is an important diagnostic tool for detecting vascular and visceral injuries following blunt trauma. Improved spatial resolution and quicker examination time, current multislice scanners, acute extravasation of contrast, and multiple parenchymal injuries can be accurately detected and managed timely. This also allows for appropriate planning of surgery and angiography with or without embolization or coiling. There is also increasing trend of conservative management based on various clinical and imaging findings such as site and size of bleeding. Low-density isolated fluid collections identified on CT can be managed conservatively whereas high-density collection and hematoma need to be carefully monitored or imaged to look for occult causes of bleed or vascular injury.

Hemodynamically Unstable Patients

Immediate fluid resuscitation with volume replacement along with rapid clinical evaluation is the first goal of patients who present with major trauma and shock or hemodynamic instability. If these patients do not respond to medical and fluid resuscitation, patient should be taken straight to the operating room.

Hemodynamically Stable Patients

Hemodynamically stable patients or patients who were initially unstable but have since responded to initial resuscitation should be addressed separately. In these patients, it needs to be decided if urgent surgery or close follow-up is needed. CT is now an important part of the decision making tool, e.g. active extravasation, perforation of hollow viscera, or major vascular injury of aorta/inferior vena cava (IVC) or their major branches. Patients even though they are hemodynamically stable may require surgery or intervention. Conversely, stable patients even with a large amount of hemoperitoneum and isolated organ injury may need only angiography with embolization and need not undergo surgery.

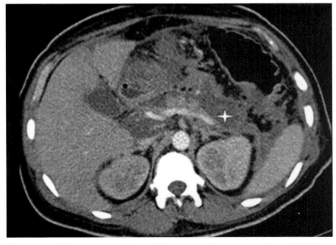

Fig. 1 Axial contrast-enhanced computed tomography (CT) in a patient who presented with high-grade fever showing ruptured liver abscess in the posterior segment of the right lobe of liver

ULTRASOUND AND PLAIN ABDOMINAL RADIOGRAPHS

Focused assessment with sonography for trauma (FAST) allows for rapid bedside diagnosis of abdominal fluid, pleural effusion, pneumothorax, and pericardial fluid; however, negative FAST scan in the relevant clinical setting has limited use and all patient now undergo CT for further evaluation. Role of FAST is now diminishing apart from a quick bedside screening modality.

Cross table lateral C-spine, chest X-ray anteroposterior (AP) on table and X-ray pelvis are part of acute trauma protocol in most emergency situations. These help to immediately identify acute severe bony injuries, example pneumothorax and complex pelvic fracture for triaging the patient.

Computed Tomography

- Computed tomography is extremely useful in triaging patients toward urgent surgery therapeutic angiography or conservative close observation
- The images should be carefully evaluated on Picture Archiving and Communication System (PACS), to identity subtle organ/bone injury and pneumoperitoneum
- Active hemorrhage on CT can lead to either arteriography plus embolization or surgery to control the bleed
- Computed tomography signs of pancreatic injury are often subtle but important; these patients may need immediate surgery or close observation for signs of complication.
- Signs of rare duodenal perforation are typical but subtle such as extraluminal air or fluid in the retroperitoneum or periportal region.
- Even if the CT is negative for gut injury but clinical suspicion is high, surgical exploration or laparoscopy, or a period of observation plus repeat CT may be used to further evaluate the patient.
- Computed tomography has a very high negative predictive value and normal CT can be safely used to discharge patients to home.

Patients with Hematuria

Imaging of the bladder must be considered in all patients with hematuria and pelvic fracture to exclude bladder rupture. An indwelling Foley catheter can easily be used to perform CT cystography by retrograde instillation of diluted contrast using drip infusion technique. Other clinical indicators where bladder injury must be excluded on imaging include inability to void, suprapubic pain/tenderness, clots in urine/low urine output, if gross blood is from urethral meatus rule out urethral injury.

Small Bowel Obstruction

- Computed tomography has high accuracy for distinguishing small bowel obstruction (SBO) from an adynamic small-bowel ileus and for identifying the cause of obstruction.
- Patients with a suspected high-grade obstruction do not require any oral contrast medium because the nonopacified fluid in the bowel provides adequate intrinsic contrast.
- An intravenous (IV) contrast is preferable for routine CT imaging of a suspected SBO, in part to demonstrate whether the bowel is perfusing normally or is potentially ischemic, and, in a minority of cases to provide information about the potential etiology, such as Crohn disease and neoplasm.
- However, in patients who cannot receive IV contrast due to an allergy or renal dysfunction, noncontrast CT appears to have comparable accuracy for diagnosing or excluding SBO.
- Computed tomography is very useful for assessing SBO complications, namely ischemia and strangulation, as well as conditions that lead directly to both obstruction and ischemia if untreated (i.e. closed-loop SBO).
- Mesenteric edema and interloop fluid/fat stranding are danger signs for early surgery to be considered **(Fig. 2)**.

Conventional Enteroclysis and Computed Tomography Enteroclysis

Computed tomography based or conventional imaging, where small bowel is directly distended, is being increasingly used in intermittent or low-grade SBO. There is increasing

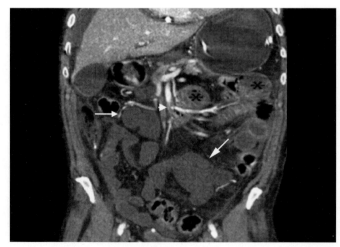

Fig. 2 Coronal images contrast-enhanced CT showing nonenhancing bowel wall (arrows) and clot in superior mesenteric artery (SMA) (arrowhead)

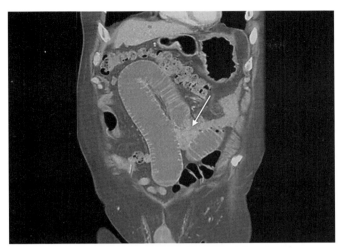

Fig. 3 Small bowel obstruction due to recurrent ovarian cancer, arrow shows solid serosal tumor implant causing recurrent obstruction

evidence that enteroclysis can distinguish sites and causes of low-grade and high-grade SBO, as well as identify adhesions from obstructing neoplasms or other etiologies (**Fig. 3**).

Gastrointestinal Bleed

- Upper gastrointestinal bleeding (UGIB) by definition occurs proximal to the ligament of Treitz, originating from the esophagus, stomach or duodenum. Typically, UGIB will present with hematemesis or with melena. If brisk, UGIB can also result in hematochezia, which is the presenting sign in 15% of cases of UGIB. The most common etiologies are duodenal ulcer, gastric erosions, gastric ulcer, varices, Mallory-Weiss tears, esophagitis, duodenitis, neoplasm, stomal marginal ulcer, esophageal ulcer and other/miscellaneous including angiodyplasia or vascular malformations, with some patients having multiple sources of bleeding.
- Patients with presumed UGIB should first be examined by upper endoscopy as it successfully identifies the source of hemorrhage in 95% of cases and provides prognostic information regarding rebleeding, the need for surgery, the level of hospital care required, and mortality. CT is used in selected clinical situations when UGI endoscopy is negative.
- Acute lower gastrointestinal (LGI) tract bleeding is defined as bleeding into the small bowel distal to the ligament of Treitz, or bleeding into the large bowel. It may present as either melena or hematochezia, depending on the site. Causes of LGI bleeding include inflammatory bowel disease, neoplasms, stress ulcers, surgical anastomoses, vascular lesions such as angiodysplasia and diverticulitis.
- Diagnostic options include colonoscopy, Tc-99m red blood cell (RBC) scan, CECT, MRI, and transcatheter arteriography. Therapeutic options can be facilitated by transcatheter arteriography, colonoscopy, and surgery.

Active Bleeding in a Hemodynamically Stable Patient

- Computed tomography angiography can detect bleeding as low as 0.3 mL/min is now replacing nuclear medicine studies. Variant anatomy, vessel occlusion which might influence transcatheter intervention, cause of bleeding, lesions unfavorable for embolization so that they can directly go to surgery can all be identified on CT angiography.
- Hemodynamically unstable patient who is actively bleeding, or required more than 5 units of blood or there is ongoing significant bleeding even though colonoscopy recognized the site of bleeding and treatment was attempted on endoscopy.
- Arteriography should be attempted as it identifies the source of lower GI bleeding. Catheter-directed treatment can be directly attempted at the demonstrated site of bleeding.

Jaundice

- Ultrasound reveals dilated bile duct in obstructive jaundice.
- Computed tomography is useful for predicting tumor extension and potential resectability. Dynamic multiphase CECT can evaluate causes of obstructive jaundice and level of obstruction.

Magnetic Resonance Imaging

Magnetic resonance imaging and magnetic resonance cholangiopancreatography (MRCP) allow for accurate visualization of the biliary tree, patency of biliary confluence. MRCP can show the three-dimensional anatomy of pancreatic and biliary duct. MRCP is most sensitive for detection of biliary calculi. MRCP can allow for planning of endoscopic retrograde cholangiopancreatography (ERCP) versus percutaneous drainage in patients with hilar biliary obstruction. MRI and MRCP are also recommended in pregnant women in suspected biliary obstruction due to lack of ionizing radiation. Dynamic MRI like dynamic CT can provide detailed evaluation of the arterial and venous vascular anatomy and evaluation/staging of local pathology and distant staging.

Endoscopic Ultrasound

Endoscopic ultrasound (EUS) is useful for tissue sampling as fine needle aspiration (FNA) possible.
- Endoscopic ultrasound is now used in addition to ERCP, it can identify small distal biliary ductal calculi, provides for local staging of periampullary neoplasm.

- Endoscopic ultrasound also allows for tissue sampling; FNA under USG guidance can also be done
- For cross-sectional imaging, CECT and/or MRI are both equally good.
- When the cause of jaundice cannot be identified on imaging, then parenchymal process or liver infiltration needs to be excluded.
- Liver biopsy is the next step in diagnosis.

Pancreatitis

The use of MRI in evaluating patient with acute pancreatitis is gaining acceptance:
- To evaluate the bile duct stones and pancreatic duct disruption
- It can also effectively evaluate morphologic changes to the pancreas and peripancreatic regions similar to that of MDCT.
- Solid debris is better identified on MRI—this can help to characterize and identify postpancreatitis collection from other cystic lesions.
- EUS and ERCP in patients with acute pancreatitis are used to confirm or refute choledocholithiasis and subsequent stone removal.
- Anatomic anomalies such as pancreas divisum and pancreatic duct stricture or stones can also be identified.

Hematuria

Causes of hematuria include calculi, infection, trauma, coagulopathy, neoplasms, etc. If the patients have risk factors such as occupational exposure to chemicals cigarette smoking, or irritative voiding symptoms, a full urologic evaluation for urothelial carcinoma is recommended even if urine analysis shows three RBC per high power field. In patients with renal parenchymal disease, such as glomerulonephritis, acute tubular necrosis, glomerulonephropathy, and acute kidney injury, USG is sufficient. Also, if there is history of vigorous exercise, or urological procedures, infection or viral illness, initial imaging workup is also not very helpful. However, if there is persistent chronic hematuria in the above populations of patients, it warrants further workup that probably should include imaging.

Following major trauma, dedicated imaging as explained below tailored to the urinary tract is suggested:
- Ultrasound is used as a screening tool and for further triaging patients who might require cross-sectional imaging. CT urography—it can diagnose small renal masses, image the upper collecting system, and identify small stones and calculi. MR urography is a reasonable alternative but it cannot detect small calculi and stones.
- USG is recommended initially and for follow-up in patients with papillary necrosis and medullary sponge kidney. Cystoscopy is recommended if computed tomography urography (CTU) is unremarkable.
- Rarely, angiography should be considered for diagnosis and therapeutic intervention for vascular disorders such as arteriovenous malformations, aneurysms, or obstruction of a calyx from overlying artery (Fraley's syndrome)
- Noncontrast CT remains the investigation of choice for evaluating the stone burden as 99% of stones are radiopaque on CT.

Urinary Tract Infection

- Imaging studies are required for diagnosis and to plan management. Clinically healthy patient need no studies if they respond to therapy within 72 hours. If no response, CT abdomen and pelvis is study of choice; can identify calculi renal and perinephric abscess.
- If the response to therapy in diabetics and immunocompromised patients is not prompt then CECT is recommended. USG is useful in identifying pyonephrosis.
- Computed tomography should be ordered sooner in adults with earlier complications. MRI is an alternative if CECT is contraindicated. Imaging can identify a treatable condition in patients with frequent relapses and reinfections.

Acute Kidney Injury

- Ultrasound should be initially performed in patients presenting with undiagnosed renal failure, the small and echogenic kidneys suggest long-standing process and unlikely to improve, or sometimes correctible cause such as obstruction. Renal length on USG is used to estimate renal size. Renal cortical thickness measured by USG in patients with chronic renal failure (CRF) correlates estimated glomerular filtration rate (eGFR).
- Acute renal failure is also a presentation in a patient with obstructed renal transplant. If USG is negative, MRI or nonenhanced CT should be obtained to look for retroperitoneal mass, lymphadenopathy, fibrosis, calculi, etc.

Renal Transplant

- Ultrasound is used for initial evaluation, follow-up and image-guided interventions in patients with renal transplant.
- Renal artery thrombosis or renal vein thrombosis can be detected with renal USG in the perioperative period, as well as flow can be monitored following renal artery stenting or angioplasty. Postbiopsy arteriovenous fistulas can be promptly identified on USG.
- The indications of USG include identification of postoperative fluid collections, guiding aspiration to differentiate urinoma, abscess, and lymphocele from liquefied hematoma.

CHEST AND CARDIOVASCULAR EMERGENCIES

Aortic Dissection

Computed tomography angiography is recommended for evaluating acute or chronic dissection. Precontrast images allow for identification of aortic calcification and intramural hematoma. Type A dissection can involve the coronaries, reported in up to 15% of patients **(Fig. 4)**.

Transesophageal echocardiography (TEE) is not routinely used in the acute setting if the CT angiography has provided of all the relevant information.

However, MRI is not possible in acute setting as well as where acute coronary syndrome may be a differential diagnosis; TEE is operator-dependent and does not allow for evaluation of branch vessel and visceral organ involvement, extent of distal aortic involvement. It is, however, an adjunct in bedside situation in ICU, hemodynamically unstable patients for evaluating the valves, cardiac wall motion, any luminal clots as a roadmap before urgent surgery with equivocal findings on CT at aortic root.

Pulmonary Embolism

Computed tomography pulmonary angiography is an investigation of choice, combined with CT venography. It also improves the sensitivity of detecting deep vein thrombosis (DVT). CT pulmonary angiography can also identify right ventricular dysfunction or has effect on patient management; for example, massive pulmonary embolism may require institution of thrombolytic therapy.

Pneumonia

In all cases of suspected pneumonia, chest radiography should be obtained. However, in severe pneumonia, CT is indicated to guide; for example, loculated pleural drainage, biopsy. CT can identify the extent of lung involvement and lymphadenopathy; however, it cannot identify the underlying pathogenic organism. Patients with severe pneumonia in ICU setting may be monitored on radiographs.

Blunt Chest Trauma

- Blunt trauma is a significant cause of mortality in younger adults. The thoracic trauma can show pleural, pulmonary, musculoskeletal, and mediastinal findings.
- The most common thoracic injury is a rib fracture while acute aortic injury or dissection is most life-threatening.
- Chest AP radiograph, AP pelvic radiograph, and lateral horizontal-beam cervical spine radiograph are quickly used to screen patients and triage injuries.
- Patients with blunt trauma are often intubated and already have other lines and tubes inserted as well.
- Misplaced lines and tubes can be identified on AP chest radiograph. Contrast-enhanced chest CT is recommended in patients with high-mechanism, altered mental status, distracting injuries abnormal chest radiographs, or clinically suspected thoracic injury.

Acute Chest Pain

- In emergency department, CT coronary angiography can be advised to patient with low or intermediate risk factors in whom electrocardiography (ECG) and cardiac enzymes are normal.
- Stress echocardiography (using dobutamine) in low/intermediate risk acute coronary syndrome (ACS) is helpful in focal/regional wall motion abnormalities. Subclinical left ventricular aneurysm, pseudoaneurysm, effusion and valvular dysfunction can be evaluated. This can be a bedside procedure.
- Transesophageal echocardiography is a specialized bedside investigation to rule out aortic dissection. TEE can identify valvular dysfunction and intracardiac thrombus; however, it is invasive and is generally not indicated in acute chest pain.
- Magnetic resonance imaging is limited in its utility in acute setting because of limited equipment ability and long scan times not possible in unstable patients.

Hemoptysis

Bronchiectasis, lung malignancies, and bronchitis are the three most common causes. Bronchitis is a clinical and endoscopic diagnosis. Bronchiectasis and lung malignancy require CECT. MDCT angiography can identify and help to plan bronchial arteriography by providing bronchial artery anatomical mapping identifying site of bleeding. Massive hemoptysis in cases such as TB (tuberculosis), bronchiectasis, bronchogenic carcinoma, and aspergillomas can be controlled by bronchial embolization.

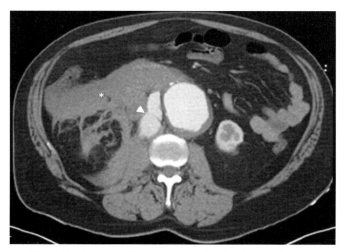

Fig. 4 Ruptured aortic aneurysm contrast-enhanced images showing active contrast extravasation

NEUROLOGIC AND SPINAL EMERGENCIES

Acute Headache

In most centers, initial screening is done with CT or MRI.

Acute subarachnoid hemorrhage (SAH) should be further investigated with magnetic resonance angiography (MRA), and/or computed tomography angiography (CTA) followed by catheter angiography if required. CTA is preferred because it is a quick investigation and is noninvasive. Advise head MRI if headache is of trigeminal autonomic origin.

If the patient has mechanical temporomandibular joint (TMJ) symptoms such as clicking, crepitus, pain and tenderness localize to at least one TMJ, MRI is indicated; CT can evaluate degenerative change. MRA of the cranial arteries can evaluate inflamed segments, aneurysms of the superficial cranial arteries and allow for diagnosis as well as follow-up.

New headache with focal neurologic deficit or papilledema, headache associated with cough, exertion, or sexual activity—intracranial pathology must be urgently excluded contrast-enhanced MRI with or without MRA and magnetic resonance venography (MRV) is the investigation of choice.

Acute Stroke/Suspected Acute Cerebrovascular Event

It is important to accurately and rapidly diagnose acute stroke. Parenchymal microhemorrhages are better seen on MRI; however, thrombolytic therapy including recombinant tissue plasminogen activator (rTPA) is based on CT findings rather than MRI. CT should be used to exclude hemorrhage in the context of 3-4.5 hours therapeutic window for administering rTPA.

Computed tomography perfusion and CT angiography are used to discriminate between infarct and penumbra. CT can quickly identify acute hemorrhage and vascular occlusive lesions; it is therefore preferred in some centers over MRI.

Head Trauma

Computed tomography can quickly identify bony injuries; parenchyma subarachnoid subdural or epidural hemorrhage identifies intracranial mass effect **(Fig. 5)**. It is performable with other medical and life-support devices. Multi-planar reformates and three-dimensional reconstruction can improve identification of subtle fractures and hemorrhages.

Magnetic resonance imaging is more sensitive than CT in detecting all stages of hemorrhage. In particular, nonhemorrhagic contusions, injuries in posterior fossa, brainstem and diffuse axonal injury (DAI) are better evaluated on MRI. MRI is, however, incompatible with certain medical devices; acquisition times are longer and emergency availability is not universal.

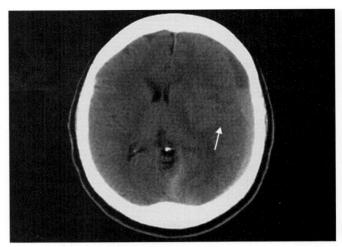

Fig. 5 Noncontrast computed tomography (NCCT) showing left subdural hematoma with effacement of the left lateral ventricle

Head Seizures

Magnetic resonance imaging with or without intravenous contrast as well as MRA/MRV remain the investigation of choice.

Imaging of the Dizzy Patient

Urgent imaging is not required in cases of classical history of benign paroxysmal positional vertigo (BPPV) or vestibular neuritis. However, if there is asymmetric hearing loss, causes of dizziness are unclear; imaging should be considered.

Magnetic resonance imaging with gadolinium contrast is recommended for evaluating the dizzy patient. Gadolinium-enhanced MRI can easily identify cerebellopontine angle lesions such as vestibular schwannomas and meningiomas. MRI can identify acute or chronic ischemic disease. CT is better for imaging the bony labyrinth.

ABNORMAL VAGINAL BLEEDING

- Transvaginal ultrasound (TVUS) is highly recommended for depiction of endometrial pathology especially in postmenopausal women.
- Focal heterogeneity or/and eccentric thickening are suspicious findings and warrant further biopsy.
- Focal heterogeneity or eccentric thickening of the endometrium detected at TVUS always should be further investigated regardless of endometrial thickness to exclude endometrial pathology.
- Transvaginal ultrasound can help to identify focal lesions within the endometrium such as polyps and submucosal fibroids, which may lead to sampling error and a negative biopsy result.

- Color and duplex Doppler US is of added value in uterine and endometrial pathology.
- Blood flow within an intracavitary lesion rules out retained blood clot.

MULTIDETECTOR COMPUTED TOMOGRAPHY IN A POLYTRAUMA PATIENT

Multislice CT in a polytrauma patient lends itself to multiple images to be reviewed by radiologist. There are certain patterns which however must be identified, for example abdominal wall tears, skin lesions and chance fractures along with bowel or mesenteric injury fall in the remit of seat belt syndrome. In transverse process, fractures abdominal injuries are seen in as many as 50% patients. Injury to gallbladder (GB) and pancreas is rare, so are injuries of the first through third ribs and aorta, these are often following high-energy trauma.

Following direct impact with steering wheel or the dashboard there are multiple associations of chest wall deformities, pneumothorax, vascular injuries, and associated contusions. There are in addition fractures of shoulder girdle, spine, pelvis, and the sternum. There is a high risk of crushing the solid abdominal organs between the anterior abdominal wall and spine or posterior thoracic cage.

Shear injuries (tear at fixed points of appointment) arise from differential movement of fixed and mobile structures. In the GI tract, shear forces result in injury to jejunum and duodenum at the ligament of Treitz. Vascular shear injuries can involve the mesenteric root, the aorta, and solid organ pedicles. Burst injuries of the hollow viscera, stretching and injuring of the diaphragm occur following sudden increases in intraluminal pressure resulting from compression and sudden increase in abdominal pressure.

Three-dimension reconstruction (recon) of the images allows for identifying orientation of the joint alignment, bony fragments, and appropriate surgical planning.

Multiphasic images allow for characterization of vascular injuries. Pseudoaneurysm is seen as round pooled contrast beyond the lumen following aortic opacification. It retains a constant round shape in all phases. Arterial extravasation spreads out and may have higher attenuation than the aorta on delayed phase images.

Chest Injuries

It is third most common site of traumatic injury and involves 20–25% of all motor collision-related deaths. Most patient with chest trauma die at crash scene.

Life-threatening aortic injuries range from subtle intimal damage to active extravasation. Less severe injuries may lead to thromboembolic events—therefore anticoagulation is often indicated. Dissection, is identified as intimal flaps, often associated with pseudoaneurysm, seen as an eccentric irregular outpouching of contrast material or a sudden change in caliber that is sometimes referred to as pseudocoarctation. Endovascular repair is the treatment of choice. The classical location of aortic injury is at the aortic isthmus, where the ligamentum arteriosum attaches. Aortic root and diaphragmatic crus are the other locations.

Mediastinal hematoma can result from injury to the vasa vasorum, sternal or spinal injuries. Sometimes periarterial hematoma in the superior mediastinum may be a sign of a great vessel injury.

Injuries of the pulmonary arteries, intrathoracic IVC, and heart are rarely seen at CT because of high at site mortality.

Head: Computed tomography head can detect contusion, bleeding, herniation, and infarction. Facial bone fractures can be better evaluated with 3D reformats to facilitate surgical planning.

Abdomen

Computed tomography scan of abdomen with contrast able to detect various injuries of abdominal cavity.

Hepatic injuries: Around 25% of patients with polytrauma have hepatic injury. Mortality rates can reach up to 80% especially if IVC or hepatic veins are injured. Around 90% of hemodynamically stable patients are treated conservatively. CT is able to identify extension of laceration to hepatic veins, associated vascular complications, such as acute extravasation and pseudoaneurysm which may require embolization.

Splenic injuries: Blunt splenic injury can be identified on CT in up to 98% of patients.

Renal injuries: CT scan identifies shattered kidney, vascular occlusion, and pedicular avulsion, these warrant urgent surgical exploration. Microcatheterization with superselective embolization can effectively control bleeding. Traumatic occlusion on CT should be promptly identified for the surgeon to immediately take corrective surgical action. Delayed images can differentiate between urinoma and hematoma and should be obtained if there is significant renal injury.

Urine leakage can also be identified on delayed images—usually treated conservatively. Stent placement is warranted in leakage lasting more than 2 weeks, transection of the ureteropelvic junction, seen as lack of ureteral contrast material distal to the injury, surgical treatment is suggested.

Pancreatic injuries: Pancreatic injuries are rare with 16–20% mortality. Early mortality is from massive hemorrhage, while delayed mortality is usually following sepsis form pseudocyst, fistula or abscess. Pancreatic neck may be related to injuries of portal vein, splenic vein, and IVC. Pancreatic duct injury must be carefully looked for. Specific signs of pancreatic injury are laceration, fluid separating splenic vein from pancreas, transection or fracture. Deep lacerations involve more than 50% of pancreatic thickness. MRCP is useful in evaluating the injuries of the pancreatic duct.

Injuries of Hollow Abdominal Viscera

Focal bowel thickening, discontinuous bowel wall with hematoma, localized extraluminal air are suspicious of bowel wall injury; however, diffuse bowel wall thickening is nonspecific and can be seen in volume overload. Imaging findings on CT in pediatric patients may show CT features of impending shock; pediatric patients can remain normotensive despite significant blood loss. Active mesenteric bleeding and abrupt occlusion or irregular vascular narrowing impending infarction and microperforation require acute intervention. Mechanical ventilation however may lead to extraluminal air.

PLAIN RADIOGRAPHY IN COMMON FRACTURES: MUST FOR EVERY TRAUMA PHYSICIAN

- A fracture is break or crack in the continuity of bone which can be either complete or incomplete.
- Fractures can be acute pathological fractures, traumatic, or stress. Traumatic fractures can be either complete, incomplete, displaced, undisplaced closed/simple open/ compound.
- Depending on orientation, fractures can be oblique fractures, spiral fractures, comminuted fractures (2 or more fragments), transverse fractures, compression/ crush fractures and depressed (in skull).
- When articular surfaces are wholly displaced, joint is dislocated and apposition is lost. A joint is: Subluxated when articular surfaces retain some contact and are partly displaced. Dislocation can occur with or without fracture.

Avulsion fractures: Pulling off or avulsion of bone fragment at site of attachment of ligaments or tendons—adolescent, growth center are prone to avulsion injuries, hyperplastic callus which forms during the healing phase can sometimes mimic a bone forming tumor.

Two views at right angles orthogonal planes are must for all fractures and dislocations. Degree of deformity is better seen by two views. All long bone fractures must also cover the joint above and below. Some fractures such as scaphoid may require additional imaging.

Spinal trauma: Radiographs are obtained without or minimal patient movement following trauma. There is a large range of spinal fractures; stable fracture is one where the spinal alignment and the position of the vertebra are maintained without immobilization. Unstable fracture is one where if immobilization is not offered, there could be deterioration in position and progressive neurological compromise. MRI and CT are increasingly being used to evaluate the bony fractures and soft tissues injuries involving the ligament, muscles, and intervertebral disk.

Hip Fracture: Dislocations of the Hip

Common in the elderly due to osteoporosis. Posterior, central, and anterior fracture dislocation. Delayed treatment can result in a vascular necrosis. Posterior dislocation is the most common and associate with fracture of the posterior rim of acetabulum **(Figs 6A and B)**.

Fractures of the femur, tibia, fibula: Bedside X-ray can be done to detect fracture in trauma patients. Oblique, spiral, comminuted, and transverse fractures can occur at any site.

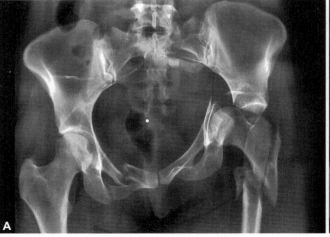 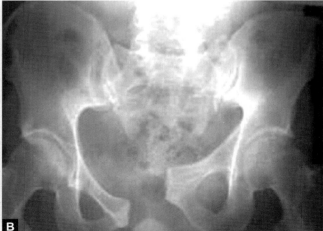

Figs 6A and B Severe shear injury leading to disruption and diastasis of pubic symphysis and right sacroiliac (SI) joint

CONCLUSION

Imaging plays an important role in emergency specially in polytrauma patient. With the advent of modern technique like CT scan, liberal use of contrast enhanced CT scan is used in polytrauma patient. This allows better selection of patient for surgery; also provide better monitoring of patient in whom nonsurgical approach has been decided. Multidetector computed tomography scan (MDCT) protocol is important for every emergency department. Multidetector CT scan not only detect visceral injury but also the active bleeding source by contrast extravasation, there for many author suggest whole body CT scan for polytrauma patient and it can be done while resuscitation also.

BIBLIOGRAPHY

1. Addiss DG, Shaffer N, Fowler BS, et al. The epidemiology of appendicitis and appendectomy in the United States. Am J Epidemiol. 1990;132:910-25.
2. Ahvenjarvi L, Niinimaki J, Halonen J, et al. Reliability of the evaluation of multidetector computed tomography images from the scanner's console in high-energy blunt-trauma patients. Acta Radiol. 2007;48(1):64-70.
3. American College of Radiology. ACR Appropriateness Criteria®: Head Trauma - Child. [online] Available from https://acsearch.acr.org/docs/3083021/Narrative/. [Accessed February 2017].
4. Amsterdam EA, Kirk JD, Bluemke DA, et al. Testing of low-risk patients presenting to the emergency department with chest pain: a scientific statement from the American Heart Association. Circulation. 2010;122(17):1756-76.
5. Balthazar EJ. CT diagnosis and staging of acute pancreatitis. Radiol Clin North Am. 1989;27:19-37.
6. Barrios C, Malinoski D, Dolich M, et al. Utility of thoracic computed tomography after blunt trauma: when is chest radiograph enough? Am Surg. 2009;75(10):966-9.
7. Bernardin B, Troquet JM. Initial management and resuscitation of severe chest trauma. Emerg Med Clin North Am. 2012;30(2):377-400.
8. Bogdanoff BM, Stafford CR, Green L, et al. Computerized transaxial tomography in the evaluation of patients with focal epilepsy. Neurology. 1975;25(11):1013-7.
9. Boudiaf M, Soyer P, Terem C, et al. CT evaluation of small bowel obstruction. Radiographics. 2001;21:613-24.
10. Bowen A. The vomiting infant: recent advances and unsettled issues in imaging. Radiol Clin North Am. 1988;26(2):377-92.
11. Brink M, Deunk J, Dekker HM, et al. Added value of routine chest MDCT after blunt trauma: evaluation of additional findings and impact on patient management. Am J Roentgenol. 2008;190(6):1591-8.
12. Cappell M. Acute pancreatitis: etiology, clinical presentation, diagnosis and therapy. Med Clin North Am. 2008;92:889-923.
13. Caruso PA, Johnson J, Thibert R, et al. The use of magnetic resonance spectroscopy in the evaluation of epilepsy. Neuroimaging Clin N Am. 2013;23(3):407-24.
14. Casas JD, Diaz R, Valderas G, et al. Prognostic value of CT in the early assessment of patients with acute pancreatitis. Am J Roentgenol. 2004;182:569-74.
15. Chan O. ABC of Emergency Radiology. New Jersey, United States: Wiley Blackwell; 2013.
16. Chun JY, Belli AM. Immediate and long-term outcomes of bronchial and non-bronchial systemic artery embolisation for the management of haemoptysis. Eur Radiol. 2010;20(3):558-65.
17. Conneely MF, Hacein-Bey L, Jay WM. Magnetic resonance imaging of the orbit. Semin Ophthalmol. 2008;23(3):179-89.
18. Cremaschi P, Nascimbene C, Vitulo P, et al. Therapeutic embolization of bronchial artery: a successful treatment in 209 cases of relapse hemoptysis. Angiology. 1993;44(4):295-9.
19. Dave BR, Sharma A, Kalva SP, et al. Nine-year single-center experience with transcatheter arterial embolization for hemoptysis: medium-term outcomes. Vasc Endovascular Surg. 2011;45(3):258-68.
20. Demehri S, Rybicki FJ, Desjardins B, et al. ACR Appropriateness Criteria((R)) blunt chest trauma—suspected aortic injury. Emerg Radiol. 2012;19(4):287-92.
21. Dillman JR, Kappil M, Weadock WJ, et al. Sonographic twinkling artifact for renal calculus detection: correlation with CT. Radiology. 2011;259(3):911-6.
22. Easton JD, Saver JL, Albers GW, et al. Definition and evaluation of transient ischemic attack: a scientific statement for healthcare professionals from the American Heart Association/American Stroke Association Stroke Council; Council on Cardiovascular Surgery and Anesthesia; Council on Cardiovascular Radiology and Intervention; Council on Cardiovascular Nursing; and the Interdisciplinary Council on Peripheral Vascular Disease. The American Academy of Neurology affirms the value of this statement as an educational tool for neurologists. Stroke. 2009;40(6):2276-93.
23. Endo H, Inoue T, Ogasawara K, et al. Quantitative assessment of cerebral hemodynamics using perfusion-weighted MRI in patients with major cerebral artery occlusive disease: comparison with positron emission tomography. Stroke. 2006;37(2):388-92.
24. Eyler WR, Clark MD. Dissecting aneurysms of the aorta: roentgen manifestations including a comparison with other types of aneurysms. Radiology. 1965;85(6):1047-57.
25. Farquhar C, Ekeroma A, Furness S, et al. A systematic review of transvaginal ultrasonography, sonohysterography and hysteroscopy for the investigation of abnormal uterine bleeding in premenopausal women. Acta Obstet Gynecol Scand. 2003;82(6):493-504.
26. Ferzoco LB, Raptopoulous V, Silen W. Acute diverticulitis. N Engl J Med. 1998;338:1521-6.
27. Fuhrman GM, Simmons GT, Davidson BS, et al. The single indication for cystography in blunt trauma. Am Surg. 1993;59(6):335-7.
28. Furukawa M, Kashiwagi S, Matsunaga N, et al. Evaluation of cerebral perfusion parameters measured by perfusion CT in chronic cerebral ischemia: comparison with xenon CT. J Comput Assist Tomogr. 2002;26(2):272-8.
29. Gastaut H, Gastaut JL. Computerized transverse axial tomography in epilepsy. Epilepsia. 1976;17(3):325-36.
30. Haidary A, Bis K, Vrachliotis T, et al. Enhancement performance of a 64-slice triple rule-out protocol vs 16-slice and 10-slice multidetector CT-angiography protocols for evaluation of aortic and pulmonary vasculature. J Comput Assist Tomogr. 2007;31(6):917-23.
31. Hanbidge A, Buckler P, O'Malley M, et al. From the RSNA refresher courses: imaging evaluation for acute pain in the right upper quadrant. Radiographics. 2004;24:1117-35.

32. Ostenen H, Pettersson H. WHO Manual of Diagnostic Imaging, 1st edition. Geneva, Switzerland: World Health Organization; 2002.
33. Hernanz-Schulman M. Imaging of neonatal gastrointestinal obstruction. Radiol Clin North Am. 1999;37(6):1163-86.
34. Soliman HH. Value of triple rule out CT in the emergency department. The Egyptian Journal of Radiology and Nuclear Medicine. 2015;46(3):621-7.
35. Huber-Wagner S, Lefering R, Qvick LM, et al. Effect of whole-body CT during trauma resuscitation on survival: a retrospective, multicentre study. Lancet. 2009;373:1455-61.
36. Hulka CA, Hall DA, McCarthy K, et al. Endometrial polyps, hyperplasia, and carcinoma in postmenopausal women: differentiation with endovaginal sonography. Radiology. 1994;191(3):755-8.
37. Jackson GD. New techniques in magnetic resonance and epilepsy. Epilepsia. 1994;35 Suppl 6:S2-13.
38. Jacobs J, Birnbaum B, Macari M, et al. Acute appendicitis: Comparison of helical CT diagnosis—focused technique with oral contrast material versus nonfocussed technique with oral and intravenous contrast material. Radiology. 2001;220:683-90.
39. Johnson TR, Nikolaou K, Wintersperger BJ, et al. ECG-gated 64-MDCT angiography in the differential diagnosis of acute chest pain. AJR Am J Roentgenol. 2007;188(1):76-82.
40. Kaewlai R, Avery LL, Asrani AV, et al. Multidetector CT of blunt thoracic trauma. Radiographics. 2008;28(6):1555-70.
41. Kaewlai R, Nazinitsky K. Acute colonic diverticulitis in a community-based hospital: CT evaluation in 138 patients. Emerg Radiol. 2007;13:171-9.
42. Khalil A, Fartoukh M, Parrot A, et al. Impact of MDCT angiography on the management of patients with hemoptysis. Am J Roentgenol. 2010;195(3):772-8.
43. Kidwell CS, Warach S. Acute ischemic cerebrovascular syndrome: diagnostic criteria. Stroke. 2003;34(12):2995-8.
44. Kim HC, Yang DM, Jin W, et al. Added diagnostic value of multiplanar reformation of multidetector CT data in patients with suspected appendicitis. Radiographics. 2008;28:393-406.
45. Kirkpatrick AW, Sirois M, Laupland KB, et al. Prospective evaluation of hand-held focused abdominal sonography for trauma (FAST) in blunt abdominal trauma. Can J Surg. 2005;48(6):453-60.
46. Knudson MM, McAninch JW, Gomez R, et al. Hematuria as a predictor of abdominal injury after blunt trauma. Am J Surg. 1992;164(5):482-5.
47. Lai V, Tsang WK, Chan WC, et al. Diagnostic accuracy of mediastinal width measurement on posteroanterior and anteroposterior chest radiographs in the depiction of acute nontraumatic thoracic aortic dissection. Emerg Radiol. 2012;19(4):309-15.
48. Leite NP, Pereira J, Cunha R, et al. CT evaluation of appendicitis and its complications: imaging techniques and key diagnostic findings. Am J Roentgenol. 2005;185:406-17.
49. Levine JA, Neitlich J, Verga M, et al. Ureteral calculi in patients with flank pain: correlation of plain radiography with unenhanced helical CT. Radiology. 1997;204(1):27-31.
50. Lieu TA, Grasmeder HM 3rd, Kaplan BS. An approach to the evaluation and treatment of microscopic hematuria. Pediatr Clin North Am. 1991;38(3):579-92.
51. Lilien LD, Srinivasan G, Pyati SP, et al. Green vomiting in the first 72 hours in normal infants. Am J Dis Child. 1986;140(7):662-4.
52. Maglinte D, Balthazar E, Kelvin F, et al. The role of radiology in the diagnosis of small bowel obstruction. Am J Roentgenol. 1997;168:1171-80.
53. Maglinte DT, Sandrasegaran K, Lappas JC, et al. CT enteroclysis. Radiology. 2007;245:661-71.
54. McMahon MA, Squirrell CA. Multidetector CT of aortic dissection: a pictorial review. Radiographics. 2010;30(2):445-60.
55. Messiou C, Chalmers AG. Imaging in acute pancreatitis. Imaging. 2004;16:314-22.
56. Miller FH, Keppke AL, Dalal K, et al. MRI of pancreatitis and its complications. Am J Roentgenol. 2004;183:1637-44.
57. Mortele KJ, Wiesner W, Intriere L, et al. A modified CT severity index for evaluating acute pancreatitis: improved correlation with patient outcome. Am J Roentgenol. 2004;183:1261-5.
58. Nicolaou S, Kai B, Ho S, et al. Imaging of acute small bowel obstruction. Am J Roentgenol. 2005;185:1036-44.
59. Raby N, Burman L, Lacy GD, et al. Accident and Emergency Radiology: A Survival Guide, 3rd edition. Philadelphia: Saunders Elsevier; 2014.
60. Nural MS, Elmali M, Findik S, et al. Computed tomographic pulmonary angiography in the assessment of severity of acute pulmonary embolism and right ventricular dysfunction. Acta Radiol. 2009;50(6):629-37.
61. Oner S, Oto A, Tekgul S, et al. Comparison of spiral CT and US in the evaluation of pediatric urolithiasis. JBR-BTR. 2004;87(5):219-23.
62. Pedrosa I, Levine D, Aimee DE, et al. MR imaging evaluation of acute appendicitis in pregnancy. Radiology. 2006;238:891-9.
63. Pereira J, Sirlin C, Pinto P, et al. Disproportionate fat stranding: a helpful CT sign in patients with acute abdominal pain. Radiographics. 2004;24:703-15.
64. Rao P, Rhea J, Novelline R, et al. Helical CT technique for the diagnosis of appendicitis: prospective evaluation of a focused appendix CT examination. Radiology. 1997;202:139-44.
65. Restrepo L, Jacobs MA, Barker PB, et al. Assessment of transient ischemic attack with diffusion- and perfusion-weighted imaging. Am J Neuroradiol. 2004;25(10):1645-52.
66. Riccabona M, Avni FE, Blickman JG, et al. Imaging recommendations in paediatric uroradiology: minutes of the ESPR workgroup session on urinary tract infection, fetal hydronephrosis, urinary tract ultrasonography and voiding cystourethrography, Barcelona, Spain, June 2007. Pediatr Radiol. 2008;38(2):138-45.
67. Rubinshtein R, Halon DA, Gaspar T, et al. Impact of 64-slice cardiac computed tomographic angiography on clinical decision-making in emergency department patients with chest pain of possible myocardial ischemic origin. Am J Cardiol. 2007;100(10):1522-6.
68. Rybkin A, Thoeni R. Current concepts in imaging of appendicitis. Radiol Clin North Am. 2007;45:411-22.
69. Schwartz ES, Dlugos DJ, Storm PB, et al. Magneto-encephalography for pediatric epilepsy: how we do it. Am J Neuroradiol. 2008;29(5):832-7.
70. See TC, Ng CS, Watson CJE, et al. Appendicitis: spectrum of appearance on helical CT. Br J Radiol. 2002;75:775-81.
71. Sekimoto M, Takada T, Kawarada Y, et al. JPN guidelines for the management of acute pancreatitis: epidemiology, etiology, natural history and outcome predictors in acute pancreatitis. J Hepatobiliary Pancreat Surg. 2006;13:10-24.

72. Shankar S, van Sonnenberg E, Silverman SG, et al. Imaging and percutaneous management of acute complicated pancreatitis. Cardiovasc Intervent Radiol. 2004;27:567-80.
73. Shanmuganathan K. Multi-detector row CT imaging of blunt abdominal trauma. Semin Ultrasound CT MR. 2004;25(2):180-204.
74. Sheiman L, Levine M, Levin A, et al. Chronic diverticulitis: clinical, radiographic, and pathological findings. Am J Roentgenol. 2008;191:522-8.
75. Shi AA, Lee SI. Radiological reasoning: algorithmic workup of abnormal vaginal bleeding with endovaginal sonography and sonohysterography. Am J Roentgenol. 2008;191(6 Suppl):S68-73.
76. Siewert B, Raptopoulos V, Liu S, et al. CT predictors of failed laparoscopic appendectomy. Radiology. 2003;229:415-20.
77. Singh A, Danrad R, Hahn PF, et al. Imaging of the acute abdomen and pelvis: acute appendicitis and beyond. Radiographics. 2007;27:1419-31.
78. Sizemore AW, Rabbani KZ, Ladd A, et al. Diagnostic performance of the upper gastrointestinal series in the evaluation of children with clinically suspected malrotation. Pediatr Radiol. 2008;38(5):518-28.
79. Smith JK, Kenney PJ. Imaging of renal trauma. Radiol Clin North Am. 2003;41(5):1019-35.
80. Smith P, Bakos O, Heimer G, et al. Transvaginal ultrasound for identifying endometrial abnormality. Acta Obstet Gynecol Scand. 1991;70(7-8):591-4.
81. Solinas L, Raucci R, Terrazzino S, et al. Prevalence, clinical characteristics, resource utilization and outcome of patients with acute chest pain in the emergency department. A multicenter, prospective, observational study in North-Eastern Italy. Ital Heart J. 2003;4(5):318-24.
82. Strasberg SM. Clinical practice. Acute calculous cholecystitis. N Engl J Med. 2008;358:2804-11.
83. Strouse PJ. Disorders of intestinal rotation and fixation ("malrotation"). Pediatr Radiol. 2004;34(11):837-51.
84. van der Meer RW, Pattynama PM, van Strijen MJ, et al. Right ventricular dysfunction and pulmonary obstruction index at helical CT: prediction of clinical outcome during 3-month follow-up in patients with acute pulmonary embolism. Radiology. 2005;235(3):798-803.
85. Vaphiades MS. Imaging the neurovisual system. Ophthalmol Clin North Am. 2004;17(3):465-80.
86. Warach S, Kidwell CS. The redefinition of TIA: the uses and limitations of DWI in acute ischemic cerebrovascular syndromes. Neurology. 2004;62(3):359-60.
87. Wei SC, Ulmer S, Lev MH, et al. Value of coronal reformations in the CT evaluation of acute head trauma. Am J Neuroradiol. 2010;31(2):334-9.
88. Williams GJ, Hodson EH, Isaacs D, et al. Diagnosis and management of urinary tract infection in children. J Paediatr Child Health. 2012;48(4):296-301.
89. Zacharia TT, Nguyen DT. Subtle pathology detection with multidetector row coronal and sagittal CT reformations in acute head trauma. Emerg Radiol. 2010;17(2):97-102.

CHAPTER 91

Disaster and Mass Casualty Management in Emergency

Devendra Richhariya, TS Srinath Kumar, Tamorish Kole

INTRODUCTION

In India about 60% of land is vulnerable to earthquakes, 16% of land is vulnerable to drought, 12% of land is vulnerable to floods, 8% of land is vulnerable to cyclones, these calamities normally result in deaths, injuries, and property damage that cannot be managed through the routine procedures and resources of government **(Figs 1A to E)**. Emergency planning is an integral part of the overall loss control program. It is important for effective management of an accident or incident to minimize losses to people and property, both in and around the facility. Following steps are important to minimize the losses:
- The reliable and early detection of an emergency and careful planning
- The coordination along with efficient trained personnel
- Resources for handling emergencies
- Appropriate emergency response actions
- Effective notification and communication facilities
- Proper training of concerned personnel
- Regular mock drill or rehearsal
- Regular review and updation of plan.

DEFINITIONS

Disaster is defined as per Disaster Management Act, 2005:
"A catastrophe, mishap, calamity or grave occurrence in any area, arising from natural or man-made causes, or by accident or negligence which results in substantial loss of life or human suffering or damage to, and destruction of property, or damage to, or degradation of environment and is of such a nature or magnitude as to be beyond the coping capacity of the community of the affected area".

Disaster is defined as any occurrence that causes damage, economic disruption, loss of human life, and deterioration in health and health services on a scale sufficient to warrant an extraordinary response from outside the affected area or community.

A serious disruption of the functioning of a community or a society causing widespread human, material, or environmental losses which exceed the ability of the affected community or society to cope using its own resources (United Nations Office for Disaster Risk Reduction).

EXAMPLES OF DISASTERS

Various examples of disasters are as follows:
- Road traffic accidents
- Air crash
- Bullet and blast injuries
- Collapse of a building
- Fire
- Communal riots
- Terrorist attacks
- Floods
- Earthquakes
- Tsunami
- Epidemics
- Nuclear/biological/chemical warfare.

CLASSIFICATION OF DISASTERS

Disasters can be classified as man-made and natural **(Table 1)**.

Various examples of natural disasters have been shown in **Figure 2**.

TERMINOLOGY RELATED TO DISASTER

- *Hazard*: A potentially damaging physical event, phenomenon, and/or human activity, which may cause the loss of life or injury, property damage, social and economic disruption or environmental degradation.

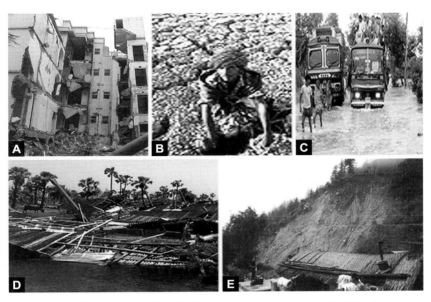

Figs 1A to E Hazard vulnerability in India. (A) 60% of area prone for earthquake; (B) 16% of area prone for drought; (C) 12% of area is prone for floods; (D) 8% of area prone for cyclone; (E) 3% of area prone for landslides

Table 1 Classification of disasters	
Man-made disaster	*Natural disaster*
• *Civil disturbances*: Riots, explosion, and demonstrations • *Warfare*: Conventional warfare (bombardment, blockage, and siege) • *Nonconventional warfare*: Nuclear, biological and chemical warfare (NBC), terrorism • *Refugees*: Forced movement of large number of people usually across frontiers • *Accidents*: Transportation calamities (land, air, and sea), collapse of building, dams, and other structures, mine disasters, fire, poison gas panic • *Technological failures*: Nuclear power station, leak at a chemical plant, break down of a public sanitation system	• *Meteorological*: Storms (cyclones, hailstorms, hurricanes, typhoons, and snow storms) • Cold spells, heat, waves, droughts • *Topographical disasters*: Avalanches, landslides, and floods • *Geological disasters*: Earthquakes, tsunamis, volcanic eruptions • *Biological disasters*: Insect swarms (locust) and epidemics of communicable diseases

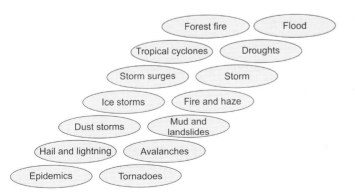

Fig. 2 Various examples of natural disasters

- *Vulnerability*: It is a condition or sets of conditions that reduces people's ability to prepare for, withstand or respond to a hazard.
- *Capacity*: Those positive condition or abilities which increase a community's ability to deal with hazards.
- *Risk*: The probability that a community's structure or geographic area is to be damaged or disrupted by the impact of a particular hazard, on account of their nature, construction, and proximity to a hazardous area.

FACTORS CONTRIBUTING TO DISASTER

Various factors contributing to disaster are:
- The scale of hazard is too big
- Vulnerabilities are too great

- Capacity is insufficient
- The risk is too high, so emergencies cannot be managed locally, and the communities may not be able to handle the situation.

> Hazard + vulnerability = Increase in disaster risk
> Increase in capacity = Decrease in disaster risk

DISASTER MANAGEMENT CYCLE

Disaster management cycle is shown in **Flow chart 1**. The terms used to represent disaster management cycle include:
- *Response*: Actions taken immediately following the impact of a disaster when exceptional measures are required to meet the basic needs of the survivors.
- *Relief*: Measures that are required in search and rescue of survivors, as well as to meet the basic needs for shelter, water, food, and healthcare.
- *Recovery*: The process undertaken by a disaster-affected community to fully restore itself to predisaster level of functioning.
- *Rehabilitation*: Actions taken in the aftermath of a disaster to:
  - Assist victims to repair their dwellings
  - Reestablish essential services
  - Revive key economic and social activities.
- *Reconstruction*: Permanent measures to repair or replace damaged dwellings and infrastructure and to set the economy back on course.
- *Development*: Sustained efforts intended to improve or maintain the social and economic well-being of a community.
- *Prevention*: Measures taken to avert a disaster from occurring, if possible (to impede a hazard so that it does not have any harmful effects).
- *Mitigation*: Measures taken prior to the impact of a disaster to minimize its effects (sometimes referred to as structural and nonstructural measures). "Structural and nonstructural measures undertaken to limit the adverse impact of natural hazards, environmental degradation, and technological hazards" are:
  - Structural measures refer to any physical construction to reduce or avoid possible impacts of hazards, which include engineering measures and construction of hazard-resistant and protective structures and infrastructure, like construction, hazard-resistant house construction, planting mangroves, drainage channels, water conservation measures, etc.
  - Nonstructural measures refer to policies, awareness, knowledge development, public commitment, and methods and operating practices, including participatory mechanisms and the provision of information, which can reduce risk and related impacts.
- *Preparedness*: Measures taken in anticipation of a disaster to ensure that appropriate and effective actions are taken in the aftermath.

DISASTER MANAGEMENT

It is a collective term encompassing all aspects of planning for preparing and responding to disasters. It refers to the management of the consequences of disasters. Fundamental of disaster management is to do the greatest possible good for possibly greatest number of affected people. Emergencies and disasters can strike without warning. Each individual with a disability has unique circumstances and needs. There will likely be problems with drinking water, electricity, and other utilities. When large-scale disasters strike, most assistance is provided by one citizen to another. Emergency medical services (EMS), police, and fire resources will not be able to reach everyone right away. In the last few years, we have seen that disaster also simultaneously destroys health facilities, besides other infrastructures. A comprehensive disaster preparedness strategy is required and its components are following:
- Hazard, risk, and vulnerability assessments
- Response mechanisms and strategies
- Preparedness plans
- Coordination
- Information management
- Early warning systems
- Resource mobilization
- Public education, training, and rehearsals
- Community-based disaster preparedness.

National disaster management structure approved by Government of India is shown in **Flow chart 2**.

Hospital Disaster Management Committee

Hospital disaster management committee includes:
- Chairman
- Medical Superintendent
- Additional Superintendent or DMS
- Heads of Departments like Emergency, Surgery, Orthopedics, Medicine, Laboratory, and Radiology
- Heads of Operation Theater, Security, Store/logistics in-Charge
- Blood Bank Officer

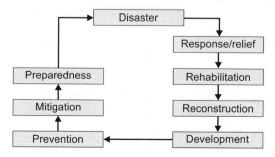

Flow chart 1 Disaster management cycle

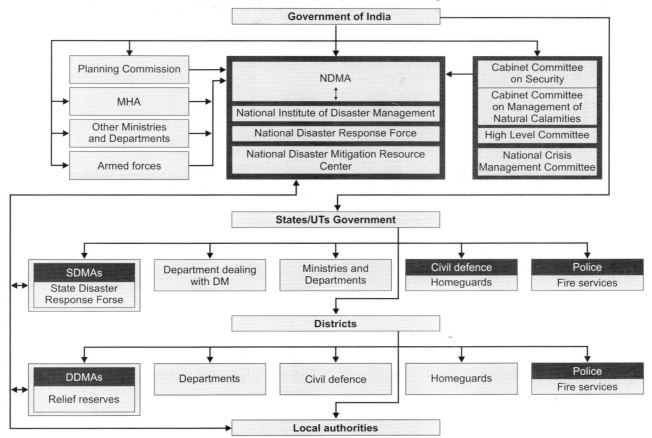

Flow chart 2 Pictorial representation of National Disaster Management Structure

- Nursing Superintendent
- Ambulance.

INCIDENT COMMAND SYSTEM

Incident command system (ICS) is an emergency management system for hospitals that helps to unify responding agencies and personnel. Medical disaster can quickly lead to chaos and confusion and ICS provides medical facilities with an organized management structure that promotes immediate, focused direction of activities during a disaster and allows for prompt resumption of normal operations. Various component of the ICS are shown in **Flow chart 3**.

Advantages of Incident Command System

- A logical, predictable management structure
- Clearly defined roles and responsibilities
- Distribution of work lessens liability
- Prioritization of duties
- Facilitation of communication via common language
- Thorough documentation of actions taken
- Flexibility and adaptability

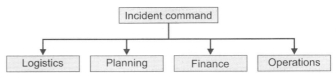

Flow chart 3 Incident command system

- Position-driven system not person-driven
- Promotes financial recovery.

Responsibilities of Incident Command System (Table 2)

- Create an Emergency Operations Center
- Prepare Department of Kits
- Plan how and when to activate ICS
- Implementation and Training.

Roles of Incident Commander

Roles of incident commander are as follows:
- Administration
- Planning

Table 2 Overall responsibilities of incident command system

Logistic (provide support)	Planning (prepare action plan)	Finance (cost accounting and procurement)	Operations (direct tactical action)
Responsible for acquisition and maintenance of facilities, services, personnel equipment, and materials	• Collect, analyze, display information • Prepare incident action plan • Maintain situation and resource status • Maintain incident documentation • Prepare demobilization • Promote continuity of operations	• Monitors incident costs • Maintains financial records • Administers procurement contracts	Carry out the medical objective to the best of their ability

Table 3 Important command officers and their roles

Public Information Officer	Safety Officer	Liaison Officer
Provide information to the news media, serves as the one central point for information dissemination	Monitors the facility and anticipates, detects, and corrects unsafe situations	Functions as incident contact person for representatives from other assisting and cooperating agencies

- Logistic
- Operation
- Public information
- Safety
- Liaison.

Important Command Staff

Trained staff are required to carry out the various responsibilities of incident command. Incident command staff and their roles are shown in **Table 3**.

Establishing the Emergency Operation Center

Emergency operation center (EOC) serves as central command post during an emergency, generally established outside the emergency department. It should be large enough for key people and support staff. It should be located in a safe area, near washrooms, food service, etc.

How to Activate and When to Activate Incident Command System?

- Determine who will activate the ICS
- Notification to hospital personnel
- Briefing to all core members regarding assignments and clear immediate direction
- Activation of ICS should be announced using standardized codes, such as "Disaster Code" or "Code Triage".

Creating the Additional Capacity for Disaster

- Utilize all available beds
- *Additional bed capacity*: Vacant beds, day care beds, preoperative beds, trolley beds, folding beds, floor beds
- Patient can be discharged for whom elective surgery is planned
- Patients requiring domiciliary/OPD care
- Utility areas (side rooms, galleries, and seminar rooms, etc.) can also be used.

Logistic Support System for Emergency Operation Center

There should be separate stock for routine day-to-day emergencies and for disaster. Inventory should include:
- All essential medicines
- Dressing materials
- Splints
- Disinfectants
- Vaccines
- Emergency trays
- Surgical supplies
- Resuscitation room
- Resuscitation kit
- Electrocardiogram, defibrillator
- Ventilators
- Suction machine
- Oxygen
- Endotracheal (ET) tubes
- Stretchers
- Wheel chairs
- Linen, blankets, etc.

Challenges during Disaster Management

Different challenges faced during disaster management are as follows:
- Additional bed space
- Biological warfare or chemical warfare

- Temporary isolation ward
- Barrier nursing, universal precaution
- Additional OT tables
- Cancel routine or elective surgery
- Monitor consumption of essential drugs and supplies
- Ensure adequate supply
- Documentation
- MLCs (medicolegal cases)
- Crowd management
- Media management
- Proper identification, tagging documentation of dead
- Creating temporary morgue
- Maintaining the essential services: water, power supply, emergency lights, waiting area, etc.

MASS CASUALTY

When an unexpectedly large number of injured or ill persons need emergency medical care at the same time is mass casualty. The aim in a mass casualty situation is to "Do the best for the most, not Everything for Everyone" and "doing the best for the most".

Goal: To apply trauma triage principles in multiple patient scenarios.

The grading of the mass casualty is done as follows:
- *Grade I*: 10–15 victims
- *Grade II*: 16–30 victims
- *Grade III*: More than 30 victims.

Triage

"Triage" is French word meaning "to sort or select" (sorting of differing grades of wool and later coffee beans).
- Napoleon's surgeon Baron Larrey applied the principle to the assessment and treatment of the injured
- To sort into categories based on an assessment of:
  - *A B C D E's in vitals*: The "ABCDE" of primary survey is, in essence, to identify the life-threatening conditions and institution of life-preserving therapies by priority based on their injuries, vital signs, and injury mechanisms **(Box 1)**.

Disaster Triage

Objective of disaster triaging is focused on the critically ill patients saving the maximum number of lives with limited medical resources and doctors.

Box 1 ABCDE approach in triage

- Airway maintenance with cervical spine control
- Breathing and ventilation
- Circulation/hemorrhage control
- Disability/neurological status
- Exposure/environmental control

Simple Triage and Rapid Transport System (START) (Flow chart 4)

- *Principle*: Tag—Treat—Transfer....
- *The objective is to*: Locate, identify and tag priority-one patients who require immediate care and transportation
- "*Triage tags*" applied to patients, make one's task of sorting much easier, are of four different colors—red, yellow, green, and black. Triage tag: fold to show appropriate color on outside
- Priority patients are those with a good chance of good survival
- *START*: Four categories **(Fig. 3)**
  - *Immediate*: Life threatening, requires immediate care
  - *Delayed*: Urgent care, but can delay for 1 hour
  - *Minor*: "Walking wounded", can delay for 3 hours
  - *Deceased*: Mortally wounded, no care required
- START system focuses on three areas:
  - Respirations
  - Pulse rate and quality
  - Mental status
- *Goal*: Correction of life-threatening condition—airway or breathing problem and profuse bleeding
- To summarize—keep it simple.

Mass Casualty Triaging Rescue

Similar to traffic signal light color
- *Red*: Red bleeder, polytrauma, cannot move as in red-light signal of traffic
- *Yellow*: Urgent
- *Green*: Walking wounded
- *Black*: Brought dead.

Percentage of different categories of patients in mass casualty:
- *Red*: 1–5%
- *Yellow*: 5–10%
- *Green*: 80%
- *Black*: 1–5%.

How to identify so many unknowns?
- Name
- Mass unique health identification number (UHID) from EHIS—X series
- *Marks of identification*: Tattoo, scar, etc.
- *Belongings*: Purse, clothes, driving license, identification card, etc.
- *Typical injuries*: Amputation.

Mass Casualty Incident

Situation may be one or combination of:
- Biological
- Nuclear
- Fire
- Chemical

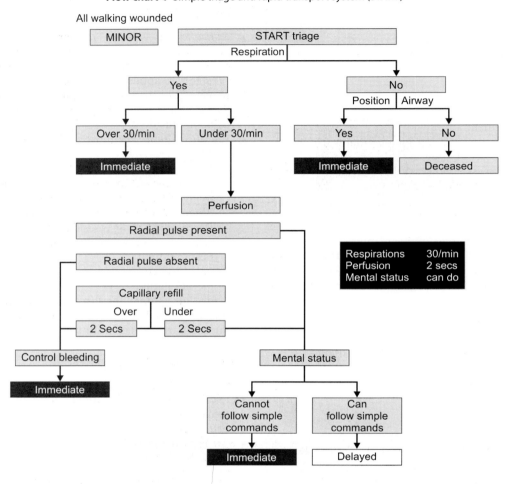

Flow chart 4 Simple triage and rapid transport system (START)

- Explosion or natural event
- Natural disaster with mass casualty incident.

Simulation Exercise for Emergency Department Staff

A simulation exercise of mass casualty management should be carried out preferably every 6 months for ED staff to test the every requirement of the drill. Various steps of the drill and debriefing is done and corrective action is taken if any gap is found. Various steps for simulation exercise for mass casualty management are discussed in **Table 4**.

Examples of Mass Casualties

Some examples of mass casualties are as follows:
- School bus accident in Jaipur (2013) killed 23 students
- Train collisions in Bangalore (2015) killed 100 people
- *Earthquake*: Multistory building collapse, e.g. in Nepal (2015)
- Stampede in Jagannath Puri Rath Yatra (2015)
- Fire in cinema hall in Uphar Mall, Delhi (1997)
- School bus drowning in river in Goa (2012)
- *Electrocution by lightening*: Rainy season in Vadodara (2013)
- Industrial hazard in Bhopal MIC gas disaster (1984)
- Mass Hooch tragedy, e.g. Ahmedabad (2009) by illicit liquor
- Floods during heavy rainfall, e.g. Chennai floods in 2015
- Midday meal poisoning in school in Bihar (2013).

EMERGENCY DEPARTMENT PREPAREDNESS FOR CHEMICAL AND RADIOLOGICAL DISASTER

Disasters like earthquake, landslide, road traffic accidents, hurricane, etc. are more common than chemical and radiological disaster but it is essential to have planning for chemical and radiological events because they have potential for major disruption to clinical care and to create hazardous consequences like chaos and confusion.

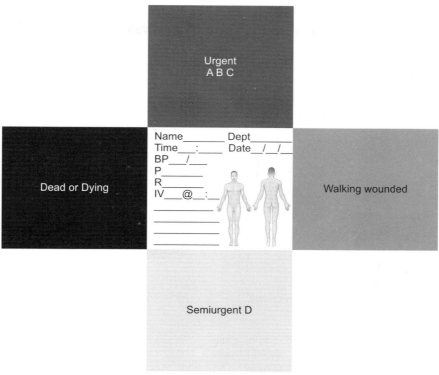

Fig. 3 Four categories of simple triage and rapid treatment

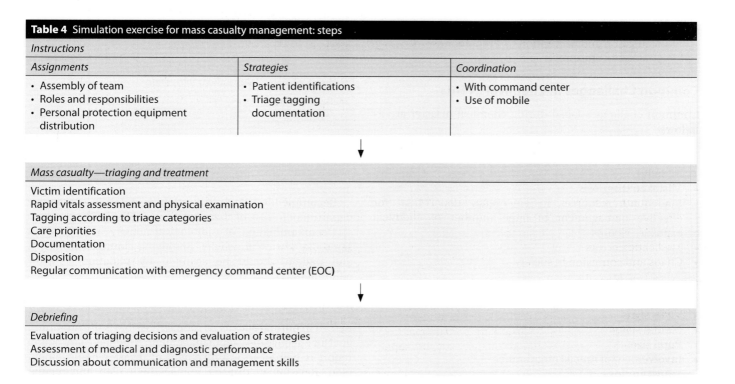

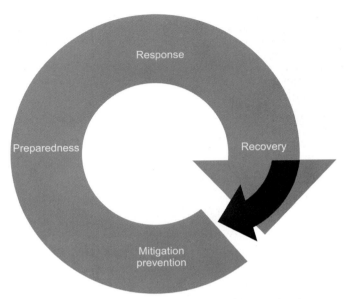

Fig. 4 Components for management of chemical and radiological disaster

Table 5 is showing various chemical and radiological agents can cause mass casualty. Hospital should have trained decontamination team area with shower and stoking of antidotes for toxicants within emergency department. Components for management of chemical and radiological disaster (disaster management cycle) are the same like any other disaster (already discussed earlier) **(Fig. 4)**.

Mitigation and prevention → Preparedness → Response → Recovery

Common Challenges in Chemical Events

Common challenges faced during chemical disaster are as follows:
- Failure to identify the offending agents for hours or days
- Medical team gives only supportive care (act blindly initially)
- Mistaken diagnosis
- Inadequate resources in emergency department for effective management of large number of chemical exposure victims
- Medication errors
- Chaos and confusion in society.

Offending chemical agents can be identified by following observations:
- Vitals signs
- Mental status
- Pupil size
- Involvement of mucus membranes
- Lungs findings
- *Skin examination*: Look for burn moisture color.

Table 5 Common offending agents in mass chemical and radiological exposures

Toxins	Common features	Examples
Irritant gases	Irritation of eye, ear, nose, and throat, wheezing breathlessness, chest pain, and tightness	Ammonia, chlorine, nitrogen dioxide, phosgene
Chemical burns	Painful skin, mucous membrane irritation	Hydrochloric acid
Organophosphate (cholinergic) Insecticide	Pinpoint pupil, eye pain, breathlessness, wheezing, drooling of saliva, vomiting, diarrhea, seizure, coma	Organophosphate, carbamate insecticides
Solvent	Headache, nausea, confusion, syncope	Pain, thinners, lubricants, methylene chloride
Metabolic poisoning	Unconsciousness, hypotension, cardiac arrest	Cyanide hydrogen sulfide
Radioactive material	Vomiting, delayed-onset skin manifestations	

Table 6 Recommended stock of antidotes in emergency department

Atropine 1 mg/mL	16 mg
Dextrose 50%	100 mL
Diazepam 5 mg/mL	40 mg
Hydroxocobalamin plus sodium thiosulfate	4 kits
Methylene blue	8 units
Naloxone 1 mg/mL	16 mg
Pralidoxime 1 g vial	10 mg
Prussian blue 500 mg capsules	12 capsules

Recommended stock of antidote is stored in emergency department in case of chemical disaster **(Table 6)**.

Decontamination of radiological activity is to be dealt same like chemical activity. Removing clothes, showering, and patient should be scanned by radiation detector equipment.

SUMMARY

Return to normal activity as soon as possible is the important goal for effective disaster management. A detailed after action report is helpful in improvement of disaster management plan. Revision of disaster management plan and regular mock drills should be conducted.

BIBLIOGRAPHY

1. American College of Emergency. Guidelines for Crisis Standards of Care during Disasters in 2013, by American College of Emergency Physicians.
2. Ciottone GR, Biddinger PD, Darling RG, et al. Ciottone's Disaster Medicine, 2nd edition. Amsterdam, Netherlands: Elsevier Publications; 2015.
3. Indian gazette notification. (2015). Indian gazette notification 2015, Ministry of Road Transport and Highways (MoRTH) notified the "Good Samaritan" guidelines. [online] egazette website. Available from *egazette.nic.in/WriteReadData*/2015/164095.pdf [Accessed February, 2017].
4. Marx J, Hockberger R, Walls R. Rosen's Emergency Medicine Concepts and Clinical Practice, 8th edition. Philadelphia: Saunders; 2013.
5. National Disaster Management Authority. National Disaster Management Authority (NDMA) guidelines under DM act 2005. [online] NDMA website. Available from *www.ndma.gov.in/en/disaster.html* [Accessed February, 2017].
6. Partridge RA, Proano L, Marcozzi D, et al. Oxford American Handbook of Disaster Medicine, 1st edition. Oxford, UK: Oxford University Press; 2012.

Section 15

Toxicology

- **Assessment and Management of Poisoning**
  VV Pillay

- **Organophosphate and Carbamate Insecticides Poisoning**
  VV Pillay

- **Aluminum Phosphide Poisoning**
  Vivekanshu Verma, Devendra Richhariya

CHAPTER 92

Assessment and Management of Poisoning

VV Pillay

DIAGNOSTIC CONSIDERATIONS

A poisoning case can present to a doctor or hospital in any one of a number of ways. Broadly, there are four types of presentation:
1. *Fulminant*: Produced by a massive dose. Death occurs very rapidly, sometimes without preceding symptoms, the patient appearing to collapse suddenly.
2. *Acute*: Produced by a single dose or several small doses taken in a short period. Onset of symptoms is abrupt.
3. *Chronic*: Produced by small doses taken over a long period. Onset is insidious.
4. *Subacute*: Characterized by a mixture of features of acute and chronic poisoning.

The majority of poisoned patients presenting to the casualty (emergency) department are victims of acute exposure. Most of them are usually coherent enough to tell the doctor what the problem is, and indeed what they have taken or been exposed to. However, in an unconscious or uncooperative patient the diagnosis will have to be made on the basis of circumstantial or third-party evidence. It is important to interrogate the persons accompanying the patient (relatives, friends, ambulance personnel, etc.) and to contact his or her family doctor as soon as possible. In spite of all this, unfortunately, in a significant proportion of cases the diagnosis remains uncertain. This is because unlike in other clinical conditions arising out of natural disease, there are only a very few syndromes (*toxidromes*)* characterized by specific signs and symptoms **(Box 1)**. In most cases, the poisoned patient presents with one or more of the following nonspecific features:
- Impairment of consciousness
- Respiratory or cardiovascular depression
- Dehydration due to vomiting or diarrhea
- Hypothermia
- Convulsions
- Cardiac arrhythmias.

However, there are some valuable clues afforded on detailed clinical examination which can help narrow down the differential diagnosis. Most of these will be dealt with in a subsequent section (general management), but a few are discussed here for the sake of convenience.
- *Ocular clues*: Several drugs or poisons affect the pupils of the eyes producing either miosis or mydriasis. A few produce nystagmus. These have been laid out in **Table 1**. Normally, both the pupils are equal in size, 3–4 mm under typical conditions, round, and react directly as well as consensually to increased light intensity by constriction. Pupillary constriction also occurs as part of the near reflex when a person focuses on near objects. All these functions result from the balance between cholinergic innervation of the iris sphincter (constrictor) by the oculomotor nerve, and sympathetic innervation of the radial muscle of the iris (dilator). Mydriasis can occur due to increased sympathetic stimulation by endogenous catecholamines or from systemic or ocular exposures to sympathomimetic drugs. Mydriasis can also result from inhibition of cholinergic-mediated pupillary constriction. Because pupillary constriction (miosis) in response to light is a major determinant of pupil size, blindness from ocular, retinal, or optic nerve disorders also leads to mydriasis. Miosis can result from increased cholinergic stimulation, or inhibition of sympathetic dilation. Other ocular manifestations along with their respective causes are mentioned in **Table 2**.

---

*Some toxicologists prefer to restrict the term "toxidrome" to a group of signs and symptoms that is consistently encountered in relation to a specific toxin, for e.g., paracetamol, salicylates, methanol, carbon monoxide, etc.

Box 1 Toxidromes (toxic syndromes)

Anticholinergic syndrome
Causes: Antihistamines, antiparkinsonian drugs, atropine, scopolamine, amantadine, antipsychotic drugs, antidepressants, antispasmodics, skeletal muscle relaxants, many plants (especially *Datura*), and fungi (e.g. *Amanita muscaria*).
Symptomatology: Delirium, tachycardia, dry hot skin, mydriasis, myoclonus, urinary retention, decreased bowel sounds, convulsions, and arrhythmias

Cholinergic syndrome
Causes: Organophosphates, carbamates, parasympathomimetic drugs, and some mushrooms
Symptomatology: Confusion, CNS depression, salivation, lacrimation, urinary and fecal incontinence, vomiting, sweating, fasciculations, seizures, miosis, pulmonary edema, and tachycardia/bradycardia

Sympathomimetic syndrome
Causes: Cocaine, amphetamines, upper respiratory decongestants (phenylpropanolamine, ephedrine, and pseudoephedrine).
Symptomatology: Paranoia, delusions, tachycardia, hypertension, hyperpyrexia, sweating, mydriasis, seizures, and arrhythmias.

Sedative-hypnotic syndrome
Causes: Opiates, barbiturates, benzodiazepines, ethanol, methaqualone, meprobamate, ethchlorvynol, glutethimide, and clonidine
Symptomatology: Miosis, hypotension, bradycardia, hypothermia, CNS depression, hyporeflexia, coma, and convulsions (rarely)

Opioid syndrome
Causes: Morphine, codeine, pethidine (meperidine), pentazocine, buprenorphine, propoxyphene, tramadol, butorphanol, dextromethorphan, diphenoxylate, loperamide, heroin, and fentanyl
Symptomatology: Miosis, hypotension, bradycardia, bradypnea, hypothermia, CNS depression, hyporeflexia, decreased peristalsis, mild diaphoresis, urinary retention (occasionally) coma, and convulsions (rarely)

Salicylate syndrome
Causes: Salicylic acid, methyl salicylate, homosalate (homomenthyl salicylate), trolamine salicylate, acetyl salicylic acid, sodium salicylate, sodium aminosalicylate, bismuth subsalicylate, mesalamine (5-aminosalicylic acid), olsalazine (sodium azodisalicylate), sulfasalazine (salicylazosulfapyridine), diflunisal, and benorylate (4-acetamidophenyl-o-acetylsalicylate)
Symptomatology: Tachycardia, tachypnea, hyperthermia, sweating, delirium, decreased peristalsis, tinnitus, and convulsions

Hallucinogen syndrome
Causes: LSD (lysergic acid diethylamide), phencyclidine, ketamine, designer drugs: MDA (*adam*), MDEA (*eve*), MDMA (*ecstasy*), α-methyl fentanyl, tryptamines (dimethyl tryptamine, psilocin, psilocybin), mescaline, and cannabinoid
Symptomatology: Tachycardia, hypertension, hyperthermia, agitation, psychotic behavior, miosis or mydriasis, and hallucinations

Serotonin syndrome
Causes: Drugs that inhibit serotonin breakdown (nonselective MAOIs, e.g. phenelzine, moclobemide, clorgyline, isocarboxazid), drugs that block serotonin reuptake (SSRIs, e.g. fluoxetine, citalopram, paroxetine, fluvoxamine, and sertraline; as well as cocaine, dextromethorphan, pethidine, pentazocine, clomipramine, trazodone, and venlafaxine), serotonin precursors or agonists (LSD, tryptophan), drugs that enhance serotonin release (cocaine, amphetamines, lithium, mirtazapine, and buspirone)
Symptomatology: Tachycardia, hypertension, hyperthermia, tachypnea, agitation, confusion, mydriasis, sweating, flushed skin and mucosa, tremor, myoclonus, hyperreflexia, rigidity, and trismus

Ethanol withdrawal syndrome
Cause: Withdrawal reaction in an alcoholic
Symptomatology: Tachycardia, hypertension, hyperthermia, tachypnea, agitation, confusion, disorientation, mydriasis, sweating, diarrhea, tremor, and convulsions

Opioid withdrawal syndrome
Cause: Withdrawal reaction in an opiate/opioid addict
Symptomatology: Tachycardia, hypertension, fever, anxiety, mydriasis, sweating, vomiting, diarrhea, rhinorrhea, and piloerection

Abbreviations: CNS, central nervous system; MDA, methylenedioxyamphetamine; MDEA, methylenedioxyethamphetamine; MDMA, methylenedioxymethamphetamine; SSRIs, selective serotonin reuptake inhibitors.

- *Olfactory clues*: Some poisons have distinctive odors which may be perceived in the vicinity of a poisoned patient, especially in the breath. Some important examples are mentioned in **Table 3**.
- *Dermal clues*: Some poisons have characteristic dermal manifestations in acute toxicity, while certain others demonstrate skin signs on chronic exposure **(Table 4)**. Unexpected dermal manifestations can occur from ingestion of chemicals such as kerosene.[1] Therapeutic drugs can produce irritant dermatitis even in nontoxic doses, e.g. antibiotics, phenothiazines, sulfonamides, nonsteroidal anti-inflammatory drugs (NSAIDs), etc.
- *Oral clues*: Careful examination of the mouth can afford valuable information about the etiology of poisoning in some cases **(Table 5)**.

Table 1 Drugs or poisons producing pupillary changes

Miosis	Mydriasis	Nystagmus
Barbiturates	Alcohol (constricted in coma)	Alcohol
Benzodiazepines	Amphetamines	Barbiturates
Caffeine	Antihistamines	Carbamazepine
Carbamates	Carbon monoxide	Phencyclidine
Carbolic acid (phenol)	Cocaine	Phenytoin
Clonidine	Cyanide	
Methyldopa	*Datura* (atropine)	
Nicotine	Ephedrine	
Opiates		
Organophosphates		
Parasympathomimetics		

Table 2 Toxic ophthalmological manifestations

Feature	Cause
Diplopia	Barbiturates, cannabis, ethanol, opiates, phenytoin, tetracycline, and vitamin A
Blurred vision	Alcohol, anticholinergics, botulism, ethanol, lithium, MAOIs, and methanol
Altered color perception	Cannabis, CO, digitalis, hydrocarbons, ibuprofen, and nalidixic acid
Corneal deposits	Chloroquine, vitamin D
Oculogyric crisis	Phenothiazines, butyrophenones, and metoclopramide
Optic neuritis	Chloroquine, digitalis, disulfiram, ergot, heavy metals, methanol, penicillamine, and quinine

Abbreviation: MAIOs, monoamine oxidase inhibitors.

Table 3 Diagnostic odors

Odor	Substance
Acetone (apple-like)	Chloroform, ethanol, isopropanol, and lacquer
Acrid (pear-like)	Chloral hydrate, paraldehyde
Bitter almond	Cyanide
Burnt rope	Marijuana (Cannabis)
Coal gas	Carbon monoxide (CO)
Disinfectant (hospital odor)	Carbolic acid, creosote
Garlicky	Arsenic, dimethyl sulfoxide, organophosphates, phosphorus, selenium, tellurium, and thallium
Mothballs	Camphor, naphthalene
Musty (fishy)	Aluminum phosphide, zinc phosphide
Rotten egg	Carbon disulfide, disulfiram, hydrogen sulfide, mercaptans, and N-acetylcysteine
Shoe polish	Nitrobenzene
Vinegar	Acetic acid
Wintergreen	Methyl salicylate

Table 4 Dermal manifestations of poisoning

Acute		Chronic	
Poison/Drug	Feature	Poison/Drug	Feature
Datura, atropine	Dry, hot skin	Heroin, barbiturates, morphine, and phencyclidine	Needle marks
Organophosphates, salicylates, arsenic, LSD, and dinitrophenol	Profuse sweating	Bromides, iodides, coal tar products, and phenytoin	Acne, brown color
Carbon monoxide(CO)	Cherry pink color	Arsenic	Rain drop pigmentation, hyperkeratosis, and exfoliative dermatitis
Cyanide	Brick-red color	Chlorinated hydrocarbons	Eczematous dermatitis
Barbiturates, CO, imipramine, methadone, and nitrazepam	Blisters	Chloroquine, busulfan, clofazimine, phenothiazines, and phenytoin	Dark pigmentation
Warfarin	Petechiae and purpuric spots	Bromides, iodides, oral contraceptives, penicillin, salicylates, and tetracycline	Erythema nodosum
Clonidine, ergot, niacin, sympathomimetics, and theophylline	Flushing		

Abbreviation: LSD, lysergic acid diethylamide.

Table 5 Drug-induced oral manifestations

Feature	Drug/Poison
Glossitis	Trimethoprim-sulfamethoxazole, diclofenac, naproxen, metronidazole, amoxicillin, erythromycin, and piroxicam
Stomatitis	Cytotoxic drugs, penicillamine, gold salts, and gentian violet dye
Sialadenitis	Phenylbutazone, isoproterenol, nitrofurantoin, and iodine
Parotitis	Methyldopa, clonidine, phenyl and oxyphenbutazone, and thioridazine
Gingival hyperplasia	Phenytoin, sodium valproate, phenobarbitone, nifedipine, diltiazem, and verapamil
Pigmentation	Cisplatin, oral contraceptives, and antimalarials
Dental discoloration	Fluorides, tetracycline, chlorhexidine, and iron tonic syrups
Dental caries	Cough and vitamin syrups, antibiotic suspensions
Xerostomia	Antipsychotics, tricyclics, antihistamines, anticholinergics, anticonvulsants, narcotics, diuretics, and centrally-acting antihypertensives
Sialorrhea	Parasympathomimetics, iodides

GENERAL MANAGEMENT OF POISONING

- *Stabilization*: The initial survey should always be directed at the assessment and correction of life-threatening problems, if present. Attention must be paid to the airway, breathing, circulation, and depression of the central nervous system (CNS) (the *ABCD* of resuscitation).
- *Evaluation*: If the patient is not in crisis, i.e. he is alert with normal speech and pulse; proceed to a complete, thorough, and systematic examination. As far as treatment is concerned, the emphasis should be on basic supportive measures.
- *Decontamination*: This is with reference to skin or eye decontamination, gut evacuation and administration of activated charcoal.
- *Poison elimination*: Depending on the situation, this can be accomplished by diuresis, peritoneal dialysis, hemodialysis, hemoperfusion, etc.
- *Antidote administration*: Unfortunately, antidotes are available for less than 5% of poisoning.[2]
- *Nursing and psychiatric care*: General nursing care is especially important in comatose patients and those who have been incapacitated by the poison. Since some cases of poisoning leave behind persisting sequelae, adequate follow-up for a period of time may be necessary. Psychiatric intervention is frequently essential in suicidal overdose.
- *Special precautions in poisoned pregnant patient*: A not too frequent conundrum facing a physician is how to manage

a poisoned or overdosed pregnant patient. It is important that some guidelines are kept in mind.

STABILIZATION

Assessment

Airway and Breathing

Symptoms of airway obstruction include dyspnea, air hunger, and hoarseness. Signs comprise of stridor, intercostal and substernal retractions, cyanosis, sweating, and tachypnea.

Normal oxygen delivery requires adequate hemoglobin oxygen saturation, adequate hemoglobin levels, normal oxygen unloading mechanisms, and an adequate cardiac output. Increasing metabolic acidosis in the presence of a normal partial pressure of arterial oxygen (PaO_2) suggests a toxin or condition that either decreases oxygen carrying capacity (e.g. CO, methemoglobinemia), or reduces tissue oxygen (e.g. cyanide, hydrogen sulfide).

The immediate need for assisted ventilation has to be assessed clinically, but the efficiency of ventilation can only be gauged by measuring the blood gases. Retention of carbon dioxide [partial pressure of arterial carbon dioxide ($PaCO_2$) >45 mm Hg or 6 Kpa], and hypoxia (PaO_2 <70 mm Hg or 9.3 Kpa) inspite of oxygen being given by a face mask are indications for assisted ventilation.

A simple method of assessing respiratory status consists of determining the minute volume by a Wright respirometer **(Fig. 1)**. If this is more than 4 L/min, there is no need for ventilation. However, it must be borne in mind that ventilatory function can fluctuate and may deteriorate suddenly. **Table 6** lists some substances which are known to cause respiratory depression. Some drugs stimulate the respiratory center: amphetamines, atropine, cocaine, and salicylates. Some drugs are associated with noncardiogenic pulmonary edema, characterized by severe hypoxemia,

Table 6 Toxic respiratory depression

Failure of respiratory center	Failure of respiratory muscles
Antidepressants	Neuromuscular blocking agents
Antipsychotics	Nicotine
Ethanol	Organophosphates
Opiates	Shellfish poisoning
Sedatives	Snake bite (Cobra)
	Strychnine

Table 7 Agents causing noncardiogenic pulmonary edema

Amphetamines	Nonsteroidal anti-inflammatory drugs
Anticoagulants	Opiates (especially heroin)
Aspirated oil, talc	Oxygen toxicity
Beta-blockers	Radiation
Calcium channel blockers	Salicylates
Carbon monoxide	Sulfonamides
Cocaine	Thiazide diuretics
Cytotoxic and immunosuppressive drugs	Tricyclic antidepressants
Irritant gases	

bilateral infiltrates on chest X-ray, and normal pulmonary capillary wedge pressure **(Table 7)**.[3]

Some drugs cause or exacerbate asthma. The most important among them include NSAIDs, antibiotics like penicillins, cephalosporins, tetracycline, and nitrofurantoin, cholinergic drugs, chemotherapeutic drugs, and some diuretics.

Circulation

Several drugs produce changes in pulse rate and blood pressure **(Table 8)**, while others induce cardiac arrhythmias and heart block **(Table 9)**.

Depression of Central Nervous System

This is generally defined as an unarousable lack of awareness with a rating of less than 8 on the *Glasgow Coma Scale* (GCS; Appendix 1). However, the European Association of Poison Centres and Clinical Toxicologists have the opinion that this scale while being very useful for trauma patients is inappropriate for acute poisoning. For those clinicians accustomed to applying the GCS to all patients with altered mental status, assigning a score to the overdosed or poisoned patient may provide a useful measure for assessing changes in neurologic status, but in this situation, the GCS should never be used for prognostic purposes, because complete

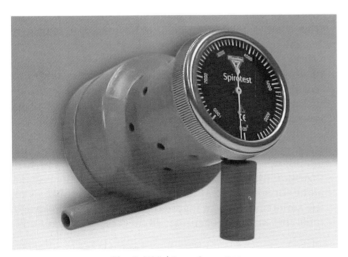

Fig. 1 Wright respirometer

Table 8 Drugs associated with disturbances in pulse rate and blood pressure

Tachycardia and normotension	Tachycardia and hypotension	Tachycardia and hypertension	Bradycardia and hypotension	Bradycardia and hypertension
Antihistamines, caffeine, cannabis, lomotil (atropine and diphenoxylate), thyroxine	Carbon monoxide, cyanide, phenothiazines, and theophylline	Amphetamines, cocaine, phencyclidine, phenylpropanolamine	Clonidine, levodopa, MAOIs, organophosphates, opiates, tricyclic antidepressants	Phenylpropanolamine

Abbreviations: MAOIs, monoamine oxidase inhibitors

Table 9 Drug or toxin-induced arrhythmias

Sinus bradycardia or Atrioventricular block	Sinus tachycardia
Alpha-adrenergic drugs, beta-blockers, carbamates, cardiac glycosides, organophosphates, tricyclic antidepressants	Amphetamines, anticholinergics, antihistamines, carbon monoxide, cocaine, phencyclidine, phenothiazines, theophylline, tricyclic antidepressants

recovery from properly managed toxic-metabolic coma despite a low GCS is the rule rather than the exception.

Several other scales have been proposed, including *Reaction Level Scale, Comprehensive Level of Consciousness Scale (CLOCS), Coma Recovery Scale, Innsbruck Coma Scale, Reed's Classification,* etc. but the predictive value of all these scales remains to be ascertained.[4] A practical guide that can be easily applied and is quite reliable is mentioned in **Table 10**, which also has the additional advantage that it takes into account not only CNS depressants producing true coma, but also CNS stimulants which produce coma only in the last stage.

There are numerous causes for coma of which one of the most important is acute poisoning. A number of substances can induce coma **(Table 11)**, and it will require a great deal of astuteness and expertise to pinpoint the poison. Before proceeding to an elaborate exercise in diagnosis however, it may be desirable to first ascertain for sure that the patient is really comatose and not just pretending (*psychogenic or hysterical coma*). This is often encountered in cases of "*suicide gesture*" in contrast to "*attempted suicide*". The former is an attention drawing gambit, where there is no real intention of ending one's life. The telltale fluttering eyelids, the patient who is half-walked, half-dragged in by relatives, an elaborate suicide note, a phone call to a friend or relative informing them of the act, pill bottles strewn about, all may point to such a suicide gesture. In addition, the signs and symptoms manifested by the patient usually are out of proportion to the ingestion itself.

So the question is, how does the doctor humanely determine whether the coma is true or fake? Several methods have been recommended of which the following constitute barbaric acts and must never be employed:
- Pinching nipples or genitals, or repeatedly pinching any part of the body
- Slapping the face hard, repeatedly
- Cotton pledgets or sterile applicator tips soaked with ammonia solution being inserted into the nostrils.*

Instead, the following steps are recommended:
- Perform a quick physical examination with particular attention to the breathing, vital signs, and the gag reflex. If these are normal, the coma is almost certainly psychogenic. Another indication is a tightly clenched jaw when attempts are made to open the mouth. However, first rule out seizure disorders.
- A useful technique is to lift the patient's hand directly above his face and letting it drop. A psychogenic etiology is almost a certainty if the hand falls gently to his side, rather than obeying the law of gravity and landing on the face. Pinching the shoulder may also be tried, but must not be repeated more than twice. Some clinicians advocate rubbing the patient's sternum with the knuckles of the clenched fist.[5]
- The key to successfully manage a patient with psychogenic loss of consciousness is to avoid humiliating the patient in front of either relatives, friends, or hospital staff. Making it known (loudly) to the patient that friends and relatives are waiting outside, and that the poison should be "wearing off about now", explaining what has to be done and why in a firm, nonemotional tone, and avoiding physical abuse or humiliation will often enable the patient to "regain consciousness" over a period of a few minutes with his dignity and self-respect intact!
- If the patient resists all the above maneuvers and the attending doctor is sure that he is dealing with a known ingestion that is harmless, it is better to leave the patient alone for sometime. If however there is any doubt as to the seriousness of the ingested substance, gastric lavage must be initiated ensuring all necessary precautions.

---

*Can cause severe alkali burns.

CHAPTER 92 Assessment and Management of Poisoning

Table 10 Grading the severity of central nervous system intoxication

	Depressants		Stimulants
Grade	Features	Grade	Features
0	Asleep, but can be aroused	-----	------------
1	Semicomatose, withdraws from painful stimuli, reflexes intact	1	Restlessness, irritability, insomnia, tremor, hyperreflexia, sweating, mydriasis
2	Comatose, does not withdraw from painful stimuli, reflexes intact	2	Confusion, hypertension, tachypnea, tachycardia, extrasystoles
3	Comatose, most reflexes lost, no depression of CVS or respiration	3	Delirium, mania, arrhythmia, and hyperpyrexia
4	Comatose, reflexes absent, respiratory and/or circulatory failure	4	Convulsions, coma, and circulatory collapse

Table 11 Toxic causes of coma

• *Hypoxia*
   – Displacement of oxygen in blood and tissues
   – Carbon monoxide
   – Agents causing methemoglobinemia
   – Acetanilide
   – Aniline dyes
   – Methane
   – Chlorates
   – Dinitrophenol
   – Nitrites
	• Displacement of oxygen in the atmosphere
	 • Carbon dioxide
	 • Butane
	 • Propane
	 • Methane

• *Acidosis*
   – Ethylene glycol
   – Isopropanol
   – Methanol
   – Paraldehyde
   – Salicylates	

• *Depression of CNS*
   – Alcohols: Ethanol, methanol, isopropanol
   – Anticonvulsants
   – Antidepressants
   – Antihistamines
   – Barbiturates
	Benzodiazepines
	 Bromides
	 Chloral hydrate
	 Opiates
	 Phenothiazines

• *Hypoglycemia*
   – Ethanol
   – Hypoglycemic drugs
   – Insulin
   – Isoniazid
   – Salicylates	

• *Enzyme inhibition*
   – Cyanide
   – Heavy metals
   – Organophosphates	

• *Postictal*
   – Amphetamines
   – Cocaine
   – Chlorinated hydrocarbons
   – Hallucinogens
   – Withdrawal from alcohol, sedatives, etc.	

• *Other causes* – Food poisoning: Botulism, mushrooms, shellfish, snake bite, etc.	

Abbreviation: CNS, central nervous system.

In the final analysis, this is probably the best of all methods to truly "awaken" a hysterical patient.*

Management

Respiratory Insufficiency

- First establish an open airway:
  - Remove dentures (if any)
  - Use the chin lift and jaw thrust, to clear the airway obstructed by the tongue falling back
  - Remove saliva, vomitus, blood, etc. from the oral cavity by suction or finger-sweep method
  - Place the patient in a semiprone (lateral) position
  - If required, insert an endotracheal tube
- If ventilation is not adequate, begin artificial respiration with Ambu bag.
- *Oxygen therapy*: This is done to raise the PaO_2 to at least 45-55 mm Hg (6.0-7.3 Kpa). Begin with 28% oxygen mask. Depending on the response as assessed by periodic arterial gas analysis, either continue with 28% or progress to 35%. If the condition is relentlessly deteriorating, consider *mechanical ventilation*.

Circulatory Failure

- Correct acidemia, if present.
- Elevate foot end of the bed (*Trendelenburg position*)
- Insert a large bore peripheral intravenous (IV) line (16 gauge or larger), and administer a fluid challenge of 200 mL of saline (10 mL/kg in children). Observe for improvement in blood pressure over 10 minutes. Repeat the fluid bolus if blood pressure (BP) fails to normalize and assess for signs of fluid overload.** Hemodynamic monitoring should be considered in those adult patients who do not respond to 2 L of infusion and short-term low-dose vasopressors such as dopamine and norepinephrine.
- Obtain an electrocardiogram (ECG) in hypotensive patients and note rate, rhythm, arrhythmias, and conduction delays.***
- In patients who do not respond to initial fluid challenges, monitor central venous pressure and hourly urinary output. Patients with severe hypotension may need more sophisticated hemodynamic monitoring (pulmonary artery catheter and intra-arterial pressure monitoring).
- Vasopressors of choice include dopamine and norepinephrine. The doses are as follows:
  - *Dopamine*: Add 200 mg (1 ampoule usually) to 250 mL of 5% dextrose in water to make a solution of 800 µg/mL. Begin with 1-5 µg/kg/min (maximum being 15-30 µg/kg/min), and titrate the dose to maintain systolic BP between 90 mm Hg and 100 mm Hg. Monitor BP every 15 minutes.
  - *Norepinephrine*: Add 8 mg (2 ampoules usually) to 500 mL of 5% dextrose solution to make a concentration of 16 µg/mL. Start at 0.5-1 mL/min and titrate to a clinical response. Monitor BP every 5-10 minutes until a clear trend is established.

ECG Changes and Cardiac Arrhythmias[6]

Obtain an ECG, institute continuous cardiac monitoring and administer oxygen. Evaluate for hypoxia, acidosis, and electrolyte disturbances (especially hypokalemia, hypocalcemia, and hypomagnesemia).

- *Abnormal P wave*: Clinically, abnormalities of the P wave occur with xenobiotics that depress automaticity of the sinus node, causing sinus arrest and nodal or ventricular escape rhythms (e.g. calcium channel blockers). The P wave is absent in rhythms with sinus arrest, e.g. xenobiotics that produce vagotonia such as cardioactive steroids and cholinergic agents. A notched P wave suggests delayed conduction across the atrial septum and is characteristic of quinidine poisoning. P waves decrease in amplitude as hyperkalemia becomes more severe until they become indistinguishable from the baseline.
- *Abnormal PR interval*: Xenobiotics that decrease inter-atrial or AV nodal conduction cause marked lengthening of the PR segment until such conduction completely ceases. At this point, the P wave no longer relates to the QRS complex; this is AV dissociation, or complete heart block. Some xenobiotics suppress AV nodal conduction by blocking calcium channels in nodal cells, as does magnesium. Although the therapeutic use of digoxin, as well as early cardioactive steroid poisoning, causes PR prolongation through vagotonic effects, direct electrophysiologic effects account for the bradycardia of poisoning.
- *Abnormal QRS complex*: In the presence of a bundle-branch block, the two ventricles depolarize sequentially rather than concurrently. Although, conceptually, conduction through either the left or right bundle may be affected, many xenobiotics preferentially affect the right bundle. This effect typically results in the left ventricle depolarizing slightly more rapidly than the right. The consequence on the ECG is both a widening of the QRS complex and the appearance of the right ventricular electrical forces that were previously obscured by those of the left ventricle. These changes are a result of the effects of a xenobiotic that blocks fast sodium channels, e.g. cyclic antidepressants, quinidine and other type IA and

---

*Do not resort to this method as a routine in all psychogenic cases of coma. Gastric lavage is a potentially risky maneuver that can have grave consequences.
**Rales, S_3, heart gallop, neck vein distension.
***PR > 0.2 second, QRS > 0.1 second, or QT interval > 50% of PR interval.

IC antiarrhythmic agents, phenothiazines, amantadine, diphenhydramine, carbamazepine, and cocaine. An apparent increase in QRS duration and morphology, which is actually an elevation or distortion of the J point called a J wave or an Osborn wave, is a common finding in patients with hypothermia. Hypermagnesemia is also associated with a widening the QRS duration and a slight narrowing of the QRS complex may occur with hypomagnesemia. Significant elevation in the serum concentrations of potassium may also cause widening and distortion of the QRS complex.

- *Abnormal ST-segment*: Displacement of the ST-segment from its baseline typically characterizes myocardial ischemia or infarction. The subsequent appearance of a Q-wave is diagnostic of myocardial infarction. Patients who are poisoned by xenobiotics that cause vasoconstriction, such as cocaine, are particularly prone to develop focal myocardial ischemia and infarction. However, any poisoning that results in profound hypotension or hypoxia may also result in ECG changes of ischemia and injury. In this situation, the injury may be more global involving more than one arterial distribution. Diffuse myocardial damage may not be identifiable on the ECG because of global, symmetric electrical abnormalities. In this situation, the diagnosis is made by other noninvasive testing, such as by echocardiogram or by finding elevations in serum markers for myocardial injury (e.g. troponin). Many young, healthy patients have ST-segment abnormalities that mimic those of myocardial infarction. The most common normal variant is termed "early repolarization" or "J-point elevation", and is identified as diffusely elevated, upwardly concave ST-segments, located in the precordial leads and typically with corresponding T waves of large amplitude. The J point is located at the beginning of the ST-segment just after the QRS complex. The Brugada ECG pattern is characterized by terminal positivity of the QRS complex and ST-segment elevation in the right precordial leads. The Brugada pattern is found in some patients with mutations of the gene that codes for a sodium channel subunit. These patients are at risk for sudden death, but a similar ECG pattern often occurs in patients who are poisoned by sodium channel blocking xenobiotics, including TCAs, cocaine, class IA (procainamide), and class IC (flecainide, encainide) antiarrhythmic agents. Sagging ST-segments, inverted T waves, and normal or shortened QT intervals are characteristic effects of cardioactive steroids, such as digoxin on the ECG. Changes in the ST-segment duration are frequently caused by abnormalities in the serum calcium concentration. Hypercalcemia causes shortening of the ST-segment through enhanced calcium influx during the plateau phase of the cardiac cycle speeding the onset of repolarization. For practical purposes this effect is more commonly identified by reduction of the QTc. In patients with hypercalcemia, the morphology and duration of the QRS complex and T and P waves remain essentially unchanged. Xenobiotic-induced hypercalcemia may result from exposure to antacids (milk-alkali syndrome), diuretics (e.g. hydrochlorothiazide), cholecalciferol (vitamin D), vitamin A, and other retinoids. Hypocalcemia causes prolongation of the ST-segment and QTc.
- *Abnormal T wave*: Isolated peaked T waves are usually evidence of early hyperkalemia. Hyperkalemia initially causes tall, tented T waves with normal QRS, QTc, and P wave. As the measured potassium rises to 6.5–8 mEq/L, the P wave diminishes in amplitude and the PR and QRS intervals prolong. Progressive widening of the QRS complex causes it to merge with the ST-segment and T wave, forming a "sine wave". ECG changes of hyperkalemia may occur following chronic exposure to potassium-sparing diuretics, ACE inhibitors, or potassium supplements. Peaked T waves also occur following myocardial ischemia and may also be confused with early repolarization effects. Consequently, the ability to properly identify electrolyte abnormalities by electrocardiography is often limited. Hypokalemia typically reduces the amplitude of the T wave and, ultimately, causes the appearance of prominent U waves. Lithium similarly affects myocardial ion fluxes and causes reversible changes on the ECG that may mimic mild hypokalemia.
- *Abnormal QT interval*: A prolonged QTc reflects an increase in the time period that the heart is vulnerable to the initiation of ventricular arrhythmias. An early after depolarization (EAD) occurs when a myocardial cell spontaneously depolarizes before its repolarization is complete. If this depolarization is of sufficient magnitude, it may capture and initiate a premature ventricular contraction, which itself may initiate ventricular tachycardia, ventricular fibrillation, or torsades de pointes. Xenobiotics that cause sodium channel blockade prolong the QT duration by slowing cellular depolarization during phase zero. Thus, the QT duration increases because of a prolongation of the QRS complex duration, and the ST-segment duration remains near normal. Xenobiotics that cause potassium channel blockade similarly prolong the QT, but through prolongation of the plateau and repolarization phases. This specifically prolongs the ST-segment duration. Hypocalcemia is caused by a number of xenobiotics, including fluoride, calcitonin, ethylene glycol, phosphates, and mithramycin. Arsenic poisoning may cause prolongation of the QTc and torsades de pointes. The mechanism is unknown, although either a direct dysrhythmogenic effect or an autoimmune myocarditis is postulated.
- *Abnormal U wave*: Abnormal U waves are typically caused by spontaneous after depolarization of membrane potential that occurs in situations where repolarization is prolonged. EAD occurs in situations where the

prolonged repolarization period allows calcium channels (which are both time and voltage dependent) to close and spontaneously reopen because they may close at a membrane potential that is above their threshold potential for opening. In this situation, the opening of the calcium channels produces a slight membrane depolarization that is identified as a U wave. Delayed after depolarization occurs when the myocyte is overloaded with calcium, as in the setting of cardioactive steroid toxicity. The excess intracellular calcium can trigger the ryanodine receptors on the myocyte sarcoplasmic reticulum to release calcium, causing slight depolarization that is recognized as a U wave. If the U waves are of sufficient magnitude to reach threshold, the cell may depolarize and initiate a premature ventricular contraction. Transient U-wave inversion can also be caused by myocardial ischemia or systemic hypertension.

- *Tachyarrhythmias*: Sympathomimetic agents such as cocaine and amphetamines increase sympathetic tone, producing sinus tachycardia and enhancing AV nodal conduction. Sinus tachycardia may be the first manifestation of exposure to a sympathomimetic agent. However, other supraventricular or ventricular dysrhythmias may develop if an abnormal rhythm is generated in another part of the heart. Similarly, xenobiotics that antagonize acetylcholine released from the vagus nerve onto the sinus node enhance the rate of firing, producing sinus tachycardia, e.g. belladonna alkaloids, antihistamines, and tricyclic antidepressants. Certain xenobiotics are more highly associated with ventricular tachyarrhythmias following poisoning. Those that alter myocardial repolarization and prolong the QTc predispose to the development of after depolarization-induced contractions during the relative refractory period (R on T phenomena), which initiates ventricular tachycardia. If torsades de pointes is noted, this is undoubtedly the mechanism, and the QTc should be carefully assessed and appropriate treatment initiated. Alternatively, xenobiotics that increase the adrenergic tone on the heart, either directly or indirectly, may cause ventricular arrhythmias. Whether a result of excessive circulating catecholamines observed with cocaine and sympathomimetics, myocardial sensitization secondary to halogenated hydrocarbons or thyroid hormone, or increased second messenger activity secondary to theophylline, the extreme inotropic and chronotropic effects cause arrhythmias. Altered repolarization, increased intracellular calcium concentrations, or myocardial ischemia can cause the arrhythmia. Additionally, xenobiotics that produce focal myocardial ischemia, such as cocaine or ephedrine, can lead to malignant ventricular arrhythmias. Bidirectional ventricular tachycardia is associated with severe cardioactive steroid toxicity and results from alterations of intraventricular conduction, junctional tachycardia with aberrant intraventricular conduction, or, on rare occasions, alternating ventricular pacemakers. The only other xenobiotic that commonly causes this arrhythmia is aconitine.
- *Bradyarrhythmias*: Sinus bradycardia with an otherwise normal ECG is characteristic of xenobiotics that reduce central nervous system outflow, e.g. benzodiazepines, ethanol, and clonidine. Calcium channel blockers, beta-blockers, and cardioactive steroids are the leading causes of sinus bradycardia and conduction disturbances. The bradycardia produced by cardioactive steroids is typically accompanied by signs of "digitalis effect", including PR prolongation and ST-segment depression.
- *Management issues*: Lignocaine and amiodarone are generally first-line agents for stable monomorphic ventricular tachycardia, particularly in patients with underlying impaired cardiac function. Sotalol is an alternative for stable monomorphic ventricular tachycardia. Amiodarone and sotalol should be used with caution if a substance that prolongs the QT interval and/or causes torsades de pointes is involved in the overdose. Unstable rhythms require cardioversion. Atropine may be used when severe bradycardia is present and premature ventricular contractions (PVCs) are thought to represent an escape complex.
    - **Lignocaine**
        - *Dose*
            - *Adult*: 1–1.5 mg/kg IV push. For refractory VT/VF an additional bolus of 0.5–0.75 mg/kg can be given over 3–5 minutes. Total dose should not exceed 3 mg/kg or more than 200–300 mg during a 1 hour period.[6] Once circulation has been restored begin maintenance infusion of 1–4 mg/min. If arrhythmias recur during infusion repeat 0.5 mg/kg bolus and increase the infusion rate incrementally (up to a maximum of 4 mg/minute).
            - *Child*: 1 mg/kg initial bolus IV; followed by a continuous infusion of 20–50 µg/kg/min.
        - *Lignocaine preparation*: Add 1 g of lignocaine to 250 mL of dextrose 5% in water to make a 4 mg/mL solution. An increase in the infusion rate of 1 mL/min increases the dose by 4 mg/min.

Central Nervous System Depression

Hoffman and *Goldfrank* reviewed data from 1966 to 1994 on the treatment of poisoned comatose patients and came to the conclusion that in every case where the identity of the poison was unknown, the following three antidotes (*coma cocktail*) must be administered:[7]

1. *Dextrose*: 100 mL of 50% solution
2. *Thiamine* (Vitamin B_1): 100 mg — All given IV
3. *Naloxone*: 2 mg

For a child, thiamine is not recommended, and the dextrose should be more dilute (20–25%). If IV access is a problem, naloxone can be given intramuscularly or even endotracheally.

The rationale for the Coma Cocktail is that a significant proportion of poisoned comatose patients in whom the identity of the poison is unknown, comprise cases of overdose from opiates, alcohol, and hypoglycemic agents. Even if a particular case is not due to any of these causes, administration of these antidotes is relatively harmless.* Physostigmine must not be a part of the cocktail, since even though coma from anticholinergic excess is also relatively common, physostigmine which is the antidote for it, produces serious side effects such as seizures. It should be administered (2 mg IV for an adult, and 0.5 mg in the child) only if there are unequivocal signs of anticholinergic excess.

Analeptics such as caffeine, picrotoxin, doxapram, nikethamide, etc. which were previously advocated as "restorative remedies" to stimulate respiration in comatose patients must also not be used since they offer no substantial benefit, and instead can lead to intractable seizures and agitation.

In addition to the coma cocktail, all patients with depressed mental status should receive 100% oxygen in a mask, (high flow, 8–10 L/min).

The history alone is not a reliable indication of which patients require naloxone, hypertonic dextrose, thiamine, and oxygen. Instead, these therapies should be considered for all patients with altered mental status, unless specifically contraindicated. The physical examination should be used to guide the use of naloxone. If dextrose or naloxone is indicated, sufficient amounts should be administered to exclude and/or treat hypoglycemia or opioid toxicity, respectively.

Attributing an altered mental status to alcohol because of its odor on a patient's breath is potentially dangerous and misleading. Small amounts of alcohol and its congeners generally produce the same breath odor as do intoxicating amounts. Conversely, even when an extremely high blood ethanol concentration is confirmed by the laboratory, it is dangerous to ignore other possible etiologies of an altered mental status; chronic alcoholics may be awake and seemingly alert with ethanol concentrations in excess of 500 mg/dL, a concentration that would result in coma and possibly apnea and death in a nonalcoholic patient.

The metabolism of ethanol is fairly constant at 15–30 mg/dL/hr. Therefore, as a general rule, regardless of the initial blood alcohol concentration, a presumably "inebriated" comatose patient who is still unarousable 3–4 hours after arrival should be considered to have structural CNS damage (head trauma) and/or another toxic-metabolic etiology for the alteration in consciousness, until proven otherwise. Careful neurologic evaluation supplemented by a head CT scan is frequently indicated in such a case. This is especially important in dealing with a seemingly intoxicated patient who appears to have only a minor bruise, as the early treatment of a subdural or epidural hematoma or subarachnoid hemorrhage is critical to a successful outcome.

In the final analysis, it must be stated that there is increasing dissatisfaction among toxicologists with regard to the true benefits of the coma cocktail, and the view is gaining ground that it has no place in practice.

EVALUATION

In all those poisoned patients where there appears to be no immediate crisis, a detailed and thorough clinical examination should be made with special reference to the detection and treatment of any of the following abnormalities.

Hypothermia

The signs and symptoms of hypothermia are summarized in **Table 12**,** while the drugs which produce hypothermia are mentioned in **Box 2**. It is essential to use a low reading rectal thermometer. Electronic thermometers with flexible probes are best which can also be used to record the esophageal and bladder temperatures.

Treatment

- *Rewarming*: For mild cases, a warm water bath (115° F) is sufficient until the core temperature rises to 92° F, when the patient is placed in a bed with warm blankets. The rate of rewarming should not exceed 5° F/hr. Heating the inspired air is recommended by some as very effective in raising the core temperature. Others advocate gastric lavage with warmed fluids, or peritoneal lavage with warmed dialysate.
- In addition, it may be necessary to correct other associated anomalies such as hypotension, hypoventilation, acidosis, and hypokalemia.

Hyperthermia

Oral temperature above 102° F is referred to as hyperthermia. If it exceeds 106° F (which is very rare), there is imminent danger of encephalopathy. In a few individuals there is a genetic susceptibility to hyperthermia, especially on exposure to skeletal muscle relaxants, inhalation anesthetics, and even

---

*If the comatose patient happens to be an opiate addict, naloxone can trigger a withdrawal reaction. Also, preliminary animal and human evidence suggests that glucose-containing IV solutions should be avoided in patients at risk for cerebral ischemia, impending cardiac arrest, or severe hypotension, or those receiving cardiopulmonary resuscitation.

**All units of temperature are expressed in Fahrenheit. To convert into the Celsius scale, subtract 32 and multiply by 5/9.

Table 12 Signs and symptoms of hypothermia

System	Features		
	Mild (95°F–90°F)	Moderate (90°F–82.4°F)	Severe (< 82.4°F)
CNS	Amnesia, dysarthria impaired judgment	Drowsiness, mydriasis, paradoxical undressing, hallucinations	Coma, loss of ocular reflexes
CVS	Tachycardia progressing to bradycardia, raised BP	Atrial and ventricular arrhythmias, lowered BP, J wave on ECG	Severe hypotension, bradycardia, asystole
Respiratory system	Tachypnea followed by decrease in minute volume, bronchospasm	Hypoventilation	Pulmonary edema, apnea
Renal and endocrine systems	Cold diuresis, shivering	Increased renal blood flow	Decreased renal blood flow, oliguria, poikilothermia
Musculoskeletal system	Increased muscle tone followed by fatiguing, anoxia	Hyporeflexia, rigidity	No motion, peripheral areflexia

Abbreviations: BP, blood pressure; CNS, central nervous system; CVS, cyclic vomiting syndrome; ECG, electrocardiogram.

Box 2 Drugs producing hypothermia

- Alcohols
- Hypoglycemics
- Antidepressants
- Opiates
- Barbiturates
- Phenothiazines
- Benzodiazepines
- Sedative-hypnotics
- Carbon monoxide

Table 13 Agents inducing hyperthermia

Muscular hyperactivity	Increased metabolic rate	Impaired thermoregulation
• Amphetamines • Antidepressants • Cocaine • MAO inhibitors • Phencyclidine • Strychnine • Withdrawal (alcohol/opiates)	• Dinitrophenol • Salicylates • Thyroid hormones	• Anticholinergics • Antihistamines • Antipsychotics • Ephedrine • Phenylpropanolamine • Phenothiazines

Abbreviations: MAO inhibitors, monoamine oxidase inhibitors.

local anesthetics—*malignant hyperthermia*.[8] This should be distinguished from *neuroleptic malignant syndrome*, which is also characterized by high fever apart from other neurological signs, but is the result of adverse reaction to antipsychotic or neuroleptic drugs, and has no genetic basis. **Table 13** lists some of the important toxicological causes of hyperthermia along with postulated mechanism. Complications include coagulopathy, rhabdomyolysis, renal failure, and tachyarrhythmias.

Treatment

- Remove all clothes, and pack the neck and groin with ice
- Immersion in cold water bath (77°F) is very effective but dangerous in the elderly and in heart patients
- Stop cooling measures when core temperature falls below 102°F, and nurse the patient in bed in a cool room
- Administration of dantrolene may be beneficial in some cases
- Do not use antipyretic drugs like paracetamol. They are ineffective.

Acid–Base Disorders

Serum electrolytes to evaluate for metabolic acidosis should be obtained if there is any possibility of mixed ingestion or uncertain history.[9]

The diagnosis of these acid-base disorders is based on arterial blood gas, pH, $PaCO_2$, bicarbonate, and serum electrolyte disturbances. It must be first determined as to which abnormalities are primary and which are compensatory, based on the pH **(Table 14)**. If the pH is less than 7.40, respiratory or metabolic alkalosis is primary.

In the case of metabolic acidosis, it is necessary to calculate the *anion gap*. The anion gap is calculated as follows:

$$(Na^+ + K^+) - (HCO_3^- + Cl^-)$$

Normally this translates as:

$$140 - (24 + 104) = 12 \text{ mmol/L } (Range: 12–16 \text{ mmol/L})$$

If the anion gap is greater than 20 mmol/L, a metabolic acidosis is present regardless of the pH or serum bicarbonate concentration. Several poisons are associated with increased anion gap (*Gap acidosis*), while others do not alter it (*nongap acidosis*).[10] The common causes for the various acid-base disorders are mentioned in **Table 15**.

Table 14 Acid–base disorders

Disorder	Parameter	Value	Interpretation
Acute respiratory alkalosis	pH PaCO$_2$ HCO$_3$	7.50 29 mm Hg 22 mmol/L	Alkalemia Respiratory alkalosis Normal
Acute respiratory acidosis	pH PaCO$_2$ HCO$_3$	7.25 60 mm Hg 26 mmol/L	Acidemia Respiratory acidosis Normal
Chronic respiratory acidosis with metabolic compensation	pH PaCO$_2$ HCO$_3$	7.34 60 mm Hg 36 mmol/L	Normal Respiratory acidosis Metabolic compensation
Metabolic alkalosis	pH PaCO$_2$ HCO$_3$	7.50 48 mm Hg 36 mmol/L	Alkalemia Respiratory compensation Metabolic alkalosis
Metabolic acidosis	pH PaCO$_2$ HCO$_3$	7.20 21 mm Hg 8 mmol/L	Acidemia Respiratory compensation Metabolic acidosis

Table 15 Causes of acid–base disorders

Type of disorder	Causes	
Acute respiratory alkalosis	Anxiety, hypoxia, lung diseases, CNS disease, pregnancy, sepsis, hepatic encephalopathy, drugs—salicylates, catecholamines, progesterone, etc.	
Acute respiratory acidosis	CNS depression, acute airway obstruction, neuromuscular disorders (myopathies, neuropathies), severe pneumonia or pulmonary edema, impaired lung motion (hemothorax, pneumothorax)	
Chronic respiratory acidosis with metabolic compensation	Chronic lung disease, chronic neuromuscular disorders, chronic respiratory center depression	
Metabolic alkalosis	Normal or high urinary chloride Cushing's disease, Conn's syndrome, steroid administration, diuretic administration, alkali overdose	Low urinary chloride Vomiting, past use of diuretics, post-hypercapnia
Metabolic acidosis	Non-gap Diarrhea, renal tubular acidosis, carbonic anhydrase inhibitors, aldosterone inhibitors, post-hypocapnia, bromism, iodism, and secondary to hyperkalemia, hypercalcemia	Gap* Methanol Uremia Diabetes Paraldehyde, phenformin Idiopathic lactic acidosis, iron, isoniazid Ethanol, ethylene glycol Salicylates, solvents, starvation

*The important causes can be remembered by the acronym MUDPIES. A more elaborate mnemonic which accounts for all the causes is as follows: I Love Chocolate Raspberry Truffle MUDPIES, the first five words standing for Ibuprofen, Lithium, Carbon monoxide, cyanide, and caffeine, Respiratory dysfunction, and Toluene.

Wrenn has characterized the rise in anion gap and the fall in bicarbonate with a numerical value, the *delta gap*.[11]

Delta gap = Rise in anion gap − decrease in HCO_3.

If the delta gap is more than +6, a metabolic acidosis is usually present, and if it is less than −6, a hyperchloremic acidosis is usually present.

Osmolal (Osmole) Gap[12]

This is a very useful parameter to check for the presence of some common toxic causes of metabolic acidosis: *m*ethanol, *e*thanol, *d*iuretics (mannitol, sorbitol, glycerine), *i*sopropanol, and *e*thylene glycol.* The osmolal gap is obtained by deducting the *calculated* osmolality of serum from the *measured* serum osmolality.** The latter should be determined by freezing point depression osmometer and never by vapor pressure determination, which would volatilize alcohols.

The calculated osmolality is obtained by the following formula:

$$\text{Calculated osmolality (mOsm)} = 2Na^+(mEq/L) + \frac{BUN (mg\%)}{2.8} + \frac{Glucose (mg\%)}{18}$$

Osmolal gap = Freezing point measured osmolality − calculated osmolality.

The normal serum osmolality is 280–295 mOsm. If the measured osmolality is more than 10 mOsm greater than the calculated osmolality, the presence of any of the above mentioned toxic substances should be suspected. However, it is to be noted that in the case of methanol and ethylene glycol poisoning the osmolal gap may be normal in the late stages when these substances are completely metabolized.[13]

Treatment of metabolic acidosis:

The drug of choice is sodium bicarbonate (**Box 3**). It is widely considered to be the best antidote for acidosis of almost any etiology.

Convulsions (Seizures)

There are several drugs and poisons which cause convulsions (**Table 16**). Improper treatment or mismanagement can lead to status epilepticus which is a life-threatening condition. Toxic convulsions may broadly be divided into three categories:
1. Those that respond to standard anticonvulsant treatment (typically a benzodiazepine).
2. Those that either require specific antidotes to control seizure activity or that do not respond consistently to standard anticonvulsant treatment, such as isoniazid-induced seizures requiring pyridoxine administration.
3. Those that may appear to respond to initial treatment with cessation of tonic-clonic activity, but which leave the patient exposed to the underlying, unidentified toxin or to continued electrical seizure activity in the brain, such as CO or hypoglycemia.

Treatment

- Administer oxygen by nasal cannula or mask
- Position patient's head for optimal airway patency
- Establish IV line
- Begin drug therapy with benzodiazepines (**Table 17**). Either lorazepam (0.1 mg/kg) at a rate of 2 mg/min, or diazepam (0.2 mg/kg) at a rate of 5 mg/min can

---

Box 3 Sodium bicarbonate

Uses
- Salicylate overdose (to alkalinize urine)
- Tricyclic antidepressant overdose (to alkalinize blood)
- Correction of metabolic acidosis (especially in methanol and ethylene glycol poisoning)
- Adjuvant in poisoning with barbiturates, phenothiazines, cocaine, and carbamazepine
- Drug or toxin-induced myoglobinuria
- As stomach wash for iron poisoning
- Possible use in lactic acidosis, diabetic ketoacidosis, and cardiac resuscitation

Formulation
50 mL ampoules of 8.4 and 7.5% solution containing 50 and 44.6 mEq of sodium bicarbonate respectively

Dose
Add 2–3 ampoules of 8.4% $NaHCO_3$ to 1 L of 5% dextrose in water, infused intravenously over 3–4 hours. In pediatric patients, add 1–2 mEq $NaHCO_3$/kg in 15 mL/kg 5% dextrose on 0.45% normal saline over 3–4 hours.
   Check urine pH in 1 hour. It should be at least 7.5, preferably 8. Maintain alkalinization with continuous infusion of 100–150 mEq in 1 L of 5% dextrose in water at 150–200 mL/hr
   Half of this dose suffices for a child

Mechanism of action
- Alters drug ionization of weak acids. Alkalinization of blood prevents movement of ionized drug within the tissues. Cellular membranes are impermeable to ionized compounds.
- Changes sodium gradients and partially reverses the fast sodium channel blockade seen
- Titrates acid, and reverses life-threatening acidemia

Dangers
- Can precipitate fatal arrhythmia if given in the presence of hypokalemia.
- Can result in alkalemia, if administered negligently.

---

*Can be remembered by the mnemonic (acronym): ME DIE.
**Osmolality refers to solute/Kg of solvent, while osmolarity refers to solute/L of solution.

Table 16 Toxic causes of convulsions

During toxicity		During withdrawal
• Amphetamines • Anticholinergics • Antidepressants • Antihistamines • Caffeine • Camphor • Carbon monoxide • Chlorinated hydrocarbons • Cholinergics	• Cocaine • Cyanide • Heavy metals • Isoniazid • Organophosphates • Strychnine • Sympathomimetics • Xanthines (theophylline)	• Barbiturates • Benzodiazepines • Ethanol • Methaqualone • Opiates

Table 17 Common drugs used to treat status epilepticus

Dose (mg/kg)	Diazepam	Lorazepam	Phenytoin	Phenobarbitone
Adult IV dose	0.15–0.25	0.1	15–20	20
Pediatric IV dose	0.1–1.0	0.05–0.5	20	20
Pediatric per rectal dose	0.5	–	–	–
Maximum IV rate	5	2	50	100
Duration of action (hours)	0.25–0.5	>12–24	24	>48
Side effects				
CNS depression	10–30 min	Several hours	None	Several days
Respiratory depression	Occasional	Occasional	Infrequent	Occasional
Hypotension	Infrequent	Infrequent	Occasional	Infrequent
Cardiac arrhythmias	–	–	Occasional	–

Abbreviations: CNS, central nervous system; IV, intravenous.

be administered IV. If status persists, administer 15–20 mg/kg phenytoin at 50 mg/min (adults), or 1 mg/kg/min (children) by IV. Phenytoin is incompatible with glucose containing solutions. The IV should be purged with normal saline before phenytoin infusion.

If status still persists, administer 20 mg/kg phenobarbitone IV at 100 mg/min. If this measure also fails, give anesthetic doses of phenobarbitone, pentobarbitone, thiopentone, or halothane. In such cases obviously, ventilatory assistance and vasopressors become mandatory.

• Monitor ECG, hydration, and electrolyte balance. Watch out for hypoglycemia and cerebral edema.

Agitation

Several drugs and poisons are associated with increased aggression which may sometimes progress to psychosis and violent behavior **(Table 18)**. This is especially likely if there are other predisposing factors such as existing mental disorder, hypoglycemia, hypoxia, head injury, and even

Table 18 Drugs associated with agitation and psychosis

During toxicity		During withdrawal
• Amphetamines • Anticholinergics • Antidepressants • Benzodiazepines (paradoxical agitation) • Cannabis • Cocaine	• Corticosteroids • *Datura* (atropine) • Digitalis • Ethanol • Hallucinogens	• Barbiturates • Ethanol • Opiates

anemia and vitamin deficiencies.[14] *Delirium** is the term which is often used to denote such acute psychotic episodes, and is characterized by disorientation, irrational fears, hyperexcitability, hallucinations, and violence. *Dementia* refers to a more gradual decline in mental processes mainly resulting in confusion and memory loss, and though it is often organic in nature due to degenerative diseases, there are some drugs which can cause this especially on chronic

---

*Also seen in high fever, insanity, anxiety, and shock.

exposure.[15] Elderly patients are more vulnerable. Dementia due to drugs is usually reversible.

Treatment

Delirium is managed by chlorpromazine, diazepam, or haloperidol. Caution is however necessary, since sedation which is inevitable with these preparations may sometimes result in more harm than benefit. **Table 19** outlines measures for managing a violent patient in the casualty [emergency department (ED)].

Movement Disorders

Exposure to several drugs and toxins can result in a wide variety of movement disorders ranging from full blown Parkinson's disease to isolated tremors.

- *Parkinsonism*: The most frequent culprits are phenothiazines and major tranquillizers, though there are several others which have been implicated **(Table 20)**. Symptoms of Parkinsonism usually appear in the first 3 months of exposure and may be indistinguishable from idiopathic Parkinson's disease.
- *Motor neuron disease*: **Table 21** lists the various types of toxin-induced motor neuron disease and the possible cause.
- *Myopathies*: Drug-induced myopathies may result from a direct toxic effect which may be local (e.g. injection of drug into muscle), or more diffuse when the drug is taken systemically. Repeated injections of antibiotics or drugs of addiction often lead to severe muscle fibrosis and contractures (*myositis fibrosa, myositis ossificans*). Clofibrate and aminocaproic acid can cause an *acute necrotizing myopathy* with myoglobinuria and renal failure. Other drugs that can induce toxic myopathies include succinylcholine, halothane, corticosteroids, chloroquine, D-penicillamine, alcohol, phenytoin, thiazide diuretics, amphotericin, procainamide, penicillin, and lipid-lowering drugs. Environmental causes include exposure to silica, certain types of food (e.g. adulterated rapeseed oil), and medical devices such as silicone implants.[16]
- *Akathisias, Dystonias, Chorea and Tardive Dyskinesia*: Tricyclic antidepressants, monoamine oxidase inhibitors, fluoxetine, lithium, buspirone, and levodopa are the

Table 19 Tranquilization of the violent patient

Type of violent behavior	Therapeutic measure
Schizophrenia (or any other psychosis)	Lorazepam 2–4 mg IM, combined with haloperidol 5 mg IM
Extreme agitation	Lorazepam 2–4 mg IM, every hour
Personality disorder	Lorazepam 1–2 mg orally every 1–2 hrs, Or 2–4 mg IM, every 1–2 hrs
Alcohol withdrawal	Chlordiazepoxide 25–50 mg orally, as required, Or lorazepam 2 mg orally
Cocaine/amphetamine toxicity	Diazepam 10 mg every 8 hrs orally or IM
Phencyclidine toxicity	Diazepam 10–30 mg orally, or Lorazepam 2–4 mg, or haloperidol 5 mg IM

Abbreviation: IM, intramuscular.

Table 20 Drug-induced Parkinsonism

Agent	Source
Antidepressants	Psychiatric medication
Carbon monoxide	Occupational, environmental
Carbon disulfide	Occupational
Hydrogen cyanide	Occupational
Lithium	Psychiatric medication
Manganese	Occupational
Mercury	Occupational
MPTP	Drug abuse
Paraquat	Herbicide
Phenothiazines	Antiemetic
Reserpine	Antihypertensive
Tranquilizers (major)	Psychiatric medication

Abbreviation: MPTP, N-methyl-4-phenyl-1, 2, 3, 6-tetrahydropyridine.

Table 21 Motor neuron disorders

Disorder	Cause	Geographic location
Lathyrism	Chickling pea (*Lathyrus sativus* seed) Toxin: Beta-N-oxalyl-amino-L-alanine (BOAA)	Africa and Asia
Amyotrophic lateral sclerosis	Lead, mercury, manganese, selenium	No specific area
Leather Workers' MND	Solvents	United Kingdom
Mantakassa	Cassava Toxin: Cyanogenic glycosides	Northern Mozambique
Konzo	Cassava Toxin: Cyanogenic glycosides	East Africa

Abbreviation: MND, motor neuron disorders.

principal causes of drug-induced *akathisia*.[17] This is characterized by extreme restlessness with constant movement and muscular quivering. *Dystonia* usually manifests as facial grimacing or torticollis, and is mainly associated with phenothiazines, butyrophenones, metoclopramide, tricyclic antidepressants, phenytoin, and chloroquine. *Chorea*, which causes involuntary writhing movements of limbs is most commonly seen with anticonvulsants (especially phenytoin), anabolic steroids, amphetamines, levodopa, and sometimes with cimetidine, ethanol, and cocaine.

Phenothiazines and metoclopramide are most often the culprits in drug-induced *tardive dyskinesia*, which is characterized by stereotyped, slow, and rhythmic movements.

- *Myasthenic crisis*: This refers to a sudden onset of severe muscular weakness, and may be precipitated by aminoglycosides, polymyxin, penicillamine, tetracycline, quinidine, lidocaine, quinine, curare, succinylcholine, procainamide, and some opiates.
- *Fasciculations*: Fasciculations are contractions of muscle fibers within an individual motor unit, and appear as twitching of affected muscles. **Box 4** lists the major toxicological causes of fasciculations.
- *Tremor*: Drug-induced tremors are of several types **(Table 22)**.

Treatment of Movement Disorders

Most of the movement disorders induced by toxins or drugs are dose and duration related. Withdrawal of the incriminating agent commonly results in recovery. The usual measures undertaken in the management of the respective drug overdose (or abuse) must be instituted wherever applicable.

Table 23 will serve as a quick reference source for common culprits of drug- or toxin-induced movement disorders.

Electrolyte Disturbances

- *Hyperkalemia (i.e. potassium level >5.5 mEq/L)*: The causes include digitalis, β_2-antagonists, potassium-sparing diuretics, NSAIDs, fluoride, heparin, succinylcholine, and drugs producing acidosis. Manifestations include abdominal pain, diarrhea, myalgia, and weakness. ECG changes are important—tall, peaked T waves, ST-segment depression, prolonged PR interval, and QRS prolongation. In severe cases there is ventricular fibrillation.
  Treatment: Glucose, insulin infusion, sodium bicarbonate, and calcium gluconate. Hemodialysis and exchange resins may be required.
- *Hypokalemia (i.e. potassium level <3.5 mEq/L)*: The causes include β_2-agonists, theophylline, insulin, chloroquine, caffeine, dextrose, loop diuretics, thiazide diuretics,

Box 4 Toxic causes of fasciculations

- Amphetamines
- Lithium
- Barium salts
- Manganese
- Black widow spider bite
- Mercury
- Caffeine
- Nicotine
- Camphor
- Phencyclidine
- Cholinergic excess
- Quaternary ammonium compounds
- Cocaine
- Scorpion sting
- Fluorides
- Shellfish poisoning
- Hypoglycemics
- Strychnine
- Lead

Table 22 Drug-induced tremor	
Type	Cause
Resting (most pronounced at rest)	• Antipsychotic drugs like chlorpromazine promazine haloperidole • GI motility drugs like metoclopramide domperidone • Other drugs like antiepileptics calcium channel blocker
Postural (most pronounced in an outstretched hand)	Beta-agonists, phenytoin, valproic acid, tricyclics, lithium, arsenic, alcohol withdrawal, amphetamines, caffeine, cocaine, theophylline, and CO
Kinetic (most pronounced with movement)	Chronic alcoholism, mercury, lithium, and acute sedative-hypnotic overdose
Choreoid (repetitive writhing movements of hands)	Anticholinergics amantadine bromocriptine and manganese
Dystonic (muscle group spasms)	Neuroleptics, antiemetics, cocaine, and chloroquine

Table 23 Drug-induced movement disorders at a glance

Drug	Disorders
Amoxapine	Parkinsonism
Amphetamines	Hyperkinetic movements
Antihistamines	Orofacial dystonia, myoclonic jerking
Butyrophenones	Parkinsonism, orofacial dystonia, opisthotonus, trismus
Caffeine	Myoclonic jerking
Carbamazepine	Orofacial dystonia
Carbon monoxide	Parkinsonism
Monoamine oxidase inhibitors	Rigidity, opisthotonus
Nicotine	Flaccid fasciculations
Organophosphates	Flaccid fasciculations
Pethidine	Tremor, muscle jerking
Phencyclidine	Generalized rigidity, trismus, orofacial dystonias, twitching
Phenothiazines	Orofacial and other dystonias
Phenytoin	Choreoathetosis
Strychnine	Rigidity, opisthotonus, trismus
Tricyclic antidepressants	Twitching, myoclonic jerking

oral hypoglycemics, salicylates, sympathomimetics, drug-induced gastroenteritis, and metabolic acidosis. Manifestations include muscle weakness, paralytic ileus, and ECG changes—flat or inverted-T waves, prominent U waves, ST-segment depression. In severe cases there is AV block and ventricular fibrillation.
Treatment: Oral or IV potassium.

- *Hypernatremia (i.e. sodium level more than 150 mEq/L)*: The causes include colchicine, lithium, propoxyphene, rifampicin, phenytoin, alcohol, mannitol, sorbitol, sodium salts, excessive water loss, IV saline solutions, and salt emetics.
Treatment: Water restriction with or without loop diuretics.
- *Hyponatremia (i.e. sodium level <130 mEq/L)*: The causes include carbamazepine, chlorpropamide, NSAIDs, amitriptyline, biguanides, sulfonylureas, captopril and other angiotensin-converting-enzyme (ACE) inhibitors, lithium, imipramine, oxytocin, and excessive water intake.
Treatment: Hypertonic saline.
- *Hypocalcemia (i.e. calcium level <4 mEq/L)*: The causes include hydrogen fluoride, oxalates, aminoglycosides, ethanol, phenobarbitone, phenytoin, theophylline, and ethylene glycol.

Treatment: Calcium gluconate IV (10% solution, 10 mL at a time, slowly).
Drug-induced hypercalcemia is uncommon.

DECONTAMINATION

Eye

Irrigate copiously for at least 15–20 minutes with normal saline or water. Do not use acid or alkaline irrigating solutions. As a first-aid measure at home, a victim of chemical burns should be instructed to place his face under running water or in a shower while holding the eyelids open. During transportation to hospital the face should be immersed in a basin of water (while ensuring that the patient does not inhale water!).

Skin

Cutaneous absorption is a common occurrence especially with reference to industrial and agricultural substances such as phenol, hydrocyanic acid, aniline, organic metallic compounds, phosphorus, and most of the pesticides. The following measures can be undertaken to minimize absorption*:

- Exposed persons should rinse with cold water and then wash thoroughly with a non-germicidal soap. Repeat the rinse with cold water
- Corroded areas should be irrigated copiously with water or saline for at least 15 minutes. Do not use "neutralizing solutions"
- Remove all contaminated clothes. It is preferable to strip the patient completely and provide fresh clothes, or cover with clean bedsheet
- Some chemical exposures require special treatment:
  - Phenolic burns should be treated by application of polyethylene
  - Phosphorus burns should be treated with copper sulfate solution
  - For hydrofluoric acid burns, use of intradermal or intra-arterial calcium gluconate decreases tissue necrosis
- For tar, bitumen, or asphalt burns, first irrigate the affected skin with cold water and then clean and apply solvents such as kerosene, petrol, ethanol, or acetone. However, since these substances cannot only be locally cytotoxic, but also be absorbed through the skin, it is preferable to use mineral oil, petrolatum, or antibacterial ointments in a petrolatum base. Prolonged irrigating applications may be required. The most effective and safest solvent is said to be *Medi-Sol (De-Solvit)*.** This preparation consists of 70% petroleum distillate (aliphatic hydrocarbon), 25% limonene (orange oil), and 1% dioctyl sodium sulfosuccinate (surfactant).[18]

---

*For potentially toxic substances subject to skin absorption, health personnel should wear impermeable gloves and gowns.
** Not available as a ready preparation in India.

Gut

The various methods of poison removal from the gastrointestinal tract include:
- Emesis
- Gastric lavage
- Catharsis
- Activated charcoal
- Whole-bowel irrigation
- Surgery and endoscopy.

Emesis

The only recommended method of inducing a poisoned patient to vomit is administration of *syrup of ipecacuanha* (or *ipecac*), and ironically it is not easy to procure it in India. However, the initial enthusiasm associated with the use of ipecac in the 1960s and 1970s in western countries has declined substantially in recent years owing to doubts being raised as to its actual efficacy and safety. A study using the Toxic Exposure Surveillance System (TESS) database evaluated the effect of home use of syrup of ipecac on the rate of referral to EDs across the United States. The study found that there was no reduction in ED use nor any improvement in patient outcome from home administration of syrup of ipecac.[19] Based on these findings and other data, the American Academy of Pediatrics published its policy statement on poison treatment in the home, concluding that syrup of ipecac should no longer be used as a standard home treatment in cases of poisoning.[20] *The current consensus is that syrup of ipecac must NOT be used, except in justifiable circumstances.*

Syrup of Ipecac*

- *Source*: Root of a small shrub (*Cephaelis ipecacuanha* or *C. acuminata*; **Fig. 2**) which grows well in West Bengal.
- *Active principles*: Cephaeline, emetine, and traces of psychotrine.
- *Indications*: Conscious and alert poisoned patient who has ingested a poison not more than 4–6 hours earlier
- *Mode of action*:
  - Local activation of peripheral sensory receptors in the gastrointestinal tract.
  - Central stimulation of the chemoreceptor trigger zone with subsequent activation of the central vomiting center
- *Dose*: 30 mL (adult) or 15 mL (child) followed by 8–16 ounces, i.e. 250–500 mL approximately, of water. The patient should be sitting up. If vomiting does not occur within 30 minutes, repeat the same dose once more. If there is still no effect, perform stomach wash to remove not only the ingested poison but also the ipecac consumed.

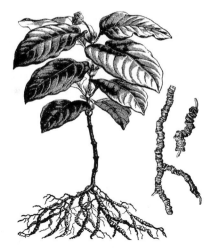

Fig. 2 *Cephaelis ipecacuanha*

However, the therapeutic doses of ipecac recommended above are not really harmful.
- *Contraindications*:
  - *Relative*:
    - Very young (less than 1 year), or very old patient
    - Pregnancy
    - Heart disease
    - Bleeding diathesis
    - Ingestion of cardiotoxic poison
    - Time lapse of more than 6–8 hours
- *Absolute*:
  - Convulsions, or ingestion of a convulsant poison
  - Impaired gag reflex
  - Coma
  - Foreign body ingestion
  - Corrosive ingestion
  - Ingestion of petroleum distillates, or those drugs which cause altered mental status (phenothiazines, antihistamines, opiates, ethanol, benzodiazepines, and tricyclics)
  - All poisons which are themselves emetic in nature
- *Complications*:
  - Cardiotoxicity (bradycardia, atrial fibrillation, myocarditis)
  - Aspiration pneumonia
  - Esophageal mucosal or Mallory-Weiss tears (due to protracted vomiting).

Other emetics: The only other acceptable method of inducing emesis that is advocated involves the use of *apomorphine*. Given subcutaneously, it causes vomiting within 3–5 minutes by acting directly on the chemoreceptor trigger zone. The recommended dose is 6 mg (adult), and 1–2 mg (child). Since

---

*Not to be confused with *fluid extract of ipecac*, which was formerly used as an amebicide and is very toxic.

apomorphine is a respiratory depressant it is contraindicated in all situations where there is likelihood of CNS depression.

In some cases, *stimulation of the posterior pharynx* with a finger or a blunt object may induce vomiting by provoking the gag reflex. Unfortunately, such mechanically induced evacuation is often unsuccessful and incomplete, with mean volume of vomitus about one-third of that obtained by the other two methods.

Obsolete emetics: The use of *warm saline* or *mustard water* as an emetic is not only dangerous (resulting often in severe hypernatremia), but also impractical since many patients, especially children refuse (fortunately) to drink this type of concoction and much valuable time is lost coaxing them to do so. One tablespoon of salt contains at least 250 mEq of sodium, and if absorbed can raise the serum level by 25 mEq/L in for instance, a 3-year-old child. It is high time that the use of salt water as an emetic be deleted once and for all from every first-aid chart or manual on poisoning.

Copper sulfate induces emesis more often than common salt, but significant elevations of serum copper can occur leading to renal and hepatic damage. It is also a gastrointestinal corrosive.

Zinc sulfate is similar in toxicity to copper sulfate, and has in addition a very narrow margin of safety.

Gastric Lavage (Stomach Wash)

The American Academy of Clinical Toxicology, and the European Association of Poison Centres and Clinical Toxicology have prepared a draft of a position paper directed to the use of gastric lavage, which suggests that gastric lavage should NOT be employed routinely in the management of poisoned patients.[21] There is no certain evidence that its use improves outcome, while the fact that it can cause significant morbidity (and sometimes mortality) is indisputable. Lavage should be considered only if a patient has ingested a life-threatening amount of a poison and presents to the hospital within 1–2 hours of ingestion.

But in India, very often caution is thrown to the wind and the average physician in an average hospital embarks on gastric lavage with gusto the moment a poisoned patient is brought in. A sad commentary on the existing lack of awareness and a reluctance to change old convictions in spite of mounting evidence against the routine employment of such "established procedures". With the advent of Poison Control Centres, and provision of enhanced emphasis on toxicology in the undergraduate medical curriculum framed by the Medical Council of India, there is hope of a change in attitude in the years to come.[22]

- *Indications*: Gastric lavage is recommended mainly for patients who have ingested a life-threatening dose, or who exhibit significant morbidity and present within 1–2 hours of ingestion. Lavage beyond this period may be appropriate only in the presence of gastric concretions, delayed gastric emptying, or sustained release preparations. Some authorities still recommend lavage up to 6–12 hours post-ingestion in the case of salicylates, tricyclics, carbamazepine, and barbiturates.
- *Precautions*:
  - Never undertake lavage in a patient who has ingested a nontoxic agent, or a nontoxic amount of a toxic agent.
  - Never use lavage as a deterrent to subsequent ingestions. Such a notion is barbaric, besides being incorrect.
- *Contraindications*:
  - *Relative*: Hemorrhagic diathesis, esophageal varices, recent surgery, advanced pregnancy, ingestion of alkali, coma.
  - *Absolute*: Marked hypothermia, prior significant vomiting, unprotected airway in coma, and ingestion of acid or convulsant or petroleum distillate, and sharp substances.
- *Procedure*:
  - Explain the exact procedure to the patient and obtain his consent. If refused, it is better not to undertake lavage because it will amount to an assault, besides increasing the risk of complications due to active noncooperation.
  - Endotracheal intubation must be done prior to lavage in the comatose patient.
  - Place the patient head down on his left lateral side (20° tilt on the table).
  - Mark the length of tube to be inserted (50 cm for an adult, 25 cm for a child.).*
  - The ideal tube for lavage is the *lavacuator* (clear plastic or gastric hose).
  - In India, however, the *Ewald tube* **(Fig. 3)** is most often used which is a soft rubber tube with a funnel at one end. Whatever tube is used, make sure that the inner diameter corresponds to at least 36–40 French size.** A nasogastric tube used for gastric aspiration is inadequate and should never be used. In a child, the diameter should be at least 22–28 French, [*Ryle's tube* may be sufficient **(Fig. 4)**].
  - The preferred route of insertion is oral. Passing the tube nasally can damage the nasal mucosa considerably and lead to severe epistaxis.
  - Lubricate the inserting end of the tube with vaseline or glycerine, and pass it to the desired extent. Use a mouth gag so that the patient will not bite on the tube.
  - Once the tube has been inserted, its position should be checked either by air insufflation while listening over

---

*Alternatively, mark off the length corresponding to the distance between the xiphoid process and the bridge of the nose of the patient.
**Each unit on the French scale equals 0.3 mm.

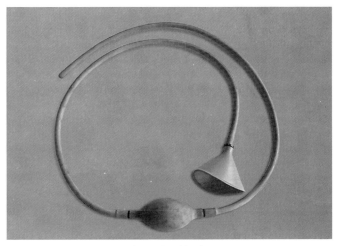

Fig. 3 Ewald tube
Source: Dr Anu Sasidharan

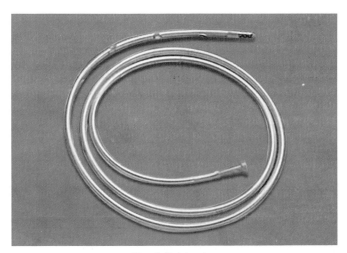

Fig. 4 Ryle's tube

the stomach, or by aspiration with pH testing of the aspirate, (acidic if properly positioned).
- Lavage is carried out using small aliquots (quantities) of liquid. In an adult, 200–300 mL aliquots of warm (38°C) saline or plain water are used. In a child, 10–15 mL/kg body weight of warm saline is used each time. Water should preferably be avoided in young children because of the risk of inducing hyponatremia and water intoxication. It is advisable to hold back the first aliquot of washing for chemical analysis.
- In certain specific types of poisoning, special solutions may be used in place of water or saline **(Table 24)**.
- Lavage should be continued until no further particulate matter is seen, and the efferent lavage solution is clear. At the end of lavage, pour a slurry of activated charcoal in water (1 g/kg), and an appropriate dose of an ionic cathartic into the stomach, and then remove the tube.
- **Complications**:
  - Aspiration pneumonia.*
  - Laryngospasm
  - Sinus bradycardia and ST elevation on the ECG
  - Perforation of stomach or esophagus (rare).

Catharsis

Catharsis is a very appropriate term when used in connection with poisoning, since it means purification. It is achieved by purging the gastrointestinal tract (particularly the bowel) of all poisonous material.

Table 24 Solutions for gastric lavage

Poison	Solution
Most poisons (known or unknown)	Water or saline
Oxidizable poisons (alkaloids, salicylates, etc.)	Potassium permanganate (1:5000 or 1:10000)*
Cyanides	Sodium thiosulfate (25%)
Oxalates	Calcium gluconate
Iron	Desferrioxamine (2 g in 1 L of water)

Controversial; can aggravate the condition of the patient.

The two main groups of cathartics** used in toxicology include:
1. *Ionic or saline*: These cathartics alter physicochemical forces within the intestinal lumen leading to osmotic retention of fluid which activates motility reflexes and enhances expulsion. However, excessive doses of magnesium-based cathartics can lead to hypermagnesemia which is a serious complication.
   The doses of recommended cathartics are as follows:
   - *Magnesium citrate*: 4 mL/kg
   - *Magnesium sulfate*: 30 g (250 mg/kg in a child)
   - *Sodium sulfate*: 30 g (250 mg/kg in a child).
2. *Saccharides*: Sorbitol (D-glucitol) is the cathartic of choice in adults because of better efficacy than saline cathartics,

---

*If this occurs, give hydrocortisone 3–4 mg/kg IV, oxygen as necessary, broad spectrum antibiotics, and arrange for physiotherapy. Treat wheezing with bronchodilators.
**Not the same as laxatives or purgatives! A laxative is an agent which promotes soft formed or semifluid stool within a few hours or days. A cathartic promotes rapid, watery evacuation within 1 to 3 hours. Purgatives induce even stronger evacuation.

but must not be used as far as possible in young children owing to risk of fluid and electrolyte imbalance (especially hypernatremia). It occurs naturally in many ripe fruits and is prepared industrially from glucose, retaining about 60% of its sweetness. Sorbitol is used as a sweetener in some medicinal syrups, and the danger of complications is enhanced in overdose with such medications when sorbitol is used as a cathartic during treatment.

Dose of sorbitol: 50 mL of 70% solution (adult)

Efficacy of catharsis: While cathartics do reduce the transit time of drugs in the gastrointestinal tract, there is no real evidence that it improves morbidity or mortality in cases of poisoning.[23] At present there is no indication for the routine use of cathartics as a method of either limiting absorption or enhancing elimination. A single dose can be given as an adjunct to activated charcoal therapy when there are no contraindications and constipation or an increased gastrointestinal transit time is expected.

Contraindications:
- Corrosives
- Existing electrolyte imbalance
- Paralytic ileus
- Severe diarrhea
- Recent bowel surgery
- Abdominal trauma
- Renal failure.

Oil-based cathartics should never be used in poisoning since they increase the risk of lipoid pneumonia, increase the absorption of fat-soluble poisons, and inactivate medicinal charcoal's effects when administered along with them. The last mentioned reason also applies to conventional laxatives, and hence they are also not recommended in poisoning.

Activated (Medicinal) Charcoal

A number of studies have documented clearly the efficacy of activated charcoal as the sole decontamination measure, while emesis and lavage are increasingly associated with relative futility.[24,25] The remarkable utility of this substance in poisoning was in fact demonstrated dramatically and publicly by the French pharmacist Touery way back in 1930, when he ingested a large dose of strychnine mixed with 15 g of activated charcoal, and suffered no ill effects at all!

But overall, as is true for the other methods of gastrointestinal decontamination, there is a lack of sound evidence of its benefits as defined by clinically meaningful endpoints. This opinion is reflected both in the consensus statements and in the overall trend toward no decontamination as shown in TESS data.[26] The consensus opinion concluded that a single dose of activated charcoal should not be administered routinely in the management of poisoned patients and, based on volunteer studies, the effectiveness of activated charcoal decreased with time, providing the greatest benefit within 1 hour of ingestion.[27] There was no evidence that the administration of a single dose of activated charcoal improved clinical outcome. Additionally, it is generally accepted that unless either airway protective reflexes are intact (and expected to remain so) or the patient's airway has been protected, the administration of activated charcoal is contraindicated.

Activated charcoal is a fine, black, colorless, tasteless powder (**Fig. 5**) made from burning wood, coconut shell, bone, sucrose, or rice starch, followed by treatment with an activating agent (steam, carbon dioxide, etc.). The resulting particles are extremely small, but have an extremely large surface area. Each gram of activated charcoal works out to a surface area of 1,000 square meters. Recently in the USA, a new superactivated charcoal has been introduced in the market with a surface area nearly double the current formulations.

- *Mode of action*: Decreases the absorption of various poisons by adsorbing them on to its surface (**Figs 5 and 6**). Activated charcoal is effective to varying extent, depending on the nature of substance ingested (**Table 25**).

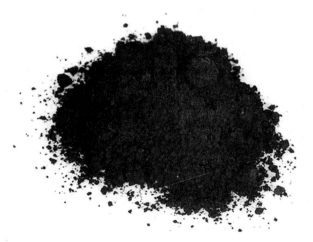

Fig. 5 Activated charcoal

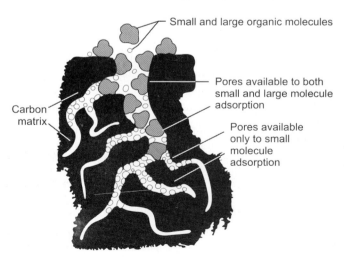

Fig. 6 Activated charcoal (diagrammatic)

Table 25 Adsorption of toxins to activated charcoal

Well adsorbed		Moderately adsorbed	Poorly adsorbed
Aflatoxins	Cimetidine	Antidiabetic drugs	Alcohols
Amphetamines	Dapsone	Kerosene	Carbamates
Antidepressants	Digitalis	Paracetamol	Corrosives
Antiepileptics	NSAIDs	Phenol	Cyanide
Antihistamines	Opiates	Salicylates	Ethylene glycol
Atropine	Phenothiazines		Heavy metals
Barbiturates	Quinine, Quinidine		Hydrocarbons
Benzodiazepines	Strychnine		Organophosphates
Beta-blockers	Tetracycline		
Chloroquine	Theophylline		

Abbreviation: NSAIDs, nonsteroidal anti-inflammatory drugs.

- *Dose*: The optimal activated charcoal dose is theoretically the minimum dose that completely adsorbs the ingested xenobiotic and, if relevant, that maximizes enhanced elimination. The results of *in vitro* studies show that the ideal activated charcoal-to-xenobiotic ratio varies widely, but a common recommendation is to deliver an activated charcoal-to-xenobiotic ratio of 10:1 or 50–100 gram of activated charcoal to adult patients, whichever is greater (1 g/kg of body weight). This amount from a theoretical perspective will adsorb 5–10 gram of a xenobiotic, which should be adequate for most typical poisonings. In children, the recommended dose is 0.5–2 g/kg of body weight.

Add four to eight times the quantity of water to the calculated dose of activated charcoal, and mix to produce a slurry or suspension*. This is administered to the patient after emesis or lavage, or as sole intervention. The slurry should be shaken well before administration.

Multiple-dose activated charcoal: The use of repeated doses (amounting to 150–200 gram of activated charcoal) has been demonstrated to be very effective in the elimination of certain drugs such as theophylline, phenobarbitone, quinine, digitoxin, phenylbutazone, salicylates, carbamazepine, methotrexate, and dapsone. This can be accomplished safely by giving the activated charcoal through a nasogastric tube over 4–8 hours. The actual dose of activated charcoal for multiple dosing has varied considerably in the available medical literature, ranging from 0.25 g/kg–0.5 g/kg every 1–6 hours to 20–60 g for adults every 1, 2, 4, or 6 hours. The total dose administered is more important than frequency of administration. A recent single-blind, randomized, placebo-controlled trial was designed to assess the efficacy of multiple-dose activated charcoal (MDAC) in the treatment of patients with yellow oleander poisoning. This clinical study demonstrated that MDAC (defined as 50 g of activated charcoal every 6 hours for 3 days) effectively reduced life-threatening cardiac dysrhythmias, deaths, and the need for ICU admission.[28]

- *Disadvantages*:
  - Unpleasant taste**
  - Provocation of vomiting
  - Constipation or diarrhea
  - Pulmonary aspiration
  - Intestinal obstruction (especially with multiple-dose activated charcoal)
- *Contraindications*:
  - Absent bowel sounds or proven ileus
  - Small-bowel obstruction
  - Caustic ingestion
  - Ingestion of petroleum distillates.

Whole-bowel Irrigation (Whole-gut Lavage)

This is a method that is being increasingly recommended for late presenting overdoses when several hours have elapsed since ingestion. It involves the instillation of large volumes of a suitable solution into the stomach in a nasogastric tube over a period of 2–6 hours producing voluminous diarrhea. Previously, saline was recommended for the procedure but it resulted in electrolyte and fluid imbalance. Today, special solutions are used such as PEG-ELS (i.e. polyethylene glycol

---

*It does not dissolve in water.
**It is gritty or sand-like in consistency, and has an unappetizing look, being black in color. This has led to many formulations to increase palatability. Bentonite, carboxymethyl cellulose, and starch have been used as thickening agents, while cherry syrup, chocolate syrup, sorbitol, sucrose, saccharin, ice cream, and sherbet have been tried as flavoring agents. However, improvement in palatability and patient acceptance have been negligible.

and electrolytes lavage solution combined together, which is an isosmolar electrolyte solution), and PEG-3350 (high molecular weight polyethylene glycol) which are safe and efficacious, without producing any significant changes in serum electrolytes, serum osmolality, body weight, or hematocrit.

- *Indications*:
  - Ingestion of large amounts of toxic drugs in patients presenting late (>4 hrs postexposure)
  - Overdose with sustained-release preparations
  - Ingestion of substances not adsorbed by activated charcoal, particularly heavy metals
  - Ingestion of foreign bodies such as miniature disk batteries (button cells), cocaine-filled packets (*body-packer syndrome*), etc.
  - *Ingestion of slowly dissolving substances*: Iron tablets, paint chips, bezoars, concretions, etc.
- *Procedure*: Insert a nasogastric tube into the stomach and instil one of the recommended solutions at room temperature, at a rate of 2 L/hr in adults, and 0.5 L/hr in children. The patient should preferably be seated in a commode. The use of metoclopramide IV (10 mg in adults, 0.1–0.3 mg/kg in children) can minimize the incidence of vomiting. The procedure should be continued until the rectal effluent is clear, which usually occurs in about 2–6 hours.

  There is some evidence against the simultaneous administration of activated charcoal with whole-bowel irrigation, since PEG-ELS has been shown to reduce the adsorptive capacity of activated charcoal in vitro.
- *Complications*:
  - Vomiting
  - Abdominal distension and cramps
  - Anal irritation
- *Contradictions*: Gastrointestinal pathology such as obstruction, ileus, hemorrhage, or perforation.

Endoscopy and Surgery

Over the years, a few case reports have presented mixed results for the endoscopic removal of drug packets from the stomach of (cocaine or heroin) body packers.[29] At present, this method is not generally recommended because of concerns about packet rupture. However, under exceptional circumstances, there is certainly a precedent for attempting this procedure in a highly controlled setting such as an ICU or operating room.

In rare cases of massive iron overdoses where emesis, orogastric lavage, and gastroscopy failed, gastrotomy was performed. There are some reports of the successful use of laparoscopic-assisted gastrotomy in the treatment of iron overdose.[30] The significant clinical improvement and postoperative recovery indicated that surgery in these particular cases was the correct approach.

ELIMINATION

Attempts at enhancing of the elimination of a xenobiotic from a poisoned patient are advisable after techniques to inhibit absorption such as gastric lavage, activated charcoal, or whole-bowel irrigation have been accomplished. Of the various methods employed, hemodialysis, hemoperfusion, and hemofiltration are considered extracorporeal therapies because xenobiotic removal occurs in a blood circuit outside the body. These methods are used infrequently because current methods of intensive supportive care keep the overall mortality rate low in poisoned patients who reach the hospital. Because these elimination techniques are not without adverse effects and complications, they are indicated in only a relatively small proportion of patients.

The various methods of eliminating absorbed poisons from the body include the following:
- Alkaline diuresis
- Extracorporeal techniques:
  - Hemodialysis
  - Hemoperfusion
  - Peritoneal dialysis
  - Hemofiltration
  - Plasmapheresis
  - Plasma perfusion
  - Cardiopulmonary bypass.

Indications for Enhanced Elimination

- Patients who fail to respond adequately to full supportive care, e.g. those with intractable hypotension, heart failure, seizures, metabolic acidosis, arrhythmias, etc. Some xenobiotics which can cause such life-threatening toxicity include theophylline, lithium, salicylates, or toxic alcohols.
- Patients in whom the normal route of elimination of the xenobiotic is impaired, e.g. those with renal or hepatic dysfunction.
- Patients in whom the amount of xenobiotic absorbed or its high concentration in serum indicates that serious morbidity or mortality is likely. Xenobiotics in this group include ethylene glycol, lithium, methanol, paraquat, salicylate, and theophylline.
- Patients with concurrent disease or in an age group (very young or old) associated with increased risk of morbidity or mortality from the overdose. An example is a patient with both severe underlying respiratory disease and chronic theophylline poisoning.
- Patients with concomitant electrolyte disorders that could be addressed by hemodialysis. An example is the lactic acidosis associated with metformin toxicity.

ALKALINE DIURESIS

Most drugs taken in overdose are extensively detoxified by the liver to produce inactive metabolites which are voided

in the urine. Sometimes hepatic degradation produces active metabolites, but the secondary compounds are then converted to nontoxic derivatives. Under these circumstances, enhancing diuresis is inappropriate. The procedure should be undertaken only if the following conditions are satisfied:
- A substantial proportion of the drug is excreted unchanged
- The drug is distributed mainly in the extracellular fluid
- The drug is minimally protein-bound.

Principle

Most drugs are weak electrolytes and exist partly as undissociated molecules at physiological pH. The extent of ionization is a function of the ionization constant of the drug (Ka for both acids and bases), and the pH of the medium in which it is dissolved. Ionization constants are usually expressed in the form of their negative logarithm, pKa. Hence the pKa scale is analogous to the pH notation: the stronger an acid the lower its pKa, and the stronger a base the higher its pKa. The relationship between pKa and the proportion of total drug in ionized form is represented by the Henderson-Hasselbalch equation:

$$\text{For weak acids, } pH - pKa = \log \frac{\text{(ionized drug)}}{\text{(nonionized drug)}}$$

$$\text{For weak bases, } pH - pKa = \log \frac{\text{(nonionized drug)}}{\text{(ionized drug)}}$$

Thus, when pKa = pH, the concentrations of ionized and nonionized drugs are equal. Cell membranes are most permeable to substances that are lipid soluble and in the nonionized, rather than the ionized form. Thus, the rate of diffusion from the renal tubular lumen back into the circulation is decreased when a drug is maximally ionized. Because ionization of weak acids is increased in an alkaline environment, and that of basic drugs is increased in an acid solution, manipulation of the urinary pH enhances renal excretion.

Alkaline diuresis is most useful in the case of salicylates, phenobarbitone, chlorpropamide, formate, diflunisal, fluoride, methotrexate, and the herbicide 2,4-dichlorophenoxyacetic acid (2,4-D). These weak acids are ionized at alkaline urine pH and tubular reabsorption is thereby greatly reduced. Alkalinization is achieved by the IV administration of sodium bicarbonate, 1-2 mEq/kg infused over 3-4 hours. The goal is to increase urinary pH to 7-8.

This degree of alkalinization may be difficult if metabolic acidosis and acidemia are present, as often is the case with salicylate poisoning. In this situation, bicarbonate (administered as the sodium salt) is consumed by titration of plasma protons before it can appear in the urine. On the other hand, salicylate poisoning often causes respiratory alkalosis as well. In that case, where partial pressure of carbon dioxide (PCO_2) is low, raising serum bicarbonate, equivalent to the induction of metabolic alkalosis, may lead to profound, life-threatening alkalemia. Finally, the risk of extracellular fluid volume overload with sodium bicarbonate administration is the same as with the administration of 0.9% NaCl. Hypernatremia may also ensue after administration of hypertonic sodium bicarbonate. Urinary excretion of bicarbonate will also be associated with urinary potassium losses, so serum potassium concentration should be monitored frequently and KCl given liberally as long as glomerular filtration rate (GFR) is not impaired. A further complication of alkalemia is a decrease of ionized calcium, which becomes bound by albumin as protons are titrated off serum proteins; if this occurs, tetany may occur. If these complications can be identified and dealt with judiciously and safely, the renal clearance of salicylate can increase fourfold as urine pH increases from 6.5-7.5 with alkalinization.

Increasing urine pH by decreasing proximal tubular bicarbonate reabsorption via administration of carbonic anhydrase inhibitors such as acetazolamide is not recommended. Although elimination of a xenobiotic may be increased, metabolic acidosis will ensue unless ample sodium bicarbonate is also administered.

Alkalinization is also used to increase the solubility of methotrexate and thereby prevent its precipitation in tubules when patients are given high-dose folinic acid rescue therapy. Precipitation of sulfonamide antibiotics with renal stones or renal failure can also be prevented by alkalinization. Extracellular fluid volume expansion with 0.9% NaCl and $NaHCO_3$ administration also protects the kidneys from the toxic effects of myoglobinuria in patients with extensive rhabdomyolysis.

Acid diuresis is no longer recommended for any drug or poison, including amphetamines, strychnine, quinine or phencyclidine.

EXTRACORPOREAL TECHNIQUES

Hemodialysis

Hemodialysis was first used in 1913 in experimental poisoning, but was not applied clinically until 1950, when it was used for the treatment of salicylate overdose. It was widely employed in the subsequent two decades accompanied by much adulatory reportage of its efficacy in medical journals. However, the popularity of hemodialysis has declined since then owing to authentic observation of its lack of utility in several types of poisoning, and the high incidence of complications such as infection, thrombosis, and air embolism.

The principle of hemodialysis is the same as other methods of dialysis; it involves diffusion of solutes across a semipermeable membrane. Hemodialysis utilizes countercurrent flow, where the dialysate flows in the opposite direction to blood flow in the extracorporeal circuit. Countercurrent flow maintains the concentration gradient across the membrane at a maximum and increases the efficiency of the dialysis.

Fluid removal (ultrafiltration) is achieved by altering the hydrostatic pressure of the dialysate compartment, causing free water and some dissolved solutes to move across the membrane along a created pressure gradient.

All drugs are not dialysable, and so it must be ensured before embarking on this procedure that the following conditions are satisfied:[31]
- The substance should be such that it can diffuse easily through a dialysis membrane
- A significant proportion of the substance should be present in plasma water or be capable of rapid equilibration with it
- The pharmacological effect should be directly related to the blood concentration.

Box 5 outlines the various factors in a toxin which can affect the outcome of hemodialysis. Extensive plasma protein binding, insolubility in water, and high molecular weight are the three most important factors in making hemodialysis ineffective.

If the percentage of free drug in the plasma divided by the apparent volume of distribution Vd (per kg body weight) is greater than 80, 6 hours of hemodialysis will remove a significant amount of a drug.[32] But, if this is less than 20, a very insignificant amount is removed.

$$\frac{\% \text{ free drug}}{Vd \text{ (L/Kg)}} > 80 = 20\text{--}50 \text{ \% removed by hemodialysis}$$

$$\frac{\% \text{ free drug}}{Vd \text{ (L/Kg)}} < 20 = 10 \text{ \% removed by hemodialysis}$$

Procedure

In hemodialysis, three primary methods are used to gain access to the blood: (1) an IV catheter, (2) an arteriovenous fistula (AV) or, (3) a synthetic graft. The type of access is influenced by factors such as the expected time course of a patient's renal failure and the condition of his or her vasculature. Catheter access (CVC or central venous catheter), consists of a plastic catheter with two lumens (or occasionally two separate catheters) which is inserted into a large vein (usually the vena cava, via the internal jugular vein or the femoral vein) to allow large flows of blood to be withdrawn from one lumen, to enter the dialysis circuit, and to be returned via the other lumen

The three basic components of hemodialysis are the *blood delivery system*, the *dialyzer* itself, and the *composition and method of delivery of the dialysate*. For acute hemodialysis, catheters are placed in a peripheral vein and passed into the inferior vena cava (**Fig. 7**). Blood from one is pumped to the dialyzer (usually by a roller pump) through lines that contain equipment to measure flow and pressure within the system. Blood returns through the second catheter. The femoral vein is preferable, but subclavian, internal jugular or other peripheral veins are also acceptable, though they have

Box 5 Factors affecting the efficacy of hemodialysis

- Molecular weight
- Charge
- Lipid protein binding
- Volume of distribution
- Tissue binding
- Total body clearance

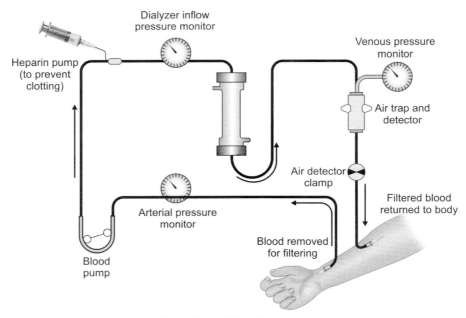

Fig. 7 Hemodialysis (schematic)

slightly higher rates of such complications as pneumothorax and arterial puncture. Hemostasis after catheter removal is also more easily achieved at the femoral site. Dialysis begins at a blood flow rate of 50–100 mL/min, and is gradually increased to 250–300 mL/min, to give maximal clearance. The original dialyzers were of the *coil type*. Later, the flat plate or *kill type* of dialyzer was developed. The most recent type which is becoming increasingly popular is the *hollow fiber*, in which the membrane is spun into fine capillaries.

In poisoned patients, hemodialysis is usually performed for 4–8 hours. Assuming that the patient's serum potassium concentration is normal, a standard bicarbonate-based dialysate with a potassium concentration of 3 or 4 mEq/L and a calcium concentration of 3 mEq/L, flowing at 600–800 mL/min, is sufficient. If dialysis is performed in a dialysis unit, the dialysate is a mixture of a concentrate with $NaHCO_3$ and highly purified water, usually derived by reverse osmosis (RO) or deionization. Dialysis procedures done in intensive care units should use portable RO machines to generate the water for mixing, but in the past tap water has been periodically used.

Indications for Hemodialysis

Hemodialysis may be considered in those patients not responding to standard therapeutic measures while treating a dialyzable toxicant (*vide infra*). It may also be considered a part of supportive care whether the toxicant is dialyzable or not in the following situations: Stage 3 or 4 coma, or hyperactivity caused by a dialyzable agent which cannot be treated by conservative means, marked hyperosmolality which is not due to easily corrected fluid problems, severe acid-base disturbance not responding to therapy, or severe electrolyte disturbance not responding to therapy. Consequently, hemodialysis is preferred for poisonings characterized by these disorders, if clearance rates resulting from hemoperfusion and hemodialysis are relatively similar. Examples include salicylate poisoning which is often associated with metabolic acidosis, and propylene glycol toxicity, which is often associated with lactic acidosis, especially in the presence of renal or hepatic impairment.

- *Best indications*: Dialysis should be initiated, regardless of clinical condition, in the following situations–after heavy metal chelation in patients with renal failure, and following significant ethylene glycol or methanol ingestion.
- *Very good indications*: Dialysis is usually effective in patients with severe intoxications with the following agents:
  - Lithium
  - Phenobarbitone
  - Salicylates
  - Theophylline.
- *Fairly good indications*: Dialysis may be initiated following exposure to the following agents, if clinical condition deems the procedure necessary (patient deteriorating despite intense supportive care)
  - Alcohols
  - Amphetamines
  - Anilines
  - Antibiotics
  - Boric acid
  - Barbiturates (short-acting)
  - Bromides
  - Calcium
  - Chlorates
  - Chloral hydrate
  - Ethanol
  - Iodides
  - Isopropanol
  - Isoniazid
  - Meprobamate
  - Paraldehyde
  - Fluorides
  - Potassium
  - Quinidine
  - Quinine
  - Strychnine
  - Thiocyanates.
- *Poor indications*: Dialysis can be considered as a supportive measure in the presence of renal failure, following exposure to:
  - Paracetamol
  - Antidepressants
  - Antihistamines
  - Belladonna alkaloids
  - Benzodiazepines
  - Digitalis and related glycosides
  - Glutethimide
  - Opiates
  - Methaqualone
  - Phenothiazines
  - Synthetic anticholinergics.

Complications

- *Infection (including AIDS, hepatitis B)*: Nosocomial bacteremia can occur if central lines are left in place for prolonged periods; central lines should be removed after 5 days at most. Femoral venous lines should always be removed in patients who are out of bed.
- Thrombosis
- Hypotension
- Air embolism
- Bleeding (due to use of heparin as a systemic anticoagulant)
- Hemodialysis increases the elimination of some drugs administered therapeutically, such as folic acid and other water-soluble vitamins and antibiotics. Doses of these drugs should be increased during dialysis or administered immediately afterwards.

Table 26 Toxins removed by hemoperfusion (more efficiently than hemodialysis)	
Amanitin	Paracetamol
Barbiturates (all categories)	Paraquat
Carbon tetrachloride	Phenols
Chloral hydrate	Phenylbutazone
Chlorpromazine	Promethazine
Dapsone	Propoxyphene
Diazepam	Quinidine, quinine
Digoxin	Salicylates*
Diphenhydramine	Theophylline
Organophosphates	Tricyclic antidepressants

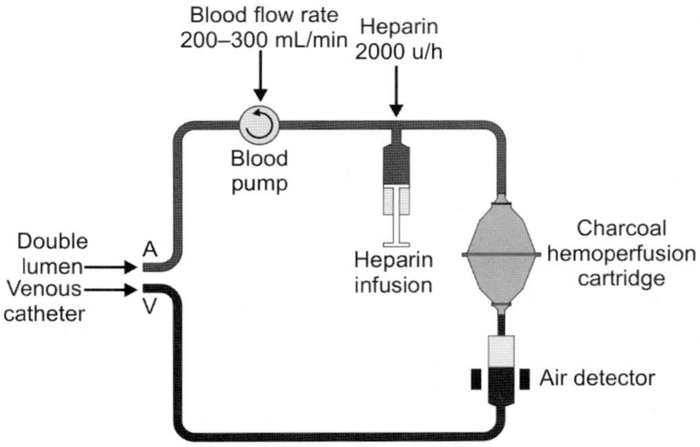

Fig. 8 Hemoperfusion circuit

Hemoperfusion

In general, if a xenobiotic is adsorbed by activated charcoal, charcoal hemoperfusion clearance will exceed that of hemodialysis. Today, the technique is increasingly becoming popular since it is capable of removing many of the toxins that are not removed well by hemodialysis **(Table 26)**.

Procedure

Blood is pumped through a cartridge containing a very large surface area of sorbent, either activated charcoal or carbon. The sorbent is coated with a very thin layer of polymer membrane such as cellulose acetate, heparin-hydrogel, or polyHEMA (2-hydroxyl methacrylate). The membrane prevents direct contact between blood and sorbent, improves biocompatibility, and helps to prevent charcoal embolization. There may be a further theoretical advantage to the heparin-hydrogel coating to diminish platelet aggregation. The adsorptive capacity of the cartridge is reduced with use because of deposition of cellular debris and blood proteins, and saturation of active sites by the xenobiotic in question. Estimation of residual adsorptive capacity by serial serum levels is usually not practical because of time delays in obtaining results. The cartridge should therefore be changed after 2 hours of use. As with hemodialysis, patients must be anticoagulated with heparin, and regional heparinization of the cartridge is possible if full anticoagulation is undesirable. Hemoperfusion is usually performed for 4–6 hours at flow rates of 250–400 mL/min. The characteristics of xenobiotics that make them amenable to hemoperfusion differ from those for hemodialysis in the important respect that hemoperfusion is not limited by plasma protein binding.

The hemoperfusion circuit is shown diagrammatically in **Figure 8**.

Although hemoperfusion has historically been considered the preferred method to enhance the elimination of carbamazepine, phenobarbital, phenytoin, and theophylline, recent improvements in hemodialysis technology, such as high-flux membranes, may make older comparisons of hemodialysis and hemoperfusion clearance rates obsolete.[32] Hemodialysis and hemoperfusion have been performed in series for procainamide, thallium, theophylline, and carbamazepine overdoses, with greater apparent clinical efficacy than with either procedure alone. In this technique, blood circulates first through the hemodialysis membrane, and then through the charcoal cartridge. If blood traverses the dialysis membrane first, some of the xenobiotic is dialyzed, and the activated charcoal cartridge has less drug to adsorb.

Complications

- Bleeding (because of heparinization)
- Air embolism
- Infection
- Thrombocytopenia
- Hypocalcemia
- Hypotension

A new concept in sorbents for poisonings is that of albumin dialysis. The patient's blood flows through a hollow-fiber hemodialyzer. The dialysate bathing the fibers contains human serum albumin that serves as a sorbent to bind the xenobiotic of interest and maintain levels of the free xenobiotic at zero. A steep concentration gradient from blood to dialysate is established so that even highly protein-bound xenobiotics can be removed from the plasma. The membrane is impermeable to albumin which remains in the dialysate. The albumin is reprocessed by passing through an activated charcoal cartridge as well as an anion exchanger so that it can then be recirculated. A current proprietary version of this procedure is called molecular adsorbents recirculating system (MARS), manufactured in Germany by Teraklin. The procedure was used successfully to improve the mortality associated with hepatic encephalopathy and liver failure.[33]

Peritoneal Dialysis

Although widely available, peritoneal dialysis today is almost never recommended for detoxification. In general, it is only 10–25% as effective as hemodialysis, and often only slightly more effective than forced diuresis. It is also time-consuming, requiring 24 hours for successful completion as compared to the 2–4 hours cycles of hemodialysis and hemoperfusion. The only advantages are that it does not require anticoagulation and uses minimal equipment.

Procedure

Peritoneal dialysis works on the same principle as hemodialysis, allowing the diffusion of toxins from mesenteric capillaries across the peritoneal membrane into the dialysate dwelling in the peritoneal cavity. It involves the placing of a stylet catheter at the bedside under local anesthesia, or the surgical insertion of a Tenckhoff catheter in the abdomen. Dialysate fluid is instilled, and 1–2 liters is exchanged each hour.

Complications

- Pain
- Hemorrhage (from vascular laceration)
- Perforation of viscus
- Bacterial peritonitis
- Arrhythmias
- Volume depletion or overload
- Pneumonia
- Pleural effusion
- Hyperglycemia
- Electrolyte imbalance.

Hemofiltration

Hemofiltration is performed similar to hemodialysis except that the blood is pumped through a hemofilter. An arteriovenous pressure difference induces a convective transport of solutes through a hollow-fiber flat-sheet membrane. This allows a substantial flow of plasma water, and a high permeability to compounds with molecular weight less than 40,000. The procedure can be done intermittently at high ultrafiltrate rates of up to 6 L/hr, or continuously at rates of 100 mL/hr (continuous arteriovenous hemofiltration, or CAVH) **(Fig. 9)**. The latter is preferred in the treatment of poisoning. The main advantage of hemodiafiltration is that it can remove compounds of large relative molecular weight (4,500–40,000). Such compounds include aminoglycoside antibiotics and metal chelates (such as iron-desferrioxamine). CAVH is also useful in poisoning with lithium, methanol, ethanol, and ethylene glycol.

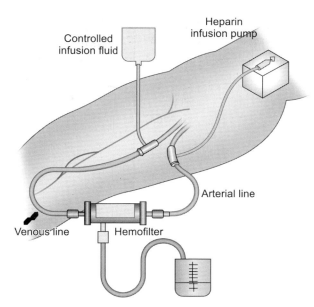

Fig. 9 Continuous arteriovenous hemofiltration

Hemodiafiltration

This is a combination of hemofiltration with hemodialysis. It has been undertaken very rarely, and nothing much is known as to its actual advantages, if any.[34]

Plasmapheresis

Plasmapheresis is a technique of separating cellular blood components from plasma **(Fig. 10)**. The cells are resuspended in either colloids, albumin, or fresh-frozen plasma, and then reinfused. It is very effective in eliminating toxic substances but exacts a heavy toll: a part of the patient's plasma proteins are sacrificed in the process. Plasmapheresis has been used in cases of overdose with theophylline, carbamazepine, amanita, mercury, hemlock, etc. but serious complications greatly limit its utility.

Complications

- *Bleeding disorders*: Disseminated intravascular coagulation (DIC) and thrombocytopenia
- *Hypercoagulation*: Cerebral thrombosis, pulmonary embolism, and myocardial infarction
- Anaphylaxis
- *Fluid overload*: Hypertension and congestive heart failure
- Infection
- Vessel perforation and air embolism
- *Dysequilibrium syndrome*: Vomiting and hypovolemia

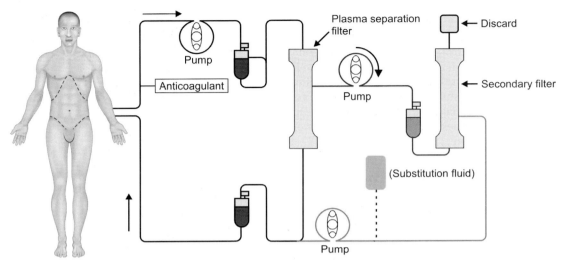

Fig. 10 Plasmapheresis circuit

- *Citrate toxicity*: Paresthesias, tetany, chills, and arrhythmias
- Convulsions
- Metabolic alkalosis.

Plasma Perfusion

This is a combination of plasmapheresis and hemoperfusion, and has rarely been used in poisoning.

Cardiopulmonary Bypass

This is another rarely used experimental procedure in the treatment of poisoning, and has been shown to be useful in certain cases of overdose involving cardiac depressants such as verapamil and lidocaine.[35]

ANTIDOTE ADMINISTRATION

In the majority of cases of acute poisoning, all that is required is intensive supportive therapy with attention to all the details mentioned in the preceding pages of this chapter. Specific antidotes are rarely necessary, besides the fact that only a few genuine antidotes exist in actual practice, though there is no denying the dramatic results that can be achieved with some of them in appropriate circumstances. Proper antidotal therapy can be lifesaving in some situations.

Antidotes work in any one of a number of ways. Common modes of action are as follows:
- *Inert complex formation*: Some antidotes interact with the poison to form an inert complex which is then excreted from the body, e.g. chelating agents for heavy metals, prussian blue for thallium, specific antibody fragments for digoxin, dicobalt edetate for cyanide, etc.
- *Accelerated detoxification*: Some antidotes accelerate the detoxification of a poison, e.g. thiosulfate accelerates the conversion of cyanide to nontoxic thiocyanate, acetylcysteine acts as a glutathione substitute which combines with hepatotoxic paracetamol metabolites and detoxifies them.
- *Reduced toxic conversion*: The best example of this mode of action is provided by ethanol which inhibits the metabolism of methanol to toxic metabolites by competing for the same enzyme (alcohol dehydrogenase).
- *Receptor site competition*: Some antidotes displace the poison from specific receptor sites, thereby antagonizing the effects completely. The best example is provided by naloxone, which antagonizes the effects of opiates at stereospecific opioid receptor sites.
- *Receptor site blockade*: This mode of action is best exemplified by atropine which blocks the effects of anticholinesterase agents such as organophosphates at muscarinic receptor sites.
- *Toxic effect bypass*: An example of this type of antidotal action is provided by the use of 100% oxygen in cyanide poisoning.

Table 27 represents a list of genuine antidotes recommended in toxicological practice today. In addition, there are certain therapeutic agents which are not antidotes as per the accepted definition, but which through their importance and sometimes specific role in the treatment of poisons, border on the concept of "antidotes". **Table 28** represents a list of such substances. Unfortunately in India, cumbersome governmental regulations and a lack of economic incentives for manufacturers have restricted availability of a substantial number of these lifesaving drugs.[36] As a result, doctors still use some substances which are more

Table 27 Specific antidotes

Antidote	Main indication	Other applications
Amyl nitrite	Cyanide	Hydrogen sulfide
Antivenom (snake-polyvalent)	Snakebite due to common cobra, common krait, Russells viper and saw-scaled viper	Related species of snakes
Ascorbic acid	Organic peroxides (osmium)	--------------
Atropine	Cholinergic agents	--------------
Aurintricarboxylic acid (ATA)	Beryllium	--------------
Benzylpenicillin	Amanitins	--------------
β-aminopropionitrile	Acids	--------------
Botulinum antitoxin (ABE-trivalent)	Botulism	--------------
Calcium salts (gluconate, chloride)	Oxalates, fluorides, and ethylene glycol	Calcium antagonists, and hypomagnesemia
L-carnitine	Valproic acid	
Dantrolene	Malignant hyperthermia	Malignant neuroleptic syndrome
Desferrioxamine	Iron, aluminum	Paraquat
Diazepam	Chloroquine	--------------
Dicobalt edetate	Cyanide	--------------
Digoxin-specific antibody fragments (Digibind, Digifab)	Digitalis glycosides	Other cardioactive steroids
Dimercaprol	Arsenic	Copper, gold, and mercury
4-dimethylaminophenol (4-DMAP)	Cyanide	Hydrogen sulfide
EDTA (ethylenediaminetetra acetic acid; calcium disodium edetate or versenate)	Lead	
Ethanol	Methanol, ethylene glycol	--------------
Flumazenil	Benzodiazepines	--------------
Folinic acid (leucovorin)	Methotrexate, methanol	--------------
Glucagon	Beta-blockers	Calcium channel blockers
Glucose	Insulin	--------------
Guanidine	Botulism	--------------
Hydroxocobalamin	Cyanide	--------------
Isoprenaline	Beta-blockers	--------------
Magnesium sulfate (injection)	Cardioactive steroids and hydrofluoric acid	Hypomagnesemia
Methionine	Paracetamol	--------------
4-methylpyrazole (fomepizole)	Ethylene glycol and methanol	Disulfiram, coprin
N-Acetylcysteine	Paracetamol	Amanitin, Other causes of liver failure
N-Acetylpenicillamine	Mercury	--------------
Naloxone	Opiates	Clonidine
Neostigmine	Peripheral anticholinergics	--------------
Octreotide	Oral hypoglycemics	
Oximes	Organophosphates	--------------

Contd...

Contd...

Antidote	Main indication	Other applications
Oxygen	Cyanide, carbon monoxide, hydrogen sulfide	-------------
Oxygen (hyperbaric)	Carbon monoxide	Cyanide, hydrogen sulfide, and carbon tetrachloride
Penicillamine	Copper	Gold, lead, and mercury
Pentetic acid (DTPA)	Radioactive metals	-------------
Phentolamine	Alpha adrenergics	MAOI interactions, cocaine, adrenaline (epinephrine), and ergot alkaloids
Physostigmine	Central anticholinergics	-------------
Phytomenadione (Vitamin K_1)	Coumarin derivatives (especially warfarin)	Anticoagulant rodenticides (especially bromadiolone)
Potassium hexacyanoferrate (Prussian Blue)	Thallium	-------------
Propranolol	Beta-adrenergics	-------------
Protamine sulfate	Heparin	-------------
Pyridoxine (Vitamin B6)	Isoniazid	Ethylene glycol, gyrometrine, and hydrazines
Sodium nitrite	Cyanide	Hydrogen sulfide
Sodium nitroprusside	Ergotism	-------------
Sodium salicylate	Beryllium	-------------
Sodium thiosulfate	Cyanide	Bromate, chlorate, and iodine
Starch	Iodine	
Succimer (DMSA)	Lead, mercury	Arsenic
Tocopherol	Carbon monoxide	Oxygen toxicity
Toluidine blue	Methemoglobinemia	-------------
Trientine (triethylenetetramine)	Copper	-------------
Unithiol (DMPS)	Arsenic	Copper, nickel, lead, cadmium, mercury

Abbreviations: DMSA, dimercaptosuccinic acid; DMPS, 2,3-dimercapto-1-propanesulfonic acid; MAOI, monoamine oxidase inhibitors.

readily available as antidotes, but are generally considered obsolete or even dangerous in Western countries **(Table 29)**. It is imperative that medical professionals strive to phase out these obsolete drugs, while working out strategies to make genuine antidotes more readily available.

NURSING AND PSYCHIATRIC CARE

Nursing Care

This is especially important in comatose patients, and involves the following measures:
- Attention to pressure points to prevent the development of decubitus ulcers—hourly turning, a pillow between the legs, use of a ripple mattress if available, etc.
- In the absence of spontaneous blinking, avoid exposure keratitis by methylcellulose eye drops, and if necessary, secure the eyelids with adhesive tape.
- Change bed linen frequently if it gets soaked with urine or stained with feces.
- Urinary incontinence can be managed with a sheath urinal for a male, but for a female, an indwelling silastic catheter inserted with aseptic precautions is necessary.
- Inhalation of gastric contents is a frequent problem which can lead to pneumonitis. This can be prevented by positioning the patient semiprone with the head slightly dependent, and intubating if necessary.
- Adequate bronchial toilet is essential, with regular aspiration of secretions.

Psychiatric Care

A significant proportion of overdose cases comprise suicide attempts. After medical stabilization, the most important aspect of management consists of psychiatric counseling in order to prevent recurrence of suicide ideation once the patient has been discharged.

Any patient who has taken an overdose or manifests suicidal ideation should get psychosocial assessment and support as early as possible. The initial evaluation can be performed prior to a total clearing of the patient's sensorium, but a final assessment should not be made unless the patient is completely alert. Recognition that the patient is possibly suicidal, with a precise analysis of the potential for suicide, is essential. Carefully analyzing the patient's psychologic state (*depressed, uncooperative, unresponsive, agitated, anxious, violent, or psychotic*) will allow for a realistic appraisal of the psychosocial alternatives with respect to immediate and long-term treatment, disposition, and continued follow-up, or outpatient care.

It is estimated that among adolescents, suicide accounts for a third of all unnatural deaths, while in college students, suicide is the second leading cause of unnatural death.[37] According to one survey, oral ingestions account for 78% of the cases, 13% are inhalational, while 5% are due to parenteral intake.[38] Patients suffering from depression commit suicide 50 times more frequently than the general population. Alcoholics and chronic dialysis patients have a suicide rate six times higher than the population at large. After the age of 40 years, the suicide rate begins to climb, with a dramatic increase after 65 years. Women attempt suicide three times more often than men, but men are more successful by a ratio of 3:1.

Significantly, 75% of all those who commit suicide do so shortly after seeing a doctor. Usually it is the family physician, not a psychiatrist who sees these patients, many of whom clearly need psychiatric support. With prompt recognition and referral, many suicides may be prevented. A patient with a past history of previous suicide attempts, vague health problems of recent onset, recent surgery, alcoholism, drug abuse, and mental unsoundness (especially psychosis), is at high risk. Stress is also a major factor leading to suicide ideation; recent bereavement, loss of a job, financial loss, etc. are well recognized as trigger factors. Hypochondriasis, pessimism, hopelessness, and other signs of depression may signal a potential suicide and should alert the clinician.

Unfortunately, there are a number of misconceptions about suicide. For example, many people believe that those who talk about suicide will never actually commit suicide and those who resort to frequent suicide "gestures" are not really serious. However, studies show that of all those who successfully commit suicide, 80% have threatened to do so in the past, and may have even made previous attempts. It is therefore essential that every patient who talks about suicide

Table 28 Adjunctival antidotes

Agent	Indication
Activated charcoal	For most poisons (Refer Table 25)
Benztropine	Dystonia
Chlorpromazine	Psychotic states
Corticosteroids	Acute allergic reaction, laryngeal edema
Diazepam	Convulsions
Diphenhydramine	Dystonia
Dobutamine	Myocardial depression
Dopamine	Myocardial depression, vascular relaxation
Epinephrine	Anaphylactic shock, cardiac arrest
Furosemide	Fluid retention, left ventricular failure
Glucose	Hypoglycemia
Haloperidol	Psychotic states
Heparin	Hypercoagulability
Lidocaine	Ventricular arrhythmias
Mannitol	Cerebral edema, fluid retention
Methylene blue (1%)	Methemoglobinemia
Noradrenaline (Norepinephrine)	Hypotension
Oxygen	Hypoxia
Pancuronium	Convulsions
Promethazine	Allergic reactions
Salbutamol	Bronchoconstriction
Sodium bicarbonate	Metabolic acidosis

Table 29 Obsolete antidotes

Agent	Indication
Copper sulfate	Phosphorus
Cysteamine	Paracetamol
Diethyldithiocarbamate	Thallium
Fructose	Ethanol
Levallorphan	Opiates
Nalorphine	Opiates
Silibinin	Amanitin
Tocopherol	Paraquat
Universal antidote	Ingested poisons

- Passive physiotherapy may be advisable to prevent stiffness and muscle atrophy.
- Prophylactic antibiotics, if necessary.

or who presents with a suicide gesture no matter how trivial, should be referred to a psychiatrist before leaving the ED.

Today, psychosocial assessment has become an important component in the comprehensive evaluation of toxicologic emergencies. It has to be initiated in every case by interviewing collateral sources (accompanying family members or friends), before talking to the patient himself. Delay in obtaining psychosocial information can have serious consequences, for example, in cases where an overdosed adult patient may have small children who were left unattended.

SPECIAL PRECAUTIONS IN POISONED PREGNANT PATIENT

In general, a successful outcome for both mother and fetus is dependent on optimum management of the mother, and proven effective treatment for a seriously poisoned mother should never be withheld based on concerns regarding the fetus.[39]

- *Physiological issues*: A pregnant woman's total blood volume and cardiac output are raised through the second trimester and into the later stages of the third trimester. This means that signs of hypoperfusion and hypotension will manifest later than they would in a woman who is not pregnant and when they do, uterine blood flow may already be compromised. For these reasons, the possibility of hypotension in the pregnant woman must be more aggressively sought and, if found, more rapidly treated. Maintaining the patient in the left-lateral decubitus position will help prevent supine hypotension resulting from impairment of systemic venous return by compression of the inferior vena cava. The left-lateral decubitus position is also the preferred position for gastric lavage, if deemed necessary. Because the tidal volume is increased in pregnancy, the baseline pCO_2 will normally be lower by approximately 10 mm Hg. Appropriate adjustment for this effect should be made when interpreting arterial blood gas results.
- *Antidotal issues*: In general, antidotes should not be used if the indications for use are equivocal. On the other hand, antidotes should not be withheld if their use may reduce potential morbidity and mortality. Risks and benefits of either decision must be considered.
  - For example, reversal of opioid-induced respiratory depression calls for the use of naloxone, but in an opioid-dependent woman, naloxone can precipitate acute withdrawal, including uterine contractions and possible induction of labor. Very slow, careful, IV titration starting with 0.05 mg naloxone may be indicated, unless apnea is present, cessation of breathing appears imminent, or the partial pressure of oxygen (pO_2) or O_2 saturation is already grossly inadequate. In these instances, naloxone may have to be administered in higher doses (i.e. 0.4–2.0 mg), or assisted ventilation provided, or a combination of assisted ventilation and small doses of naloxone used.
  - A paracetamol overdose is a serious maternal problem when it occurs throughout pregnancy, but the fetus is at greatest risk in the third trimester. Although paracetamol crosses the placenta easily, N-acetylcysteine has somewhat diminished transplacental passage. During the third trimester, when both the mother and the fetus may be at substantial risk from a significant paracetamol overdose, immediate delivery of a mature or viable fetus may need to be considered.
  - In contrast to the situation with paracetamol, the fetal risk from iron poisoning is less than the maternal risk. Because desferrioxamine is a large charged molecule with little transplacental transport, it should never be withheld out of unwarranted concern for fetal toxicity when indicated to treat the mother.
  - Carbon monoxide poisoning is particularly threatening to fetal survival. The normal pO_2 of the fetal blood is approximately 15–20 mm Hg. Oxygen delivery to fetal tissues is impaired by the presence of carboxyhemoglobin, which shifts the oxyhemoglobin dissociation curve to the left, potentially compromising an already fragile balance. For this reason, hyperbaric oxygen (HBO) is recommended for much lower carboxyhemoglobin concentrations in the pregnant, as compared to the nonpregnant woman.

CONCLUSION

The assessment and management of the unknown exposure and poisoning can be diagnostically and therapeutically challenging. The diagnosis may be complicated by the possibility of multiple-drug ingestion. Life-saving supportive care is the priority over the identification of the poison.

The history and physical examination, most of time can provide the clues to the appropriate diagnosis. Poisoning can present with variety of clinical symptoms, including abdominal pain, vomiting, tremor, altered mental status, seizures, cardiac dysrhythmias, and respiratory depression. The drug or toxin can be identified by a careful history, a targeted physical examination, and commonly available laboratory tests.

Consultation with a regional poison center or clinical toxicologist early in the care of poisoned patient can have a profound impact on the management and disposition of such patients. The prognosis and clinical course of recovery of a patient poisoned by a specific agent depends largely on the quality of care delivered within the first few hours in the emergency setting.

REFERENCES

1. Sadananda Naik B, Jyothi CS. Isolated skin lesions without systemic manifestations following kerosene ingestion. J Indian Soc Toxicol. 2007;3(2):21.

2. Pillay VV. Misconceptions about antidotal therapy of poisoning and overdose. Amrita J Med. 2011;7(2):4-11.
3. Lee-Chiong T Jr, Matthay RA. Drug induced pulmonary oedema and acute respiratory syndrome. In: Camus P, Rosenow EC III (Eds). Drug-induced and Iatrogenic Respiratory Disease. Florida: CRC Press, Taylor & Francis Group; 2010.
4. Pillay VV. Comprehensive Medical Toxicology, 2nd edition. Hyderabad, India: Paras Medical Publisher. 2008.
5. Pillay VV. Modern Medical Toxicology, 4th edition. New Delhi: Jaypee Brothers Medical Publishers; 2013.
6. Love JN, Enlow B, Howell JM, et al. Electrocardiographic changes associated with beta-blocker toxicity. Ann Emerg Med. 2002;40:603-10.
7. Hoffman RS, Goldfrank LR. The poisoned patient with altered consciousness: Controversies in the use of a "coma cocktail". JAMA. 1995;274:562-9.
8. Litman RS, Rosenberg H. Malignant hyperthermia: update on susceptibility testing. JAMA. 2005;293(23):2918-24.
9. Chabali R. Diagnostic use of anion and osmolal gaps in pediatric emergency medicine. Pediatr Emerg Care. 1997;13(3):204-10.
10. Ellenhorn MJ. Medical Toxicology: Diagnosis and Treatment of Human Poisoning, 2nd edition. 1997. Baltimore: Williams and Wilkins; 1997. p. 49.
11. Wrenn K. The Delta gap. An approach to mixed acid-base disorders. Ann Emerg Med. 1990;19(11):1310-3.
12. Purssell RA, Lynd LD, Koga Y. The use of the osmole gap as a screening test for the presence of exogenous substances. Toxicol Rev. 2004;23(3):189-202.
13. Aabakken L, Johnsen KS, Rydningen EB, et al. Osmolal and anion gaps in patients admitted to an emergency medical department. Hum Exp Toxicol. 1994;13(2):131-4.
14. Mofenson HC, Carraccio TR. The agitated, violent, or acutely psychotic patient. PP/T Review Nassau County Medical Centre Regional Poison Control Centre. 1992;11:301-6.
15. Pillay VV. Adverse neuropsychiatric effects of therapeutic drugs. J Applied Med. 1997;23:385-90.
16. Plotz PH, Rider LG, Targoff IN, et al. Myositis – immunologic contributions to understanding cause, pathogenesis, and therapy. Ann Intern Med. 1995;122:715-25.
17. Sabaawi M, Holmes TF, Fragala MR. Drug induced akathisias: subjective experience and objective findings. Milit Med. 1994;159(4):286-91.
18. Material Safety Data Sheet. De-Solv-It Solution. (2011). [online] Available from *http://www.rcr.com.au/media/pdf/desolvit_datasheet.pdf*. [Accessed February, 2017].
19. Bond GR. The role of activated charcoal and gastric emptying in gastrointestinal decontamination: A state-of-the-art review. Ann Emerg Med. 2002;39(3):273-86.
20. American Academy of Pediatrics Committee on Injury, Violence, and Poison Prevention: Poison treatment in the home. Pediatrics. 2003;112(5):1182-5.
21. Vale A. Gastric lavage. In: Proceedings, Meeting of American Academy of Clinical Toxicology; European Association of Poison Centres and Clinical Toxicologists, and American Academy of Poison Control Centres. Vienna; 1994.
22. Sharma BR, Harish D, Sharma AK, et al. Management of toxicological emergencies at different health care levels – A comparative study. J Indian Soc Toxicol. 2005;1(2):23-30.
23. Albertson TE, Owen KP, Sutter ME, et al. Gastrointestinal decontamination in the acutely poisoned patient. Int J Emerg Med. 2011;4:65.
24. Christophersen AB, Levin D, Hoegberg LC, et al. Activated charcoal alone or after gastric lavage: A simulated large paracetamol intoxication. Br J Clin Pharmacol. 2002;53:312-7.
25. Thakore S, Murphy N. The potential role of prehospital administration of activated charcoal. Emerg Med J. 2002;19:63-5.
26. Chyka PA, Seger D. Position statement: single-dose activated charcoal. American Academy of Clinical Toxicology; European Association of Poisons Centres and Clinical Toxicologists. J Toxicol Clin Toxicol. 1997;35:721-41.
27. Kulig K. Initial management of ingestion of toxic substances. N Engl J Med. 1992;326:1677-81.
28. de Silva HA, Fonseka MM, Pathmeswaran A, et al. Multiple-dose activated charcoal for treatment of yellow oleander poisoning: A single-blind, randomised, placebo-controlled trial. Lancet. 2003;361:1935-8.
29. Choudhary AM, Taubin H, Gupta T, et al. Endoscopic removal of a cocaine packet from the stomach. J Clin Gastroenterol. 1998;27:155-6.
30. Haider F, De Carli C, Dhanani S, et al. Emergency laparoscopic-assisted gastrotomy for the treatment of an iron bezoar. J Laparoendosc Adv Surg Tech. 2009;19(Suppl 1):141-3.
31. Engbersen R, Kramers C. Enhanced extracorporeal elimination of valproic acid in overdose. Netherlands J Med. 2004;62(9):307-8.
32. Palmer BF. Effectiveness of hemodialysis in the extracorporeal therapy of phenobarbital overdose. Am J Kidney Dis. 2000;36:640-3.
33. Mitzner SR, Stange J, Klammt S, et al. Extracorporeal detoxification using the molecular adsorbent recirculating system for critically ill patients with liver failure. J Am Soc Nephrol. 2001;12(Suppl 17):S75-S82.
34. Bellomo R, Kearly Y, Parkin G, et al. Treatment of life threatening lithium toxicity with continuous arteriovenous haemodiafiltration. Crit Care Med. 1991;19:836-7.
35. Carmona MJC, Pereira VA, Malbouisson LMS, et al. Effect of cardiopulmonary bypass on the pharmacokinetics of propranolol and atenolol. Braz J Med Biol Res. 2009;42(6):574-81.
36. Pillay VV. Toxicology sans antidotes: The grim Indian scenario. J Karnataka Medicolegal Soc. 1998;7(1):11-6.
37. Ernst DC. The suicidal patient. Top Emerg Med. 1992;14:45-55.
38. Andrzejowski JC, Myint Y. The management of acute poisoning. Br J Intensive Care. 1998:97-102.
39. Pillay VV. Maternal and foetal poisoning: A new dimension to toxicology. J Applied Med. 1994;20(8):619-20.

APPENDIX

GLASGOW COMA SCALE

The *Glasgow coma scale* or *GCS* is a neurological scale which aims to give a reliable, objective way of recording the conscious state of a person, for initial as well as subsequent assessment. A patient is assessed against the criteria of the scale, and the resulting points give a patient score between 3 (indicating deep unconsciousness) and 15 (relatively normal). GCS was initially used to assess level of consciousness after head injury, and the scale is now used by first aid, emergency medical services (EMS) and doctors as being applicable to all acute medical and trauma patients **(Table A1)**.

The scale comprises three tests: eye, verbal, and motor responses. The three values separately as well as their sum are considered. The lowest possible GCS (the sum) is 3 (deep coma or death), while the highest is 15 (fully awake person).

- *Best eye response (E)*: There are four grades starting with the most severe:
  1. No eye opening
  2. Eye opening in response to pain (*patient responds to pressure on the patient's fingernail bed; if this does not elicit a response, supraorbital and sternal pressure or rub may be used*)
  3. Eye opening to speech
  4. Eyes opening spontaneously.
- *Best verbal response (V)*: There are five grades starting with the most severe:
  1. No verbal response
  2. Incomprehensible sounds (*moaning, but no words*)
  3. Inappropriate words (*random speech, but no conversational exchange*)
  4. Confused (*patient responds to questions coherently but there is some disorientation and confusion*).
  5. Oriented (*patient responds coherently and appropriately to questions such as the patient's name and age, where they are and why, the year, month, etc.*).
- *Best motor response (M)*: There are six grades starting with the most severe:
  1. No motor response
  2. Extension to pain (*abduction of arm, internal rotation of shoulder, pronation of forearm, and extension of wrist-decerebrate response*)
  3. Abnormal flexion to pain (*adduction of arm, internal rotation of shoulder, pronation of forearm, and flexion of wrist-decorticate response*)
  4. Flexion or withdrawal to pain (*flexion of elbow, supination of forearm, flexion of wrist when supraorbital pressure applied; pulls part of body away when nailbed pinched*)
  5. Localizes to pain (*purposeful movements towards painful stimuli; e.g. hand crosses midline and gets above clavicle when supraorbital pressure applied*)
  6. Obeys commands (*patient does simple things as asked*).
- *Interpretation*: Individual elements as well as the sum of the score are important. Hence, the score is expressed in the form "GCS 9 = E2 V4 M3 at 07:35".

Generally, brain injury is classified as:
- *Severe*: GCS less than or equal to 8
- *Moderate*: GCS 9–12
- *Minor*: GCS greater than or equal to 13.

The GCS has limited applicability to children, especially below the age of 36 months (where the verbal performance of even a healthy child would be expected to be poor). Consequently the *Pediatric GCS*, a separate yet closely related scale, was developed for assessing younger children.

Table A1 Glasgow coma scale

Feature observed	Score
Eye opening	
• Spontaneous	E4
• To speech	3
• To pain	2
• Nil	1
Best motor response	
• Obeys	M6
• Localizes	5
• Flexes (withdrawal)	4
• Flexes abnormally (decorticate rigidity)	3
• Extends (decerebrate rigidity)	2
• Nil	1
Best verbal response	
• Oriented	V5
• Confused conversation	4
• Inappropriate words	3
• Incomprehensible sounds	2
• Nil	1

FURTHER READING

1. Pillay VV. Comprehensive Medical Toxicology, 2nd edition. Hyderabad, India: Paras Medical Publisher; 2008.
2. Teasdale G, Jennett B. Assessment of coma and impaired consciousness. A practical scale. Lancet. 1974;2:81-4.

CHAPTER 93

Organophosphate and Carbamate Insecticides Poisoning

VV Pillay

PESTICIDES

Pesticides are compounds that are used to kill or repel pests which may be insects, rodents, fungi, nematodes, mites, ticks, molluscs, and unwanted weeds or herbs. They include substances which prevent, destroy, repel, or mitigate any pest, or are used as a plant regulator, defoliant, or desiccant.

CLASSIFICATION

- *Insecticides*: Compounds which kill or repel insects and related species, e.g. organophosphates, carbamates, organochlorines, diethyltoluamide (DEET), and pyrethrum and its derivatives (pyrethroids).
- *Rodenticides*: Compounds which kill rats, mice, moles, and other rodents, e.g. anticoagulants (bromadiolone), thallium, vacor, phosphorus, alpha-naphthyl-thiourea (ANTU), cholecalciferol, arsenic, barium carbonate, bromethalin, fluoroacetamide, sodium monofluoroacetamide, red squill, strychnine, and zinc phosphide.
- *Herbicides*: Compounds which kill weeds, e.g. acrolein, dalaphon, glyphosate, paraquat, diquat, atrazine, propazine, simazine, nitrofen, trichloroacetic acid, and chlorophenoxy compounds.
- *Fungicides*: Compounds which kill fungi and moulds, e.g. thiocarbamates, captan, captafol, bavistin, vitavax, hexachlorobenzene, and sodium azide.
- *Nematicides*: Compounds which kill nematodes (i.e. worms), e.g. ethylene dibromide.
- *Acaricides*: Compounds which kill mites, ticks and spiders, e.g. azobenzene, chlorobenzilate, tedion, and kelthane.
- *Molluscicides*: Compounds which kill molluscs such as snails and slugs, e.g. metaldehyde.
- *Fumigants*: Methyl bromide, phosphine, aluminum phosphide, naphthalene, paradichlorobenzene, dichloropropene, and hydrogen cyanide.
- *Miscellaneous pesticides*: Neonicotinoid compounds, phthalic acid diamides (flubendiamide),[1] compounds of lead, copper and mercury, nicotine, rotenone, sabadilla, tetrachloroethylene, trichloroethane, dinitrophenol, dinitrocresol, dinitrobutylphenol, pentachlorophenol, chlorfenson, chloralose and fipronil. Dioxins, which are present as contaminants of some herbicides, also can produce toxicity.

In this chapter, only organophosphorus compound (organophosphate) and carbamate insecticide poisoning will be discussed.

ORGANOPHOSPHORUS INSECTICIDE POISONING

Organophosphorus insecticides (hence forth referred to as organophosphates for the sake of convenience) are among the most popular and most widely used insecticides in India. **Table 1** lists common varieties along with respective brand names.

Physical Appearance

These compounds are available as dusts, granules, or liquids. Some products need to be diluted with water before use, and some are burnt to make smoke that kills insects.

Usual Fatal Dose

*Toxicity Rating**

The following compounds are extremely toxic (*LD50: 1–50 mg/kg*), or highly toxic (*LD50: 51–500 mg/kg*)–Chlorfenvinphos,

---
*Partly as per the Insecticide Rules, 1971.

Table 1 Common organophosphate compounds	
Generic name	Brand name
Acephate	Acemil, Acet, Acetaf, Agrophate, Asataf, Dhanraj, Hilfate, Hythane, Orthene, Ortran, Sicothene, Starthene, Torpedo
Anilofos	Aniloguard, Arozin, Dhanudan
Chlorfenvinphos	Birlane, Chlorfenvinphos
Chlorpyrifos	Agrofas 20, Calban, Chlorofos 20, Classic, Coroban, Cyfos, Daspan, Dermite, Dermot, Dhanuchlor, Dhanvan, Dursban, Force, Gilphos, Hildan, Hyban 20, Lasso, Lethal, Nuchlor, Phors 20, Primaban, Radar, Roban, Ruban 20, Sicobon, Strike, Suchlor, Tafaban, Tefaban, Tricel
Cyclopyriphos	Duramet
Demeton methyl	Metasostox
Diazinon	Agroziron, Basudin, Bazanon, Ditaf, Suzinon, Tik 20, Zionosul 50
Dichlorvos	Agrovan 76, Agro 76 EC, Bangvas, Cockroach killer, Dash, DDVP, Divap, Divisol, Madhuvun, Nuvan, Nuvasul 76, Paradeep, Savious, Vapona, Vapox, Vegfru
Dimethoate	Agrodimet 30, Agromet 30EC, Bangor 30EC, Corothate, Cropgor 30, Cycothate, Cygon, Devigor, Dimethoate, Dimex, Entogor, Hexagor, Hygro 30, Klex Dimethoate, Krogar, Methovip, Milgor, NB Dimethoate, Paragor, Parrydimate, Primogor, Ramgor, Rogor, Tagor, Tara 909, Tara Dimex Sulgor, Tka 30, Unigor, Vijaygor, Vikagor
Ediphenphos	Hinosan, Nukil
Ethion	Challenge, Demite, Dhanumit, Dhan-unit, Ethion, Ethione, Ethiosul 50, Fosmit, Mit 505, Mitex, Miticil, Mitvip, Phostech, RP-thion, Tafethion, VegFru Fosmite, Volathin
Fenitrothion	Accothion, Agrothion, Danathion, Fenicol, Fenitrosul, Folithion, Sicothoin, Sumithion, Vikathion
Fenthion	Agrocidin, Baytex, Fenthiosul, Labaycid, Lebaycid, Lebazate
Formothion	Anthio
Iprobenfos	Tagkite
Malathion	Agromal, Bharat, Celthion, Cython, Dhuthione, Finit, Himalaya, Kathion, Licel, Madhuthione, Maladan, Maladol, Malafil, Malathione, Malazene, Primothion, Sulmathion, VegFru Malatox
Methyl parathion	Antirepellant,* Agropara, Agrotex, Ekatox, Folidol, Folidol-M, Harvest Kempar, Kilex-M, Metacid, Metapar, Metpar, Milphor, Paracrop, Paradol, Parahit, Parataf, VegFru Paratox
Monocrotophos	Atom, Azodrin, Balwan, Corophos, Entophos, Hilcrone, Luphos, Macrophos, Microphos, Monocil, Monochrovin, Monochrome, Monocron, Monocrown, Monocyl, Monodhan, Monokem, Monostar, Monovip, Nuvacron, Phoskill, Sicocil, Sufos, Unicron
Oxydemeton methyl	Dhanuciytax, Hexasystox, Hymox, Knock Out, Metaciyta, Metasystox
Phenthoate	Agrofen, Delsan, Elsan, Guard, Phentox
Phorate	Anuphorate, Croton, Dhan, Dhang, Dragnet, Fortan, Glorat, Luphate, Phorachem, Phoratox, Phrotax, Thimate 10G, Thimet, VegFru Foratox, Vijayphor, Volphor
Phosalone	Zolone
Phosmet	Phosmite
Phosphamidon	Agromidon 85, Bangdon 85, Bilcran 85, Cildon, Delphamidon, Demacron, Demecron, Dimecron, Directon, Eagle, Entecron 85, Hildon, JK Midon, Midon, Phamidon, Phosul, Rilon, Sudon, Sumidon, Vimidon
Phoxim	Phoxin
Primiphos methyl	Acetellic
Profenfos	Carina, Curacrone, Polytrine, Profex
Quinalphos	Agroquin, Agroquinol, Bayrusil, Chemlox, Coroqueen, Dhanulux, Dyalux, Ekalux, Fact, Flash, Kilex, Quenguard, Quick, Quinal, Quinaltof, Quinseed 25, Silofos, Solux, Vazara, Vikalux
Temephos	Abate 50EC, Farmico's
Thiometon (Morphothion)	Agrothimeton, Ekatin
Triazophos	Hostathion, Sutathion, Triphos, Truso
Trichlorphon	Dipterex

*Caution: The same brand name may refer to lindane.

Chlorpyriphos, Demeton, Diazinon, Dichlorvos, Dimethoate, Disulfoton, Edifenphos, Ethion, Fenitrothion, Fensulfothion, Fenthion, Fonophos, Formothion, Methyl Parathion, Mevinphos, Monocrotophos, Oxydemeton Methyl, Phenthoate, Phorate, Phosphamidon, Quinalphos, tetraethyl pyrophosphate (TEPP), and Thiometon.

The following compounds are moderately toxic (*LD50: 501–5,000 mg/kg*), or slightly toxic (*LD50: more than 5,000 mg/kg*)—Abate, Acephate, Coumaphos, Crufomate, Famphur, Malathion, Phenthoate, Primiphos Methyl, Ronnel, Temephos, Triazophos, and Trichlorphon.

Even in cases where treatment was begun early with atropine and oximes, mortality in organophosphate poisoning is generally to the extent of 7–12%.[2]

Toxicokinetics

Organophosphorus compounds are very well absorbed from the lungs, gastrointestinal (GI) tract, skin, mucous membranes, and conjunctiva following inhalation, ingestion, or topical contact. Even percutaneous exposure can cause severe toxicity. The difficulty in removing these compounds from the skin and clothing may explain some chronic poisonings, and inadequate skin and respiratory protection during pesticide application is responsible for most of the remainder. Most organophosphate insecticides are lipophilic. Adipose tissue gradually accumulates the highest levels. Cholinergic crisis may recur in patients when unmetabolized organophosphate agents are mobilized from fat stores. The more lipophilic compounds such as fenthion and chlorfenthion are particularly likely to cause this phenomenon.

Peak levels of most organophosphate insecticides are measured around 6 hours after oral ingestion in man. Although serum half-lives of these compounds range from minutes to hours, prolonged absorption or redistribution from fat stores may allow for measurement of circulating insecticide concentrations for up to 48 days.

Organophosphorus insecticides are metabolized by various mixed function oxidases in the liver and intestinal mucosa, though the exact pathways are not yet clearly understood. The phosphorylating ability of these substances is lost when any of the side chains are hydrolyzed. Certain indirect-acting compounds are activated to a more toxic compound by this initial metabolism. Particularly lipophilic organophosphate compounds may be protected from metabolism by fat storage, markedly prolonging their elimination half-life. Inactive metabolites of these compounds are excreted in the urine.

Recent studies have suggested possible relationship between human serum paraoxonase (PON) activity and susceptibility to acute and chronic effects of organophosphate poisoning.[3] Paraoxonase is an A-esterase that can hydrolyze the active (oxon) metabolites of some organophosphate compounds. Some animal models of organophosphate poisoning demonstrate protection from toxicity when exogenous PON is administered, and greater susceptibility to poisoning when enzyme-deficient animals are exposed. Some authors have postulated that genetic polymorphisms in human PON activity may lead to variations in interindividual susceptibility to some organophosphate insecticides.[4]

Mode of Action (Figs 1 and 2)

Organophosphates are powerful inhibitors of acetylcholinesterase which is responsible for hydrolysing acetylcholine to choline and acetic acid after its release and completion of function (i.e. propagation of action potential). As a result, there is accumulation of acetylcholine with continued stimulation of local receptors and eventual paralysis of nerve or muscle.* Although organophosphates differ structurally from acetylcholine, they can bind to the acetylcholinesterase molecule at the active site and phosphorylate the serine moiety. When this occurs, the resultant conjugate is infinitely more stable than the acetylcholine-acetylcholinesterase conjugate, although endogenous hydrolysis does occur. Depending on the amount of stability and charge distribution, the time to hydrolysis is increased. Phosphorylated enzymes degrade very slowly over days to weeks, making the acetylcholinesterase essentially inactive.

Figure 3 represents the basic formula for organophosphorus compounds. The "X" or "leaving group" determines the main characteristics of the compound and is useful in classifying organophosphates into four main groups:

1. *Group 1*: Compounds contain a quaternary nitrogen at the X position and are called phosphorylcholines. These chemicals originally developed as chemical warfare agents are powerful cholinesterase inhibitors and can also directly stimulate cholinergic receptors, because of their structural resemblance to acetylcholine (ACh). Example—echothiophate iodide.
2. *Group 2*: Compounds are called fluorophosphates because they possess a fluorine molecule as the leaving group. Like group 1 compounds, these compounds are volatile and highly toxic, making them also well suited for chemical warfare. Examples—dimefox, sarin, mipafox.
3. The leaving group of group 3 compounds is a cyanide molecule or a halogen other than fluorine. Examples, cyanophosphates such as tabun.
4. The fourth group is the broadest and comprises various subgroups based on the configuration of the R_1 and R_2

---

*Acetylcholine is the neurotransmitter at pre- and postganglionic parasympathetic synapses, sympathetic preganglionic synapses, and at the neuromuscular junction.

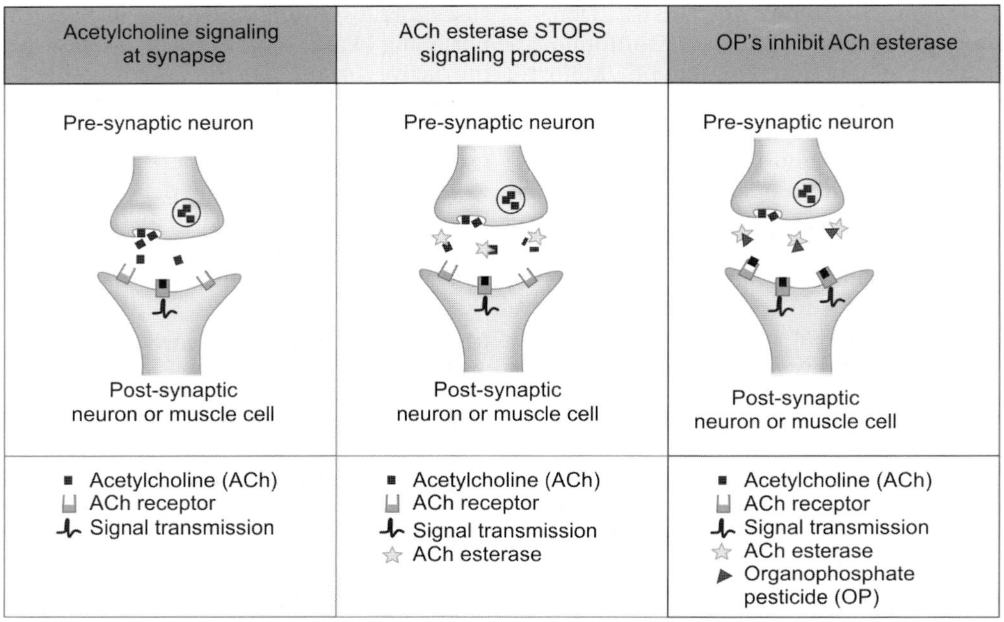

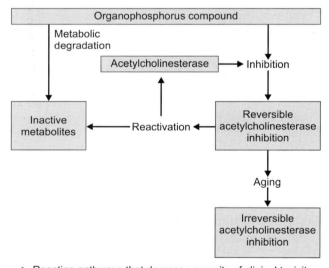

Fig. 1 Mode of action—organophosphate pesticides

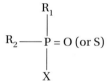

Fig. 3 Basic formula of organophosphate compound

Fig. 2 Organophosphates: Reaction pathways

→ Reaction pathways that decrease severity of clinical toxicity
→ Reaction pathways that induce or prolong clinical toxicity by acetylcholinesterase inhibition
Reactivation occurs spontaneously, which can be increased by administration of an oxime

groups with the majority falling into the category of either a dimethoxy or diethoxy compound. Most of the insecticides in use today fall into this last class.
- *Leaving group*:
  - *Dimethoxy*: Azinphos-menthyl, bromophos, chlorothion, crotoxyphos, dicapthon, dichlorvos, dicrotophos, dimethoate, fenthion, malathion, mevinphos, parathion-methyl, phosphamidon, temephos, and trichlorfon
  - *Diethoxy*: Carbophenothion, chlorfenvinphos, chlorpyriphos, coumaphos, demeton, diazinon, dioxathion, disulfoton, ethion, methosfolan, parathion, phorate, phosfolan, and TEPP
  - *Other dialkoxy*: Isopropyl paraoxon and isopropyl parathion
  - *Diamino*: Schradan
  - *Chlorinated and other substituted dialkoxy*: Haloxon
  - *Trithioalkyl*: Merphos
  - *Triphenyl and substituted triphenyl*: Triorthocresyl phosphate (TOCP)
  - *Mixed substituent*: Crufomate and cyanofenphos.

Direct-acting organophosphate insecticides can inhibit acetylcholinesterase (AChE) without being structurally altered by the body. However, many organophosphates, such as parathion and malathion, are "indirect" inhibitors or prodrugs requiring partial metabolism (to paraoxon and malaoxon, respectively) within the body to become active.

Most of the indirect inhibitors undergo desulfuration in the intestinal mucosa and liver following absorption to form the more active phosphate or "oxon" metabolites. The active form is a more potent cholinesterase inhibitor. The covalent bond is completed as the leaving group of the organophosphates insecticide is split off by AChE, resulting in a stable but reversible bond between the remaining substituted phosphate of the organophosphates compound and AChE, effectively inactivating the enzyme. Although the splitting of the choline-enzyme bond in normal ACh metabolism is completed within microseconds, the severing of the organophosphates compound-enzyme bond can be prolonged. In organophosphates poisoning, the complex becomes irreversibly bound during the next 24–72 hours when one of the R groups leaves the phosphate molecule. This step is termed "aging".[5] As this occurs, the enzyme can no longer spontaneously hydrolyse and becomes permanently inactivated.[6] De novo synthesis of AChE is required to replenish its supply once aging has occurred.

Apart from acetylcholinesterase, organophosphates exert powerful inhibitory action over other carboxylic ester hydrolases such as chymotrypsin, plasma cholinesterase (pseudocholinesterase), hepatic carboxylesterase, paraoxonases, and other nonspecific proteases. It has been proposed that delayed peripheral neuropathy caused by organophosphates is due to phosphorylation of some esterase(s) other than acetylcholinesterase, such as neurotoxic esterase, also known as neuropathy target esterase (NTE). Neuropathy caused by inhibition of NTE may develop 2–5 weeks after an acute poisoning.[7]

Clinical Features

Acute Poisoning

Patients with massive ingestions can become symptomatic very quickly, sometimes within 5 minutes following ingestion, and deaths have occurred within 15 minutes of ingestion. Most victims however become symptomatic in about 8 hours of exposure and virtually all within 24 hours. Delays usually occur with compounds requiring metabolic activation, such as malathion or highly lipid-soluble agents such as fenthion. Symptoms may last for variable periods of time, again based on the exact compound and the nature of the exposure. For example, lipophilic compounds such as dichlofenthion can cause cholinergic excess for several days following ingestion.

*Cholinergic excess**: Muscarinic effects (hollow organ parasympathetic manifestations):

Common manifestations include bronchoconstriction with wheezing and dyspnea, cough, pulmonary edema, vomiting, diarrhea, abdominal cramps, increased salivation, lacrimation, and sweating, bradycardia, hypotension, miosis, and urinary incontinence. Excessive salivation, nausea, vomiting, abdominal cramps, and diarrhea are common muscarinic effects, and have been reported even following the cutaneous absorption of organophosphate. Bradycardia and hypotension occur following moderate-to-severe poisoning. Bronchorrhea can be so profuse that it mimics pulmonary edema even when the lungs are not edematous.

Nicotinic effects (autonomic ganglionic and somatic motor effects due to stimulation of nicotinic adrenal receptors and postganglionic sympathetic fibers): Fasciculations, weakness, hypertension, tachycardia, and paralysis. Mydriasis has been reported in as many as 13% of cases, presumably from nicotinic stimulation of sympathetic receptors.[8] Muscle weakness, fatiguability, and fasciculations are very common.

Hypertension can occur in up to 20% of patients.[9] Tachycardia is also common. Cardiac arrhythmias and conduction defects have been reported in severely poisoned patients. ECG abnormalities may include sinus bradycardia or tachycardia, atrioventricular and/or intraventricular conduction delays, idioventricular rhythm, multiform premature ventricular extrasystoles, ventricular tachycardia or fibrillations, torsades de pointes, prolongation of the PR, QRS, and/or QT intervals, ST-T wave changes, and atrial fibrillation.

Bronchodilation and urinary retention can occur as a result of sympathetic activity on smooth muscle.

Rarely, patients may present only with paralysis from nicotinic effects without any other initial signs and symptoms suggestive of organophosphate toxicity.[10] This is more common with chemical warfare organophosphate compounds (sarin, tabun, soman, etc.).

Central nervous system (CNS) effects: Restlessness, headache, tremor, drowsiness, delirium, slurred speech, ataxia, and convulsions. Coma supervenes in the later stages. In a review of 16 cases of pediatric organophosphate poisoning, all 16 children developed stupor and/or coma.[11]

Death usually results from respiratory failure due to weakness of respiratory muscles, as well as depression of central respiratory drive.[12] Acute lung injury (noncardiogenic pulmonary edema) is a common manifestation of severe poisoning. Acute respiratory insufficiency, due to any combination of CNS depression, respiratory paralysis, bronchospasm, acute respiratory distress syndrome (ARDS), or increased bronchial secretions, is the main cause of death in acute organophosphate poisonings.[13] Metabolic acidosis has occurred in severe poisonings.[14]

---

*Two mnemonics which help in remembering the main manifestations are 1. DUMBELS—**D**iarrhea, **U**rination, **M**iosis, **B**ronchospasm, **E**mesis, **L**acrimation, **S**alivation; 2. SLUDGE and the Killer Bees—**S**alivation, **L**acrimation, **U**rination, **D**iarrhea, **G**astric distress, **E**mesis and **B**ronchospasm, **B**ronchorrhea and **B**radycardia.

A characteristic kerosene—like odor is often perceptible in the vicinity of the patient since the solvent used in many organophosphate insecticides is some petroleum derivative such as aromax.

The Peradeniya Organophosphorus Poisoning (POP) Scale is predictive of death, necessity for mechanical ventilation, and the required total atropine dose over the first 24 hours.[15] This scale rates 5 clinical variables, each on a 0 to 2 scale: miosis, muscle fasciculations, respirations, bradycardia, and level of consciousness.

It is important to note that:

- In a given case, there may be either tachycardia or bradycardia; hypotension or hypertension.
- Miosis while being a characteristic feature may not be apparent in the early stages. In fact mydriasis is very often present, and hence treatment should not be delayed if there is absence of pupillary constriction.[16,17] Blurred vision may persist for several months.
- Ocular exposure can result in systemic toxicity. It can cause persistent miosis in spite of appropriate systemic therapy, and may necessitate topical atropine (or scopolamine) instillation.[18]
- Exposure to organophosphate vapors rapidly produces symptoms of mucous membrane and upper airway irritation and bronchospasm, followed by systemic symptoms if patients are exposed to significant concentrations.
- While respiratory failure is the most common cause of death, other causes may contribute including hypoxia due to seizures, hyperthermia, renal failure, and hepatic failure. Nephrotoxicity has been postulated to be a matter of concern in some cases of organophosphate poisoning which is often not paid due attention by the attending physician.[19]
- Unequal sympathetic stimulation of myocardial cells and interactions with potassium channels and the Na^+/Ca^{++} exchanger in the myocardial cell membrane are probably responsible for the occasional prolonged QTc interval. This prolongation in QTc interval can be associated with polymorphic ventricular tachycardia (torsades de pointes). Finally, hypotension may occur because of stimulation of vascular receptors by excessive circulating ACh. Patients with organophosphate poisoning and QTc prolongation are more likely to develop respiratory failure and have a worse prognosis than patients with normal QTc intervals.[20] Patients with organophosphate poisoning who develop PVCs (premature ventricular contractions) are more likely to develop respiratory failure and have a higher mortality rate than patients without PVCs.
- Because liquid preparations are usually dissolved in a hydrocarbon aspiration frequently results following ingestion in severe poisoning and can lead to hydrocarbon pneumonitis.
- Excessive adrenergic influences on metabolism cause glycogenolysis with hyperglycemia and ketosis that may be mistaken for diabetic ketoacidosis.[21] Hypoglycemia can also occur, although the mechanism is unclear. Increased sympathetic activity usually precipitates white blood cell demargination, resulting in leukocytosis.
- Elevations of hepatic enzymes can occur following organophosphate pesticide exposures.

Sequelae:

- An *intermediate syndrome* sometimes occurs 1–4 days after poisoning due to long-lasting cholinesterase inhibition and muscle necrosis. This phenomenon was first described in 1987, and is termed the "intermediate syndrome" because it occurs in between the periods of acute and delayed toxicity.[22] It is more common with chlorpyrifos, dimethoate, monocrotophos, parathion, sumithion, fenthion, fenitrothion, ethyl parathion, methyl parathion, diazinon, malathion, trichlorfon, and methamidophos. Redistribution of these lipophilic pesticides and their metabolites from adipose tissue may be responsible,[23] and the syndrome may resolve when the body burden of these metabolites diminishes and cholinesterase levels normalize. Main features include muscle weakness and paralysis. The most commonly affected muscles are the facial, extraocular, palatal, respiratory, and proximal limb muscles. Paralytic signs include inability to lift the neck or sit up, ophthalmoparesis, slow eye movements, facial weakness, difficulty swallowing, limb weakness (primarily proximal), areflexia, respiratory paralysis, and death. There is growing speculation that intermediate syndrome may result from inadequate oxime therapy,[24] although more recent case reports question this theory.[25] One recent study suggests that the occurrence of intermediate syndrome strongly correlates with the initial degree of cholinergic crisis, and appears to be a continuum with the neuromuscular paralysis resulting from the early stages of poisoning.[26] The study suggests that muscle injury during early cholinergic crisis may progress to intermediate syndrome. Electromyograms will often show tetanic fade in these patients, and suggest both presynaptic and postsynaptic involvement. However, repetitive nerve stimulation may not always accurately predict the occurrence or severity of intermediate syndrome, but may be beneficial in determining the need for mechanical ventilation. Once it sets in, the intermediate syndrome will have to be managed by supportive measures, since it does not respond to oximes or atropine. However, because some reports correlating pralidoxime dose and intermediate syndrome suggest that insufficient dosing may play a part, it is recommended that pralidoxime infusion be reinstituted at 500 mg/h when intermediate syndrome is suspected. The weakness and paralysis commonly resolve in 5–18 days. In one study from India, up to one-third of admissions of organophosphate poisoning in a major hospital developed intermediate syndrome.[27]

- A *delayed syndrome* (now called *delayed encephalopathy and neuropathy syndrome*) sometimes occurs 1–4 weeks after poisoning due to nerve demyelination, and is characterized by flaccid weakness and atrophy of distal limb muscles or spasticity and ataxia. A mixed sensory-motor neuropathy usually begins in the legs, causing burning or tingling, then weakness. Severe cases progress to complete paralysis, impaired respiration and death. The nerve damage of organophosphate-induced delayed neuropathy is frequently permanent. This disorder appears to result from inhibition of an enzyme within nervous tissue named neurotoxic esterase or neuropathy target esterase. Symptoms seem to be initiated by the phosphorylation of this enzyme, or perhaps of some related compound, followed by aging of the complex. Such neuropathies may even result from exposure to organophosphate compounds that do not inhibit red blood cell (RBC) cholinesterase or produce clinical cholinergic toxicity. Pathologic findings demonstrate effects primarily on large distal neurons, with axonal degeneration preceding demyelination. Organophosphates that have been associated with delayed neuropathy in humans include chlorophos, chlorpyrifos, dichlorvos, dipterex, ethyl parathion, fenthion, isofenphos, leptophos, malathion, mecarbam, mephosfolan, merphos, methamidophos, mipafox, trichlorofon, trichloronate, and TOCP (tri-ortho-cresyl phosphate).[28] Electromyograms and nerve conduction studies may be helpful in diagnosing the delayed syndrome by identifying the type of neuropathy (such as axonopathy, myelinopathy or transmission neuropathy) and differentiating it from similar presentations such as Guillain-Barré syndrome. Recovery of these patients is variable and occurs over months to years with residual deficits common.
- Hyperamylasemia is occasionally reported in cases of severe organophosphate pesticide poisoning, and although pancreatitis may result from spasm of the sphincter of Oddi, hyperamylasemia is most often the result of salivary gland stimulation and not the result of pancreatic dysfunction. Parathion ingestion has resulted in fatal hemorrhagic pancreatitis. Diazinon has also been implicated. Hemoperfusion is said to be beneficial if this occurs.
- Patients poisoned with highly lipid soluble organophosphates such as fenthion have rarely developed extrapyramidal effects including dystonia, resting tremor, cogwheel rigidity, and choreoathetosis. These effects began 4–40 days after acute organophosphate poisoning and spontaneously resolved over 1–4 weeks in survivors.
- It is important to note that children may have different predominant signs of organophosphate poisoning than adults. In some studies of children poisoned by organophosphate or carbamate compounds, the major signs and symptoms were CNS depression, stupor, flaccidity, dyspnea, and coma. Other classical signs of organophosphate poisoning such as miosis, fasciculations, bradycardia, excessive salivation and lacrimation, and GI symptoms were infrequent.[29]

Chronic Poisoning

It usually occurs as an occupational hazard in agriculturists, especially those who are engaged in pesticide spraying of crops. Route of exposure is usually inhalation or contamination of skin. The following are the main features:
- *Polyneuropathy*: Paresthesias, muscle cramps, weakness, and gait disorders.
- *CNS effects*: Drowsiness, confusion, irritability, and anxiety.
- *Sheep farmers disease*: Psychiatric manifestations encountered in sheep farmers involved in long-term sheep-dip operations.[30]
- A study of 24 agricultural workers revealed significantly lower cancellous bone area and bone formation at cellular and tissue level in workers with long-term exposure to organophosphates compared with healthy age-matched controls.[31]
- Organophosphate poisoning has been associated with a variety of subacute or delayed onset chronic neurological, neurobehavioral, or psychiatric syndromes. One author has termed these "chronic organophosphate-induced neuropsychiatric disorder" (COPND) and noted that the standard hen neurotoxic esterase test is not sufficient to detect which organophosphates can cause this condition.[32] Signs and symptoms include confusion, psychosis, anxiety, drowsiness, depression, fatigue, and irritability. Electroencephalographic changes may be noted and can last for weeks. Single photon emission computed tomography (SPECT) scanning may reveal morphologic changes in the basal ganglia. Although no specific treatment is effective, most psychological abnormalities resolve within a year.
- A cluster of congenital anomalies has been reported in a Hungarian village where pregnant women were believed to have consumed trichlorfon contaminated fish during pregnancy. Of 15 live births, 11 (73%) had congenital abnormalities and six were twins. Other likely causes (known teratogenic factors, familial inheritance, consanguinity) were excluded.[33] Abnormalities included Down syndrome (4 births), ventricular septal defect and pulmonary atresia, congenital inguinal hernia, stenosis of the left bronchus, anal atresia, choanal atresia, cleft lip, and Robin sequence.
- In a pesticide exposure study in children, a significant association was found between risk of non-Hodgkin lymphoma and increased frequency of reported pesticide use in the home, professional exterminations within

the home, and postnatal exposure. Higher risks were found in both young (younger than 6 years of age) and older children, for T-cell and B-cell lymphomas; for lymphoblastic, large cell, and Burkitt morphologies. In addition, there was a higher risk for non-Hodgkin lymphoma with occupational exposure to pesticides.[34]

- Some studies indicate a link between Parkinson's disease and chronic exposure to organophosphate insecticides.[35] The structures of some of these compounds are similar to that of known neurotoxins like 1-methyl-4-phenyl-1,2,3,6-tetrahydropyridine (MPTP). Some individuals may have a possible genetic susceptibility. In some cases of acute exposure to organophosphate compounds, there have been reports of self-limited movement disorders resembling Parkinson that resolve over weeks to months. Although statistics derived from some epidemiologic studies suggest the connection,[36] others studies have failed to find an association between organophosphate compounds and parkinsonism.[37]

There are some organophosphates which are extremely potent but do not find place as insecticides; instead they have been used in chemical warfare. These include sarin, tabun, soman, etc.

Diagnosis

Depression of Cholinesterase Activity

Plasma cholinesterase (butyrylcholinesterase) metabolizes various xenobiotics including succinylcholine and cocaine. Erythrocytes contain a form of AChE (red blood cell cholinesterase or RBC cholinesterase) that is structurally similar to the enzyme found in neuronal tissue. Inhibition of either RBC cholinesterase or plasma cholinesterase serves as markers for cholinesterase inhibitor poisoning, but the extent of inhibition of these enzymes does not correlate well with the severity of poisoning. There is also tremendous interindividual and interchemical variability in the degree and duration with which organophosphate insecticides affect various cholinesterases.

After significant exposure, plasma cholinesterase activity usually falls first, followed rapidly by RBC cholinesterase. By the time patients present with acute symptoms, levels of both cholinesterase activities have usually fallen well below baseline values, and often have fallen below detectable limits. Plasma cholinesterase activity usually recovers before RBC cholinesterase activity, often returning to normal within a few days. However, plasma cholinesterase activity is less specific for exposure than RBC cholinesterase activity. The former can be lowered significantly in patients with a number of disorders, including hereditary deficiency of the enzyme, malnutrition, hepatic parenchymal disease, chronic debilitating illnesses and iron-deficiency anemia. In fact, day-to-day variation in the activity of this enzyme in healthy individuals may be as high as 20%.

Red blood cell cholinesterase activity is more reliable because the AChE in red blood cells is true AChE. It is generally suggested that clinical organophosphate pesticide poisoning can be said to have occurred when RBC cholinesterase activity falls to below 50% of baseline values.[38]

However, there are several pitfalls in interpreting cholinesterase laboratory values. Firstly, it is AChE inhibition in nervous tissue that causes toxicity and RBC and plasma cholinesterase activity may not always reflect neuronal enzyme activity. Organophosphate insecticides vary in their ability to inhibit both enzymes. Because these tests are only markers of neuronal enzyme inhibition, this variation may lead to some patients presenting highly symptomatic after minimal reductions in RBC or plasma cholinesterase, although others can be asymptomatic after losing 50% activity. It is also well known that there is a wide normal range of RBC and plasma cholinesterase activity, which allows for patients with high normal values to suffer significant falls in cholinesterase activity, yet still register near normal levels of cholinesterase activity on laboratory assay.

Red blood cell cholinesterase regenerates more slowly than AChE found in neurons. To completely replenish the RBC AChE supply, the red blood cells in circulation at the time of the organophosphate insecticide exposure must be replaced, or pralidoxime administered. An average of 66 days may be necessary for RBC cholinesterase activity to recover following severe inhibition and activity may take up to 120 days to return to normal. The patient may have completely recovered neuronal activity of AChE and resolved all cholinergic symptoms, yet still have low RBC cholinesterase laboratory values. For this reason, in subacute poisoning with organophosphate compounds, it is difficult to accurately predict the actual time of onset or duration of exposure when only the RBC cholinesterase activity is known. In fact, the ability of RBC cholinesterase activity to serve as a historical marker for excessive exposure to organophosphate insecticides provides the basis for monitoring the activity of this enzyme in pesticide workers.

It is important to note that depressed RBC cholinesterase activity may be the result of exposures or conditions other than insecticide poisoning, such as in therapy with antimalarial agents such as chloroquine and pernicious anemia. Genetic and circadian variations are also common with daily fluctuations within the same individual as high as 10%. Additionally, levels are normally slightly lower in children younger than 4 months of age, probably increasing as hepatic function matures. Oral contraceptives raise RBC cholinesterase activity.

Blood samples for cholinesterase activity must be obtained in the appropriate blood tubes. Tubes containing fluoride will permanently inactivate the enzyme, yielding falsely low activity levels, and should not be used. Specimens for RBC cholinesterase must be drawn into tubes containing a chelating anticoagulant such as ethylenediaminetetraacetic acid (EDTA) to prevent clot formation. Plasma cholinesterase does not require an anticoagulant and can be drawn into a tube without chelators or anticoagulants.

Table 2 gives an overview of the benefits and disadvantages of estimating RBC and plasma cholinesterase levels in suspected organophosphate or carbamate pesticide poisoning.

Plasma cholinesterase usually recovers in a few days or weeks; red blood cell cholinesterase recovers in several days to 4 months depending on severity of depression. Some studies have found plasma cholinesterase to have no significant association with either the mortality or as a means to assess the need for patients requiring ventilator support.[39]

P-nitrophenol Test

P-nitrophenol is a metabolite of some organophosphates (e.g. parathion, ethion) and is excreted in the urine.

Procedure: Steam distill 10 mL of urine and collect the distillate. Add sodium hydroxide (2 pellets) and heat on a water bath for 10 minutes. Production of yellow color indicates the presence of p-nitrophenol. The test can also be done on vomitus or stomach contents.

Levels of alkyl phosphates such as diethyl phosphate (DEP) and dimethyl phosphate (DMP) may be more sensitive markers of exposure.

Atropine Challenge Test

An atropine sulfate challenge may be helpful in diagnosing cholinergic poisoning in a patient who presents with findings suggestive of this disorder, but in whom no history is available to suggest excessive exposure to an organophosphate or carbamate insecticide. In an individual not exposed to significant amounts of insecticide a test dose of 1–5 mg of atropine (adult), or 0.05 mg/kg (children) should produce classic antimuscarinic findings such as mydriasis, tachycardia, and dry mucous membranes. Conversely, the persistence of cholinergic signs and symptoms after an atropine challenge strongly suggests the presence of organophosphate compound or carbamate poisoning. However, some patients suffering from mild-to-moderate anticholinesterase poisoning may respond to these doses of atropine. Therefore, the reversal of cholinergic findings does not exclude poisoning by one of these compounds.

Electromyogram

Repetitive nerve stimulation testing is an accurate method of quantifying AChE inhibition at the neuromuscular junction.[40] Spontaneous repetitive potentials or fasciculations following single-nerve stimulation resulting from persistent ACh at nerve terminals can be a sensitive indicator of AChE inhibition at the motor endplate, and may be useful in the early diagnosis of organophosphate or carbamate poisoning. This kind of evaluation may also be of benefit in early detection of rebound cholinergic crisis caused by continued insecticide absorption or redistribution from adipose tissue or onset of an intermediate syndrome.[40]

Thin Layer Chromatography

The presence of an organophosphate in a lavage, or vomit, or gastric aspirate sample can also be determined by thin layer chromatography (TLC). The sample is extracted twice with 5 mL of petroleum ether, and the extract is washed with distilled water. It is then dried in steam compressed air, reconstituted in methanol, and spotted on silica gel-coated TLC plate along with the standard and run in a mixture of petroleum ether and methanol (25:1). After the solvent has travelled a considerable distance, the plate is dried and exposed to iodine vapor. The RF is compared with that of the standard.

Table 2 Comparison of red blood cell (RBC) and plasma cholinesterase assays in organophosphate (OP)/carbamte poisoning

	RBC cholinesterase	Plasma cholinesterase
Advantage	More reliable	Easier to measure, declines faster
Site	RBC (reflects CNS gray matter, motor end plate)	Central nervous system (CNS) white matter, plasma, liver, pancreas, heart
Regeneration (untreated)	1%/day	25–30% in first 7–10 days
Normalization (untreated)	35–49 days	28–42 days
Use	Unsuspected prior exposure with normal plasma cholinesterase	Acute exposure
False depression	Pernicious anemia, hemoglobinopathies, antimalarial treatment, oxalate blood tubes	Liver dysfunction, malnutrition, hypersensitivity reactions, drugs (succinylcholine, codeine, morphine), pregnancy, genetic deficiency

Ancillary Investigations

There may be evidence of:
- Leukocytosis (with relatively normal differential count)
- High hematocrit
- Anion gap acidosis
- *Hyperglycemia or hypoglycemia*: Hypoglycemia can be recalcitrant to treatment.[41]
- Elevation of serum creatine kinase.

In every case monitor electrolytes, electrocardiograph (ECG), and serum pancreatic isoamylase levels in patients with significant poisoning. Patients who have increased serum amylase levels and those who develop a prolonged QTc interval or PVCs are more likely to develop respiratory insufficiency and have a worse prognosis. If pancreatitis is suspected, an abdominal CT-scan can be performed to evaluate diffuse pancreatic swelling. If respiratory tract irritation is present, monitor chest X-ray. Many organophosphate compounds are found in solution with a variety of hydrocarbon-based solvents. Aspiration pneumonitis may occur if these products are aspirated into the lungs. Bronchopneumonia may develop as a complication of organophosphate-induced pulmonary edema. High performance thin layer chromatography (HPLC) technique can be used to identify several organophosphate compounds in human serum.

Treatment

Determine plasma or red blood cell cholinesterase activities. Depression in excess of 50% of baseline is generally associated with severe symptoms (*vide supra*). The initial treatment for a patient exposed to organophosphate compounds must be directed at ensuring an adequate airway and ventilation, and at reversing excessive muscarinic effects. Seizures must be treated with standard anticonvulsants such as benzodiazepines or barbiturates.

Decontamination

- If skin spillage has occurred, it is imperative that the patient be stripped and washed thoroughly with soap and water.
  Procedure:
    - Shower is preferable. Make the patient stand (if he is able to) under the shower, or seated in a chair.
    - Wash with cold water for 5 minutes from head to toe using nongermicidal soap. Rinse hair well.
    - Repeat the wash and rinse procedure with warm water.
    - Repeat the wash and rinse procedure with hot water.

Treating personnel should protect themselves with water-impermeable gowns, masks with eye shields and shoe covers. Neoprene or nitrile gloves must be used, if available. Double-gloving with standard vinyl gloves may be protective for short intervals. Although alcohol-based soaps are sometimes recommended to dissolve hydrocarbons, these products can be difficult to find, and immediate skin cleansing should be the primary goal. It must be noted that skin absorption can also result from contact with organophosphate compounds in vomitus and diarrhea. Oily insecticides may be difficult to remove from thick or long hair, even with repeated shampooing, and shaving scalp hair may be necessary. Exposed leather clothing or products should be discarded because decontamination is very difficult once impregnation has occurred.

- If ocular exposure has occurred, copious eye irrigation should be done with normal saline or Ringer's solution. If these are not immediately available, tap water can be used.
- In the case of ingestion, stomach wash can be done, though this is often unnecessary because the patient would have usually vomited by the time he is brought to hospital. Activated charcoal can be administered in the usual way even though evidence is lacking as to its efficacy in organophosphate poisoning. One dose (1 g/kg) may be sufficient.

Decontamination of spills: A variety of methods have been described for organophosphate spill decontamination, most of which depend on changing the pH to promote hydrolysis to inactive phosphate diester compounds. The rate of hydrolysis depends on both the specific organophosphate compound involved and the increase in pH caused by the detoxicant used.

- *Caution!*: Do not use a mixture of bleach and alkali for decontaminating acephate organophosphates. This can cause release of toxic acetyl chloride, acetylene, and phosgene gas. Spills of acephate organophosphates should be decontaminated by absorption and scrubbing with concentrated detergent.
- Treatment of the spilled material with alkaline substances such as sodium carbonate (washing soda), sodium bicarbonate (baking soda), calcium hydroxide (slaked or hydrated lime, or lime water), and calcium carbonate (limestone) may be used for detoxification.
- Chlorine-active compounds such as sodium hypochlorite (household bleach) or calcium hypochlorite (bleaching powder, chlorinated lime) may also be used to detoxify organophosphate spills.
- Disposal of large quantities or contamination of large areas may be regulated by various governmental agencies and reporting may be required.

Antidotes

Atropine: Atropine, a competitive antagonist of acetylcholine at the muscarinic postsynaptic membrane and in the CNS, will block the muscarinic manifestations of organophosphate poisoning.

Pralidoxime: This is a nucleophilic oxime which helps to regenerate acetylcholinesterase at muscarinic, nicotinic, and CNS sites. Actually, human studies have not substantiated the benefit of oxime therapy in acute organophosphate poisoning, but they are widely used. Most authors advocate the continued use of pralidoxime in the clinical setting of severe organophosphate poisoning.[42]

The antidotes for organophosphates have been discussed in detail in **Box 1**.

Supportive measures: Maintain airway patency and oxygenation. Suction secretions. Endotracheal intubation and mechanical ventilation may be necessary. Monitor pulse oximetry or arterial blood gases to determine need for supplemental oxygen.
- Administer intravenous (IV) fluids to replace losses.
- *Oxygenation/intubation/positive pressure ventilation*: To minimize barotrauma and other complications, use the lowest amount of positive end-expiratory

Box 1 Antidotes for organophosphates

Atropine
Mode of action: Blocks the muscarinic manifestations of organophosphates. However, since atropine affects only the postsynaptic muscarinic receptors, it has no effect on muscle weakness or paralysis.
Diagnostic dose: Organophosphate-poisoned patients are generally tolerant to the toxic effects of atropine (dry mouth, rapid pulse, dilated pupils, etc.). If these findings occur following a diagnostic atropine dose, the patient is probably not seriously poisoned.
Diagnostic dose: Adult— 1 mg intravenously or intramuscularly; *Child*: 0.25 mg (about 0.01 mg/kg) intravenously or intramuscularly.
Therapeutic dose: 1–2 mg IV or IM (adult); 0.05 mg/kg IV (child); every 15 minutes until the endpoint is reached, i.e. drying up of tracheobronchial secretions. Pupillary dilatation and tachycardia are not reliable indicators of the endpoint. Atropine can also be administered as an IV infusion after the initial bolus dose, at a rate of 0.02 to 0.08 mg/kg/hr. Once the end point has been reached, the dose should be adjusted to maintain the effect for at least 24 hours.[43] Atropinization must be maintained until all of the absorbed organophosphates have been metabolized. This may require administration of 2–2,000 milligrams of atropine over several hours to weeks. Large doses of atropine are often needed to reverse the bronchospasm, bronchorrhea, bradycardia, and heart block associated with severe organophosphate (OP) pesticide toxicity. Some patients with mild symptoms need only 1 or 2 mg of atropine to reverse cholinergic toxicity, but the moderately poisoned adult commonly requires total doses as large as 40 mg or more. Severe poisonings may necessitate even higher doses. Some adults have received over 1,000 mg of atropine in 24 hours (with adequate pralidoxime dosing) without demonstrating antimuscarinic effects, and total doses as high as 11,000 mg during the course of treatment have been reported.[44] Children have been managed with continuous infusions of atropine starting at 0.025 mg/kg/hr, and adult infusions of atropine can begin at 0.5–1 mg/hr and titrated as needed. Continuous infusions have been used for as long as 32 days in severely poisoned patients.[45]

Atropine therapy must be withdrawn slowly to prevent recurrence or rebounding of symptoms, often in the form of pulmonary edema. This is especially true of poisonings from lipophilic organophosphates such as fenthion.

Precautions:
- Many parenteral atropine preparations contain benzyl alcohol or chlorobutanol as preservatives. High-dose therapy with these preparations may result in benzyl alcohol or chlorobutanol toxicity. Preservative-free atropine preparations are available, and should be used if large doses are required.
- The half-life of atropine is significantly longer in children under 2 years and adults over 60 years; the rate of administration in these patients should be adjusted accordingly.
- Effects of overdosing with atropine include fever, warm dry skin, inspiratory stridor, irritability, and dilated and unresponsive pupils.
- A urinary catheter should be inserted in all atropinized patients to prevent urinary retention.
- If atropine supplies are exhausted during therapy, other antimuscarinic agents like diphenhydramine may be used.

Endpoint: "Atropinization" is said to have occurred when the patient exhibits dry skin and mucous membranes, decreased or absent bowel sounds, tachycardia, reduced secretions, no bronchospasm and mydriasis. Reduction or disappearance of pulmonary secretions is the most important target in atropine therapy and can be guided by following lung sounds and oxygenation. Tachycardia is not a contraindication to atropine therapy. Although the pupils are often helpful in gauging the need for atropine, the miosis encountered in severe ingestions and by direct ocular exposure to OP insecticides may respond only to topical ophthalmic atropine. Conversely, a positive pupillary response alone should not be used to discontinue further therapy.
Adverse effects: Atrial arrhythmias, A-V dissociation, multiple ventricular ectopics, photophobia, raised intraocular pressure, hyperpyrexia, hallucinations, and delirium.

Glycopyrrolate
When antimuscarinic central nervous system (CNS) toxicity becomes evident, yet peripheral cholinergic findings necessitate the administration of more atropine (e.g. bradycardia, bronchorrhea, vomiting), glycopyrrolate bromide can be substituted for atropine because its quaternary ammonium structure limits CNS penetration.[46,47] The initial IV dose of glycopyrrolate for adults is 1–2 mg, repeated as needed, and in children 0.025 mg/kg up to adult doses. As with atropine, much higher doses of glycopyrrolate may be required to stabilize patients with severe poisoning.

Contd...

Pralidoxime (Pyridine-2-aldoxime methiodide; 2-PAM)
Structurally, pralidoxime is 2-hydroxyiminomethyl-1-methylpyridinium chloride.

Mode of action: It is usually given along with atropine. Although phosphorylated acetylcholinesterase (AChE) undergoes hydrolytic regeneration at a very slow rate, this process can be markedly enhanced by using an oxime such as pralidoxime hydrochloride (2-PAM). In addition to rejuvenating AChE, pralidoxime may also reverse toxicity by directly inactivating free OP molecules and by exhibiting an apparent antimuscarinic effect on nervous tissue.[48] Regeneration of AChE lowers ACh concentrations to normal levels, reversing both muscarinic and nicotinic effects. An immediate rise in RBC cholinesterase activity is often noted after the administration of pralidoxime.

Pralidoxime competes for the phosphate moiety of the organophosphorus compound and releases it from the acetylcholinesterase enzyme, thereby liberating the latter and reactivating it. Most phosphorylated AChE will usually be "aged" within 24–48 hours of exposure. Pralidoxime is unable to rejuvenate active enzyme from the OP compound-AChE complex that has undergone aging. Therefore, pralidoxime therapy is most effective if started early in the course of toxicity. The actual rate of aging, however, varies significantly among OP compounds. While it is advisable to begin pralidoxime therapy within 48 hours of poisoning, it can be administered even much later with beneficial effects. Circulating OP pesticide concentrations have been measured for as long as 48 days after exposure, either because of prolonged absorption from the GI tract, or redistribution from fat stores.[45] Therefore, some AChE may still be undergoing new inhibition for days or weeks after exposure in symptomatic patients, and such inhibition may be reversible by pralidoxime.[49] Some reports support this theory by recording dramatic effects in reversing paralysis, weakness, and cholinergic symptoms even after late administration of pralidoxime.[22,50]

Pralidoxime is not equally effective in reversing cholinergic symptoms in all types of OP compound poisonings. It is particularly effective in reversing toxicity from parathion, diazinon, methyl parathion, TEPP, dimethoate, and dichlorvos but dimethoxy compounds, such as malathion and methyl demeton may be more resistant to reversal.[51]

Till recently, pralidoxime was said to be contraindicated in carbamate poisoning because experiments with carbaryl (*Sevin*) suggested a worsening of symptoms when it was administered. However, studies have pointed out that while pralidoxime is not a necessary adjunct to atropine in carbamate overdose, it may be beneficial in some cases.[5]

Dose: For adults—1–2 g in 100–150 mL of 0.9% sodium chloride, given IV over 30 minutes. This can be repeated after 1 hour, and subsequently every 6–12 hours, for 24–48 hours. Alternatively, a 2.5% concentration of pralidoxime can be given as a loading dose followed by a maintenance dose. Serious intoxication may require continuous infusion of 500 mg/hr in adults. Many workers feel that this high-dose therapy minimises the incidence of complications such as the Intermediate Syndrome.[52] Maximum dose should not exceed 12 g in a 24-hour period. Infusion over a period of several days may be necessary and is generally well tolerated. Although minimal serum concentrations of 4 mcg/mL are estimated to be necessary for maintenance of enzyme reactivation, the degree of reactivation may be dependent on the specific identity and concentrations of both oxime and OP compound. Bolus dosing of pralidoxime every 4–8 hours is ineffective in maintaining these levels, and therefore a constant infusion appears to be more appropriate.[53] Present recommendations for adults are to begin the maintenance infusion at 250–500 mg/h, titrating to symptoms. Alternative dosing by weight reported in other studies suggests using 4–5 mg/kg as a loading dose over 15–30 minutes, followed by a continuous infusion of 2–4 mg/kg/h to maintain serum concentrations.[54]

The WHO currently recommends an initial bolus of at least 30 mg/kg, followed by an infusion of more than 8 mg/kg/hr.

For children—20–40 mg/kg to a maximum of 1 g/dose given IV, and repeated every 6–12 hours for 24–48 hours. Alternatively, IV infusion can be resorted to at a rate of 9–19 mg/kg/hr.

Adverse effects: Side effects of pralidoxime are usually minimal at normal doses. Severely poisoned patients have received 500 mg/hr for weeks without adverse effects.[45] Rapid infusion can cause mild cholinergic effects because of transient blockade of AChE and has resulted in neuromuscular blockade and central respiratory depression.[55] Occasional visual complaints are also reported in patients receiving pralidoxime. Rapid administration can cause tachycardia, laryngospasm, and even cardiac or respiratory arrest. Other adverse effects include drowsiness, vertigo, headache, and muscle weakness.

- It is generally not advised for the treatment of carbamate overdose, especially carbaryl.
- In cases where intravenous administration is not possible, pralidoxime can be given intramuscularly as an initial dose of 1 gram or up to 2 grams in cases of very severe poisoning. Recent research in animals suggests that oral dosing of pralidoxime and atropine may also improve survival.[56]
- In some countries obidoxime is used instead of pralidoxime, though it does not appear to be superior to the latter. It is apparently favored over pralidoxime in clinical practice in Belgium, Israel, The Netherlands, Scandinavia, and Germany, and is the only oxime available in Portugal.
- Several investigators have started suggesting that oximes have only a limited role in organophosphate poisoning, and successful management is possible without employing them at all, though this view is not shared by some other workers in the field.[57,58]

Diazepam
Several studies demonstrate that administering diazepam along with oximes in the treatment of OP nerve agents (sarin, soman, tabun, VX) or OP pesticides can increase survival and decrease the incidence of seizures and neuropathy.[59] Diazepam can also decrease cerebral morphologic damage resulting from OP compound-induced seizures. Some investigators suggest that diazepam may also help attenuate OP-induced respiratory depression by minimizing the overstimulation of central respiratory centers caused by OP insecticides.[60]

Dose: For adults—5–10 mg IV slowly, every 15 minutes, up to a maximum of 30 mg.
For children—0.25–0.4 mg/kg IV slowly, every 5–10 minutes, up to a maximum of 10 mg.
If diazepam is ineffective, phenytoin or phenobarbitone can be used instead.

pressure (PEEP) possible while maintaining adequate oxygenation. Use of smaller tidal volumes (6 mL/kg) and lower plateau pressures (30 cm water or less) has been associated with decreased mortality and more rapid weaning from mechanical ventilation in patients with ARDS.[61]
- The following drugs are contraindicated: Parasympathomimetics, phenothiazines, antihistamines, and opiates. Do not administer succinylcholine (suxamethonium) or other cholinergic medications. Prolonged neuromuscular blockade may result when succinylcholine is administered after organophosphate exposure.
- Treat convulsions with benzodiazepines or barbiturates.
- Antibiotics are indicated only when there is evidence of infection.
- Hemoperfusion, hemodialysis, and exchange transfusion have not been shown to affect outcome or duration of toxicity in controlled trials of organophosphate poisoning.

Prevention of further exposure: After the patient has recovered, he should not be re-exposed to organophosphates for at least a few weeks since he is likely to suffer serious harm from a dose that normally would be harmless, owing to alteration of body chemistry.[62]

Following acute poisoning, patients should be precluded from further organophosphate exposure until sequential RBC cholinesterase (AChE) levels have been obtained and confirm that AChE activity has reached a plateau. Plateau has been obtained when sequential determinations differ by no more than 10%.[63] This may take 3–4 months following severe poisoning.

Treatment of pregnant victim: Therapeutic choices during pregnancy depend upon specific circumstances such as stage of gestation, severity of poisoning, and clinical signs of mother and fetus. The mother must be treated adequately to treat the fetus. A severely poisoned patient with a late gestation viable fetus may be a candidate for emergency cesarean section. The fetus may require intensive care after birth. Pralidoxime chloride is recommended for use in the pregnant patient to counteract muscle weakness. Both atropine and pralidoxime are pregnancy class C drugs, and therefore not contraindicated outright.

Glycopyrrolate: Unlike atropine, glycopyrrolate usually does not readily cross the placenta and would not directly affect fetal poisoning. However, the fetus may be best served by treating the mother to retain good respiratory function and fetal oxygenation.[64]

Autopsy Features[65]

External:
- Characteristic odor (garlicky or kerosene-like)

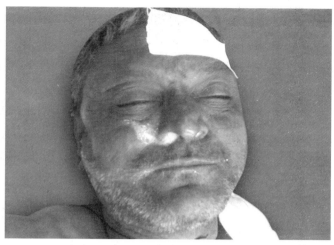

Fig. 4 Greenish frothy fluid oozing out of mouth and nose—dichlorvos poisoning
Source: Dr Swapnil Agarwal.

- Frothing at mouth and nose. Some compounds may impart a characteristic discoloration, e.g. greenish in dichlorvos poisoning **(Fig. 4)**
- Cyanosis of extremities
- Constricted pupils

Internal:
- Congestion of GI tract; garlicky or kerosene-like odor of contents.
- Pulmonary and cerebral edema
- Generalized visceral congestion.

A useful sign in mortuaries infested with flies is that some of these flies after settling on an opened body (dead of organophosphate poisoning) may themselves subsequently die and land on the autopsy table. It is also pertinent to remember that organophosphates resist autolysis and can be easily detected even in putrefied bodies.

CARBAMATES

They are as popular as organophosphates in their role as insecticides (and fungicides) and share a number of similarities. Only the differentiating features will be discussed. Indian brands are listed in **Table 3**.

Usual Fatal Dose

*Toxicity Rating**

The following are extremely toxic (*LD50: 1–50 mg/kg*) or highly toxic (*LD50: 51–500 mg/kg*): Aminocarb, Bendiocarb, Benfuracarb, Carbaryl, Carbofuran, Dimetan, Dimetilan, Dioxacarb, Formetanate, Methiocarb, Methomyl, and Oxamyl, Propoxur.

---
*Partly as per the Insecticide Rules, 1971.

Table 3 Common carbamates	
Generic name	Brand name
Aldicarb	Aldrin, Temik
Carbaryl	Agrovin, Agroyl, Bangvin 50, Caravet, Corovin, Hexavin, Kevin 50, Kilex Carbaryl, Sevidal, Sevin 50, Sujacarb, Sulfarl 50
Carbaryl + Gamma benzene hexachloride (BHC)	Sevidol
Carbofuran	Agrofuron 3G, Carbocil 3, Carburan, Crane, Furadan 3G, Hexafuran, VegFru Diafuran
Carbosulfan	Marshal
Fenobucarb	Merlino
Methomyl	Astra, Dunet, Lannate, Lannet, Mathoyl
MPMC (Xylylcarb)	Bipuin
MTMC (Metolcarb)	Emisan
Propoxur	Baygon, Isocarb, Protox Bait
Thiodicarb	Larvin

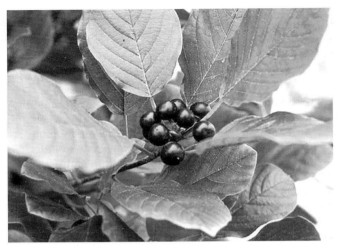

Fig. 5 *Physostigma venenosum*: Calabar bean

The following are moderately toxic (*LD50: 501–5,000 mg/kg*) or slightly toxic (*LD50: more than 5,000 mg/kg*): Aldicarb, Bufencarb, Isoprocarb, MPMC (3,4-dimethylphenyl N-methylcarbamate), MTMC (3-methylphenyl N-methylcarbamate), and Pirimicarb.

Mode of Action and Clinical Features

Carbamates were discovered in the 19th century when it was observed that the Calabar bean (*Physostigma venenosum Balfour*) **(Fig. 5)** was being used in tribal rituals in West Africa.[66] These beans were imported to Great Britain in 1840, where in 1864, Jobst and Hesse isolated an active alkaloid they named "physostigmine". This alkaloid was first medicinally used to treat glaucoma in 1877. In the 1930s, the synthesis of aliphatic esters of carbamic acid led to the development and introduction of carbamate pesticides, marketed initially as fungicides. In 1953, the Union Carbide Corporation developed and first marketed carbaryl, the very same insecticide that being manufactured at the notorious plant in Bhopal, during the methyl isocyanate tragedy in 1984.

As described in the previous chapter, those cholinesterase-inhibiting (anticholinesterase) insecticides that contain phosphorus are collectively termed organophosphorus compounds, while those that contain the OC=ON linkage are termed carbamates. Most carbamate insecticides are N-methyl carbamates derived from carbamic acid. Medicinal carbamate compounds include physostigmine, pyridostigmine, and neostigmine. Drugs such as meprobamate and various urethanes are also carbamate derivatives, but they do not inhibit cholinesterase.[66] Thiocarbamate fungicides and herbicides (e.g. maneb, zineb, nabam, and mancozeb) also do not inhibit AChE and do not produce cholinergic excess.

Carbamates (like organophosphates) are inhibitors of acetylcholinesterase, but carbamylate the serine moiety at the active site instead of phosphorylation. This is a reversible type of binding and hence symptoms are less severe and of shorter duration. Aging cannot occur since the carbamate-AChE bond hydrolyzes spontaneously, reactivating the enzyme. As such, the duration of symptoms in carbamate poisoning is generally less than 24 hours. As a result, both morbidity and mortality are limited when compared to organophosphate poisoning. Also, since carbamates do not penetrate the CNS to the same extent as organophosphates, CNS toxicity is likewise much less. With respect to all other clinical manifestations, there is general similarity between carbamates and organophosphates.

Carbamates are well absorbed across skin and mucous membranes, and by inhalation and ingestion. Peak serum levels of some compounds are generally achieved in 30–40 minutes following ingestion. Most carbamates undergo hydrolysis, hydroxylation, and conjugation in the liver and intestinal wall with 90% excreted in the urine within 3 days. There are two main pharmacokinetic differences between carbamates and organophosphate compounds. First, carbamates do not easily cross into the CNS. CNS effects are thus limited, although CNS dysfunction may still occur in massive ingestion (especially aldicarb),[66] or from hypoxia secondary to pulmonary toxicity and paralysis. Second, the carbamate-cholinesterase bond does not "age" as in organophosphate compound poisoning; thus, it is reversible with spontaneous hydrolysis occurring usually within several hours. Carbamates are rapidly metabolized. Most of them are rapidly hydrolyzed by liver enzymes to methyl carbamic acid and a variety of low toxicity phenolic substances. These metabolites may sometimes be measured in urine as long as 2–3 days after significant pesticide absorption.

Miosis, a muscarinic effect, is characteristic of severe and moderately severe poisonings, but may appear late.[67] Miosis was the most common symptom seen (57%) in a retrospective observational study of 54 children admitted to a pediatric intensive care unit following anticholinesterase (carbamate and organophosphate) poisoning.[68] Pupil dilation may occur as a nicotinic effect and may be present in up to 10% of patients.[44]

Sinus tachycardia with ST segment depression may occur early in the course of poisoning. Repolarization abnormalities may occur and are generally transient. Complete heart block has been reported.[69]

Dyspnea is a common manifestation of carbamate exposure. Chest tightness, bronchospasm, increased pulmonary secretions, and rales may develop secondary to muscarinic effects. Acute lung injury (pulmonary edema) is a potential clinical manifestation of severe carbamate poisoning and is attributed to the muscarinic action of the insecticide. Contributing factors to the development of pulmonary edema include bradycardia and weakened cardiac contraction from an accumulation of acetylcholine on the cardiovascular system. Hypoxia may develop due to increasing capillary permeability.

Headache, dizziness, blurred vision, tremor, paresis, mental depression, coma, delayed neuropathies, various dystonias, weakness, muscle twitching, and convulsions have all been reported with carbamate poisoning. In an outbreak of gastroenteritis reported in patrons of a Thai restaurant, it was discovered that the food had been seasoned with methomyl-contaminated salt. Patients reported dizziness (72%), headache (52%), and chills (48%). Dizziness, lightheadedness or a feeling of disequilibrium were reported as the initial symptom in 51 cases (48%).[70] Children may be more likely to develop CNS depression, convulsions, and hypotonia than the typical cholinergic syndrome. Absence of classic muscarinic effects has been reported in several children intoxicated with carbamate insecticides. The presence of either a cardiac arrhythmia or respiratory failure is associated with a higher incidence of fatal poisoning.

Delayed neuropathies are not usually associated with carbamate insecticides. One reason for this difference is presumed to be that "aging" of the neuropathy target esterase pesticide complex is a requirement for neuronal degeneration. Paradoxically, studies suggest that subgroups of carbamates may actually bind neuropathy target esterase and exert a protective effect against more toxic organophosphates compounds. However, cases of possible delayed neuropathy associated with carbamates have been reported.[71] These cases involve ingestion of carbaryl, m-tolyl methyl carbamate, and carbofuran, include both sensory and motor tracts, and tend to resolve over 3–9 months. Electromyography (EMG) findings in these subjects are variable. The symptoms are similar to those seen with organophosphates. Behavioral toxicity following carbamate exposure is extremely rare.

Acute pancreatitis has been reported with propoxur.[72]

Combined toxicity of organophosphate and carbamate compounds can cause multiple complications, e.g. parkinsonism, thrombocytopenia, intermediate syndrome and neuropsychiatric manifestations (COPIND) during acute phase, and treatment can be complicated.[73]

Diagnosis

Carbamates inhibit neuronal and RBC AChE and plasma cholinesterase. However, the relative rapidity with which spontaneous decarbamylation of cholinesterase takes place may result in the measurement of relatively normal RBC cholinesterase activity despite severe cholinergic symptoms if the assay is not performed within several hours of sampling. In vitro decarbamylation has been found to be promoted by dilution of the sample. The carbamylated sample should be stored undiluted and refrigerated or frozen. As in the case with organophosphates pesticide poisoning, the wide "normal" range of cholinesterase values may make interpretation of cholinesterase activity difficult at times when the patient's baseline values are unknown. Unlike organophosphates pesticides, carbamates generally do not cause persistent depressed RBC and plasma cholinesterase activities.

Rotenberg et al. (1995) propose an assay technique to distinguish between carbamate and organophosphate poisoning.[74] Carbamylated cholinesterase activity follows a nonlinear kinetic pattern over time, whereas phosphorylated enzyme activity is linear. At inhibition of greater than 40%, the nonlinear pattern characteristic of carbamates is easily mapped.

The atropine challenge test as described for diagnosis of organophosphates pesticide poisoning (in the previous section) can be done in carbamate poisoning also.

One technique for assessing absorption of the principal N-methyl carbamate compounds is measurement of specific phenolic metabolites in urine. For example, carbaryl (alpha-naphthol), carbofuran (carbofuranphenol), and propoxur (isopropoxyphenol).

Chest X-ray should be obtained in all symptomatic patients. The major cause of morbidity and mortality in carbamate insecticide poisonings is respiratory failure and associated pulmonary edema.

Treatment

An important differentiating point from organophosphates is that oximes are generally not recommended, while atropine can be given. Especially in carbaryl poisoning, oxime therapy can lead to the production of a carbamylated oxime which

may be a more potent acetylcholinesterase inhibitor than carbaryl itself. With other carbamate insecticides (particularly aldicarb), oximes may be a useful adjunct to atropine therapy.[75] The current consensus is that pralidoxime can be used in conjunction with atropine for specific indications as follows:
- Life-threatening symptoms such as severe muscle weakness, fasciculations, paralysis, or decreased respiratory effort
- Continued excessive requirements of atropine
- Concomitant organophosphate and carbamate exposure.

Fortunately, because of the rapid hydrolysis of the carbamate-AChE complex, symptoms, including weakness and paralysis, usually resolve within 24–48 hours without pralidoxime therapy. However, administering pralidoxime to a poisoned patient in a cholinergic crisis is appropriate when it is not known whether the patient is suffering from organophosphate or carbamate pesticide poisoning. If the poisoning is from a carbamate pesticide, pralidoxime therapy may not be necessary, but if used, should not prove detrimental. Second, significant inhibition of RBC cholinesterase and plasma cholinesterase by carbamates generally does not last for more than 1–2 days, assuming absorption is complete. Patients exposed to carbamates usually have normal values by the time of discharge. There are no reported cases of recurrent or delayed poisonings following carbamate insecticide poisoning. Therefore, repeating cholinesterase tests after patients are asymptomatic are usually unnecessary.

In all cases, administer atropine in repeated doses intravenously until atropinization is achieved (indicated by drying of pulmonary secretions).

Adult dose: 2–4 mg IV every 10–15 minutes.

Pediatric dose: 0.05 mg/kg IV every 10–15 minutes.

Convulsions can be controlled with a benzodiazepine (diazepam or lorazepam). If they persist or recur, administer phenobarbitone.

REFERENCES

1. Gouda HS, Prasad MDR, Honnungar RS, et al. Flubendiamide-entry of a new insecticide into the field of clinical toxicology. J Indian Soc Toxicol. 2010;6(2):45-6.
2. Bawaskar HS, Joshi SR. Organophosphate poisoning in agricultural India—status in 2005. J Assoc Physicians India. 2005;53:422-4.
3. Akgur SA, Ozturk P, Solak I, et al. Human serum paraoxonase (PON1) activity in acute organophosphorous insecticide poisoning. Forensic Sci Int. 2003;133:136-40.
4. Furlong CE, Li WF, Richter RJ, et al. Genetic and temporal determinants of pesticide sensitivity: Role of paraoxonase (PON1). Neurotoxicology. 2000;21:91-100.
5. Pillay VV. Modern Medical Toxicology, 4th edition. New Delhi: Jaypee Brothers Medical Publishers (P) Ltd.; 2013.
6. Taylor P. Anticholinesterase agents. In: Hardman JG, Limbird LE, Molinoff PB, et al. (Eds). Goodman and Gilman's The Pharmacological Basis of Therapeutics, 9th edition. New York: McGraw-Hill, Health Professions Division; 1996. pp. 161-76.
7. Moretto A, Lotti M. Poisoning by organophosphorus insecticides and sensory neuropathy. J Neurol Neurosurg Psychiatry. 1998;64:463-8.
8. Etzel RA, Forthal DN, Hill RH Jr, et al. Fatal parathion poisoning in Sierra Leone. Bull World Health Organ. 1987;65:645-9.
9. Agarwal SB. A clinical, biochemical, neurobehavioral, and sociopsychological study of 190 patients admitted to hospital as a result of acute organophosphorus poisoning. Environ Res. 1993;62:63-70.
10. Rajasekaran D, Subbaraghavalu G, Jayapandian PJ. Guillain-Barre syndrome due to organophosphate compound poison. J Assoc Physicians India. 2009;57:714-5.
11. Lifshitz M, Shahak E, Sofer S. Carbamate and organophosphate poisoning in young children. Pediatr Emerg Care. 1999;15:102-3.
12. Takahashi H, Kojima T, Ikeda T, et al. Differences in the mode of lethality produced through intravenous and oral administration of organophosphorus insecticides in rats. Fundam Appl Toxicol. 1991;16:459-68.
13. Nair PM, Javad H, Al-Mandhiry ZA. Organophosphate poisoning in children—atropine, pralidoxime or both (letter)? Saudi Med J. 2001;22:814-5.
14. Rubio CR, Felipe Fernández C, Manzanedo Bueno R, et al. Acute renal failure due to the inhalation of organophosphates: successful treatment with haemodialysis. Clin Kidney J. 2012;5(6):582-3.
15. Senanayake N, Sanmuganathan PS. Extrapyramidal manifestations complicating organophosphorous insecticide poisoning. Hum Exp Toxicol. 1995;14:600-4.
16. Eddleston M, Buckley NA, Eyer P, et al. Management of acute organophosphorus pesticide poisoning. Lancet. 2008;371(9612):597-607.
17. Futagami K, Hirano N, Iimori E. Severe fenitrothion poisoning complicated by rhabdomyolysis in psychiatric patient. Acta Med Okayama. 2001;55:129-32.
18. Aaron CK. Organophosphates and carbamates. In: Shannon MS, Borron SW, Burns M (Eds). Clinical Management of Poisoning and Drug Overdose, 4th edition. New York: Elsevier Science; 2006.
19. Singh B, Menezes RG, Bharadwaj DN. Toxic nephropathies of anticholinesterase compounds. J Indian Soc Toxicol. 2008;4(1):31-8.
20. Chuang FR, Jang SW, Lin JL, et al. QTc prolongation indicates a poor prognosis in patients with organophosphate poisoning. Am J Emerg Med. 1996;14:451-3.
21. Meller D, Fraser I, Kryger M. Hyperglycemia in anticholinergic poisoning. Can Med Assoc J. 1981;124:745-8.
22. Yang CC, Deng JF. Intermediate syndrome following organophosphate insecticide poisoning. J Chin Med Assoc. 2007;70(11):467-72.
23. Sudakin DL, Mullins ME, Horowitz BZ, et al. Intermediate syndrome after malathion ingestion despite continuous infusion of pralidoxime. J Toxicol Clin Toxicol. 2000;38:47-50.
24. De Bleecker JL. Intermediate syndrome: Prolonged cholinesterase inhibition. J Toxicol Clin Toxicol. 1993;31:197-9.
25. Khan S, Hemalatha R, Jeyaseelan L, et al. Neuroparalysis and oxime efficacy in organophosphate poisoning: A study of butyrylcholinesterase. Hum Exp Toxicol. 2001;20:169-74.

26. John M, Oommen A, Zachariah A. Muscle injury in organophosphorous poisoning and its role in the development of intermediate syndrome. Neurotoxicology. 2003;24:43-53.
27. Palimar V, Arun M, Mohan Kumar TS, et al. Intermediate syndrome in organophosphorus poisoning. J Indian Acad Forensic Med. 2005;27:28-30.
28. Meggs WJ. Permanent paralysis at sites of dermal exposure to chlorpyrifos. J Toxicol Clin Toxicol. 2003;41:883-6.
29. van Heel W, Hachimi-Idrissi S. Accidental organophosphate insecticide intoxication in children: a reminder. Int J Emerg Med. 2011;4(1):32.
30. Stephens R, Spurgeon A, Calvert IA, et al. Neuropsychological effects of long-term exposure to organophosphates in sheep dip. Lancet. 1995;345:1135-9.
31. Compston JE, Vedi S, Stephen AB, et al. Reduced bone formation after exposure to organophosphates (letter). Lancet. 1999;354:1791-2.
32. Jamal GA. Neurological syndromes or organophosphorous compounds. Adv Drug React Toxicol Rev. 1997;16:133-70.
33. Czeizel AE, Elek C, Gundy S, et al. Environmental trichlorfon and cluster of congenital abnormalities. Lancet. 1993;341:539-42.
34. Buckley JD, Meadows AT, Kadin ME, et al. Pesticide exposures in children with non-Hodgkin lymphoma. Cancer. 2000;89:2315-21.
35. Stephenson J. Exposure to home pesticides linked to Parkinson disease. JAMA. 2000;283:3055-6.
36. Engel LS, Checkoway M, Keifer MC, et al. Parkinsonism and occupational exposure to pesticides. Occup Environ Med. 2001;58:582-9.
37. Taylor CA, Saint-Hilaire MH, Cupples LA, et al. Environmental, medical and family history risk factors for Parkinson's disease: A New England-based case control study. Am J Med Genet. 1999;88:742-9.
38. Rajapakse BN, Thiermann H, Eyer P, et al. Evaluation of the Testmate ChE (cholinesterase) field kit in acute organophosphorus poisoning. Ann Emerg Med. 2011;58(6):559-64.e6.
39. Vaidyanathan R, Ashoka HG, Kumar GN Pramod. Management of organophosphorus compound poisoning—a one year experience in a tertiary care hospital. J Indian Soc Toxicol. 2012;8(1):38-42.
40. Benson BJ, Tolo D, McIntire M. Is the intermediate syndrome in organophosphate poisoning the result of insufficient oxime therapy? J Toxicol Clin Toxicol. 1992;30:347-9.
41. Sheth Sanket P, Vaishnav Bhalendu, Desai Devangi. Recurrent hypoglycemia in organophosphorus compound poisoning—an unusual complication. J Indian Soc Toxicol. 2011;7(2):22-3.
42. Singh S, Chaudhry D, Behera D, et al. Aggressive atropinisation and continuous pralidoxime (2-PAM) infusion in patients with severe organophosphate poisoning: Experience of a northwest Indian hospital. Hum Exp Toxicol. 2001;20:15-8.
43. Sundaray NK, Kumar JR. Organophosphorus poisoning: Current management guidelines. Medicine Update. 2010;20:420-5.
44. Clark RF. Insecticides: organic phosphorus compounds and carbamates. Goldfrank's Toxicological Emergencies, 7th edition. New York: McGraw-Hill Professional; 2002. pp. 1346-60.
45. Gerkin R, Curry SC. Persistently elevated plasma insecticide levels in severe methylparathion poisoning [abstract]. Vet Hum Toxicol. 1987;29:483-4.
46. Robenshtok E, Luria S, Tashma Z, et al. Adverse reaction to atropine and the treatment of organophosphate intoxication. Isr Med Assoc J. 2002;4:535-9.
47. Kumaran SS, Chandrasekaran VP, Balaji S, et al. Combined atropine and glycopyrrolate in organophosphate poisoning: The right solution for an old problem? J Indian Soc Toxicol. 2007;3(1):32-5.
48. Koplovitz I, Mento R, Matthews C, et al. Dose-response effects of atropine and HI-6, treatment of organophosphorus poisoning in guinea pigs. Drug Chem Toxicol. 1995;18:119-36.
49. Willems JL, De Bisschop HC, Verstraete AG, et al. Cholinesterase reactivation in organophosphorus poisoned patients depends on the plasma concentrations of the oxime pralidoxime methylsulphate and of the organophosphate. Arch Toxicol. 1993;67:79-84.
50. De Bleeker JL. Multiple system organ failure: Link to intermediate syndrome indirect. J Toxicol Clin Toxicol. 1996;34:249-50.
51. Gallo MA, Lawryk NJ. Organic phosphorus pesticides. In: Hayes WJ, Laws ER (Eds). Handbook of Pesticide Toxicology. San Diego, CA: Academic Press. 1991. pp. 917-1090.
52. Shivakumar S, Raghavan K, Ishaq RM, et al. Organophosphorus poisoning: A study on the effectiveness of therapy with oximes. J Assoc Physicians India. 2006;54:250-1.
53. Medicis JJ, Stork CM, Howland MA, et al. Pharmacokinetics following a loading plus a continuous infusion of pralidoxime compared with the traditional short infusion regimen in human volunteers. J Toxicol Clin Toxicol. 1996;34:289-95.
54. Willems JL, Langenberg JP, Verstaete AG, et al. Plasma concentrations of pralidoxime methylsulphate in organophosphorus poisoned patients. Arch Toxicol. 1992;66:260-6.
55. Eyer P. The role of oximes in the management of organophosphorus pesticide poisoning. Toxicol Rev. 2003;22:165-90.
56. Bowls BJ, Freeman Jr JM, Luna JA, et al. Oral treatment of organophosphate poisoning in mice. Acad Emerg Med. 2003;10:286-8.
57. Cherian MA, Roshini C, Visalakshi J, et al. Biochemical and clinical profile after organophosphorus poisoning—A placebo controlled trial using pralidoxime. J Assoc Physicians India. 2005;53:427-31.
58. Dawson A. Organophosphates: New antidotes from old drugs. J Indian Soc Toxicol. 2006;2(1):4.
59. Kusic R, Jovanovic D, Randjelovic S, et al. HI-6, in man: Efficacy of the oxime in poisoning by organophosphorus insecticides. Hum Exp Toxicol. 1991;10:113-8.
60. Dickson EW, Bird SB, Gaspari RJ, et al. Diazepam inhibits organophosphate-induced central respiratory depression. Acad Emerg Med. 2003;10:1303-6.
61. The Acute Respiratory Distress Syndrome Network. Ventilation with lower tidal volumes as compared with traditional tidal volumes for acute lung injury and the acute respiratory distress syndrome. N Eng J Med. 2000;342:1301-8.
62. Henry J, Wiseman H Pesticides. Management of Poisoning: A Handbook for Health Care Workers. Geneva: World Health Organization; 1997. pp. 115-53.
63. Irwin RS, Rippe JM. Irwin and Rippe's Intensive Care Medicine, 6th edition. Philadelphia: Lippincott Williams & Wilkins; 2008.
64. Haddad LM, Winchester JF. Clinical Management of Poisoning and Drug Overdose, 2nd edition. Philadelphia, PA, USA: WB Saunders Co.; 1990.

65. Tomy M. A clinico-biochemical study of levels of serum acetylcholinesterase enzyme in insecticidal poisoning. 1996; MD dissertation, University of Calicut, India.
66. Taylor P. Anticholinesterase agents. In: Hardman JG, Limbird LE, Gilman AG (Eds). Goodman and Gilman's The Pharmacological Basis of Therapeutics, 10th edition. New York: McGraw-Hill, Medical Pub. Division; 2001. pp. 175-91.
67. Tracqui A, Flesch F, Sauder P, et al. Repeated measurements of aldicarb in blood and urine in a case of nonfatal poisoning. Hum Exper Toxicol. 2001;20:657-60.
68. Verhulst L, Waggie Z, Hatherill M, et al. Presentation and outcome of severe anticholinesterase insecticide poisoning. Arch Dis Child. 2002;86:352-5.
69. Siegal D, Kotowycz MA, Methot M, et al. Complete heart block following intentional carbamate ingestion. Can J Cardiol. 2009;25:e288-90.
70. Buchholz U, Mermin J, Rios R, et al. An outbreak of food-borne illness associated with methomyl-contaminated salt. JAMA. 2002;288:604-10.
71. Yang PY, Tsao TCY, Lin JL, et al. Carbofuran-induced delayed neuropathy. J Toxicol Clin Toxicol. 2000;38:43-6.
72. Singh S, Parthasarathy S, Sud A, et al. Acute pancreatitis following propoxyfur (Baygon) ingestion. J Assoc Physicians India. 2003;51:78-9.
73. Jyothi VS, Dhage SS, Pai R, et al. Multiple unusual complications in a single patient with combined organophosphate-carbamate pesticide exposure. J Indian Soc Toxicol. 2011;7(1):47-50.
74. Rotenberg M, Almog S. Follow up of carbamate-exposed workers: Pitfalls in measurement of cholinesterase activity. Abstract No.131. J Tox Clin Tox. 1995;33(5).
75. Burgess JL, Bernstein JN, Hurlbut K. Aldicarb poisoning. A case report with prolonged cholinesterase inhibition and improvement after pralidoxime therapy. Arch Intern Med. 1994;154:221-4.

CHAPTER 94

Aluminum Phosphide Poisoning

Vivekanshu Verma, Devendra Richhariya

INTRODUCTION

Aluminum phosphide (AlP)—solid fumigant, tablets of AlP most commonly used as insecticides and rodenticides—is also referred to as "rice tablets", "wheat pill", celphos, and alphos **(Figs 1A and B; Table 1)**.

PECULIAR FEATURES

Peculiar features of AlP poisoning are as follows:
- It is kept as tablets which are used in grain storage after harvesting.
- It is found to be the most common cause of acute poisoning in India.
- It was also found to be the most common cause of suicidal death in north India.
- It shows a distinct male preponderance in the lower socioeconomic strata and in rural areas, probably due to the heavy social stress burden in this group.
- A positive history of ingestion is the basis of diagnosis in most cases.
- The presence of typical clinical features, garlicky odor from the mouth and highly variable arrhythmias in a young patient with shock and no previous history of cardiac disease points toward AlP.
- Unfortunately, its widespread use has been associated with a galloping rise in the incidence of AlP poisoning. Recent studies have indicated that the number of deaths so far have exceeded the number of fatalities in the Bhopal gas tragedy.

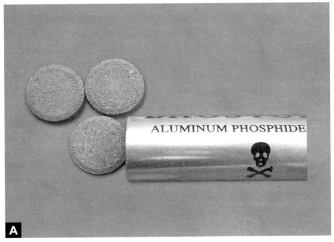
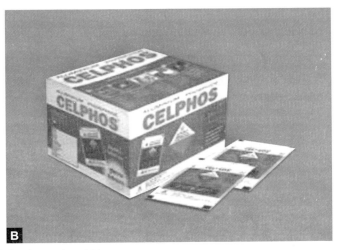

Figs 1A and B Usage of aluminum phosphide

Table 1 Comparison of aluminum phosphide and organophosphates

	AlP	OPC
Compound of phosphorus	Metallic salt of phosphorus	Organic compound of phosphorus
Available	Tablets/powder	Liquid form dissolved in kerosene
Pesticide	Fumigant in closed grain storage	Spray on open crops
Fatal	Cardiotoxic and cellulotoxic	Neurotoxic and respiratory failure
Life-saving treatment	IABP to support circulation	Intubation and mechanical ventilation
Antidote	Nil	Atropine and pralidoxime
Fatal period	Within hours	Within hours
Fatal dose	1 tablet (3 g)	10–15 mL
Smell	Mousy odor	Kerosene like noxious smell

Abbreviations: AlP, aluminum phosphide; OPC, organophosphates compound; IABP, intra-aortic balloon pump.

MECHANISM

Flow chart 1 describes the mechanism of AlP toxicity.

CLINICAL FEATURES

Clinical features of AlP poisoning are:
- The presenting symptoms depend on the route of administration.
- Poisoning by inhalation produces irritation of mucous membrane, dizziness, easy fatigability, nausea, vomiting, headache, and diarrhea in mild exposure.
- Ataxia, numbness, paresthesia, muscle weakness, paralysis, diplopia, and jaundice result from moderate degree of exposure.
- In severe cases of inhalational poisoning, the patient presents with acute respiratory distress syndrome (ARDS), congestive cardiac failure, convulsion, and coma.
- Nausea, vomiting, and abdominal pain are the earliest symptoms that appear after ingestion.
- Gastrointestinal (GI) symptoms present in moderate to severe poisoning are excessive thirst, abdominal pain, and epigastric tenderness while cardiovascular abnormalities seen are profound hypotension, dry pericarditis, myocarditis, acute congestive heart failure, and arrhythmias.
- Involvement of the respiratory system may lead to dyspnea, which may progress to type I or II respiratory failure.
- Nervous system manifestations include headache, dizziness, altered mental status, convulsion, acute hypoxic encephalopathy, and coma.
- A rare finding in AlP poisoning is pseudo-shock syndrome due to impaired fluid distribution which results in microcirculatory failure.
- Cardiac arrhythmias, respiratory failure, metabolic acidosis, and requirement of mechanical ventilation are poor prognostic markers with AlP poisoning **(Flow chart 2)**.
- Electrocardiogram (ECG) abnormalities: Most probably due to hypomagnesemia caused by cardiotoxic effect of phosphine.
- Absence of antidote for AlP
- Mortality rates are very high due to AlP toxicity (about 40–100%).

DIAGNOSIS

Diagnosis of AlP poisoning involves the following:
- A positive history of ingestion is the basis of diagnosis in most cases. The presence of typical clinical features, garlicky odor from the mouth and highly variable arrhythmias in a young patient with shock and no previous history of cardiac disease points toward AlP poisoning.
- Confirmation can be done by the *Silver Nitrate Test*. In this test, 5 mL of gastric aspirate and 15 mL of water are put in a flask and the mouth of the flask is covered by filter paper impregnated with 0.1 N silver nitrate. The flask is heated at 50°C for 15–20 minutes. If phosphine is present the filter paper turns black. For performing the test on exhaled air, the silver nitrate impregnated filter paper is placed on the mouth of the patient and the patient is asked to breathe through it for 15–20 minutes, blackening of the paper indicates the presence of phosphine in breath. The sensitivity of the test is 100% and 50% vis-à-vis gastric fluid and exhaled air, respectively.
- However, the most specific and sensitive method for detecting the presence of pH in blood or air is gas chromatography.
- For spot sampling of phosphine in air, detector tubes and bulbs are available commercially.

Flow chart 1 Mechanism of aluminum phosphide toxicity

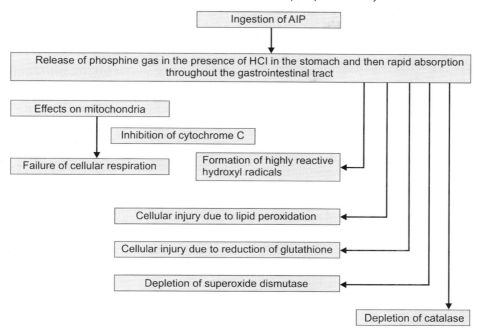

Flow chart 2 Effect of aluminum phosphide on cardiovascular system causing hypotension and arrhythmia

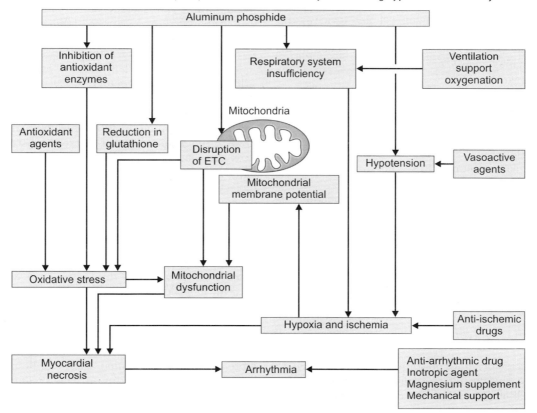

LABORATORY INVESTIGATIONS IN ALUMINUM PHOSPHIDE POISONING

Laboratory investigations in AlP poisoning comprise of the following:
- Laboratory evaluation is mainly done to assess the prognosis.
- Leukopenia indicates severe toxicity.
- Increased SGOT (serum glutamic oxaloacetic transaminase) or SGPT (serum glutamic-pyruvic transaminase) and metabolic acidosis indicate moderate to severe ingestional poisoning.
- Electrolyte analysis shows decreased magnesium while potassium may be increased or decreased.
- Measurement of plasma renin is significant as its level in blood carries a direct relationship with mortality and is raised in direct proportion to the dose of pesticide.
- The serum level of cortisol is usually found to be decreased in severe poisoning.

MANAGEMENT

Two important steps, resuscitation of shock and supportive measures, should be taken as soon as possible. In management, the main objective is to provide oxygenation, ventilation, and circulation till phosphine is excreted. Specific management toward AlP toxicity includes reducing absorption of phosphine, reducing cellular toxicity, and increasing excretion through kidney and lungs.

"Point of care" bedside devices in emergency department are useful for managing AlP poisoning:
- Electrocardiogram
- Arterial blood gas (ABG)
- Ultrasonography (USG) of chest and heart two-dimensional echo
- CARD test for cardiac enzymes
- Portable chest X-ray
- Intra-aortic balloon pump (IABP) for supporting failing heart
- Portable mechanical ventilator after intubation in refractory shock
- No role of mouth-to-mouth artificial ventilation as it can cause inhalational poisoning to rescuer, use bag and mask instead
- No role of noninvasive bi-level positive airway pressure ventilation (BiPAP) in poisoning as phosphine gas fumes are coming in breaths of poisoned victim.

Suspected Case of Alphos Poisoning

In case of suspicion of alphos poisoning:
- Take personal protection measures, including full face mask and rubber gloves during decontamination
- Secure airway, intravenous (IV) access preferably central venous pressure (CVP) and send routine investigations
- Gut decontamination with $KMnO_4$ (1:10,1000), vegetable or coconut oil (within 6 hours)

Emergency Department Management

Emergency department management of AlP poisoning includes the following **(Flow chart 3)**:
- After ingestion, effectiveness of gut decontamination primarily depends on the duration of exposure of poison and should be done as early as possible.
- To reduce the absorption of phosphine, gastric lavage is done with coconut oil.
- Gastric lavage with normal saline or distil water is contraindicated as phosphine gas is liberated from AlP on coming in contact with water.
- Intravenous access should be established and 2-3 L of normal saline is administered within the first 8-12 hour.
- Low dose dopamine (4-6 μg/kg/min) is given to keep systolic blood pressure more than 90 mm Hg.
- Hydrocortisone 200-400 mg every 4-6 hour is given intravenously to combat shock, reduce the dose of dopamine, check capillary leakage in lungs (ARDS), and to potentiate the responsiveness of the body to endogenous and exogenous catecholamines.
- Oxygen is given for hypoxia. ARDS requires intensive care monitoring and mechanical ventilation.
- A cathartic (liquid paraffin) is given to accelerate the excretion of AlP and phosphine.
- Antacids and proton pump blockers are added for symptomatic relief.

Potassium permanganate (1:10,000) can be used for gastric lavage as it oxidizes phosphine to nontoxic phosphate. There is no well-proven basis to conclude that $KMnO_4$ is efficient against AlP poisoning. Slurry of activated charcoal also helps to adsorb phosphine from the GI tract in most of the literature. Activated charcoal has a wide internal surface area consisting of pores (10-20 Å). It efficiently adsorbs toxins of moderate molecular weight (100-800 Da). The molecular weight of AlP is about 58 Da, therefore, role of activated charcoal in AlP poisoning is again doubtful as liberated phosphine cannot be detoxified.

Magnesium sulfate helps in scavenging free radicals through glutathione (GSH) recovery, hence, is effective as parenteral antioxidant in this poisoning as well as has been tried for its general membrane stabilizing effect in cardiac cells. It is observed that dose-related mortality rates in patients treated with and without $MgSO_4$ are not significantly different. Magnesium is weak antiarrhythmic agent and may be useful in controlling few supraventricular arrhythmia and more potent antiarrhythmic agent can be used. Adequate hydration and renal perfusion with IV fluid enhance the excretion through urine.

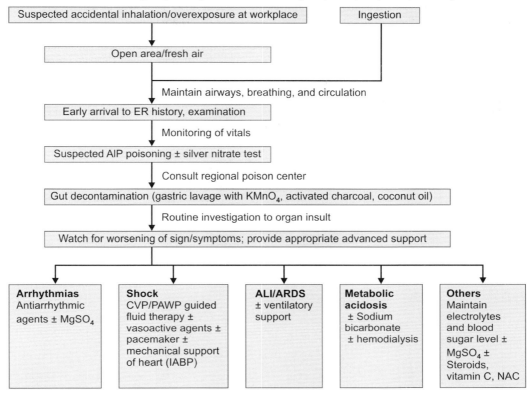

Flow chart 3 Emergency management of aluminum phosphide/phosphine poisoning

Abbreviations: AlP, aluminum phosphide; CVP, central venous pressure; PAWP, pulmonary artery wedge pressure; IABP, intra-aortic balloon pump; ECLS, extracorporeal life support; ALI/ARDS, acute lung injury/acute respiratory distress syndrome; NAC, n-acetylcysteine.

Watch for Worsening of Signs and Symptoms

Worsening of signs and symptoms includes:
- *Shock*: Fluid therapy with 2–3 L normal saline in first 8 hours to maintain CVP of 12–14 cm saline.
- *No response*: Low dose dopamine (4–6 µg/kg/min) is given to keep systolic blood pressure more than 90 mm Hg.
- *Refractory hypotension*: Consider IABP.

INTRA-AORTIC BALLOON PUMP IN ALUMINUM PHOSPHIDE POISONING

Role of IABP in AlP poisoning:
- The role of advanced measures like use of IABP to mechanically support the heart has been practiced in tertiary care hospitals.
- The role of advanced measures like use of IABP to mechanically support the heart has been demonstrated in toxic myocarditis with refractory shock due to AlP poisoning. IABP can mechanically support the heart, decrease the afterload, and improve perfusion to the vital organs and coronary arteries.
- The possibility of beneficial effect of extracorporeal life support (ECLS) as a supportive measure for intractable circulatory collapse.
- Extracorporeal membrane oxygenation (ECMO) is a novel technique for supplying oxygen and it may have a beneficial role in management of AlP poisoning.

CONCLUSION

Aluminum phosphide poisoning has high mortality rate due to nonavailability of specific antidote. Only possible measures to save the life in poisoning with unexposed form of AlP are supportive.

BIBLIOGRAPHY

1. Chefurka W, Kashi KP, Bond EJ. The effect of phosphine on electron transport in mitochondria. Pest Biochem Physiol. 1976;6:65-84.
2. Chugh SN, Arora V, Sharma A, Chugh K. Free radical scavengers and lipid peroxidation in acute aluminium phosphide poisoning. Indian J Med Res. 1996;104:190-3.
3. Chugh SN, Ram S, Chugh K, Malhotra KC. Spot diagnosis of aluminium phosphide ingestion: an application of a simple test. J Assoc Physicians India. 1989;37(3):219-20.

4. Chugh SN. Aluminium phosphide poisoning with special reference on its diagnosis and management [Review article]. J Med Assoc Clin Med. 1995:1:20-2.
5. Grover A, Bansal S. Aluminium phosphide poisoning. Manual of medical emergencies, 1st edn. New Delhi:M M Healthcare; 1997.pp. 76-9.
6. Lall SB, Peshin SS, Seth SD. Acute poisonings. A ten years retrospective hospital based study. Ann Natl Acad Med Sci (India). 1994;30:35-9.
7. Sepaha GC, Bharani AK, Jain SM, Raman PG. Acute aluminium phosphide poisoning. J Indian Med Assoc. 1985;83(11):378-9.
8. Singh S, Sharma BK, Wahi PL, Anand BS, Chugh KS. Spectrum of acute poisoning in adults (10 years experience).J Assoc Physicians India. 1984;12(7):561-3.
9. Singh S, Wig N, Chaudhary D, Sood NK, Sharma BK.Changing pattern of acute poisoning in adults: experience of a large North-West Indian Hospital (1970-1989). J Assoc Physicians India. 1997;45(3):194-7.
10. Siwach SB, Singh H, Jagdish, Katyal VK, Bhardwaj G. Cardiac arrhythmias in aluminium phosphide poisoning studied by on continuous holter and cardioscopic monitoring. J Assoc Physicians India. 1998;46(7):598-601.

SECTION 16

Environmental Emergencies

- **Management of Animal Bite Cases**
  Ashok Mishra
- **Snake Bite**
  Narendra Nath Jena, Devendra Richhariya
- **Heat Stroke**
  Sharad Manar, Taif Nabi, Pooja Kataria
- **Drowning**
  Vivekanshu Verma, Atul Bansal, Devendra Richhariya
- **Emergency Management of Burns**
  Aditya Aggarwal, Vimalendu Brajesh, Sukhdeep Singh, Umang B Kothari, Rakesh K Khazanchi
- **Electrical Injuries**
  Basar Cander

CHAPTER 95

Management of Animal Bite Cases

Ashok Mishra

INTRODUCTION

Management of animal bite cases is mandatory to protect against the risk of rabies which is an acute fatal encephalomyelitis caused by an RNA virus under the Genus *Lyssavirus* and family *Rhabdoviridae*. It is the most important viral zoonosis of warm-blooded animals like dogs, cats, jackals, etc. recognized today because of its global distribution, incidence, veterinary and human health costs and extremely high case fatality rate.[1]

Most of the mortality due to rabies is from Asia and Africa with 56% of the deaths estimated to occur in Asia and 44% in Africa. Human rabies is mainly caused by dog bites and annual incidence of bite in India is 1.7%.[2] Human rabies is endemic in India. According to a recent WHO estimate, globally 55,000 deaths occur every year; of these, 20,000 (36%) occur in India.[3] In India, there are 17.4 million exposures to animal bites each year.[4] Rabies is transmitted to man usually by bites or licks of rabid animals.[5]

Rabies now features among the 17 identified neglected tropical diseases (NTDs) by the WHO.[6] The acute viral infection is characterized by inflammation of the central nervous system. When the disease occurs in man, the most characteristic symptom is fear of water (hydrophobia) which develops due to painful spasms of the muscles of deglutition. Rabies is an extremely dangerous disease with a frequently long incubation period, highly distressing symptoms and as a rule, a lethal outcome. The violent symptoms associated with the illness and usual inevitability of death makes it one of the most terrifying diseases.[7]

Rabies or hydrophobia is probably the oldest recorded infection of mankind. Even today, it is as frightening a disease as it was in the past.

Sushruta, the famous Indian Physician, observed this condition in dogs, foxes, etc. which manifests as a state of confusion, drooping of tail and lower jaw and profuse salivation. He emphasized that this condition was fatal, once clinical symptoms became apparent.[8]

Dr Louis Pasteur in 1885 developed the first antirabies vaccine[9] which was first administered on July 6, 1885 to Joseph Meister, the young boy who had been severely bitten 14 times by a rabid dog.[10] After Jenner and his concept of protection against smallpox, rabies vaccine was the third vaccine developed in history, long before recognition of the nature of viruses.[11]

CURRENT SCENARIO

September 28 is being observed as World Rabies Day. This viral disease which is almost invariably fatal kills 50,000–70,000 people per year.[12] Around the world, rabies kills around 100 children every day because they cannot afford the vaccine. In Africa and Asia alone, the disease threatens 3.3 billion people—just under half the world's population.[13]

More than 99% of all human deaths from rabies occur in the developing world, and rabies still remains a neglected disease throughout most of Asia.[14] Asia accounts for more than 90% of all rabies deaths with nearly 31,500 deaths and 40–60% of all animal bites occurring in children under 14 years.[15] Dog bites are the primary source of human infection in all rabies endemic countries in the region and account for 96% of human rabies cases. The annual incidence of suspect bites from rabid dogs is 6.5 per million humans in Asia.[16]

India, Bangladesh, and Myanmar are high rabies endemic among the South-East Asian countries.[17] The estimated number of human rabies deaths in Asia is approximately 30,000–40,000 annually (20,000 in India, 2,000 in Bangladesh, remainder in the rest of Asia).[18]

In India, about 15 million people are bitten by animals, mostly dogs (91.5%) every year and need postexposure prophylaxis (PEP).[19] The incidence of animals bites in 17.4 per 1,000 population. A person is bitten every 2 seconds, and someone dies from rabies every 30 minutes.[4]

Cats are the second most common source of human rabies exposures in Asia and virus samples collected from Asian rabid cats and other domestic animals revealed only canine street virus strains.[20]

PATHOPHYSIOLOGY OF THE CONDITION

Agent Factors

Agent

The causative agent (Lyssavirus type 1) is a very small (size 120 × 80 nm), bullet shaped, i.e. round at one end and flat at another, neurotropic RNA containing virus **(Fig. 1)**. The virus is present in the saliva of rabid animals, saliva of human rabies patients, and also in the urine in low titers. Upon biting, scratching or licking on broken skin and intact mucous membrane, the virus enters the body, multiplies locally in the tissues and muscles, and then travels to brain at the speed of 3–10 mm/hour via neurotropic nerves. There it affects the brain stem function, causing hydrophobia (fear of water), aerophobia (fear of breeze) and/or photophobia (fear of light) and finally resulting in respiratory paralysis and death.[21] Virus is highly resistant against cold, dryness and decay and can remain infectious for weeks in dead bodies.

The virus recovered from naturally occurring cases of rabies is called "Street virus". It is pathogenic for all mammals and shows a long variable incubation period (20–60 days in dogs). Serial brain-to-brain passage of the street virus in rabbits modifies the virus such that its incubation period is progressively reduced until it becomes constant between 4–6 days. Virus isolated at this stage is called a "fixed virus". A fixed strain of virus is one that has a short, fixed, and reproducible incubation period (4–6 days) when injected intracerebrally into suitable animals. It does not form Negri bodies. The fixed virus is used in the preparation of antirabies vaccine.[5]

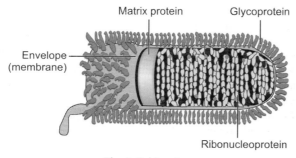

Fig. 1 Rabies virus

Reservoirs of Infection

Rabies exists in three epidemiological forms:
1. *Urban rabies*: The transfer of infection from wildlife to domestic dogs results in the creation of urban cycle while is maintained by dog and is responsible for 99% of human cases in India.
   Cats can also be the source of human infection.
2. *Wild life rabies*: Wild life or sylvatic rabies is perpetuated by the jackal, fox, hyena, etc. In South Africa, the disease is enzootic in the mongoose. These animals maintain a cycle amongst themselves and transmit the infection to dogs and domestic animals. Man may contract rabies through intrusion into this wild life cycle of rabies.
3. *Bat rabies*: In some Latin American countries like Brazil, Venezuela, Mexico, Trinidad, Tobago and parts of USA the vampire bat is an important host and vector of rabies. They can transmit rabies to animals and humans. This form of rabies is responsible for killing hundreds of thousands of cattle annually. Human are affected while sleeping outdoors. Recently, rabid bats have been found in Germany, Denmark, and Holland but not reported in India. Rabies virus is probably transmitted between vampire bats by either bite or aerosol.[5]

Source of Infection

The source of infection for man is the saliva of rabid animals. In dogs and cats, the virus may be present in the saliva for 3-4 days (occasionally 5-6 days) before the onset of clinical symptoms and during the course of illness till death.[5] Only half of rabid animals have virus in saliva so the probability of getting rabies following the bite of a rabid canine is 50%.[22]

Carrier States

In rare cases, carrier states have also been reported where the animal although apparently healthy, has transmitted the disease.[23]

Host Factors

All warm-blooded animals including man are susceptible to rabies.[5] Incidence of rabies is maximum in children aged less than 15 years. Bites around head and neck are most dangerous. Veterinary workers, animal handlers, forest staff, hunters, field naturalists and laboratory staff working with rabies virus are much more vulnerable for exposure to rabies virus.[5,22]

Mode of Transmission

Animal Bites

In India, most of the human rabies cases occur due to bite of a rabid dog. There is also possibility of contracting rabies through the bites of cats, monkey, horses, sheep, goat, etc. As a prerequisite to transmission, the saliva of the biting animal must contain the virus at the time of bite.

Licks

Licks on abraded skin and mucosa (abraded or unabraded) can transmit the disease. In rare instances, the disease may be transmitted through bone splinter or other object contaminated with saliva of a rabid animal.

Aerosols

Aerosol (respiratory) transmission can occur in two ways, either in caves harboring rabid vampire bats or in the laboratory where aerosols created during homogenization of infected animal brains can infect laboratory workers.

Person-to-Person

Man-to-man transmission, although rare, is possible either through bite by a hydrophobia patient or through corneal or organ transplants.[5]

Incubation Period

The incubation period in man is highly variable, commonly 3–8 weeks following exposure (may be up to 3 months),[22] but it may vary from 4 days to many years.[5]
The incubation period depends on number of factors:
- Site of the bite
- Severity of the bite
- Number of wounds
- Amount of virus injected, i.e. virus inoculum
- Species of the biting animal
- Protection provided by clothing, and
- Treatment undertaken, if any.

In general, incubation period is shorter in severe bites, bites on head and neck region, upper extremities and also bites by wild animals. In no other communicable disease is the incubation period so variable and dependent on so many factors as in rabies.[5]

Pathogenesis

The live virus, once introduced through the epidermis or mucous membrane, multiplies and ascends centripetally up the peripheral nerves to the central nervous system resulting in generalized encephalomyelitis. Once the virus reaches the CNS, it multiplies exclusively in the gray matter and then spreads centrifugally along autonomic nerves to other tissues including salivary glands and cornea **(Fig. 2)**.[22]

The pathognomonic lesion is an intracytoplasmic eosinophilic inclusion body commonly known as Negri bodies. These Negri bodies are seen only with infection of "Street virus" and not with "fixed virus".[22]

So far, the virus has not been isolated from the blood of rabies patients and hence the hematogenous route of spread is ruled out.[7]

In rabies, there is no initial viremia and the virus is not accessible to the normal immune mechanism of the body. The viremia or the stimulation of the normal immune mechanism is only during the end stages of the fatal disease therefore the role of naturally acquired infection is practically nonexistent.[24]

CLINICAL PRESENTATION

Clinical Features in Man

Rabies in man is known as hydrophobia in general. The disease can be divided into different stages:
- *Prodromal stage*: The disease begins with prodromal symptoms like fever, headache, myalgia, sore throat, and vomiting. There is pain and tingling or numbness at the site of bite in about 80% of cases. It is the most important complaint at this time and is related to the multiplication of virus at the local site. This stage may last for 3–4 days.[5,22]
- *Stage of acute encephalitis*: This stage is characterized by excessive motor activity and agitated behavior. There is widespread excitation and stimulation of nervous system involving the sensory, the motor, and the sympathetic and mental systems. There are symptoms of confusion, hallucination, muscle spasms, and convulsions. There is exaggerated sensitivity to noise, light, touch or currents of air. Autonomic symptoms like increased perspiration, salivation, lacrimation, pupillary dilatation, and hypotension are present. Hypoxia and hyperventilation progress to hypoventilation and repeated apnea.[5,22]
- *Stage of brainstem dysfunction*: Now the characteristic symptom of hydrophobia appears which is pathognomonic of rabies and is absent in animals. This fear of water is due to painful, violent, involuntary contraction of diaphragm, respiratory, laryngeal and pharyngeal muscles, initiated by swallowing of liquids. Progressively, even the sight, smell or sound of liquids can precipitate spasm of muscles of deglutition. More than 80% patients succumb to the disease during this stage. Death is due to respiratory arrest, convulsions or choking. Rest of the patients may progress to next stage.[5,22]
- *Stage of paralysis*: Paralytic symptoms can occur at any time during the course of illness. Now the muscle spasms cease and there is apathy, stupor, coma, and generalized flaccidity. Death occurs due to hypoxia or heart failure. Occasionally, rabies may present as Guillain-Barré type of ascending paralysis. This may be seen with bite of a vampire bat or in patients who have received postexposure prophylaxis against the disease.[22]
- *Death*: Once the symptoms develop, the disease is fatal and the patient dies within 2 weeks.[22]

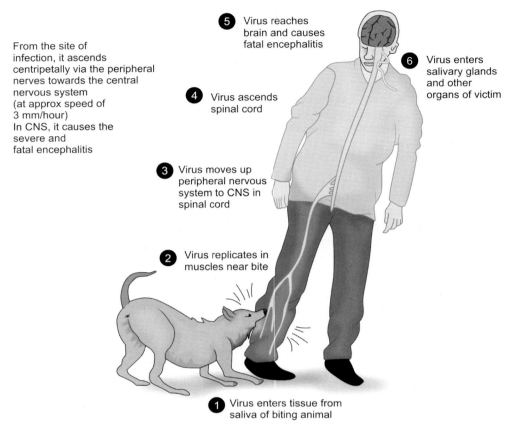

Fig. 2 Pathogenesis of rabies

There are no quarantine restrictions for a rabies patient. However, since the saliva, urine or tears, etc. may contain the virus; all the persons coming in contact should be immunized against rabies. Transmission from man-to-man, though uncommon is possible.[7]

Diagnosis

The *clinical diagnosis* can be possible on the basis of classical signs and symptoms. Hydrophobia is pathognomonic of rabies. There is history of animal bite.[5,22]

Laboratory Diagnosis

The laboratory tests are not routinely done for the management of animal bite cases, as these are not cost effective for management purposes and have limited availability in specific centers of big cities.

Several biological samples like saliva, cerebrospinal fluid (CSF), skin biopsies containing hair follicles collected at the nape of neck, extracted hair follicles, tears and urine can be used. Positive results of viral RNA in samples should be confirmed by sequencing to avoid false positives. Sensitivity of testing only one skin biopsy/patient is more than or equal to 98% but by collecting and testing three serial daily saliva samples per patient, it is possible to achieve maximal, i.e. 100% sensitivity.[25] Fluorescent antibody test is a very reliable test nowadays and can establish the diagnosis within a few hours. If the brain is negative by this test, a person need not be treated. Fluorescent antibody titers in clinical rabies are more than 1:10,000 which help to differentiate between rabies and vaccine reaction.

Rabies-specific ELISA (enzyme-linked immunosorbent assay) technique: ELISA techniques for detection of rabies antigen or anti-rabies IgG are rapid, easy to use and safe.[25]

Fluorescent antibody test can be performed on corneal impressions. After 7–10 days of illness, virus-neutralizing antibodies appear in the serum and CSF which can be measured by the Rapid Fluorescent Focus Inhibition Test (RFFIT) or ELISA.[23] Histopathologically, the necrosed ganglia, demyelinized cord sheaths, glial proliferation and Negri body inclusions are typical feature for a specific encephalomyelitis due to rabies.[7]

Differential Diagnosis

Before the appearance of hydrophobia and in those cases where it does not manifest, rabies needs to be differentiated from other clinical conditions such as tetanus (Lockjaw), encephalitis, hysteria, acute polyneuritis, poliomyelitis, and belladonna poisoning.

RABIES IN DOGS

Clinical Features in Dogs

Two clinical forms of manifestation are known in dogs:
1. *Furious rabies*: Dog behaves abnormally and becomes very restless. Gradually, it becomes dangerously aggressive with a tendency to bite objects, animals, and man indiscriminately and without provocation. There is profuse salivation due to paralysis of muscles of deglutition and tone of bark changes due to partial paralysis of vocal cords. Generalized convulsions followed by muscular incoordination and paralysis of muscles of trunk and extremities are seen at the terminal phase of illness.[26]
2. *Dumb rabies*: It is characterized by predominantly paralytic clinical features. The excitation phase, if present, tends to be very short. Progressive paralysis starts with head and neck region. Animal has difficulty in swallowing.[26] The dog withdraws itself from being disturbed and lapses into a stage of sleepiness and dies in about 3 days.[5]

Once the symptoms of rabies develop in an animal, it rarely survives more than a week.[5]

Observation of an animal for 10 days from the day of biting for signs of rabies is applicable for dogs and cats only and not for other domestic or wild animals. The rationale for observation is that if these animals are having infective saliva with rabies virus, they will show signs of disease in the next 3–5 days and die subsequently in another 3–5 days.[21]

MANAGEMENT OF A CASE OF HUMAN RABIES (HYDROPHOBIA)

Although no specific treatment for rabies is available, a case has to be managed according to following procedure:
- The patient should be sedated and kept in a quiet room, with shades drawn on windows. No external stimuli like noise, bright light, etc. should be present which may lead to convulsions. Patient should be treated symptomatically and proper hydration and diuresis should be maintained. Intensive respiratory and cardiac therapy is given.
- The nursing attendants and all persons coming in contact with the patient should be adequately protected as these patients are potentially infectious.
- The intensive care and nursing support are a must for rabies patients and there are seven cases of human rabies on record who survived this dreaded disease.[24]

Prevention of Human Rabies

Postexposure Prophylaxis for Rabies

Human rabies is essentially a fatal disease once the clinical signs develop, although 100% preventable. Rabies PEP consists of thorough wound care along with administration of modern antirabies vaccine and rabies immunoglobulin. This is highly effective if carried out systematically and diligently. If a person has received pre-exposure prophylaxis (PrEP), then it eliminates the need for rabies immunoglobulin (RIG) in case of an exposure.[27] The key to survival is administration of PEP as soon as possible. A patient with category III exposure needs thorough wound cleansing and a first dose of vaccine along with rabies immunoglobulin on the day of bite or day of reporting. The vaccination is done according to one of the WHO approved schedules to achieve a serum antibody titer of more than 0.5 IU/mL, which is considered acceptable according to WHO.[28] In case of any confusion regarding exposure it is always better to give over treatment rather than under treatment for prevention of rabies.

Assessment of exposure: According to WHO, assessment and management of rabies exposure have been discussed in **Table 1**.

Observation period: Immunization must be initiated immediately after every bite. Observation of dog/cat for signs of rabies for at least 10 days is important as well as valid. We can modify the treatment regimen (from postexposure to pre-exposure) if the dog/cat survives 10 days of observation.

We start the modern antirabies vaccine [cell culture vaccine (CCV)] according to WHO schedule on the day of bite by dog/cat or as soon as the patient reports. That is considered day "0". Then the vaccine is given on day "3" and "7" as per schedule. If the dog/cat is alive and normal till the 10th day then the remaining doses are not given.[25] Alternatively, after giving the first and second doses on days "0" and "3", the third dose of day "7" may be deferred if the dog/cat is healthy on day 7. It is further deferred to day 14 if the dog/cat is alive and healthy for 10 days. Then the patient is given the option of converting the present postbite/postexposure vaccination into a modified preventive/pre-exposure vaccination by giving the third dose of vaccine either on day 21 or day 28.[24] As the three doses confer immunity for a duration of 1 year, so it is advisable to give a booster dose after 1 year. Thus, we convert the postexposure schedule to pre-exposure schedule. It is further emphasized that the observation period of 10 days is valid for dogs and cats only and not for any other animals because of the variability in the period of infectivity in other animals' saliva.

Table 1	Management of rabies exposure in rabies endemic countries*		
		Recommended treatment	
WHO category	Nature of contact	Unknown, sick, proven or wild mammal	Healthy animal
I	Petting, teeding, licking on healthy skin, no mucous membrane exposure	None	None+
II	Superficial scratch, lick on broken skin	Modern tissue culture Rabies vaccine	Modern tissue culture Rabies vaccine++
III	Single or multiple transdermal bites or scratches at an location, or lick over mucous membrane	Modern rabies vaccine and Rabies immunoglobin (RIG)	Modern rabies vaccine and Rabies immunoglobin (RIG)

Important considerations:
+This is a good time to start pre-exposure vaccination. Particularly in children and others likely to have repeated animal contact, such as postmen, vets and others that are at a risk of dog bites.
++Start full treatment on first day and discontinue vaccine, if animal is alive and well on day 10, or if it has been found rabies negative on reliable laboratory examination. Encourage patient to return for another dose of vaccine on day 21, so that a full pre-exposure series has been completed.
Note: If there is significant delay in presentation or if the patient is immunosuppressed, it may appropriate to double the first dose of vaccine. Administration of two ampoules of vaccine, one in each arm, on day 0.
*Adapted from International Journal of Infectious Diseases 1997;1:140.

Wound care and treatment: Proper wound care is a very important step as it may bring down the risk of infection to the extent of 50–70%. This step is however often neglected. Our objective is to reduce the virus deposited at the site of bite as much as possible. The wound treatment must be done immediately or as early as possible after the bite. The steps are as follows:
- Gentle washing of the wound using a detergent soap, preferably under running tap water for at least 10 minutes.[7,21]
- Application of household antiseptics like povidone iodine, 40–70% alcohol or 0.01% aqueous solution of iodine can be done.[5]
- In some extensive deep wounds, the exploration of wound followed by debridement, removal of dirt and dead tissue may be required in a hospital setting and sometimes under anesthesia.[29]
- *Suturing must be generally avoided as a rule* as it may lead to the risk of inoculation of virus deep into the wound. However, if it cannot be avoided, it should be done as late as possible, from several hours up to 1 or 2 days.[5] The suturing should be loose and minimum possible stitches should be given. Before the suturing equine rabies immunoglobulins (ERIG) or human rabies immunoglobulins (HRIG) should be infiltrated into the wound.
- *Generally, animal bite wound should not be dressed or bandaged* and if unavoidable, it should be loose and not occlusive.
- Proper tetanus prophylaxis and wherever necessary, systemic antibiotics to prevent wound sepsis should be given.
- The use of any local applicant or irritant like turmeric, neem, red chilli, lime, plant juices, coffee powder, coin, etc. should be discouraged or avoided as these will propel the virus deeper into the wound causing nerve infection, encephalitis, and death.[5,21]

Administration of modern antirabies vaccine: The vaccine against rabies is a liquid or dried preparation of fixed virus inactivated by a suitable method.[30]

In India, mainly three types of modern CCV are available which are:
1. Human diploid cell vaccine (HDCV)
2. Purified chick embryo cell vaccine (PCECV)
3. Purified vero cell rabies vaccine (PVRV)

Dose: 1 mL. Intramuscular (IM) for HDCV and PCECV and 0.5 mL IM for PVRV irrespective of age of person.

All CCV can be stored at 2–8 °C and never to be stored in freezer compartment.

Indications: All cases of animal bites irrespective of severity of exposure require the same number of injections and dose per injection. The category III requires simultaneous administration of RIGs.[26]

Site for IM injection: The deltoid region is ideal site for injection (anterolateral aspect of mid-thigh in young children). Gluteal region is not recommended due to the amount of fat present there which retards the absorption of vaccine and interferes with the optimal antibody production and immune response.[26]

The use of modern, inactivated, purified CCV with a potency of at least 2.5 IU per single intramuscular dose should be done according to one of the following WHO schedules:[5]

- *Intramuscular schedule*: The most widely used is WHO Essen Schedule on day 0, 3, 7, 14 and 28 with an optional dose on day 90.
  Abbreviated multisite IM schedule (Zagreb schedule), i.e. the 2-1-1 regimen (one dose of CCV IM in right arm and one in left arm on day 0, one dose on day 7 and one dose on day 21), although WHO approved, is however not approved by Drug Controller General of India and hence should not be used in our country.[26]
- *Intradermal schedule*: This schedule has been recommended by WHO to reduce the cost of postexposure treatment with CCV. This has been approved by Government of India also. This should only be used where adequately trained staff is present well versed in technique and maintenance of cold chain and storage of supplies. The regimen currently in use is known as the updated Thai Red Cross Schedule. In this schedule, one dose of vaccine in a volume of 0.1 mL is given intradermally at two different lymphatic drainage sites, usually the right and left upper arms, on day 0, 3, 7, and 28. This updated Thai Red Cross Schedule (2-2-2-0-2) has been adopted in India.[26]

It is important to know that the IM dose of PVRV is 0.5 mL and that of PCECV is 1 mL. Still as per the recommendations of WHO, the ID dosage of all rabies vaccines uniformly is 0.1 mL.[24]

Regarding adverse effects, properly prepared CCV have not been associated with any serious adverse effects. Some people may complain of localized edema and redness, sore arm, headache, nausea, malaise, and fever.[5,26]

Switch over from one CCV to other is not encouraged as good immune response is best achieved with same brand/type of vaccine.[26] However, in case of nonavailability of same type/brand switch over can be done.

Administration of rabies immunoglobulin for passive immunization: The RIGs or ARS (antirabies serum) are ready-made antirabies antibodies providing passive immunity and immediate protection. Even the best of modern vaccines take 10–14 days to elicit the protective antibody titer of more than 0.5 IU/mL of serum and therefore RIGs cover this vulnerable period in category III exposure.[21]

The combination of antirabies vaccine and RIG is almost 100% effective "at prevention" of clinical symptoms and disease; however, attempts to use vaccine or RIG after the onset of symptoms have not been successful.[28] Some salient points related with use of RIG should always be kept in mind. These are:
- The RIG should be administered in all individuals with category III exposure and in those with category II exposure who are immunodeficient.
- The RIG is administered only once and as soon as possible after the initiation of PEP. RIG is not indicated beyond the 7th day after the first antirabies vaccine dose.
- The dose of human RIG is 20 IU/kg body weight and for equine RIG, 40 IU/kg body weight.
- All of the RIG, or as much as anatomically possible, should be administered into or around the wound site/s.
- Remaining RIG, if any, should be injected IM at a site distant from the site of vaccine administration. RIG may be diluted to a volume sufficient for all wounds to be effectively and safely infiltrated. There are no scientific grounds for performing a skin sensitivity test prior to ERIG administration.[19] So, it is not mandatory.

Rabies immunoglobulin should be immediately given after exposure to inhibit viral spread because vaccination needs time to induce a humoral response. RIG can be diluted with normal saline whenever the calculated dose (20 IU/kg body weight for HRIG subject to a maximum of 1,500 IU and 40 IU/kg body weight for ERIG subject to a maximum of 3,000 IU) is inadequate to infiltrate all wounds without previous dilution. However, the overall dose of HRIG or ERIG should not be increased because it may interfere with vaccination and may lead to reduced rate of seroconversion.[28]

Pre-exposure Prophylaxis

It is recommended for high-risk groups like laboratory staff handling the rabies virus and infected material, physicians and paramedics attending the hydrophobia cases, veterinarians, animal handlers and catchers, wild life wardens, pet owners and travellers from rabies-free to rabies-endemic areas.[5,26]

Pre-exposure prophylaxis should consist of three 1 mL IM or 0.1 mL ID doses of CCV, one dose each given on day 0, 7, and 28 with one booster after 1 year. Persons in high-risk group should have their neutralizing antibody titers checked every 6 months. If it is less than 0.5 IU/mL a booster dose of vaccine should be given. These persons after successful PrEP, if get exposed to rabies virus irrespective of time interval between previous vaccination and re-exposure require only two booster doses of CCV on day 0 and 3 without any RIG, whatever be the category of exposure or bite.[26]

Management of Re-exposure following Pre-exposure or Postexposure Prophylaxis with Cell Culture Vaccine

In case of re-exposure anytime, if a person has previously received complete pre-exposure prophylaxis of three doses with one booster after 1 year or postexposure prophylaxis of five doses with a potent CCV, should be given only two booster doses, IM or ID on days 0 and 3 but no RIG is necessary in them (WHO, 2002).[26]

CONTROL OF RABIES

As the major source of infection is dog, the control of dog population along with their mass immunization in the shortest possible time remains the most logical approach for the control of this dreaded disease. A canine rabies control program has been launched by the Ministry of Agriculture.[22] This type of program should incorporate three basic elements:

1. Epidemiological surveillance
2. Control of dog population
3. Mass immunization of dogs by giving primary vaccination at 3 months of age and booster 1 year later and then every year.

Nowadays safe oral vaccines have become available and can be used for mass immunization. Oral immunization can cover 75% of dog population.[22,26]

Oral vaccination of wild animals with attenuated as well as recombinant vaccines by using "oral vaccine baits" has successfully reduced and controlled wild life rabies in foxes in some countries of Europe like Germany, Switzerland, etc. and also in Canada.[5,31]

Health Education

Health education of public regarding prevention and control of rabies and management of animal bite is crucial to save lives. It is a real tragedy that this disease, which is 100% preventable, is still a major cause of mortality in developing countries.

Indications for Doubling the First Dose of Cell Culture Vaccine

In some situations, it becomes necessary and appropriate to double the first dose of antirabies CCV, whatever route or schedule is used. These are:

- In patients with underlying chronic disease (e.g. liver cirrhosis)
- In patients who are severely malnourished.
- In patients, reporting for treatment after a delay of 48 hours or more
- In patients who are congenitally immunodeficient or suffering from acquired immunodeficiency syndrome
- In patients taking immunosuppressive drugs (including corticosteroids, antimalarials, and anticancer drugs)
- In patients with very high degree of exposure or extensive wounds, i.e. on head, neck, face, hands, and genitals, etc. following bites by suspect or proven rabid animals or by wild animals like fox, jackal, mongoose, etc.
- In patients where RIG is indicated but unavailable.[24,31]
- *Pregnancy and lactation*: There are no contraindications regarding the use of modern CCV for postexposure prophylaxis during pregnancy and lactation.
- *Extremes of age*: The dose of CCV is not dependent on age and weight. The dose is exactly the same from pediatric to geriatric age group.[27,31]
- If a dog is vaccinated against rabies, it cannot suffer from or transmit the disease. But in view of questionable maintenance of cold chain it is very difficult to say that a vaccinated dog is immune against rabies unless it is confirmed by a serological test. However, a modern tissue culture vaccine of adequate potency, if given regularly to dog following strict schedule should prove to be sufficiently protective.
- Consumption of raw milk of any suspected rabid animal (cow, buffalo, goat, etc.) shall be considered and treated as category III exposure. Boiling of milk destroys the rabies virus.
- Proper cooking of meat destroys the virus but raw meat can transmit the virus.
- If a person presents after a considerable delay of weeks to months with a history of animal bite, it is mandatory to give complete course of postexposure treatment including infiltration of wound site with RIG in view of the 100% mortality with this disease. It may be appropriate to double the first dose of vaccine.

SUMMARY: IMPORTANT POINTS TO REMEMBER

- The saliva of rabies patients contains rabies virus and is infective; hence, in case of suspicion about contact with saliva of a rabies patient during kissing the contact requires rabies postexposure vaccination. If ulcers are present in the mouth, then immunoglobulins should be advised by IM route.
- Rabies virus is present in the semen and to some extent in vaginal secretions. In some male patients, priapism and in both male and female patients increased libido may be observed. Hence, to the healthy contact, a complete course of postexposure vaccination should be given. If abrasion on penis or vagina, RIG is to be given by IM route.
- There have been some instances of failure even after complete course of antirabies treatment. During discussions at WHO and other expert committee meetings it was found that the efficacy and immunogenicity of modern CCV were never in doubt but failures were either due to delay in getting vaccination or RIG was not used or there was already immunosuppression in patients.
- There is no contraindication of giving antirabies vaccine along with EPI/pediatric vaccines in case of postexposure vaccination; however, an interval of 3–4 weeks between the two types of vaccines is advisable in case of PrEP.
- Modern antiretroviral (ARV) can be safely given to children having chickenpox, measles or any other eruptive fevers.
- If during antirabies vaccination, any dose is missed then patient is counseled regarding strict adherence to schedule and schedule is completed as soon as possible.
- No dietary restrictions are required during vaccination but alcohol, tobacco, gutka, and smoking must be avoided.
- There is no single shot antirabies vaccine till date and a full course of antirabies vaccination does not guarantee or provide lifelong immunity against the disease.

Rabies is still a very dreadful as well as dreaded disease. Strict measures to control or eliminate the disease in domestic as well as wild animals must be taken if we are ever to achieve mastery over this deadly virus.

In conclusion, cases of human rabies would be extremely rare if all patients knew whom to approach for treatment in case of bite, if antirabies vaccine and serum were readily available and if the postexposure treatment was strictly and diligently carried out following the guidelines.[26,32]

REFERENCES

1. Nandi S, Kumar M. Global perspective of rabies and rabies related viruses: a comprehensive review. Asian J Anim Vet Adv. 2011;6:101-16.
2. Chawan VS, Tripathi RK, Sankhe L, et al. Safety of equine rabies immunoglobulin in grade III bites. Indian J Community Med. 2007;32(1):73-4.
3. Sudarshan MK, Ashwath Narayan DH, Ravish HS. Is the skin sensitivity test required for administering equine rabies immunoglobulin? Natl Med J India. 2011;24:80-2.
4. Sudarshan MK. Association for Prevention and Control of Rabies in India, Assessing the burden of rabies in India: WHO sponsored national multi-centric rabies survey (May 2004). Assoc Prev Control Rabies India J. 2004;6:44-5.
5. Park K. Park's Textbook of Preventive and Social Medicine, 21st edition. Jabalpur, Madhya Pradesh, India: Banarsidas Bhanot Publishers; 2011. pp. 250-7.
6. WHO: the world health report, Geneva. World Health Organisation 1996; 57.
7. WHO: the health situation in South-East Asia Region. New Delhi Regional office of SEAR 1994-7.
8. Gode GR. Treatment of human rabies, problems and possibilities. In: Kaul HL (Ed). Advances in Anaesthesiology. Proceeding of Vth Asian and Australian Congress of Anaesthesiology. New Delhi: Sagar Publishers; 1978. pp. 229-303.
9. King AA, Turner GS. Rabies: a review. J Comp Pathol 1993;108:1-39.
10. Perrin P, Lafon M, Sureau P. Rabies vaccines from Pasteur's time up to experimental subunit vaccines today. In: Plotkin S (Ed). Viral Vaccines. New York: Wiley-Lisss Inc.; 1990. pp. 325-45.
11. Wu X, Smith TG, Rupprecht CE. From brain passage to cell adaptation: the road of human rabies vaccine development. Expert Rev Vaccines. 2011;10(11);1597-608.
12. Rupprecht CE, Gibbons RV. Prophylaxis against Rabies. N Engl J Med. 2004;351 (25): 2626-35.
13. King AA, Turner GS. Rabies: a review. J Comp Pathol. 1993;108:1-39.
14. WHO Expert Committee on Rabies, 8th report. Geneva:World Health Organisation, 1992;TRS 824.
15. Meslin FX, Briggs D. Re: preventing the incurable: Asian rabies experts advocate rabies control. Vaccine. 2006;24(47-48):6807.
16. Briggs DJ, Dreesen DW, Wunner WH. Vaccines. In: Jackson AC, Wunner WH, eds. Rabies. San Diego, USA: Academic Press, 2002;371-400.
17. Gongal G, Wright AE. Human rabies in the WHO Southeast Asia region: forward steps for elimination. Adv Prev Med. 2011;2011:383870.
18. Human rabies prevention – United States, 1999: Recommendations of the Immunisation Practices Advisory Committee (ACIP). MMWR Recomm Rep. 1999;48(RR1):1-21.
19. WHO Publication. Rabies vaccines: WHO position paper—recommendations. Vaccine. 2010;28(44):7140-2.
20. Nicholson KG. Rabies. Lancet. 1990;335:1201-5.
21. Sudarshan MK. Rapid consult on rabies prevention. In: Sudarshan MK (Ed). A Communication. Gurgaon, India: McMillan Medical Communication; 2010.
22. Gupta P, Ghai OP. Text Book of Preventive and Social Medicine, 2nd edition. CBS Publishers; 2007.
23. Human rabies prevention – United States, 1999: Recommendations of the Immunisation Practices Advisory Committee (ACIP). MMWR Recomm Rep. 1999;48 (RR1):1-21.
24. Sudarshan MK. Rabies prophylaxis. Gurgaon: McMillan Medical Communications; 2012.
25. Dacheux L, Wacharapluesadee S, Hemachudha T, et al. More accurate insight into the incidence of human rabies in developing countries through validated laboratory techniques. PLoS Negl Trop Dis. 2010;4(11):e765.
26. Lal S, Adarsh, Pankaj. Textbook of Community Medicine, 2nd edition. New Delhi: CBS Publishers; 2009.
27. Shantavasinkul P, Wilde H. Postexposure prophylaxis for rabies in resource-limited/poor countries. Adv Virus Res. 2011;79:291-307.
28. Both L, Banyard AC, van Dolleweerd C, et al. Passive immunity in the prevention of rabies. Lancet Infect Dis. 2012;12(5):397-407.
29. Batra RK, Kaul HL. Rabies—Pathophysiology and Current Status of Management. J Gen Med. 1994;6(4).
30. Cabasso VJ, Loofbourow JC, Roby RE, Anuskiewicz W. Rabies immune globulin of human origin: preparation and dosage determination in non-exposed volunteer subjects. Bull World Health Organ. 1971;45:303-15.
31. IJCP Medinews. Rabies Emerging Trends. New Delhi: An IJCP Group Publication; 1998.
32. Wasi C, Chaiprasithikul P, Thongcharoen P. Progress and achievement of rabies control in Thailand. Vaccine. 1997;15:S7-11.

CHAPTER 96

Snake Bite

Narendra Nath Jena, Devendra Richhariya

FACTS ABOUT SNAKE BITE

- India—highest snake bite mortality in the world (WHO).
- WHO —estimates 83,000 snake bites per annum with 11,000 deaths.
- In India most of which are nonpoisonous and 13 known species are poisonous cobra, Russell viper, saw scaled viper and common krait are common poisonous snakes capable of causing life threatening symptoms.
- 55% of victims are age 17 to 27 years.
- Ethanol intoxication was present in 30-60% of bitten victims.
- 15% victims had previous snake bites.
- 45% are dry bites.
- Seasonal incidence—rainy season.
- Venomous bites and stings—by snakes and scorpions due to immigration from soil pits and hole filled with water flooding during rains and floods, forcing reptiles out of their homes.
- Fatalities are high because victims not reaching hospital in time for definitive treatment, continue to adopt harmful first aid practices
- Antidotes—antisnake venoms.

IDENTIFICATION OF VENOMOUS AND NONVENOMOUS SNAKE (FIGS 1A AND B)

- Snake can be differentiated on the basis of anatomy of head pupil fangs and tail.
- Venomous snake has triangular head, elliptical pupil, venom apparatus and single row tail.
- Nonvenomous snake has rounded head and pupil, double row tail and no venom apparatus.

CLASSIFICATION OF VENOMOUS SNAKE

- ***Elapidae (neurotoxic)*** e.g. cobra, king cobra spitting cobra and kraits—the cobra and krait producing neuroparalysis like ptosis, external ophthalmoplegia, dysphagia, flaccid quadriparesis, neck muscle weakness, respiratory paralysis which becomes fatal. Responds well with antisnake venom, but patient may die before reaching the hospital as symptoms starts very fast .
- ***Viperidae (Hemotoxic)*** e.g. Russell viper, saw scaled viper, pit viper—viper causes bleeding and coagulation disorders. Symptoms starts late patient reaches the hospital with multiorgan involvement, critical care including ventilator support are required till organ recovery.

COMPONENTS OF SNAKE VENOM

- Snake venom is acidic, specific gravity—1.030–1.070, and water soluble.
- Lethal dose of cobra venom 0.12 g, kraits venom 0.06 g, Russell viper venom 0.15 g
- Snake venom is combination of enzymatic and non-enzymatic polypeptide.

Zinc metalloproteinase: Damage vascular endothelium, causing bleeding.

Hyaluronidase: Help in spreading the venom.

Procoagulant enzyme: Promotes consumption coagulopathy and bleeding. Blood will not clot.

Phospholipase A2 (lecithinase): It damages mitochondria, red blood cell, leukocytes, platelets, peripheral nerve endings, skeletal muscle, vascular endothelium, and other membranes, and produces presynaptic neurotoxicity

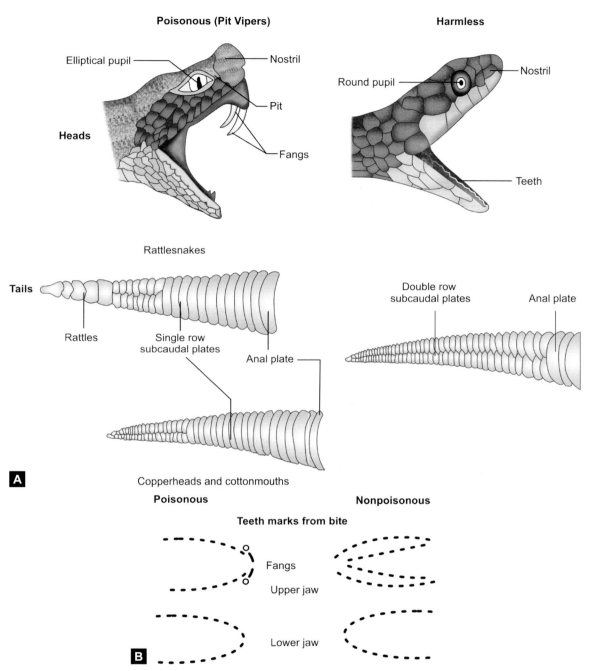

Figs 1A and B Difference between poisonous and nonpoisonous snake

Protiolytic enzyme (metalloproteinases, endopeptidases, hydrolases, polypeptide): Proteolytic enzyme responsible for edema bruising, blistering and necrosis at the site of bite.

Mechanism of Action Snake Venom

Krait and Russell's viper has presynaptic neurotoxin that means acetylecholine release is inhibited from the presynaptic membrane, so recovery is slow and delayed and depends on regeneration of terminal axons. while cobra venom has postsynaptic neurotoxin that means cobra toxins bind to acetylecholine receptors and produce neuromuscular blockade. Anticholinesterases reverse the neuromuscular blockade, thus neostigmine useful in cobra but not in krait and viper.

CLINICAL FEATURES OF SNAKE BITE

Generalized Features
- Nausea, vomiting, abdominal pain
- Dizziness, faintness, drowsiness
- Visual disturbances
- Collapse, hypotension, shock, arrhythmias
- Pulmonary edema
- Chemosis

Local Features
- Fang marks **(Fig. 2A)**
- Local pain, bleeding, bruising, blister necrosis **(Fig. 2B)**
- Lymphangitis
- Enlargement of lymph node.

Systemic Features

Bleeding disorders: Bleeding from bite marks, epistaxis, hemoptysis, hematemesis, hematuria.

Neurological symptoms: Dizziness drowsiness ptosis, dysphagia, dysphasia, flaccid paralysis.

Renal symptoms: Myoglobinuria, oliguria/anuria, acute renal failure hyperkalemia.

Endocrine symptoms: Shock and hypoglycemia due to acute pituitary infarction resulting acute onset insufficiency.

MANAGEMENT OF SNAKE BITE

Stepwise approach is adopted in management of snake bite which includes:
- *Prehospital care* which includes first aid and transfer to hospital.
- *Hospital care* includes rapid assessment and resuscitation, pain management, laboratory test and specific measures like anti-snake venom.
- *Supportive care* includes treatment of bitten part, rehabilitation, and treatment of chronic complications.

First Aid

Numerous first aid methods are popular in the society regarding snake bite and are provided to patient before reaching the hospital. Common first aid methods popular in community are local incisions at the site, sucking the venom out of the wound, tying the cloth (tourniquets) around the limb, local application of chemicals and herbs but most of them are useless and dangerous, and these first aid methods are not recommended.

Recommended first-aid methods are:
- Snake bite individuals are very anxious. Reassurance should be given to the victims.
- Immobilization of patient is important. Patient should be in comfortable position and affected limb should be immobilized with splint or slings.
- Any attempts of giving incisions, rubbing, cleaning, massage, application of herbs or chemicals increases absorption of the venom into blood.

Transfer to Hospital

- The patient should be transported to hospital as quickly as possible in safe and comfortable manner. Movement of the bitten limb should be minimized.
- Patients should be placed in the recovery position, in case they vomit.

Rapid Assessment and Resuscitation

Patient should be assessed immediately in triage. Airway assessment should be priority. Tracheal intubation and initiation of mechanical ventilation helpful in patient with respiratory distress and bulbar palsy. Early critical care

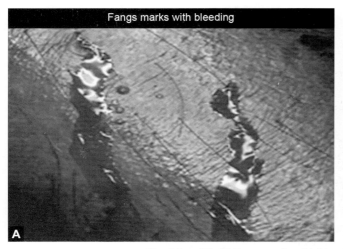 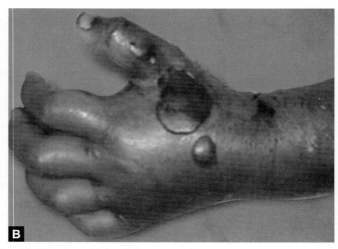

Figs 2A and B (A) Fangs marks with bleeding; (B) Blistering with local tissue necrosis

support for multiorgan failure patient. Antitetanus toxoid and antibiotics for preventing wound sepsis.

Pain Management

- Oral paracetamol, tramadol are recommended
- NO aspirin/NSAID (nonsteroidal anti-inflammatory)

Supportive Diagnostic Features and Laboratory Tests for Snake Bite in Emergency Department

Signs of Systemic Envenomation

- Cobra and krait—paraplegia, drooping of saliva, ptosis, drowsiness, gasping state.
- Viper—hemoptysis, hematuria, hematemesis, bitten-wound bleeding and disseminated intravascular coagulation (DIC).
- Electrocardiography (ECG)—bradycardia, AV block with ST-elevation.
- Arterial blood gases (ABG)—hypoxemia, respiratory acidosis (need for ventilator), hyperkalemia, renal metabolic acidosis (impending ARF).
- Coagulation screen—prothrombin time (PT) prolonged.
- Cardiac enzymes—creatine phosphokinase (CPK) increase.
- Bedside—20 min WBCT (whole blood clotting time).
- Urine visual examination—discolored urine in hematuria, proteinuria, myoglobinuria.
- Anuria—sign of ARF—need of dialysis.
- Additional test helpful in differential diagnosis are blood and urine toxic screen. Opiates and heroine can give rise to acute neurotoxic respiratory arrest.

20WBCT

- Reliable bedside test of coagulation
- Establishing the clotting capability in snake bite
- Keep the venous blood in glass tube for 20 min, if blood is liquid even after 20 min the blood is not coagulable and this indicate coagulopathy. The test should be carried out every 30 min from admission for 3 hours then hourly **(Fig. 3)**.

Neostigmine Test: Cobra Bite

- Despite the fact that the neostigmine test (neostigmine 0.5 mg IM with atropine 0.6 mg IV) was actually an Indian discovery, it is still poorly used in India.
- Reverse respiratory failure and neurotoxic symptoms.
- Use of atropine to mitigate the hypersecretory condition that develops with the use of neostigmine.
- Cobra venom is alpha-bungarotoxin, which reversibly blocks postsynaptic acetylcholine receptors.
- *Neostigmine*: 0.5–2.5 mg in adults and 0.025 mg/kg in children IV infused over 5 minutes.
- Give concurrent administration of atropine 0.6–1.2 mg IV in adults and 0.01 mg/kg of atropine IM or SC in children.
- The use of oral formulations of neostigmine is not routinely used in poisoned patients.

Differential Diagnosis: Acute Flaccid Paralysis

- Acute flaccid paralysis (AFP) surveillance in children—for polio
- AFP in farmer—neurotoxic snake bite
- AFP in elderly—acute stroke

SPECIFIC TREATMENT

Anti-snake Venom (ASV)

- Anti-snake venom (ASV) is the specific of treatment.
- Polyvalent ASV, effective against four common poisonous snake in India; no monovalent ASVs are available.

Indications for Anti-snake Venom

- If following features develops in patient with suspected or proven snake bite.
- Rapid developing swelling in more than half of the affected limb, enlarged and tender lymph node.

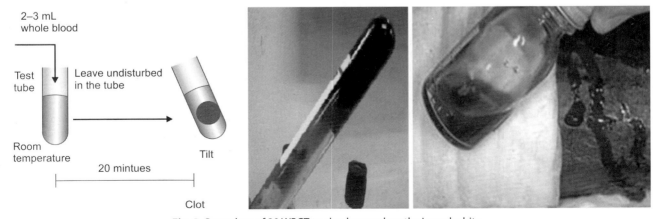

Fig. 3 Procedure of 20 WBCT to check coagulopathy in snake bite

- *Coagulation abnormalities*: Epistaxis hemoptysis hematuria and gum bleeding.
- *Neurotoxic features*: Ptosis, ophthalmoplegia, regurgitation, nasal voice bulbar palsy.
- *Cardiotoxic feature*: Hypotension, shock, arrhythmia
- *Acute kidney injury (renal failure)*: Features of rhabdomyolysis hyperkalemia dark brown urine, oliguria or anuria, raised urea creatinine.

Anti-snake Venom Administration

- Types of ASV—polyvalent— liquid/dry lyophilized
- Dose in victim is same in all—child, pregnancy, and elderly.
- ASV anaphylaxis—there is no recommendations of test dose. Premedication with—antihistamine and hydrocortisone but no evidence that this regimen is effective in preventing the ASV reaction.
- Keep injection adrenaline 0.5 mg 1:1,000 ready. Physician should be ready to handle this situation
- Shelf life of liquid ASV—2 yrs at 4°C.
- 8–10 vials ASV to be administered over one hour.
- Intravenous "push" injection and intravenous infusion are recommended.
- Anaphylactic reaction should be managed with antihistamine hydrocortisone and adrenaline. After recovery from the anaphylaxis, ASV can be started slowly for 10–15 min under close monitoring.
- Next clotting test should be done at 6 hours because the liver unable to clear clotting factors in less than 6 hours
- Signs of recovery are spontaneous bleeding from various site usually stops, blood starts clotting (20 WBCT), urine color become normal, recovery in shock and rise in blood pressure.
- Feature of postsynaptic neurotoxic (cobra bite) improves within hours but presynaptic neurotoxic feature (krait bite) takes linger time to improve.
- Repeat the dose of ASV (½ or 1 full dose) if WBCT is >20 minutes and continue it every 6 hourly till normal coagulation. Other criteria for repeating the dose are presence of neurotoxic and/or cardiotoxic feature after 1–2 hours of ASV injection.
- Neostigmine (anticholinesterase) is helpful in postsynaptic neurotoxin by cobra bite; if neurologic symptoms improves by administering 0.5–2 mg IV then it should be continued ½ hourly over next 8 hours. Neostigmine not useful in presynaptic neurotoxin like common krait and viper bite.
- *Late presentation of snake bite victims:* Sometimes snake bite patient present late in emergency department after several days. Anti-snake venom only neutralize unbound venom so perform the 20WBCT test if coagulopathy present then give 8–10 vials of ASV.
- If respiratory failure or ptosis is present give ASV to ensure no unbound venom is present in blood.

Indications for Intensive Care Admission in Snake Bite

- Respiratory failure
- Acute renal failure due to rhabdomyolysis needs hemodialysis.
- Bleed in brain.
- Disseminated intravascular coagulation.
- Encephalopathy, paralysis and coma.
- Hypotension and shock.
- Tetanus and cellulitis
- Compartment syndrome and gangrene.

RECENT ADVANCES IN SNAKE BITE MANAGEMENT

- Tranexamic acid—helpful in bleeding victims.
- If prothrombin time is prolonged, vitamin K is indicated.
- Enzyme-linked immunosorbent assay (ELISA) of blood venom levels and for detecting venom antigens for identifying snake.
- Monovalent FAB (fragment antigen binding) ASV—still not available for Indian snakes.
- Immunoglobulin FAB fragments which neutralize and bind venoms allowing them to be redistributed and taken away from the target tissues and subsequently eliminated.
- Hemodialysis to detoxify blood from venom as snake venom is dialyzable poison.

BIBLIOGRAPHY

1. API Textbook of Medicine, 10th edition, 2014.
2. Goldfrank's Toxicologic Emergencies, 10th edition, 2015.
3. Harrison Principles of Internal Medicine, 19th edition, McGraw Hills 2015.
4. Medical Law Cases for Doctors—The Medical Law Reporter of India. 2015:9.
5. Modi's Medical Jurisprudence and Toxicology, 23rd edition 2012 Lexis Nexis.
6. National Snake bite Management Protocol, 2009 by Director General Health Services, Ministry of Health and Family welfare, Government of India.
7. Oxford Textbook of Medicine 5th edition 2010.
8. Pillay's Textbook of Modern Medical Toxicology 4th edition, Jaypee Publishers, 2013.
9. Snake bite Mortality in India: A Nationally Representative Mortality Survey. Published in 2011 Dr Bijayeeni Mohapatra. *http://journals.plos.org/plosntds/article?id=10.1371%2Fjournal.pntd.0001018.*
10. WHO's List of top 10 Neglected Tropical Diseases includes snake bite. *http://www.who.int/neglected_diseases/diseases/en/.*

CHAPTER 97

Heat Stroke

Sharad Manar, Taif Nabi, Pooja Kataria

INTRODUCTION

Heat stroke is a common medical emergency in tropical areas, clinically diagnosed as a core temperature more than 40°C with central nervous system dysfunction or multiorgan dysfunction Core temperature is at which blood perfusion of hypothalamus and vital organs of body like heart and brain are maintained. Normal core body temperature is 36–37.5°C and rectal temperature being the closest approximation.

Heat stroke is one of the important treatable causes of multiple organ failure resulting from thermoregulatory failure. Heat stroke problem in tropics is increasing with rise of global warming. In India, northern and western parts are worst affected due to heat stroke. Exertion-induced heat stroke cases are reported in military recruits. In spite of advances in the treatment, mortality due to heat stroke remains high.

Heat stroke can be classified as:
- Classical heat stroke
- Exertional heat stroke.

CLASSICAL HEAT STROKE

It usually affects older age group with limited mobility and/or chronic diseases, and individual vulnerable to excessive environmental temperature and humidity. Laboratory feature like respiratory alkalosis is common.

EXERTIONAL HEAT STROKE

It is usually seen in young healthy individual who overexert in the heat and humidity. Respiratory alkalosis with lactic acid, rhabdomyolysis, renal failure, disseminated intravascular coagulation (DIC) and hyperuricemia can be frequently seen.

RISK FACTORS FOR HEAT STROKE

- Male sex
- Obesity
- Poor physical conditions
- Lack of acclimatization
- Diuretic therapy
- Dehydration
- Febrile illness
- Alcohol abuse
- Skin diseases that affect sweating
- Drugs impairing normal thermoregulatory response
- Past history of heat stroke.

PATHOPHYSIOLOGY

Heat stress and hyperthermia induces acute phase reactant and heat stroke proteins which lead to heat stroke. Direct cytotoxicity of heat, inflammatory and coagulation responses of the host result in alteration in microcirculation and consequent damage to vascular endothelium and tissues. Increased permeability due to ischemia may lead to endotoxin release, resulting in excessive production of inflammatory cytokines, endothelial cell activation, and release of nitric oxide and endothelin. Endotoxins leak into circulation and enhance the acute phase response, leading to increased production of pathogenic cytokines and nitric oxide. Both cytokines and nitric oxide can interfere with thermoregulation and precipitate hypothermia, hypotension, and heat stroke **(Flow chart 1)**.

Heat stroke causes failure of normal cardiovascular adaptation to heat, acute physiological alteration, and progression to multiorgan dysfunction due to hyperthermia by increasing metabolic demand, circulatory failure, and hypoxia.

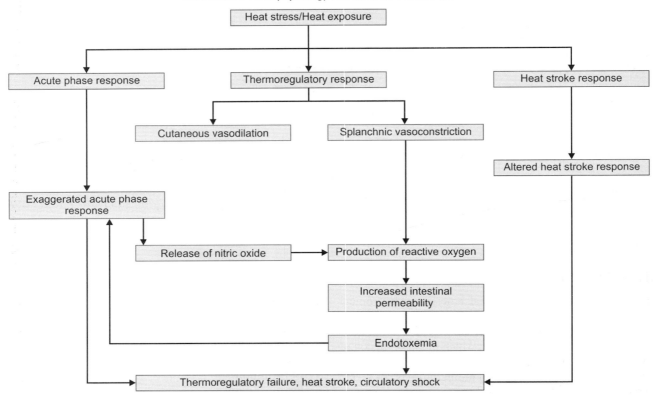

Flow chart 1 Pathophysiology of heat stress or heat exposure

CLINICAL FEATURES

- *Early features*: Temperature more than 40°C, dry skin, extreme fatigue, headache, high fever, vomiting, and diarrhea.
- *Respiratory symptoms*: Tachypnea including acute respiratory distress syndrome (ARDS).
- *Cardiovascular symptoms*: Tachycardia, hypotension, and shock.
- *Central nervous system*: Altered mental status including violent behavior, confusion, convulsion, and coma.
- Renal and liver failure coagulopathy rhabdomyolysis.

LABORATORY FINDINGS

- Hemoconcentration and leukocytosis
- Blood urea nitrogen (BUN) with dyselectrolytemia
- Hypoglycemia
- Proteinuria, tubular cast, and myoglobinuria
- *Arterial blood gas (ABG)*: Respiratory alkalosis (along lactic acidosis in exertional heat stroke)
- *Coagulation profile*: Thrombocytopenia, raised bleeding and clotting time, fibrinolysis, and rhabdomyolysis
- Hyperuricemia
- Raised CK-MB suggests myocardial damage
- *Electrocardiogram (ECG)*: Nonspecific ST changes, prolongation of QT interval.

COMPLICATIONS

- Acute renal failure
- Shock
- Brain cell damage
- ARDS
- DIC
- Multiorgan failure.

Other conditions present with high core temperature:
- Malignant hyperthermia
- Neuroleptic malignant syndrome
- Anticholinergic poisoning
- Thyroid storm
- Cerebral malaria
- Sepsis
- Meningitis.

TREATMENT

Supportive treatment and rapid cooling is the main stay of treatment.

Start cooling the patient in prehospital setting as soon as possible to reduce the core temperature to about 39°C. Move the patient to a cooler place, remove his or her clothing and initiate external cooling. Apply cold packs on the neck, axilla, and groin. Position an unconscious patient to lateral position, clear the airway, administer oxygen, and give intravenous normal saline.

The cooling process **(Fig. 1)** must be continued when the patient is being transported to the hospital. There are several cooling methods like fanning and spraying cold water on a completely undressed patient. Other cooling methods like cold intravenous fluids, gastric and bladder lavage by cold water also reduce the core temperature. Large volume of fluids and correction of electrolyte imbalance is important and should be managed in intensive care unit. There is no proven drug that lowers the core temperature in heat stroke patient. Diazepam is used to treat the seizures in heat stroke patients.

Treatment in Hospital

- Diazepam to control seizures
- Elective intubation to protect airway and to keep oxygenation SpO_2 (peripheral capillary oxygen saturation) >90%.
- Refractory hypotension should be treated with vasopressin
- Management of hyperkalemia to prevent life-threatening cardiac arrhythmias
- In rhabdomyolysis patients, management of life-threatening complication in intensive care unit
- Degree and duration of hyperthermia is important for recovery of patients. Complete neurological recovery is achieved in most of the patients, but residual brain damage may occur in 20% of patients with high mortality and morbidity. Cerebellum is the most susceptible to thermal damage.

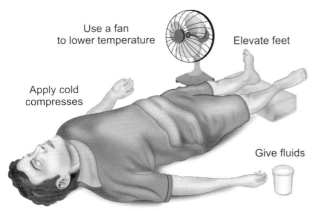

Fig. 1 First aid for heat stroke

HEAT EXHAUSTION

Heat exhaustion is not a life-threatening condition. Patients may present with weakness, malaise, dizziness, nausea, vomiting or sometime heat syncope (after standing long period of time in heat). Patient looks tired, sweaty, tachycardia, with normal sensorium and core temperature. Diagnosis is based on clinical presentation. Laboratory tests are needed to rule out hypoglycemia, acute coronary syndrome, and infections.

Treatment

Keep the patient on a flat surface in a cool environment. Sometimes, oral rehydration therapy may not be effective so start intravenous fluid and correction of electrolyte imbalance. Rate and volume of intravenous fluid should be titrated according to response, age, and underlying morbidity usually 1–2 L of crystalloid solution is required.

Table 1 shows differentiating features of heat exhaustion and heat stroke.

PROGNOSIS

Mortality remains high in heat stroke (10–50%) even with advanced care. Poor prognostic indicators are persistent body temperature more than 39°C despite all cooling measures taken.

- Resistant hyperthermia to cooling methods
- Prolonged comatose shock state
- Pulmonary edema
- Lactic acidosis
- Acute kidney injury (AKI) and hyperkalemia
- Higher levels of liver enzyme.

PREVENTION

- The risk of heat stroke can be minimized with appropriate measures
- Avoid overheating and dehydration
- Take plenty of oral liquids to prevent dehydration

Table 1 Differentiating features of heat exhaustion and heat stroke	
Heat exhaustion	**Heat stroke**
• Heavy sweating • Heavy thirst • Panting/rapid breathing • Rapid pulse • Headache • Blurred vision • Exhaustion, weakness • Clumsiness • Confusion • Dizziness or fainting • Cramps	• No sweating • Red or flushed, hot dry skin • Any symptom of heat exhaustion but more severe • Difficult breathing • Pinpoint pupils • Bizarre behavior • Convulsions • Confusion • Collapse

- Light and loose fitting clothes cool body by allowing perspiration to evaporate
- Light color cap or hat prevents head and neck from warming
- Avoid vigorous exercises in hot and open areas.

BIBLIOGRAPHY

1. Bouchama A. Heatstoke: A new look to ancient disease. Intensive care med. 1995;21:623-5.
2. Giercksy T, Boberg KM, Farstad IN, et al. Severe liver failure in exertional heat stroke. Scand J Gastroenterol. 1999;34(8): 824-7.
3. Heat-related illnesses, deaths, and risk factors—Cincinnati and Dayton, Ohio, 1999, and United States, 1979–1997. MMWR Morb Mortal Wkly Rep. 2000;49:470-3.
4. Heled Y, Rav-Acha M, Shani Y, et al. The "golden hour" for heatstroke treatment. Mil Med. 2004;169(3):184-6.
5. Hong J, Lai Y, Chang C, et al. Successful treatment of severe heatstroke with therapeutic hypothermia by a noninvasive external cooling system. Ann Emerg Med. 2012;59:491-3.
6. India Spend. "61% Rise in heat-stoke deaths over decade". May 27, 2015. Retrieved 26 June 2015.
7. McGugan EA. Hyperpyrexia in the emergency medicine department. Emergency Medicine Australasia. 2001;13(1):116-20.
8. Moseley PL. Heat shock proteins and heat adaptations of the whole organism. J Appl Physiol (1985). 1997;83(5):1413-7.
9. Proulx CI, Ducharme MB, Kenny GP. Effect of water temperature on cooling efficiency during hyperthermia in humans. J Appl Physiol (1985). 2003;94(4):1317-23.
10. Reuters. "India heat wave: death toll passes 2,500 as victim families fight for compensation". 2 June 2015. Retrieved 26 June 2015.
11. Sakurada S, Hales JR. A role of gastrointestinal endotoxins in enhancement of heat tolerance by physical fitness. J Appl Physiol (1985). 1998;84(1):207-14.
12. Slovis CM. Features and outcomes of classical heat stroke. Ann Intern Med. 1999;130:614.
13. Wyndham CH, Strydom NB, Cooke HM, et al. Methods of cooling subjects with hyperpyrexia. J Appl Physiol. 1959; 14(5):771-6.

CHAPTER 98

Drowning

Vivekanshu Verma, Atul Bansal, Devendra Richhariya

INTRODUCTION

According to WHO drowning is defined by "Drowning is the process of experiencing respiratory impairment from submersion/immersion in liquid". Drowning is a leading cause of accidental death around the world, especially in children and young adults. More important, it is a disease that can be prevented through improved public education and treated appropriately through a simple understanding of the underlying pathophysiology (**Fig. 1**). The primary cause of systemic injury in drowning patients is hypoxemia, and its correction should be the focus of prehospital and emergency department (ED) resuscitation and treatment. Once the condition is stabilized, the disposition of a patient can be determined by physical examination findings and response to treatment with patients displaying mild symptoms able to be safely discharged after a short period of observation.

There are an estimated 8 million nonfatal drowning worldwide each year, many of which may lead to severe morbidity.

Risk factors in all age groups are as follows (**Box 1**):
- Inability to swim
- Seizure disorder

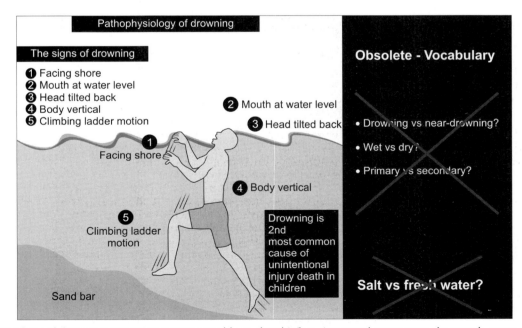

Fig. 1 Pathophysiology of drowning: Drowning person not able to clear his/her airway and water enter the mouth, some amount of water swallowed and spat out, person cannot hold the breath more than 1 minute and water is aspirated into the lungs if the person is not rescued water aspiration continues hypoxia leads to apnea and loss of consciousness and finally asystole

- Cardiovascular disease
- Substance abuse
- Trauma (diving in shallow water, boating).

The primary cause of morbidity and mortality in drowning is hypoxia. In addition, the actual volumes of water commonly aspirated are much smaller than originally postulated. Therefore, a resuscitative strategy focused on expelling water from the lungs, instead of reversing hypoxia, will do more harm than good.

Box 1 Risk factors for drowning by age

Infants and toddlers
- Unsupervised bath time
- Bath seats
- Caucasian ethnicity
- Residential pools
- Low and middle income families

Children and adolescents
- Underlying medical conditions
- Access to open bodies of water
- Unsupervised swimming
- African-American ethnicity
- Male sex
- Autism spectrum disorders

Teenagers and adults
- Underlying medical conditions
- Intoxication
- Trauma
- Tourism
- Swimming alone

All ages
- Cardiac arrhythmia syndromes
- Epilepsy

STAGES IN DROWNING

Stages in drowning have been shown in **Flow chart 1**.

SYMPTOMS IN DROWNING

The patient of drowning may present with wide range of symptoms. Patient may be completely asymptomatic, or may present with mild cough dyspnea or pulmonary. Patient may be confused or present with coma. Patient may present in ED in cardiac arrest state.

It is important to categorize the symptoms according to severity which is helpful in management as shown in **Box 2**.

COMPLICATIONS OF DROWNING

Multisystem effects of drowning have been shown in **Table 1**.

MANAGEMENT OF DROWNING

Management of drowning has been shown in **Flow chart 2**.

In general, all drowning patients should receive initial resuscitative efforts. In general, a submersion time longer than 10 minutes or resuscitation time longer than 25 minutes has been shown to correlate with death or survival with poor neurologic outcome.

If there is high suspicion for cervical spine injury (witnessed diving or fall from height, known ethanol ingestion, facial trauma), appropriate precautions should be taken with in-line stabilization, application of cervical collar as long as it does not delay intubation.

Therapeutic hypothermia has been shown to be of benefit in cardiac arrest, and case reports have suggested similar outcomes for victims of submersion. This should be initiated only after proper resuscitation, with a focus on ventilation, and only in facilities with the proper policies, equipment,

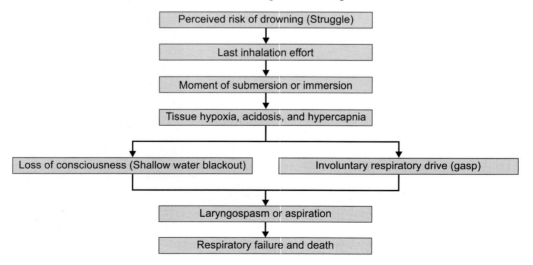

Flow chart 1 Stages of drowning

Box 2 Severity of symptoms and their management

Asymptomatic
- Full vital signs, including temperature and pulse oximetry
- Chest X-ray
- Discharge with precautions or observe 4–6 hours

Mild symptoms
- Full vital signs, temperature, oxygen PRN
- Bronchodilator
- Chest X-ray, electrolytes
- Treat mild hypothermia
- Observe 6–24 hours

Moderate-to-severe symptoms
- Full vital signs, temperature, oxygen PRN, telemetry
- Chest X-ray, electrolytes, CBC, coagulation studies
- Consider NIPPV or intubation with PEEP
- Volume support, treat hypothermia
- Supportive care and admission

Cardiopulmonary arrest
- ACLS
- Post-arrest temperature management
- Consider ECMO

Abbreviations: CBC, complete blood count; NIPPV, noninvasive positive pressure ventilation; PEEP, positive end-expiratory pressure; ACLS, advanced cardiovascular life support; ECMO, extracorporeal membrane oxygenation.

Table 1 Complication of drowning

Pulmonary	Edema, V/Q mismatch, hypoxemia, ARDS
Neurologic	Anoxic encephalopathy, traumatic brain/cord lesions
Acid/base	Metabolic acidosis
Cardiac	Decreased cardiac output, dysrhythmia, infarction
Renal	Azotemia

and training to initiate and maintain the hypothermia for 24–48 hours.

Extracorporeal membrane oxygenation (ECMO) has received increased attention in the literature for the treatment of drowning patients. If available, this may be considered for severe or refractory hypothermia or hypoxemia.

When highly contaminated water is involved (e.g. sewage), prophylactic antibiotics may be considered. Their use is indicated after initial resuscitation in the presence of clinical evidence suggesting pneumonia, and should be guided by bronchoalveolar sampling.

The possibility of toxicologic conditions also should be investigated with appropriate toxicologic screens performed.

Prognosis in Drowning Victims

The most consistent prognostic indicator found in the literature is duration of submersion, and this highlights the pivotal role that hypoxia plays in the injury process. Other factors that have been found to have some prognostic value are:

- Delay in initiation of cardiopulmonary resuscitation (CPR)
- Delay in arrival of emergency medical services (EMS)
- Need for prolonged resuscitation
- Low Glasgow Coma Scale score (less than or equal to 5)
- pH < 7
- Asystole on arrival to the ED.

PREVENTION OF DROWNING

Expert and research studies suggests following measure to prevent the drowning:

- Unnecessary accumulated water should be drained from bucket pond
- Apply flood control measures in flood prone area

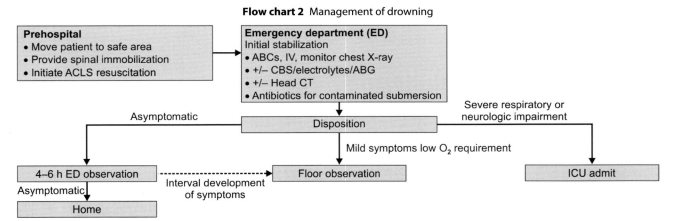

Flow chart 2 Management of drowning

Abbreviations: ABG, arterial blood gas; ACLS, advanced cardiovascular life support; CBC, complete blood count.

- Mandatory fencing and rules for swimming pools
- Apply safety signs and warning flags
- Encourage to learn swimming and water safety skills
- Swim in area with lifeguards
- Use of grills over water well
- Constant and closely supervise children who are near water
- Learn about use of life jacket
- Knowledge about first aid CPR

CONCLUSION

According to WHO, drowning is the second most common cause of unintentional death after road-traffic accident, estimated problem is even bigger as data are not available or unreliable from most of the countries. Drowning problem is more common in children aged 1–14 years and male persons. Alcohol and epilepsy are important risk factors for drowning. Drowning associated with multiple complications like ARDS renal failure hypoxic encephalopathy. Management includes cardiopulmonary resuscitation, and intensive care unit management including therapeutic hypothermia and ECMO. Prevention is important aspect to decrease the morbidity, mortality and economic burden on the society.

BIBLIOGRAPHY

1. Ludes B, Fornes P. Drowning in: Forensic Medicine: Clinical and Pathological Aspects. Payne-James J, Busuttil A, Smock W (Eds), Greenwich Medical Media. 2003. pp. 247-57.
2. Modell JH. Prevention of needless deaths from drowning. South Med J. 2010;103:650-3.
3. Oehmichen M, Hennig R, Meissner C. Near-drowning and clinical laboratory changes. Leg Med (Tokyo). 2008;10:1-5.
4. Szpilman D. Near-drowning and drowning classification: a proposal to stratify mortality based on the analysis of 1831 cases. Chest. 1997;112:660-5.
5. Warner D, Knape J. Recommendations and consensus brain resuscitation in the drowning victim. In: Bierens JJLM (Ed). Handbook on Drowning: Prevention, Rescue, and Treatment. Berlin: Springer-Verlag. 2006. pp. 436-9.

CHAPTER 99

Emergency Management of Burns

Aditya Aggarwal, Vimalendu Brajesh, Sukhdeep Singh, Umang B Kothari, Rakesh K Khazanchi

INTRODUCTION

Burns constitute a severe form of trauma which can be associated with significant morbidity and mortality. World Health Organization (WHO) estimates that more than 3 lakh people die due to burn injuries.[1] Every year with many more pushed into a life with severe disabilities and disfigurement.[1,2] Low- and middle-income countries carry the maximum burden of burn-related mortality and morbidity. Burns affect the people of productive age groups and are the only form of trauma where incidence is more in females.[1] Most of the risk factors for burn injuries are preventable and the mortality and morbidity can be minimized with proper care.

CLASSIFICATION

Burns can be classified in multiple ways depending upon the cause and depth.

Depending on the Cause[3,4]

Most of the burns are accidental with assaults and attempted suicides making up the less common causes. Depending upon the agents causing the burns, they can be classified as follows:
- *Thermal burns*: This is the most common type of burns. These are caused due to contact with flame, a hot liquid or a hot object.
- *Chemical burns*: These are caused due to contact with a chemical agent which may either be an acid or an alkali. Most common agents are sulfuric acid present in toilet cleaners and sodium hypochlorite present in bleach **(Fig. 1)**.
- *Electrical burns*: They are further divided into two types, low voltage (<1,000 Volts) or high voltage (>1,000 Volts) burns. Electric burns may occur due to flame caused by

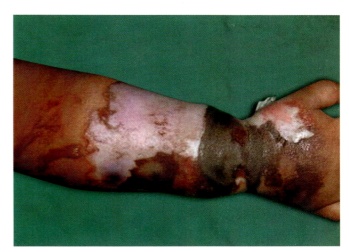

Fig. 1 A case of chemical (sulfuric acid) burns on the hand of a child. These are generally deep and will require surgical management for healing

an electric arc (flash burns). These may be associated with other injuries occurring due to fall or due to violent muscle contractions. Spine, especially cervical spine, may be injured due to fall or due to muscle contractions and needs to be protected till injury has been ruled out. Electric burns may also cause cardiac arrhythmias. The surface wound is generally smaller as compared to the internal damage with extensive muscle necrosis. There may also be derangement of renal parameters due to myonecrosis. Lightning burns are also considered as a part of electric burns **(Fig. 2)**.
- *Radiation burns*: These may be caused due to prolonged exposure to sunlight (sunburns) or due to ionizing radiation like X-rays, following radiotherapy or as a result of nuclear fallout. Sunburns are generally superficial but

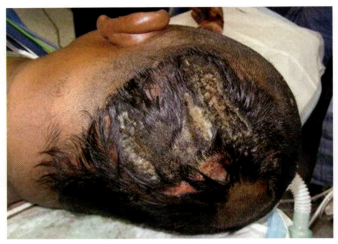

Fig. 2 A case of electric burns on the scalp. In these deep burns underlying tissue necrosis is generally more than what is apparent on the surface

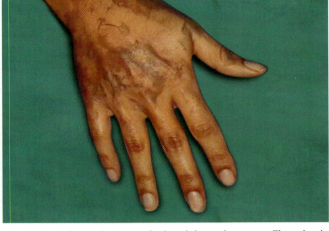

Fig. 3 First-degree burns on the hand due to hot water. These heal spontaneously without any scarring

the extent varies from person to person depending upon the skin type. Burns due to ionizing radiation may vary from just erythema to a weeping raw area depending upon the dose and the duration of exposure. Radiation burns are treated in the same way as any other burn.

Depending on the Depth[3,5-7]

Depending upon the layers of the skin involved, burns can be classified into four degrees. Exact assessment of the depth may not be possible immediately after the event and is better assessed after 48–72 hours. Good resuscitative efforts may limit the progression of superficial burns to deeper burns.

First-degree Burns

They involve just the epidermis and appear red and dry. They are painful and generally heal in 5–10 days without any scarring. Sunburn is an example of a first-degree burn **(Fig. 3)**.

Second-degree Burns

They can be distinguished from a first-degree burn by running a gloved finger on the burn wound. If the area feels slippery (due to separation of the epidermis from the dermis: Nikolsky's sign),[4] it is likely to be a second-degree burn. These are further subdivided into two types:
- *Second-degree superficial burn*: These involve the epidermis and the papillary dermis and are characterized by blisters with clear fluid. They appear red, moist, blanch on touch and are very painful. These generally heal in 10–14 days with no scarring. Inadequate resuscitation or infection can convert a second-degree superficial burn into a deeper one **(Figs 4A and B)**.
- *Second-degree deep burn*: These extend into the deeper (reticular) dermis. The burn wound appears dry, whitish or pale yellowish and mottled. There is minimal or no blanching on touch. There may be a few thick-walled blisters. These are generally painless with the patient experiencing some discomfort in the area. These wounds, if let to heal spontaneously, take weeks to heal and heal with scarring and contracture formation and are better managed by excision and grafting **(Fig. 5)**.

Third-degree Burns

These involve the entire dermis and extend into the subcutaneous tissue. The area appears leathery white and there is no blanching. The wound is painless as the nerves get destroyed. These areas are best managed by excision and grafting **(Fig. 6)**.

Fourth-degree Burns

In this type, the entire skin and subcutaneous tissue is involved with the depth reaching up to the underlying muscle or bone. The area appears black and charred, dry and is painless. These burns may lead to amputation of the affected limb **(Fig. 7)**.

ASSESSMENT AND MANAGEMENT

The care of the burns patient should start at the time of the burn. This is discussed as prehospital care and care in the hospital. If the patient does not receive any prehospital

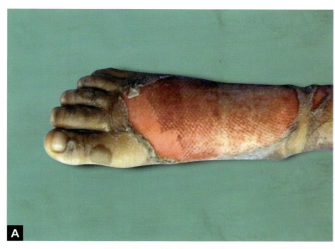
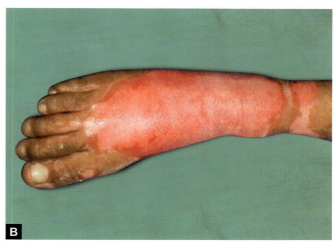

Figs 4A and B Second-degree superficial burns on the dorsum of the foot showing ruptured blisters. (A) Patient before the removal of dead skin. (B) Patient after removal of the dead skin

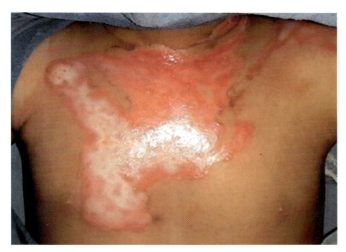

Fig. 5 Second-degree deep area (whitish) along with second-degree superficial (pinkish) burns due to spillage of hot tea on the chest. The deeper areas will heal with scarring

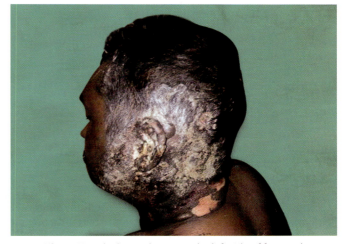

Fig. 7 Fourth-degree burns on the left side of face and scalp due to electric burns

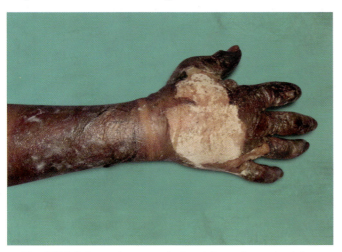

Fig. 6 Third-degree burns on the hand due to firecracker injury

care than these steps need to be followed after arrival in the hospital.

Prehospital Care[4,8,9]

- The first thing that needs to be done is to remove the patient from the site of harm. If the person is on fire, the flames need to be extinguished with water, if available, or by wrapping in a blanket or the person can roll on the ground to put out the fire.
- All constricting objects, pieces of jewelry should be removed.
- In case of scald, all the wet clothing needs to be removed as prolonged contact may lead to deeper burns.
- The burnt area should be washed with cool water till the burning sensation persists. Ice-cold water should not be used as it may cause hypothermia, vasoconstriction, and deeper burns.

- In case of chemical burns, the area needs to be washed with copious amounts of water to wash off the entire chemical taking care that the chemical does not run off to the unburnt areas. In case of powders, the extra powder or chemical should be brushed off and bigger pieces of powder or chemical removed with forceps before washing. No attempt should be made to neutralize the acid with an alkali and vice versa as it can cause more heat production and deeper burns. If the eyes are involved than they need to be irrigated with copious amounts of water and an ophthalmology consultation will be required after the patient reaches the hospital.
- In case of bitumen (coal tar) burns, no attempt should be made to remove the bitumen but irrigation with water should be done till there is no burning sensation. Bitumen should be allowed to separate on its own and removal to be done only, if it is compromising the airway or circulation of any part.
- The patient should be wrapped in a clean sheet or a blanket before taking to a hospital to prevent hypothermia. The burn wound may be wrapped in cling film (not to be used in chemical burns or facial burns) before transportation, taking care that it is not wrapped too tight.

Hospital Care

Initial Assessment

After arrival in the hospital, history should be taken with regards to the cause, time, and duration of contact with the source of burn and any care received so far for the burn injury. If the patient has any comorbidities like diabetes, hypertension, and coronary disease than that need to be recorded as they may have a bearing on the final outcome. Known allergies and any medication that the patient is having also need to be recorded. Status of tetanus immunization, if known, should also be noted.

- The initial assessment is like in any case of trauma and involves assessment of airway, breathing, and circulation. If the patient has not received any prehospital care then the previously mentioned interventions need to be undertaken. A quick initial survey of the patient should be carried out to assess for the type, extent, and depth of the burn wounds and inhalational injury should be ruled out. Associated injuries should also be looked for and managed accordingly. The nature of burn flame, scald, contact, chemical, radiation, etc. should be assessed as the management may vary accordingly.
- The presence of inhalational burns also needs to be assessed. The presence of the following may indicate presence of inhalational injury **(Fig. 8)**.[4,10,11]
    - Deep burns on the face
    - Singed facial and nasal hair
    - Hoarseness of the voice
    - Expectoration of carbonaceous sputum
    - Wheezing
    - Intraoral burn.

This assessment can be done at the site of injury by the paramedical staff or after arrival at the hospital. There should be a low threshold for intubation in such patients as increased airway edema after fluid resuscitation may make it difficult to gain access to the airway. The initial X-ray may be normal but as the changes progress, X-ray may show bronchial thickening, peribronchial cuffing, interstitial edema and atelectasis.[10] If available fiber optic bronchoscopy may be done and is considered to be the "Gold Standard" for diagnosis of inhalational injury.[10] These patients should be started on humidified oxygen inhalation.

- The extent of the burnt surface area is an important predictor of the prognosis and guides fluid resuscitation and the decision to refer to a specialist burns center. It is expressed as a percentage of the total body surface area (TBSA). The most commonly used methods are the Wallace rule of nines **(Fig. 9)** and the Lund and Browder charts **(Fig. 10)** with the latter being more complex but more accurate.[7] The percentage body surface area of the various body parts varies with age and necessary adjustments need to be made accordingly while calculating the burnt surface area. The Lund and Browder chart is more accurate for children as it accounts for the change in percent area of various parts with age.[7] The palmar surface of the hand and fingers account for about 0.8% of TBSA and this fact can be used as a rough estimate of the burnt surface area especially for smaller percentage of burns.[7]
- Depth of the burns wound also guides management and helps in predicting prognosis. It may not be possible to assess the depth correctly at the time of presentation with

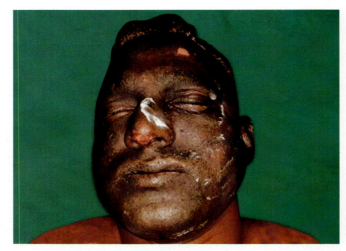

Fig. 8 Deep burns on the face showing singed hair. These patients are likely to have inhalational injury

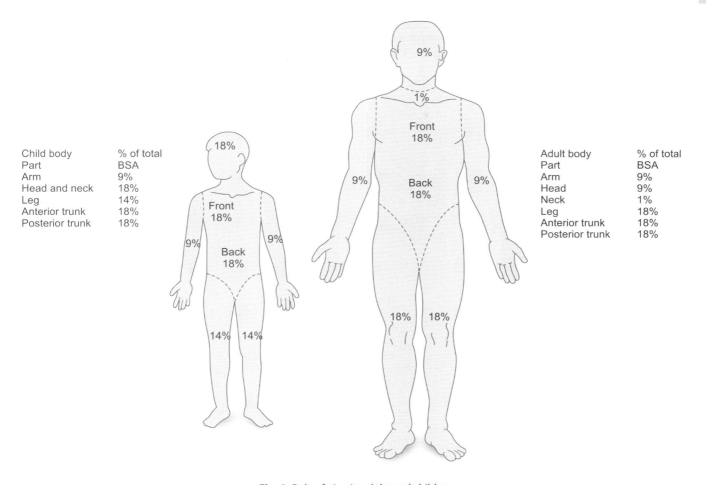

Fig. 9 Rule of nine in adults and children

the exact depth becoming evident in 48–72 hours. Some superficial areas may become deep if the patient does not receive adequate resuscitation or if infection occurs. The depth is assessed as mentioned earlier. A simple clinical way to differentiate between superficial and deep burns is to check for bleeding and pain on pin prick with brisk bleeding indicating a superficial burn, delayed bleeding meaning a deep dermal burn and no bleeding meaning a full thickness burn.[7] Similarly presence of pain indicates a superficial burn and its absence means a deeper burn **(Table 1)**.

- The severity of the burn has also been graded by the American Burn Association. This grading is based on the age of the patient, TBSA, depth of the burn, burns in specific anatomical regions and associated injuries. Three classes have been described as minor, moderate, and major burn **(Table 2)**. Minor burns may be managed at home, moderate at a hospital, and major ones requiring admission in a specialized burns center.

Management in Hospital

The initial management is the same as in any trauma case. The life-threatening conditions need to be excluded or managed as per Trauma Care Protocols (C-A-B approach). Burns patients rarely present with shock and if in shock then other causes like cardiac cause, severe associated orthopedic trauma or in long-standing cases, sepsis should be ruled out. In patients suspected of inhalational injury, humidified oxygen inhalation should be started. If available, fiber-optic bronchoscopy should be performed for both diagnosis and for airway toileting. There should be a low threshold for intubation in such cases and if required tracheostomy should be considered. High frequency percussive ventilators or high frequency oscillatory ventilators are recommended to be used in such patients. Tetanus prophylaxis is recommended in patients who have not had a tetanus vaccine in the last 5 years.[4] Systemic antibiotics are generally not started as the burn wound is sterile and gets colonized only after 48–72 hours.

806 SECTION 16 Environmental Emergencies

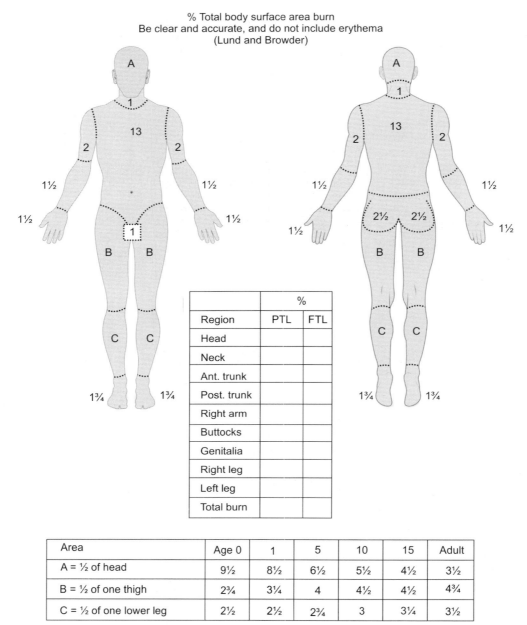

Fig. 10 Lund and Browder charts
Abbreviations: PTL, partial thickness loss; FTL, full thickness loss.

Routine investigation like a hemogram, renal and liver function tests should be ordered. If inhalational burns are suspected then an X-ray of the chest and arterial blood gas analysis should also be done. In electric burns, ECG and cardiac assessment is also needed along with urine analysis. Once the assessment of the patient has been completed, the management of the burn is to be initiated and it can be discussed under the following heads.

Fluid Management

As burnt patients lose a lot of fluid from the burn wounds, fluid resuscitation is critical for successful management. There is a shift of fluid from the intravascular to the extravascular space. Fluid management is essential to maintain circulatory volume and perfusion of vital organs. Adult patients with more than 15% burns and children with more than 10% of

Table 1 Assessment of the depth of burns[15]

Type	Layers involved	Appearance	Texture	Sensation	Healing time	Prognosis
Superficial (first degree)	Epidermis	Red without blisters	Dry	Painful	5–10 days	Heals well Repeated sunburns increase the risk of skin cancer later in life
Superficial partial thickness (second degree)	Extends into superficial (papillary) dermis	Redness with clear blister. Blanches with pressure	Moist	Very painful	less than 2–3 weeks	Local infection/cellulitis but no scarring typically
Deep partial thickness (second degree)	Extends into deep (reticular) dermis	Yellow or white. Less blanching. May be blistering	Fairly dry	Pressure and discomfort	3–8 weeks	Scarring, contractures (may require excision and skin grafting)
Full thickness (third degree)	Extends through entire dermis	Stiff and white/brown No blanching	Leathery	Painless	Prolonged (months) and incomplete	Scarring, contractures, amputation (early excision recommended)
Fourth degree	Extends through entire skin, and into underlying fat, muscle and bone	Black charred with eschar	Dry	Painless	Requires excision[10]	Amputation, significant, functional, impairment and in some cases, death

Table 2 Criteria and classification of burns

Criteria	Minor burn	Moderate burn	Severe burn
Total body surface area (TBSA) (%)	• All first-degree burns <10% adults <5% children or elderly • <2% for third degree	• Second-degree burns 10–20% adults 5–10% in children or elderly • 2–5% for third degree	• All first-degree burns >20% adults >10% children and elderly • >5% for third degree
Type of burn injury		• Low-voltage burn • Suspected inhalation injury	• High-voltage burn • Chemical burn • Known inhalational injury
Location		Circumferential burn	• Clinically significant burn to face, eyes, ears, genitalia, over joints
Coexisting conditions		• Concomitant medical problem predisposing to infection (e.g. diabetes, sickle cell anemia)	• Significant associated injuries (e.g. fracture, other major trauma)
	Outpatient management	*Inpatient management*: Consider referral to burn center	Referral to burn center

Source: Modified from Singer AJ, Dagum AB. Current management of acute cutaneous wounds. N Engl J Med. 2008;359(10):1037-46.

TBSA should be started on intravenous fluids.[7] Burns less than that can be managed with oral rehydration. Two large bore intravenous lines should be secured in patients requiring intravenous fluids preferably through unburnt skin.[4,12-14] All patients requiring intravenous fluids also should have a Foley catheter put to measure urine output and direct fluid therapy.[4]

Various formulae have been suggested to assess the volume requirement but none is perfect. The most commonly used formula is the Parkland formula as given in **Box 1**.[7]

Parkland formula uses Ringer's lactate (RL) as the fluid to be used in the first 24 hours as it has almost the same electrolyte concentration as the plasma. 24-hour area

Box 1 Parkland formula

Parkland formula for burns resuscitation:
- Total fluid requirement in 24 hours =
  4 mL× [total burn surface area (%) × body weight (kg)]
- 50% given in first 8 hours
- 50% given in next 16 hours

Children receive maintenance fluid in addition, at hourly rate of:
- 4 mL/kg for first 10 kg of body weight plus
- 2 mL/kg for second 10 kg of body weight plus
- 1 mL/kg for >20 kg of body weight

End point:
- Urine output of 0.5–1.0 mL/kg/hr in adults
- Urine output of 1.0–1.5 mL/kg/hr in children

counted from the time of burn and not from the time of presentation in the hospital. In children RL with 5% dextrose is preferred as children have low glycogen reserves.[15] There is no consensus regarding the use of colloids in the first 24 hours.[4] At some centers colloids are used after 8 hours as the shift from the intravascular space is decreasing, most wait for 24 hours before introducing colloids as leakage of colloids into the interstitial space will lead to increase in tissue edema. The authors suggest using colloids after 24 hours. In electric burns, the fluid requirements are significantly high and are calculated as 9 mL × (burnt body surface area in %) × (weight in kg).[7] The aim is to have a urine output of 1.5–2 mL/kg/hr so as to avoid acute renal failure due to rhabdomyolysis. Inhalational burns also have a higher fluid requirement. After 24 hours colloids are used as 0.5 mL × (burnt body surface area in %) × (weight in kg) with a dextrose containing crystalloid being given as 1.5 mL × (burnt body surface area in %) × (weight in kg). Preferred colloid in children is fresh frozen plasma and in adults, albumin or synthetic starches can be used.

Parkland and the other formulae serve purely as guidelines for fluid resuscitation. Fluid requirement needs to be adjusted according to the urine output and other clinical parameters like pulse rate and blood pressure.[7] Whereas use of less fluid causes hypoperfusion, excessive fluid use causes increased tissue edema and tissue hypoxia. The phenomenon of *fluid creep* has been described by Pruitt as increased tissue edema and its antecedent complications, including abdominal compartment syndrome, due to use of excessive fluid for resuscitation.

Wound Management

Management of the burns wound varies according to its depth. Other than the first-degree burns which may be left open with topical applications, all other wounds should be covered with a dressing. The aim of dressing is to promote healing and prevent wound desiccation, prevent or treat infection and provide comfort to the patient.

First-degree burns can be managed by cleaning the area with soap and water and application of a bland moisturizing ointment or lotion 4 hourly. These need to be protected from sunlight by physical (hats/caps/full-sleeved clothes) and chemical (sunscreens) means.[4] Topical antimicrobial ointments like neomycin, mupirocin, fucidin or silver sulfadiazine (SSD) may be used to prevent infections as it may lead to conversion of a superficial to a deeper burn. These may also be used for burn wounds of greater depths. SSD is a routinely used ointment for burn wounds and it should be applied as at least 1 cm thick layer on the wound.[4] Daily dressing is required with washing and cleaning of the wound before each application of SSD. It should not be used for patients allergic to sulfa drugs, patients with glucose-6-phosphate dehydrogenase (G6PD) deficiency, in pregnancy and infants and on the face (as it causes permanent staining of the skin).[16] It is also known to cause transient neutropenia on the 3rd or 4th day of use which generally settles spontaneously even with continued use.[4]

Second-degree burns generally present with blisters. Although the management of blisters is debatable with some advising leaving the blisters as such and some advising their rupture and removal of dead skin. At our center we generally deroof the blisters and remove the dead skin and dress the wound either with collagen (dry or wet) and an absorbent dressing on top or an absorbent dressing such as hydrocolloid or alginate dressing. These dressings stick onto the wound and come off as the wound gets epithelialized. With these, daily dressing is not required and only the outer dressing needs to be changed every 3–4 days or earlier if it gets soaked. Collagen and alginate dressings are avoided in wounds more than 48–72 hours old as by that time colonization of the burn wound has happened and chances of infection are more and in such situations antimicrobial or silver impregnated dressings are preferred.[4] Clearing of the blisters in children and in adults with larger burnt areas requires general anesthesia. Various silver impregnated dressings are also available and have been recommended but we limit their use to infected wounds. If these dressings are not available, a non-adherent paraffin impregnated dressing like Jelonet or Bactigras can be used as a contact layer with an absorbent cotton dressing on top.

Deep burns will generally require excision and grafting and may be dressed with a nonadherent dressing (Jelonet or Bactigras) covered with absorbent cotton dressing. Collagen has no role in deeper burns and should be avoided.

Splintage of the burnt area not only provides comfort to the patient but also helps in preventing contractures. If there are burns around the neck a cervical collar should be given. In burns involving the hands splint should be given in functional position of the hand. Foot drop splint should be considered in patients with burns around the legs and those who are likely to be in bed for long. Axilla (in 90° abduction) and elbow (in full extension) also need to be splinted in patients with involvement of these areas. Limb elevation helps in reducing edema and pain and improves healing (**Fig. 11**).[4]

Patients with deep circumferential burns of the chest or of the extremities may need escharotomies if there is difficulty in breathing or there is circulatory compromise of the extremities. This can be done bedside with the help of an electrocautery or a scalpel with the risk of bleeding being more with the use of scalpel.[4] Adrenaline containing local anesthetic solution may be infiltrated along the proposed line of incision and the incisions made to release the tight skin. The deep fascia need not be cut unless there is presence of a compartment syndrome.[4] The markings for the escharotomy are as shown in the **Figure 12**. This procedure carries the risk of injury to the ulnar nerve at the elbow, superficial branch of the radial nerve at the wrist, the great saphenous vein and nerve near the ankle and the common peroneal nerve near the neck of fibula and therefore should not be taken lightly.[4]

CRITERIA FOR REFERRAL TO A SPECIALIZED BURN CENTER[17]

Burn injuries that should be referred to a burn center include:
- Partial thickness burns greater than 10% of TBSA
- Burns that involve the face, hands, feet, genitalia, perineum, or major joints
- Third-degree burns in any age group
- Electrical burns including lightning injury
- Chemical burns
- Inhalation injury
- Burn injury in patients with pre-existing medical disorders that could complicate management, prolong recovery, or affect mortality.

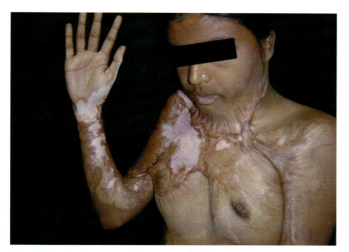

Fig. 11 Lack of proper splintage can lead to contractures across the joint surfaces. These are difficult to manage and lead to significant morbidity to the patients

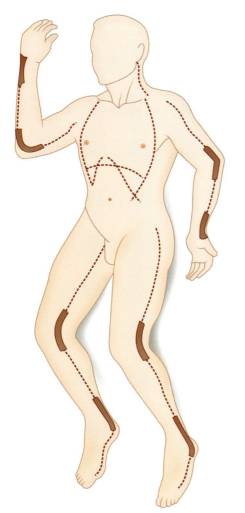
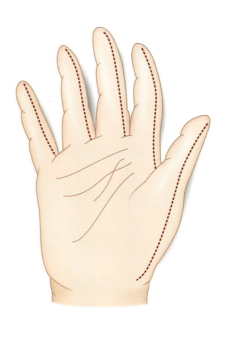

Fig. 12 The incisions for escharotomy with sites of potential injury to the vital structures

- Any patient with burns and concomitant trauma (such as fractures) in which the burn injury poses the greatest risk of morbidity or mortality. In such cases, if the trauma poses the greater immediate risk, the patient may be initially stabilized in a trauma center before being transferred to a burn unit. Physician judgment will be necessary in such situations and should be in concert with the regional medical control plan and triage protocols.
- Burnt children in hospitals without qualified personnel or equipment for the care of children.
- Burn injury in patients who will require special social, emotional, or rehabilitative intervention.

REFERENCES

1. Krug E. A WHO plan for burn prevention and care. Geneva: WHO. 2008.
2. Shankar Gowri, Naik Vijaya A, Rajesh Powar, et al. Epidemiology and Outcome of Burn Injuries. J Indian Acad Forensic Med. 2012;34(4):312-14.
3. Wikipedia. (2003). Burns. [online] Available from *https://en.wikipedia.org/wiki/Burn* [Accessed January, 2017].
4. John Greenwood, Sheila Kavanagh. First Aid and Emergency Management of Adult Burns, 2011 Practice Guidelines, Royal Adelaide Hospital-The Burns Unit.
5. Cartotto R. Fluid Resuscitation of the Thermally Injured Patient. Clin Plast Surg. 2009;36(40):569-81.
6. Monstrey S, Hoeksema H, Verbelen J, et al. Assessment of burn depth and burn wound healing potential. Burns. 2008;34(6):761-9.
7. Hettiaratchy S, Papini R. Initial management of a major burn: II--assessment and resuscitation. BMJ. 2004;329(7457):101-3.
8. Shrivastava P, Goel A. Pre-hospital care in burn injury. Indian J Plast Surg. 2010;43:S15-S22.
9. Allison K, Porter K. Consensus on the prehospital approach to burns patient management. Emerg Med J. 2004;21(1):112-4.
10. Greenhalgh DG. Topical Antimicrobial Agents for Burn Wounds. Clin Plastic Surg. 2009;36(4):597-606.
11. Lafferty KA, et al. (2016). Smoke Inhalation Injury. [online] Available from *http://emedicine.medscape.com/article/771194-overview*.
12. Palmieri TL. What's New in Critical Care of the Burn-Injured Patient? Clin Plast Surg. 2009;36(4):607-15.
13. Adaira Landry, Heike Geduld, Alex Koyfman, et al. An overview of acute burn management in the Emergency Centre. African J Emerg Med. 2013;3(1):22-9.
14. Tintinalli JE, Stapczynski JS, John MO, et al. Tintinalli's Emergency Medicine: A Comprehensive Study Guide, 8th edition. In: Tintinalli JE (Ed). New York: McGraw-Hill Companies; 2010. pp. 1374-86.
15. Sharma RK, Parashar A. Special considerations in paediatric burn patients. Indian J Plast Surg. 2010;43:S43-50.
16. Greenhalgh DG. Topical Antimicrobial Agents for Burn Wounds. Clin Plastic Surg. 2009;36(4):597-606.
17. Resources for Optimal Care of the Injured Patient, Committee on Trauma, American College of Surgeons Excerpted from Guidelines for the Operation of Burn Centers; 2006. pp. 79-86.

CHAPTER 100

Electrical Injuries

Basar Cander

INTRODUCTION

Although electricity has longstanding existence in nature; it has come to our lives from the 1800s and become one of the main structures of our daily lives in this era. Today, we live with electricity every minute of every day and it is now impossible to maintain our daily lives without it. Besides its major benefits, this common type of energy has created a new form of trauma which was not existed in ancient medicine: electrical injuries. Although this type of injury is not very common, it has a wide spectrum of impact from a simple exposure to severe traumas that occasionally may lead to death. This type of injuries which we can consider within the context of traumas is an important part of emergency medicine education and takes an important place in education of medical branches. Electrical injuries influence a number of medical fields from surgery to nephrology and cardiology depending on the form of injury. Therefore, particularly physicians working in the field of emergency medicine need to know well about electrical injuries.

Approximately 1,000 deaths per year are due to electrical injuries in the United States, with a mortality rate of 3–5%.

PATHOPHYSIOLOGY OF THE CONDITION OR DESCRIPTION

Electrical injury occurs due to the direct contact of a person with electrical current. First skin and then viscera and muscles are affected depending on severity of the impact. The human body is a very good conductor of electricity, thus paving the way for conducting current through the skin to the internal organs. Electrical injuries are a trauma and should be assessed from the forensic aspect.

Numerous factors affect the severity of electric shock including voltage, strength of current, exposure time, source, type of current and the route via which the current travels in the body. For example, the power of electricity used in workplaces is higher than that used in houses, thus electrical injuries occurring in workplaces are more hazardous. Similarly, if the route through which the electrical current goes is related to the heart, rhythm disorders are more likely to occur.

Voltage, also called electromotive force, is a quantitative expression of the potential difference in charge between two points in an electrical field. The greater the voltage, the greater the flow of electrical current. The electrical voltage used in workplaces is higher than that used in houses with voltage value differs between 110 and 220 volt (V) in houses while it can reach to 100,000 V in workplaces in the electrical industry.

Electric current, a flow of moving electrical charge particles, is another critical factor. It reflects the electric charge transferred through a section over a time. Although its unit is ampere (A), the current affecting human body is measured in milliamperes (mA). Detrimental effects of electric current deepen as the current increases **(Table 1)**. Even ventricular fibrillation may develop in exposure to a current between 50 mA and 100 mA.

Table 1 Effect of current increases with increase in current

Effect	Current (mA)
Tingling sensation/perception	1–4
Let-go current—Children	3–4
Let-go current—Women	6–8
Let-go current—Men	7–9
Skeletal muscle tetany	16–20
Respiratory muscle paralysis	20–50
Ventricular fibrillation	50–120

In addition, the injury mechanism is affected by whether the current is in alternative or direct form. Alternative current (AC) is generally used in houses and offices, while direct current (DC) is used in workplaces. AC is three times more dangerous than DC of the same voltage. Whereas, since electric voltage used in industry is much higher, in general industrial injuries are more serious.

The effect of electricity on tissues is also related to the resistance of the tissue type. Different tissues have different resistance. The resistance in the muscles, nerves, and vessels is lower, thus these structures in the body better conduct electricity. Whereas the resistance of the bones, adipose tissue, and tendons is higher, making them to less conductive of electricity.

Another issue is the exposure time to electric current. In general, a longer exposure to high-voltage increases the damage done by electricity to the tissues. The route via which electricity travels in the body also affects the form of injury. A current directly exerting its effect toward the heart and thorax may lead to cardiac arrhythmias and myocardial damage. Direct transmission of electric current to the brain may cause cerebral damage, respiratory arrest, and paralysis. A current which runs toward the eye region may cause cataract. Therefore, the route via which electricity travels affects the way of injury. Electrical exposure creates damage in the body through three main mechanisms including direct tissue damage, thermal injury, and mechanical injury.

CLINICAL PRESENTATION

The first intervention to be made in the case of electric shock is airway, breathing, and circulation (ABC), namely to provide a security cordon by taking ABC under control. Cardiac arrest, respiratory arrest, coma, and burns in various degrees may be encountered in severe cases. The priority in these severe cases is to perform the resuscitative procedures. The cases of arrest due to electric shock are intervened in concordance with Advanced Cardiovascular Life Support (ACLS) guidelines. After completion of the resuscitative intervention, it is now turn of receiving history.

History is of paramount importance and should be taken in detail from the patient themselves, their families, and eyewitnesses. Scene of the accident, type of the electric source, whether it was a residential or industrial source, time of exposure and history of falling from height should be learned in details as much as possible. Whether the voltage and electric current are in direct or alternative form influence the severity of injury.

In physical examination, injuries caused by falls, especially head trauma and consciousness should be sought. Inlet and outlet holes of the electric current should be detected and the pathway which the current has followed should be found with inspection. Furthermore, burns occurred and their degrees should be determined.

Electrical burns may affect whole body beginning from the skin, causing various organ dysfunctions.

Skin Injuries

Electric current first affects the skin, resulting in thermal injury and burns in various degrees. This type of injury is most commonly seen in the hands where the most frequent sequelae are observed. Skin injuries should be assessed in conjunction with soft tissue injuries. The location where most severe burns occur is the site of direct contact or the ground contact point. Various burns may be developed depending on the voltage of the current.

The site of contact and the tissue beneath it is influenced more in high-voltage injuries. The injury may be painless due to necrosis and small amount of bleeding may be observed.

Arc Burns

When an arc of current passes from an object of high to low resistance, it creates a high temperature pathway that causes skin lesions at the site of contact with the source and at the ground contact point (not always the feet). These areas typically have a dry parchment center and a rim of congestion around them. There will be clues to the internal pathway taken by the arc based on the location of these surface wounds, whereas burns in low-voltage are usually related to the longer duration of contact. This type of injury may be seen in a wide range from simple erythema to all tissue burns.

A specific type of skin burn is a mouth burn, which is generally seen in children under the age of four years. This type of burn is caused especially by biting electrical cables. Edema and eschar may be seen. Bleeding due to arterial invasion may be observed in the late period. In such cases, airway management takes the priority.

Cardiac Injuries

Cardiac injury is the most important injury of electrical injury. It may lead to mortal rhythms ranging from asystole to ventricular fibrillation. Asystole is more common in high-voltage AC or DC currents, while cardiac arrest due to ventricular fibrillation may be seen in low-voltage AC injuries. Therefore, ventricular fibrillation may be observed in the domestic electric injuries. Again, cardiac arrhythmias have been reported to be frequently seen in low-voltage currents. Several arrhythmias may develop such as sinus tachycardia, reversible prolonged QT, and transient ST elevation. Patients having a normal initial electrocardiogram (ECG) are less likely to develop late arrhythmias.

Respiratory Injuries

Respiratory arrest is in general related to the respiratory center in the brain, because the lungs are less affected by electric current.

Neurologic Injuries

Altered level of consciousness may be seen ranging from temporary blackout to amnesia and coma. These pathologies may be resulted from trauma or direct electric current. Intracranial hemorrhage developing as a result of blunt trauma should be ruled out in the event of impaired consciousness. Neurological disorders often develop due to blunt trauma; however, it may also occur from the direct effect of electric current. A very severe current may impact the cerebral cells, causing respiratory arrest. Blackout, short-term memory loss, and lack of concentration may be seen in high-voltage injuries. Seizures may also be observed due to electric shock.

Vertebral fractures and related damage of various degrees may be seen as a result of trauma. Therefore, vertebral fractures should be ruled out in the presence of trauma. Neurological symptoms may also exist in the early or late period without trauma. Limb weakness and paresthesias may be seen in the early period. These symptoms are usually temporary and will spontaneously resolve over time. Descending paralysis and transverse myelitis have been reported in the late period.

Musculoskeletal Injuries

Traumatic fractures and compartment syndrome due to burns may occur due to electric shock. Distal pulse, motor, and sensory function should be carefully assessed in the event of suspected compartment syndrome. The diagnosis should be established through pressure measurement, if necessary. This condition may require early surgical consultation and fasciotomy.

Head Injuries

Especially in high-voltage injuries, the head is one of the common inlet sites of electric current. This may also lead to cervical spine injury. Several types of injury may be seen including cataract and facial burns.

MANAGEMENT

Investigations

Laboratory and Radiologic Evaluation

Except for minor injuries, the following investigations should be carried out in all patients with electrical injuries:

- Complete blood count
- Electrolyte level including sodium, potassium, and chloride
- Serum myoglobin test
- Blood urea nitrogen creatinine level should be performed due to the risk of rhabdomyolysis
- Urinalysis with special attention to myoglobinuria, myoglobin is important in terms of rhabdomyolysis. Some studies demonstrate the association of myoglobin with arrest and compartment syndrome
- Creatine kinase (CK) level is high especially in the case of massive muscular injuries and may also be a marker of rhabdomyolysis. Having the initial value is important to determine amounts of the subsequent rises
- Creatine kinase-MB and troponin may be elevated in electrical injuries. Elevation in these markers is seen especially in cases of electric current passing through thoracic trace
- Brain natriuretic peptide (BNP) has been reported in several studies to be raised in various types of electrical injuries
- Arterial blood gases should be studied in severe electrical injuries
- Other investigations including the levels of alanine aminotransferase (ALT), aspartate aminotransferase (AST), amylase, and low-density lipoproteins (LDL) levels should be carried out in patients considered to have a severe blunt injury.

Imaging

- Cranial tomography imaging should be ordered in patients with level of consciousness or those with head trauma which is not minor.
- Computed tomography (CT) should be performed in the events of seizures or neurologic deficit.
- Chest X-ray should be considered in the cases of respiratory distress and blunt trauma.
- Cervical spinal imaging—cervical MRI or tomography—should be ordered if there is the possibility of cervical trauma.
- Abdominal USG (ultrasonography) or tomography should be considered in compliance with the general trauma guidelines in the case of blunt abdominal trauma and in unconscious patients.

Treatment

First Aid

The priority in electrical accidents is the safety of the rescuer. Because of the conductivity of the human body, the rescuer may also be exposed to electric current. Therefore, electric current must be shut down and the current buttons must be switched off, if it could be done safely. Trying to rescue a person who is near high-voltage current is dangerous. First, the current must be shut down. Next, the emergency medicine system should be immediately activated (via phone). If electric current cannot be cut-off, the patient must be moved away from the scene utilizing nonconductor materials and taken to the safe zone. ABC control must be then performed with basic life support given as required. In the case of burns, the clothes must be taken off to prevent any contact. Burn first aid must be carried out. Considering that the patient might have experienced trauma, interventions should be done by sparing the cervical and lumbar regions. Advanced trauma life support (ATLS) and advanced cardiac life support (ACLS) protocols should be performed in association with the events of arrest.

In Emergency Department

Airway should be maintained and intravenous access should be established. Cervical stabilization should be obtained. The patient should be oxygenized in the case of hypoxia and monitored.

Fluid Therapy

The most important problem in the early period in both thermal and electrical burns is dehydration and shock status that develop due to the fluid which is lost from the damaged skin or passes into the intracellular space. Fluid resuscitation should be initiated and titrated according to urine output. In the cases of myoglobinuria or severe burns, fluid should be administered so as to provide urine output at a rate of 0.5–1 mL/kg/h. Furosemide or mannitol can be given for myoglobin diuresis. Fluid resuscitation should be performed with normal saline or Ringer's lactate. Urine alkalization can also be used in order to increase myoglobin output. Sodium bicarbonate ($NaHCO_3$) should be administered at a serum pH of 7.5. Tetanus immunization should be provided in the cases of open wounds or burns. Specific treatment methods should be applied for the concomitant injuries. Monitoring should be continued for 24–48 hours in arrhythmias or cardiac exposure.

Intracompartment pressure measurement would be appropriate if compartment syndrome is suspected. Patients requiring fasciotomy should be identified by this way and fasciotomy should be performed in the presence of compartment syndrome.

Patients having high-voltage injury and severe burns should be treated in burn units. These patients should be referred to burn units in compliance with the burn care protocols. Analgesics should be added to treatment in case of pain. If the pain is severe, opioids may be needed.

In electrical injuries due to low-voltage, the patient can be discharged directly from the ED if physical examination is normal and the patient is asymptomatic. Asymptomatic patients who are not pregnant, have no known heart disorders, and who have had only brief exposure to domestic electric current usually have no significant acute internal or external injuries that would necessitate admission and can be discharged.

Cardiac monitoring for 6–12 hours is indicated for patients with the following conditions:
- Arrhythmias
- Chest pain
- Any suggestion of cardiac damage
- Pregnancy (possibly)
- Known heart disorders (possibly).

Patients with minor burns or symptoms of moderate severity can be discharged following 12 hours observation in the emergency department (ED) and if the laboratory outcomes are normal. If the symptoms continue in this period, observation time may be prolonged until the symptoms are resolved. Patients who have severe symptoms such as cardiac arrest, altered level of consciousness, hypoxia, arrhythmias, burns, and trauma should be hospitalized for treatment.

Procedure Technique

Fasciotomy

It should be performed in the presence of compartment syndrome which is considered in the following conditions and the definite diagnosis is established with pressure measurement method:
- Tension and tenderness in the extremity
- Pain
- Numbness
- Hypoesthesia.

Central Venous Catheterization

It is appropriate in shock, over dehydration conditions, and severe burns. Jugular or femoral region can be preferred.

SUMMARY

Electrical injuries are important emergencies that may be encountered in a wide spectrum of manifestations ranging from simple injuries to fatal arrhythmias and burns. This type of injury requires following both ATLS and ACLS guidelines. Protective measures are paramount importance in electrical injuries. Safety in first aid gains more importance because of the electrical conductivity of the human body. Primary treatment consists of the prevention of complications with fluid resuscitation and cardiac monitoring. Simple cases can be discharged directly from EDs, but patients with severe symptoms must be hospitalized and electrical burns must be referred to burn units in compliance with relevant guidelines.

BIBLIOGRAPHY

1. Andrews CJ, Cooper MA, ten Duis HJ, Sappideen G. The pathology of electrical and lightning injuries. In: Wecht CJ (Ed). Forensic Sciences, Chapter 23A, Release 19 update NY: Matthew Bender & Co, 1995.
2. Cander B, Dur A, Koyuncu F, et al. The Demographical Characteristic and Affecting Factors on Length of Stay in Hospital Due to Electrical Injuries. Akademik Acil Tıp Dergisi. 2010;2:72-4.
3. Claudet I, Marechal C, Debuisson C, et al. Risk of arrhythmia and domestic low-voltage electrical injury. Arch Pediatr. 2010;17(4):343-9.
4. Cooper MA. Emergent Care of Lightning and Electrical Injuries. Semin Neurol. 1995;15(3):268-78.
5. Dalay C Travma. Electrical Burns. In: Ertekin C, Taviloğlu K, Güloğlu R Kurtoğlu M (Eds). İstanbul Medikal Yayıncılık. pp. 594-601.
6. Daniel P Runde. Electrical Injuries. Available from: *http://www.merckmanuals.com/professional/injuries-poisoning/electrical-and-lightning-injuries/electrical-injuries.* [Accessed March 2017].
7. Gjorgje Dzhokic, Jasmina Jovchevska, Artan Dika. Electrical Injuries: Etiology, Pathophysiology and Mechanism of Injury. Macedonian Journal of Medical Sciences. 2010;1(2):54–58.
8. Jensen PJ, Thomsen PE, Bagger JP, et al. Electrical injury causing ventricular arrhythmias. Br Heart J. 1987;57(3):279-83.
9. Kym D, Seo DK, Hur GY, et al. Epidemiology of electrical injury: Differences between low- and high-voltage electrical injuries during a 7-year study period in South Korea. Scand J Surg. 2015;104(2):108-14.
10. Luz DP, Millan LS, Alessi MS, et al. Electrical burns: a retrospective analysis across a 5-year period. Burns. 2009;35(7):1015-9.
11. Nazire Belgin Akıllı, Ramazan Köylü, Bekir Opuş, et al. Thalamic Infarct due to Electrical Injury. JAEMCR. 2014;5: 244-6.
12. Price TG, Cooper MA. Electrical and lightning injuries. In: Marx JA, Hockberger RS, Walls RM, Adams J, Rosen P (Eds). Rosen's Emergency Medicine: Concepts and Clinical Practice, 8th edition. Philadelphia: Elsevier Mosby; 2014. pp. 142.
13. Robb M, Close B, Furyk J, et al. Review article: Emergency Department implications of the TASER. Emerg Med Australas. 2009;21(4):250-8.
14. Spies C, Trohman RG. Narrative review: Electrocution and life-threatening electrical injuries. Ann Intern Med. 2006;145(7):531-7.
15. Strote J, Walsh M, Angelidis M, et al. Conducted electrical weapon use by law enforcement: an evaluation of safety and injury. J Trauma. 2010;68(5):1239-46.
16. Tracy A Cushing. Electrical Injuries in Emergency Medicine. [online] Medscape website. Available from: *http://emedicine.medscape.com/article/770179.* [Accessed March 2017].
17. Zipes DP. TASER electronic control devices can cause cardiac arrest in humans. Circulation. 2014;129(1):101-11.

Index

Page numbers followed by *b* refer to box, *f* refer to figure, *fc* refer to flowchart and *t* refer to table

A

Abbey pain scale 12
Abdomen 21, 602, 610, 668, 693, 699
    acute 498, 503, 504
    plain X-ray 425, 448
    ultrasound of 421*f*
Abdominal trauma, blunt 647, 648, 653, 693
Abortions
    complete 498
    incomplete 498
    previous spontaneous 502
    threatened 498
Abrasion 25, 26
Abscess 465, 537
    formation 515
    intraperitoneal 421*f*
    peritonsillar 100, 465
    prostatic 465
    retropharyngeal 100
    septal 100
Absorption atelectasis 170
Acaricides 753
Accidents, bicycle 629
Acephate 754
Acetaminophen 175
Acetanilide 723
Acetazolamide 161
Acetic acid 719
Acetoacetate 160
Acetylcholinesterase 756
Acetylsalicylic acid 213
Acid
    base disorder 158, 159, 159*t*, 728, 729*t*
        analysis of 159
    diuresis 741
    fast bacilli 331
    suppression 395
Acidemia 729
Acidosis 91, 493, 723, 729
    metabolic 159, 160, 162, 368, 435, 729, 749, 799
    respiratory 159, 729
Aclidinium 33
Acne 720
Acquired immunodeficiency syndrome 364
Addison's disease 432
Adenoids 100

Adenoma
    bronchial 315
    metastasis, pituitary 492
Adenomyosis 498
Adenosine 241
Adrenal crisis, acute 490, 491, 492*b*, 492*fc*, 493*t*
Adrenal gland
    basic anatomy of 490
    division of 490*t*
    physiology of 490
Adrenal insufficiency, causes of 492*t*
Adrenaline 220
Adsorbents recirculating system 744
Adult respiratory distress syndrome 668
Advanced cardiac life support 3, 84, 97*fc*, 348, 516, 517, 799, 812, 814
    cardiac arrest algorithm 95
    survey 92
Advanced trauma life support 3, 84, 612, 626, 637, 646, 656, 814
Aerobic gram-negative bacilli 539
Aflatoxins 739
Agitation 365, 367, 731
Air embolism 247, 743-745
Airway 73, 83, 101, 118, 311, 317, 324, 348, 373, 516, 606, 624, 626, 812
    assessment 18, 101*f*
    breathing 21
    disease, obstructive 285
    maintenance 606
    management 99, 101, 102*f*, 603, 632
    obstruction 100, 161, 603
        causes of 100
        signs of 324
    opening pressure 142
    pressure 142, 143
    smooth muscles 114
    stent 315
    surgical 102, 103, 106
Akathisia 732, 733
Alanine aminotransferase, levels of 813
Albuterol nebulization 585
Alcohol 193, 474, 719, 723, 728, 739, 743
    abuse 160, 364, 793
    benzodiazepines 367
    intoxication 365
    withdrawal 732
Aldosterone 490, 491

inhibitors 729
    resistance 435
    role of 491*b*
    secretion, reduced 435
Alkalemia 729
Alkali overdose 729
Alkaline diuresis 740, 741
Alkalosis 91, 400
    metabolic 159, 160, 162, 729, 746
    refeeding 162
    respiratory 149, 159, 160, 162, 729, 794
Allergic interstitial nephritis, acute 446
Allergic reactions 749
Allergy 610
    history 17
Allograft rejection 446
All-trans-retinoic acid 589
Alpha-adrenergic drugs 722
Alpha-naphthyl-thiourea 753
Alphos poisoning 774
Alprazolam 361
Alteplase 221
Aluminum phosphide 719, 771, 772, 772*t*, 773*fc*, 775
    poisoning 771, 774, 775
    toxicity 773*fc*
    usage of 771*f*
Alveolar
    arterial oxygen gradient 323
    hemorrhage, diffuse 577
    pressure 142, 143
    proteinosis 324
Amanitin 744, 749
Ambu bag 101, 102*f*
Amenorrhea 493
American Academy of Clinical Toxicology 736
American College of Surgeons 417
American Diabetes Association and Endocrine Society 473
American Heart Association 91, 92, 93*fc*, 95, 97*fc*
American Pancreatic Association 404
American Society of Echocardiography 286
American Urological Association 468
Amikacin 454, 539
Aminoglycosides 162, 442, 454, 586
Aminophylline 267, 333
Amiodarone 96, 241, 243, 304

Amitriptyline 361
Ammonia levels 368
Amoxapine 734
Amoxicillin 720
Amphetamines 249, 719, 721-723, 728, 731, 733, 734, 739, 743
    toxicity 732
Ampicillin 539
Amyl nitrite 747
Amyloidosis 577
Amyotrophic lateral sclerosis 732
Anal
    fissure 174
    irritation 740
Analgesics, nonopioid 175
Anaphylaxis 118, 330, 446, 571, 745
Anemia 194, 330, 493, 558, 569, 587
    acute 368
        microangiopathic 253
            hemolytic 250
        pernicious 465
        severe 112, 201
Anesthesia 674
    topical airway 102
Aneurysm 74
    atherosclerotic 257
    left ventricular 278
    partially coiled 382f
Angina 250
    stable 188
    unstable 184, 186, 205, 207, 209t, 212t
    worsening 252
Angiodysplasias 393
Angioedema 330, 570, 571t
Angiography 638
    coronary 201
Angioplasty, high risk 222
Angiostrongylus cantonensis 537
Angiotensin converting enzyme 474, 485
    inhibitors 227, 229, 253, 264, 299, 309, 442, 485, 570
Angiotensin receptor blocker 227, 229, 442, 474, 548
Aniline 743
    dyes 723
Anilofos 754
Animal bite 682, 780
    cases, management of 779
Anion gap
    acidosis 480, 762
    concept 160
Ankle-brachial index 683
Anorexia 412, 420, 438, 493
Anoxia 533
Anterior cord syndrome 629
Antiarrhythmic drugs 217
Antibiotics 20, 333, 408, 446, 529, 529t, 568, 569, 625, 718, 743
    intravenous 21
Antibody fragments, digoxin-specific 747

Anticholinergic 333, 365, 367, 447, 719, 720, 722, 728, 731
    agents 104
    long-acting 333
    poisoning 794
    short-acting 333
    syndrome 718
Anticholinesterase 766
Anticoagulants, types of 266
Anticoagulation therapy, monitoring 267
Anticonvulsants 568, 625, 720, 723
Antidepressants 447, 721-723, 728, 731, 732, 739, 743
Antidiabetic drugs 739
Antidiarrheal drugs 529, 530
Antidote 747, 748, 762
    administration 720, 746
Antiemetics drugs 530
Antiepileptic 365, 739
    drugs 533, 534
Anti-Epstein-Barr nuclear antigen 540
Antigen, prostatic specific 464
Anti-glomerular basement membrane disease 316
Antihistamines 719, 720, 722, 723, 728, 731, 734, 739, 743
Antihypertensive 383, 732
    drugs, hypotensive action of 368
Antimalarials 720
Antimicrobial therapy 129, 454
Antineoplastic agents 439
Antineutrophil cytoplasmic antibodies 447, 576
Antinuclear antibody 374, 570
Antiparkinsonism 365
Antiphospholipid syndrome 345, 575, 577
Antipsychotics 721, 728
Antipyretics 338
Anti-rape laws 87
Anti-snake venom 791
    administration 792
Antistreptolysin O 460
Anti-viral capsid antigen 540
Anuria 791
Anxiety 162, 186, 324, 330, 367, 729
    disorders 193
Aorta
    abdominal 285f
    arch of 262f, 263f
    ascending 262f, 555
    coarctation of 249
    descending 555, 555f
    dilatation of 256f, 260
    inflammatory disease of 257
    repair 394
    severe coarctation of 556
Aortic aneurysm 183, 319
    abdominal 197
Aortic arch 370, 556
    interruption 555f
    vessel occlusion 260

Aortic dissection 74, 183, 184, 186, 197, 217, 249, 256, 262f, 263, 273, 284, 290, 297, 347, 697
    acute 174, 250, 253, 257, 260t, 285f, 297
    ascending aorta diagnostic of 261f
    classification of 257f
    subacute 257
    surgical management of 264
    traumatic 259f
Aortic graft 315
Aortic injury 641
Aortic regurgitation 260, 261, 285
    immediate paravalvular 301
    paravalvular 301
    severe 258f
Aortic root 258f, 285f
Aortic rupture 257, 264
Aortic stenosis 85, 183, 197
    critical 556
    severe 290
Aortic ulcer, penetrating 297
Aortic valve
    closure of 222f
    cusps 258f
    disease 183
    regurgitation 257, 261
    replacement 304
    sclerotic 289
Aortic valvular heart disease 257
Aortic wall 258f
Aortoarteritis 257
Aortobronchial fistula 315
Aortoenteric fistula 394
Aortography 262
Aortopulmonary window 556, 557
Apathy 20
Aphasia 20
Apical ventricular septal rupture 288f
Apnea 728
Appendage thrombus, left atrial 289
Appendectomy 415
    laparoscopic 411, 415, 415t, 416f
Appendicitis 74, 368, 412
    acute 174, 410, 411f, 413f, 414b, 414fc, 503, 692
    anatomical position of 410f
    chronic 416
    division of 416f
    perforated 412, 415
    recurrent 416
    signs of 412t
    symptoms of 412t
Arc burns 812
Arformoterol 333
Arm
    breast upper chest, swelling of 581
    sensory loss of 20
Arrhythmia 118, 193, 201, 213, 273, 301, 303, 304, 330, 368, 438, 553, 557, 559, 745, 746, 773fc, 790, 792, 814
    atrial 728

Index

cardiac 197, 273, 435, 717, 724
   supraventricular 217
   toxin induced 722t
   unstable 437
Arsenic 720
Arterial blood 219
   gas 125, 147, 158, 160, 169, 170, 199, 332, 337, 368, 420, 774, 791, 794, 799
      analysis 158, 160, 374
      levels 609
Arterial catheterization, pulmonary 315
Arterial hypertension, refractory 264
Arterial oxygen
   partial pressure of 125, 127, 164, 164t, 165
   saturation 331
   tension 322
Arterial pressure index 683
Arteriography 448, 684
Arteriovenous malformation 315, 319, 377, 556
Arteritis
   infectious 537
   temporal 363
Artery 446
   catheter, pulmonary 219, 220
   innominate 315
   pulmonary 262, 316, 556
   radial 158
   selection of 158
   spinal 319
   thrombosis, renal 448
   wedge pressure, pulmonary 775
Arthralgia 438, 493
Arthritis
   reactive 577
   rheumatoid 576f, 577
   septic 577
Ascites 110, 226, 330
Ascorbic acid 747
Aspartate aminotransferase 813
Aspiration 138, 324
   pneumonia 336, 735, 737
Aspirin 175, 267, 361, 394
Assist control ventilation 146f
Assisted reproductive technologies 502
Asterixis 324, 365
Asthma 137, 144, 241, 324, 329, 329t, 330, 341
   acute 164, 329, 329t
      exacerbation of 328, 347
      severe 143
   bronchial 148, 328, 330
   family history of 329
Ataxia 20
Atelectasis
   adhesive 170
   radiological signs of 170
Atenolol 241

Atheroembolism 446, 449
Atherosclerosis 249, 370
Atlantoaxial dislocation 577
Atresia 100
   pulmonary, pulmonary 554
Atrial
   fibrillation 193, 234, 239, 240, 266, 274, 275, 276f, 297, 301, 303, 370, 484, 735
   flutter 240, 275, 561f
   myxoma, large 290
   natriuretic peptide 309
   pressure, right 219
   septal defects 193, 289, 371
Atrioventricular
   block 722
   nodal re-entrant tachycardia 275f
   node 238
   reciprocating tachycardia 275f
   reentrant tachycardia 193, 239, 240, 561
Atropine 712, 719, 720, 722, 731, 739, 747, 762, 763
   challenge test 761
Attack, acute 362
Aurintricarboxylic acid 747
Auscultation 105, 260
Australasian triage scale 11
Autoimmune 336
   adrenalitis 492
   diseases 405
   hemolytic anemia 577
Automated external defibrillator 95b, 96f, 387, 388, 516
Autonomic system 465
Axial contrast-enhanced computed tomography 693f
Axonal injury, diffuse 623, 698
Azotemia 250, 799
   prerenal 448
Aztreonam 539

B

Back trauma 492
Bacterial
   cystitis 465
   fragments removal 443
   infection 446, 469
   meningitis 536, 537fc, 539t
   peritonitis 400, 745
Bacteriuria 452
Bacteroides 412
Bag mask ventilation 103
Balanitis 465
Balloon size, selection of 222t
Barbiturates 568, 625, 719, 720, 723, 728, 731, 739, 743, 744
Barcelona declaration 23
Barium salts 733
Barotrauma 138
Basal bolus regimen 544

Basal septum 283f
Basic life support 91, 516
Bat rabies 780
Beck's triad 559
Belladonna alkaloids 743
Benzodiazepine 364, 365, 400, 719, 723, 728, 731, 739, 743
Benztropine 749
Benzylpenicillin 747
Beriberi 558
Beta-blocker 435, 559, 721, 739
   therapy 558
Bevacizumab therapy 316
Bicarbonate 161
   anion 112
   serum 159
   therapy 482
Bicuspid aortic valve 257
Bilharziasis 465
Biomedical waste management 1998 77
Biopsy 341
   renal 448
   transbronchial 341
Birth and Death Act, registration of 77
Birth
   forceps-assisted 510f
   vacuum-assisted 510f
Bismuth cholestyramine 530
Bisphosphonates 269, 439
Bites 681
Black widow spider bite 733
Bladder
   catheterization 515
   injury 652f
   stone 464
   tumor 464
Bleeding 589, 744
   amount of 316
   cause of 316
   disorders 112, 498, 745, 790
   gastrointestinal 393, 400, 695
   per vaginum, treatment of 501
   rapid control of 21
   requiring re-exploration 301
Blood
   ammonia testing 401
   and blood product administration 130
   bank, responsibility of 154
   clot 447
   count, complete 19, 156, 332, 396, 420, 447, 460, 468, 528, 554, 570, 799, 813
   culture 20
   examination 528
   flow
      pulmonary 553f
      renal 114, 728
   gas
      monitoring 331
      normal values of 161t

glucose
    level 86
    self-monitoring of 546
grouping 420
investigations 499
loss 110
    volume of 498
pH 159
picture, complete 425
pressure 13, 20, 73, 86, 113, 117, 123, 196, 197, 250, 259, 260, 330, 331, 374, 549, 548, 663, 722t, 728
    ambulatory 201
    diastolic 248, 374
    high 383
    low diastolic 111
    management 378
    monitoring, noninvasive 102
    systolic 13, 19, 122, 130, 206, 208, 248, 374, 600
    target 249t
products 153
test 267, 347
transfusions 395
    citrated 439
    massive 439
urea nitrogen 406, 447, 448, 493, 794
volume expansion 556
Bloodstream 452
Blunt trauma, multiple 643
Body
    fluid compartments 110
    mass index 297, 299
    surface
        area 147
        pressure 142, 143
Boerhaave's syndrome 186
Bolam's test 41f
Bone
    marrow
        aspiration 3
        transplantation 587
    pain 438
Boric acid 743
Botulinum antitoxin 747
Botulism 723
Bounding pulse 111
Bowel
    diseases cholecystitis 183
    ischemia 427, 577
    obstruction, low small 424
    perforation 577, 693
    signs of strangulation of 427
    sounds 420
    surgery 738
Brachial artery injury 658f
Bradbury-Eggleston syndrome 198
Bradyarrhythmias 217, 233, 273, 276, 553, 561, 726
Bradycardia 193, 197, 241, 304, 324, 367, 438, 487, 722, 728, 735
    symptomatic 250
Brain
    abscess 365, 536
    cell damage 794
    computed tomography scan of 374
    hemorrhage, symptomatic 379
    imaging 401
    injuries 492, 626
        mild traumatic 623
        moderate traumatic 623
        pattern of 623, 623t
        penetrating 625
        severe traumatic 623
    metastasis 581, 584
    natriuretic peptide 813
    stem infarction 372
    tumor 365, 465, 533
Brainstem dysfunction, stages of 781
Braunwald classification system 209, 209t
Breath
    shortness of 285, 329
    sound 337
    types of 14
Breathing 73, 118, 311, 318, 348, 373, 516, 606, 607, 624, 626, 721, 812
    assessment of 18
    physiology of 142
    spontaneously 143, 144
    work of 136, 146
Breathlessness 239, 325, 581
Breech presentation 513
Bridging vein injury 623
Brittle nails 439
Bromides 720, 723, 743
Bromism 729
Bronchial artery 316, 319
    embolization 319
Bronchiectasis 315, 324
    cystic shadows suggestive of 317f
    left upper lobe 318f
Bronchioles, obstruction of 337
Bronchoconstriction 252, 749
Bronchodilators 333
    short-acting 333
Bronchoscopy 315, 317, 318, 320
Bronchospasm 112, 439
Brown-Séquard syndrome 630
Bruise 25, 26
    fresh 26
B-type natriuretic peptide 214
Bulbocavernosus reflex 467
Bullet and blast injuries 704
Bundle branch block 239, 275, 276f, 277f, 279t
    left 199, 206-208, 217, 220, 274, 278, 279, 279f
    right 199, 242, 275, 279
Burkitt's lymphoma 588
Burns 26, 100, 107, 111, 324, 446, 671, 809
    classification of 807t
    deep 804f
    friction 685f
    depth of 807t
    electric 174, 801, 802f, 803f, 809
    emergency management of 801
    first-degree 802
    flash 801
    fourth-degree 802
    injury 26, 27t, 809
        types of 807
    intraoral 804
    phenolic 734
    radiation 801
    second-degree 802, 803f
    thermal 169, 174, 801
    third-degree 802, 803f, 809
Burst fractures 630, 631, 631f
Busulfan 720
Butane 723
Butyrophenones 719, 734
Bypass open heart surgery 222

C

Caffeine 193, 719, 722, 731, 733, 734
Cairo-bishop classification system 584b
Calcineurin inhibitors 442
Calcitonin 439, 585
Calcium 112, 743
    channel blocker 217, 721
    disodium edetate or versenate 747
    gluconate 734, 737
    malabsorption 439
    salts 747
    serum 447
    sign 260
Calculi 447
Camphor 719, 731, 733
Campylobacter 526
    jejuni 526
Canadian Cardiovascular Society 213
    Angina Score 299
Canadian triage scale 11
Canal defect, complete atrioventricular 556
Cancers 498
    metastatic 394
Cannabis 719, 722, 731
Cannula, intravenous 153
Cape triage score 11
Capillary wedge pressure, pulmonary 112, 208
Capnography 105, 609
Captopril 250, 251
Carbamates 719, 722, 739, 753, 765
    poisoning 761t
Carbamazepine 535, 568, 719, 734
Carbapenem 454, 586
Carbaryl 766
Carbofuran 766
Carbolic acid 719
Carbon
    dioxide 322, 723

tension 158
    partial pressure of 147, 159, 170, 554
disulfide 732
    monoxide 164, 330, 363, 719-723, 728, 731, 732, 734
        poisoning 169, 365
    tetrachloride 744
Carbonaceous sputum 804
Carbonic anhydrase inhibitors 729
Carbosulfan 766
Carboxyhemoglobin 164, 363
Carcinoma 423, 447
    catamenial 341
    infection 447
Card test 774
Cardiac
    arrest 438, 749
        algorithm 97fc
        management of 91
        maternal 515, 516, 517f
    biomarkers 269, 271
    chest pain, ischemic 184
    disease 329, 552
    emergency 562
        causes of 553t
    enzyme 368, 774
    examination 187
    failure 112
        congestive 144
    free wall rupture 217
    glycosides 722
    index 130, 208
    injury 640, 812
        blunt 640
        penetrating 640
    markers 213
    output 114, 117
        monitoring of 112
    perforation 247
    resynchronization therapy 245
    sounds, reduced 487
    surgery 301, 307
    syncope 197
    tamponade 117, 197, 247, 280, 288, 290, 330, 559t, 581, 583, 610f
    trauma 217
    tumors 289, 290
Cardioembolic stroke, causes of 289f
Cardioembolism 371
Cardiomyopathy 118, 193, 217, 330
    arrhythmogenic right ventricular 242
    hypertrophic 203, 217, 240, 278
    idiopathic dilated 277f
    postpartum 12
Cardiopulmonary
    arrest 144
    bypass 301, 303, 309, 740, 746
    resuscitation 93, 97, 311, 341, 515, 517, 640
        cycles of 93

Cardiorenal syndrome 228
Cardiorespiratory system 365
Cardiotoxicity 735
Cardiovascular
    collapse 347, 555
    diseases 187, 248, 798
    dysfunction 484
    system 114, 115, 773fc
        examination 357
Carotid 20
    artery 370, 371
        imaging 374
    sinus
        hypersensitivity 198
        massage 201
        syncope 197
Cartilage, septal 677f
Catamenial hemoptysis 316
Catastrophic antiphospholipid syndrome 575, 578
Catecholamines 490, 729
Catharsis 735, 737, 738
Catheter
    ablation 240
    knotting 247
Cauda equina
    syndrome 583, 630
    tumors 465
Cefepime 539
Cefoperazone 454
Cefotaxime 539
Ceftazidime 539
Ceftriaxone 454, 539
Celiac disease 548
Cell culture vaccine 783
Central cord syndrome 630
Central nervous system 125, 353, 355, 365, 368, 386, 486, 487, 532, 536, 537, 590, 622, 718, 720, 728, 731, 794
    depression 161, 367, 721, 723, 726
    disease 162
    effects 484, 757
    examination 357
    infections 536
    injury, acute 375f
    intoxication, grading severity of 723t
Central venous access devices 587
Central venous pressure 112, 119, 128, 130, 218, 219, 420, 774, 775
    oxygen saturation of 130
Central vertigo 355
Cephaelis ipecacuanha 735f
Cephalosporin 568, 586
Cerebellar
    Artery
        anterior inferior 20
        posterior inferior 20
    signs 486
Cerebral
    artery 376f, 377f

        anterior 20, 372
        middle 20, 372, 376
        posterior 372, 382f
        stroke 376f
    blood flow 622
    edema 112, 749
    hemorrhages 533
    infarction 250, 533
    ischemia 380
    malaria 794
    malperfusion 258
    perfusion pressure 622
    thrombosis 745
    vasoconstriction 622
Cerebritis 537
    lupus 577
Cerebrospinal fluid 363, 522, 536, 537, 539, 539t, 540, 587, 625, 675
    drainage 625
    examination 368
Cerebrovascular
    accident 161, 360, 374, 577
    disease 484
    episode 465
Cerebrum
    basal cistern ventricles 623
    tentorium falx 623
Cervical
    artery dissection 371
    collars 632f
    pregnancy 506
    spine
        and neck 610
        immobilization 657f
        injury 107, 632
        protection 606, 608f
        radiograph of 657
        stabilization of 603
        tenderness 21
Cervix 447
Cesarean delivery 515
Cheek lacerations 675
Chemical
    burns 801, 809
    disaster 710
        management of 712f
    injuries 26
    pleurodesis 342
Chemosis 790
Chest 610
    compression 96f, 311, 517f
        high-quality 94b
    decompression 21
    discomfort 239
    drain insertion 342, 342f
    heaviness 239
    injuries 319, 699
    pain 183, 184t, 186t, 188, 189fc, 190fc, 814
        acute 183, 295, 697
        causes of 183 183f, 183t

evaluation 296*fc*
locations of 186*f*
noncardiac 184
nonischemic causes of 184
pleuritic 347
substernal 170
roentgenogram 259*f*, 260
syndrome, acute 186
trauma
blunt 315, 697
penetrating 315
tube
insertion 174, 340, 341, 603
management 642
selection of 342
wall 324, 330
deformity 162
injuries 638
syndromes 186
trauma 324
X-ray 337, 341, 420, 421*f*, 553*f*, 554, 555*f*, 560*f*, 637
periodic 247
Chick embryo cell vaccine, purified 784
Chills 337, 746
Chin-lift maneuver 607*f*
Chlamydia
pneumoniae 337
trachomatis 502
Chlamydophila psittaci 337
Chloral hydrate 719, 723, 743, 744
Chloramphenicol 539
Chlorates 723, 743
Chlordiazepoxide 732
Chlorfenvinphos 754
Chlorhexidine 720
Chloride 267, 747
Chlorine 112
Chloroform 719
Chloroquine 719, 739
Chlorpromazine 361, 744, 749
Chlorpyrifos 754
Choanal atresia 100
Cholangiopancreatography, postendoscopic retrograde 404
Cholecystitis, acute 692
Cholera 528, 529
Cholesterol, high 383
Cholinergic syndrome 718
Cholinesterase activity, depression of 760
Chorea 732, 733
Chromatography, thin layer 761
Chvostek's sign 407, 439
Cimetidine 739
Cinacalcet 439
Ciprofloxacin 454, 539
Circulation 73, 83, 118, 318, 348, 373, 516, 606, 607, 624, 626, 721, 812
assessment of 18
Cirrhosis 399, 431, 446

Cisplatin 585, 720
Citrate toxicity 746
Clavicular fractures 639
Clean lacerated wound 670
Clevidipine 251, 252
Clinical establishment Act 49, 77, 517
Clofazimine 720
Clonazepam 535
Clonidine 250, 251, 253, 719, 720, 722
withdrawal 249
Clopidogrel 267
therapy 213
Closed-loop obstruction 427
Clostridium difficile 408, 587
colitis 693
Clotting time, activated 302, 303
Clumsy hand dysarthria 372
Cluster headache, treatment of 361
Coagulation irregularities 439
Coal tar products 720
Cobra bite 791
Cocaine 193, 316, 719, 721-723, 728, 731-733
Coccidioides immitis 537
Code trauma 601, 602
advantages of 604
team members 602, 603*t*
Codeine 176, 361
Cognitive defects 308
Colchicine overdose 439
Cold extremities 111
Colicky pain 424
Colitis 693
Collapse 790
Collar sign 652*f*
Coma 250, 324, 367, 626, 719, 728
hysterical 722
psychogenic 722
recovery scale 722
status 487
toxic causes of 723*t*
Comatose 368
shock state 795
Compartment syndrome 169, 657, 658
abdominal 138
pathophysiology of 659*fc*
Compression 446
fracture 630, 631*f*
ultrasonography 348
Computed tomography 17, 21, 214, 261, 263, 308, 317, 373, 375, 376, 401, 404, 414, 453, 454, 459, 460, 476, 537, 582, 587, 588, 625, 646, 652*f*, 684, 692, 694
abdomen 368
angiographic cross-section 262*f*
angiography 201, 348, 698
contrast enhanced 21, 693
enteroclysis 694
scan 150, 340, 603, 657, 648, 650

severity index 406
urography 458, 696
Confusion 324, 362, 438, 626
assessment method 367
post-traumatic 624
Confusional state, acute 364, 364*fc*, 365, 367, 368*t*
Congestion
evidence of 226
pulmonary 219
Congestive heart failure, acute 263, 553, 556
Conjugate eye deviation 20
Conn's syndrome 249, 729
Connective tissue
disease 341
disorder 257, 258
Consciousness 21
clouding of 365
loss of 624
scale, comprehensive level of 722
transient loss of 196, 200
Constipation 400, 424, 438, 464, 487, 493, 585
Constitutes medical negligence 41
Consumer protection Act 77
Continuous glucose monitoring
devices 477
system 546*f*
Contraception 502
Control mode ventilation 145*f*
Contusion 25
parenchymal 623
pulmonary 639
Conus medullaris 465
Convulsions 532, 717, 730, 746, 749
toxic causes of 731*t*
Cool extremities 227
Copper sulfate 736, 749
Cord
compression 590
lesions 799
Cornea, protection of 674
Corneal deposit, pulmonary 241
Coronary
artery 206, 260
bypass grafting 120, 213, 214, 219-222, 295, 301
disease 183, 208, 209, 214, 226, 266, 281, 295, 300, 577
left 556
spasm 278
care unit 7
computed tomography 294, 295, 295*t*
angiography 294
intervention, percutaneous 120, 213, 220
syndrome, acute 22, 183, 186, 190, 197, 205, 211*b*, 250, 269, 270, 270*fc*, 273, 281, 294, 295, 297, 301, 307, 330, 331, 697

vascular supply, typical distribution of 282f
Corpus luteum cyst, ruptured 503
Corrosives 738, 739
Cortex, adrenal 490
Corticosteroid 129, 267, 333, 731, 749
    high dose 583
    systemic 333
    therapy, adjunctive 538
Corticotropin hormone, adrenal 491
Cortisol 474
Costochondritis 186, 347
    arthritis 183
Cosyntropin 492
Cotrimoxazole 568
Cough 337, 347, 582, 720
    pleural effusion 577
Counter-pressure maneuvers 202f
Coupled plasma filtration adsorption 443, 444
Cramps 740
Cranial nerves 357
Craniotomy, decompressive 625
Cranium 668
C-reactive protein 23, 122, 210, 330, 337, 406
Creatine kinase 211
    myocardial band 209, 210
Creatinine, serum 309, 442
Cremasteric reflex 467
Cricoid cartilage 99
Cricothyroidotomy 106
    kit 102, 106
    percutaneous 103, 106, 106f
    surgical 102, 103, 106
Criminal law (amendment) Act 87
Crisis
    adrenal 492
    hypertensive 250, 259, 577
Crohn's disease 423
Crufomate 756
Cryptococcus neoformans 537
Crystalloids 129
Cullen's sign 405
Cushing's disease 729
Cushing's reflex 623
Cushing's syndrome 249
Cut-off sign 426f
Cyanide 719, 720, 722, 723, 731, 739
    toxicity 252
Cyanoacrylates 688
Cyanofenphos 756
Cyanosis 325, 347, 553, 553f, 554fc
    peripheral 324
    respiratory causes of 554t
Cyanotic spell 557, 558
Cyclic vomiting syndrome 728
Cyclophosphamide 585
Cyclopyriphos 754
Cyclosporine 249

Cysteamine 749
Cystic fibrosis 341
Cystitis 452, 457
    tubercular 465
Cystocele 464
Cystography 652f
Cystoscopy, role of 459
Cysts 100
    hydatid 319
    ruptured 12
Cytokine removal 443
Cytomegalovirus 449, 693
Cytotoxic drugs 217, 720

D

Dalteparin 131
Dantrolene 747
Dapsone 739, 744
Dark pigmentation 720
Day time sleeping 365
Deafness, ipsilateral 20
Debakey classification 256
Debris 447
Decompression
    nasogastric 427
    sickness 169
Decontamination 720, 734
Deep vein thrombosis 112, 126, 131, 266, 269, 270, 345, 347, 378, 577, 697
Dehydration 110, 112, 118, 364, 365, 400, 420, 425, 526, 527, 527t, 528, 528b, 529t, 717, 793
    assessment of 527
    degree of 527t
    severe 112
Dehydroepiandrosterone acetate 490
Delirium 364, 438, 731
    previous episode of 364
Delivery, modes of 510f
Dementia, advance 364
Demeton methyl 754
Dental
    caries 720
    discoloration 720
Deoxyribonucleic acid 505
Depression 368, 439
    psychosis 493
    severe 368
Dermatitis
    eczematous 720
    exfoliative 720
Dermatologic emergencies 567, 567t
Dermis 571
Desferrioxamine 737, 747
Dextran 112
Dextrose 712, 726
    normal saline 111, 112
Diabetes 112, 383, 447, 493, 548t, 729
    control and complications trial 541, 542

    diagnosis of 541t
    education 548
    etiological classification of 542b
    insipidus 434b, 435, 435t, 446
        causes of 434fc
        complete central 435
    management 541, 542, 548
    mellitus 205, 206, 217, 226, 308, 339, 442, 453, 465, 473, 478, 542, 543
    pediatric 543t
    types of 542b
Diabetic ketoacidosis
    classification of 480t
    pathogenesis of 479fc
Dialysate, delivery of 742
Diaphoresis 184, 324, 367
Diaphragmatic injury
    signs of 652f
    X-ray of 651f
Diarrhea 110, 111, 161, 400, 431, 446, 493, 526-528, 528b, 529t, 530t, 529, 717, 729
    acute 526
    assessment of 527, 527t
    dysentery 526
    management of 528
    patterns of 526
    persistent 526, 529
    severe 738
    types of 526t
    watery 526
Diazepam 712, 732, 744, 747, 749, 764
Diazoxide 253
Diclofenac 175, 176, 361, 720
Dicobalt edetate 747
Diethoxy 756
Diethyl phosphate 761
Diethyldithiocarbamate 749
Diethylstilbestrol exposure 502
Diethyltoluamide 753
Dieulafoy's lesions 393
Digibind 747
Digifab 747
Digitalis 193, 731, 739, 743
    toxicity 241, 279
Digoxin 217, 241, 563t, 744
Diltiazem 241, 720
Dimercaprol 747
Dimercaptosuccinic acid 748
Dimethoate 754
Dimethoxy 756
Dimethyl sulfoxide 719
Dinitrophenol 723, 728
Diphenhydramine 744, 749
Diphtheria 100
Diplopia 719
Dipyridamole 267
Disaster 21
    classification of 704, 705t
    examples of 704

management cycle 706, 706fc
natural 705, 705f
radiological 710
triage 709
Disease modifying antirheumatic drugs 267
Disequilibrium 353
Dissection 446
  chronic 257
  flap
    extension of 258f
    presence of 260
Disseminated intravascular coagulation 123, 315, 589, 793
Distal sodium, reduced 435
Distension, abdominal 420, 740
Distress, respiratory 164, 337
Disulfiram 719
Diuretics 162, 228, 253, 400, 720
  administration 729
  like furosemide 585
  therapy 793
Diverticulosis 394
Diverticulum 419
Dix-Hallpike maneuver 357
Dix-Hallpike test 356, 357, 357f
Dizziness 239, 252, 790
  types of 353t
Dobutamine 114, 220, 230, 749
Docetaxel 585
Domestic violence 12, 185
Dopamine 96, 114, 125, 130, 220, 230, 724, 749
Doppler signs 288
Dorsal
  free flap 685f
  hand skin avulsion 685f
  horn 173
  split-skin graft 685
Double-lumen endobronchial tube 318f
Drainage, gastrointestinal 427
Dropsy 315
Drowning 797
  complications of 798, 799t
  management of 798, 799fc
  pathophysiology of 797f
  prevention of 799
  stages of 798fc
Drowsiness 728, 790
Drug and Cosmetic Act 77
Drug and Magical Remedies Act 77
Drugs
  abuse 732
  therapy 240
  toxicity 368
Dry
  hairs 487
  heat 26
  mucus membrane 367, 527
  powder inhaler 334
  skin 367, 439

Dumb rabies 783
Dye allergy 319
Dyselectrolytemia 588, 794
Dysequilibrium syndrome 745
Dysfunction, gastrointestinal 484
Dyslipidemia 548
Dysphagia 439
Dysplasia
  arrhythmogenic right ventricular 199, 243, 277f, 295
  bronchopulmonary 170
  fibromuscular 249
Dyspnea 184, 250, 259, 285, 337, 347, 487
  acute 330b
  management of 332fc
  severity of 331fc
Dysraphic lesions 465
Dysrhythmias 114, 301, 799
Dystonia 732, 733, 749

E

Ear 614
  bites 681
  laceration 675
    complex 676f
Earthquake 13, 704
Eaton-Lambert syndrome 162
Ebstein's anomaly 240
Echinococcosis 465
Echo virus 538
Echocardiogram 374
Echocardiography 201, 289
  role of 281
  two-dimensional 305
Eclampsia 12, 250, 253
Ectopic pregnancy 74, 174, 498, 502-504
  management of 503
  previous 502
  ruptured 12, 504
  signs of 503
  surgical management of 500
  symptoms of 503
Edema 100, 226, 447, 571
  cardiogenic pulmonary 137
  generalized 112, 487
  mucosal 149
  periorbital 581, 619f
  pulmonary 161, 250, 324, 330, 347, 368, 443, 450, 728, 790, 795
Ediphenphos 754
Ehlers-Danlos syndrome 257
Ejection fraction 208, 282
  left ventricular 214, 217, 226
Elapidae 788
Elastic recoil pressure 143
Elbow dislocation, posterior 666f
Electrocardiogram 188, 194, 197, 199, 205, 206, 208, 209, 213, 214, 218, 219, 233, 238, 240, 247, 260, 273, 274b, 277f, 279, 281, 294, 300, 307, 331, 332, 348f, 368, 373, 374, 375, 375f, 486, 552, 554, 556, 584, 640, 724, 728, 774, 794, 812
  monitoring 609
Electroencephalogram 386, 533f
Electrolyte 368, 425, 431, 432, 568
  correction 558
  disturbance 162, 733
  imbalance 194, 273, 400, 420, 431, 569, 745
  serum 480
Electromyogram 761
Emergency department
  care 508
  design 6
  function 6
  management 774
  preparedness 710
  thoracotomy 643
Emergency medical services 596, 706
Emergency severity index 11
Emesis 735
Empiric antibiotics options 586t
Empyema 537
  extradural 536
Enalaprilat 251, 252
Encephalitis 144, 162, 365, 368, 536, 781
Encephalopathy 399
  anoxic 799
  hypertensive 249, 250, 253, 365, 450
End-diastolic pressure, left ventricular 217, 218
Endocarditis 371
  nonbacterial thrombotic 290
Endocrine systems 728
Endometrial ablation 501
Endometriosis 502
  thoracic 341
Endometritis 515
Endopeptidases 789
Endoscopic signs 394
Endoscopy 735, 740
  therapeutic 395
Endothelial dysfunction 442
Endothelium 256
Endotoxins 443
Endotracheal
  intubation 104
  tube 83, 101, 102, 135
    connection 169f
Energy, low 597
Enterococcus faecalis 453
Environment Protection Act 77
Enzyme-linked immunosorbent assay technique 270, 782
Ephedrine 114, 115, 719, 728
Epidemic Diseases Act 77
Epigastric pain, chronic 394

Index

Epiglottis 100
Epilepsy 531*f*
   surgery 388
Epinephrine 95, 96, 114, 230, 474, 749
Epley's maneuver 357
Epley's repositioning method 358*f*
Ergot 720
   derivatives 362
Ertapenem 454
Erythema nodosum 720
Erythrocyte 587
   sedimenation rate 337, 363, 374, 570
Erythromycin 568, 720
Escherichia coli 412, 422, 453, 465, 491, 526, 537
Esmolol 251, 252, 264
Esophageal
   detectors 105
   injuries 641
   rupture 185
   varices 394
Esophagitis 185
Esophagogastroduodenoscopy 396
Esophagus, perforated 186
Estrogen progesterone therapy 501
Ethambutol 568
Ethanol 161, 405, 719, 721, 723, 729, 731, 743, 747, 749
   withdrawal syndrome 718
Ethion 754
Ethosuximide 535
   valproate 535
Ethylene glycol 160, 161, 723, 729, 739
Ethylenediaminetetraacetic acid 747
Etomidate 104
Etoposide 585
Ewald tube 736, 737*f*
Exacerbation, acute 32, 137, 169, 330
Excessive bleeding, management of 303*fc*
Exercise 435, 547
Expiratory positive airway pressure 137
Exposure, assessment of 783
Extensor tendon
   injury 685*f*
   repair 685*f*
External defibrillator 92, 246*f*
Extracorporeal
   life support 775
      membrane oxygenation 220-222, 326, 799
      techniques 741
      therapies 443
Extractable nuclear antigens 576
Extraglottic devices 103, 105
Extrapyramidal syndrome 577
Extremities 21, 118, 668
Eye 617, 734
   examination of 674
Eyebrow lacerations
   assessment of 674
   management of 674
Eyelid 688
   laceration of 619*f*

F

Face 679
   complicated laceration of 670*f*
   mask 101
   sensory loss of 20
Facemask 165
   simple 167, 167*f*
Facial
   bones 615*f*
   expression 174
   injuries 621*fc*, 680*f*
   lacerations
   motor, ipsilateral 20
   nerve
      injury 680*f*
      palsy 20, 680*f*
   repair 680*f*
      deep 688
      superficial 688
   skin 678
      avulsion 676*f*
   trauma 612, 632
Faintness 790
Familial hypocalciuric hypercalcemia 438
Fangs marks 790*f*
Fascicular block
   left anterior 279
   left posterior 279
Fasciculations 367, 733
   toxic causes of 733*b*
Fasciitis, necrotizing 567, 570, 570*f*
Fasciotomy 814
Fasting glucose, impaired 541
Fat embolism syndrome 662
Fatal accident 603
Fatigue 439, 493, 585
   diaphragmatic 324
   weight loss 577
Febrile
   neutropenia 581, 585, 588*fc*
   seizure 531, 532
      pathophysiology of 533*f*
Fecal
   flora, modulation of 402
   impaction 464
Felbamate 535
Femoral artery 158
   injury 658*f*
Femur
   fractures, bilateral 664*f*
   shaft fracture 667*f*
Fenobucarb 766
Fenoldopam 251, 252, 309
Fenoterol 333
Fentanyl 105

Fenthion 754
Fetal heart
   rate 511
   tones 514
Fever 110, 194, 337, 420, 521, 523, 538, 575, 693
   arthritis 577
   high-grade 693*f*
   of unknown origin 291
   rheumatic 240
   treatment of 524
Fiberoptic
   bronchoscope 102
   intubation 103, 107, 107*f*
Fibrinolysis 794
Fibrinolytic therapy 221
Fibroids 498
Fibroplasia, retrolental 170
Fibrosis 447
   pulmonary 324
Fine needle aspiration 695
Finger in ear test 614*f*
Fingertip injury, multiple 685*f*
Firecracker injury 803*f*
Fistula
   bleeding, arteriovenous 450
   bronchopleural 342
   gastrointestinal 110
Five-tier triage scales 11, 11*t*
Flaccid muscles 629
Flaccid paralysis, acute 791
Flail chest 162, 324, 330, 602, 638
Flank pelvis 21
Flecainide 241
Flexion 666*f*
Flow resistance pressure 143
Fluid 424, 568
   administration 220
   and electrolyte
      imbalance 567
      replacement 427
   deficit 111
   indications of 110
   intravenous 111*t*, 112*t*, 427
   levels, multiple 425, 426*f*
   management 481, 806
   overload 745
   removal 443
   responsive hypotension 20
   restriction 400
   resuscitation 20, 442, 625, 668*t*
   retention 749
   therapy 20, 120, 407, 814
      monitoring 111
      principles of 110
   volume, distribution of 110*fc*
Flumazenil 747
Flunarizine 361
Fluorescence in situ hybridization 587
Fluoride 475, 720, 733, 743

Fluoroquinolones 454, 568, 586
Flurbiprofen 361
Focal neurologic deficit 624, 626, 632
Fogarty's catheter 319f
Foley's catheterization 452, 626, 652f
Folinic acid 747
Food poisoning 723
Foot
    crush injury of 686f
    dorsum of 803f
Forced expiratory volume 331
Formoterol 333
Formothion 754
Foscarnet 439
Fosfomycin 454
Fosphenytoin 388
Fossa lesions, posterior 625
Fournier's gangrene 567
Four-tier triage scales 11
Fracture 631, 637
    acetabulum 667f
    avulsion 700
    care 656
    depressed 620f, 625
    femur 700
    fibula 700
    long bone 657, 662
    management of 656
    multiple 657, 667
    neck talus 661f
    proximal long bone 602
    rib 330, 347, 638
    shoulder 667f
    sternal 639
    tibia 700
    types of 630, 631t
    wedge 631
Francisella tularensis 337
Fresh frozen plasma 156, 267, 302, 303, 589
Fructose 749
Fumigants 753
Fundoscopy 250
Fungal 492
    ball 447
    infections 446
    meningitis 539t
Fungicides 753
Furious rabies 783
Furosemide 585, 749

G

Gabapentin 535
Gallstones 405, 423
Gamma
    aminobutyric acid 400
    benzene hexachloride 766
Gap acidosis 728
Gas 424
    fluid levels, multiple 425
    gangrene, treatment of 169

Gaskin all-fours maneuver 513
Gastric
    catheters 609
    distention 138
    lavage 735, 736, 737t
    pressure 138
Gastroenteritis 427, 526
Gastroesophageal reflux 186
    disease 185, 526
Gastrointestinal
    bleeding
        lower 394, 395
        upper 393-395, 695
    tract 755
        acute lower 695
Gastrotoxic medications 394
Gatifloxacin 539
Gelatin 112
Genetic factors protein C 345
Gentamicin 539
Gentian violet dye 720
Gingival hyperplasia 720
Gland, adrenal 490
Glasgow coma scale 11, 19, 21, 86, 122, 124,
    142, 330, 367, 536, 599, 599t, 600,
    609t, 622, 624, 625, 632, 721
Glass cut injury 683f
    forearm 684
Glaucoma 363
Global Registry of Acute Coronary Events
    206, 213
Glomerular
    filtration rate 214, 228, 445, 458, 486,
        741
    injury 446
Glomerulonephritis 449
    acute 577
    poststreptococcal 460
    primary 249
Glossitis 720
Glucagon 474, 476, 747
Glucocorticoids 439, 490
    therapy, long-term 491
    secrets 490
Glucokinase 543
Gluconate 747
Gluconeogenesis 491
    lipolysis 491
Glucose 432, 476, 539, 747, 749
    6-phosphate dehydrogenase deficiency
        808
    control 308
    normal plasma concentration of 473
    tolerance, impaired 541
Glutethimide 743
Glycemic control 126, 130, 546t
    monitoring of 545
Glyceryl trinitrate 307
Glycopyrrolate 763, 765
Glycopyrronium 333

Glycosides, cyanogenic 732
Gnathostoma spinigerum 537
Goldman septal elevator 614f
Goodpasture syndrome 316
Gout 577
Graft versus host disease 590, 590fc
Granulomatosis 316
    diseases 447
Graves' disease 484
Gravid uterus, retroverted impacted 464
Great arteries 233
    complete transposition of 554
Great vessels, transposition of 555
Grievous hurt 26
Guanidine 747
Guillain-Barré syndrome 161, 464, 465, 577
Guitar pick sign 620, 620f
Gunshot wounds 646
Gustilo-Anderson open fracture
    classification 661t
Gusto risk score 210t
Gut obstruction 693

H

Haemophilus influenza 336, 523, 539
Hair removal 673
Hallucination 365, 367, 723, 728, 731
    syndrome 718
Haloperidol 367, 749
Hamman's sign 330
Hand wash, procedure of 76f
Harmless acute pancreatitis score 405
Hashimoto's encephalopathy 488
Head 699
    computed tomography of 538, 619
    impulse test 356, 356f
    injuries 174, 365, 603, 632, 643, 813
    seizures 698
    tilt chin lift maneuver 103, 103f
    trauma 149, 622, 698
        high risk 624
        low risk 624
        management of 624
        medium risk 624
    up tilt table test 201
Headache 170, 250, 252, 324, 360, 362, 438,
    538, 581
    acute 360, 362, 363, 698
        subarachnoid 173
    classification of 360fc
    cluster 361
    primary 360
    secondary 362, 362t
    worsening 624
Health education 786
Heart 370
    attack 74, 201
    block 241, 252
        complete 562f
        congenital 199

computed tomography angiography of 294
disease 383
   congenital 193, 315, 552, 554
   coronary 184
   ischemic 240, 394
   rheumatic 240, 557f
   structural 197, 241
dysfunction, right 349
failure 162, 184, 201, 226, 252, 253, 269, 271, 315, 345, 365, 368, 394, 431
   acute 226, 226f
   chronic 226
   congestive 112, 137, 193, 205, 207, 210, 241, 250, 308, 339, 446, 484, 485, 557, 745
   decompensated 310, 330
   drug-induced 222
function, low 201
rate 13, 86, 113, 114, 184, 206, 208, 233, 330, 331, 394, 561t
   fast 297
   high 20
valve
   mechanical 370
   prosthetic 285
Heat
   exhaustion 795, 795t
   exposure, pathophysiology of 794fc
   stress, pathophysiology of 794fc
   stroke 793, 795t
      classical 793
      exertional 793, 794
      first aid for 795f
Heavy alcohol use 394
Helmet removal technique 632
Hemadsorption 443
Hematemesis 315
Hematochezia, severe 396, 396fc
Hematocrit 309
Hematologic disorders 446
Hematoma 107, 247, 447, 456, 457, 515, 694, 696
   epidural 365, 623, 625
   extradural 307
   hyperechoic 620f
   intramural 297
   retrobulbar 620f
   septal 613f
   subcapsular 651f, 652f
   subdural 307, 623-625
Hematuria 459
   confirmation of 456
   gross 456, 459
   microscopic 456, 457, 459
   nonglomerular 458
   persistent 457, 460
   transient 460
   urologic evaluation of 459fc

Hemianopsia, contralateral homonymous 20
Hemiparesis, ataxic 372
Hemo thorax 161
Hemoadsorption 443
Hemoconcentration 794
Hemodiafiltration 745
   continuous 443
      arteriovenous 443
      venovenous 443
Hemodialysis 439, 740, 741, 742b, 742f, 743
   continuous 443
      arteriovenous 443
      venovenous 443
Hemodynamic
   instability 213, 308
   stability 20, 498
Hemofiltration 740, 745
   continuous 443
      arteriovenous 745f
Hemoglobin 446
Hemoglobinuria 456
Hemogram, complete 368
Hemolysis, elevated liver enzymes, and low platelet count 250
Hemolytic uremic syndrome 460, 527
Hemoperfusion 740, 744
   circuit 744f
Hemopneumothorax, traumatic 342
Hemoptysis 315, 317f, 347, 697
   management of 320fc
   massive 315
Hemorrhage 154, 162, 197, 250, 330, 368, 378, 446, 515, 515, 745
   acute subarachnoid 380, 381f, 698
   adrenal 491, 492
   antepartum 12, 250
   control 21, 606, 607, 608fc
   gastrointestinal 569
   hypertensive 380
   intracerebral 249, 253, 380
   intracranial 381
   major external 21
   parenchymal 381
   postpartum 12, 498
   primary postpartum 515
   pulmonary 324, 577
   subarachnoid 197, 360, 365, 375f, 377, 380f, 382fc, 381, 623
Hemosiderosis, idiopathic 316
Hemothorax 247, 342, 343, 559t, 602, 638, 642
Hemotympanum 614f
Heparin 131, 208, 266, 267, 749
   neutralize 302
Hepatic
   artery aneurysm, rupture of 577
   encephalopathy 368, 399, 400b, 400t, 401, 401b, 402, 729

   classification of 399t
   treatment of 401b
failure 162, 368, 394
injury 699
   grading scale 651, 651f
   scan 647f
Hepatitis 743
Hepatobiliary disease 693
Hepatocellular disease 399
Hepatorenal syndrome 446
Herbicide 732, 753
Hernia 423, 720
   diaphragmatic 342
   strangulation of 427
Herpes
   simplex virus 538
      encephalitis 465
   zoster 185, 567
      virus 465
Heterophil antibody 540
Hiatus hernia 183
High flow oxygen therapy 326
High performance thin layer chromatography 762
Hip dislocation, posterior 666f, 667f
Hip
   dislocations of 700
   fracture 700
Hirschsprung's disease 527
His bundle 238
His-Purkinje system 280
Histoplasma capsulatum 537
Homocysteine 374
Hong Kong four level field triage system 11
Hormone
   adrenal 491t
   adrenocorticotropic 510
   antidiuretic 431, 434
   deficiency 475
   replacement therapy 345
Horner's syndrome 20
Hospital disaster management committee 706
Human
   bites 681
   diploid cell vaccine 784
   immunodeficiency virus 42, 405, 492, 538
   organs transplantation Act 77
   rabies
      immunoglobulins 784
      prevention of 783
Humidification 165
Hyaluronidase 788
Hybrid ventilators 137
Hydralazine 251-253, 378
Hydration 439
Hydrocarbons 719, 739
   chlorinated 720, 723, 731
Hydrocephalus 465

Hydrocortisone 333, 585
Hydrogen
  cyanide 732
  ion 91
  sulfide 719
Hydrolases 789
Hydrophobia 783
Hydroxocobalamin 747
  plus sodium thiosulfate 712
Hygroma 100
Hyperadrenergic states 253
Hyperalimentation 161
Hyperamylasemia 759
Hyperbaric oxygen therapy 169
Hypercalcemia 273, 405, 434, 446, 729
  actue 446
  drug-induced 734
  investigation of 438t
  less common causes of 438t
  management of 439t
  signs of 438t
  symptoms of 438t
  treatment of 585t
Hypercalciuria 438
Hypercapnia 324, 368
Hypercatabolic state 569
Hyperchloremic nongap acidosis 160
Hypercoagulation 745
Hyperglycemia 365, 368, 435, 480, 575, 745, 762
Hyperglycemic hyperosmolar states 478
Hyperinsulinism, endogenous 474
Hyperkalemia 91, 273, 280f, 432, 433, 435t, 443, 493, 585, 729, 733, 795
  management of 436fc
  treatment of 432
Hyperkalemic periodic paralysis 435
Hyperkeratosis 720
Hyperlipidemia 405
Hypernatremia 112, 432, 734
Hyperosmolality 435
Hyperoxia test 553
Hyperparathyroidism, tertiary 438
Hyperphosphatemia 438, 439, 585
Hyperpigmentation 493
Hyperpnea 367
Hypersensitive carotid sinus syndrome 234
Hypersensitivity 112, 368
  pneumonitis 324
Hypertension 206, 207, 217, 218, 226, 240, 259, 324, 367, 438, 548, 558, 722, 745, 757
  cause of 558
  idiopathic pulmonary 285
  malignant 248, 449
  portal 394, 399
  postoperative 248
  pregnancy-induced 249
  prevention of 308
  pulmonary 183, 185, 319, 446, 577

rebound 252
  refractory 264, 775
  severe pulmonary 290
  stages of 248t
  upper extremity 638
Hypertensive crisis, secondary causes of 249t
Hypertensive emergencies 248, 250b, 251, 252t
  clinical outcomes of 250b
Hyperthermia 365, 367, 446, 727, 728t, 795
  malignant 728, 794
Hyperthyroidism 194, 558
Hypertonic saline 625
Hypertrophy, left ventricular 240, 278
Hyperuricemia 585, 794
Hyperventilation 159, 330, 367, 439
Hyperviscosity syndrome 581, 583
Hypervitaminosis
  A 438
  D 438
Hypoalbuminemia 364, 439
Hypocalcemia 273, 434, 533, 558, 585, 734, 744
  causes of 439t
  mild 436
  severe 436
  signs of 439t
  symptoms of 439t
Hypochloremia 493
Hypoesthesia 814
Hypoglycemia 111, 194, 365, 368, 374, 473, 474t, 475, 477, 533, 547, 723, 749, 762, 794
  causes of 474b
  mild 493
  noninsulinoma pancreatogenous 474, 476
Hypoglycemic disorder 477
Hypokalemia 91, 162, 273, 400, 425, 433, 437, 733
  causes of 437t
  conditions of 437t
  severe 112
  severity of 435, 435t
  signs of 437t
  symptoms of 437t
  treatment of 437t
Hypomagnesemia 162, 439
Hyponatremia 111, 112, 365, 368, 400, 431, 431t, 493, 533, 734
  causes of 431, 431t
  dilutional 432
  diseases of 431t
  investigation of 432b
  management of 433fc
Hypoparathyroidism 439, 558
Hypoperfusion 370, 446
Hypophosphatemia 162, 438
Hypoplastic left heart syndrome 556

Hyporeflexia 728
Hypotension 122, 126, 138, 164, 241, 252, 259, 287, 324, 325, 349, 394, 420, 493, 638, 722, 743, 744, 749, 773fc, 790, 792
  intractable 307
  orthostatic 197, 201, 252
  permissive 608
  persistent 643
  severe 728
Hypothermia 80, 91, 365, 388, 405, 425, 487, 511, 606, 625, 717, 727
  drugs producing 728b
  signs of 728t
  symptoms of 728t
  therapeutic 798
Hypothyroid coma 486, 487b
Hypothyroidism 486fc, 548, 558
Hypoventilation 159, 170, 323, 728
Hypovolemia 91, 117, 446, 585, 745
  signs of 608fc
Hypoxemia 99, 170fc
  severe 319
  treatment of 169
Hypoxemic respiratory failure, acute 137
Hypoxia 20, 99, 162, 324, 365, 368, 723, 729, 749
  anemic 165
  cytotoxic 165
  hypoxic 80, 165
  normoxic 164
  types of 164, 165t
Hysterectomy 500

I

Ibuprofen 175, 176, 361, 719
Ibutilide 241
Iliac fossa, right 425
Imipramine 720
Implantable cardioverter defibrillators 203, 243
Incident command system 707
Incubation period 781
Indacaterol 333
Indian Laws for Patient's Safety 77
Indian laws, list of 77b
Indian Medical Association 51
Indian Medical Council Act 77
Indian Medical Council Regulation 77
Indian Penal Code 26, 87
Indomethacin 474
Infarction 693, 799
  adrenal 491, 492
  pituitary 492
  pulmonary 315
Infection 20, 100, 111, 336, 364, 405, 446, 451, 465, 484, 502, 567, 743-745
  acute 577
  enteroviral 540

focus of 523
minimizing risk of 674
prevention of 129, 247
reservoirs of 780
systemic 484, 526
Inferior vena cava 287, 648, 693
Infertility 493, 502
Inflammation 329, 446
Inflammatory bowel disease 527
Infraorbital rim 612
Inhalation injury 809
Injection
    intravenous 176
    subcutaneous 176
Injuries 674
    abdominal 649*f*
    blunt 19, 623
    countercoup 33, 623
    degloving 657
    diaphragmatic 641
    duration of 25
    electrical 811
    gravity of 26
    lightning 809
    location of 671
    long bone 19
    mechanical 25
    mechanism of 596, 629, 650*f*, 671
    modes of 605*f*
    nature of 25
    neurologic 813
    penetrating 603, 623, 626, 649*f*
    primary 597
    secondary 597
    severe mechanism of 602
    severity score 600
    spinal 603
    tertiary 597
    time of 671
    urethral 609*fc*
Innsbruck coma scale 722
Inotropes 113, 115, 116
Insecticides 753
Inspiratory
    flow patterns, types of 145*f*
    positive airway pressure 137
Inspired oxygen, fraction of 127, 147, 164, 167, 168, 310
Institute of Neurological Disorders and Stroke 373
Insulin 474, 475, 723
    deficiency 435
    deficient diabetes 474
    delivery devices 545
    dose 543
    independent glucose utilization 475
    injection sites 545, 545*f*
    regimen 544
    secretagogues 474
    storage 545
    subcutaneous 482
    therapy 481, 542
    types 543
Insulinoma 474
Intensive care unit 7, 19, 92, 122, 137, 142, 220, 303, 322, 329, 334, 338, 378, 401, 404, 448, 486, 601
Interface attachments, types of 136*f*
Interleukin 23, 590
Intermittent positive pressure ventilation 305
International Association of Pancreatology 404
International Society for Pediatric and Adolescent Diabetes 546
Interstitial nephritis, acute 449
Interstitium 324
Intervertebral disk disease 465
Intervertebral disk space 634
Intestinal obstruction 423, 425
    acute 427
    management of 427, 427*fc*
Intra-aortic balloon
    counterpulsation 120, 121, 307
    pump 22, 218, 220, 221, 222*f*, 772, 774, 775
Intramuscular injection 176
Intrauterine
    device 502
    growth restriction 577
Intravascular volume depletion 446
Intravenous
    fluids, classification of 111
    therapy 438
    tissue plasminogen activator 24
Intubation, rapid sequence 103, 104
Intussusception 423, 427, 527
Iodides 720
Iodine 720
Ipratropium 333
Iprobenfos 754
Iron tonic syrups 720
Irrigation 673
Ischemia 222, 537
    lower limb 263
    mesenteric 263, 307, 423, 577
    onset of 425
    renal 263, 577
Ischemic stroke
    acute 379
    causes of 370
    workup, complete 374
Isolated musculoskeletal chest pain syndrome 185
Isoniazid 161, 723, 731, 743
Isoprenaline 114, 115, 747
Isopropanol 719, 723, 743
Isopropyl alcohol 160
Isoproterenol 720
Itching 571

J

Janani Suraksha Yojana 508, 517
Jaundice 368, 695
Jaw thrust 103, 103*f*
    maneuver 607*f*
Jervell and Lange-Nielsen syndrome 561*f*
Jet ventilator 102
Joint 174
    commission international 36, 173
    dislocations 174
Jugular venous pressure 111, 118, 226, 260, 347, 584

K

Kangaroo technique 511
Kerosene 739
Ketamine 104
Ketoacidosis 482
    alcoholic 161
    diabetic 110, 161, 330, 478, 482, 547
Ketoconazole 439
    etomidate 492
Ketogenesis 479
Ketoprofen 175
Ketosis 543
Kidney 452
    disease 112, 441
        acute 435
        chronic 364, 435, 442, 445, 450, 689
        improving global outcomes 445*t*
    end-stage 441
    failure, acute 420
    function 368
        test 499
    injury
        acute 301, 309, 368, 441, 448, 445, 445*t*, 446*t*, 448*t*, 696, 792, 795
    molecule 442, 448
Klebsiella pneumoniae 336, 422
Knee dislocation 667*f*
Kyphoscoliosis 162, 324

L

Labetalol 250-252, 378
Labor, stages of 508*b*
Laceration 25, 618, 671*t*
    closure of 686
    parameters 688
Lacrimation 367
Lactate
    dehydrogenase, elevated 302
    liver enzyme 20
    serum 23
Lactation 786
Lactic acidosis 20, 161, 324, 795
    idiopathic 729
Lamotrigine 535, 568

Laparoscopic salpingectomy, technique
    of 504
Laparotomy 647
Laryngeal
    edema 749
    inlet 100, 100f
    mask airway 101, 102, 102f, 105, 105f
    trauma 100
    tube airway 101, 105, 106f
Laryngopharynx 99
Laryngoscope 101
Laryngospasm 439, 737
Laryngotracheobronchitis 100
Lateral uterine displacement method 517f
Lathyrism 732
Le Fort fractures, types of 616f
Lead 733
    dislodgement 247
Leg
    fasciotomy of 660f
    sensory loss of 20
Legionella pneumophila 336
Lepra reaction 571
Lethargy 585
    seizures 528
Letones, serum 480
Leucovorin 747
Leukemia 446, 588
Leukocytes 587
Leukocytosis 368, 420, 762, 794
Leukopenia 368
Leukostasis 588
Leukotriene receptor antagonists 333
Levallorphan 749
Levetiracetam 388, 535
Levodopa 722
Levofloxacin 454
Levosalbutamol 33
Licorice 162
Lidocaine 749
Ligament of Treitz 699
Lignocaine 104, 726
    preparation 726
Limb
    ataxia, ipsilateral 20
    elevation 808
    fractures 174
    injuries 346, 682
        clinical evaluation of 683t
    ischemia 258, 259
    threats 657
    trauma 656f
Linezolid 586
Lip 677
    laceration, complex 677, 680f
Lipid protein binding 742
Lipoproteins, low density 813
Listeria monocytogenes 539
Lithium 438, 719, 732, 733, 743
Liver
    biopsy 341

disease 112
    end-stage 364
    severe 394
enzyme 795
failure 533
    failure, acute 399
function test 330, 368, 405, 499
transplantation 402
Lobar consolidation 336
Lomotil 722
Loperamide activated charcoal 530
Lorazepam 732
Low capacity systems 165
Low cardiac
    ejection fraction 371
    output syndrome 301
Low perfusion, evidence of 227
Lower urinary tract
    causes 447
    symptoms 463, 464
Ludwig angina 100
Lumbar puncture 3, 363, 368, 538
Lund and Browder charts 806f
Lung 315
    abscess 315
    cancer 315
        inoperable 319
    collapse, retrocardiac 555f
    contusion 324, 330
    disease
        chronic 729
        restrictive 161
    diseases 729
        interstitial 341
    injuries 639
        acute 775
        penetrating 640
        transfusion related 324
    marking, absence of 341
    parenchyma 315, 324
    pressure 142
    protective mechanical ventilation 130
    resection 324
    tumor 330
Lupus
    erythematosus 249, 575, 577
    nephritis protinuria hematuria 577
Lyme disease 465
Lymph nodes 447
Lymphoma 446
Lysergic acid diethylamide 720

M

Macroglossia 487
Magills forceps 101
Magnesium 435
    citrate 737
    infusion 388
    sulfate 737, 747
    therapy 482

Magnetic resonance
    angiography 374, 448, 698
    cholangiopancreatography 695
    imaging 21, 74, 150, 250, 262, 374, 376,
        400, 404, 454, 476, 499, 533, 538,
        583, 626, 635, 639, 684, 692, 695
    sagittal section 263f
    urography 454, 458
    venography 698
Malaise 337
Malaria 365
Malathion 754
Malignancy 185, 336, 346
    gastrointestinal 464
    hypercalcemia of 581, 584, 585t
Malignant
    disease 439
    pleural effusion 342, 581, 584
Mallampati classification 101, 102f
Mallampati score 103
Mallory-Weiss tear 394, 735
Malnutrition 364
Malperfusion, evidence of 263
Malpractice claims 38f
Manchester triage scale 11
Mandible 99, 615
Manganese 732, 733
Mangled extremity 657, 662
    severe score 663t
Mannitol 160, 625, 749
Marfan syndrome 257
Mask fit 166
Mass casualties, examples of 710
Massive adrenal hemorrhage, bilateral 491
Mastitis 12, 515
Maturity-onset diabetes of young 542, 543
Maxilla examination 616f
Maxillofacial trauma 100
Mean arterial pressure 113, 114, 124, 125,
    128, 130, 219b, 220, 309, 450, 622
Meatal stenosis 464
Mechanical ventilation 142, 143, 144, 144b,
    162, 174, 326, 334, 341, 342
    types of 144
Meclofenamate sodium 175
Mediastinal widening 260, 261f
Medical Council Act 77
Medical Council of India 178
Medical Termination of Pregnancy Act 77
Medicolegal
    case 25, 27
        procedure of 35f
    record
        completion of 27
        components of 27
Medium capacity systems 165
Medullary syndrome, lateral 372
Membrane, prolonged rupture of 515
Memory deficit, short-term 365
Meniere's disease 357

Meningitis 144, 162, 363, 365, 533, 536, 368, 540, 794
   aseptic 577
   chronic 537
   subacute 537
Meningococcemia 567
Meningomyelocele 465
Mental
   Health Act 77
   health disorders 6
   retardation 535
   status 13, 21
      acute onset 367
Meprobamate 743
Mercaptans 719
Merci retriever 380*f*
Mercury 732, 733
Meropenem 454, 539
Mesenteric artery, superior 694*f*
Mesoappendix, dissection of 416*f*
Mesothelioma 297
Metalloproteinases 789
Metaprolol 241, 361
Metastasis 315, 492
Methadone 720
Methane 723
Methanol 160, 161, 719, 723, 729
Methaqualone 731, 743
Methemoglobinemia 252, 723, 749
Methicillin-resistant *Staphylococcus aureus* 129
Methionine 747
Methomyl 766
Methotrexate therapy 505
Methyl parathion 754
Methyl salicylate 719
Methyldopa 253, 719, 720
Methylene blue 712, 749
Methylenedioxyamphetamine 718
Methylenedioxymethamphetamine 718
Methylprednisolone 333
Methylxanthines 333
Methysergide 361
Metoclopramide 361, 719
Metoprolol 241
Metronidazole 720
Microbiology 331, 337, 453
Micrognathia 100
Midazolam 105, 388
Migraine 361, 362, 365
Milk-alkali syndrome 438
Milrinone 220, 230
Mimicking acute respiratory distress syndrome 170
Mineralocorticoid 491
   secrets 490
Minoxidil 253
Minute ventilation 147, 149
Miosis 367, 717, 719
Miscarriage 503, 577

Mitral
   annular calcification 289
   inflow late diastolic velocity 286
   regurgitation 209, 213, 219, 220, 222, 285, 301
      acute 223
      severe 557*f*
   stenosis 285, 315
   valve
      disease 183, 184
      valve prolapse syndrome 240
Mixed acid-base disorder 159
Mixed venous oxygen 220
   low 323
   saturation 219
Modern antirabies vaccine, administration of 784
Modified early warning score 12, 13*t*
Moist heat 26
Molecular weight heparin, low 131, 266, 267, 348, 378
Molluscicides 753
Monoamine oxidase inhibitors 719, 728, 734, 748
Monocrotophos 754
Morphine 176, 365, 400, 720
Morphothion 754
Mortality, trimodal pattern of 601
Motor neuron
   disease 732
   disorders 732*t*
Motor vehicle
   accidents 596
   collision 629
Mouth
   floor of 100
   pressure 142
Movement disorders 732
   drug-induced 734*t*
   treatment of 733
Moxifloxacin 539
Mucous membrane
   drying of 170
   losses 446
Multidetector computed tomography 693, 699
   scan 397, 701
Multifocal atrial tachycardia 193, 239, 240
Multiorgan
   failure 794
   involvement 575
Multiple
   organ dysfunction syndromes 601
   sclerosis, multiple 447, 465
Multisystem trauma 595
Multivessel coronary artery disease 217
Murmur, systolic 638
Muscle
   cramps 439
   fibers, arrangement of 283*f*

   protein catabolism 491
   spasm, local 629
   weakness 438, 439, 585
Muscular
   hyperactivity 728
   spasm 183
Musculoskeletal
   examination 188
   injuries 813
   pain 186
   symptoms 187
Myalgia 493
Myasthenia gravis 144, 162
Myasthenic crisis 733
Mycetoma 315, 319
Mycobacterium tuberculosis 537
Mycoplasma 336, 337
   pneumoniae 337
Mydriasis 367, 717, 719, 728
Myelitis 536
Myocardial
   contusion 217
      aortic stenosis 222
   deformation 283*f*
   depression 749
   dysfunction, reversible 224
   infarction 117, 118, 184, 186*f*, 205, 206, 208-210, 217, 217*f*, 218, 222, 226, 244, 245, 266, 270, 275, 276*f*, 288, 288*f*, 289*f*, 294, 347, 368, 427, 484, 577, 745
      acute 23, 164, 173, 186, 206, 206*t*, 208*t*, 216, 226, 250, 256, 277*f*, 278*f*, 365, 395
      left ventricular 219
   ischemia 183, 184*t*, 253
      nonfatal 212*t*
   oxygen demand 169
   perforation 247
Myocarditis 117, 186, 217, 224, 226, 577, 735
Myoclonic jerks 324
Myoglobin 446
   test, serum 813
Myoglobinuria 456, 794
Myopathy, necrotizing 732
Myositis
   fibrosa 732
   ossificans 732
Myxedema 273, 368
   coma 486
      pathogenesis of 487*fc*
   madness 486

N

Nabumetone 175
N-acetylcysteine 309, 747
N-acetylpenicillamine 747
Nafcillin 539

Nail bed 684f, 688
    blood return 118
    injury 684f
Nalidixic acid 719
Nalorphine 749
Naloxone 712, 726, 747
Naphthalene 719
Naproxen 175, 176, 361, 568, 720
Narcotic Drugs and Psychotropic Substances Act 77
Nasal
    cavity 99
    deformity 104
    infection 104
    injury, complicated 677f
    prongs 101, 165, 166f, 167
        working of 167t
    stuffiness 170
    trauma classification 613
Nasogastric tube 395, 396
    loss 446
    placement 341
Nasolacrimal duct injuries 675, 676f
Nasopharyngeal airway 101, 102, 102f, 104
Nasopharynx 99
National Academy of Clinical Biochemistry 211
National Diabetes Surveillance Program 478
National disaster management structure 707fc
National Glycohemoglobin Standardization Program 541
National Institutes of Health Stroke Scale 379f
National Standard for Ambulances in India 86
National Tuberculosis Control Programme 331
Nausea 170, 184, 250, 252, 362, 367, 412, 420, 438, 585, 790
Neck 21, 100
    infection, deep 330
    pain 538, 656, 657
    surgery 107
    trauma 100, 330
Needle cricothyroidotomy 103, 106
Neglected tropical diseases 779
Negri bodies 781
Neisseria meningitidis 523, 537, 539
Nematicides 753
Neonatal advanced life support 3, 517
Neonatal cardiac emergencies 552
Neostigmine 747, 791
    test 791
Nephrocalcinosis 438
Nephrolithiasis 438, 447
Nephropathy
    contrast 450
    obstructive 450

Nephrostomy, percutaneous 450
Nephrotic syndrome 446
Neprilysin inhibitor 229
Nesidioblastosis 474
Nesiritide 229
Neurocardiogenic syncope 197
Neuroleptic malignant syndrome 728, 794
Neurological disorders 577
Neuromuscular disorders 162
Neuropathy
    autonomic 465
    diabetic 464
    syndrome 759
Neurovascular damage, digital 683f
Neutral protamine hagedorn 544
Neutropenia 596t
Neutrophil
    count, absolute 586, 586t
    extracellular trap 123
    gelatinase-associated lipocalin 442, 448
New York Heart Association Classification 299
Niacin 720
Nicardipine 251, 252
    infusion 378
Nicotine 719, 721, 733, 734
    deficiency 365
Nifedipine 720
Nikolsky's sign 802
Nitrazepam 720
Nitrites 723
Nitrobenzene 719
Nitrofurantoin 454, 720
Nitrogen dioxide toxicity 316
Nitroglycerin 209, 229, 251-253
Nitroprusside 229, 253
Nocturia 438
Nodal reentrant tachycardia 193
Nomenclature 159
Nonanion gap acidosis 161
Noncontrast computed tomography 624f, 698f
    image of epidural hematoma 624f
Nonislet cell tumor 474
Non-malignant granulomatous disease 438
Nonpoisonous snake 789f
Non-rebreathing mask 166, 167f, 168
Non-ST
    elevation acute
        coronary syndrome 207, 213
        myocardial infarction 205, 208
    elevation myocardial infarction 186, 273, 281
    segment elevation myocardial infarction 207, 270
Nonsteroidal anti-inflammatory drugs 267, 361, 393, 394, 442, 446, 447, 465, 524, 570, 638, 718, 721, 739
Nonsulfonylureas 474
Nontyphoidal salmonella 526

Nonvenomous snake 788
Noradrenaline 220, 749
Norepinephrine 96, 114, 130, 230, 724, 749
Normocarbia, maintenance of 308
Normoxia, maintenance of 308
Nose 100, 613
    bimanual digital palpation of 613f
    lacerations 675
Numerical rating scale 12
Nursing Council Act, 1946 77
Nutrition 126, 407, 568
Nystagmus 355, 719

O

Obesity 107, 297, 345, 346, 383, 543
    hypoventilation syndrome 137
    massive 324, 330
    morbid 107
Obstruction
    acute 423, 427
    chronic 423
    complete 427
    recurrent 695
    simple 423
    strangulated 423
    subacute 423
Obstructive
    airway disease, chronic 149, 273
    lung disease, chronic 331
    pulmonary disease, chronic 135, 142, 144, 150, 161, 164, 170, 184, 308, 322, 324, 328-330, 339, 340, 341, 347, 349, 485
    sleep disease, chronic 328
Obturator sign 412
Octreotide 747
Ocular
    reflexes, loss of 728
    scan 620f
Oculogyric crisis 719
Ofloxacin 454
Olfactory clues 718
Oliguria 20, 250, 728
Olodaterol 333
Oncologic emergencies, classification of 581t
One-hand technique 104, 104f
Open appendectomy 415
Open fractures 657, 659
    impending 661
Opiates 104, 367, 719, 721-723, 728, 731, 739, 743, 749
Opioid withdrawal syndrome 718
Optic neuritis 241, 719
Oral
    anticoagulants 267
    antidiabetics 299
    antihypertensive agents 251t
    cavity 100

clues 718
contraceptive 720
   pills 500
glucose tolerance test 541
hypoglycemic drugs and insulin 473
manifestations, drug-induced 720t
mucosa 612, 688
rehydration therapy 528
Orbit 617
Organ
   dysfunction 20
   hypoperfusion 601
Organic brain syndrome 577
Organochlorines 753
Organophosphate 330, 720-723, 731, 734, 739, 744, 753, 756f, 761t, 763b, 772t
   compound 754t, 772
      basic formula of 756f
      induced neuropsychiatric disorder, chronic 759
      pesticides 756f
Organophosphorus insecticide poisoning 753
Organs, movement of 648
Oropharyngeal airway 101, 102, 102f, 104
Oropharynx 99
Orthopedics 19
Orthopnea 226
Orthostasis 198
Osborn wave 280
Osmolal gap 160, 730
Osmotic diuresis 446
Osteoarthritis 576f
Osteopenia 438
Osteoporosis 438
Outflow tract obstruction 217
Out-of-hospital cardiac arrest 91, 92
Ovarian
   cancer, recurrent 695f
   cyst 464
   hemorrhagic cyst, ruptured 498
   pregnancy 505
   torsion 503
Ovary 447
Oxacillin 539
Oxcarbazepine 535
Oximes 747
Oxitropium 333
Oxydemeton methyl 754
Oxygen 748, 749
   amount of 167
   delivery of 311
   devices 164, 166fc
   displacement of 723
   flow rates 166
   inhalation 341
   mask 165
   partial pressure of 161, 554
   requirement, assessment of 170fc
   saturation 119
   source 101
   tension 158
   therapy 164, 166fc, 333, 338
      goals of 169
      long-term 169
      monitoring 170t
   toxicity 169, 721
Oxygenation, assessment of 160
Oxyhemoglobin saturation 158

P

P wave
   abnormal 724
   characteristic of 238
Pacemaker
   dysfunction 435
   malfunction 197
   mediated tachycardia 194
Packed red blood cell 156, 311
Pain 20, 173, 259, 260, 263, 457, 659, 745, 814
   abdominal 12, 259, 250, 420, 438, 493, 650f, 790
   acute 172
      abdominal 693
   assessment of 11, 173
   categories 172
   chronic 172
   constant 425
   control 407
      failure 174
   management 18, 367, 569, 603, 791
      acute 172
   nociceptive 172, 172f
   pathway 173f
   persistent 264
   psychogenic 172
   relief 672, 674
   rib 185
   signals, inhibition of 173
   site of 424f
   treatment of 174, 176t
Palatal weakness, ipsilateral 20
Palpate
   entire face 612
   peripheral pulses 683
Palpitations 193
Pamidronate 585
Pancreatic injuries 699
Pancreatitis 74, 183, 368, 438, 577, 585, 693, 696
   acute 174, 273, 278, 404, 405, 407, 427, 439
Pancuronium 749
Panic attacks 193
Papillary
   fibroelastomas 290
   muscle 288f
      dysfunction 217
      rupture 223
Papilledema 250, 324
Papilloma 100
Paracetamol 176, 361, 739, 743, 744, 749
Paradox, abdominal 324
Paradoxical
   agitation 731
   embolism 289, 290
Paraldehyde 161, 719, 723, 729, 743
Paralysis 435, 629, 659
   stages of 781
Paralytic ileus 423, 585, 738
Paranasal sinus 588
Paraphimosis 464
Paraproteinemia 446
Parasympathomimetics 719, 720
Parathyroid hormone 435, 438
Parenchymal lesions 625
Paresthesias 435, 659, 746
Parkinson's disease 368, 465, 732
Parkinsonism, drug-induced 732t
Parkland formula 807, 807b
Parotid duct injury 676f
Parotitis 720
Paroxysmal
   positional vertigo, benign 354, 355, 359, 698
   supraventricular tachycardia 239, 274, 275f
Partial rebreathing 166
   mask 166, 168
Partial thromboplastin time, activated 267, 302, 377, 498
Parturition 484
Patent
   ductus arteriosus 555
   foramen ovale 289, 371
Peak expiratory flow rate 331
Pedestrian accidents 597
Pediatric
   advanced life support 3
   cardiac emergencies 552, 557
   pain scale 174t
   trauma score 599
Pelvic
   endometriosis 341
   examination 540
   fractures 657
   inflammatory disease 498, 502, 503
   mass 464
   organ prolapse 464
   scan 648f
   surgery, previous 502
   volume 668f
Pelvis 668
   fracture 664
   unstable 602
Pemphigus vulgaris 570
Penicillamine 719, 720, 748
Penicillin G 539
Penile trauma 466

Peptic ulcer 394, 438
  disease 186, 393
Peradeniya organophosphorus poisoning 758
Percutaneous transluminal coronary angioplasty 221, 295
Perforation
  gastrointestinal 419
  peritonitis, stages of 419
Pericardial
  diseases 446
  effusion 260, 273, 450
  tamponade 305, 306f, 557, 559
Pericarditis 183, 184, 186, 577
Perimortem cesarean section delivery 516
Perineal cellulitis 515
Periorbital
  injury, complex 676f
  laceration, complex 676f
Peripheral
  capillary oxygen saturation 73, 164, 164t, 170
  vascular
    disease 308
    resistance 114
Peritoneal
  dialysis 450, 740, 745
    acute 443
    peritonitis 451
Peritonitis 419b, 420b, 423, 427
  etiology of 422t
  medication of 422t
  perforation 419, 420
  postoperative 419
  primary 419
  secondary 419
  signs of 425
  tertiary 419
  types of 422t
Permanent junctional reciprocating tachycardia 240
Personality disorder 732
Pesticides 753
Pet dog bite 682f
Pethidine 734
Pharyngeal infection 330
Pharynx 100
Phencyclidine 249, 719, 720, 722, 728, 733, 734
  toxicity 732
Phenformin 729
Phenobarbitone 720, 743
Phenol 719, 739, 744
Phenothiazines 193, 718-720, 722, 723, 728, 732, 734, 739, 743
Phenthoate 754
Phentolamine 251, 252, 748
Phenylbutazone 568, 720, 744
Phenylephrine 114, 115, 220
  hydrochloride 559

Phenylpropanolamine 722, 728
Phenytoin 388, 439, 535, 568, 719, 720, 734
Pheochromocytoma 194, 249, 438
Philadelphia collar 632f
Phimosis 464
Phlebitis, local 252
Phorate 754
Phosalone 754
Phosphamidon 754
Phosphates 439, 447
Phosphodiesterase-4 inhibitors 333
Phosphorus 719, 749
  burns 734
Photon emission computed tomography 759
Photophobia 538
Photosensitivity erythematous rashes over skin 577
Phoxim 754
Phrenic
  nerve stimulation 247
  palsy 161
Physostigma venenosum 766f
Physostigmine 748
Phytomenadione 748
Piperacillin 586
Piroxicam 175, 720
  diclofenac 568
Pizotifen 361
Placenta
  abruption of 515
  previa 498, 515
Placental abruption 498
Plasma
  biomarkers 442
  cholinesterase 761t
  exchange 443
  osmolality 480
  perfusion 740, 746
  tonicity 431
Plasmapheresis 740, 745
  circuit 746f
Platelets 587
Pleurisy 186, 297
Pneumomediastinum 330
Pneumonia 144, 162, 184, 186, 297, 315, 324, 330, 331, 336, 347, 365, 368, 400, 478, 529, 693, 697, 745
  acute 337t
  atypical 324
  classification of 336
  community-acquired 336, 338
  evaluation of 338fc
  hospital-acquired 336
  lupus 577
  nosocomial 336
  pleuritis 183
  treatment of 337
  ventilator associated 336
Pneumonitis 336

Pneumoperitoneum 427, 653, 653f
Pneumothorax 161, 183, 184, 247, 297, 330, 331, 340, 342, 343, 347, 559t, 602, 642
  classification of 341t
  complicated 342
  etiology of 341t
  size of 341
  small 341
  spontaneous uncomplicated 342
  treatment of 341
P-nitrophenol test 761
Poikilothermia 659, 728
Pointing sign 412
Poisoning
  acute 757
  assessment of 717
  chronic 759
  dermal manifestations of 720t
  general management of 720
  management of 717
Poisonous snake 789f
Poliomyelitis 465
Polyangiitis 316
  nodosa 249
Polyarthritis 575
Polycystic ovary 498
  syndrome 542
Polydioxanone 688
Polydipsia 435, 438, 585
Polyglandular autoimmune syndromes 492
Polymerase chain reaction 337
Polymorphic ventricular tachycardia 242, 276
Polymorphonuclear neutrophils 539
Polyneuropathy 759
Polypeptide 789
Polyps 498
Polytrauma 19, 21, 74, 595, 603, 605f, 624, 657, 667
Polyurea 438, 585
Portosystemic shunt 399
Positive airway pressure
  bilevel 135, 774
  continuous 135, 147, 166, 325, 332, 334
  nasal mask, continuous 169f
Positive end-expiratory pressure 136, 148, 150, 302, 325, 799
Positive pressure ventilation 763
  noninvasive 135-137, 166, 332, 799
Positron emission tomography 583, 587
Postcardiac surgery 257
Postchest surgery 342
Postgastric bypass hypoglycemia 474
Posthypercapnia 162
Posthypocapnia 161, 729
Postintubation laryngeal edema 324
Postparathyroidectomy 439
Post-thrombolytic management 378
Post-traumatic tattooing 671f

Postural orthostatic tachycardia syndrome 198, 201
Potassium 112, 267, 743
    hexacyanoferrate 748
    permanganate 737
    replacement 482
Pralidoxime 712, 763, 764
Prazosin 251
Pre-cardiac surgery evaluation 299
Pre-Conception and Pre-Natal Diagnostic Techniques Act 77
Precordial catch syndrome 186
Prednisolone 333, 585
Pre-exposure prophylaxis 785
Pregnancy 100, 330, 345, 346, 414, 453, 484, 497, 729, 786, 814
    toxemia of 446
Pre-natal diagnostic technique 36
Pressure
    chronic retention, high 467
    control 145f
    gradients 143t
    intra-abdominal 149
    intracranial 149, 625, 625b
    intraocular 363
    intrapleural 142
    intrapulmonary 142
    regulated volume control 147
    support ventilation 135, 136, 147, 147f, 334
    systemic 316
    time product 136
Presyncope 353
Primidone 535
Prinzmetal's angina 184
Procainamide 241
Procalcitonin 24, 122
    serum 23
Profenofos 754
Progesterone 162, 729
    serum 503
Progestin therapy 501
Progressive oliguria 227
Promethazine 361, 744, 749
Prominent taut triceps tendon 666f
Promyelocytic leukemia, acute 589
Propafenone 241
Propane 723
Propofol 625
    infusion 388
Propoxyphene 361, 744
Propranolol 264, 361, 748
Prostaglandin therapy 556
Prostate 447
    transurethral resection of 468
Prostatic
    hyperplasia, benign 463, 464
    hypertrophy, benign 447
Prostatitis 465
Protamine sulfate 748

Protein 539
Proteinuria 250, 794
Proteolytic enzyme 789
Prothrombin time 156, 267, 374
Protiolytic enzyme 789
Proton pump inhibitors 395
Proximal coronary artery 261
Pruritus 585
Prussian blue 712, 748
Pseudoaneurysm, femoral 247
Pseudohemoptysis 315
Pseudohyperkalemia 432, 435
Pseudohypoglycemia 475
Pseudohypoparathyroidism 439
Pseudomembranous colitis 527
Pseudomonas 491
    aeruginosa 129
Psoas sign 412
Psoriasis 439
Psychiatric
    care 749
    medication 732
    symptoms 187
    syncope 198
Psychosis 438, 577, 731t, 732
Pubic
    ramus fracture 609f
    symphysis, diastasis of 667, 700f
Pulmonary edema
    acute 253
    noncardiogenic 721t
Pulmonary embolism 74, 117, 118, 162, 183, 184, 186, 247, 266, 284, 294, 295, 297, 330, 345, 345b, 346, 347, 347b, 347t, 348, 348f, 577, 697, 745
    acute 270, 273, 278
    massive 197, 290
    pathophysiology of 346f
Pulmonary vein flow 286
    diastolic velocity 286
Pulp
    laceration 684f
    repair 684f
Pulse
    oximetry 609
    pressure 118
        narrow 20, 111, 227
    rate 73
Puncture wounds 681
Purkinje fibers 238
Pyelography, intravenous 448, 458
Pyelonephritis 452
    acute 452
    chronic 249
Pylephlebitis 412
Pyoderma gangrenosum 567, 569, 570
Pyrexia 412
    tachycardia hypotension 425
Pyridoxine 748
Pyuria 452

Q

QRS complex, abnormal 724
Q-sofa score 123f, 124f
QT interval, abnormal 725
Quadriparesis 20
Quaternary ammonium compounds 733
Quinalphos 754
Quinidine 739, 743, 744
Quinine 474, 719, 739, 743, 744
Quinolone antibiotics 474

R

Rabies 673, 783
    control of 785
    endemic countries 784t
    pathogenesis of 782f
    virus 780f
Radiation 721
Radical pelvic surgery 465
Radiculopathy, thoracic 186
Radiological disaster, management of 712f
Radionuclide scan 454
Radiosensitive tumors 583
Rain drop pigmentation 720
Raised intracranial pressure, prevention of 308
Random donor platelets concentrate 156
Rapid assessment
    components of 18fc
    team 7
Rapid fluorescent focus inhibition test 782
Rapidly progressive glomerulonephritis 577
Rasmussen's aneurysm 316
Raynaud's phenomenon pericarditis 577
Reaction level scale 722
Recombinant tissue plasminogen activator 698
Rectocele 464
Red blood cell 21, 396, 447, 460, 695, 759, 761t
Red cell transfusion 155, 435
Reed's classification 722
Reflex
    syncope 197
        management of 202t
    tachycardia 252
Refractory
    angina despite aggressive medical therapy 213
    osteomyelitis, chronic 169
Rehabilitation, posthospital 596
Rehydration therapy 528
Renal disease 441, 458
Renal failure 112, 161, 226, 394, 400, 438, 439, 445, 475, 533, 738, 792
    acute 112, 250, 253, 441, 794
    advanced 431
    chronic 696
Renal function test 330, 420, 468

Renal injury 649f, 652, 652f, 699
  scale 649, 649f
Renal replacement therapy 126, 309, 443
  continuous 443
  indications of 443
Renal systems 728
Renal tubular acidosis 161, 439, 729
Renal vasoconstriction 446
Renal vein thrombosis 449
Replacement fluids 111
Reserpine 732
Respiration 21
Respiratory
  acidosis
    acute 161, 729
    chronic 161, 729
  center depression, chronic 729
  crepts 118
  disorder 159
    metabolic compensation of 159
  distress syndrome, acute 126, 130, 143, 144, 149, 150, 165, 322, 324, 325, 330, 775, 794
  failure 250, 301, 312, 322, 324b, 365
    acute 137, 322, 326
    hypercapnic 164, 324
    hypoxemic 164, 322, 323
    postoperative 310
    types of 310
  high rate 20
  illness, chronic 328
  infection, upper 515
  injuries 813
  insufficiency 724
  muscles, failure of 721
  rate 13, 73, 86, 123, 147, 331, 600
  system 728
    pressure gradients of 142f
  tract infection, upper 355
Resting skin tension lines 674
Resuscitation 18, 607
  hypotensive 608
Retinal detachment 620f
Retinopathy 548
  hypertensive 249
Retroperitoneal mass 464
Revised trauma score 599, 600t
Rhabdomyolysis 161, 438, 439, 450, 794
Rheumatoid arthritis, acute 174
Rheumatological disorder 575, 575f
Rhinosporidiosis 100
Rib fractures, multiple 602, 638
Richmond agitation sedation scale 367
Rifampin 539
Right lower quadrant pain 692
Ringer's lactate 19, 111, 112, 807
  solution 154
Ring-of-fire appearance 411f
Road and air ambulance, disadvantages of 82b

Road traffic accident 632f, 672f, 676f, 678f, 680f, 685, 686f, 687f, 704
Rockall scoring system 394, 394b
Rocky Mountain spotted fever 567
Rocuronium 105
Rodenticides 753
Roller machine injury 685f
Rollover collisions 597
Romberg test 356
Rotary wing air transfer 78f, 81f
Rotavirus vaccine 526
Roundworm mass 423
Rovsing's sign 412
Rule of nine 805f
Ryle's tube 167, 737f

S
Sacral agenesis 465
Sacroiliac joint 667, 700f
Saddle anesthesia 630
Salazine 568
Salbutamol 333, 749
Salicylate 161, 162, 175, 330, 720, 721, 723, 728, 729, 739, 743, 744
  syndrome 718
Salivation 367
Salmeterol 333
Salmonella 529
  enteritidis 523
  gastroenteritis 527, 529
Salpingectomy 504
Salt triage scheme 16fc
Sarcoid 446
Sarcoidosis 492
  histiocytosis hemochromatosis 492
Scalp 677
  avulsion 678f, 679f
  defect 679f
  wound 625
Scapular fracture 639
Schistosomiasis 447
Schizophrenia 732
Scleritis 577
Scleroderma 446
Scleromalacia perforans 577
Sclerosis, systemic 249
Scorpion sting 733
Seat belt
  fractures 630, 631, 632f
  sign 650
Sedative hypnotic syndrome 718
Seizures 250, 324, 365, 367, 439, 577, 626, 730
  causes of 534, 534t
  classification of 532fc
  partial 535
  post-traumatic 624
  prevention of 308
Selective serotonin reuptake inhibitors 267, 718

Selenium 719
Sensation, loss of 629
Sensorimotor 372
Sensory
  dysfunction 629
  loss 20
Sepsis 19, 20t, 110, 118, 122, 125, 130, 162, 330, 365, 441, 446, 478, 569, 729, 794
  assessment of 123f
  cascade 20
  development of 122fc
  evaluation 23
  fluid therapy of 129
  induced-myocardia dysfunction 224
  kills 128
  management of 127, 128b
  mortality rate of 124f
  protocols, management of 125
  puerperal 12
  severe 20, 23, 122f
  sources of 441
  symptoms 126f
Septic
  portal vein thrombosis 412
  shock, fluid management of 130fc
Sequential organ failure assessment score 125t
Serotonin
  noradrenaline reuptake inhibitors 267
  syndrome 718
serum beta-human chorionic gonadotropin 503
Sexual assault cases 27
Sexually transmitted disease 42
Sheep farmers disease 759
Shellfish poisoning 721, 733
Shigella 529
  dysentery 529
Shock 20, 110, 115, 116, 144, 164, 216, 223, 438, 491, 553, 775, 790, 792, 794
  anaphylactic 117, 749
  cardiogenic 115, 121, 144, 216, 217b, 217f, 217t, 218fc, 218t, 220t, 221fc, 222, 222t, 349, 365, 446
  causes of 118t
  distributive 116, 121
  electric 516
  etiopathophysiology of 117
  hemorrhagic 144, 273, 378
  hypovolemic 111, 111t, 112, 115, 120
  initial assessment of 119fc
  management of 20, 113fc, 118, 120fc
  obstructive 115, 121
  overview of 117
  pathophysiology of 125fc
  septic 111t, 113fc, 117, 122, 123f, 124, 124f, 125, 127fc, 128fc, 144, 425, 439
  severe dehydration 528

spinal 629
syncope 493
types of 118t, 119, 119f, 119t, 216f
Shoulder 664
   dislocation, anterior 665f
   dystocia, general management of 512
   external rotation of 665f
   posterior dislocation of 665f
Shrinking lung syndrome 577
Shy-Drager syndrome 198, 465
Sialadenitis 720
Sialorrhea 720
Sick sinus syndrome 193, 234, 240
Sickle cell disease 186
Silibinin 749
Simple triage and rapid transport system 709, 710fc
Sinoventricular rhythm 280f
Sinus 612
   arrest 234
   bradycardia 233, 561, 722, 737
   node 238, 240
      abnormalities of 233
      dysfunction 277f
   pause 234
   rhythm 277f, 278f, 280f
      electrocardiogram of 275f
   tachycardia 193, 239, 274, 278f, 279f, 722
Skeletal injury, serious 657
Skin 26, 400, 446, 577, 734
   degloving of 661f
   discoloration 241
   diseases 793
   failure, acute 567
   injuries 812
   intraoral 678
   rashes 575
Skull
   base fracture 626
   fracture 624
Sleep apnea, obstructive 135, 137
Small bowel
   injury 653, 653f
   obstruction 423, 424, 426f, 694, 695f
Snake bite 721, 723, 788, 790, 791f, 792
   management of 790, 792
   victims, late presentation of 792
Snake venom, components of 788
Society of Thoracic Surgeons 309
Sodium 112
   bicarbonate 730b, 749
   chloride 130
   glucose co-transporter 478
   nitrite 748
   nitroprusside 251, 252, 264, 748
   salicylate 748
   sulfate 737
   thiosulfate 737, 748
   valproate 720
Soft tissue 634

edema 620f
infections 400
Solid serosal tumor implant 695f
Somatic pain 172
Somatostatin analogs 395
Sorbitol, dose of 738
Sore throat 170
Sotalol 241
Speckle tracking echocardiography 282
Spills, decontamination of 762
Spina bifida occulta 465
Spinal cord 21, 635
   compression 581, 582, 583f, 590
   hematoma 465
   injury 161, 447, 629
      prevention of 635
   trauma 465, 634
Spinal injury
   modes of 629
   sites of 631f
   types of 630f
Spinal trauma
   clues of 629
   emergency evaluation of 634
Spine 668
   boards 633
   pain 632
   thoracic 639
   trauma
      radiological evaluation of 634
      X-ray of 635f
Spironolactone 161
Splenic CT injury grading scale 651
Splenic injury 650f, 651f, 699
Split-mix regimen 544
Spondyloarthritis 577
Spontaneous pneumothorax
   primary 184, 340, 341
   secondary 340, 341
ST elevation myocardial infarction 205, 273, 281
Stabilization 720, 721
Stagnant hypoxia 165
Stanford classification 257
Staphylococcal skin syndrome 567
Staphylococcus
   aureus 129, 336, 523, 570
   infections 491
   saprophyticus 453
Starvation 729
Status epilepticus 365, 386, 387, 387t, 388, 388t, 389, 531, 532, 731t
   causes of 533
   convulsive 386
   management of 387
   nonconvulsive 386
   refractory 386, 388, 388t
Stenosis 296f
   critical pulmonary 554
   severe pulmonary 290
   spinal 465

Sterilization 502
Steroids 365, 394, 585
   administration 729
   induced psychosis 575
Stevens-Johnson syndrome 567-569, 569f
Stomach wash 736
Stomatitis 720
Stool polymorphonuclear neutrophils 528
Street virus 780, 781
Streptococcus
   agalactiae 539
   pneumoniae 129, 523, 537
   viridans 412
Streptokinase 221
Stress
   cardiomyopathy 184
   testing, noninvasive 212
   ulcer 126
Stroke 19, 20fc, 24, 74, 144, 263, 301, 307, 308, 330, 345, 365, 368, 372, 383fc, 464, 577
   acute 370, 370f, 371, 371b, 374, 374b, 375, 376, 376f, 698
   clinical features of 20t
   cryptogenic 383, 383fc
   hemorrhagic 380
   irreversible 263
   ischemic 112, 249, 266, 370, 371t, 378
   management 372
   syndromes, types of 372
   volume 112, 113
Strychnine 721, 728, 731, 733, 734, 739, 743
ST-segment elevation
   myocardial infarction 206t, 208, 217
   noninfarction causes of 278b
Stump appendicitis 412
Stupor 438
Subcutaneous insulin infusion, continuous 542, 544, 547
Substance abuse 185, 798
Subtraction angiography, digital 308, 376, 377f
Succinylcholine 105
Sudden death 347, 557
Suicide gesture 722
Sulfadoxine 568
Sulfonamides 474, 568, 718, 721
Sulfonylurea 474
   receptor 474
Sulfuric acid 801f
Sumatriptan 361
Sunburns 801
Sunken
   eyes 527
   fontanelle 527
Super-refractory status epilepticus 388, 388t
Supine roll test 356
Supracondylar fracture humerus 658f
Supraglottic devices 103, 105
Supraorbital rim 612

Supraventricular tachycardia
    preexcited 276
    treatment of 240
Surgery 319, 346, 349, 397, 400, 446, 735, 740
    abdominal 419
    gastrointestinal 19
    route of 504
    thoracic 19
Suturing equine rabies immunoglobulins 784
Sweating 110, 367
Swinging heart 288
Sympathomimetics 367, 731
Synchronized intermittent mandatory ventilation 146, 146f
Syncope 184, 196, 236, 263, 290, 349, 582
    mimics 196
    neurologic 198
    risk stratification of 200fc
    types of 197f
Syndrome of inappropriate antidiuretic hormone 432, 433, 585
Systemic envenomation, signs of 791
Systemic inflammatory response syndrome 20, 122, 405, 420, 420f, 601

T

T wave, abnormal 725
Tabes dorsalis 465
Table fan injury 686f
Tachyarrhythmias 238, 239fc, 273, 274, 303, 553, 559, 726
    classification of 274fc
    narrow complex 240fc
Tachycardia 20, 24, 197, 239, 240, 240t, 252, 324, 337, 367, 420, 650f, 722
    monomorphic ventricular 242, 275
    narrow complex 560
    supraventricular 195, 201, 238-241, 274, 561f
Tachypnea 20, 334, 337, 577
Takayasu arteritis 558
Takotsubo cardiomyopathy 184
Tamponade, echocardiographic signs of 305
Tardive dyskinesia 732, 733
Tazobactam 586
Tellurium 719
Temephos 754
Temperature 13
    high 20
    low 20
Temporary pacing 244
    complications of 246, 247b
    procedure 245
    pulse generator 246f
    types of 244
Temporomandibular joint 698
    dislocation 617, 617f
        traditional method of 618f

Tenderness, abdominal 425
Tendon injury 672
Tenecteplase 221
Tension
    headache 361
        treatment of 361
    pneumothorax 117, 118, 186, 301, 304, 340, 610f
Terbutaline 333
Terrorist attacks 704
Tetanus toxoid 673
Tetany 439, 746
Tetracycline 267, 719, 720, 739
Tetralogy of Fallot 554
Texidor's twinge 186
Thallium 719
Theophylline 193, 267, 333, 720, 722, 731, 739, 743, 744
    toxicity 438
Thermoregulation, impaired 728
Thermoregulatory dysfunction 484, 567
Thiamine 365, 726
Thiazide diuretics 431, 438, 721
Thiocyanates 743
Thiodicarb 766
Thiometon 754
Thiopental sodium 388
Thioridazine 720
Thoracentesis 341
Thoracic aorta, descending 262, 262f, 263f
Thoracoplasty 324
Thoracotomy 643b
Thorax 21
Thready pulse 111
Three-tier triage scales 11
Thresher injury 686f
Thrombasthenia 315
Thrombectomy, mechanical 380
Thrombocytopenia 267, 315, 368, 577, 744, 745, 794
Thrombocytosis 368
Thromboelastography 303
Thromboembolism 446
    pulmonary 484
Thrombolysis 206, 377
    concept of 377f
    in myocardial infarction risk score 206
        calculation of 207f
    intra-arterial 379
Thrombophlebitis 515
Thromboplastin, partial 302
Thrombosis 370, 446, 743
    episode, acute 575
Thrombotic thrombocytopenic purpura 577
Thrombus, left ventricular 289
Thyroid
    dysfunction 241, 365, 498
    emergencies 483
    function test 368, 432
    gland hormones, pathophysiology of 483f

hormone 728
    replacement 488
    nodules, autonomous 484
    stimulating hormone 483, 548, 570
    storm 368, 483, 484b, 484t, 794
Thyrostatic 485
    drugs, withdrawal of 484
Thyrotoxic storm 485f
Thyrotoxicosis 438
Thyroxine 483, 722
Tiagabine 535
Tiotropium 333
Tissue
    adhesives 687
    binding 742
    catabolism 435
    defect, large 671
    hypoxia, conditions of 164
    transglutaminase 548
Tobramycin 539
Tocopherol 748, 749
Toluidine blue 748
Tongue 679, 688
    blade test 617f
    laceration of 619f, 680f
Tonic-clonic status epilepticus, generalized 534t
Topical bronchoscopic therapy 318
Topiramate 535
Toraymyxin 444
Torsades de pointes 561f
Total anomalous pulmonary venous connection 555, 556
Total parenteral nutrition 131
Total weak acid buffers 162
Toxic
    conversion, reduced 746
    epidermal necrolysis 567, 568, 568t, 569f
    exposure surveillance system 735
    ingestion 330
    megacolon 527
    ophthalmological manifestations 719t
    respiratory depression 721t
    substance 365
    syndromes 718b
Toxicity rating 753, 765
Toxicokinetics 755
Toxidromes 717, 718b
Toxin
    adsorption of 739t
    drugs 217
    endogenous 446
T-piece 168
Trachea 100
Tracheal obstruction 100
Tracheal tube 318f
    erosion of 315
Tracheobronchial injuries 640
Tracheoinnominate fistula 319
Tracheomalacia 100

Index

Tracheostomy 341
    tube 135
Tramadol 175, 176
Tranexamic acid 21
Transairway pressure 142, 143
Transalveolar pressure 143
Transcutaneous pacing 246
Transesophageal echocardiography 261, 263, 284, 301, 697
Transfusion protocol, massive 153, 154, 156, 156fc
Transient ischemic attack 198, 210, 355, 372, 374, 577
Transjugular intrahepatic portosystemic shunt 395
Transplantation of Human Organs Act 77
Transpulmonary pressure 142, 143
Transthoracic
    echocardiography 260, 284
    needle aspiration 315, 341
    pressure 142, 143
Transtubular potassium gradient 432
Transvaginal ultrasound 503, 698
Transvenous pacing 244, 245
Transverse myelitis 465, 577
Trauma 13, 19, 65, 100, 107, 111, 118, 174, 257, 342, 365, 405, 419, 446, 465, 484, 498, 798
    abdominal 646, 653, 654f, 738
    blunt 596, 648
    complex 657
    mortality 605
    multiple 19
    penetrating 597, 648
    scoring system 599
    spinal 629, 632, 633f, 700
    system, basics of 595
    team 19
        activation criteria, modified 602
    thoracic 637
Traumatic brain injury 601, 622, 622fc, 625t
    pathophysiology of 622
Treacher Collins syndrome 100
Tremor 241, 439
    drug-induced 733t
Trendelenburg position 724
Treponema pallidum 537
Triage early warning score 12, 13t
Triazophos 754
Trichlorphon 754
Tricuspid
    endocarditis 315
    regurgitation 219, 285
    valve injury 247
Tricyclic antidepressants 721, 722, 734, 744
Trientine 748
Triethylenetetramine 748
Triiodothyronine 483
Trimethoprim-sulfamethoxazole 454, 539, 720

Triorthocresyl phosphate 756
Triple rule out protocol 297, 297b
Tripod fracture 615f
Triptans 362
Troponins 211
Trousseau's sign 407, 439
True volume depletion 431
Truncus arteriosus 556, 557
Tuberculosis 315, 427, 447, 697
    fungal infection 492
    meningococcal disease 492
Tubo-ovarian abscess 503
Tubular necrosis, acute 447, 449
Tubulointerstitial injury 446
Tumor 10, 447, 693
    atrial 217
    intra-abdominal 447
    lysis syndrome 581, 584, 584b, 585t, 587-589, 589fc
    mass compressing superior vena cava 582f
    necrosis factor 538, 590
Two-hand technique 104, 104f

U

U wave, abnormal 725
Ulcer 419
    disease 183, 394
Ultrasound 103, 105, 107, 453, 499
    abdomen 420
Umbilical cord prolapse 514
    management of 514fc
Unithiol 748
Upper limb 174
    crush injury 656f
Urea 432
    cycle 399
Uremia 161, 368, 729
Uremic encephalopathy 450
Ureteral ligation 447
Ureterojejunostomy 435
Ureteropelvic shunt 161
Urethra 452
Urethral valves, posterior 447
Urethritis 452, 465
Uric acid 446, 447
Urinary
    biomarkers 442
    bladder 452
    calculi 503
    catheters 609
    indices 448
    retention 367
        acute 463, 464, 464t, 465t, 466t, 467, 468fc
        bladder 365
        postoperative 465
        pregnancy-associated 465
    sodium concentration 432
    tract extrinsic causes, upper 447

    tract infections 365, 400, 452, 453, 457, 460, 465, 478, 515, 521, 529, 696
        classification of 452
        management of 454
    tract intrinsic causes, upper 447
    tract obstruction 453
Urine
    anion gap 160
    culture 453, 458
    cytology 458
    examination 456, 528
    leakage 699
    output, low 20
    routine microscopy 447
    visual examination 791
Urodynamic parameters 464
Urolithiasis 464
Uropathy, obstructive 368
Urosepsis 452, 453
Urticaria 570, 571
Uterine
    artery embolization 500
    bleeding, dysfunctional 498
    curettage 500, 502
    displacement 516
    fibroid 464
    inversion 498
    prolapse 464
Uterus 447
Uveitis 577

V

Vacuum-assisted closure 662
Vagal maneuver 240
Vaginal
    bleeding 12, 497
        abnormal 698
    breech delivery maneuvers 513
    lichen
        planus 465
        sclerosis 465
    pemphigus 465
Valproate 361, 388, 535
Valsalva square wave 226
Valve surgery 308
Valvular
    disease 118, 194, 226, 446
    dysfunction 330
    heart disease 217, 285
    pulmonary stenosis, severe 555
Vancomycin 539, 568, 586
Varicella zoster virus 465
Vasa previa 498
Vascular
    injury 657, 667f, 684
        amputation 603
    relaxation 749
    resistance
        pulmonary 119

systemic 113, 119
surgery 19
Vasculature, pulmonary 324
Vasculitis 370, 446, 449, 571, 571f, 575, 577, 578
Vasoactive
   agents 113, 220
   drugs 114t, 120
      pharmacology of 114t
Vasopressin 220, 230
Vasopressor 113, 115, 116, 129, 442
Vasovagal syncope 201
Veins 446
Vena cava syndrome, superior 581
Venography 448
Venomous snake 788
   classification of 788
Veno-occlusive disease, pulmonary 324
Venous
   hypertension, pulmonary 557f
   thromboembolic disease 23
   thromboembolism 131, 345
   thrombosis 247, 345
Ventilation 95b, 148, 603, 606, 607
   dual modes of 147
   initiation of 147
   intermittent mandatory 146
   modes of 144
   noninvasive 135, 137, 311, 325, 332, 334
Ventricular
   arrhythmia 217, 222, 247, 728, 749
   complexes, premature 241
   contractions, premature 726
   drain, external 382
   dysfunction 556, 557
   ejection fraction, right 220
   end-diastolic pressure, right 217, 218
   fibrillation 203, 304
   hypertrophy 217
   myocardial infarction, right 219, 220, 223, 285, 287
   septal
      defects 193, 556
      rupture 217, 222, 223, 288
   tachyarrhythmias 290
   tachycardia 238-241, 274, 276f, 277f, 304
      nonsustained 201
      pulseless 97
      stable 304
      unstable 304
Ventriculitis 537
Venturi
   device 168f
   principle 168f
   system 168
Verapamil 241, 720
Verbal pain score 12
Vermilion border 677, 679f
Vero cell rabies vaccine, purified 784
Vertebral
   arteries 371

bodies spine process 634
column 21
Vertigo 353
   acute 354, 359fc
   peripheral 355, 355t
Very high-capacity systems 165
Vesicoureteral reflux 453
Vessel
   atherosclerosis, large 371
   disease, small 370
   large 446
   perforation 745
   vasculopathy, small 371
Vestibular nucleus, connections of 354f
Vestibulo-ocular reflex 356
Video laryngoscope 102, 103, 107, 107f
Video-assisted thoracic surgery 643
Vinblastine 585
Vincristine 585
Violent behavior, types of 732
Viperidae 788
Viral
   culture 540
   infections 446
   meningitis 540
Virchow's triad 345, 346t
Viscera, abdominal 700
Visceral malperfusion 258
Viscus, perforation of 745
Vision
   blurred 719
   loss, sudden 577
Visual
   analogue scale 12
   disturbances 790
   field defects 250
Vital signs 13, 187, 330
Vitamin
   A 719
   B12 365
      deficiency 493
   B6 748
   D 435, 719
      deficiency 439, 558
      supplementation 436
   K1 748
   syrups 720
Vitiligo 493
Vocal cord paralysis 324
Voice, hoarseness of 582, 804
Volar skin graft 685f
Volvulus 423
Vomiting 94, 110, 111, 162, 170, 184 250, 252, 362, 367, 400, 420, 424, 431, 438, 446, 493, 526, 530t, 585, 624, 717, 740, 745, 790
   causes of 526
   persistent 528
   severe 110
Vulvovaginitis, acute 465

W

Wall Motion Score Index 282
Wallenberg's syndrome 20, 372
Warm extremities 111, 324
Waste disposal 77f
Water deprivation test 435t
Weaning 138, 170, 222
Wedge pressure, pulmonary 219
Wegener's granulomatosis 316
Wells score 347, 347b
Wernicke's encephalopathy 365
Wheezing 439, 804
Whipple's triad 473
White blood cell 20, 523, 528, 539, 583
Whole bowel irrigation 735, 739
Wide complex tachycardia 241
Wide pulse pressure 111, 259
Wild life rabies 780
Wolff-Parkinson-White syndrome 199, 239-241, 273, 280f
Wong-Baker faces pain rating scale 12, 174f
Wound 670
   care 684, 784
   characteristics 681
   closure 681
   extent of 672
   infection 12
   management 673, 808
   medicolegal classification of 25
   preparation 73
   primary closure of 673f
   triage 689fc

X

Xanthines 731
Xerostomia 720

Y

Young stroke 575

Z

Zinc
   metalloproteinase 788
   phosphide 719
   sulfate 736
Zoledronic acid 585
Zona
   fasciculata 490
   glomerulosa 490
   reticularis 490
Zonisamide 535
Zygoma 675
Zygomatic arch 612